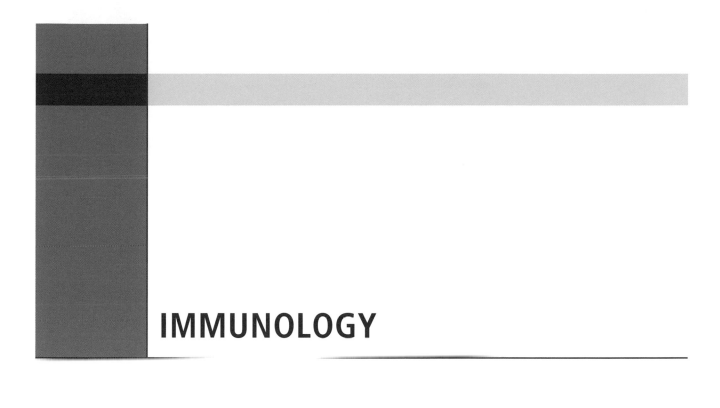

# IMMUNOLOGY

# IMMUNOLOGY

## UNDERSTANDING THE IMMUNE SYSTEM

## Second Edition

**Klaus D.**

Microbiology and Immunology Section
Department of Biological Sciences
Virginia Tech
Blacksburg, Virginia

**⊛WILEY-BLACKWELL**

A John Wiley & Sons, Inc., Publication

*Library of Congress Cataloging-in-Publication Data is available.*

978-0-470-08157-0

Printed in United States of America.

10 9 8 7 6 5 4 3 2 1

*10/0/09*

*To*

*Kathleen, Heather and Scott and Devon and Ayden,*
*and Colleen and Jim and Cameron*

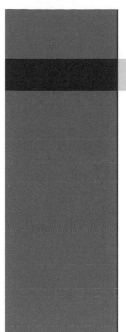

# CONTENTS

# PREFACE

Since the last edition, the science of immunology has continued its astonishing pace of new discoveries. It has seen extraordinarily productive investigations of the body's immune mechanism, particularly in innate immunity that not too many years ago was considered a back-water of immunology. This conversion is illustrated by the impressive growth in our understanding of Toll-like receptor function in innate immunity. A new chapter devoted to innate immunity has been added. The explosion in the characterization of immune cell signal transduction pathways has revealed the sophisticated mechanisms used by these cells to control not only their actions but also others. The once thought random movement of immune cells has given way to a picture of precise movement that is orchestrated by chemokines and their receptors. The seemingly endless discoveries of new T cell subsets, the resurrection of "suppressor" T cells to a new guise called T regulatory cells, and the too-numerous-to-count accessory secondary-signal molecules needed for all these cells to interact reinforce the extent to which the immune system goes to control the development of effector immune responses. The second edition of this book has been significantly revised to include these and other rapidly expanding areas of immunology, and to reinforce the connection between topics some chapters have been combined. To fully appreciate the "reason" for having an immune system—provide protection against microbes—one must have a basic knowledge of pathogens, how they cause disease, how they have evolved to evade the immune system, and the bolstering of the immune system to counteract pathogens. Toward this end, the new Chapter 17 has been added. Furthermore, all the second edition book figures have been colorized, most have been revised, and where applicable have a stepped-out format. Because knowledge of the immune system accumulates so rapidly, it is impossible for even the most dedicated researcher/instructor, let alone a student, to be familiar with all the advances in this field. The next few years will probably witness no slowing of this pace. The consequence is that a one-semester immunology course taught at the advanced undergraduate level (consisting of accelerated juniors, seniors, and some graduate students) is becoming a staple curricular offering at virtually every college and university. The extraordinary growth of immunology as an academic discipline is unrivaled by few other fields. The second edition of *Immunology: Understanding the Immune System* is still an introductory text that grew out of the shared interests of former students and the author in examining ways to answer four frustrating complaints: (1) "I don't know the direction the chapter is taking me"; (2) "What am I expected to learn from the reading?"; (3) "This new information is overwhelming me; I need mental breathers within the chapter to reassess the material just covered"; (4) "I need to know if I comprehend the material and be able to test my knowledge of the material before an exam!" The second edition continues to remedy these problems. The second edition of *Immunology: Understanding the Immune System* assumes that the reader or student has a working knowledge of organic chemistry, cell biology, and microbiology. At times, chapters present experimental data/foundations and on discussions of the concepts that led to these experiments, particularly for topics that explain the basic principles of how the immune system works. This should be useful both to students with only a passing interest and to those planning further study.

As in the first edition, the first chapter (especially the latter part) is a mini-version of the book. Once students finish this chapter, they will have an overall view of immunology as each new topic is introduced. The remaining 16 chapters are organized into the following sequence: Chapters 2 through 6 discuss the immune system's cells and organs, innate immunity, and antigens and antibodies—where and how the participants of the immune system work, the first line of defense in the form of natural resistance, the substances that induce an immune response, the immune substances that are induced, the interactions between the two (serology: methods used to test for the immune substances that are induced), and the genes that code for receptors called antibodies. Chapters 7 through 11 discuss immunobiology—the location of genes that control the immune response, how these genes allow immune cells to communicate with each other, how T cells recognize antigen and become activated, what molecules immune cells release once they are activated by antigen, what events are involved in the cellular interactions required for the development effector responses, how the immune response is downregulated, how lymphocytes are selected to tolerate self-constituents, and how antigen-antibody interactions and antigen directly start the complement system that leads to enhanced protective events and destruction of antigen. Chapters 12 through 16 discuss immunopathology (the immune system is not infallible)—problems encountered due to antibodies, T cells, reactions against innocuous substances or intracellular organisms, reactions against self, and reactions against helpful nonself tissues and organs. Also discussed is the failure of the immune system to respond to harmful self and how the immune response is modulated, both from within and acquired means. Lastly, the completely new Chapter 17 gets at the heart of the immune system, how it counteracts pathogens, what pathogens do to evade the immune system, and immunization approaches to augment immunity.

In particular chapters, such as those dealing with genetics, cellular interactions, and tumor immunology, but also generally throughout the text, emphasis is placed on the experimental basis for our acceptance of important concepts. Describing a moderate amount of experimental evidence greatly deepens our appreciation of the concepts presented.

The reference value of the book is enhanced by a selected list of further readings presented at the end of each chapter. The material at the end also heightens this book's value as a reference: an extensive glossary and an appendix, which includes a list of human CD molecules, and particularly the lengthy index.

Any endeavor of this magnitude is never done alone, and the writing of the second edition is no exception. The exception will be my inability to articulate my indebtedness to all who contributed. Beyond a simply sincere thank you, here goes the rest. Throughout the preparation of this book, I have become deeply indebted to many friends and colleagues for discussing the book with me and for their invaluable constructive criticisms and information. First, to Dr. Carol J. Burger, again volunteering to review material. I am happy to say that Carol and others, who devoted many hours to the book in order to provide extensive technical advice, are still my friends. For advice on specific points, I thank Dr. Noel R. Krieg again, now emeritus Alumni Distinguished Professor, American Society for Microbiology Carski Awardee, and fellow author, who graciously supply me with unused text that we thought would be used in another book. To say the least, I received valuable help from many sources, the too-many-to-count reviewers, who shared their expertise with me by critically reviewing chapters of the book; the staff of John Wiley & Sons, Inc., who kept it a pleasurable experience; and particularly Thomas H. Moore (better known as Thom, not only senior editor, but also, what luck, he could speak and write German), the responsible editor through the writing of the book. And thank you to Thom's great staff, particularly Melissa Yanuzzi, for their help. To Virginia Tech, for allowing me a sabbatical and the many individuals who directly or indirectly furthered this project, thanks. Appreciation is extended to the students who have passed through 30 plus years of my classes not realizing that I would take to heart their complaints about the difficulty of learning immunology. The writing of the second edition continues to be inspired by them and was created in an attempt to make learning this field more palatable for beginners. My hope is that the second edition will provide a solid foundation and in turn, inspire students to continue their studies of immunology. A substantial thanks goes to the big _Generator_ _Of_ _D_iversity for bringing me through this project. Let me end with a tribute to my wife, Kathleen, to whom this work is dedicated as a small expression of my gratitude for her love and acute criticism, which were always encouraging.

KLAUS D. ELGERT

*Blacksburg, Virginia*

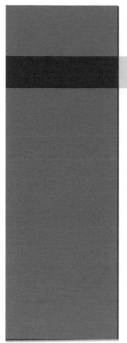

# NOTE TO READER

Immunology is not an easy discipline. It is as complex as the natural system it scrutinizes. However, just a brief dose of the basics of immunology will prepare you for the many upcoming, seemingly formidable concepts that you will be required to understand. The way to this "dose" is through the (highly recommended) reading of the first chapter and especially the *Overview* starting on page 15, which represents an expanded outline that emphasizes the basics, or the big picture. The *Overview* is a mini-version of the book and is written in less technical language. The prudent reader will find that *the time invested early avoids the need to invest a disproportionately large amount of time later*. One chapter cannot describe *all* the interrelationships of immunology that influence a topic. If the reader, however, first views immunology on the *Overview* big screen, how the topic under discussion fits into the surrounding act becomes apparent.

Reading an immunology text for the first time, you might be overwhelmed by the bewildering array of terms and complex abbreviations. This book will help you move yourself into the land of immunology. By learning to speak the language, you begin to think in immunologic terms, and the learning comes easily. When first introduced, important terms are fully defined and presented in **boldface** type. Words that are to be focused on and remembered are presented in *italics*.

The book's brief CONTENTS expands as each chapter begins with a detailed *Chapter Outline* that serves as both a road-map and a survey of things to come. The Chapter Outline is followed by a list of *Objectives* or "take-home" lessons that the reader should comprehend.

Other support systems are used within each chapter. *Footnotes* provide descriptive comments about specific passages in the text. At major chapter breaks, *Mini Summaries* allow the reader to concisely reinforce the material and mentally "switch gears" to the next topic. Each chapter concludes with a *Summary* that contains highlighted terms. The summaries will help you recall and reinforce the information just covered; they should not be used as *the* tool to learn the material. If you read only certain parts of the chapter, the result may be reminiscent of the oft-told Hindu/Buddhist fable of the six blind men who examined different parts of an elephant. Because they did not examine the whole animal, they came up with six different descriptions.

To better comprehend the material just read and prepare for an exam, review questions are provided in the *Self-Evaluation* section at the end of each chapter. The Self-Evaluation section includes key terms, multiple-choice questions, and short-answer essay questions. In lieu of answer keys, the page numbers for answers to the multiple-choice questions are provided.

Although immunology is still a young science, it has become vast and complex. To obtain greater clarification through additional study or to satisfy a desire to learn more about the chapter's topic, a section called *Further Readings* appears at the end of each chapter. The extensive *Glossary* and an *Appendix* are located at the back of the book.

As you progress from one chapter to the next, remember to be like the mythical Phoenix, *rising renewed and ready to begin again*.

# CHAPTER ONE

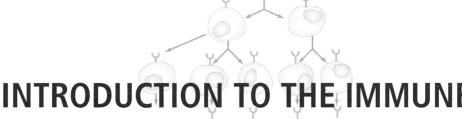

# INTRODUCTION TO THE IMMUNE SYSTEM

## CHAPTER OUTLINE

1. Immunology as a science has a brief history.
2. Innate immunity in vertebrates is constitutive and lacks immunologic memory; it protects through multiple mechanisms.
   a. External innate immunity, natural barriers to infection, prevents the penetration of pathogens into tissues.
   b. Internal innate immunity offers many forms of protection after pathogens enter the body.
3. Adaptive immunity in vertebrates that is achieved through experience because of either recovery from disease or medical intervention.
   a. Adaptive immunity is humoral, cell-mediated, or both.
   b. Adaptive immunity can be active or passive.
4. Clonal selection of lymphocytes explains diversity, specificity, and memory.
5. The immune system has two levels of development.
6. The architecture and mechanisms of the immune system are varied and complex: an overview.

## OBJECTIVES

The reader should be able to:

1. Begin to speak immunology by learning the vocabulary.
2. Appreciate the two functions of the immune system.
3. Gain perspective on immunology's historical foundations.
4. Distinguish between innate immunity and adaptive immunity.
5. Discuss how clonal selection explains the immune system's ability to recognize millions of antigens.
6. Follow the development of the immune system in a species and within an individual member of a species.
7. Understand the basic structural and functional components of the immune system.

---

The body is a citadel under relentless siege from disease-causing agents (such as bacteria or viruses) and cancer cells. The counterattack, or **immunity** (L. *immunis*, free of burden) originally denoted freedom from some kind of service to the Roman state; now, in medical terms, it denotes freedom from disease. Vertebrate animals acquire immunity against these challengers because of the cells and molecules that make up the body's defense system—*the immune system*. Successful immunity depends on the successful collaboration of these cells, which leads to many new cells and molecules that match up with and counteract each challenger. This activity constitutes the *immune response*. In an anthropomorphic sense, the immune system identifies invaders as either friends or enemies and subsequently directs its various components either "to pass in peace" or "to seek and destroy." Our health depends on the accuracy of such decisions. Furthermore, the immune system can "remember" invaders (a characteristic that we exploit when we are vaccinated) so efficiently that there are no symptoms. Because of the protection it provides, the immune system is vital to an organism's livelihood. Vertebrate animals lacking functional immune systems are without defense and consequently perish.

However, a dark side to the immune system's behavior exists. In some instances, the efficiency of the immune system can actually be harmful to the organism it is designed to protect. Sometimes the immune system responds negatively to an innocuous substance or a life-saving organ transplant. Whether an immune response leads to protection or disease, the mechanisms of recognition and response are the same. The single-mindedness of the immune system does not allow it to distinguish between good and bad foreign substances, or foreign substances it is better off leaving alone. The immune system also can cause destruction of what is thought to be nonself tissue but is really normal self-tissue. This aberration can lead to autoimmune diseases. At the opposite end of the immune spectrum, deficiencies in the ability to mediate immune responses can lead to life-threatening infections or cancer. Fortunately, as our knowledge of immunology increases, we are learning how to safely modify or prevent undesirable or augment missing immune responses.

*The immune system has two primary functions: (1) recognition of, and defense against, foreign substances and (2) establishment of immunosurveillance.* Receptor-ligand interaction, the lock-and-key complementarity mechanism, instigates the conveyance of signals called *signal transduction;* the signals follow a pathway of intracellular molecule interactions that ends with the consequence of the signal—activation of the immune cell and destruction of the invader. The recognition of a foreign substance protects against disease, but immunity is not restricted to pathogens (disease-causing organisms). We develop immunity against many harmless substances. In some cases, immunity also can be harmful to the host. Allergies and autoimmune diseases are the classical examples of detrimental immune responses. The second major function of the immune system is surveillance. Surveillance consists of the recognition and destruction of mutant cells that can become cancerous. The incidence of malignant diseases is much lower than predicted by the frequency of abnormal cell generation. A depressed immune surveillance system (caused by immunodeficiency diseases or by chemotherapy-induced immunosuppression) can lead to the appearance of some types of cancer.

The increase in basic immunologic information has dramatically advanced during the past century and particularly during roughly the past five decades. In addition to allergy therapy, autoimmune disorder treatments, and increased organ transplantation efficacy, the rise in knowledge has allowed the development of vaccines to prevent infectious disease and of new methods to detect and treat cancer, and somatic gene therapy for immunodeficiency diseases. The prospect of being able to bolster failing immune defenses in different clinical situations is truly epochal. Also, scientists have used immunologic discoveries in the laboratory to identify pathogens facilitating the diagnosis and prevention of disease, product or package tampering; and in fundamental studies of cell biology, such as identifying different protein substances in cell cytoplasm. Deciphering the complex molecular pathways of immune cell activation will continue to provide mechanistic understandings needed to target molecules in dysfunctional immune cells. Human genome sequencing data combined with immunologic data are being exploited through the science of bioinformatics and its subdisciplines to determine gene function on a whole-organism scale. Assigning function to immune system-associated genes will allow us to generate a key for deciphering the type and nature of immune responses—furthering our understanding of the immune system through these approaches boggles the imagination.

Keeping infectious microbes out, destroying them once they enter, and doing the same for self-infectious cells like cancer cells is the immune system's mission. This chapter introduces the complex and sensitive system of checks and balances that permit (when provoked) the development of an immune response.

# IMMUNOLOGY AS A SCIENCE HAS A BRIEF HISTORY

**Immunology**, *or the science that studies the structure and functioning of the immune system*, began long before anyone knew about disease-causing microbes or even that individuals had an immune system that protected the body against disease. Immunology began through efforts to understand, and to intervene in, states of disease. The Greek historian of the Peloponnesian War, Thucydides (430 B.C.), recorded that during the plague of Athens only those persons who recovered from the disease could nurse the sick because they did not catch the disease a second time. During the 15th century, the Arabs and the Chinese translated this knowledge into a crude form of clinical practice by infecting individuals with material from the pustules of smallpox patients. The intentional infection usually gave the infected person a mild form of the disease and induced immunity. It was not risk free, between 1 and 2% of those deliberately infected died as compared to 30% who died when they contracted smallpox naturally. Furthermore, the mild form of the disease that the patient contracted could spread, causing an epidemic. This practice of using unmodified pathogen became established in Western Europe in 1718 when Lady Mary Wortley Montagu (the wife of the English ambassador in Constantinople) performed this technique, called **variation** (L. *variola*, smallpox), on her children. Variation was modified by Edward Jenner, an English physician, in 1796 and his results on *vaccination* were published in 1798—the birth of Immunology. Although he knew nothing about the immune system, Jenner observed that dairymaids who contracted cowpox from cows rarely contracted smallpox. Jenner reasoned that the mild cowpox disease protected an individual against the killer smallpox. He tested this hypothesis by inoculating an 8-year-old boy with fluid from a dairymaid's cowpox pustule and later inoculated the boy with smallpox (variation). The experiment proved successful because the boy was protected from smallpox. Thus, Jenner is credited with the technique of **vaccination**[1] (L. *vacca*, cow),

---

[1]Vaccination is the process of using noninfectious substances to do harmlessly what the body does after recovering from a disease—establish resistance.

which replaced variation. Because cowpox and smallpox viruses were structurally similar, the immune system could not differentiate between the look-alikes. The flip side would be that the immune system *does* distinguish between the two. The similar structures allowed for cross-reactive protection to smallpox with cowpox vaccine. Effective vaccination programs eradicated the smallpox virus in 1979 from the face of the earth.

A century later, Louis Pasteur formulated the germ theory of disease. This theory declared that disease is caused by microorganisms rather than by an imbalance of body humors or the position of the moon. Although Pasteur was the founder of bacteriology, he was much more interested in preventing the diseases caused by microorganisms than in studying the microorganisms themselves. To induce immunity to microbes, Pasteur used **vaccines** (he called them vaccines in honor of Jenner). These substances contain components from infectious organisms that stimulate immunity (but not disease), which protects against reinfection by those organisms. The **attenuation of virulence** (*elimination or reduction of disease-causing potential*) was achieved in two ways: aging of cultures and variation of culture temperature. Pasteur showed (accidentally at first) that the causative agents of chicken cholera and rabies lost their virulence when maintained in culture for long periods of time but still could induce immunity. Pasteur also showed that temperature attenuated *Bacillus anthracis* (the causative agent of anthrax). The vaccines against chicken cholera, rabies, and anthrax are called **attenuated vaccines**. Later, two other types of immunizing agent vaccines were introduced: **killed vaccines** (*suspensions of killed bacteria or viruses*) and **toxoids** (*attenuated bacterial toxins*) (see Chapter 17). Pasteur's many contributions to the discipline, in particular his development of the rabies and chicken cholera vaccines, marked the beginning of modern scientific immunology. There are new categories of vaccines, they include: *subunit, glycoconjugate, recombinant*, and *nucleic acid vaccines* (see Chapter 17).

At the time of Pasteur, the underlying mechanisms of adaptive immunity were unknown. Building on Pasteur's achievements, the new field of immunology began developing in two directions. Efforts continued to extend the range of diseases treated by vaccination and to find new ways of preparing these vaccines; simultaneously, bacteriologists began trying to explain the mechanisms responsible for immunity. The evolution of immunology from the 19th century to the 1930s can be summarized as follows: (1) separating immunity into two divisions, (2) identification of the principal mediators of immunity, (3) recognition of the detrimental side of immunity, (4) description of the main human blood groups, and (5) observation that a host normally cannot induce immunity to its body constituents.

At the turn of the 20th century, immunologists were trying to answer the question "How is protection mediated?" Two camps arose: the humoralists lead by Paul Ehrlich, who pushed the idea that soluble (so-called "humoral" cell-free) molecules mediated immunity, based on the induction of antitoxin and bactericidal activity in serum, and the cellularists lead by Elie Metchnikoff, who believed innate phagocytic cells (which he called *macrophages*) mediated immunity, based on ingestion and digestion of microorganisms—the humoral (adaptive) immunity and the cell-mediated (innate) immunity camps. (Ehrlich and Metchnikoff shared the 1908 Nobel Prize, largely to call a truce in a divisive war.) A US microbiologist by the name of Wright brought the two camps together. He showed that humoral molecules (non-antibodies now known as *complement* and considered part of innate immunity) enhanced cellular phagocytic immune responses. Cell-mediated immunity as mediated by T cells, along with humoral immunity mediated by antibodies, are now both considered part of adaptive immunity, while innate immunity is mediated in part by phagocytic cells. The humoral arm of adaptive immunity dominated until the mid-1940s, when Gowens brought back cells, but they were lymphocytes. It took until the mid-1990s to integrate the adaptive and innate systems—which are jointly needed for the resolution of most infections.

The first three principal mediators described were: (1) the phagocytic cells (actively internalize foreign substances), (2) antibodies (mark foreign substances for destruction), and (3) complement (plasma proteins that "complement" antibody activity). At the same time that these mediators were identified, the hallmark of immunity, specificity, was described. Immunologically, specificity means that the antibody or immune cell that protects you from measles will not protect you from mumps. However, antibody that protects one person from a specific disease can be transferred to another and protect that person from the same disease. These early results showed that the body is capable of producing specific antibodies when invaded by infectious agents. In the 1920s, the dangers of immunity were recognized by Arthus, Dale, and others, who found that such diseases as hay fever and poison ivy are immunologically based. For example, when certain people are exposed to pollen, their bodies make a specific antibody that overreacts and produces responses like hay fever. In the 1940s, scientists finally realized that an injured or absent immune system eliminates protection against disease-causing agents.

The discovery by Karl Landsteiner in 1900 of the three main human blood groups (A, B, and O) showed that immunologic reactions could affect tissues. Red blood cells can differ from person to person; if a wrong blood type is transfused, an immune response called a *transfusion reaction* occurs. A naturally occurring equivalent arises during childbirth when an Rh incompatibility occurs between the fetus and the mother. (Landsteiner also discovered Rh red blood cell markers.) If the mother becomes immunized to the fetus's red blood cells, the resulting antibodies can destroy the fetus's red cells. This disease is called *hemolytic disease of the newborn*.

Ehrlich observed another important characteristic of the immune system early in the 20th century. He noted that our bodies do not normally produce antibodies against our own tissues; he called this phenomenon *horror autotoxicus* (fear of self-poisoning). Currently, it is called *immunologic tolerance*. The maintenance of this peaceable coexistence of immune cells and other body cells, or self-tolerance, is the balancing feature of the immune system, preventing the continual initiation of autoimmune diseases.

During World War II, urgent medical problems shifted emphasis from immunochemistry to immunobiology and helped to develop immunology into a major discipline of basic science that delved into problems of infectious disease, allergy, maternal-fetal interactions, immunologic tolerance, immunologic deficiency diseases, autoimmunity, transplantation, and cancer. This shift in interest is illustrated by the research on immunologic tolerance. The experimental basis for an understanding of tolerance was provided in 1946 by Ray Owen, who observed that some nonidentical twin cattle were incapable of an immune response against their nonidentical sibling. These cattle had shared a common blood supply during fetal development because of a birth defect. Because they were of differing types, the expectation had been that the components of each other's blood would elicit immune responses. From these observations, Peter Medawar (1953) designed an experiment in which he exposed fetal animals to foreign skin cells and thus deliberately induced tolerance to foreign skin grafts. He also showed that tolerance was specific because these animals as adults still rejected unrelated skin grafts. Others helped to show that cells of the immune system are responsible for the rejection of grafts. The work of Snell and others in the 1930s on the genetics of graft rejection showed that the problem of transplantation was partly genetic and that inherited tissue markers recognized by the immune system that distinguish self from nonself frequently lead to graft rejection. A self-arising transplant, or cancer, also was shown to have unique markers that can be recognized as foreign. This discovery of tumor-specific immune responses produced an entirely new area of medicine, immunotherapy, and opened a major subdiscipline of immunology called *tumor immunology.*

One of the most significant findings during the late 1940s involved the recognition of the importance of certain white blood cells (*lymphocytes*), which can be activated to perform many biologic functions. Most of contemporary immunology starts in the 1960s and is devoted to studies dealing with the activation, proliferation, and differentiation of lymphocytes and the functions that these lymphocytes are then able to perform and molecules lymphocytes can make; characterizing these molecules lead to the discovery of how antibody and T cell antigen receptor (TCR) diversity was generated, and the *in vitro* production of pure copies of antibody and TCRs. This knowledge of immune cells and the previous knowledge of antibodies formed the basis for the separation of adaptive aspects of immunology into its classical and current divisions *humoral (antibodies)* and *cellular (immune [T] cells) immunology.* The recognition that two types of lymphocytes were responsible for this division led to an explanation of how lymphocytes recognize foreign substances and the needed "immune response" genes, their trafficking to sites of collaboration, their mechanisms of collaboration and subsequent activation pathways, and the ever increasing number of elements in this collaboration, leading to the realization that the immune system infrastructure was, and continues to be, much more varied and complex than originally appreciated.

It was not until the mid-1990s that the divisiveness of the early 1900s ended when a link between innate and adaptive immunity was discovered—the discovery of Toll-like receptors (TLRs) and their associated functions provided the connection. It suggested that innate immunity was not only a first line of defense but that it incited adaptive immunity into action, and like adaptive immunity it could be divided into humoral and cellular parts.[2]

---

[2]For more information on the benchmark developments in immunology see the "Pillars in Immunology" series in *The Journal of Immunology* starting in July of 2004.

# INNATE IMMUNITY IN VERTEBRATES IS CONSTITUTIVE AND LACKS IMMUNOLOGIC MEMORY; IT PROTECTS THROUGH MULTIPLE MECHANISMS

Initially, the term *immunity* only implied resistance to disease because infectious diseases were the main cause of death in humans. Early immunologists focused primarily on the development of immunity to infectious agents. Contemporary immunologists investigate all aspects of the immune response, and, as a result, immunity has acquired a much broader meaning.

Spore-forming bacteria can be considered capable of immune responses because they produce spores when confronted with hostile conditions. However, immunologists evaluate the specialized responses of vertebrate hosts. *When foreign substances such as bacteria, viruses, fungi, or parasites are introduced into a vertebrate host, the host either (1) nonspecifically clears the infectious agent using preformed components or (2) produces specific cells and molecules directed against the foreign invader. The combined responses are traditionally called an* **immune response**. The foreign invader that induces and reacts with immune cells and the molecules it induced (such as antibodies) is called an *antigen*. These two responses, or two kinds of immunity—innate and adaptive—are the abbreviated subject of the pages that follow. A general comparison between innate and adaptive is illustrated in Figure 1-1 and Table 1-1. *The distinction revolves around the mechanisms and receptors used for immune recognition, that is, how the immune system senses infection and how it eradicates infection while spuring self-tissues.*

**Innate immunity** *(also called natural resistance) operates relatively nonspecifically during the early phases of an immune response without a need for prior exposure.* Innate immune system recognition is mediated by *pattern recognition receptors (PRRs)*, which recognize conserved shared classes of molecules produced by pathogens called *pathogen-associated molecular patterns (PAMPs)* (detailed in Chapter 3); PAMPs are not restricted to pathogens all microbes express them. These PAMPs are not found in host tissues and cells. Pattern recognition receptor engagement with infectious agents activates nonspecific cells and molecules. This interaction signals the host that a microbial pathogen has been encountered, drives

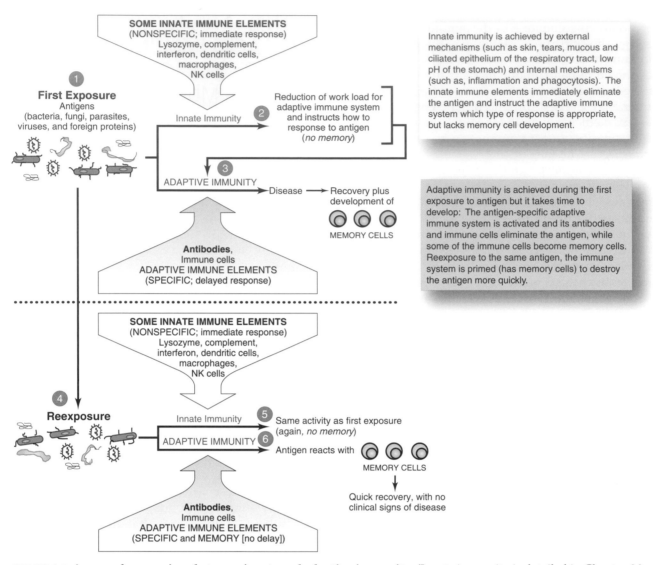

**FIGURE 1-1  A general comparison between innate and adaptive immunity**. (Innate immunity is detailed in Chapter 3.)

**TABLE 1-1** Innate and Adaptive Immunity

| Property | Innate Immune System | Adaptive Immune System |
|---|---|---|
| Receptors | Germline-encoded | Antigen receptors are products of somatic DNA recombination |
| Mechanism for recognition | Nonspecific (conserved molecular patterns: LPS, mannan, glycans) | Specific (details of molecular structure: proteins, peptides, carbohydrates) |
| Effector components | Preformed | Selected |
| Activation time of effectors | Immediate | Delayed |
| Immunologic memory | No | Yes |
| Distinguishing self from nonself components | Perfect | Imperfect (autoimmune diseases) |

LPS, Lipopolysaccharides.

the maturation of these nonspecific cells, clears the pathogen, and eventually leads to the activation of the adaptive immune response. Innate immunity serves as the first line of defense and includes both external and internal constitutive responses. External defenses occur in those areas of the body exposed to the outside environment (the contact areas for pathogens). Internal defenses come into play when the pathogen has penetrated the external defenses; the host creates an inhospitable or lethal environment to microbes. The major component of these internal processes is *inflammation. Taken together, the components of innate immunity are preformed* (the components are present before challenge), *standardized* (the response magnitude is consistent), *without memory* (the host does not realize it has been reexposed to the same invader), and relatively *nonspecific* (targets commonly shared microbe antigens). The latter antigens are unique to microorganisms and the receptors that recognize them do not recognize host molecules—a perfect system that recognizes only foreign antigens (pathogens) and ignores self components.

## External Innate Immunity, Natural Barriers to Infection, Prevents the Penetration of Pathogens into Tissues

External, innate immunity (skin, body secretions, and mucous membranes) prevents the penetration of pathogens into host tissues (see Figure 3-2). Intact skin prevents penetration of most pathogens; exceptions include *Treponema pallidum* and *Schistosoma mansoni* (the causative agents of syphilis and schistosomiasis, respectively). *T. pallidum* is acquired through sexual contact, attaches to host cells by coating itself with fibronectin, and invades intact mucous membranes or abraded skin by boring through them. *S. mansoni* can be acquired by contact with water containing the infective forms, which penetrate the skin by means of enzymes that break down the skin. Skin also secretes lactic acid and fatty acids that act as bacteriostatic agents by lowering skin pH. Tears protect the eye by providing a washing action. Tears also contain a hydrolytic enzyme against Gram-positive bacteria called *lysozyme*. If pathogens are inhaled, mucus and the ciliated epithelium of the respiratory tract act as filters. If pathogens are swallowed, mucus in the digestive tract prevents adsorption and penetration of pathogens into cells. The low pH in the stomach kills organisms, and the normal flora of the lower intestine inhibits the attachment of pathogens. Similar components and mechanisms are in place in the urogenital tract.

## Internal Innate Immunity Offers Many Forms of Protection After Pathogens Enter the Body

If a pathogen breeches the external innate defenses and invades the tissues, internal defense mechanisms provide protection. Internal, innate immunity includes three general mechanisms: (1) *physiologic barriers*, (2) *phagocytosis*, and (3) *inflammation*. Physiologic barriers offer inhospitable environments to pathogens. These barriers include body temperature and oxygen tension. For example, chickens are resistant to anthrax because of their high body temperature. If their temperature is lowered, they become susceptible. Anaerobic organisms (such as *Clostridium perfringens*, the causative agent of gangrene) cannot grow in tissues where oxygen concentrations are high. Microorganisms themselves also can activate physiologic barriers called *complement proteins* that mediate cell lysis and enhance phagocytosis. Virally infected host cells release *interferons*, which interfere with the replication of viruses that have infected neighboring cells.

A more effective innate internal defense is phagocytosis. **Phagocytosis** *involves the engulfment and destruction of pathogens and particulate matter by cells of the* **mononuclear phagocyte system**. The cells that make up this network are the *mononuclear phagocytic cells* (*monocytes* and *macrophages*). These cells also provide help during adaptive immunity. Monocytes and macrophages are called *professional phagocytes*—professional in the sense that their primary role is phagocytosis. Phagocytic cells, the first line of internal defense, respond immediately and without specificity (see Figure 3-11). Macrophages ingest and digest whole bacteria and even injured and dead host cells. Macrophages constitutively express receptors for polysaccharides found on bacteria; these receptors facilitate phagocytosis. Also, during phagocytosis, macrophages release powerful chemical molecules, called *monokines* (generically called *cytokines*), such as tumor necrosis factor-$\alpha$ (TNF-$\alpha$), interleukin-1 (IL-1), and IL-6 that activate many nonspecific protective effects through the inflammatory response. However, phagocytosis against soluble antigens (such as toxins) is poor.

Another important group of professional phagocytic cells, filled with granules containing potent digestive chemicals, not included in the mononuclear phagocyte system are the *polymorphonuclear neutrophilic leukocytes*, or *neutrophils* for short (so named because they exhibit large, lobed nuclei). These cells are arbitrarily excluded from the mononuclear phagocyte system because they are not participants in normal specific immune induction reactions; they only internalize microorganisms for digestion, not for subsequent presentation to other immune cells. Along with their phagocytic activity, neutrophils are the main source for small peptides called *defensins* and *cathelicidins*. These peptides have a broad antimicrobial spectrum and exert nonspecific cytotoxic activity against a wide range of normal and malignant targets.

The third group of paraprofessional phagocytes is *dendritic cells*, which are a specialized group of cells that are inefficient at clearing infectious microbes but are highly efficient at presenting antigens to T lymphocytes—a bridge between innate and adaptive immunity.

Another set of granule-filled, lymphocyte-like cells called *natural killer (NK) cells* are not phagocytic but contribute to innate immunity through nonspecific defense against virus-infected body cells and tumor cells without need for prior exposure and clonal expansion. In addition to their killing abilities, they produce the immunoregulatory cytokines interferon-$\gamma$ and TNF-$\alpha$, which stimulate dendritic cell maturation and activation, the activation of macrophages, and drive the development of certain adaptive immune cells. *Natural-killer T (NKT) cells*, a cross between a NK cell and a T cell, exhibit rapid cytolytic activity and cytokine production without need for priming and clonal expansion—early responders important in the initation and regulation of immune responses.

The other component of the internal innate defenses is a complex group of reactions leading to **inflammation**. Pathogen insult and chemical mediators that are released during the host's attempt to clear the pathogen and repair the associated tissue damage initiate the inflammatory response. Inflammation (literally, "setting on fire") of a particular body region is indicated by the suffix *-itis*; for example, inflammation of the tonsils is called *tonsillitis*, and inflammation of the appendix is called *appendicitis*. The four cardinal signs of inflammation were described by the Roman physician Celsus roughly 2000 years ago. The four distinct symptoms that always accompany short-term, or acute, inflammation are redness, swelling, heat, and pain. Two hundred years after Celsus's description, another physician, Galen, added a fifth sign, loss of function. *Inflammation collectively involves a series of vascular events that serve as a defense mechanism. Inflammation includes (1) clotting mechanism activation, (2) increased blood flow, (3) increased capillary permeability, and (4) enhanced influx of phagocytic cells* (see Chapter 3).

Innate immunity serves as a rapid response system for sensing and clearing infections caused by pathogens. If the system fails to contain a pathogen, vertebrates use an additional immune recognition strategy called *adaptive*, or *acquired* or *specific, immunity*. Adaptive immunity kicks in later and permits the host to recognize and respond to a specific invader and is marked by an enhanced response on repeated exposures to the invader. Nonetheless, both innate and adaptive immune defenses work together to enhance each other's effects. Innate mechanisms reduce the workload and set the stage for adaptive defenses, and adaptive mechanisms amplify and focus innate defenses.

---

**MINI SUMMARY**

The immune system has two primary functions: (1) recognition of and defense against foreign substances and (2) immunosurveillance. The components of external and internal innate immunity are preformed, standardized, without memory, and nonspecific. When external defenses such as skin, secretions, and mucous membranes fail to prevent invasion by pathogens, internal innate defenses such as temperature, oxygen tension, phagocytosis, and inflammation control infections. To accomplish this, the innate immune system depends heavily on neutrophils, macrophages, dendritic cells, NK cells, and NKT cells for host defense. Collectively, innate immunity reduces the workload for the immune system's specific defenses and sets the stage for adaptive immunity.

---

# ADAPTIVE IMMUNITY IN VERTEBRATES THAT IS ACHIEVED THROUGH EXPERIENCE BECAUSE OF EITHER RECOVERY FROM DISEASE OR MEDICAL INTERVENTION

**Adaptive** (also called **acquired** or **specific**) **immunity** *develops during a host's lifetime and is based partly on the host's experiences, such as stimulated by tissues-invading microbes—in turn, the immune system adjusts to the microbe's presence* (see Table 1-1). This exposure process is called **immunization**. Adaptive immunity is the surveillance mechanism of vertebrates that *specifically* recognizes foreign *antigens* and *selectively* eliminates them, and on reencountering the antigens has an enhanced response. The recall response is often so efficient that no symptoms appear. This activity is organized around two classes of specialized cells, T cells and B cells, and their somatically generated, structurally unique, specific receptors. Once a host has been exposed to a specific disease, the host will develop specific immunity and will probably not catch the disease again. This section briefly describes the six major characteristics of adaptive immunity: *(1) specificity, (2) inducibility, (3) diversity, (4) memory, (5) distinguishing self from nonself*, and *(6) self-limiting*.

The persistence of a foreign antigen in a host initiates, or induces, adaptive immunity. The recognition of and response to the antigen are highly specific, each lymphocyte is endowed with a unique receptor—a lock and key complementarity, although immune specificity is not absolute. **Cross-reactions** *happen when adaptive immunity to one substance gives immunity to another substance.* The earlier example of cowpox exposure causing immunity to smallpox illustrates cross-reactive protection. This cross-reactivity is due to the physical similarity of the agents. If there was no immunity to a foreign substance before exposure, immunity to that substance can be induced by that substance. In fact, there is an opulence, or diversity, to the immune system's resources once the system is induced. It can recognize and mount a unique response to a seemingly endless variety $(10^9)$ of antigens. This diversity is the result of a matching number of antigen receptors. Two or three types of gene segments, randomly assembled during B- and T-cell development by a series of DNA-rearrangement events, encode the antigen-binding portions of these receptors. Once immunity has been acquired, reexposure to the same antigen leads to a rapid and more effective immune response called a *secondary immune response. The ability of the immune system to remember antigenic intrusion is called* **immunologic memory** (in contrast, innate immunity lacks specificity for unique protein structures and memory). Although the immune system can respond to at least $10^9$ different foreign antigens, it is unresponsive to, or tolerant of, self-antigens present in that individual. A breakdown in the maintenance of self-tolerance can lead to autoimmune disease. When the antigen has been brought under control, the immune response is downregulated through antigen removal, antagonistic cytokine production, limiting immune cell activity by regulatory cells, and feedback regulation of the induced response.

How does the immune system accomplish an adaptive immune response? It divides it into phases or functional steps: antigen recognition (the cognitive phase), lymphocyte activation (a two signal event), and antigen elimination (effector phase). The successful completion of these phases leads to decline of the immune response (homeostasis) and memory. The antigen recognition phase requires direct contact (ensures specificity) between the antigen and the counterpart receptor on a clone of antigen-specific lymphocytes. This engagement leads to the activation phase, which requires two distinct but synergistic signals: the first signal is antigen and the second signal is a series of costimulators and cytokines. The second signal results from the interaction of innate immune system components with microbes and injured cells. The result of the activation phase events is the proliferation and differentiation of lymphocytes into effector cells, which produce effector molecules or mediate effector functions directly and memory cells. The effector molecules (antibodies) and cells (T lymphocytes) neutralize and eliminate extracellular (such as bacteria) and intracellular (such as viruses) antigens, respectively. Once antigen is removed the immune system returns to a resting state. Any remaining antigen-specific effector cells die by apoptosis.

## Adaptive Immunity Is Humoral, Cell-Mediated, or Both

Vertebrates possess two types of adaptive immunity based on the components the immune system uses to mediate immunity (Figure 1-2). **Humoral immunity**[3] *is mediated by antigen-specific blood proteins called <u>antibodies</u>* (see Chapter 4). Antibodies are secreted only by plasma cells (the daughter cells of *bone marrow–derived B <u>lymphocytes</u>*). This immunity protects against circulating extracellular antigens such as bacteria, microbial exotoxins, and viruses in their extracellular phase; that is, antibodies normally interact with circulating antigens but are unable to penetrate living cells. Humoral immunity's concomitant counterpart during an immune response is **cell-mediated immunity**. *This immunity is mediated by antigen-specific cells called <u>thymus-derived</u>, or <u>T</u>, lymphocytes; there are at least two main subpopulations of T cells: T helper ($T_H$) cells and T cytotoxic ($T_C$) cells* (see Chapter 2). Cell-mediated immunity protects against intracellular parasites, such as viruses, and is important in the rejection of organ transplants and tumor cells. Because activated, antigen-specific B and T lymphocytes eliminate antigen, they are called *effector*

---

[3]The word *humoral* is used because plasma cells secrete antibodies into the body's fluids, or humors.

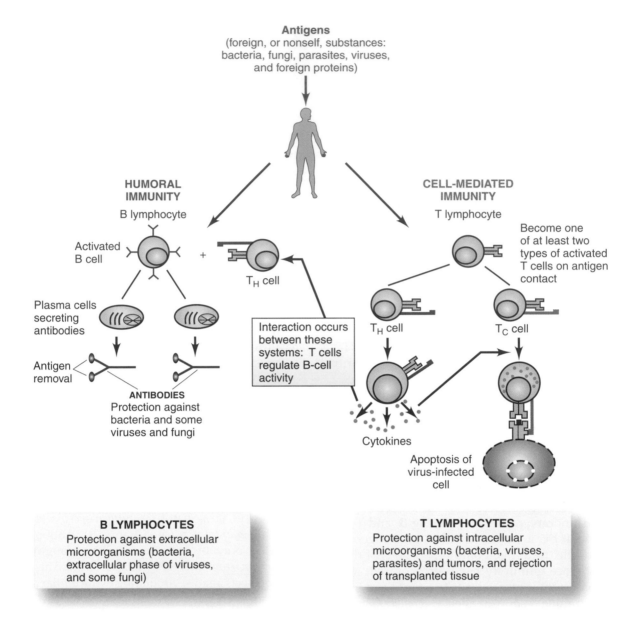

**FIGURE 1-2  The two types of adaptive immunity—humoral and cell-mediated**. When antigens such as bacteria or some viruses are introduced into a host, the host responds by producing antibodies that bind the introduced antigens and lead to their elimination. This response to antigens constitutes the *humoral immune response*. When an antigen is unreachable by antibodies or a virus-infected cell, the host can rally cytotoxic T ($T_C$) cells that can specifically react with and destroy the virus-infected cell; this response is known as the *cell-mediated immune response*. To develop into plasma cells or $T_C$ cells, these cells need help from helper T ($T_H$) cells and their cytokines.

*cells*. B cell–derived plasma cells act as effector cells by releasing antibodies, while $T_H$ cells release communication molecules (*cytokines*) and $T_C$ cells kill target cells. Both humoral and cellular immune responses are evoked during antigen insult, although one of these two responses predominates based on the type of challenge.

## Adaptive Immunity Can Be Active or Passive

Humoral and cell-mediated adaptive immunity can each be divided into **active** and **passive immunity** (Figure 1-3). Active immunity is acquired gradually (5 to 14 days after antigen exposure), lasts for years,

Immune Sytem Hierarchy

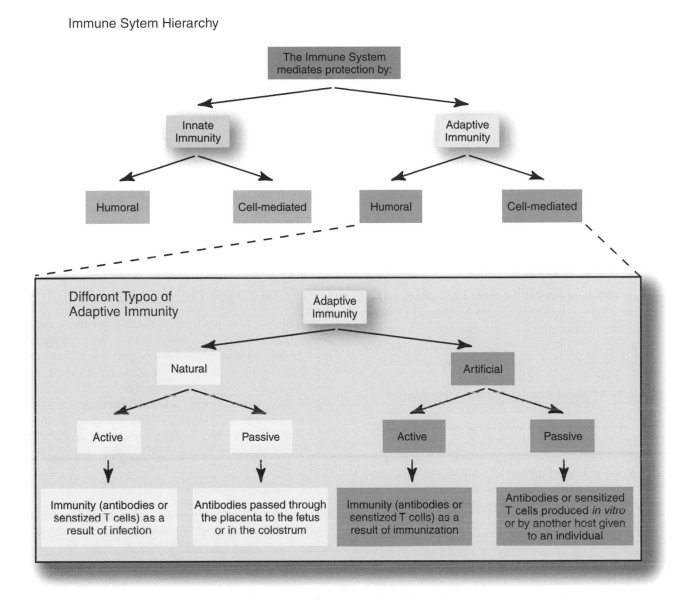

**FIGURE 1-3  A flow chart of the different types of immunity.**

and is highly protective. Passive immunity is immediate, lasts for days to months, has low to moderate protective effectiveness, and does not develop memory in the recipient. Some diseases, such as tetanus, often kill a person before immunity can be established. To avoid such a drastic result, the person can be given immediate protection by the infusion of antibodies, but the effect is short-lived and there is no immunologic memory. Both active and passive immunity can be further subdivided into *natural* and *artificial* forms. In active immunity, an individual has adaptive immunity mediated by antibodies or sensitized T lymphocytes (T cells) *formed by that individual*. If an individual is exposed to foreign

substances naturally through the environment, rather than by immunization with a vaccine, that individual acquires the *natural* rather than the *artificial* form of active immunity. In passive immunity, an individual has adaptive immunity mediated by antibodies (or sensitized T cells) *formed in another individual*. Antibodies are transferred from one host to another to confer immunity. The passage of antibodies between individuals is called *passive transfer*. *Adoptive transfer* is the passage of T cells (or any immune cells) between inbred animals of the same strain or in human bone marrow transplants to grant immunity. The passage of antibodies from the mother to the fetus across the placenta or to the infant through the colostrum is a form of natural, passive adaptive immunity. Artificial, passive adaptive immunity occurs when preformed antibodies or immune cells are given to a nonimmune individual (such as gamma globulin injections for hepatitis).

# CLONAL SELECTION OF LYMPHOCYTES EXPLAINS DIVERSITY, SPECIFICITY, AND MEMORY

As mentioned earlier, adaptive immunity revolves around two groups of lymphocytes that bind antigen using antigen-specific membrane receptors. To set the stage for clonal selection let's answer the following question: how do these receptors originate? Genetic rearrangement recombines linearly arranged groups of germline gene segments into a single, contiguous DNA sequence that encodes the antigen-binding part of B or T cell antigen receptor chains. This process occurs as B cells develop in the bone marrow and T cells develop in the thymus. The unsuccessful production of functional receptors for either cell type leads to their death in these organs. This mixing-and-matching process, the random recombination of different gene segments, leads to the huge diversity of functional genes that encode the antigen-binding domains of antigen-receptors—thus shaping our adaptive immune system to recognize and react with all antigens. This huge number of different antigen specificities is called the *immune repertoire*. Since this repertoire is randomly generated, some lymphocytes express self-antigen- reactive receptors; when these cells bind to antigen in the bone marrow or thymus, they are eliminated (*clonal deletion*) before they mature. If they escape this process, they are inhibited in the periphery (see Chapter 13).

The specificity and memory associated with adaptive immunity fall within the framework of *clonal selection*. This paradigm of immune cell origin and development is the central integrating concept in modern immunology. Clonal selection of lymphocytes provides the framework to explain the hallmarks of the immune response, which comprise (1) *diversity*, (2) *specificity*, and (3) *immunologic memory*. *Each immune cell can recognize and respond to only one antigen and the specificity of these cells is developed before the antigen is introduced*. An antigen does not induce the appearance of immune cells; rather, it *selects* preexisting antigen-specific immune cells by interacting with the cells' receptors. Thus a host exists in a preimmune state against antigens that have yet to be encountered. The group of immune cells specific for an antigen is called a *clone* of cells. Clones are derived from the same mother cell and so are identical; clones are activated after antigen selectively stimulates their antigen-specific receptors. Thus diversity and specificity result from having millions of different clones that each demonstrate unique antigen specificity, and both diversity and specificity exist before any antigen exposure. However, memory develops during clonal expansion and differentiation. *Memory cells* represent an enlarged clone of long-lived cells B or T cells that are committed to respond rapidly, or by their clonal expansion, on reexposure to the same antigen. Immunologic memory results from having more cells and cells that can immediately be directed against a previously encountered antigen; it permits a secondary immune response on reexposure to the antigen.

Many years of research led to the development of the concept known as *clonal selection*. Immunologists now know, for example, that the B cell is a "parent" cell that expresses antibody on its surface. The binding of specific antigen by surface antibodies induces the B cell to proliferate and differentiate into an antibody-secreting "daughter" cell called a *plasma cell*. The antibody secreted has the same antigen-binding specificity as when the antibody acted as a receptor molecule.

B cells are <u>selected</u> when antigen binds to membrane-bound antibody receptors specific for that antigen. This interaction, plus signals from other immune cells, causes B cells to differentiate into plasma cells that secrete antibody with the <u>same</u> specificity as their membrane-bound counterpart. This scenario for interaction is one of the basic tenets of **clonal selection** in antibody formation. It is called *selective* because antibody receptors are selected for specifically by the right antigen. B cells that bind antigens are found in an individual before the individual has been exposed to those antigens.

Realization that DNA determined protein structure changed the thinking of immunologists. If every antigen receptor specificity means a different protein molecule and each protein molecule has a unique gene, the genetic information that encodes these receptors must exist in a person's DNA before exposure to the antigen. Within a few years of the discovery of DNA structure, immunologists, particularly Burnet, outlined the **clonal selection theory** of antibody formation. Burnet's contemporized basic tenets for the clonal selection theory are summarized as follows:

1. Early in embryogenesis and throughout adult life, a host develops a large repertoire of

antibody[receptor]-forming cell precursors, or *clones* (can be B cell or T cell clones). Each clone can recognize and respond to only one unique antigen. The number of progenitor cells in each clone is small (each lymphocyte expresses a single type of receptor with a unique specificity, so at the single-cell level there is no diversity), but the collective clonal repertoire can respond to any antigen.

2. During *in utero* development and throughout adult life, a host takes inventory of self-antigen reactive cells, and these cells (Burnet called them *forbidden clones*) are deleted or functionally inhibited. "Forbidden clones" are the precursor cells capable of responding against the host's tissue antigens and therefore absence from the repertoire of mature lymphocytes. (If absent, why do we still have autoimmune diseases? This question will be answered in later chapters.)

3. Foreign antigen reacts selectively with the right high-affinity receptor-expressing, pre-existing clones and activates them. Clonal

expansion occurs, leading to differentiation into antibody[receptor]-forming cells and memory cells; all of these daughter cells will bear receptors of identical antigen specificity to the parental cells.

Clonal selection supports genetic control of the immune response (Figure 1-4) and suggests that discrete, separate genes control the tertiary structure of antibody. It also supports that the interaction of antigen with antibody receptors starts the clonal proliferation of a group of B cells genetically restricted to one antibody specificity. These cells differentiate into either memory cells or antibody-forming plasma cells. However, both antigen-independent and antigen-dependent phases of B-cell development exist. The generation of diversity that leads to antigenically committed B cells, which then can be "selected," is antigen-independent (see Chapter 6). The antigen-dependent phase of B-cell development (clonal selection) occurs only when specific antigen *chooses* the appropriate preexisting B cell (see Chapter 10).

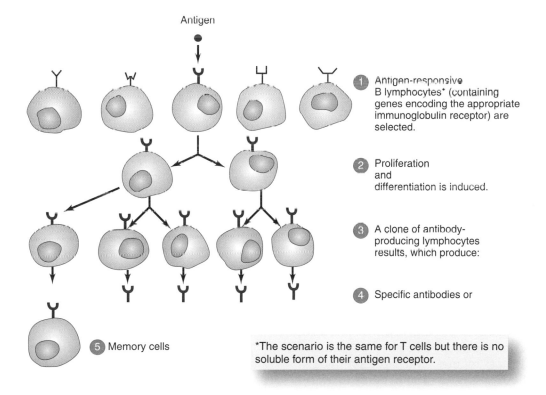

Antigen

1. Antigen-responsive B lymphocytes* (containing genes encoding the appropriate immunoglobulin receptor) are selected.

2. Proliferation and differentiation is induced.

3. A clone of antibody-producing lymphocytes results, which produce:

4. Specific antibodies or

5. Memory cells

*The scenario is the same for T cells but there is no soluble form of their antigen receptor.

**FIGURE 1-4 Model of clonal selection.** A host exists in a preimmune state because each B lymphocyte has genes that encode one specific antibody. Specific antibodies that are secreted are at first found on the surface of lymphocytes as receptors. The antigen selects the right cell and induces it to proliferate and differentiate. These activities lead to a clone of antibody-producing cells (plasma cells) that secrete specific antibody. The released antibody is an accurate reflection of its receptor counterpart. Memory cells with receptors of the same specificity also are generated.

Although discussions of clonal selection mention antibodies, this paradigm also applies to cellular immunity. T cells are selected for specific antigen by TCR interaction, inducing proliferation and differentiation of a clone of T cells into regulators of humoral immunity and regulators/effectors of cell-mediated immunity and innate immunity (see Chapter 10). Clonal selection remains the pivotal integrating concept in modern immunology and provides explanations for immunologic diversity, specificity, and memory.

# THE IMMUNE SYSTEM HAS TWO LEVELS OF DEVELOPMENT

Immune system development occurs at two levels: (1) the species level and (2) the individual level. *The developmental history of the immune system during evolution is called* **phylogeny**, *and the developmental history of the immune system in an individual within a species is called* **ontogeny**. The first antibody to appear in phylogeny is also the first to appear during immunologic development in an individual. Thus, "ontogeny recapitulates phylogeny" and vice versa.

Phagocytosis and inflammatory reactions are the most primitive signs of an immune-like system. These forms of nonspecific (innate) immunity are present in invertebrates (such as porifera [sponges], annelids [earthworms], and arthropods [insects, crustaceans]). The anti-microbial peptides and pattern recognition receptors start in arthropods. The first evidence of a vertebrate-like immune system (also called the *lymphoid system*) appears in the primitive vertebrates cyclostomes (hagfish and lamprey) that possess a diffuse system and lack distinct higher vertebrate immune structures. Hagfish and lampreys produce a high-molecular-weight antibody on exposure to foreign substances and reject foreign transplanted tissues. This antibody is comparable to a class of human antibody known as *immunoglobulin M (IgM)*. The earliest immune organ to appear in phylogeny is the thymus. The thymus is present in most primitive vertebrates such as the elasmobranches (dogfish and shark). Amphibians, reptiles, and birds produce at least two of the five classes of antibodies found in humans, mediate graft rejection, and possess B and T cells and the immune organs typical of mammals, such as the thymus, lymph nodes, and spleen.

Throughout the fetal, newborn, and young adult stages of life, the individual undergoes progressive immunologic maturation (ontogeny). The human fetus starts to develop an immune system during the first trimester of pregnancy, and serum antibody (IgM) can be detected during the second trimester. Cells responsible for nonspecific and specific immunity arise from descendants of hematopoietic stem cells. These cells are initially found in the yolk sac, but later appear in the fetal liver and finally in the bone marrow (see Chapter 2).

Because the immune system is poorly developed both in the fetus and in the newborn, the mother's antibodies provide protection. Maternal antibodies are transmitted to the fetus through the placenta during prenatal development in the womb and to the newborn through the colostrum during breast-feeding. A human newborn's lymphocytes are fully competent for cell-mediated immune responses.

In summary, the immune system develops early within species (phylogeny) and becomes progressively more sophisticated. Immune development in individuals within a species (ontogeny) occurs shortly after conception, with final maturity being reached at puberty.

## MINI SUMMARY

Adaptive immunity, whether humoral or cellular, permits the destruction of all substances (living and nonliving) within the body that are not recognized as self. The six major characteristics of adaptive immunity are (1) specificity, (2) inducibility, (3) diversity, (4) memory, (5) distinguishing self from nonself, and (6) downregulation of itself. The main cells of the adaptive immune system are B cells and T cells (and dendritic cells and macrophages). B cells are responsible for humoral immunity, and T cells confer cellular immunity. Unlike the lymphocytes, phagocytic cells (such as dendritic cells and macrophages) do not respond specifically to foreign substances but instead play required auxiliary roles. Adaptive immune responses develop in three phases: antigen recognition, lymphocyte activation, and antigen elimination. Adaptive immunity can be divided into active and passive immunity, each of which is further subdivided into natural and artificial forms. Clonal selection explains how the vertebrate immune system specifically recognizes millions of different antigens. It applies to both B and T cells and accounts for immunologic diversity, memory, and specificity. The developmental history of host immunity can be divided into phylogeny and ontogeny—innate immunity is found in all multicellular plants and animals, while adaptive immunity is found only in vertebrates.

# THE ARCHITECTURE AND MECHANISMS OF THE IMMUNE SYSTEM ARE VARIED AND COMPLEX: AN OVERVIEW

The immune system is a complex functional system consisting of diverse organs, tissues, and cells distributed throughout most of the body (Figure 1-5). Despite the system's complexity, its components are interrelated and act in a highly coordinated and specific manner when they recognize, eliminate, and remember foreign macromolecules and cells (Figure 1-6). To accomplish this task, the immune system must distinguish between *self* and *nonself* materials.

Any foreign substance (living or nonliving) that induces an immune response when introduced into a host is called an *immunogen*, or more generally, an *antigen*. Most antigens are large, complex macromolecules not recognized as self. Only small parts of antigens, called *antigenic determinants* or *epitopes*, induce and react with immune elements such as antibodies or antigen receptors on lymphocytes. Antibodies recognize antigens through their surface characteristics, particularly by the antigen's pattern or shape and

charge. The binding sites of the antibody are precisely complementary, or *specific*, for the right antigenic determinant. When antigen enters the body, it usually induces the production of antibodies that react only with that particular antigen. The immune system also has pre-existing lymphocytes expressing receptors capable of reacting with the specific antigen. The first time we are exposed to an antigen, the result is a *primary immune response*. The second exposure to the same antigen leads to a *secondary immune response*, which is much faster and stronger. This phenomenon is mediated by *immunologic memory cells* and accounts for a person's long-term immunity against infectious diseases.

Among the first cells to interact with antigen are *macrophages* ("big eaters"). As their name implies a defining feature of macrophages is their ability to internalize antigen; they are janitorial cells. These phagocytic cells internalize (called *phagocytosis*) and digest the whole antigen, displaying a small peptide portion on its surface in association with membrane self-markers. This series of events, known as *antigen processing and presentation*, manipulates the antigen into a form that can be recognized as nonself by the T lymphocyte. Thus macrophages, along with their star-shaped cousins dendritic cells, are called *antigen-presenting cells (APCs)*. Dendritic cells also

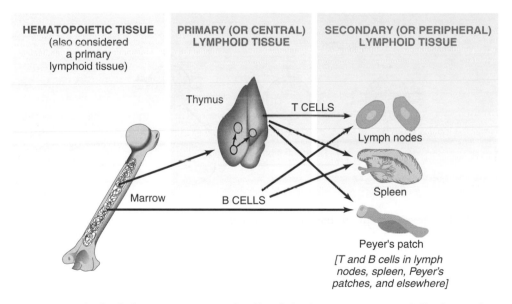

**FIGURE 1-5 Principal tissues, organs, and cells of the immune system**. Cells destined to become immune cells are produced in the bone marrow. Some of the descendants of stem cells can become lymphocytes. The classes of lymphocytes are T cells and B cells. The pre-T cells migrate to the thymus, where they multiply and mature into T cells capable of mediating an immune response. In humans, B cells complete most of their maturation in the bone marrow. Once both T and B cells are mature physically and functionally, they populate the secondary lymphoid organs.

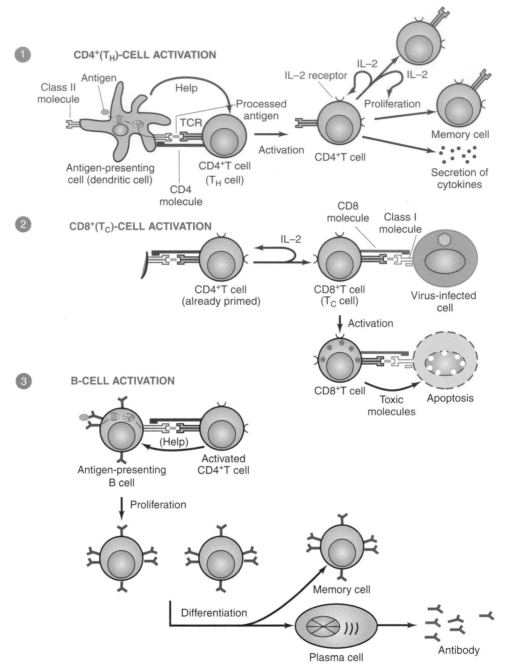

**FIGURE 1-6 Development of the immune response.** The details of this response will be discussed in subsequent chapters. When an antigen [■] is introduced into a host, antigen-presenting cells (mainly dendritic cells) process and present the antigen to CD4+ T cells (usually considered $T_H$ cells). This process and the release of interleukin-1 (IL-1), a helper cytokine, and other cytokines, activate the CD4+ T cells. Activated CD4+ T cells help themselves and CD8+ T cells (usually considered $T_C$ cells) by releasing IL-2 and interferon-γ. Activated CD8+ T cells respond in cell-mediated immunity reactions by their direct participation as effector cells. Antigen-activated B cells, after processing and presenting antigen to activated CD4+ T cells, convert to plasma cells with help through direct interaction with CD4+ T cells and by cytokines like IL-4 and IL-5. The plasma cells secrete specific antibodies against the inducing agent and thereby provide humoral immunity. Some cells become memory cells and react more rapidly to rechallenge by the same antigen. The T cell receptors (TCR) of CD4+ and CD8+ T cells recognize antigen only when associated with class II or I MHC molecules, respectively.

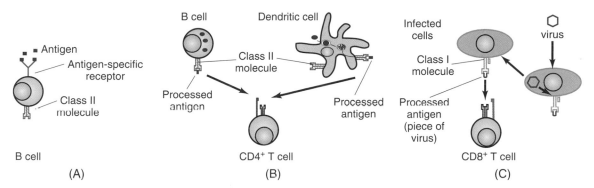

**FIGURE 1-7 Receptors for antigen recognition.** Membrane-bound antibodies, T cell antigen receptors, and MHC molecules are the three kinds of molecules used by the immune system to recognize antigen. **(A)** The B cell's antigen-specific receptor is an antibody anchored in its surface that recognizes antigen in its natural state. B cells can internalize and process antigens similar to the method used by macrophages and dendritic cells and eventually present the antigen using class II MHC molecules. MHC molecules serve as self-labels and identify a cell as belonging to that individual; these molecules permit processed antigen presentation to the appropriate T cell. **(B)** The CD4$^+$ T cell's antigen-specific receptor cannot recognize antigen in its natural state; the antigen must be processed and presented by APCs such as dendritic cells and macrophages. **(C)** The CD8$^+$ T cell's antigen-specific receptor is like that of the CD4$^+$ T cell, but it recognizes antigen bound to a class I MHC molecule, which is found on all nucleated body cells.

communicate with T cells during antigen invasion through soluble factors. The *T and B lymphocytes* are the only immunologically specific cellular components of the immune system (Figure 1-7).

T and B lymphocytes are antigen-specific thereby the mediators of adaptive immunity, but their function is under the control of innate immunity cells, *dendritic cells*—the premier APCs of which there are many types. While macrophages, in addition to being APCs, execute a wide array of functions, the related dendritic cells have developed as specialized APCs. In contrast to macrophages, dendritic cells do not use phagocytosis as a scavenger function, but as a means to process and present antigen-derived peptides to specific T cells. Dendritic cells establish themselves in an immature form in tissues, such as Langerhans' cells in the skin, where they are highly phagocytic but cannot present antigen. Upon encountering an infectious microbe in the periphery, they capture it, process it, express lymphocyte co-stimulatory molecules, migrate to lymphoid organs where they arrive as mature dendritic cells with antigen-presenting capacity—they lose their phagocytic ability and shift to APCs that can activate T cells, the initiation of primary adaptive immunity. They are more than initiators; dendritic cells are also crucial regulators of innate immune activities, in particular natural killer (NK) cell function. In turn, NK cells can influence dendritic cell activity.

A third group of lymphocytes, *NK cells*, do not recognize antigen in the same way as T and B cells and therefore are nonspecific killer cells and part of innate immunity. Unlike T and B cells, whose receptors undergo random DNA recombination or sequence diversification in somatic cells, NK cell receptors are hard-wired. NK cells use a two-receptor (killer-activating and killer inhibitory receptors) recognition strategy, they recognize normal cells and cells that lack major histocompatibility complex (MHC) class I surface molecules, which are normally expressed on all nucleated cells. Cells can sometimes lose the ability to express these MHC molecules due to either microbial interference with the expression mechanism or malignant transformation making them "abnormal." Killer-activating receptors recognize some ubiquitous surface molecules present on normal, nucleated cells, and in the absence of a blocking signal from their counterpart killer-inhibitory receptors, which recognize MHC class I molecules, the killer-activating receptors instruct NK cells to attack and kill the target cell. NK cells mediate killing by cellular cytotoxicity and production of cytokines and chemokines. They are important in attacking virus-infected cells, during the early phases of an infection. They are also efficient killers of tumor cells and thereby involved in tumor surveillance. NK cells are more than killing cells, they also can exert an immunoregulatory effect, particularly on dendritic cells.

Another group of lymphocytes with innate-like antimicrobial functions, *natural killer T (NKT) cells* are a heterogeneous subset of T cells that expresses both NK cell markers and semi-invariant $\alpha\beta$ TCRs. As NK cells, there is interplay between dendritic cells and NKT cells. Some NKT cells recognize lipid antigens, which are presented to NKT cells by dendritic cell-expressed MHC-like CD1d molecules. Selective presentation of lipids by dendritic cells induces a stronger and more prolonged NKT-cell response. Reciprocally, NKT cells can promote dendritic cell maturation. After TCR stimulation, NKT cells rapidly produce copious amounts of interferon-$\gamma$ and IL-4. In contrast to T and B cells but like NK cells, NKT cells exhibit rapid effector functions without need for priming and clonal expansion.

Cells of the immune system communicate by *cytokines*, small, "messenger" molecules that can determine the fate of an immune response. The cytokines produced by lymphocytes are called *lymphokines*, whereas macrophage-derived signals are called *monokines. Interleukins*, as the name implies, act as messengers between *leukocytes* (the general name for lymphocytes and APCs). Interleukins are a major group of cytokines. Another group of cytokines are called *chemokines*. They are a large group of low-molecular-weight molecules that mediate leukocyte chemotaxis (soluble signposts that help immune cells find their way in the body) and control the expression of leukocyte adhesion molecules (once they arrive, they stick to the surrounding cells). Chemokines play a major role in inflammatory reactions.

Although T lymphocytes originate in the bone marrow, maturation in the absence of antigen occurs in the *thymus*. Because their differentiation occurs during their residence within the thymus, these cells are called *thymus-derived (T) lymphocytes* or *T cells*. The vast majority of mature T cells express antigen receptors (abbreviated TCR) on their surfaces that are composed of an $\alpha$ chain and a $\beta$ chain, the remaining 1–5% of T cells express a $\gamma$ chain and a $\delta$ chain. Each T cell reacts only with the antigen for which its receptor is specific; the level of receptor diversity, the type of antigen, and how it is recognized differs between $\alpha\beta^+$ and $\gamma\delta^+$ T cells. T cells expressing the $\alpha\beta$ receptor cannot react against free, undigested protein antigen like B cells and their antibodies can; $\alpha\beta^+$ T cells recognize antigen-derived peptides only when they are associated with self-major histocompatibility complex (MHC) molecules on the surface of an APC or some other target cell. This interaction stimulates the T cells to proliferate and produce progeny with the same antigen specificity. Two major T cell populations exist that differ both phenotypically and functionally. One population of T cells expresses the surface molecule CD8, usually is called *cytotoxic T*

*($T_C$) cells*, and recognizes antigen on the target cell surface associated with class I MHC molecules. These MHC molecules are present on all nucleated cells and permit the $CD8^+$ T cells to recognize and destroy virally infected (any intracellular parasite-infected) cells, foreign tissues, or tumor cells. The other population of T cells expresses CD4, usually is called *helper T ($T_H$) cells*, and acts as the commander-in-chief of the immune system by providing direct and indirect help to various cellular components. $CD4^+$ T cells recognize antigen presented on the surface of APCs in association with class II MHC molecules. Unlike class I MHC molecules, class II MHC molecules are expressed only on APCs such as macrophages, dendritic cells, and B cells. Based on cytokine profiles, naïve $T_H$ cells can differentiate into at least two functional subsets during an immune response: $T_H1$ cells, which secrete interferon-$\gamma$, and $T_H2$ cells, which secrete interleukin-4. $T_H1$ and $T_H2$ cells are generally responsible for cell-mediated and humoral immunity, respectively. Recent evidence suggests that the twins may be triplets; a new $T_H$ cell subset producing interleukin-17, a previously unknown lineage of $CD4^+$ T cells, has emerged—the $T_H17$ cell. It seems to regulate tissue inflammation and, in some animal models, the development of autoimmune disease. There also are $CD4^+$ regulatory T cells

The other main class of lymphocytes is the *bone marrow-* or *bursa-derived (B) lymphocytes* or B cells. Like T cells, there are B cell subsets. B cells both originate and mature in the bone marrow (except in birds) and the spleen. Mature B cells express antibodies (the abbreviation for these antigen receptors is BCR) on their surfaces and bind free antigen with them. When the antigen is processed by its specific B cell and presented to $T_H$ cells, the B cells proliferate and differentiate. The end cells, the sole producers of antibodies, are *plasma cells* that develop elaborate internal machinery and produce large quantities of antibody also referred to as *immunoglobulins* because they are globular proteins that confer immunologic protection. A typical plasma cell can secrete antibodies at the rate of 2000 to 10,000 molecules per second for 4 or 5 days before it dies. These antibody molecules have the same binding specificity as when they were BCRs. Secreted antibodies act as circulating forms of receptors and "red flags" that mark foreign antigen for destruction. Antibodies also "butter up" antigens, thereby enhancing phagocytosis—adaptive immunity helping innate immunity. The prototype antibody is made of four chains, containing about 1300 amino acids. Two of the chains are about twice as long as the other two; they are called *heavy chains*, and the smaller ones are called *light chains*. The heavy

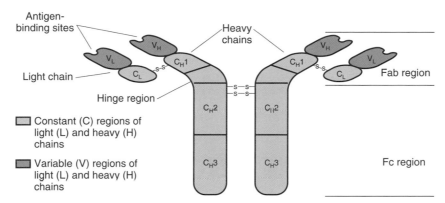

**FIGURE 1-8 Prototype structure of an antibody or immunoglobulin.** The different regions of antibodies perform different functions. The corresponding ends of each pair of adjacent light (L) and heavy (H) chains represent the two antigen-binding parts of the antibody molecule; they are called *variable*, or *V*, *regions*. These regions vary greatly in amino acid sequence among antibodies responding to different antigens and account for the *diversity of antibodies*. The other regions have constant amino acid sequences that are characteristic for each antibody class; therefore, they are called *constant*, or *C*, *regions*. They determine the class and biological function of antibodies. Light chains and $V_H$ and $C_H1$ make up the fragment for the antigen-binding (Fab) region. Other common regions of the H chain make up the fragment of the crystallization (Fc) region.

and light chains are held together by disulfide bonds, forming a Y (Figure 1-8). The ends of the Y arms are the antigen-binding sites.

Antibodies and TCRs are primary gene products. The light- and heavy-chain and TCR gene pools contain one or more constant-region genes and sets of variable gene segments (see Figure 1-9). *The variable sequences form the antigen-binding site and determine specificity.* To make a receptor molecule, light-chain and heavy-chain and TCR gene segments are selected and assembled. Because people and animals can respond to any antigen, immunologists once thought that individuals must have between 10 million and 100 million different receptor genes. However, this number is unreasonably large because human chromosomes possess only a few hundred genes that encode receptors. For example, how can a person have so few genes yet unlimited antibody diversity? Two possibilities were initially proposed; the *germline* and *somatic* mechanisms. Germline mechanisms proposed that *all* antibody genes are inherited from our parents, while the somatic mechanisms proposed that during development to a mature B cell a *few* germline antibody genes undergo some sort of somatic variation. It turns out that both mechanisms are largely correct. The important point is that the genes encoding antibodies and TCRs do not exist as one sequence of nucleotides, even though the genes encoding all other proteins are inherited intact. Rather than harboring a complete or functional set

of antibody or TCR genes, embryonic cells contain several hundred genetic bits and pieces that can be thought of as an "erector set" of antibody or TCR genes. Segments are randomly selected and by DNA recombination placed together on the DNA in each B and T cell as it becomes immunocompetent. This mixing and matching of gene segments allows each B or T cell to reassemble the parts to form its functional *composite gene* that encodes an antibody light or heavy chain (Figure 1-9) or α and β (or γ and δ) TCR chains.

Human Immunoglobulins can be divided into five classes (*IgG, IgM, IgA, IgD, and IgE*), which differ from each other in one portion of their heavy chains (Figure 1-10). Two (IgM and IgA) of the five antibody classes consist of multiples of the two light-chain and two heavy-chain structures of the prototype antibody molecule. All of the five antibody classes except IgD have distinctive and important biological functions as soluble molecules. IgG can coat microbes to promote phagocytosis and killing by immune cells. IgG is also the only class of antibody that can cross the placental barrier. IgM is known as an "early" antibody because it is the first antibody to be formed in an immune response. IgM is the largest antibody and consists of five monomeric forms of the prototype antibody. IgG and IgM, on reacting with specific antigen, activate a blood protein system (the *complement system*, which "complements" the work of antibodies) that amplifies the inflammatory and

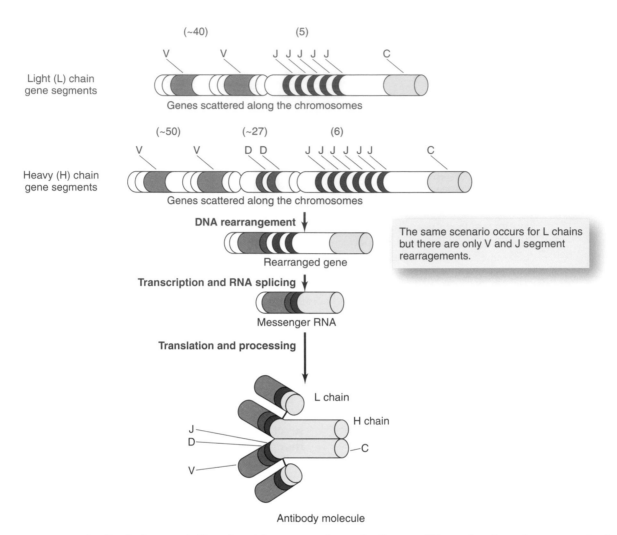

FIGURE 1-9 **Antibody (receptor) diversity.** A host can make antibodies to millions of antigens because antibody genes (listed as *rearranged gene*) that encode antibody chains are pieced together from scattered bits of DNA called *variable (V)*, *diversity (D)*, *joining (J)*, and *constant (C) segments*. (The same scenario occurs for the development of T cell receptor chain diversity.)

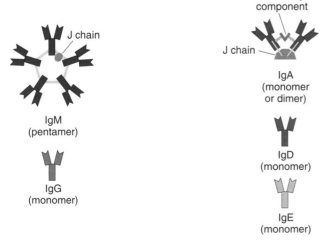

FIGURE 1-10 **Antibody classes.**

immune responses and can cause the lysis of some types of bacteria. IgA is the predominant antibody class present in the body's secretions (including those of the respiratory and gastrointestinal tracts). IgA acts as the first line of defense at the mucosal linings against invading organisms. IgE, from a human's perspective, seems to have only negative activities because its production is responsible for an overzealous response against pollen, animal dander, and dust. Such reactions against "harmless" intruders lead to the common immune disorder known as *allergy*. A positive activity of IgE is its role in immunity to certain parasites. The fifth class, IgD, is found in large quantities on the surfaces of antigen-naïve mature B cells. The function or importance of IgD in the immune response is unclear, but it is relevant during antigen-triggered B cell growth.

The humoral immune system mediates protection by several methods. Antibodies enhance phagocytosis (called *opsonization*) and can prevent a virus or toxin from attaching to a target cell (called *neutralization*). Antibodies also regulate certain nonspecific defense mechanisms, the most important of which is the *complement system*. There are three pathways of complement activation, one pathway uses antibodies, and microbes or their products activate the other two pathways. This system consists of several serum proteins that work in a sequential cascade and ultimately puncture the targeted microbes. The breakdown products of the intermediate complement components have powerful effects on blood vessels and leukocytes. The result is an amplification of the immune response.

As described in the previous paragraphs, all vertebrates possess an important genetic region called the *major histocompatibility complex (MHC)* that regulates many immunologic functions and interactions. In humans, the MHC is called the *human leukocyte antigen (HLA) complex*; in mice it is called the *H-2 complex*. The MHC contains genes that encode both *class I molecules* that are expressed on all nucleated cells, including immune cells, and *class II molecules* that are found on APCs (macrophages, dendritic cells, and B cells). Class I and class II MHC molecules exist in each species in many different genetic forms and are required by TCRs to distinguish between self and nonself cells. Specific T-cell activation occurs only when digested antigen is presented by some cell in the context of class I or II MHC molecules to a T cell that has a receptor specific for that antigen-MHC complex. This focused, or restricted, interaction is called *MHC restriction*. MHC genes also encode components of the complement system, cytokines, and molecules needed for antigen processing. Thus, the genes of the MHC help determine susceptibility to many diseases in humans and animals.

These genes and ones for antigen receptors occasionally allow for immune responses against self-antigens. *Autoimmunity* is a disease state in which the host has a destructive immune response against its own tissues. Some familiar diseases caused by autoimmunity are type I diabetes and rheumatoid arthritis. In both of these conditions, MHC genes appear to influence susceptibility. A related immunologic response, at least in the sense of reacting against tissues, is rejection of an organ transplant. The host's body recognizes the genetic differences (class I MHC molecules) on the organ transplant as foreign and eliminates the antigen by rejection and destruction.

When autoimmunity occurs, like "friendly-fire," the immune system mistakenly kills healthy body cells. When cancer occurs, body cells malfunction and replace healthy cells. Membranes of cancerous cells change slightly and subsequently appear to the immune system as nonself. If this "alien from within" eludes detection, full-blown cancer results. *Tumor immunology* investigates how the immune system handles these homegrown assailants and how to treat cancer. Because of the exquisite specificity of the immune response, one would expect that a tumor could be destroyed without changing normal tissue. Many tumors bear unique antigenic determinants, yet most human tumors elicit an ineffective antitumor immune response. Nonetheless, evidence suggests that the immune system acts as a surveillance mechanism, recognizing and destroying clinically inapparent cancers through these antigenic determinants. Tumor immunologists are trying to understand the mechanisms of the immune system's response to tumor-specific antigens through assessment of these antigens' molecular nature and cellular structure. Tumor immunologists also will have to understand the molecular basis of the immune response and of effector mechanisms in simple and highly defined antigenic systems.

The glare of the more exotic diseases of autoimmunity and cancer is dimmed when we realize we are bathed in a sea of predatory microbes, which are bent on destroying us. The immune system, an organization of cells and molecules with specialized roles in defending against infection, stands in the breach. There are two conjoined types of responses to invading microbes; innate (or natural) immune responses that are repeated irrespective of the number of times the infectious agent is encountered, whereas acquired (adaptive) responses improve on rechallenge to a given infection. To establish an infection, the pathogen must first overcome numerous surface barriers that either are directly antimicrobial or inhibit attachment of the microbe. Because the surface of skin or the mucus-lined body cavities are sparse habitats for most organisms, microbes must breach these levels of innate defenses. Any organism that breaks through this first barrier encounters formidable additional defenses, the cellular and soluble components of innate and adaptive immune responses. Innate immunity is more than a stopgap against pathogens, because after their recognition, release of phagocytic effector cells and microbiocidal molecules, and perfectly ignoring host self-tissues, it provides the necessary signals to instruct the adaptive immune system to initiate a response. In turn, the adaptive response supplies molecules that augment the innate immune response. The innate encounter and recognition of pathogens usually comes with a price; it triggers an acute inflammatory response. In the short-term, inflammation is a beneficial response to foreign challenge and associated tissue damage because it leads to the restoration of tissue structure and function. Conversely, prolonged inflammation is not a beneficial event and it contributes to the pathogenesis of many disease states. The challenge (avoiding the Jekyll and Hyde effect) remains in the development of antimicrobial treatments that harness inflammatory responses, leading to successful removal of the pathogen with limited inflammatory and autoimmune disease costs.

Despite all its specialized machinery for identifying and fighting off the continuous onslaught of microbes, the immune system occasionally fails to provide the required protection; this defect is defined as an *immunodeficiency*—a decrease in the number and function of immune cells. An immunodeficiency can be inherited, leading to primary immune deficiency diseases, or acquired through an infection (such as HIV), or it can result as a side effect of some immunosuppressive medical treatments. Irrespective of source, it leads to increased susceptibility to infections and occurrence of cancers and compromised immunotherapies such as vaccination. There are more than 120 known inherited primary immunodeficiency diseases and many of the associated genetic defects have been identified. In fact, these deficiencies have contributed greatly to our understanding of the immune system, for example, children born without a thymus, called *DiGeorge's syndrome*, provided evidence of thymic involvement in immune function long before its importance in T-cell development was known. The identification of the molecular defects that trigger immunodeficiencies and the implementation of new therapeutic modalities to correct these genetic defects are being vigorously pursuit.

The crux of the immune system is to provide protection. So as we began the chapter, stating that we are continuously surrounded by invaders—microorganisms—we end the chapter and the text with how the immune system deals with pathogens. Infectious diseases are the largest single cause of illness in the world. These diseases range from annoying, the common cold, to life threatening, AIDS. Moreover, infectious diseases are a common complication associated with therapies such as transplant immunosuppression and cancer chemotherapy, and primary or secondary immunodeficient patients. Despite the success of antibiotics and anti-microbial drugs, they have not, nor are they likely, to eliminate infectious diseases as a major health problem.

However, using the power of the immune system as a tool to control infectious disease is unmistakably obvious by the success of vaccines—the complete and near elimination of smallpox, poliomyelitis, diphtheria, pertussis, and tetanus to name a few. The continuance and expansion of vaccine prophylaxis provides promise to controlling many other infectious diseases. Whether a disease condition occurs depends on the outcome of the interaction of the microbe and its host. Anything we can do to shift the balance in favor of the host's immune system will surely lead to consequent savings in cost of medical care but more importantly reduction in human misery and dead.

# SUMMARY

*Immunity* is concerned with the recognition and disposal of nonself substances from a host; *immunology* is the study of the *immune response*, or the reaction that creates immunity. Immunology involves the study of the cells, soluble molecules, and organs responsible for this recognition and disposal; these responses, interactions, and other activities; their desirable or undesirable consequences; and the ways in which they can be augmented or dampened.

Early scientists manipulated immunity by *variolation* and *vaccination*. A *vaccine* is administered for the prevention of disease and contains either *killed* or *attenuated* microorganisms or a solution of altered toxins (*toxoids*). Genetic engineering has led to new categories of vaccines.

The integrity of the body is maintained by multiple defense systems, including immune responses. Protection against infection can be *innate* (inborn and unchanging) or *adaptive* (developed and adjusting to antigen during the lifetime of the host). Innate immunity is achieved by external mechanisms (skin, tears, mucous and ciliated epithelium of the respiratory tract, low pH of the stomach) or internal mechanisms (*inflammation* and *phagocytosis*). Inflammation involves increased blood flow to the site of injury and increased permeability of the vascular endothelium to allow access of white blood cells and serum components to the tissues. Phagocytosis, which can trigger inflammation, uses "professional" phagocytes (neutrophils, monocytes, macrophages, and dendritic cells) to remove foreign materials that have been introduced into the body. Phagocytes show no specificity, and the kind of protection they provide is different from adaptive immunity. Dendritic cells and macrophages are more than janitorial cells; they also prod the adaptive immune response into action. Nonphagocytic cells, such as NK cells and NKT cells also contribute to innate immunity.

Adaptive immunity is attributable to T and B cells that can respond *selectively* and *specifically* to a seemingly infinite number of different nonself materials; this selective specific response leads to a specific *immunologic memory*. Adaptive immunity is divided into three phases: antigen recognition, lymphocyte activation, and antigen elimination. Functionally, T cells are responsible for **cell-mediated immunity** and regulation of the immune response, while B cells are responsible for **humoral immunity**. Adaptive immunity can be divided into **active** and **passive** *immunity*.

"How are antigen receptors formed?" or "Do antigens *select* or *instruct* cells to produce receptors against the right antigen?" The first theory proposed to answer this question was the **selective theory**. It stated that an individual has all the immune cells capable of responding to any antigen and that the introduced antigen *selects* the correct cell by interacting with specific receptors (membrane antibodies or TCRs). The interaction stimulates the cell to proliferate and differentiate and eventually to produce either specific antibody or more identical T cells. The host has preexisting immune cells for all antigens. These activities now are included in the framework of the **clonal selection**. The crux of the clonal selection is that each B- or T-cell clone synthesizes an antibody or daughter cell with a unique antigen-binding site. Before encountering an antigen, the receptor molecules are inserted into the plasma membrane, where the antibodies or TCRs serve as *membrane-bound receptors*. When antigen binds them, it stimulates the B cells to divide and differentiate into plasma cells that secrete soluble antibodies with the same antigen-binding site as the receptor form of the antibodies. The soluble antibody can react with the stimulating antigen. For T cells, it leads to clones of cells with identical TCRs.

Only nonspecific innate immune mechanisms (phagocytosis) are evident among invertebrates. Primitive fishes make only IgM-like antibodies; more classes of immunoglobulins appear in advanced vertebrates. Immune cells become progressively more specialized and interactive in higher vertebrates. In this way, phylogeny repeats ontogeny; that is, the first antibody to appear in the development of a species (**phylogeny**) is also the first to appear in the development of an individual (**ontogeny**).

# SELF-EVALUATION

## RECALLING KEY TERMS

Active immunity
Adaptive immunity
Attenuation of virulence
Cell-mediated immunity
Clonal selection
Cross-reactions
Humoral immunity
Immune response
Immunity
Immunization
Immunologic memory
Immunology
Inflammation
Innate immunity
Mononuclear phagocyte system
Ontogeny
Passive immunity
Phagocytosis
Phylogeny
Vaccination
Vaccines
   Attenuated
   Killed
   Toxoids
Variolation

## MULTIPLE-CHOICE QUESTIONS

*(An answer key is not provided, but the page[s] location of the answer is.)*

1. Cowpox infection provides protection against smallpox because of (a) passive protection, (b) innate immunity, (c) cross-reactivity of causative agents, (d) similar appearance of disease, (e) none of these. *(See pages 3 and 9)*

2. A toxoid (a) reduces the toxic activity of a toxin, (b) enhances the toxic activity of a toxin, (c) does not induce immunity, (d) is not used as a form of vaccination, (e) is none of these. *(See page 3)*

3. Innate immunity is characterized by (a) a memory component, (b) an absence of specificity to commonly shared microbial antigens, (c) a primary involvement of lymphocytes, (d) no phagocytic cell involvement, (e) none of these. *(See pages 5–7)*

4. Attenuated vaccines were introduced by (a) Jenner, (b) Pasteur, (c) Metchnikoff, (d) Ehrlich, (e) Landsteiner, (f) none of these. *(See page 3)*

5. Injection of human gamma globulin to protect against hepatitis infection is an example of (a) natural, active adaptive immunity, (b) natural, passive adaptive immunity, (c) artificial, active adaptive immunity, (d) artificial, passive adaptive immunity, (e) none of these. *(See page 12)*

6. Which of the following is not a direct part of innate immunity? (a) Macrophages, (b) lysozyme, (c) antibodies, (d) mucus, (e) neutrophils, (f) none of these. *(See pages 7 and 8)*

7. Which of the following is an example of innate immunity? (a) a memory response to cowpox virus, (b) plasma cell antibody production, (c) antigen removal by respiratory tract cilia, (d) cytotoxic T cell–mediated killing of virus-infected cells, (e) antibody-induced complement activation, (f) none of these. *(See page 7)*

8. Which of the following is an example of active immunization? (a) immunization with cowpox virus vaccine, (b) immunization with anti-tetanus antibodies, (c) transfer of antibody through the mother's milk, (d) transfer of antibody across the placenta from mother to fetus, (e) none of these. *(See pages 10–12)*

9. Ontogeny recapitulates phylogeny because (a) the first antibody to appear during immunologic development in an individual is also the first to appear during immunologic development in a species, (b) the first antibody in phylogeny is IgG, (c) the fetus has passive immunity provided by the mother, (d) cell-mediated immunity is not present in the newborn, (e) of none of these. *(See page 14)*

10. The modern concept of clonal selection (a) was proposed by Ehrlich, (b) is unable to explain fetal tolerance, (c) holds that forbidden clones are suppressed by T cells, (d) violates the central dogma of molecular biology, (e) none of these. *(See pages 12–14)*

## SHORT-ANSWER ESSAY QUESTIONS

1. One of the functions of the immune system is surveillance. If surveillance is naturally or artificially suppressed, what can happen to the host?

2. Differentiate between variolation and vaccination.

3. Define vaccine and name two types of vaccines and give examples of each.

4. Discuss external and internal innate defenses.

5. What are three important characteristics that set adaptive immunity apart from innate immunity? Briefly discuss each.

6. Differentiate between humoral and cell-mediated immunity.

7. Why is active immunity better than passive immunity?

8. How does clonal selection explain receptor diversity, receptor specificity, and immunologic memory?

9. Why was the discovery of DNA structure important in describing the development of antibody-mediated immunity?

10. We exist in a preimmune state. Explain.

11. What do we mean, in an immunologic sense, when we say, "ontogeny recapitulates phylogeny"?

## FURTHER READINGS

Ada, G.L., and G. Nossal. 1987. The clonal-selection theory. *Sci. Am.* 257: 62–69.

Baxter, A.G., and P.D. Hodgkin. 2002. Activation rules: The two-signal theories of immune activation. *Nat. Rev. Immunol.* 2: 439–446.

Bibel, D.J. 1988. *Milestones in Immunology: A Historical Exploration.* Madison, WI: Science Tech Publishers.

Boehm, T., and C.C. Bleul. 2007. The evolutionary history of lymphoid organs. *Nat. Immunol.* 8: 131–135.

Chase, M.W. 1985. Immunology and experimental dermatology. *Annu. Rev. Immunol.* 3: 1–30.

Cohn, M., N.A. Mitchison, W.E. Paul, A.M. Silverstein, D.W. Talmage, and M. Weigert, 2007. Reflections on the clonal-selection theory. *Nat. Rev. Immunol.* 7: 823–830.

Cooper, E.L. 1976. Comparative immunology. *In Foundations of Immunology Series.* Englewood Cliffs, NJ: Prentice-Hall.

Danilova, N. 2007. The evolution of immune mechanisms. *J. Expt. Zool.* 306B: 496–520.

Hodgkin, P.D., W.R. Heath, and A.G. Baxter. 2007. The clonal selection theory: 50 years since the revolution. *Nat. Immunol.* 8: 1019–1026.

Jaret, P. 1986. Our immune system: The wars within. *Natl. Geogr.* 169: 702–736.

Kabat, E.A. 1983. Getting started 50 years ago—Experiences, perspectives, and problems of the first 21 years. *Annu. Rev. Immunol.* 1: 1–32.

Kabat, E.A. 1988. Before and after. *Annu. Rev. Immunol.* 6: 1–24.

Litman, G.W., J.P. Cannon, and L.J. Dishaw. 2005. Reconstructing immune phylogeny: New perspectives. *Nature Rev. Immunol.* 5: 866–879.

Mazumdar, P.M.H. 2003. History of immunology. In *Fundamental Immunology*, 5th ed. W.E. Paul, ed. Philadelphia: Lippincot Williams & Wilkins. p. 23–47.

Paul, W.E. 2003. *Fundamental Immunology*, 5th Ed. Philadelphia: Lippincott Williams & Wilkins.

Sela, M. 1987. A peripatetic and personal view of molecular immunology for one-third of the century. *Annu. Rev. Immunol.* 5: 1–19.

Silverstein, A.M. 1989. *A History of Immunology.* New York: Academic Press

Talmage, D.W. 1986. The acceptance and rejection of immunological concepts. *Annu. Rev. Immunol.* 4: 1–11.

# CHAPTER TWO

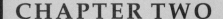

# CELLS AND ORGANS OF THE IMMUNE SYSTEM

## CHAPTER OUTLINE

1. The immune system is made up of five major kinds of cells.
   a. The genesis of immune cells starts in the bone marrow and involves a common, receptor-negative, self-renewing ancestral cell.
   b. B lymphocytes are antibody factories.
   c. T lymphocytes are a diverse group.
   d. Natural killer (NK) cells are lymphocyte like cells that are nonspecific hunter-killers.
   e. Macrophages are the "big eaters" of the immune system.
   f. Dendritic cells are innate sentinels translating innate to adaptive immunity.
2. The organs of the immune system are repositories for immune cells.
   a. Primary lymphoid organs are maturation sites for immune cells in the absence of antigen.
      1) The B-cell factories are the bone marrow and the bursa of Fabricius.
      2) The T-cell factory is the thymus.
   b. Secondary lymphoid organs are maturation sites for antigen-driven immune cells.
      1) The lymph nodes are junctional filters in the lymphatic system.
      2) The spleen is a filter in the circulatory system.
      3) The mucosa-associated lymphoid tissue (MALT) localizes antibodies at major sites of pathogen entry.

## OBJECTIVES

The reader should be able to:

1. Describe the life history, or hematopoiesis, of leukocytes.
2. Contrast B lymphocytes and T lymphocytes in terms of their origin, maturation process, location, surface structures, and role in immunity.

---

*Immunology: Understanding the Immune System, Second Edition,* by Klaus D. Elgert
Copyright © 2009 John Wiley & Sons, Inc.

3. Differentiate between helper T cells, inflammation-inducing T cells, cytotoxic T cells, and regulatory T cells.

4. Recognize the role of NK cells in immunity; describe some characteristics of NK cells.

5. Explain the phagocytic elements, or macrophages, in terms of their origin, location, and nomenclature; describe the role of macrophages in immunity.

6. Understand why dendritic cells are considered specialized antigen-capturing cells not just another phagocytic cell and be able to explain the difference.

7. Locate the different types of lymphoid tissue in the body.

8. Differentiate between primary and secondary lymphoid organs, between bone marrow and thymus, and between lymph nodes, spleen, and MALT.

9. Explain the structure of the thymus; interpret the role of the thymus in the establishment of the immune system in the body.

10. Draw a cross section of a lymph node and the spleen; explain how the structure of the lymph node and spleen are built around its lymph and blood supply, respectively.

To monitor against antigen intrusion anywhere within the body, the immune system stations throughout the body cells and tissues that constitute the **lymphoid system**, or **immune system** (Figure 2-1). The tissues are generally called **lymphoid organs** and include the bone marrow, thymus, lymph nodes, spleen, and mucosa-associated lymphoid tissue (MALT). They are called *lymphoid organs* because they are concerned with the maturation, concentration, interaction, and deployment of *lymphocytes*. Four main groups of leukocytes participate in immune responses: *lymphocytes, natural killer (NK) cells, macrophages*, and *dendritic cells* each with important roles. Some of these cells are also discussed in Chapter 3. The first part of the chapter describes the life history, structure, and function of these immune cells; the second part describes the structure and function of immune organs.

# THE IMMUNE SYSTEM IS MADE UP OF FIVE MAJOR KINDS OF CELLS

The human body's immune system stockpiles a formidable arsenal of lymphocytes and other immune cells (Table 2-1). Approximately 1% of the body's weight is made up of lymphocytes (roughly 2 trillion cells) widely dispersed throughout the body. When exposed to antigen, those cells of the correct specificity multiply to the numbers needed to counteract the antigen. To meet and destroy all the

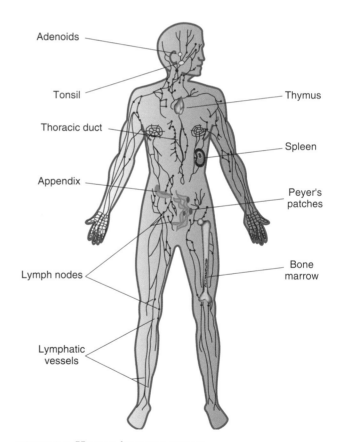

FIGURE 2-1 **Human immune system.**

antigens that the body encounters, lymphocytes must remain a dynamic cell group; their turnover per year can be equivalent to a person's body weight. Five main groups comprise the mononuclear leukocyte

**TABLE 2-1** Cell Percentages in the Blood

1. White blood cells (leukocytes)
   Polymorphonuclear (Granulocytes)
   1) Neutrophils: 50–70%
   2) Eosinophils: 1–3%
   3) Basophils: <1%
   Mononuclear
   1) Lymphocytes: 28–39%*
   2) Monocytes: 3–7%
   3) NK cells: 10–19%
2. Red blood cells (Erythrocytes)

*High percentages of lymphocytes are also found in the lymphoid organs (see Table 2-2).

pool: *bone marrow–* or *bursa of Fabricius–derived (B) lymphocytes, thymus-derived (T) lymphocytes, natural killer (NK) cells, macrophages,* and *dendritic cells* (Figure 2-2). B and T lymphocytes occupy center stage because they are the only antigen-specific cells. Their supporting cast includes specialized cells, called *antigen-presenting cells* (APCs, dendritic cells and macrophages) that display antigen-derived peptides and collaborate with them in response to antigen. Unlike dendritic cells and macrophages, the remaining cell is the nonphagocytic, lymphocyte-like NK cell. As its name implies, NK cells can directly kill virally infected host cells or tumor cells without prior exposure to them; therefore, they are primarily considered part of innate immunity. Nonetheless, they influence adaptive immunity through their production of cytokines.

## The Genesis of Immune Cells Starts in the Bone Marrow and Involves a Common, Receptor-Negative, Self-Renewing Ancestral Cell

*The bone marrow, the definitive hematopoietic tissue,* contains **pluripotent hematopoietic stem cells,** *the common ancestral cells for all blood and immune cells.*[1] These stem cells have the ability both to perpetuate themselves (self-renewal) and to differentiate to all blood and immune cell lineages; they differentiate through a series of intermediate cells that undergo lineage commitment and eventual development along a single pathway. This process is driven by molecular crosstalk between hematopoietic stem cells (HSCs) and the cellular constituents of the bone-marrow microenvironment, known as the *HSC niche.* The transition from a pluripotent HSC to a mature blood cell is called **hematopoiesis.** Before birth, the differentiation process begins in the embryonic yolk sac; after 10 weeks of gestation hematopoiesis moves to the liver and then spleen; after birth it occurs in the bone marrow. Figure 2-3 illustrates the different maturation pathways for the descendants of HSCs. Hematopoiesis occurs in an irreversible descending hierarchy, which begins with a quiescent HSC that is positive for the markers lineage marker (lin), c-kit,

---

[1]Estimates of total hematopoietic stem cells in the mouse and humans range from 1.12 to 12.5 × 10⁴ cells per host for each species.

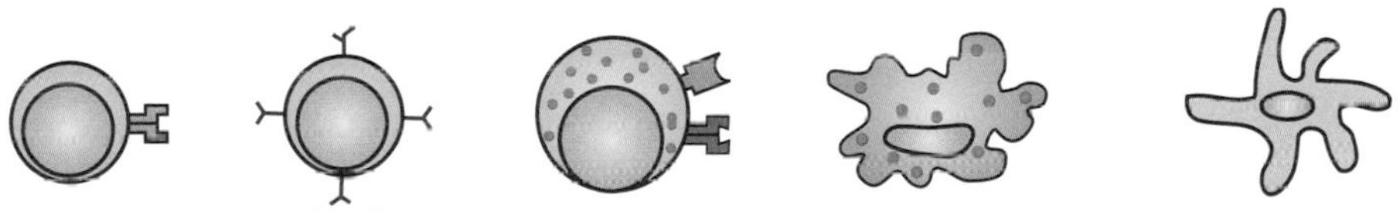

| | T cell | B cell | NK cell | Macrophage | Dendritic cell |
|---|---|---|---|---|---|
| **Antigen receptor** | TCRαβ TCRγδ | Ig | KIR & CD94-NKG2 | None (nonspecific receptors) | None (nonspecific receptors) |
| **Characteristic membrane markers** | CD3, CD4 or CD8 | Ig, CD5, CD19, CD20, CD40, CD79a, CD79b CD80/86, Class II molecules | CD16, CD56 | Class II molecules Complement receptors (CD11b, CD35) Fc receptors (CD16, CD23, CD32, CD64) CD14, CD68, CD40, CD80/86 | Class II molecules Complement receptors (CD21, CD35) Fcγ receptors CD40, CD80/86 |
| **Functions** | Cytokine secretion, cytotoxicity | Ig secretion, antigen presentation, cytokine secretion | Cytokine secretion, cytotoxicity, ADCC | Phagocytosis, antigen presentation, cytokine secretion | Antigen presentation, cytokine secretion |

**FIGURE 2-2 Lineages of lymphocytes (T cells, B cells, and NK cells), the mononuclear phagocyte, the macrophage, and the specialized phagocyte, the dendritic cell.** The NK cell is lymphocyte-like cell. Abbreviations: CD, cluster of differentiation antigen; TCR, T-cell receptor for antigen; Ig, immunoglobulin; ADCC, antibody-dependent cell-mediated cytotoxicity.

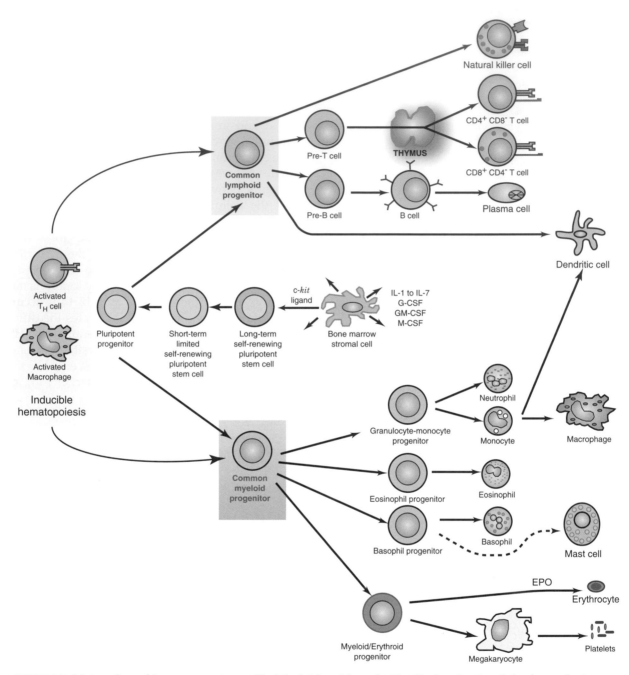

**FIGURE 2-3 Maturation of immune system cells**. Myeloid and lymphoid cells develop in adults from pluripotent (many different potentials) stem cells in the bone marrow. This development is driven by colony-stimulating factors. Nonlymphoid stem cells give rise to *elements of the peripheral blood*, such as erythrocytes, platelets, granulocytes (basophils, eosinophils, or neutrophils), and *monocytes* (precursor cells for *macrophages* and some *dendritic cells*). Lymphoid stem cells can develop along two pathways. If these stem cells migrate through the thymus, they become *T lymphocytes* or *T cells*, represented by CD4+ T and CD8+ T cells. If the lymphoid stem cells mature in the bone marrow, the cells become a population of lymphocytes, called *B lymphocytes* or *B cells*.

stem cell antigen-1 (Sca-1), and CD34. Phenotypically unique HSCs can be functionally distinguished into long-term and short-term populations. The long-term population ($lin^{-/low}$, c-kit$^+$, Sca-1$^+$, CD34$^+$) has life-long self-renewal and multi-lineage differentiation potential. The short-term population, which is derived from long-term HSCs, keeps its multi-lineage differentiation potential, but exhibits decreased self-renewal potential. The short-term HSCs give rise to pluripotential progenitors, which have lost self-renewal potential, but can differentiate into all blood- and immune-cell lineages. The self-renewing stem cell releases a cytokine called *c-kit ligand* (also called *stem cell factor*), which binds to *c-kit* encoded tyrosine kinase membrane receptors to start hematopoiesis. The earliest branching of the differentiation pathway divides the progenitor cells of B and T lymphocytes, NK cells, and some dendritic cells, the common *lymphoid progenitors*, from the common *myeloid progenitors* that give rise to the red cell and platelet (megakaryocyte) lineages, and all other types of leukocytes, the granulocytes, mononuclear phagocytes, and dendritic cells. The bone marrow also is the source of lymphocyte precursors for the thymus. In fact, the bone marrow is the source for all elements of the peripheral blood and immune cells. To maintain steady-state levels, the bone marrow supplies the body, at the rate of about 1 million cells every second, or roughly $10^{11}$ cells every day, with lymphocytes and other immune cells. To maintain steady-state levels of individual cell lineages (homeostatsis), a balance between cell proliferation and differentiation is maintained through a process called *programmed cell death*. Usually, the morphologic changes associated with this process are called *apoptosis*, where the cell shrinks, chromatin condenses, cell-membrane blebs, and DNA fragments. Eventually, the cell disintegrates into many membrane-bound apoptotic bodies, which are removed by neighboring phagocytic cells. This efficient clearing of dying cells leaves no remains to induce necrosis/inflammation.

Cytokine receptor signaling and transcription factors have instructive roles in driving lineage commitment. Bone marrow stromal cells (fat cells, endothelial cells, fibroblasts, and macrophages) influence hematopoiesis by providing a meshwork for stem cell growth and by providing either membrane-bound or diffusible cytokines. Because some of these cytokines stimulate the formation of leukocyte colonies in bone marrow cultures, they are called *colony-stimulating factors (CSFs)*. These include interleukin-3 (IL-3), granulocyte (G)-CSF, granulocyte-macrophage (GM)-CSF, macrophage

(M)-CSF, and IL-7. Hematopoietic cytokines are also produced by antigen-stimulated T cells and activated macrophages, in a process called *inducible hematopoiesis*, to restock consumed leukocytes during an inflammatory or immune response. Kidneys produce erythropoietin (EPO), which drives terminal erythrocyte development and controls erythrocyte production. Several other cytokines (IL-4 through IL-10) also affect hematopoiesis and are described in Chapter 9. The cues that specify lymphoid and myeloid fate are complex, in particular the role of transcription factors in these processes. Ikaros and PU.1 are dominant transcription factors in differentiation; they are broadly expressed in the hematopoietic system. The absence of either factor disrupts all differentiation from uncommitted progenitors with the exception of megakaryocytic-erythroid lineages in PU.1-deficient mice. Even though the loss of Ikaros most severely affects lymphoid lineages, changes are found in myeloid lineages. B cell development requires a complex set of transcription factors, namely PU.1, Ikaros, early B cell factor (EBF), E2A, and paired box protein 5 (Pax5); the inactivation of any of these factors yields a dysfunctional phenotype. The absence of either GATA-3 or Notch1 arrests T cell development at the earliest detectable T cell progenitor stage.

The common myeloid progenitors give rise to *mononuclear phagocytes* and *polymorphonuclear phagocytes*. The mononuclear phagocytes are blood monocyte-derived *macrophages* and the closely related *dendritic cells*, which can be of monocyte or lymphoid origin. Both cell types can present antigen to T cells but dendritic cells are more efficient at antigen presentation; thus, they are called *APCs* and can initiate adaptive immune responses to most pathogens by presenting pathogen-derived antigen to T cells by class II MHC molecules. Macrophages and dendritic cells are distributed throughout the body; therefore, neither cell will be far away from a microbe invasion site. Macrophages and dendritic cells are not a uniform population of cells; rather they are morphologically diverse. Of the two cell types, dendritic cells are the minority population among mononuclear phagocytes. Even though macrophages are known for their phagocytic killing of microbes, perhaps their most important functions are supervisory; they elaborate chemotactic cytokines, which recruit neutrophils (mentioned below and detailed in Chapter 3) to the site of infection.

Some leukocytes, the *granulocytes*, are responsible for general defenses (see Table 2-1). Granulocytes, like macrophages, are phagocytes and therefore capable of ingesting and destroying microbes. Also known as *polymorphonuclear leukocytes* (because their nuclei come in many shapes), granulocytes contain granules filled with potent enzymes that can digest microorganisms. Granulocytes found in the blood include neutrophils, eosinophils, and basophils, while granulocytes found in tissues consist of mast cells. The various granulocytes are named by the characteristics of their specific granules. Eosinophils, for instance, have an affinity for acidic dyes such as eosin; basic methylene blue reacts to granules in the basophil; and granules of the neutrophil stain with both.

Neutrophils are short-lived (1 to 3 days) and represent the first leukocytes to appear at an infection site. Neutrophils can be considered "kamikaze cells" because they are killed in the process of killing (see Chapter 3). Unlike neutrophils, eosinophils exhibit very limited phagocytic activity against bacteria, but they actively phagocytize antigen-antibody complexes and serve as an important defense against parasitic infestations. Basophils are the circulating counterparts of mast cells. They are not phagocytic but collect at infection sites. These cells release pharmacologically active substances that play a role in immediate hypersensitivity reactions (see Chapter 12).

**Lymphocytes** are round cells, 6 to 15 micrometers ($\mu$m) in diameter, with little cytoplasm, large round nuclei, and chromatin arranged in coarse masses. They bear the major responsibility of the adaptive immune system: the recognition, specificity, and memory functions. Lymphocytes represent 20 to 40% of the body's leukocytes and are found circulating between blood and lymphoid tissues. Lymphocytes can migrate to extravascular tissues and localize in lymphoid organs. *The two groups of nonphagocytic, morphologically indistinguishable, but functionally different lymphocytes are called* **B lymphocytes** or **B cells** and **T lymphocytes** or **T cells**; their ontogeny is shown in Figure 2-3. T cells are divided into two populations according to CD4 or CD8 cell-surface molecule expression.[2] $CD4^+$ T cells usually are considered *helper T ($T_H$) cells* and are partitioned functionally into three subsets known as $T_H1$, $T_H2$, $T_H17$, and $CD4^+$ T regulatory ($T_{reg}$) cells (see Chapter 10). $T_H1$ cells produce interferon-$\gamma$ (IFN-$\gamma$)

and promote cellular immunity whereas $T_H2$ cells produce IL-4, -5, -10, and -13 and help regulate humoral immunity and allergic responses. Recent evident suggests that the twins are triplets; T cells producing IL-17, called *$T_H17$ cells*, constitute a previously unknown lineage of $CD4^+$ T cells, which have an important function in inflammatory responses associated with autoimmunity. The remaining $CD4^+$ subset, $T_{reg}$, controls immune responses. $CD8^+$ T cells usually are considered *cytotoxic ($T_C$) cells* that also may be partitioned functionally into two subsets. *Both B cells and T cells are programmed to recognize specific antigen targets; these immune cells are the repositories of specific immunity.* Commitment to the B- and T-cell lineages is marked by irreversible DNA rearrangements in either *immunoglobulin* or *T-cell receptor (TCR)* genes, respectively. These changes in cell genotype lead to individual B cells and T cells that possess clonally distinct, antigen-specific immunoglobulins or TCRs. *B cells are responsible for the production of antibodies and mediate the humoral response, whereas T cells are responsible for the cellular immune response and helping humoral and cellular responses.* B or T cells that have not interacted with antigen are small, antigen-naïve, resting cells in the $G_0$ phase of the cell cycle; they are called *naïve cells.* Following interaction with the appropriate antigen, they are *activated* and enter the cell cycle. Activated cells differentiate into either *effector* or *memory cells,* such as antibody-producing plasma cells and cytokine-secreting effector $T_H$ cells and killing $T_C$ cells or memory B and T cells. The antigen-induced development of these cells requires nonlymphoid cells, called **accessory cells,** which are antigen-nonspecific cells such as dendritic cells and macrophages. A third group of lymphocytes are the large, granular lymphocytes called **natural killer (NK) cells,** which do not express surface markers or antigen receptors characteristic of B or T cells and whose function of "naturally" killing host target cells makes them a major cell of the innate immune system.

## B Lymphocytes Are Antibody Factories

B lymphocytes are called *B* because they were first studied in detail in the *b*ursa of Fabricius organ of chickens. *The quintessential characteristic of B lymphocytes is that their progeny cells,* **plasma cells,** *are the only cells to secrete antibodies.* Each B cell carries the genetic instructions to produce immunoglobulin (antibody) of unique antigen specificity, *which it initially expresses as membrane receptors—membrane-bound immunoglobulin (antibody) antigen-specific molecules.* Mature B cells

---

[2]CD stands for *cluster of differentiation* and refers to families, or clusters, of monoclonal antibodies that recognize different antigenic determinants on a particular lineage or differentiation stage of a cell. Thus, this CD designation is assigned to all leukocyte surface antigens, or markers, whose structures are defined. More than 325 human leukocyte CD designations have been described (see Appendix).

do *not* secrete antibody but readily differentiate into terminal nondividing effector antibody-secreting plasma cells during antigen stimulation. Plasma cells secrete millions of clonospecific antibody molecules each second—the secreted antibodies are an accurate reflection of their receptor counterparts. B cells constitute one arm of the immune system; they are responsible for humoral immunity.

Naïve (immature) B220+IgM+IgD− B cells that survive developmental checkpoints in the bone marrow enter the circulation and migrate to the spleen. The spleen is the primary recipient of immature, newly formed transitional B cells. In the spleen, the B cell either dies or undergoes a further series of structural and functional changes as it matures (Figure 2-4). These changes include passing through transitional stages T1 and T2 and subjection to additional checkpoints before becoming fully mature (see Chapter 10). Transitional B cells segregate into either a small proportion of cells that home to the splenic marginal zone (located at the border of the spleen white pulp) and remain there as naïve noncirculating marginal-zone B cells or a majority population that matures into naïve long-lived follicular B cells, which continue circulating to spleen and lymph node follicles, and to the bone marrow until they either die or encounter specific antigen and undergo antigen-dependent differentiation. These naïve, mature recirculating IgM- and IgD-expressing B cells, also called *conventional, or B2, B cells,* have an average life span that exceeds 6 weeks. They are the precursor cells for T cell-dependent B-cell responses to most protein antigens.

The most thoroughly studied surface molecules on B cells are the membrane-bound, B-cell specific immunoglobulin (Ig) classes—IgG, IgA, IgM, IgD, and IgE (see Chapter 4). From 5% to 15% of peripheral blood lymphocytes in humans express immunoglobulin. Naïve mature B cells have both IgM and IgD on their surface. Immunoglobulins allow for B-cell clonal selection by antigen and serve as the receptor molecules that recognize and react with specific antigenic determinants. The Ig receptor is called the *B cell receptor (BCR).* Surface Igs on a single B cell all have the same specificity and thus bind with only one kind of antigenic determinant. Each B cell expresses 50,000 to 150,000 Ig molecules on its surface, although the membrane Igs may consist of more than one class of Ig (usually IgM and IgD on naïve mature B cells). *Immunoglobulins can directly recognize protein, polysaccharide, glycolipid, or nucleic acid antigens in their <u>undigested</u>, or <u>natural</u>, state.* The direct engagement between the BCR and antigen or indirect engagement with $T_H$ cells causes

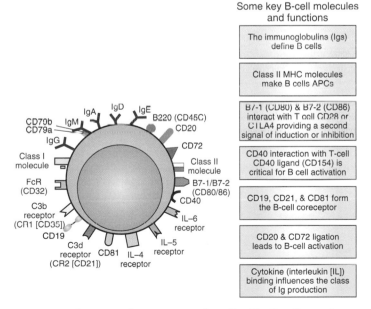

Some key B-cell molecules and functions

| The immunoglobulins (Igs) define B cells |
| --- |
| Class II MHC molecules make B cells APCs |
| B7-1 (CD80) & B7-2 (CD86) interact with T cell CD28 or CTLA4 providing a second signal of induction or inhibition |
| CD40 interaction with T-cell CD40 ligand (CD154) is critical for B cell activation |
| CD19, CD21, & CD81 form the B-cell coreceptor |
| CD20 & CD72 ligation leads to B-cell activation |
| Cytokine (interleukin [IL]) binding influences the class of Ig production |

**FIGURE 2-4 Some markers expressed on B cells.** B-cell membrane molecules include antibody classes, Fc receptors, complement receptors (C3b and C4b), receptors for T cell-derived factors, B-cell differentiation markers, and MHC proteins (class I and II MHC molecules). (All antibody classes are drawn on the same cell for illustrative purposes only.)

the activation and differentiation of antigen-specific clones of B cells, which leads to either short-lived, terminally differentiated plasma cells, long-lived plasma cells associated with survival niches such as the bone marrow, and long-lived memory cells.

Several other surface markers are important to B lymphocytes (see Figure 2-4). The Fc receptor, found on all B cells early in their development, specifically binds to the Fc, or stem, portion of IgG. The Fc receptor has a role in modulating B cell events after engagement of the BCR with antigen. Complement receptors (CD21 and CD35) are expressed on most B cells and enable B cells to bind to antigen-antibody-complement complexes. *CD5 has been used to identify B-cell subsets, B-1 B cells express CD5, and while B-2 B cells, and marginal zone B cells do not.* B-2 B cells represent most (95%) recirculating B cells in normal hosts and express both IgM and IgD, whereas B-1 B cells express only IgM. The B-1 B-cell subset is found in the peritoneal and pleural cavities, has a unique self-renewing capacity (generating naïve B-1 cells), expresses a BCR repertoire that is skewed towards recognition of T-cell-independent type 2 antigens (see Chapter 10), produces low-affinity IgM antibodies that recognize a variety of self and bacterial antigens (*polyreactive antibodies*), and rarely differentiate into memory cells. The marginal zone B-cell BCR repertoire is similar to B-1 B cells. B cells also can be defined by the expression of either CD19 or CD20, which have a role in B-cell activation. The costimulatory molecules B7-1 (CD80) and B7-2 (CD86), found on activated B cells, bind to counter-receptors on T cells. B cells also express class I and II MHC molecules that are important in the presentation of antigen to T cells. In particular, the expression of class II MHC molecules makes B cells APCs. Like MHC molecules, B cell CD40 also has a role in $T_H$-B cell interactions (see Chapter 10).

---

**MINI SUMMARY**

Five main groups of immune cells participate in immune responses: B cells, T cells, NK cells, macrophages, and dendritic cells. Under the influence of cytokines and transcription factors, bone marrow–derived pluripotent hematopoietic stem cells proliferate and differentiate through the lymphopoietic or myelopoietic pathways.

B lymphocytes are derived from bone marrow stem cells and develop mostly within the bone marrow; the final maturation steps occur in the spleen. Mature B cells express surface immunoglobulins that act as receptors for specific antigen. All antibodies on a B cell, irrespective of the classes or combinations of classes, have the same antigen specificity. Some surface molecules distinguish B-cell subsets but most are associated with the modulation of BCR-mediated responses.

---

## T Lymphocytes Are a Diverse Group

The B cell's counterpart in immunity is the T cell. The T in "T cell" comes from *t*hymus, the organ where pre-T cells migrate to and mature in. The expression of the αβ or γδ TCR, unique to T cells, is the key to calling a lymphocyte a *T* lymphocyte. Figure 2-5 shows various cell surface molecules found on T cells. *T cells are required for the full expression of immunity.* They regulate antibody production, cellular immune reactions, and killing of altered cells. T cells differ from B cells in the kind of antigen they recognize and in the way they recognize antigen. *Unlike B cells, T cells can only recognize protein antigen but cannot directly recognize it in its natural or free state; the protein antigen must be broken down and the peptide fragments bound to MHC molecules displayed on self-cells.* This focusing of T-cell antigen recognition through MHC molecules is known as *MHC restriction* (see Chapters 7 and 8). The MHC molecule-peptide complex may be displayed on APCs (such as B cells, macrophages, and dendritic cells) or virus-infected cells, graft cells, and cancer cells. When TCRs (structurally related to antibody molecules but functionally distinct) engage protein antigen in association with self-MHC molecules on the surface of a host cell, the T cells are *activated*. These T cells divide and acquire the ability to perform at least one of three different tasks:

1. T cells can act as *regulatory cells* that modulate the activities of other T cells, dendritic cells, macrophages, or B cells. Regulation can take the form of help or suppression.
2. T cells mediate cellular immunity reactions through the production of *cytokines* and *chemokines*, which promote proliferation and differentiation of T cells and attract or activate other elements of the immune system (i.e., stimulate inflammatory responses). These reactions are exemplified by inflammation (see Chapter 3), delayed-type hypersensitivity (see Chapter 12), and resistance to infection by intracellular bacteria or viruses (see Chapter 17).

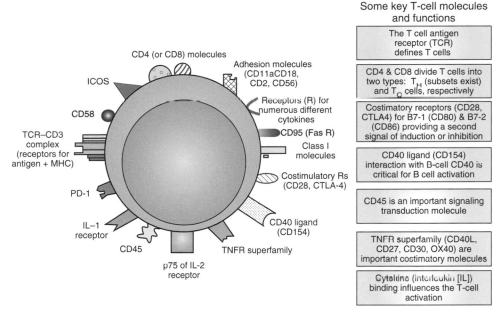

Some key T-cell molecules and functions

| The T cell antigen receptor (TCR) defines T cells |
| CD4 & CD8 divide T cells into two types: T$_H$ (subsets exist) and T$_C$ cells, respectively |
| Costimatory receptors (CD28, CTLA4) for B7-1 (CD80) & B7-2 (CD86) providing a second signal of induction or inhibition |
| CD40 ligand (CD154) interaction with B-cell CD40 is critical for B cell activation |
| CD45 is an important signaling transduction molecule |
| TNFR superfamily (CD40L, CD27, CD30, OX40) are important costimatory molecules |
| Cytokine (interleukin [IL]) binding influences the T-cell activation |

**FIGURE 2-5 Some markers expressed on T cells.** Both CD4 and CD8 are drawn on the same cell for illustrative purposes only.

3. T cells can interact directly with target cells and destroy virus-infected cells, foreign tissues, or tumor cells (see Chapter 10). As *cytotoxic cells*, T cells are the major cells involved in viral, transplantation, and tumor immunity

Bone marrow–derived T cell precursors arrive in the thymus; about 3 weeks are required for human thymocytes to migrate through the thymus. During their journey, thymic stromal cells release the thymic hormones and cytokines plus express ligands that promote the differentiation of multiple T cell subsets; they include CD4 and CD8 αβ T cells, γδ T cells that may divide into intraepithelial lymphocytes, T$_{reg}$ cells, and natural killer T cells. Thymic stromal cells and APCs (macrophages and dendritic cells) condition the MHC recognition of either class I or class II MHC molecules (see Chapter 8). Immature cortical thymocytes are rapidly dividing cells and do not show the functions associated with peripheral T cells. As the thymocytes emigrate from the cortex to the medulla, they express TCR of one of two types, αβ or γδ, associated with CD3 and ζ/η signaling molecules, and they differentiate into two distinct lineages that can be distinguished by their expression of *CD4* or *CD8* membrane molecules. Most mature T cells also express a variety of accessory molecules for costimulation, such as the CD28 family of receptors, tumor necrosis factor receptor superfamily, adhesion molecules, and many more. Eventually, thymocytes mature into one of two kinds of T cells (at least according to their expression of CD4 or CD8) that distribute themselves throughout the body (see Table 2-2):

**TABLE 2-2 Approximate Percentages of Lymphocytes in Human Lymphoid Organs**

| Lymphoid organ | T lymphocytes | | | B lymphocytes | NK cells |
| | Total | CD4$^+$ | CD8$^+$ | | |
|---|---|---|---|---|---|
| **Primary** | | | | | |
| Bone marrow | 10 | — | — | 90 | — |
| Thymus | >95 | 60–80 | 20–40 | <1 | <0.1 |
| **Secondary** | | | | | |
| Spleen | 20–30 | 70–90 | 10–30 | 40–50 | 1–5 |
| Lymph nodes | 70–80 | 60 | 20–40 | 10–20 | <1 |
| Blood | 67–76 | 38–46 | 31–40 | 11–16 | 5–10 |

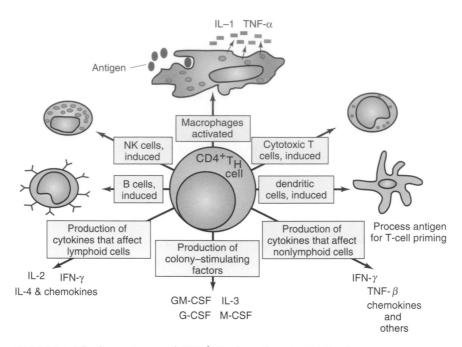

**FIGURE 2-6 The importance of CD4$^+$ T$_H$ lymphocytes in the immune response.** These cells are directly or indirectly responsible for many aspects of the immune response and for nonlymphoid cell functions.

1. **Helper T (T$_H$) cells** *are the commanders of the immune cells* (Figure 2-6) (see Chapter 10). As their name indicates: T$_H$ cells help B cells and other T cells to multiply into large clones and carry out their role in the immune response. T$_H$ cells enhance B-cell antibody production, macrophage activation, and T$_C$ cell activation. The T$_H$ cells also maintain memory and are the principal proliferative cells responding to foreign antigen associated with class II MHC molecules. T$_H$ cells are usually identified by the presence of the cell-surface molecule *CD4. CD4$^+$ T-cell preference, or restriction, for class II MHC molecules is related to the direct binding of CD4 to regions of the APC's class II MHC molecule* (see Chapters 7 and 8). CD4$^+$ T cells are subdivided further into four subsets (T$_H$1, T$_H$2, T$_H$17, and T$_{reg}$ cells) based on their pattern of cytokine secretion and functional activities (see Chapter 10). CD4$^+$ T cells account for 55 to 70% of all T cells.

    Naïve T$_H$ cell TCR engagement of the appropriate antigen-class II MHC molecule complex triggers activation followed by rapid clonal expansion and programmed differentiation, leading to clone of antigen-specific effector cells. These cells secrete numerous cytokines that can activate B cells, T cells, and many other immune and nonimmune cells. The type of antigen exposure and interactions with APCs drives the T$_H$ cell differentiation process; the resulting cells have unique cytokine profiles, which force immune responses to be highly polarized. Naïve T$_H$ cells can differentiate to at least three functional classes during an immune response: *type 1 T helper (T$_H$1), T$_H$2, and T$_H$17 cells* (see Chapter 10). T$_H$1, T$_H$2, and T$_H$17 cells preferentially support cell-mediated (type 1 response) or humoral (type 2 response) immunity, and inflammation, respectively. T$_H$1 cells secrete IFN-γ, interleukin-2 (IL-2), and tumor necrosis factor-β (also called *lymphotoxin*); T$_H$2 cells secrete IL-4, -5, -10, and 13; and T$_H$17 cells secrete IL-17.

2. **Cytotoxic T (T$_C$) cells** *are the hand-to-hand combat troops of the immune cells* (see Chapter 10). *They are responsible for killing virus-infected cells, transplanted tissue, and cancer cells.* T$_C$ cells kill a target cell either by latching on to the cell's surface and injecting chemicals called *perforin* and *granzymes* or by a mechanism involving engagement of the *Fas* cell-surface molecules, which lead to apoptosis. Unlike most T$_H$ cells, T$_C$ cells usually recognize and proliferate in response to foreign processed antigen associated with class I MHC molecules (the normal class I MHC molecules have been altered with the addition of virus-derived antigen or tumor cell development). T$_C$ cells express the *CD8* surface molecule. *CD8$^+$ T-cell preference, or restriction, for class I MHC molecules is related to the direct binding*

*of CD8 to regions of the target cell's class I MHC molecule* (see Chapters 7 and 8). Naïve $T_C$ cells, under conditions of appropriate costimulation by dendritic cells and cytokines, are activated when they encounter, through their TCR, the correct antigen-class I MHC molecule complex presented at the APC surface (called *cross-presentation*; see Chapter 10). Once activated, they differentiate into IFN-$\gamma$-secreting, effector $T_C$ cells, which kill the altered-self, target cell by apoptosis. Regarding CD8$^|$ T cells as simply cytotoxic cells is incorrect. Like CD4$^+$ T cells, CD8$^+$ T cells can be divided functionally into two possible subsets according to their cytokine secretion profiles. CD8$^+$ T cells account for 25 to 40% of all T cells. The ratio between CD4$^+$ $T_H$ cells and CD8$^+$ $T_C$ cells in normal human peripheral blood is roughly 2:1.

Even though T cells are divided into functional subsets, in practice this separation is not absolute. For example, CD4$^+$ cells, besides being helpers, can be cytotoxic, and CD8$^+$ cells may function as helpers. Nonetheless, *$T_H$ cells are generally considered as being class II restricted and CD4$^+$*; *$T_C$ cells are generally considered as being class I restricted and CD8$^+$*.

Immune responses need to be regulated; the host works to balance appropriate levels of anti-pathogen protection against inappropriate autoimmune responses. Yet it took decades to convincingly prove that there are immune cells responsible for this task, initially called *suppressor T cells*, which were never clearly characterized causing interest to dwindle—nonetheless the notion of a functional distinct subpopulation of "suppressor" cells has resurfaced as *regulatory ($T_{reg}$) cells*. Even though at least three phenotypically distinct CD4$^|$ regulatory T-cell populations have been suggested, the classic $T_{reg}$ cells are thymus-derived CD4$^+$ cells expressing CD25 (IL-2 receptor $\alpha$-chain) and the transcription factor forkhead box P3 (FOXP3), not only a key intracellular marker but a crucial developmental and functional factor for $T_{reg}$ cells—5 to 15% of CD4$^+$ T cells are *CD4$^+$CD25$^+$FOXP3$^+$ T cells ($T_{reg}$ cells)*. Although the main function of $T_{reg}$ cells appears to be autoimmune disease prevention, they curtail effector T-cell responses to infections and cancer. The latter information suggests we have not resolved the regulatory cell question, "Is it a special job or everyone's responsibility?"

In contrast to $\alpha\beta^+$ T cells, a small subset of CD4$^-$CD8$^-$CD3$^+$ T cells (1–10% of peripheral blood T cells) express the $\gamma\delta$ TCR. Much present evidence suggests that $\gamma\delta^+$ T cells function in an innate manner, even though they rearrange their TCR genes and develop a memory phenotype. Unlike $\alpha\beta^+$ T cells, $\gamma\delta^+$ T cells show less TCR diversity and do not recognize peptides processed from complex antigenic proteins by APCs; they recognize unconventional antigens such as phosphorylated microbial molecules and lipid antigens. In addition, $\gamma\delta^+$ T cells do not require presentation of these ligands in association with conventional class I and class II MHC molecules (see Chapter 7), which is supported by their absence of CD4 or CD8. The $\gamma\delta^+$ T cells are particularly enriched in the gut mucosa, within a population of lymphocytes called *intraepithelial lymphocytes* (discussed later). Because $\gamma\delta^+$ T cells are not constrained by antigen processing or MHC restriction, they can recognize a wide array of soluble protein and non-protein antigens of endogenous origins and common molecules produced by microbes. This simple recognition mechanism allows human $\gamma\delta^+$ T cells to rapidly discriminate healthy cells from altered cells and the presence of infection leading to production of a variety of proinflammatory cytokines (notably IFN-$\gamma$ and tumor necrosis factor-$\alpha$ [TNF-$\alpha$]) and/or lysis of infected cells or tumor cells—a rapid, first-line T-cell defense.

## MINI SUMMARY

Pre-T lymphocytes of the bone marrow migrate to the thymus and develop into mature T cells. T cells do not produce antibodies but are responsible for the full expression of immunity to most antigens. T cells are effector and regulatory cells. They express markers that allow for their division into subpopulations; they include mainly (1) $T_H$ cells (class II-restricted and CD4$^+$) and (2) $T_C$ cells (class I-restricted and CD8$^+$). $T_H$ cells can be further divided into subsets, $T_H1$, $T_H2$, and $T_H17$ cells, according to their cytokine production profiles. CD4$^+$ $T_{reg}$ cell subpopulation has regulatory activity. $\gamma\delta$ T cells may be part of the innate immune system.

## Natural Killer (NK) Cells Are Lymphocyte-Like Cells That Are Nonspecific Hunter-Killers

*Lymphoid-derived cells* that lack the cell surface markers characteristic of other lymphocytes and do not rearrange Ig or TCR genes are called **natural killer (NK) cells**. These cells develop normally in B- and T-cell-deficient mice and do not express antigen-specific receptors. They are not macrophages or dendritic cells, which express conserved pattern recognition receptors; NK cells do not, nonetheless NK cells represent an arm of the innate immune system. They are more closely related to lymphocytes than cells of the innate immune system. Morphologically, most NK cells are described as large granular lymphocytes, which are found in lymph nodes but they are most plentiful in the blood (roughly 15% of circulating lymphocytes), liver, and spleen. Resting, blood-circulating NK cells once activated by cytokines can migrate into inflamed or tumor tissue. NK cells mediate two types of killing functions: direct (recognize alterations in target cell class I MHC molecules) and indirect (recognition of target cell-bound antibodies) cytotoxicity. NK cells can be considered primitive $T_C$ cells that do not use the TCR to recognize antigen, and antigen recognition is not MHC-restricted as associated with $T_C$ cells. Furthermore, NK cells are unaffected by the absence or presence of antibody. However, NK cells can mediate cytotoxicity against IgG-coated target cells, a phenomenon called **antibody-dependent cell-mediated cytotoxicity** (**ADCC**). Until recently, NK cells were thought to exist in the absence of any known priming, because resting mature NK cells are constitutively armed-to-the-teeth with IFN-$\gamma$ and granules chocked full of cytotoxic mediators perforin and granzymes. Nonetheless, they required activation by type I interferons (IFN-$\alpha$ and IFN-$\beta$) or proinflammatory cytokines, such as IL-12, IL-15, and IL-18, to develop into fully functional effector cells. These cytokines are probably derived from dendritic cells. NK cell importance in immunity is as antiviral and antitumor effector cells. NK cells can kill virally infected cells and syngeneic, allogeneic, and even xenogeneic cancer cells. Hence this cytotoxicity is designated *natural immunity*, and the effector cells as *natural killer (NK) cells*. The main responsibilities of NK cells are surveillance against spontaneously arising tumors, destruction of virally infected cells and tumor cells, and restriction of tumor metastases. This is supported by using NK cell-deficient, or beige, mice, or humans that are unable to rearrange their antigen receptor genes, which are more susceptible to viral infections and transplantable tumors than are their normal counterparts. NK cells also appear to play a role in graft-versus-host disease in patients receiving bone marrow transplants (see Chapter 14). However, NK cells are not just killers. They secrete cytokines, in particular IFN-$\gamma$ and tumor necrosis factor-$\alpha$ (TNF-$\alpha$), which can activate macrophages and neutrophils and drive adaptive immune responses, and reciprocally interact with dendritic cells that produce cytokines that activate NK cells. The cross talk between dendritic cells and NK cells can mediate $T_C$ cell differentiation and NK cell activation; this interaction is integral to the development of effective antiviral immunity.

In humans, TCR$^-$CD3$^-$ NK cells make up 5 to 10% of peripheral blood lymphocytes, are described as large granular lymphocytes, and express CD16 and CD56. Coexpression of these two molecules distinguishes cells that mediate NK cell activity; however, NK cells do not express any single cell-surface molecule that is required for their function (such as the BCR that makes a B cell a B cell and the TCR that makes a T cell a T cell). Even though NK cells express distinct markers, most are also expressed by some other T cell subsets; therefore, human NK cells are usually defined as CD56$^+$CD3$^-$ cells (in mice, they are defined as NK1.1$^+$CD3$^-$ or DX5$^+$CD3$^-$ cells). The CD16 marker is equivalent to the Fc receptor for IgG and is expressed on NK cells and neutrophils but not on monocytes or B cells. CD16 is only rarely coexpressed on CD3$^+$ T cells. The CD3$^-$CD16$^+$ peripheral blood lymphocytes mediate most of the cytotoxicity. NK cells also express IL-2/-15R$\beta$. NK activity can be increased by IFN-$\alpha$, IFN-$\beta$, IL-2, IL-12, IL-15, or IL-18. High levels of IL-2 can induce NK cells to differentiate into lymphokine-activated killer cells that are more effective killers of a greater variety of targets than untreated NK cells.

T-cell receptor gene rearrangements and their transcription are used to determine the relationship between T cells and NK cells. The TCR genes are not rearranged in human CD56$^+$CD3$^-$ NK cells. Because these cells do not rearrange TCR genes, they do not recognize target cells through the TCR/CD3 complex. However, NK cell target specificity is not random. NK cells can lyse several tumor cell lines. Although NK cells can lyse virally infected cells, they do not lyse uninfected cells. Unlike B or T cells, NK cells are not regulated by any single receptor; they work by the integration of numerous signals from multiple receptors. In fact, NK cell activation is controlled by balancing between the binding of activating and inhibitory receptors with their ligands—activating receptors bind various target cell ligands while inhibitory receptors bind class I MHC molecules (see Figure 10-24 in Chapter 10). Because most cells express high levels of class I MHC molecules, they provide inhibitory signals to NK cells. The decreased, or loss of, expression of class I MHC molecules on tumor target cells and virus-infected cells and/or upregulation of ligands stimulate NK cell-mediated killing. Thus, NK cells do have receptors and do recognize MHC molecules. The difference is that

MHC recognition is a negative event. NK cells are turned off, not on, by MHC molecules. They express two types of molecules that regulate killing: the inhibitory receptors represented by three types of molecules, human killer cell immunoglobulin-like receptors (KIRs), CD94/natural-killer group 2, member A (NKG2A), and rodent Ly49; the activating receptors represented by two types of molecules NKG2D, and NKp46, NKp30, and NKp44. Although the structures and mechanisms of NK cell target recognition are different, NK cells and $T_C$ cells use similar mechanisms to kill target cells.

Lastly, NK cells acquire target specificity by using ADCC. NK cells and target cells become "cross-linked" when the Fc receptors (CD16) on the surfaces of NK cells bind the Fc portions of IgG antibodies attached to the antigenic determinants of the target cells. Interestingly, the bridging of target cells and NK cells by their Fc receptors and antibodies on the target cell is required but not enough to produce lysis. Both Fc receptor engagement and cell-cell interaction are concomitantly required for target cell lysis. Neither DNA nor protein synthesis is required for NK cell-mediated cytotoxicity. ADCC is illustrated in Figure 15-10 of Chapter 15.

Another lymphocyte-like cell has emerged as an important regulator; it is called the **natural killer T (NKT) cell** (also see Chapter 15). It is a T cell subset that draws characteristics from NK cells and T cells. Like T cells, NKT cells express αβ TCRs; however, these receptors do not react with class I or II MHC molecules but a family of MHC-like molecules, which specialize in presenting lipid antigens to T cells, called *CD1* (see Chapter 7). Furthermore, NKT cells express TCRs that are composed of invariant α chains and conventional β chains. Like NK cells, NKT cells express NK cell receptors and variable levels of CD16. Because of their self-reactivity and anti-microbial activity, their expression of NK cell receptors, and their ability to rapidly secrete large quantities of IFN-γ and IL-4, NKT cells can initiate and regulate the early stages of immune responses—provide rapid support while waiting for $T_H$ cell responses to build up.

is accomplished without sensitization and in the absence of antibody and complement. NK cells mediate cytotoxic reactions in the absence of, or decrease in, class I MHC molecule or upregulation of characteristic ligands expression on target cells. NK cells also can kill target cells by ADCC.

Another rapid responder cell is the NKT cell, which mediates killing and rapid production of cytokines in the early stages of a response to pathogens.

## Macrophages Are the "Big Eaters" of the Immune System

Macrophages were the first cell type identified that protect the host from antigenic intrusion; they were once derided as the "garbage collectors" of the immune system. During the 110-plus years since Metchnikoff discovered macrophages (also called *mononuclear phagocytes*), immunologists have realized that macrophages are important immunoregulators of humoral and cell-mediated immunity. Tissue macrophages and their precursors (monocytes) are part of the **mononuclear phagocyte system** because they share a common lineage and because their primary function is phagocytosis.

Macrophages develop from a myelomonocytic stem cell through the **monoblast, promonocyte,** and **monocyte** stages until they reach the mature end-cell stage—the structurally heterogeneous **tissue macrophages** (see Figure 2-3). Before becoming tissue macrophages, they exist briefly in the bloodstream as nomadic adolescent cells called *monocytes* and constitute 3 to 7% of peripheral blood leukocytes. Once in the tissue, monocytes undergo transformation into permanently rooted tissue macrophages. *Tissue macrophages* are so called because they are seeded in a variety of guises throughout the body tissues, where they stay for 2 to 3 months. They are named according to their residency in the many tissues they inhabit (Figure 2-7). Macrophages measure 10 to 40 μm in diameter. The macrophage's morphology varies, depending on its state of activity. The membrane protein turns over rapidly (approximate half-life of 7 hr), irrespective of receptor engagement. The cytoplasm contains vacuoles, is slightly basophilic, and contains an ovoid nucleus 6 to 12 μm in diameter.

Macrophages have six characteristics: they (1) are mononuclear cells, (2) show peroxidase and esterase activity, (3) bear specific receptors for antibody and complement, (4) show phagocytic abilities (see

## MINI SUMMARY

NK cells are CD3⁻, large granular lymphocytes that express CD16 and CD56 but have no required cell surface molecule to function as a NK cell, such as is the case for B cells (the BCR) and T cells (the TCR). NK cells are capable of killing virally infected and cancerous target cells. Killing

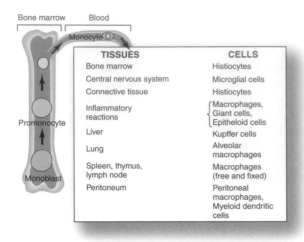

**FIGURE 2-7 Nomenclature of the monocyte lineage.**

Figure 3-11), (5) may be stimulated into a state of activation, and (6) possess a varied and prolific secretory ability. Because macrophages adhere to glass or plastic, they can be separated from nonadherent T and B cells. Unlike T and B cells, macrophages are neither clonally restricted nor antigen-specific but function instead as nonspecific *accessory cells*.

Monocytes, the blood precursors for macrophages, are heterogeneous as defined by CD14 (part of the receptor for lipopolysaccharide [LPS]), CD16 (Fc receptor for antigen-antibody complexes), and chemokine receptor expression. Circulating monocytes recruited to inflammation sites exhibit cell-surface profiles indicative of molecules known to be involved in inflammatory-cell recruitment, migrate to inflamed tissues and differentiate into macrophages and dendritic cells, and accordingly are called *inflammatory monocytes*. In contrast, monocytes that move into tissues in the absence of inflammation (steady-state conditions) switch their cell-surface molecules, enter tissues and restock tissue macrophages and myeloid dendritic cells, and are called *resident monocytes*. Tissue macrophages are heterogenous but maturation can be studied by observing CD14, Fc receptors (CD16, CD23, CD32, and CD64), C3b receptors (CD11b), CD68, and class I and II MHC molecules. There are several enzyme markers; the one most widely used is nonspecific esterase. Lysozyme and peroxidase are other useful enzyme markers. The location of peroxidase can be used to determine what stage of differentiation a macrophage is in because the peroxidase location is different for each stage, and all but resident macrophages possess peroxidase-containing granules.

*Macrophages are versatile cells that can play four roles: accessory, secretory, effector, and regulatory.*

1. Although primarily recognized for their phagocytic ability, macrophages are also accessory (supportive) cells because they participate in several other immunologic functions. Macrophages encounter and internalize antigen either by phagocytosis or by receptor-mediated endocytosis or infection and degrade most of it through lysosomal proteolysis (Figure 2-8). Some of the antigen, once processed, is reexpressed as a peptide on the macrophage surface in the context of class II MHC molecules and is presented to T cells (see Chapter 7). Macrophages exhibiting this activity are called **antigen-presenting cells** (**APC**s). Dendritic cells are the premier APCs because they initiate immune responses while macrophages participate in amplifying those responses. As nucleated cells, APCs also express class I MHC molecules; therefore, they can also display antigenic peptides associated with class I MHC molecules (see Figure 2-8 and see Chapter 7).

2. Macrophages also are important secretory cells. Over 100 macrophage-derived substances have been identified, many of which affect lymphocyte proliferation, differentiation, and effector capabilities. Macrophage-derived products include cytokines, chemokines, hydrolytic enzymes, complement components, oxygen metabolites, nitric oxide, nucleosides, and bioactive lipids (platelet-activating factor, prostaglandin $E_2$, thromboxane, leukotrienes, and so on). Other molecules derived are defined according to their function—IL-1, transferrin, TNF-$\alpha$, IL-12, and glucocorticoid-antagonizing factor. Many macrophage mediators regulate positive and negative feedback loops that affect the inflammatory response and immunologic networks. In many instances, the production of macrophage-derived molecules depends of whether macrophages are activated as described next.

3. Most macrophages are normally in a resting state, on exposure to agents that stimulate gene transcription, macrophages become larger and ruffled and have increased expression of various gene products that allow them to perform effector functions. *At this stage, they are called* **activated macrophages**. They are activated by an assortment of stimuli, but not unexpectedly as phagocytic cells, the first stimulus during an immune response is the process of phagocytosis. Macrophages can be further enhanced

by activated $T_H$ cell-derived cytokines, by inflammation-promoting chemokines, and by bacterial cell-wall components. The best-described macrophage-activating factor is IFN-$\gamma$. IFN-$\gamma$ activates macrophages to kill microorganisms and tumor cells, changes their receptor profiles, improves APC function, promotes acute inflammation, stimulates macrophage cytokine and chemokine production and receptivity, and increases their ability to activate T cells. Activated macrophages become better APCs because they express more class II MHC molecules and more accessory molecules (see Chapter 8). Activated macrophage products, such as platelet-activating factor, prostaglandins, and leukotrienes, act in concert with the cytokines TNF-$\alpha$ and IL-1 and chemokines CXCL8 to produce local inflammation

that first causes local tissue destruction and later promotes replacement by connective tissue (see Chapter 3). Activated macrophages also mediate the lysis of infected cells, allografts, and tumor cells. Macrophage-mediated cytotoxicity can be antigen-specific[3] or nonspecific. The macrophage's direct antitumor activity is probably attributable to lysis of tumor cells by macrophage-derived TNF-$\alpha$ or nitric oxide. Because macrophages are cytotoxic, widely distributed, and possess tumor infiltration

---

[3]Macrophages alone are not antigen-specific; antibody is needed to achieve antigen specificity. This process, called *antibody-dependent cell-mediated cytotoxicity (ADCC)*, was introduced earlier in the chapter and described in detail in Chapter 15.

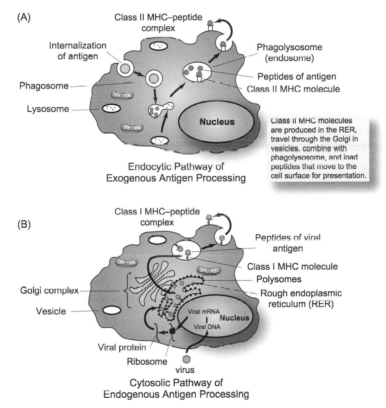

**FIGURE 2-8 Antigen processing and presentation of peptides with class II and class I MHC molecules**. (A) Antigen presentation starts when native antigen binds to an APC, followed within minutes by its internalization through phagocytosis or receptor-mediated endocytosis in clathrin-coated pits into vesicles called *phagosomes*, which fuse with lysosomes. Once in the low-pH environment of the phagolysosome (also called the *endosome*), antigen processing of the native antigen begins. (B) All nucleated cells express class I MHC molecules; therefore, APCs can also present antigenic peptide associated with class I MHC molecules, which is important in the induction of antiviral $T_C$ cell activation (see Chapter 7).

abilities, the macrophage may represent one of the primary surveillance cells against cancer. The bottom-line is that whatever macrophages are doing, they do it better when activated.

The activation of macrophages by antigens and other stimuli during an immune response functionally polarize macrophages (and dendritic cells), which in turn polarize innate and adaptive immune responses. Depending on environmental-derived signals, for example, IFN-$\gamma$ and LPS promote the orientation of macrophages to a type I direction, called a M1 (also called *classically activated macrophages*); the type number mirrors the $T_H1/T_H2$ dichotomy we mentioned above. M1 polarized macrophages drive the development of type I immune responses, which are mediated by $T_H1$ cells. Exposure to IL-4, IL-10, and IL-13 orientates macrophages to a M2 population (also called *alternatively activated macrophages*) (there are at least three proposed versions of M2 phenotype), which drives the development of type II immune responses, which are mediated by $T_H2$ cells.

4. The fourth function, regulation, helps control immune responsiveness, but the mechanisms of regulation are poorly understood. Macrophages regulate T-cell proliferation in a cell-cell contact manner and through *monokines* (macrophage-derived cytokines that enhance or inhibit other immune cell activities; see Chapter 9). Inhibitory molecules that suppress lymphocyte proliferation include prostaglandins, thymidine, arginase, toxic oxygen intermediates, nitric oxide, and IFN-$\alpha$.

### MINI SUMMARY

Macrophages are mononuclear phagocytic cells derived from myeloid stem cells in the bone marrow. The macrophage's immediate precursor cells are monocytes. Tissue macrophages are the "professional" phagocytes of the mononuclear phagocyte system. Macrophages demonstrate accessory, secretory, effector, and regulatory functions. Once activated, macrophages facilitate immune responses.

## Dendritic Cells Are Innate Sentinels Translating Innate to Adaptive Immunity

Early studies evaluating the contribution of glass and plastic adherent cells to immune responses revealed adherent star-shaped cells that were called **dendritic cells**, so named because their cytoplasm arranges into a web of long, finger-like processes that resemble nerve cell dendrites—the processes can interdigitate between lymphoid cells of lymphoid tissue, skin, and squamous epithelium. The next series of experiments showed that dendritic cells were superior stimulates of T cells later described to be due to elevated levels of class II MHC molecule and costimulator molecule expression—combined with this ability and the finger-like processes, they are potent APCs. Dendritic cells can exist in two states, as immature or mature cells with the latter cells capable of driving naïve T cell responses (that is, acting as APCs). A pathogen invades the tissue causing inflammation (see Chapter 3), tissue-residing, immature dendritic cells sampling their environment, capture the antigen (pathogen), process it, after which they migrate to secondary lymphoid tissues, en route they mature from an antigen-sampling cell to an APC. Exogenous molecules such as cytokines and microbial components, confirmed by phenotypic changes, regulate dendritic cell maturation.

As is detailed in Chapter 3, dendritic cells are part of the innate immune system cellular repertoire. They initiate immune responses to pathogens by the recognition of pathogen-associated molecular patterns that are not expressed by host cells. This recognition is mediated by pattern recognition receptors such as the Toll-like receptor (TLR) family (see Chapter 3), several of which are expressed by immature dendritic cells. Signaling through TLRs influences phagocytosis, the migration, the upregulation of class II MHC and costimulatory molecules, a switch in chemokine receptor expression, the secretion of cytokines and chemokines, and the presentation of antigens by dendritic cells to naïve T cells in lymph nodes. As innate immune system cells, dendritic cells provide direct innate defenses through antigen capturing and processing, cytokine production such as IL-12, IL-18, and type I interferons (IFN-$\alpha$ and -$\beta$), and the activation of NK cells. These properties also allow dendritic cells to take innate-retrieved information and translate it into adaptive immunity. In fact, dendritic cell–derived cytokines can bias (polarize as discussed in the preceding section) CD4$^+$ T cell activity toward a $T_H1$ response. The same cytokines can also activate NK cells, which make IFN-$\gamma$, and thereby indirectly promote $T_H1$ responses. Dendritic cells may also promote $T_H2$ responses through the expression of Notch ligands (see Chapter 3). So we can see that not only are dendritic cells efficient at inducing the activation and proliferation of naïve T cells, they fine-tune immune responses by instructing T-cell differentiation and polarization.

The developmental origin-picture of dendritic cells is fragmented; piecing together the picture is complicated because of their heterogeneity and differences between dendritic cells formed during steady-state conditions (healthy host, no infection or inflammatory stimuli) versus dendritic cells produced during inflammation. Nonetheless, as all immune cells, human dendritic cells arise from pluripotent $CD34^+$ stem cells but they do not develop from a single progenitor lineage, that is, the common myeloid progenitor (CMP) or the common lymphoid progenitor (CLP). In fact, when starting from a single CMP or a single CLP both could generate mature/conventional dendritic cells or precursors of dendritic cells. Irrespective of source, the cytokine FMS-related tyrosine kinase 3 ligand (FLT3L) is crucial for the development of dendritic cells; it regulates early hematopoiesis by binding the FLT3 receptor and stimulating the FLT3 signal transduction pathway. In the bone marrow, FLT3 expression is restricted to $CD34^+$ cells and the subset of dendritic precursor cells. FLT3 expression correlates with the short-term HSCs compartment ($Lin^-$ $Sca$-$1^-$ $c$-$Kit^+$ $FLT3^+$ cells) discussed earlier.

Despite the fact that the origin of different dendritic cells is not completely understood, they are known to be a multimember family. Dendritic cells are sparsely but widely distributed heterogeneous sentinel cells that are specialized for the capture, processing, and presentation of antigens to naïve T cells. The conversion from a continuous sampler of the surrounding antigenic environment to one of APC occurs following encounter with invading microbes, which initiates the migration of dendritic cells to draining lymph nodes. During the trip, they have upregulated class II MHC molecule and costimulatory molecule expression, so on lymph node arrival they are mature dendritic cells that can efficiently trigger receptor-specific naïve T cells. The dendritic cell categories, which go by several guises depending on their location, are summarized below.

The skin and epithelial surfaces of the respiratory and the gastrointestinal tract constitute the largest immune organ in the body and represent a major first line of defense. **Langerhans cells**, characterized by Birbeck granules and Langerin, are present in the epidermis and mucous membrane epithelia, whereas another dendritic cell is present in the dermis (interstitial dendritic cells, mentioned below). While Langerhans cells reside in the skin or epithelia they are immature sentinel cells detecting incoming skin pathogens (antigen). After taking up antigen and migrating to cutaneous-draining lymph nodes, as mature cells they move into T-cell areas of the lymph nodes, secrete chemokines that attract naïve T cells, present antigen, and induce the proliferation and differentiation of antigen-specific T cells.

Immature **interstitial dendritic cells** are found, with the exception of the brain, in all organs throughout the body within the interstitial spaces that are drained by afferent lymphatic vessels. As Langerhans cells, interstitial dendritic cells sample the surrounding environment for invading microbes, internalized and process antigen, carrying it to draining lymph nodes. Once they arrive in the lymph nodes as mature cells, they localize in the T-cell areas where they are called *interdigitating dendritic cells* because their "dendrites" extend between the T cells.

**Monocyte-derived dendritic cells** are the prototype for studies of dendritic cell development and function. The best-characterized example of a distinct dendritic cell type that is produced as a consequence of inflammation is the dendritic cells that are derived from the inflammatory monocytes (discussed earlier). The conversion is dependent on the cytokine granulocyte-macrophage colony-stimulating factor (GM-CSF). In fact, cultured monocytes exposed to GM-CSF and IL-4 differentiate into dendritic cells. As monocytes exit circulation into inflamed tissues and remain at the site they differentiate into macrophages, if they take-up antigen and migrate to draining lymph nodes, they arrive as dendritic cells and function accordingly.

The most recently described dendritic cells are the **plasmacytoid-derived dendritic cells**. The name "plasmacytoid" is used because these cells have a round morphology with an eccentric nucleus and abundant endoplasmic reticulum; however, they are non-B, non-T, nonmonocytic type cells. They correspond to a specialized cell population that produces large amounts of type I interferons (IFN-α and -β) in response to viruses, and therefore they are also called *natural interferon-producing cells*. This is not surprising because they express the pattern recognition receptors, Toll-like receptors 7 and 9 (TLR7 and TLR9), which respond to single-stranded RNA and DNA viruses, respectively (see Chapter 3). Type I interferons are also important in the activation of NK cells, which are themselves a major killer of virus-infected cells. (Nonimmune virus-infected cells can also produce type I interferons, which is taken-up by neighboring cells and blocks viral replication [see Chapter 3].)

Another type of cell with a dendritic cell morphology, the **follicular dendritic cell**, named for its exclusive location in the B cell-rich follicles of the lymph node, are not of bone marrow origin and do not function as the antigen-presenting dendritic cells described above. Follicular dendritic cells lack class II MHC molecules; thus, they do not act as APCs for T-cell activation. Follicular dendritic cells do express high levels of membrane receptors for antibody and complement. Binding of circulating antibody-antigen complexes by these receptors facilitates B-cell activation in lymph nodes. These complexes are retained on the dendritic cell membrane for extended periods of time, the length is uncertain. The antigen-antibody complexes are found coating beaded structures of the follicular dendritic cell processes, called *iccosomes*, which may play a role in the development of memory B cells within the follicle. Iccosomes bud off and may be internalized by B cells.

---

### MINI SUMMARY

The immune system needs to constantly sample the peripheral tissues for microbial invasion; dendritic cells "fill-these-shoes," because as immature cells they are designed with pattern-recognition receptors that recognize molecules expressed by microbes but not host cells; once recognized the microbes are internalized. They then convey that information to naïve T cells distant from the infection site usually found in the draining lymph nodes. Before this happens, migrating dendritic cells mature to APCs with increased levels of class II MHC and costimulatory molecules and display the antigen-MHC complex to naïve T cells localized in T-cell areas of the lymph nodes. The process of moving antigen from the periphery to where the T cells reside, is accomplished by at least four different types of dendritic cells: Langerhans cells, interstitial dendritic cells, monocyte-derived dendritic cells, and plasmacytoid dendritic cells. Unlike these dendritic cells, follicular dendritic cells lack class II MHC molecules; therefore, they are not APCs but may mediate B-cell memory.

---

# THE ORGANS OF THE IMMUNE SYSTEM ARE REPOSITORIES FOR IMMUNE CELLS

Unlike the circulatory or digestive systems, the immune system is neither contained completely within a set of organs nor controlled by a central organ like the brain; furthermore, it is not hard-wired to the brain, as is the eye or the ear. Instead, interconnected lymphoid organs serve as repositories for

mononuclear leukocytes and specialized epithelial cells. *These lymphoid organs have at least four functions: (1) to provide an environment for the maturation of the immune system's immature cells, (2) to concentrate lymphocytes into organs that drain areas of antigen insult, (3) to permit the interaction of different classes of lymphocytes with each other and professional APCs, and (4) to provide an efficient vehicle for the disbursement of antibodies and other soluble factors from lymphocytes and other immune cells.* Lymphoid organs include the *bone marrow* (more accurately described as a tissue), *thymus, lymph nodes, spleen,* and *MALT.*

Organs of the immune system can be divided into **primary** and **secondary lymphoid organs** (or tissues) (Table 2-2). Primary lymphoid organs are those with special microenvironments where *antigen-independent differentiation* of lymphocytes takes place—the *thymus* and the *bone marrow* (in birds, the *bursa of Fabricius*). The mature lymphocytes manufactured in the thymus and bone marrow are exported through the blood to the secondary lymphoid organs, the *lymph nodes, spleen,* and the *MALT.* These secondary lymphoid organs are the places where lymphocytes encounter antigen and as a result undergo *antigen-dependent differentiation.*

## Primary Lymphoid Organs Are Maturation Sites for Immune Cells in the Absence of Antigen

Immature lymphocytes must reside for a limited time in special environments where they undergo structural and functional changes. In mammals, some immature lymphocytes remain in the bone marrow; in birds, some remain in the bursa of Fabricius. In either organ, the cells are acted on by complex and incompletely understood mechanisms. Other immature lymphocytes move to the thymus (in both mammals and birds), and are acted on by thymic stromal cell-derived cytokines and by interaction with stromal (epithelial and mesenchymal) cells. Once cells have matured in the primary lymphoid organs, they are able to carry out immune responses.

### The B-Cell Factories Are the Bone Marrow and the Bursa of Fabricius

The **bone marrow** is the B-cell factory in mammals. It is the birthplace for all immune cells (in the early fetus, it is the liver and spleen). The bone marrow also provides the essential microenvironment, known as *niches*, for the antigen-independent differentiation of B cells. The bone marrow is also the site for NK cell differentiation. The bone marrow constitutes the soft tissue in the hollow shafts called the *medullary cavities* of the flat bones (iliac bones, ribs, sternum, and vertebrae) of the body and weighs about 3 kg (equal to or larger than the liver) in an averaged-sized adult. It is divided into vascular and hematopoietic compartments. The stem cells and their progeny are packed into spaces between medullary vascular sinuses all surrounded by fatty tissue. Hematopoiesis occurs in the spaces between the sinuses. What cells provide the environmental niche and drive B-cell development through the ordered series of stages is an open question. Some candidates include the osteoblasts, chemokine CXCL12-expressing reticular cells, and IL-7–expressing cells. The cellular composition of normal bone marrow is made up of 5 to 15% lymphocytes, 1% plasma cells, and 4% monocytes and megakaryocytes (the source of platelets), connective tissue cells, stromal cells, and adipocytes. Human stem cell frequency ranges from 0.7 to 8.3 HSCs per $10^8$ bone marrow cells.

As immature B cells proliferate and differentiate through different stages in the bone marrow, they are undergoing random rearrangement of antibody heavy and light chain genes, which leads to an enormous diversity of antibody receptor expression (mentioned earlier and see Chapter 6). A selection process culls B cells with defective and self-reactive antibody receptors. Culled cells are eliminated through a process called *apoptosis*. The immature IgM$^+$ B cells exit the bone marrow and enter the blood to reach the spleen, where they mature into peripheral mature B cells expressing both IgM and IgD. Once mature B cells encounter antigen, they differentiate into short-lived and long-lived plasma cells, the latter cells can return to the bone marrow.

NK cells are derived from hematopoietic stem cells; however, the definite site(s) for NK cell development is uncertain. The bone marrow is considered the primary site of NK cell generation because it provides the microenvironment and ligands required for NK cell development. This is supported by bone marrow ablation, which leads to decreased numbers and functional capabilities of peripheral NK cells.

The **bursa of Fabricius** is the B-cell factory in birds. It is a sac-like lymphoepithelial organ at the terminal portion of the cloaca in birds. To differentiate into antibody-secreting cells, pre-B lymphocytes must dwell in the bursa for a limited time. No distinct anatomic equivalent to the bursa has been found in mammals, although the bone marrow appears to be the human counterpart in a functional sense.

### The T-Cell Factory Is the Thymus

The **thymus** is a bilobed, fully developed elongated organ weighing 15 to 20 g at a human's birth. It grows rapidly during the first 2 years, then more slowly, and reaches a maximum weight of roughly 40 g at puberty. At that time, under the influence of sex hormones, it begins to involute, as shown by a drop in the cortex to medulla ratio. However, the thymus never disappears, even though the cortex becomes progressively thinner and eventually is almost completely replaced by adipose tissue. The thymus, or its remnants, remains functional throughout life but thymic T cell output is proportionally reduced and maintained at lower levels. The importance of the thymus is exhibited in humans with a congenital birth defect such as DiGeorge syndrome and in mice called *nude mice*; both lack a thymus, which leads to an absence of T cell–mediated cellular and humoral immunity and increased infections.

The thymus lies above the heart near the throat, resting on the pericardium behind the breastbone. *It is a* **lymphoepithelial organ** *created by the migration of lymphocytes from bone marrow into the epithelial rudiment during embryogenesis.* Each lobe is divided into many lobules by fibrous septae. Each lobule consists of two main compartments, called the **cortex** and the **medulla** (Figure 2-9), which are surrounded by a subcapsule zone. Both compartments have a stromal-cell network chocked full of epithelial cells, macrophages, and dendritic cells, which contribute to thymus structure and drive T-cell differentiation. The more prominent of the two is the cortex, which makes up 85 to 90% of the thymus. The mouse thymus contains about 200 million thymocytes and generates roughly 50 million new thymocytes each day. These *thymocytes*, epithelial cells, and a few macrophages tightly pack together to make up the cortex (the site of lymphocyte differentiation). The macrophages serve to eliminate thymocytes undergoing apoptosis. From 90% to 95% of the cells in the thymus are in the cortex. The cortex is further subdivided into the *subcapsular outer cortex* and the *deep cortex*. Cortical thymocytes are phenotypically and functionally immature but under the influence of stromal cell signals transduced through Notch1 receptors that switch on specific genes, they progressively differentiate into T cells within the thymic cortex. The T cells migrate to the medulla, where selection and maturation are completed, and then exit as mature T cells into the blood. The medulla makes up 10 to 15% of the thymus, is less closely packed with thymocytes than the cortex, and contains structures of tightly packed whorls of epithelial cells called *Hassall's corpuscles*. The medullary thymocytes, which comprise 5 to 10% of the thymic cells, are nearly mature or mature, immunocompetent cells in close associated with epithelial cells, macrophages, and dendritic cells and are in the process of leaving the thymus. The release of thymocytes from the thymus is slow, with only about 2% leaving the thymus each day (in mice, roughly 1 million mature T cells). The remaining cells die by apoptosis, which takes place in the cortex. Whether this high attrition rate is caused by low efficiency in the formation of functional T cells of any specificity or because of stringent culling of T cells for the right specificity is unresolved. The immune system must be extremely careful to eliminate anti-self specificities so that it targets only the correct cells for destruction (see Chapter 8).

The thymus generates and selects a repertoire of T cells to protect against infection. Like B cells, the intrathymic T-cell maturation process proceeds through a series of ordered stages where immature T cells are undergoing random rearrangement of TCR $\alpha\beta$ or $\gamma\delta$ chain genes, which leads to the generation of two distinct T-cell lineages, $\alpha\beta$ or $\gamma\delta$ chain-expressing T cells, the combination results in TCR expression with a huge diversity directed against antigen–self-MHC complexes. The majority of these cells are incapable of recognizing any antigen-MHC complex—useless cells that undergo apoptosis. Taken together, the thymus serves as an inductive environment for the switching of uncommitted stem cells to a particular T-cell lineage ($T_H$ or $T_C$ cells), as well as for keeping (positive selection) T cells that can distinguish self from nonself and deleting (negative selection) any cells that are reactive against self antigens (see Chapter 8). The entire maturation and selection process takes roughly three weeks to complete.

Small thymocytes within the cortex are in contact with cortical epithelial cells, dendritic cells, macrophages, and large epithelial cells called *nurse cells*. These cells all express high levels of class I and class II MHC molecules and produce cytokines that initiate and maintain growth and differentiation. Many cortical thymocytes specifically bind MHC molecules. These cell-cell interactions are responsible for the thymocytes' ability to recognize self-markers for future cell interactions and antigen presentation. This positive and negative selection process causes emigration of only those T lymphocytes that are endowed with specificities for foreign antigenic fragments bound to cell surface molecules encoded in the MHC (see Chapters 7 and 8).

## MINI SUMMARY

The lymphoid organs are distributed throughout the body and serve as repositories for immune cells. Primary lymphoid organs (bone marrow, bursa of Fabricius, and thymus) provide an environment for antigen-independent B- and T-cell differentiation, whereas secondary lymphoid organs (lymph nodes, spleen, and MALT) serve as sites for antigen-dependent B- and T-cell differentiation. All lymphocytes are derived from pluripotent hematopoietic stem cells in the bone marrow. Immature B cells develop mostly in the bone marrow in mammals or in the bursa of Fabricius in avian species. Immature T cells develop in the thymus.

## Secondary Lymphoid Organs Are Maturation Sites for Antigen-Driven Immune Cells

Some lymphocytes that exit the bone marrow and thymus congregate in the secondary lymphoid organs. These organs, including the *lymph nodes*, the *spleen*, and *MALT*, are locations where antigens become concentrated and where *antigen-dependent lymphocyte differentiation* occurs. The principal function of lymph nodes is to respond to antigens introduced into the tissues they drain—they convert innate immune responses to adaptive immunity. The principal function of the spleen is to respond to antigens in the blood. The MALT protects against pathogens at major entry points.

### The Lymph Nodes Are Junctional Filters in the Lymphatic System

The immune system faces a continuous challenge—respond to a large number of random antigens anywhere in the body at any given moment with naïve lymphocytes, which exist at low frequency for any given antigen. The lymphatic system and its lymph nodes (and the other secondary lymphoid organs) meet the challenge. Immune cells travel throughout the body by the circulatory and lymphatic systems (Figure 2-10). The lymphatic system is the drainage system of the body composed of blind-ended, highly permeable thin-walled capillaries and larger vessels that drain lymph from the extracellular spaces within tissues and organs and thereby recovers materials lost from the blood capillary network, invading antigens, and cells that enter the tissues spaces and returns them to the blood. The lymphatic vessels have valves that only allow unidirectional flow through the lymph nodes towards the body's core. Lymphatic vessels are absent in avascular structures such as the

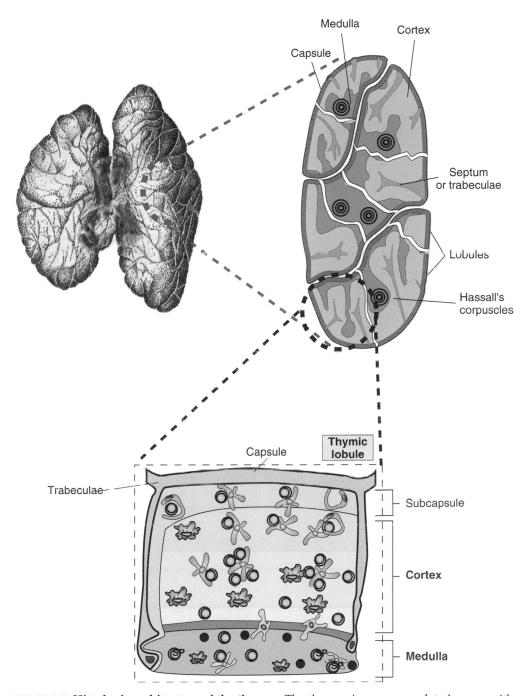

**FIGURE 2-9 Histologic architecture of the thymus.** The thymus is an encapsulated organ with septa or trabeculae extending from the capsule into the thymus. The thymus is divided into many lobules. The cortex is densely populated with rapidly dividing, immature T lymphocytes and packed with Hassall's corpuscles, while the medulla is sparsely populated with mostly nondividing T lymphocytes ready to exit the thymus. The outer cortex is the region closest to the capsule, and the inner cortex is the region closest to the medulla. (For a maturation flowchart of lymphocytes through the thymus, see Figures 8-10 and 8-11 in Chapter 8.)

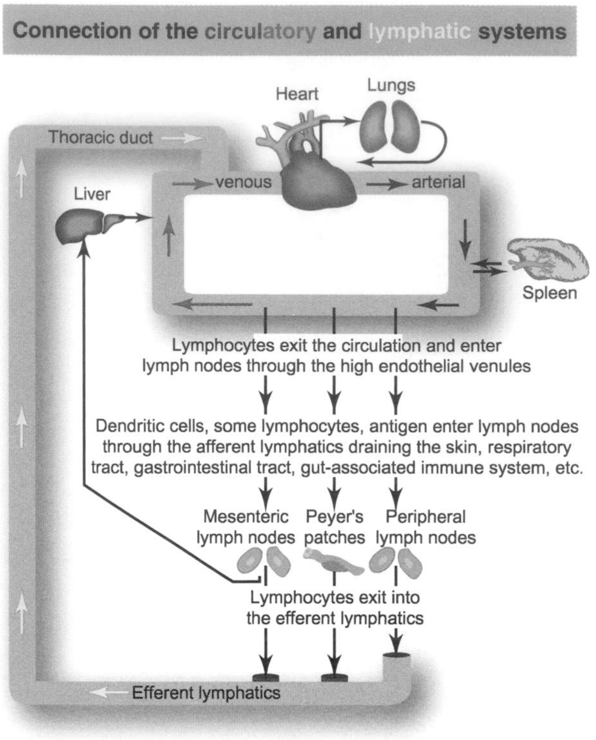

**FIGURE 2-10 Connection of the circulatory and lymphatic system**. (Adapted from A. Duijvestijn and A. Hamann. 1989. *Immunol. Today* 10:23.)

epidermis, hair, nails, cartilage, and cornea and in some vascularized organs such as the retina and probably the brain. **Lymph nodes** are small, encapsulated, lymphoreticular organs that are strategically laced along the lymphatic routes through which lymph percolates en route to its junction with the blood. Lymph nodes act primarily as filters for lymph, a straw-colored, protein-rich interstitial fluid that bathes the body's tissues; it contains antigens, antigen-bearing dendritic cells and macrophages, and memory T cells. The vessels transport lymph to the nodes, which arrives at the node through several *afferent lymphatics* on its convex side, empties into the subcapsular sinus, and percolates through the lymph node, where antigens and cells are filtered out. *The lymph nodes (1) provide a site for phagocytosis and antibody production against antigen, (2) act as a junction between the lymphatic system and the circulatory system, (3) support the induction, proliferation, and differentiation of lymphocytes, and (4) allow the recirculation of lymphocytes.* Nutrients and naïve immune cells also enter from the nodal artery and the nodal vein returns blood (not immune cells) and waste to the circulation. As the lymph is filtered, it is enriched with antibodies, cytokines, and mainly

effector T lymphocytes. Outgoing, *efferent*, lymphatic vessels merge into the thoracic duct and the right lymphatic duct, and these empty their contents into the bloodstream. Once in the bloodstream, lymph is transported throughout the body. The antibodies and effector immune cells patrol for foreign antigens and gradually drift back into the lymphatic vessels, where they begin the cycle again. We will see that this coordinated migration of the lymph nodes' cellular constituents dictates the lymph node's many responsibilities.

The diverse locations and architecture of lymph nodes hint at their functional importance during an immune response—collecting stations, libraries, for antigen visited by naïve lymphocytes. The internal appearance of a lymph node depends on whether it has recently been antigenically stimulated. A "resting" node can be morphologically divided into the **cortex, paracortex,** and **medulla** (Figure 2-11), with lymphocytes distributed mainly in the cortex and paracortex. The cortex contains spherical aggregations of B cells called **primary follicles** or **nodules**. Primary follicles consist of a network of follicular dendritic cells and $IgM^+IgD^+$ small, recirculating B cells. After antigenic stimulation, primary follicles form **secondary follicles**, consisting of a bull's-eye-like structure of concentrically packed, activated, dividing B cells that make up a **germinal center**. The follicles are the main sites of humoral responses. The areas between the follicles consist of T cells, mostly $CD4^+$ $T_H$ cells. Because B cells aggregate in the follicles of the cortex and because there is no morphologic change in the lymph node follicles following thymectomy, the cortex is called the **thymus-independent area**. The paracortical and interfollicular parts, called the *paracortex* of the cortex contain primarily $CD4^+$ $T_H$ cells and some B cells (in a ratio of 3:1). Because of this predominance of T cells in the paracortex and the drastic effects of thymectomy (or any other condition that reduces the number of T cells) on the paracortical region, this region is called the **thymus-dependent area**. This T-cell–rich area is where circulating naïve lymphocytes enter the lymph nodes and where naïve $T_H$ cells interact with dendritic cells presenting peptide-MHC complexes, starting T-cell immune responses. The third—and central—region of the node is the sparsely populated medulla, consisting of a reticular network and sinuses populated by different cell types, including medullary cords full of activated T and B cells, plasma cells, and memory T cells that arise during an ongoing immune response. Medullary sinuses coalesce into a single outgoing (efferent) lymphatic vessel.

The paracortex contains the postcapillary **high endothelial venules** (**HEVs**), only found in secondary lymphoid tissues (except for the spleen), which mediate trafficking of naïve lymphocytes from circulation into lymph nodes. The HEVs differ from ordinary venules; HEVs have a prominent perivascular sheath composed of pericytes, a thick basal lamina and a luminal layer of plump cuboidal endothelial cells (see Figure 2-11). HEVs are also unique in that they constitutively produce certain chemokines, which have a crucial role in lymphocyte trafficking to lymph nodes. Through these venules, by *extravasation* or *diapedesis*, roughly 50% of naïve T lymphocytes travel from the blood via the nodal artery into the node and are continually circulated back into the blood (Figure 2-12). This continual lymphocyte travel allows the full spectrum of lymphocyte antigen specificities available in the total lymphocyte pool to pass regularly through every lymph node, where they can meet antigen—this movement is called *lymphocyte recirculation*. This cycling can occur many times because antigen-naïve T cells have a half-life of roughly 8 weeks without ever dividing. In addition, the transient concentration of lymphocytes in the lymph nodes aids the cell-cell interactions needed for immune response

induction and regulation. Mature circulating naïve lymphocytes and endothelial cells express "gatekeeper" molecules—leukocyte and endothelial **cell adhesion molecules** (**CAMs**). Lymphocyte binding to lymph node HEVs is mediated by HEV-expressed sulfated glycosaminoglycans, collectively called *peripheral-node addressin (PNAD)*, which are ligands or CAMs for *L-selectin* (CD62L); these lymphocyte molecules are called *homing receptors* (or *selectins*). The PNAD carbohydrate-binding groups that bind L-selectin may be attached to different sialomucins on the HEVs, such as CD34 and glycan-bearing cell adhesion molecule-1 (GlyCAM-1). The molecules guiding naïve lymphocyte localization from the circulation into the lymph nodes are a family of adhesion molecules called *addressins* or *integrins* and *chemokines*—the ligands on HEVs for lymphocyte homing receptors (Figure 2-13). To trigger an immune response, a pathogen (antigen), antigen-presenting dendritic cells (an APC), and rare antigen-specific T and B lymphocytes need to meet. The T cells must first interact with mature dendritic cells (ones that have encountered antigen in the periphery) and the B cells with follicular dendritic cells, and then with each other. Tissue-invading pathogens (free antigen) and/or antigen-full

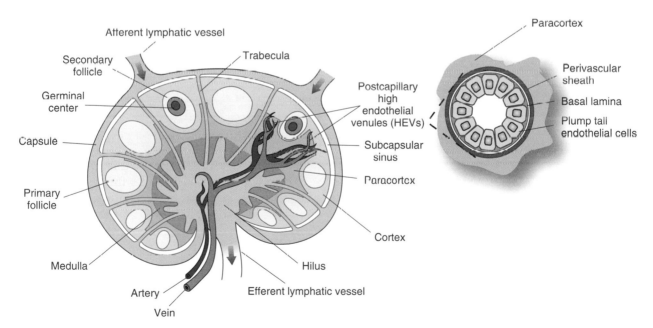

**FIGURE 2-11 Lymph node structure.** The lymph node contains three important areas: the *cortex* (thymus-independent area), containing B cells that are mostly in the follicles; the *paracortex* (thymus-dependent area), containing mostly T cells in the interfollicular areas but also some B cells; and the *medulla*, containing different cell types, including activated B cells and plasma cells. The cortex area contains dense aggregates of B cells, called *primary* and *secondary follicles*, surrounded by some T cells. Secondary follicles have foci of mitotic activity called *germinal centers*. Blood lymphocytes enter the node by traversing the walls of small, specialized veins called postcapillary *high endothelial venules (HEVs)*.

dendritic cells migrate through the lymphatic system to the draining lymph nodes (plasmacytoid dendritic cells can enter lymph nodes through HEVs), whereas naïve lymphocytes enter lymph nodes through HEVs. As lymphocytes approach and interact with HEVs, they undergo a sequential series of steps. The lymphocytes slow down and roll on the endothelium using their L-selectin as a rolling receptor; the rolling occurs through L-selectin–PNAD CD34 should read PNAD/CD34 interactions, which slows-down the movement through the HEVs. This allows T-cell integrins to be activated by HEV-produced CC-chemokine ligand 21 (CCL21) and CCL19 binding to T-cell expressed CC-chemokine receptor 7 (CCR7). The preceding activation leads to T cells binding to the HEV molecules intercellular adhesion molecule 1 (ICAM1 [CD54]) and ICAM2 (CD102) with the activated integrin lymphocyte function-associated antigen 1 (LFA1 [CD11aCD18]). Following integrin activation, the lymphocytes stop rolling, tight adhesion occurs, and they now move across the HEVs. CCL21 and CXCL12, along with CXC-chemokine ligand 13 (CXCL13), activate B cells to carry out LFA1-dependent cell adhesion and extravasation.

Once in the lymph node, naïve T cells migrate toward the paracortical region in response to CCR7–CCL21/CCL19 interactions (the dendritic cells and HEV stromal cells produce the chemokines). In contrast, naïve B cells migrate toward the follicles in response to CXCR5–CXCL13 interactions (the follicular stromal cells produce CXCL13). Once $T_H$ cells are activated, they transiently downregulate the expression of CCR7 and upregulate the expression of CXCR5, which allows them to migrate preferentially to B-cell follicles and interact with antigen-primed B cells. $CD4^+CXCR5^+$ $T_H$ cells are called *follicular B helper T cells*. In contrast, primed B cells downregulate the expression of CXCR5 and upregulate CCR7 and move to the paracortical region. The reciprocal movement of T and B cells facilitates their interaction. As B cells differentiate into plasma cells, they downregulate both CXCR5 and CCR7 expression and depart the lymph node. Most long-lived IgG-producing plasma cells upregulate CXCR4 and migrate to the bone marrow. In contrast, IgA-producing plasma cells upregulate CCR9 and CCR10 and move to mucous membranes.

The effector T cell's mission is eliminating the source of its cognate antigen, typically found in nonlymphoid tissues. Activated T cells can move to follicles to participate in B-cell activation or exit the lymph nodes. The recirculation pathways, or homing, of activated T cells (memory and effector T

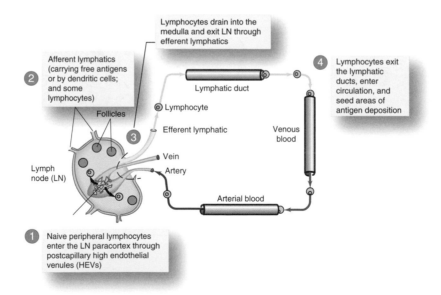

**FIGURE 2-12 Lymphocyte traffic through the lymph node**. Lymphocytes enter the lymph node through the postcapillary HEVs. These lymphocytes cross into the paracortex and exit through the medulla by way of the efferent lymphatics. The average transit time for T cells is 15 to 20 hr in a lymph node, while B cells can spend up to 30 hr in a lymph node. The lymphocytes enter the venous circulation, where the lymphatic ducts connect with veins in the neck.

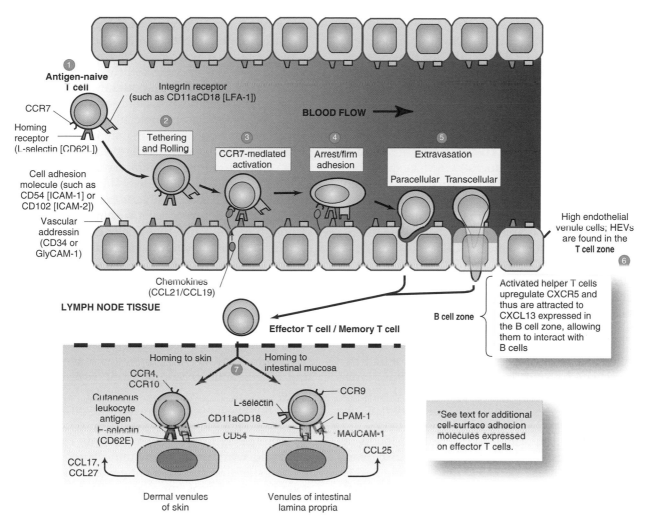

**FIGURE 2-13 A model for lymphocyte attachment and rolling, adhesion, and extravasation. (1)** Lymphocyte interaction with HEVs is with two types of adhesion molecules, the tissue-specific vascular addressins expressed (such as CD34) on certain lymphoid organs and the cell-adhesion molecules expressed (CD54 or CD102) on various cells. Recirculating naïve lymphocytes display homing receptors for specific vascular addressins. **(2–4)** Homing receptor tissue-specific interaction with HEVs leads to tethering and rolling. The rolling lymphocytes bind the CCR7 ligands CCL21 and/or CCL19, which induce conformational changes in the lymphocyte-expressing integrins that allow firm binding to the ICAM molecules. **(5)** The latter interaction allows for adhesion and extravasation into the lymph node. Lymphocytes choose between two routes of cellular transmigration (extravasation), paracellular (migrating around the HEV cells) or transcellular (piercing through the HEV cell cytoplasm) and once within the lymph node migrate to the appropriate regions. **(6)** Within lymph nodes, T cells interact with dendritic cells, leading to antigen-specific activation. **(7)** Effector T cells now express homing receptors and chemokine receptors that allow their migration into peripheral sites. The two memory T cell populations that arise—central memory T ($T_{CM}$) cells and effector memory T ($T_{EM}$) cells—have distinction homing patterns and effector functions. $T_{CM}$ cells express CCR7 and CD62L and continuously recirculate through lymph nodes, where they can respond to secondary antigen challenge. In contrast, $T_{EM}$ cells do not express either CCR7 or CD62L (they express chemokine receptors and other receptors that traffic them to appropriate target tissue), reside in nonlymphoid tissues, and mediate effector functions immediately after activation. Abbreviations: GlyCAM-1, glycosylation-dependent cell-adhesion molecule 1; ICAM, intercellular adhesion molecule; LAF-1, lymphocyte function-associated antigen 1; LPAM-1, lymphocyte Peyer's patch adhesion molecule 1; MAdCAM-1, mucosal addressin cell-adhesion molecule 1. (Adapted from A. Duijvestijn and A. Hamann. 1989. *Immunol. Today* 10:26.)

cells) to peripheral tissues are defined by the expression of several chemokine receptors and adhesion molecules (Figure 2-14). Following T-cell activation, the surface molecules very late activation molecule 4 (VLA-4), CD44, and CD11a/CD18 are upregulated. Because the ligands for these three surface markers are endothelium-associated molecules (vascular cell adhesion molecule 1 [VCAM-1; also called *CD106*], hyaluronic acid, and CD54, respectively), activated T cells are more prone to bind to other endothelial surfaces than lymph node HEVs. In fact, activated T cells release IL-4, which induces VCAM-1 expression. Therefore, these changes in surface marker expression promote the distribution and availability of lymphocyte subsets. What traffics them to the infection site is the expression of the appropriate chemokine receptors, if $T_H1$ cells they express CCR5 and CXCR3, if $T_H2$ cells they express CCR4 and CCR8. However, it is not so clear cut, for example, whether the induction of naïve T cells in lymph nodes is affected by whether the antigen was encountered in a cutaneous or intestinal environment. In the skin, venules display CCL17 and CCL27 and their counterpart effector T cells specific for cutaneous antigen express CCR4 and/or CCR10. Gut-associated effector T cells express CCR9 and lymphocyte Peyer's patch adhesion molecule 1 (LAMP-1) that responses to CCL25 and mucosal addressin cell adhesion molecule 1 (MAdCAM-1), respectively.

A group of important accessory cells found in the lymph nodes are dendritic cells (discussed earlier and in Chapter 3). Dendritic cells are large, motile, antigen-capturing, "professional" APCs that usually have several elongated pseudopodia. According to their overall initial location, dendritic cells can be divided into two groups: migratory versus lymphoid-tissue-resident dendritic cells. Irrespective of type, dendritic cells are considered immature cells before contact with antigen. Dendritic cells, sparsely but widely distributed cells, comprise about 1% of the cells in the secondary lymphoid organs and roughly 50% are lymph-node residents. They are localized strategically in the T-cell areas (called *interdigitating dendritic cells*) and the follicles (called *follicular dendritic cells*) of the lymph nodes. Mature interdigitating dendritic cells express large amounts of class II MHC and costimulatory molecules, and this expression plays a pivotal role in the presentation and induction of naïve CD4$^+$ T cells to their cognate antigen. A classic example of migratory dendritic cells are Langerhans cells, a population of skin-associated dendritic cells, which change their morphology to become interdigitating dendritic cells within the T-cell areas of lymph nodes. Langerhans cells give the immune system information regarding foreign substances that breach the skin. They pick up skin-sensitizing antigens and migrate to the draining lymph nodes. Another type of nonhematopoietic-derived dendritic cell localizes in the lymph node's B-cell follicles called *follicular dendritic cells*. It expresses no class II MHC or costimulatory molecules but high levels of CD23 (an Fc receptor) and C3 receptors, which allow them to trap antigen-antibody complexes and present them to B cells.

Lymphocyte traffic operates independent of antigen presence although antigen has profound effects on lymphocyte traffic. A lymph node can increase to 15-fold its normal size within 5 to 7 days after antigen stimulation. When antigen enters the lymph node by the afferent lymphatics, it localizes in two sites: the paracortex and the primary follicles of the cortex. In the first area of antigen localization, antigen can be trapped by macrophages and interdigitating dendritic cells, all of which are found in the paracortical region and lining of the lymphoid sinuses.

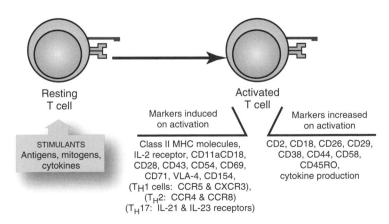

**FIGURE 2-14 Some phenotypic differences between resting and activated T cells.**

Within minutes of antigen entry, dendritic cells take up antigen, process it, and present antigen-derived fragments to antigen-specific CD4$^+$ T lymphocytes. Activated CD4$^+$ T cells localize to the follicle edges where they provide help to antigen-specific B cells that have moved out of the secondary follicles into the paracortical region; the B cells return to the follicle and promote the formation of germinal centers. The germinal center is a site devoted to maturation of antigen-activated B cells. The maturation steps include: clonal proliferation of antigen-specific B cells, somatic mutation of their immunoglobulin heavy- and light-chain genes, selection for B cells with highest affinity (called *affinity maturation*), switching of immunoglobulin classes, and differentiating into plasma cells or memory B cells. The secondary follicle, characterized by the presence of a germinal center, acquires a structure of concentric circles and contains B cells and follicular dendritic cells (Figure 2-15). The small number of antigen-activated B cells, about three for each follicle, is recruited from outside the follicle. These cells undergo exponential growth and fill the follicular dendritic network within 4 or 5 days; the germinal center lasts for 10 to 20 days. Once the network is filled, the B-cell blasts move to the center of the follicle. Antigen-naïve and recirculating small B cells are excluded from the center of the follicle and form the follicular mantle. The germinal center now takes on its characteristic bull's-eye-like structure, and over the next few hours the blast cells lose their surface antibody, now called *centroblasts*, and move to the dark zone. Proliferating centroblasts, undergoing somatic hypermutation in their antibody variable-region genes, give rise to both more centroblasts and centrocytes. The centrocytes, reexpressing surface antibody that has undergone somatic mutation, migrate to the layer surrounding the dark zone, the basal light zone, where they interact with, i.e. selected by, antigen held on the active follicular dendritic cells. Within the light zone there is considerable centrocyte apoptosis, suggesting that intense selection of somatically mutated cells is occurring. If centrocytes successfully interact with antigen, they progress to the apical light zone, where they receive differentiation signals that drive them to leave the germinal center as memory cells or plasma cells. Centrocytes failing to interact with antigen undergo apoptosis and are removed by *tingible-body macrophages*, which specialize in removing apoptotic lymphoid cells.

### The Spleen Is a Filter in the Circulatory System

The **spleen**, the largest single secondary lymphoid organ in mammals, is an ovoid filtering organ situated high in the abdomen under the diaphragm on the left side. It weights 100 to 150 grams in adults and contains roughly 25% of the body's mature lymphocytes of which 50% are B lymphocytes, 30–40% are T lymphocytes of which two-thirds are CD4$^+$ T cells and one-third are CD8$^+$ T cells. Unlike the lymph node, which filters lymph from specific areas of the body and therefore responds primarily to regional influences, the spleen filters blood and thus responds to systemic influences. It does so by receiving blood and retaining antigen, macrophages, dendritic cells, and antigen-specific T cells, B cells, and plasma cells. It also supports cell-cell interactions and allows recirculation of lymphocytes. The spleen also rids the body of old and injured red blood cells. Its structure and location leads to efficient removal of blood-borne microbes, making it the most important organ for antibacterial and antifungal immune responses.

Figure 2-16 illustrates the architecture of the spleen. The spleen is encapsulated by a coating of connective tissue; projections known as *trabeculae* form its structural matrix. Its interior is histologically divided into the **white pulp**, consisting of cylinders of lymphoid cells, and the **red pulp**, containing erythrocyte-rich blood intermingled with stromal cells, many macrophages, NK cells, and plasmablasts and plasma cells. The red pulp is the splenic blood-filtering system, which includes iron-recycling macrophages that are also involved in the removal of bacteria from the blood. Between these two areas is the **marginal zone**; which is populated by lymphocytes and macrophages. The white pulp is dispersed throughout the organ and is organized around small arteries and arterioles. The white pulp is organized into T- and B-cell compartments, surrounding the branching arterial vessels, so it resembles lymph node structure. Like in the lymph nodes, lymphocyte trafficking is controlled by specific chemokines, establishing T- and B-cell zones. Follicular dendritic cells and neighboring stromal cells produce the CXCL13 required for B cells to migrate to the B-cell zones, whereas mainly T-cell zone stromal cell-derived CCL19 and CCL21 are required for attracting T cells and dendritic cells to the T-cell zones. The thymus-dependent region is synonymous with the **periarteriolar lymphoid sheath** (**PALS**; also called the *T-cell zone*), two thirds of the T cells are CD4$^+$ and the remaining third are CD8$^+$. Follicles and their conversion to secondary follicles with germinal centers characterize the B-cell zone. In the PALS, T cells interact with dendritic cells and passing B cells, whereas in the B-cell follicles, activities are identical to those described for secondary follicles in the lymph node. Attached to

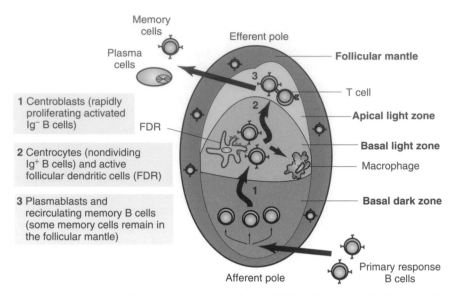

**FIGURE 2-15 The zonal pattern of a secondary follicle with a germinal center.** B cells, or centroblasts, of the dark zone are rapidly proliferating cells undergoing somatic hypermutation of their variable-region genes. These cells mature into centrocytes that reexpress membrane-bound antibody and enter the basal light zone. If centrocytes interact with follicular dendritic cell-held antigen, they move to the apical light zone. Centrocytes failing to appropriately interact with antigen die. Cells in the apical light zone are driven by differentiation signals to become memory B cells or plasma cells.

the outer region of the PALS is the marginal zone, a transit area for cells leaving circulation and moving into the PALS. It contains B cells and marginal-zone macrophages that present T-independent antigens (encapsulated bacteria) to B cells. Another unique type of macrophage is found in the marginal zone called *marginal-zone metallophilic macrophage*; its function is unknown.

Lymphocyte traffic through the spleen is completely by blood circulation. The spleen is the predominant organ in lymphocyte recirculation, moving more lymphocytes than all the lymph nodes combined. The transit time of T cells is 5 to 6 hr in the spleen; B cells spend more time. Thus, there is ample opportunity for the right lymphocytes to meet antigen localizing in the spleen. Blood-borne lymphocytes and antigens enter the spleen through the splenic trabecular artery (the spleen lacks HEVs), which courses along the capsule and into the trabeculae and empties into first the marginal zone and then the red pulp. The marginal zone is a rim of lymphocytes (CD4$^+$ T$_H$ cells and B cells) and macrophages. As antigen passes from the arteriole into the marginal zone, it is captured by the processes of interdigitating dendritic cells, processed, and presented to neighboring naïve T cells. The antigen-activated T cells, in turn activate B cells in the marginal zones, which are adjacent to the

sheath T$_H$ cells. Within 2 hr, antigen-activated B cells are found in the sheath at the periphery of primary lymphoid follicles. After 24 hr, the B cells are concentrated in the germinal centers. Antigen-activated B cells and antibodies cross from the white pulp through the marginal zone through bridging channels to the red pulp sinuses, where they are collected by veins that leave the spleen. There is also significant antibody production in the red pulp by plasmablasts that have transitioned into plasma cells under the influence of CD11c$^{hi}$ dendritic cells, leading to rapid entry of antibodies into the circulation.

### The Mucosa-Associated Lymphoid Tissue (MALT) Localizes Antibodies at Major Sites of Pathogen Entry

An additional group of nonencapsulated clusters of lymphoid tissue with immune function is the **mucosal immune system**. It is common around the membranes lining the respiratory, digestive, and urogenital tracts (gateways to the body for invading organisms). The anatomically well-organized structural components of this system are the specialized **mucosa-associated lymphoid tissue**, or **MALT**, such as the adenoids in the upper airways, tonsils in the throat, and Peyer's patches and lamina propria of the

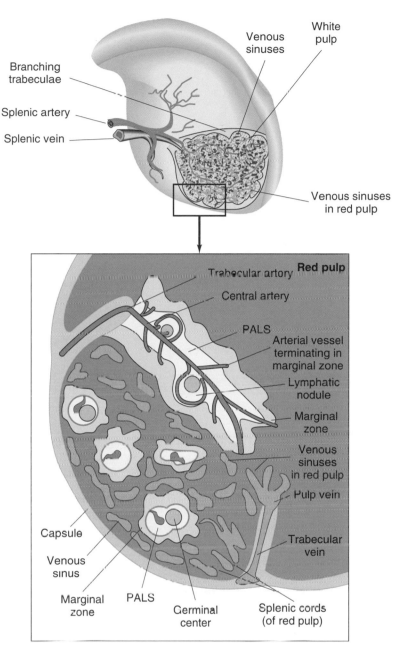

**FIGURE 2-16 Structure of the spleen.** The spleen is encapsulated by a connective tissue covering from which the trabeculae arise and project into the interior. The splenic artery enters the spleen and moves through the hilus, along the capsule, and into the trabeculae. It branches away from the trabeculae to become the small central arteries. These arteries are surrounded by densely packed layers of T-cells called the *periarteriolar lymphoid sheath (PALS)*, the thymus-dependent region. As the arteries branch further, they are generally surrounded by B-cell areas, the B cell-containing lymphoid follicles that may contain germinal centers. These areas are collectively called the *white pulp*. Lymphocytes exit from the white pulp through the marginal zone into the loosely organized *red pulp*, filtered by red pulp sinuses, where they are collected by veins leaving the spleen.

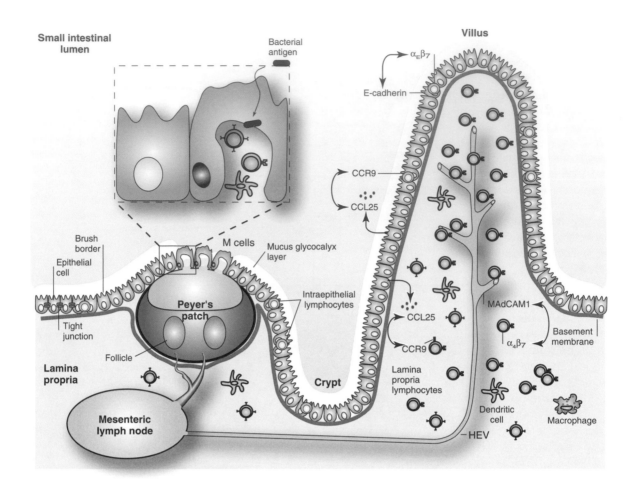

**FIGURE 2-17  Structure of GALT.** The immune system surrounding the intestinal tissues can be divided into immune-function-based compartments; the initiation compartment called the *gut-associated lymphoid tissues (GALTs)*, which includes the mesenteric lymph nodes (MLNs) and the Peyer's patches and the effector compartment, which includes the lamina propria, to which antigen-activated T cells migrate after stimulation in the initiation compartment, and the intestinal epithelium, where intraepithelial lymphocytes (IELs) reside interspersed among the luminal epithelial cells held together by tight junctions. M cells are the entry portals for antigen, they take-up luminal antigens and deliver them to the initiation compartment (see inset). Once the Peyer's patch and MLN naïve T cells are activated, they upregulate integrin $\alpha_4\beta_7$ expression, which interacts with intestinal-tissue high endothelial vessels (HEVs) that express mucosal addressin cell-adhesion molecule 1 (MAdCAM1), thereby facilitating homing to the mucosal effector compartments. Lymphocytes of the small intestine express chemokine CC receptor 9 (CCR9); thus, they are also attracted to the intestinal mucosa by chemokine CC-chemokine ligand 25 (CCL25)-producing epithelial cells of the small intestine. Epithelial cells express E-cadherin, which facilitates the tethering of $\alpha_E\beta_7$-expressing IELs to the intestinal epithelium.

small intestine. The best-characterized mucous membrane is the MALT of the gut called the *gut-associated lymphoid tissues (GALT)*. The single-cell layer of gut brush-bordered epithelium that separates the luminal antigen-rich environment ($10^{14}$ bacteria) from the sterile core of the host is a pathogen-impervious barrier held together by *tight junctions* between the cells. The flipside to this strong passive protection is that it also hampers antigen uptake by APCs; we will see below how the host resolves this.

Beneath the gut epithelial cells lies a meshwork of connective tissue called the *lamina propria*, containing various myeloid and lymphoid cells. The lamina propria includes a unique type of lymphocytes within the epithelial layer, and T cells, many IgA-producing plasma cells, macrophages, and dendritic cells scattered throughout the lamina propria, and focal accumulations of lymphocytes in the Peyer's patches (Figure 2-17). These lymphocytes first arrive from the blood, if unactivated, recirculate into the blood through draining lymphatics connected to the GALT. Once activated, mucosal tissue lymphocytes remain in the mucosal system and migrate into the surrounding laminar propria and epithelium. GALT has the histologic organization characteristic of the lymph nodes, divided into B- and T-cell zones, but antigen delivery is different. In the GALT, pathogens are ferried across the mucosa by specialized highly absorptive cells—antigen-uptake cells—called *microfold M cells*. Unlike their epithelial cell neighbors, M cells are not covered by glycocalyx; therefore, they can interact directly with luminal content through their apical surface. Furthermore, the basolateral surface of M cells is invaginated forming a pocket, which contains B cells, T cells, and dendritic cells. This invagination brings the "outside," the intestinal content, closer to the "inside," the basolateral lymphoid tissues that is, it facilitates antigen uptake. M cells cover the intestine luminal-exposed side of specialized lymphoid follicles found in the submucosa of the small intestine called *Peyer's patches*. Viewing from the luminal side of the intestine, Peyer's patches have a convex-dome structure covered with M cells. Thus, M cells can transport luminal antigen directly to the underlying subepithelial dome of the Peyer's patches for sampling by dendritic cells. Underlying the M cells are B-cell follicles separated by T cell zone segments. Like lymph node follicles, the Peyer's patch B-cell zone follicles contain dendritic cells, tingible body macrophages, and a few T cells, while the T-cell zones contain dendritic cells, macrophages, a supporting structure of stromal cells, and HEVs that deliver B and T cells. The HEVs express mucosal addressin cell-adhesion molecule 1 (MAdCAM-1), which interacts with the mucosal integrin molecule $\alpha_4\beta_7$ upregulated on naïve T cells activated by dendritic cells in the Peyer's patches and mesenteric lymph nodes. This interaction facilitates the migration of antigen-activated T cells to gut effector sites. Small intestine epithelial cells produce abundant amounts of CCL25, which binds to CCR9 expressed on most small intestine lymphocytes. CCL25 also upregulates the expression of $\alpha_4\beta_7$ on laminar propria lymphocytes. The T cells that reside as single cells in the small intestine epithelium, *intraepithelial lymphocytes (IELs)*, express the integrin molecule $\alpha_E\beta_7$, which interacts with epithelial cell-expressed E-cadherin, thereby facilitating IEL tethering to the intestinal epithelium. Most T cells are either $\alpha\beta TCR^+$ $CD4^+$ or $CD8\alpha\beta^+$ cells but a minority (1–10%) are $\delta\gamma TCR^+$ lymphocytes and most of them are represented as IELs in the intestinal epithelium or other mucosal tissues; their phenotype is $\delta\gamma TCR^+$

$CD4^-$ $CD8\alpha\beta^- CD8\alpha\alpha^+$. IEL development can be thymic-dependent or -independent and they can recognize soluble protein antigens and non-protein self-antigens. In fact, $\gamma\delta^+$ IELs do not require antigen processing or MHC-restricted antigen recognition, which means that antigen recognition diversity is not, unlike that of $\alpha\beta^+$ T cells, constrained by MHC-required binding, thereby allowing $\gamma\delta^+$ IELs to recognize a wide array of antigens. The ability to respond to common pathogen-derived moieties combined with their location makes for a highly effective antigen recognizing system.

Common functional characteristics of the MALT are their support of IgA-expressing B cells and IgA-producing plasma cells and the T cells that drive the development of these types of B cells. The MALT filters out antigens that enter in air and food or come from microorganisms growing in the intestines. The antigen-activated B lymphocytes of the MALT make secretory IgA, an antibody molecule that represents the body's first line of defense against infection by microorganisms (see Chapters 4 and 17). These B cells also make IgE as a main response to helminths.

## MINI SUMMARY

The secondary lymphoid organs (the lymph nodes and the spleen) are the sites for antigen-dependent lymphocyte differentiation. Lymph nodes are divided into the cortex, the paracortex, and the medulla, and contain lymphocytes and APCs. Lymphocytes from the bloodstream enter the lymph node through the HEVs or from the lymphatic system by the afferent lymphatics, migrate across the node, and leave by the efferent lymphatics. Following antigen exposure, primary follicles in the cortex develop into secondary, enlarged follicles that contain germinal centers. Germinal centers are the principal area for B-cell maturation and development of humoral immune responses. The patterns of recirculation are different for antigen-naïve and memory T cells. Naïve T cells localize in the lymph nodes, whereas effector memory T cells move to extravascular tissue and central memory cells remain in the lymph nodes.

The spleen filters the blood and retains antigen that enters the circulation. The spleen consists of red pulp and white pulp. T cells are located near the central arteriole, and B cells are localized within primary follicles. Primary follicles change to secondary follicles with germinal center formation following antigen stimulation. Spleen is

> responsible for removal of blood-borne pathogens, thus it is the most important organ for antibacterial and antifungal immune responses.
>
> The MALT, organized like lymph nodes but collect antigen differently, contains immune cells that protect the main portals of pathogen entry by secreting large amounts of IgA antibodies.

# SUMMARY

Five main kinds of immune cells participate in immune responses: B cells, T cells, NK cells, macrophages, and dendritic cells. *B cells* are precursors of antibody-producing plasma cells. *T cells* have regulatory and effector functions. T-cell maturation occurs in the thymus. T cells can be divided functionally and physically into *helper T cells* (usually CD4$^+$) and *cytotoxic T cells* (usually CD8$^+$). Each T cell type can be divided into subsets; the best-characterized are the $T_H1$, $T_H2$, followed by $T_H17$ and $T_{reg}$ cells. *NK cells* demonstrate cytotoxic activity and may function primarily as antitumor cells. NK cells are TCR$^-$CD3$^-$, exist in the absence of any known sensitization, and can lyse targets using *ADCC*. *Macrophages* possess phagocytic, accessory, secretory, effector (killing), and regulatory functions. Even though macrophages can internalize and reexpress antigen fragments for presentation in the context of their own class II molecules to T cells, they are considered phagocytic janitorial cells that direct surrounding cells. As immature cells with many guises, **dendritic cells** are prone to antigen-capturing, moving antigen to draining lymph nodes, en route maturing to cells that present antigen to naïve T cells, leading to their activation. Macrophages and dendritic cells that exhibit this process are called *antigen-presenting cells (APCs)*; macrophages and dendritic cells also are *accessory cells*.

The immune system's tissue architecture consists of *primary* and *secondary lymphoid organs*. The primary lymphoid organs include the *bone marrow*, the *thymus*, the *intestinal epithelium*, and the avian *bursa of Fabricius*. The secondary lymphoid organs include the *lymph nodes*, the *spleen*, and the *MALT*. The bone marrow contains *pluripotent hematopoietic stem cells*, the source of all myeloid and lymphoid cells. *Antigen-independent differentiation* of lymphocytes takes place in the primary organs. In mammals, B cells mature within the bone marrow. T-cell precursors leave the bone marrow and mature in the thymus to become T cells. Once B and T cells

mature, they leave the bone marrow or thymus and travel to secondary lymphoid organs. These are the sites for *antigen-dependent lymphocyte differentiation*. Lymph nodes are filters placed along the lymphatic ducts. B and T cells home to the lymph node follicles of the *cortex (thymus-independent area)* and *paracortex (thymus-dependent area)*, respectively. The cortex contains *primary follicles* made up of B cells. Following antigen stimulation, the primary follicles convert to *secondary follicles*, which consist of a mantle of concentrically packed B cells surrounding a *germinal center*. Lymphocytes leave the blood and enter the paracortex through the *HEVs*. Lymphocytes contact antigen through presentation of antigen by dendritic cells in the paracortical region or primary follicles of the cortex. Lymphocytes exit the lymph nodes through the *medulla* by the medullary sinuses, which coalesce into the efferent lymphatic vessel. Naïve T cells localize in the lymph nodes and can recirculate, while effector memory T cells localize in extravascular tissue and central memory cells remain in the lymph nodes. The spleen also is a secondary lymphoid organ and consists of *white pulp* (which contains the *periarteriolar lymphoid sheath*) and *red pulp*, which are separated by a *marginal zone*. The spleen filters out blood-borne pathogens, leading to humoral antibacterial and antifungal immune responses.

The *MALT* consists of secondary unencapsulated lymphoid tissue that is found in submucosal areas of the respiratory, gastrointestinal, and urogenital tracts. It provides the first-line of defense through the production of IgA antibodies.

# SELF-EVALUATION

## RECALLING KEY TERMS

Accessory cells
Activated macrophages
Antibody-dependent cell-mediated cytotoxicity (ADCC)
Antigen-presenting cells (APCs)
B lymphocytes (or B cells)
Bone marrow
Bursa of Fabricius
Cytotoxic T cells
Dendritic cells
   Interstitial dendritic cells
   Langerhans cells
   Monocyte-derived dendritic cells
   Plasmacytoid-derived dendritic cells
Germinal center
Helper T cells

Hematopoiesis
Lymph nodes
  Cortex
  High endothelial venules (HEVs)
  Medulla
  Paracortex
  Thymus-dependent area
  Thymus-independent area
Lymphocytes
Lymphoepithelial organ
Lymphoid organs
Lymphoid system (or immune system)
Macrophages
Monoblasts
Monocytes
Mononuclear phagocyte system
Mucosal immune system
  Mucosa-associated lymphoid tissue (MALT)
Natural killer (NK) cells
Plasma cells
Pluripotent hematopoietic stem cells
Primary follicles
Primary lymphoid organs
Promonocytes
Secondary follicles
Secondary lymphoid organs
Spleen
  Marginal zone
  Periarteriolar lymphoid sheath (PALS)
  Red pulp
  White pulp
T lymphocytes (or T cells)
Thymus
  Cortex
  Medulla
Tissue macrophages

## MULTIPLE-CHOICE QUESTIONS

*(An answer key is not provided, but the page[s] location of the answer is.)*

1. The periarteriolar lymphoid sheath is (a) the thymus-dependent region of the spleen, (b) the thymus-dependent region of the lymph nodes, (c) the thymus-independent region of the spleen, (d) the thymus-independent region of the lymph nodes, (e) none of these. *(See page 54.)*

2. B cells do not express (a) C3 receptors, (b) class II molecules, (c) class I molecules, (d) CD4 molecules, (e) any of these. *(See pages 33 and 34.)*

3. Cytotoxic T cells are identified by antibodies against (a) CD8, (b) CD4, (c) CD3, (d) class I molecules, (e) none or all of these. *(See pages 35 to 37.)*

4. A severe decrease in the numbers of CD4$^+$ T cells in humans is likely to lead to (a) severe decrease of humoral immune responses, (b) severe decrease of cell-mediated immune responses, (c) both *a* and *b*, (d) neither *a* nor *b*, (e) none of these. *(See pages 35 and 36.)*

5. Which of the following is/are not true concerning NK cells? (a) they have Fc receptors, (b) their activity is class II MHC-restricted, (c) they are found in beige mice, (d) they are spontaneously cytotoxic, (e) none of these. *(See pages 38 and 39.)*

6. Which of the following is/are true concerning macrophages? (a) they secrete monokines, (b) they can adhere to glass or plastic, (c) they have associated enzyme markers, (d) all of these, (e) none of these. *(See pages 39 and 41.)*

7. Immature dendritic cells are (a) efficient APCs, (b) better at antigen-uptake than mature dendritic cells, (c) characterized by their expression of class II MHC and costimulatory molecules, (d) called follicular dendritic cells, (e) all of these, (f) none of these. *(See pages 42 and 43.)*

8. If all of an animal's immune cells are destroyed, which of the following cells may reconstitute the entire immune system? (a) thymocytes, (b) bone marrow stem cells, (c) lymph node cells, (d) T lymphocytes, (e) B lymphocytes, (f) none of these. *(See pages 29 to 31.)*

9. Lymphocytes cross from the postcapillary venules into the cortical region of the lymph node because of (a) high blood pressure, (b) osmotic pressure, (c) muscle contraction, (d) the presence of receptors on lymphocytes for molecules on endothelial cells, (e) none of these. *(See pages 49 and 50.)*

10. In which of the following organs does antigen-dependent proliferation of different lymphocytes take place? (a) spleen, (b) lymph nodes, (c) *a* and *b* are correct, (d) neither *a* nor *b* is correct. *(See page 45.)*

11. In which of the following organs does antigen-independent maturation of different lymphocytes take place? (a) thymus, (b) lymph nodes, (c) bone marrow, (d) *a* and *b* are correct, (e) *a* and *c* are correct. *(See page 45.)*

## SHORT-ANSWER ESSAY QUESTIONS

1. Although the immune system has B and T cells, it has been said that "no T cells, no immunity." Explain.

**2.** Briefly describe the specific roles of helper and cytotoxic T cells in normal immunity. How do these roles correlate with CD4$^+$ T cells and CD8$^+$ T cells?

**3.** When you mix thymic cytokines with bone marrow pre-T cells, it causes the appearance of helper activity. How would you determine that this activity is mediated by mature helper T cells? *Hint*: What CD markers are present on these cells as compared to T cells found in the cortex of the thymus?

**4.** Unlike B and T cells, macrophages are neither clonally restricted nor antigen-specific. Explain. List some other distinguishing characteristics of macrophages.

**5.** A hallmark of dendritic cells is the conversion of immature sentinels to mature immunostimulatory cells. Explain.

**6.** NK cells are not MHC-restricted, at least in the classical sense. Explain. How do they kill their target cells?

**7.** Differentiate between primary and secondary lymphoid organs.

**8.** Name the three morphologic areas of the lymph node, describing the cellular composition of each. Which area is called the *thymus-dependent area*, and why? Which area is called the *thymus-independent area*, and why?

**9.** What is the significance of follicles to antigen-induced B cell differentiation?

## FURTHER READINGS

Banchereau, J., F. Briere, C. Caux, J. Davoust, S. Lebecque, Y-J. Liu, B. Pulendran, and K. Palucka. 2000. Immunobiology of dendritic cells. *Annu. Rev. Immunol.* 18:767–811.

Bendelac, A., P.B. Savage, and L. Teyton. 2007. The Biology of NKT Cells. *Annu. Rev. Immunol.* 25:297–336.

Blom, B. and H. Spits. 2006. Development of human lymphoid cells. *Annu. Rev. Immunol.* 24:287–320.

Chaplin, D.D. 2003. Lymphoid tissues and organs. In *Fundamental Immunology*, 5th ed. W.E. Paul, ed. Philadelphia: Lippincott Williams & Wilkins. p. 419–454.

Cheroutre, H. 2004. Starting at the beginning: New perspectives on the biology of mucosal T cells. *Annu. Rev. Immunol.* 22:217–246.

Girardi, M. 2006. Immunosurveillance and immunoregulation by Tδ T cells. *J. Investig. Dermatol.* 126:25–31.

Gordon, S. 2003. Macrophages and the immune response. In *Fundamental Immunology*, 5th ed. W.E. Paul, ed. Philadelphia: Lippincott Williams & Wilkins. p. 481–496.

Gordon, S. and P.R. Taylor. 2005. Monocyte and macrophage heterogeneity. *Nat. Rev. Immunol.* 5:953–964.

Hardy, R.R. 2003. B-cell development and biology. In *Fundamental Immunology*, 5th ed. W.E. Paul, ed. Philadelphia: Lippincot Williams & Wilkins. p. 159–194.

Hardy, R.R. 2006. B-1 B cell development. *J. Immunol.* 176: 2749–2754.

King, C., S.G. Tangye, and C.R. Mackay. 2008. T follicular helper (T$_{FH}$) cells in normal and dysregulated immune responses. *Annu. Rev. Immunol.* 26:741–766.

Laiosa, C.V., M. Stadtfeld, and T. Graf. 2006. Determinants of Lymphoid-Myeloid Lineage Diversification. *Annu. Rev. Immunol.* 24:206–738.

Lanier, L.L. 2005. NK cell recognition. *Annu. Rev. Immunol.* 23:225–274.

Ley, K., C. Laudanna, M.I. Cybulsky, and S. Nourshargh. 2007. Getting to the site of inflammation: The leukocyte adhesion cascade updated. *Nat. Rev. Immunol.* 7: 678–689.

Marrack, P. and J. Kappler. 2004. Control of T cell viability. *Annu. Rev. Immunol.* 22:765–787.

Mestecky, J., R.S. Blumberg, H. Kiyono, and J.R. McGhee. 2003. The mucosal immune system. In *Fundamental Immunology*, 5th ed. W.E. Paul, ed. Philadelphia: Lippincot Williams & Wilkins. p. 965–1020.

Miyasaka, M. and T. Tanaka. 2004. Lymphocyte trafficking across high endothelial venules: Dogmas and enigmas. *Nat. Rev. Immunol.* 4:360–370.

Moser, M. 2003. Lymphoid tissues & organs. In *Fundamental Immunology*, 5th ed. W.E. Paul, ed. Philadelphia: Lippincot Williams & Wilkins. p. 419–454.

Motonari, K., A.J. Wagers, M.G. Manz, S.S. Prohaska, D.C. Scherer, G.F. Beilhack, J.A. Shizuru, and I.L. Weissman. 2003. Biology of hematopoietic stem cells and progenitors: Implications for clinical application. *Annu. Rev. Immunol.* 21:759–806.

Papadimitriou, J.M., and R.B. Ashman. 1989. Macrophages: Current views on their differentiation, structure, and function. *Ultrastructural Pathology* 13:343–372.

Pillai, S, A. Cariappa, and S.T. Moran. 2005. Marginal zone B cells. *Annu. Rev. Immunol.* 23:161–196.

Poussier, P., and M. Julius. 1994. Thymus independent T cell development and selection in the intestinal epithelium. *Annu. Rev. Immunol.* 12:521–553.

Randall, T.D., D.M. Carragher, and -J. Rangel-Moreno. 2008. Development of secondary lymphoid organs. *Annu. Rev. Immunol.* 26:627–650.

Raulet, D.H. 2003. Natural killer cells. In *Fundamental Immunology*, 5th ed. W.E. Paul, ed. Philadelphia: Lippincott Williams & Wilkins. p. 365–392.

Sansonetti, P.J. 2004. War and peace at the mucosal surfaces. *Nat. Rev. Immunol.* 4:953–964.

Shortman, K. and S.H. Naik. 2007. Steady-state and inflammatory dendritic-cell development. *Nat. Rev. Immunol.* 7:19–30.

Unanue, E.R., and P.M. Allen. 1987. The basis for the immunoregulatory role of macrophages and other accessory cells. *Science* 236:551–557.

# CHAPTER THREE

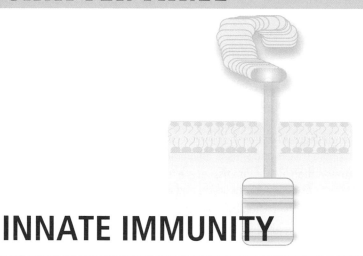

# INNATE IMMUNITY

    b. Cytokines, signaling proteins that recruit, coordinate, activate, control defensive cells, induce inflammation, and then turn off these responses or prod the adaptive immune system for a specific attack.

        1) Interferons are cytokines that mediate antiviral effects.

        2) Proinflammatory, or inflammation-promoting, cytokines orchestrate inflammation.

**6.** The biological defenses, recruitment and promotion of professional phagocytes, recognize and kill pathogens but do not spare self-tissues.

    a. Guided leukocyte migration and resulting inflammation, the seek-and-destroy mission of the immune system.

        1) The guideposts, cell-adhesion molecules, inform innate immune cells where to exit into extra-lymphoid tissues and sites of inflammation.

        2) Extravasation of cells into tissues is a regulated multistep process involving a series of coordinated interactions between leukocytes and endothelial cells.

        3) Microbe internalization by phagocytic cells triggers proinflammatory signals initiating a salutary but tissue-damaging acute inflammatory response.

## OBJECTIVES

The reader should be able to:

1. Discuss factors that could predispose a host to different levels of disease resistance.

2. Describe how pathogens could enter the body by bypassing external barriers.

3. Distinguish innate immune recognition systems; give examples of pathogen-associated molecular patterns (PAMPs) and the pattern recognition receptors (PRRs), and discuss their contributions to antimicrobial protection.

4. List the leukocytes that mediate innate immunity and differentiate how they recognize, respond to, and kill pathogens; describe phagocytosis.

5. Explain why dendritic cells are considered specialized phagocytic cells.

6. Describe the innate immune responses directed against viral pathogens; include the source and functions of interferons and the role of natural killer (NK) cells.

7. Recap the innate activation of complement, and review the functions of the components resulting from activated complement.

8. Describe the local and systemic effects of the macrophage cytokines TNF-$\alpha$, IL-1, IL-6, IL-12, and the chemokine CXCL8.

9. Explain leukocyte migration including how neutrophils adhere to endothelial cells, the adhesion molecules involved, and the coordinated interactions between neutrophils and endothelial cells in the process of extravasation.

10. Describe inflammation, including a description of the purpose of inflammation, the cells and molecules involved, and the successful outcome of the acute inflammatory process.

Our entire life is spent in contact with microorganisms. Many kinds of microbes normally inhabit the human body—harmlessly held in check by the body's defense mechanisms. If these mechanisms are weakened, however, some of these microorganisms can become opportunistic pathogens and cause disease. Other pathogenic microorganisms can invade the human body; whether a disease condition occurs depends on the outcome of the interaction between the pathogen and the immune status of the host.

In the biological world, innate immunity is the most common and basic means of warding off disease. Plants and most animals survive a hostile world of potential pathogens with only nonspecific innate resistance as their defense. Innate immunity is not completely nonspecific, as was originally thought, but can discriminate between host constituents (self) and a variety of pathogens. Only vertebrate animals are capable of acquiring specific resistance (adaptive immunity). Thus, they can be more efficient in combating infection. First, they use nonspecific innate resistance mechanisms, composed of external (the barriers of skin, mucus, cilia, and pH) and internal (cells, chemicals, and biologic) barriers, which are immediately available, against invading pathogens. Even though internal innate defenses provide a barrage of weapons from scavenger cells generically focused on invading pathogens, to specialized sentinel cells, to a complex series of circulating proteins whose components attach to the organism's surface leading to enhanced phagocytosis or the puncturing of its cell membrane, to inflammatory responses that halt the microbes early in their invasion and confine them to a localized area. Tougher microbes that evade these defenses take stronger defenses, the multiple layers of adaptive immunity, that is, in some cases, if innate immune responses are ineffective at containing invaders, they kick-in the mechanisms of specific (adaptive) immunity as reinforcement or, in the case of a persistent infection, as the ultimate means of resistance. If the combined effects of both innate immunity and adaptive immunity are unable to halt the spread of infection, the death of the host is invariably the final result. In most cases, immunologic victory means future immunity.

This chapter focuses on innate immunity's constituents, how they interact with one another to protect against invading microbes, how they recognize all microbes and perfectly distinguish between microbes and self-tissues, and the consequences of interactions between microbes and innate immune components.

# GLOBAL IMMUNITY HAS MANY COMPONENTS

When a microorganism enters body tissues and multiplies, it establishes an *infection*. Infections, caused by bacteria, viruses, fungi, and parasites, are the major cause of human disease (see Chapter 17). Depending on host susceptibility, infections range from mild respiratory illnesses like the common cold, to incapacitating conditions like chronic hepatitis and life-threatening diseases like AIDS. The state of resistance from infectious disease—**immunity**—is provided by nonspecific and specific defense systems. As mentioned in Chapter 1, when foreign substances, or *antigens*, such as bacteria, viruses, fungi, or parasites are introduced into a vertebrate host, the host either (1) uses its preformed, front-line, nonspecific defenses, innate immunity or (2) if tougher microbes pass through the front lines of defense they confront two layers of specific defenses, the cells and molecules of adaptive immunity. The combined responses are traditionally called an **immune response**.

**Innate immunity** is the sum of host defenses that exist before, and function independently of, any exposure to an invader such as a microbe; that is, innate immunity has preexisting broad specificity for different classes of microbes. Figure 3-1 compares innate immunity and adaptive immunity and their interrelationships. As the first line of a universal form of defense, the innate immune system includes both external and internal nonspecific responses. If you think of the body as a tube, external defenses are present in those areas of the body exposed to the outside environment (the contact areas for pathogens). Internal defenses come into play after the pathogen has penetrated the external defenses. As mentioned in Chapter 1, the components of innate immunity are *preformed, standardized, without memory,* and *nonspecific*. Innate and adaptive immunity do not operate independently of each other; rather, innate mechanisms reduce the workload for the immune system's specific defenses and keep infections in check until adaptive (specific) immunity can develop, whereas adaptive mechanisms supplement and augment the nonspecific defenses.

The innate immune system, present in all multicellular organisms, is the oldest host defense system. Complex multicellular organisms arose in the presence of rapidly dividing single-cell microbes. The multicellular organisms developed innate defense mechanisms to combat and protect themselves against the constant barrage of the more rapidly dividing single-cell invaders. Because the response had to be rapid and capable of distinguishing the invaders from self-tissues, the innate system focused on so-called *pattern recognition sequences*, or biologic patterns (molecules) unique to, and necessary for the survival of, microorganisms—called **pathogen-associated molecular patterns (PAMPs)**.[1] So common are these PAMPs that a limited number of receptors, called **pattern recognition receptors**

---

[1] The acronym PAMPs is somewhat of a misnomer because these "patterns" are not restricted just to pathogens but all microbes that are sensed.

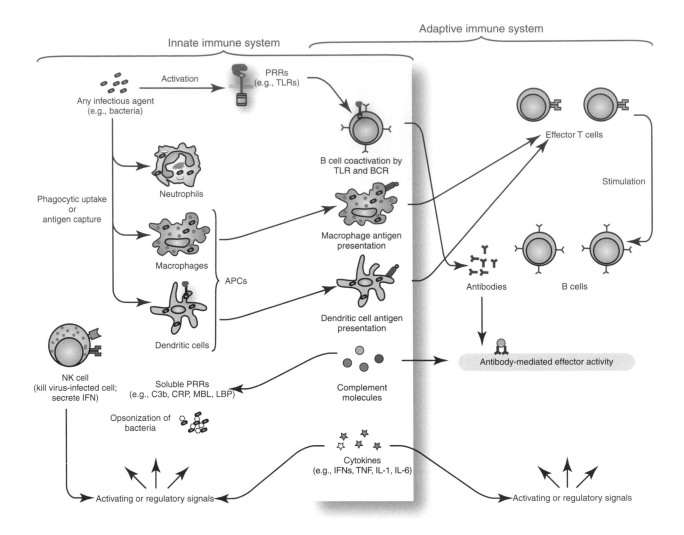

**FIGURE 3-1 The overlapping innate and adaptive immune systems**. Innate immune mechanisms are immediate, nonspecific responses to pathogens, which include antigen internalization by neutrophils, macrophages, and dendritic cells. Many of these activities depend on pattern-recognition receptors (PRRs), such as Toll-like receptors (TLRs), which recognize pathogen-associated molecular patterns (PAMPs) shared by a variety of microbes. Soluble PRRs, such as complement proteins (C3b), mannose-binding lectin (MBL), and acute phase proteins, such as C-reactive protein (CRP), contribute to innate immunity by opsonizing pathogens. Initial adaptive immune mechanisms are delayed, specific responses, which involve T cell receptors (TCRs) and B cell antibody receptors (BCR) binding specific antigens. This leads to naïve responder cell proliferation and differentiation into effector cells and memory cells. The innate and adaptive immune systems interrelate through antigen capturing by distinct antigen-presenting cells (such as dendritic cells), which by presenting antigen and costimulatory molecules to T cells generate an appropriate T-cell response. In addition, costimulation of B cells through TLRs (such as TLR9) can lead to the production of anti-self-specific antibodies. Cytokines such as interferons (IFNs), tumor necrosis factor (TNF), interleukin (IL)-1, and IL-6 stimulate innate and adaptive immune responses. Complement proteins are activated by microbes directly during innate immune responses and by specific antibodies during adaptive humoral responses.

(**PRRs**), recognize them and because the host does not express PAMPs, host tissues and cells are ignored. PAMPs and their counterparts PRRs will be discussed shortly.

---

### MINI SUMMARY

The integrity of the body is maintained by multiple defense systems, including immune responses. The two overarching divisions that mediate protection against infection are innate (inborn and unchanging) and acquired/adaptive (developed during the lifetime of the host and adjusts to the disease-causing microbe) immunity. Even though the immune system is characteristically described to consist of two distinct divisions, the innate and the adaptive, it is becoming increasingly clear that these two divisions are tightly interwoven.

---

# NUTRITION, AGE, STRESS, AND GENETIC FACTORS FRAME THE PREDISPOSING FEATURES OF HOST RESISTANCE

A host's innate immunity depends, in part, on some predisposing factors of disease resistance that are inherent in each host and in the host's environment. Either naturally resistant hosts do not provide some of the essential nutritional factors required by the microorganism for growth, or they have other defense mechanisms to resist infection by the microbe. Certain environmental factors of the host can also play a role in giving the host either resistance or susceptibility to infection. These factors include general health and state of nutrition, the host's age, and genetic factors. These environmental and genetic factors are so intertwined that it is difficult to evaluate their distinct contributions to the disease process. When susceptibility factors exceed resistance factors in the delicate balance between disease and health, disease develops.

The importance of many factors to innate immunity in the human is obvious. Poor nutrition contributes to greater disease incidence. For instance, a diet containing the required amounts of proteins and vitamins is directly related to protection from microbial disease. Dietary proteins are used to make healthy tissues and serum proteins. Protein-calorie malnutrition decreases the production of important antimicrobial effector molecules and retards immune cell functions. Vitamins promote efficient metabolism and maintain integrity of skin and membrane surfaces. Their deficiencies often exhibit significant effects on host defense. Vitamin A deficiency affects epithelial cell integrity, which can allow skin infections to occur. Vitamin $B_1$ and $B_2$ deficiencies lower aspects of adaptive immunity, and folic acid deficiencies lower antigen-specific immune cell numbers. Zinc deficiency can lead to impaired thymic development and related immune cell insufficiency. However, over-nutrition can also be harmful. Many bacteria scavenge host iron to survive; thus when iron is in short supply bacterial growth is restricted.

Age of the host also plays a role in disease susceptibility, with the very young and the very old having the highest risk of infection. In a young child, the immune system is less developed or experienced, whereas in an elderly person it is no longer as efficient. Thus young people are susceptible to "childhood diseases" such as measles and chicken pox and intestinal diseases due to the lack of the normal microbiota found in adults. The aged are more susceptible to respiratory diseases such as influenza, probably caused by a combination of age-related anatomical changes and a decline in immune responses to respiratory pathogens.

Severe physical and emotional stresses—such as sleep deprivation, fatigue, anxiety, and depression make a person more vulnerable to disease. In the stressed condition, there is enhanced production of adrenaline accompanied by altered levels of adrenal corticoid hormones; this suppresses the function of many groups of defensive cells and depresses a wide range of defense mechanisms used by the body.

Resistance to infection varies with the species of animal or plant. For example, *Yersinia pestis* is carried by ground squirrels, in which it causes no obvious disease. But when fleas move from squirrels to humans, fleabites can transmit the bacterium that causes bubonic plague. Dogs do not become infected with measles; humans do not contract canine distemper. The reason resistance varies from one species to another is not always understood. However, basic physiological and anatomical characteristics of a species can determine whether a microorganism can be pathogenic for that species. For example, because of differences in normal body temperature, many diseases of mammals do not affect fish or reptiles, and vice versa. Herbivorous animals are usually resistant to enteric diseases of carnivores—probably because herbivores have multiple stomachs and different intestinal microbiota and digestive juices. Other animals often resist diseases of the skin, to which humans are particularly susceptible, because they have more hair and thicker hides. Species resistance is an obstacle in biomedical research, because it is difficult to study diseases that cannot be reproduced in laboratory animals. Two such diseases are syphilis and cholera, which have no animal models for use in laboratory experiments.

In some cases, genetic factors make certain races of people more susceptible or more resistant than other races to a particular infection. For instance, resistance to malarial infection caused by *Plasmodium vivax* is found in West African blacks. This is attributed to the absence of a specific component on their red blood cell membranes to which the malarial parasite *P. vivax* must bind in order to invade and multiply. There are other genetic protections against malaria, including thalassemias and glucose-6-phosphate dehydrogenase deficiencies. In the 1800s, the Plains Indians of North America lost two-thirds of their population to smallpox and tuberculosis because of natural susceptibility to these diseases. They had not been previously exposed to these diseases, unlike the European settlers who survived because their ancestors were more resistant as a result of genetic selection due to prior exposure. The likely basis for these susceptibility differences probably relates to differences in major histocompatibility complex (MHC) gene composition (see Chapter 7).

---

### MINI SUMMARY

The pathogenicity of a microbe is determined both by its virulence and by host resistance factors. Predisposing factors of host resistance are those of the environment, as well as those inherent in the individual, race, or species. Environmental factors that influence host resistance and susceptibility include nutrition, the age of the host, and physical and emotional stresses, in addition to genetic factors.

---

# THE EXTERNAL FRONT-LINE DEFENSES PROVIDE NATURAL SHIELDS AGAINST THE PENETRATION OF PATHOGENS INTO TISSUES

External defense mechanisms are the first line of defense in innate immunity (summarized in Figure 3-2). Mechanical barriers created by the skin and mucous membranes, together with host secretions, and the competition of normal microbiota with pathogenic intruders for particular ecologic niches in the human body, are usually regarded as the body's first defense against invading microorganisms.

## Skin and Mucous Membranes are Mechanical Barriers to Many Microbial Pathogens

The unbroken skin and mucous membranes are effective mechanical barriers to many infectious agents. The skin consists of two distinct layers: (1) the *epidermis*, the thin outer layer, and (2) the *dermis*, the thicker deep layer. The epidermis is composed of several tightly packed layers of epithelial cells, with the outer layer composed of dead cells filled with a waterproofing protein called *keratin*. The epidermis has no blood vessels and relies on nutrients from the underlying dermis. The outermost layer of old epidermal cells are sloughed off and replaced by new cells, such that the epidermis is completely replaced every 15 to 30 days. The connective tissue-containing dermis houses blood vessels, hair follicles, sebaceous glands, and sweat glands. Associated with hair follicles are the sebaceous glands, which secrete an oily substance, called *sebum*. Sebum maintains a skin pH between 3 and 5 that inhibits the growth of most microorganisms. Bacteria that can metabolize sebum live as opportunistic pathogens on the skin, causing a severe form of acne. Saturated fatty acids are present in the skin secretions of the scalp and other hairy parts of the body. These fungistatic acids are important in the control of fungi that cause superficial skin and hair infections; therefore, areas devoid of sebaceous glands, like skin between the toes, are more susceptible to fungal infections. Other antimicrobial peptides associated with the skin are β-defensins, psoriasin, and dermcidin.

The low moisture content of the skin makes it an inhospitable environment for microorganisms. However, it is possible for some microorganisms (such as *Francisella tularensis* and certain fungi) to enter the skin through hair follicles, sebaceous glands, sweat glands, or abrasions. The bite of ticks and insects like fleas, mites, and mosquitoes can penetrate the skin and introduce pathogens into the body as they feed. For example, the malaria-causing protozoan *Plasmodium* is injected into humans when mosquitoes take a blood meal. Likewise, Lyme disease (*Borrelia burgdorferi*) is spread by the bite of ticks, and bubonic plague (*Y. pestis*) is spread by the bite of fleas.

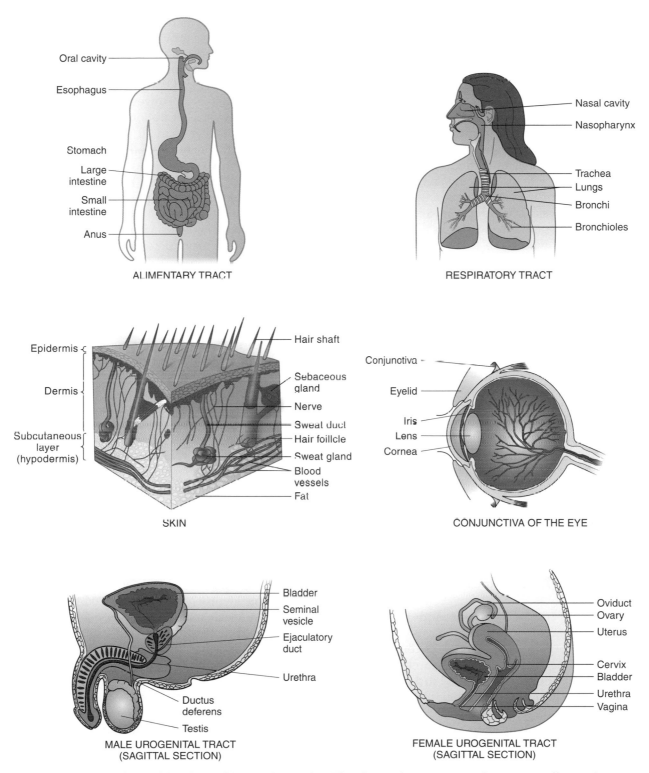

**FIGURE 3-2 The mechanical barriers of innate immunity.** The skin and mucous membranes are effective barriers between the environment and the internal components of the body. Areas of the human body lined by skin or mucous membranes are indicated.

Like the skin, mucous membranes consist of an epithelial layer and an underlying connective tissue layer. Mucous membranes line the entire respiratory, alimentary, urogenital, and reproductive tracts (see Figure 3-2). The epithelial layer of a mucous membrane secretes *mucus*, a viscous fluid that prevents the tracts from drying out and aids in the removal of microorganisms. Even though most pathogens enter through the mucous membranes, a number of nonspecific defense mechanisms prevent their entry. Mucous secretions act as immunologic glue, trapping many microorganisms until they can be removed or lose their infectivity. Mucous secretions wash away microorganisms and contain antibacterial and antiviral substances. Respiratory and alimentary tract mucous secretions (and the washings in the eye) flow to the stomach, where the acid can destroy most microorganisms.

Some microorganisms have developed ways to escape mucous-mediated defenses, allowing them to invade the body through mucous membranes. The gonorrhea-causing organism *Neisseria gonorrhoeae* displays surface projections that enable it to bind to the urogenital tract's epithelial cells and penetrate the mucous membrane. Similarly, the influenza virus expresses surface molecules that permit it to attach firmly to cells in mucous membranes, preventing the virus from being swept out by the ciliated epithelial cells. Bacterial adherence to mucous membranes involves interactions between hairlike protrusions on a bacterium (the fimbriae or pili) and certain glycoproteins or glycolipids that are expressed only by some mucous membrane epithelial cells. Differential expression of these molecules explains why some tissues are susceptible to bacterial colonization, whereas others are not.

### Respiratory Tract Is Exposed to Airborne Microbes

Lungs are full of nutrients and have many crevices for concealing microorganisms. Every day we breathe in hundreds of liters of air contaminated with dust, pollen, and microbes, yet rarely do we get lung infections. The nose is designed so that the turbulent flow of air throws these particles onto the sticky mucous nasal linings. Once particles stick, sinus filtration continues by gravity-induced mucous secretion flow. If microorganisms are inhaled, mucus, secreted by epithelial cells of the respiratory tract, entraps them. The microorganisms trapped in the tracheal mucus, in contrast to those trapped by sinus filtration, are swept upward at a rate of 10–20 mm/min by beating *cilia*, the hairlike projections of the epithelial cells that line the air passages, into the throat where

they are either expectorated or swallowed and killed in the stomach. In a healthy individual, this mucous coat clears 90% of entrapped material every hour. Similarly, mucous-entrapped microorganisms in the lung are propelled up and out to the throat by the synchronous movement of cilia lining air passages of the lung. Sneezing and coughing also expel material from these passages. However, these mechanisms have a 10-$\mu$m-size filtration limit. Even though bacteria are smaller than 10 $\mu$m, most bacteria are associated with moisture or other particles, which are larger, and thus the bacteria are filtered out. There are exceptions; for example, mucous secretions and cilia cannot remove small particles (such as floating *Mycobacterium tuberculosis*) that reach the alveoli. Smoking can paralyze cilia movement, thereby compromising a major defense of the lungs.

### Alimentary Tract Is Exposed to Ingested Microbes

Anatomically, humans are designed around a tube, open at both ends (mouth to anus). This tube is lined with mucous membranes, not by the dry protective skin cells covering the exterior of the body. From its top to its bottom, starting with the mouth, this human tube harbors a host of permanently residing microbes. The symbiotic relationship of these microbes usually does little harm to a healthy person. Regardless of how thoroughly we brush our teeth, the natural microbiota remains attached. Mouth microbes have evolved elaborate systems for sticking to oral cavity surfaces. By preventing other potential pathogens from establishing themselves, the resident microbiota help protect us. In addition, a continuous flow of fluid (saliva) through the mouth flushes loose microbes into the stomach. The tongue's movement over the teeth also washes away microbes.

The stomach is a harsh environment for most organisms. Hydrochloric acid derived from cells lining the stomach makes it highly acidic, bordering on a pH of 1. Additionally, the stomach contains proteolytic enzymes and mucus. Most microbes and their toxins are killed by this acidic environment and digested by the proteolytic enzymes. Only markedly aciduric organisms or those embedded deeply in food particles can escape the protein-precipitating capacity of stomach acidity. In fact, until fairly recently, it was thought that the stomach was sterile because of its low pH. This hypothesis changed with the discovery of the bacterium *Helicobacter pylori*. Unlike most bacteria, which cannot tolerate the stomach's acidity, *H. pylori* not only thrives in the stomach but causes ulcers and stomach cancer by initiating a chemical reaction that partially neutralizes acids and inhibits the production of digestive enzymes. It then secretes its own enzymes, which degrade the stomach's mucus lining. To make matters worse, *H. pylori* infections are often accompanied by an overgrowth of *Candida albicans*, which protects *H. pylori* against the environmental stresses of the stomach by buffering it from acids, heat, dehydration, and antibiotics.

As organisms pass into the small intestine, they encounter a slightly alkaline pH caused by the pH of the entering pancreatic and biliary fluids. These fluids contain pancreatic enzymes and bile, respectively. Along with the enzymes and detergents (bile) that digest microbes as well as food, the fluid contains secretory IgA antibody (see Chapter 4). This combination of substances, in addition to the peristaltic action of the small intestine, leads to continual purging of microorganisms. Even though the small intestine can be full of nutrients, the body's absorption system efficiently removes these nutrients from the intestine so rapidly that residential microbes have little to live on. Because the intestines are anaerobic, obligate aerobes are unable to grow there even if they survive passage through the stomach.

The large intestine is quite different from other digestive tract compartments; it collects and processes undigested material that passes through the small intestine. Bacteria, including some potential pathogens, grow robustly yet rarely invade the body. The large intestine wall is coated with a protective mucous layer that separates the contents from direct contact with the cells lining the large intestine. The normal microbiota of the large intestine evolved to live on the available nutrients in the anaerobic conditions found there. Feces are roughly 40% bacteria by weight. This large number of microbes is of great importance in controlling the population of any pathogens or potential pathogens that have survived the trip so far. The resident organisms tend to colonize the epithelial cells of mucosal surfaces. This normal microbiota usually outcompetes pathogens for attachment sites on the epithelial cell surfaces and for needed nutrients.

When the normal microbiota is suppressed, as by broad-spectrum antibiotic therapy, it upsets the natural microbial balance and allows pathogens to establish themselves. This scenario often leads to intestinal problems (such as diarrhea) until the original mix of microbes is reestablished.

### Urogenital Tract Is Exposed to Skin-Associated Microbes

The kidneys, urinary bladder (and the urine within), and ureters are sterile. Microbes are prevented from reaching the kidneys and the bladder by the slight acidity, lysozyme (see below) and urea content, and flushing action of urine and mucus. Because a women's urethra is shorter than a man's, bladder infections are more common in women.

The vagina is held at a low pH (high acidity) because of the growth of acid-tolerant Döderlein's bacilli (*Lactobacillus acidophilus*) that degrade vaginal epithelium-produced glycogen to form lactic acid. The antibacterial activity of mucus and its outward flow also remove organisms from the vagina. For example, the high acidity of the adult human vagina during the years of ovarian activity protects its membranous surfaces against colonization by many types of pathogenic microbes.

## Chemical Secretions Reinforce the Mechanical Barriers

In addition to the mechanical barriers such as skin and mucous membranes, secreted chemical substances with antimicrobial action are an important component of external defense. For instance, the mucous membranes secrete many substances, including enzymes, which can impair microbial infectivity. Specifically, **lysozyme** is an enzyme found in many body fluids and secretions such as tears and saliva. It begins a digestion of the cell walls of Gram-positive bacteria and a few Gram-negative bacteria by hydrolyzing peptidoglycan. A muramidase, lysozyme cleaves the $\beta$-1,4-glycoside bond that unites *N*-acetylglucosamine and *N*-acetylmuramic acid, the backbone of the bacterial cell wall. Lipids in Gram-negative bacterial cell walls tend to mask the substrate from lysozyme and protect these bacteria. As was discussed earlier, the sebaceous glands of the skin produce sebum, which can inhibit the growth of certain microorganisms. Stomach glands produce gastric juice, which is sufficient to kill most microorganisms. The extreme acidity or alkalinity of body fluids has a detrimental effect on many microorganisms and helps to prevent potential pathogens from entering the deeper tissues of the body.

Other antimicrobial substances that offer defense at mucosal surfaces are the mucosal *defensins* and *cathelicidins*. They are produced by epithelial cells of the mouth, the lungs, the gut, and possible the urogenital tract. At the cellular level, defensins and cathelicidins are most abundant in neutrophil granules. Mucosal defensins and cathelicidins are active against many Gram-positive and Gram-negative bacteria, fungi, and enveloped viruses. Structurally, they are made of cationic peptides that function by attaching themselves electrostatically to microbial membranes. Once attached, they form ion channels or multimeric pores that cause spillage of the microbe's contents.

Another protein with known antimicrobial activity is *lactoferrin*. It is an iron-containing protein found in milk as well as in most of the secretions that bathe the human mucosal surfaces (including bronchial mucus, saliva, nasal discharges, tears, hepatic bile, pancreatic juice, seminal fluid, and urine). It is also an important component of neutrophil (a phagocytic cell discussed shortly) granules. Its blood counterpart is *transferrin*. These proteins tie up, or chelate, available iron in the environment, thus limiting the availability of this essential mineral nutrient to invading microorganisms. Other blood defensive chemicals like *fibronectin* and *β-lysin* have antibacterial activity. Fibronectin is a large glycoprotein that binds to surface molecules of *Staphylococcus aureus* and groups A, C, and G streptococci, aiding phagocytic cells in clearing them from the body. Fibronectin is also found on oral epithelial cells to block the attachment of certain bacteria, thereby modulating the type of organism that can colonize the upper respiratory tract. Beta-lysin is a highly reactive heat-stable cationic polypeptide that is bactericidal for Gram-positive microorganisms (except streptococci). Its release from platelets during coagulation leads to killing of surrounding organisms by disrupting their cell membrane.

Hormone release or imbalance (such as in insulin diabetes) has a direct effect on susceptibility to a number of infectious diseases; for example, hormones like corticosteroids inhibit inflammatory responses. Staphylococcal, streptococcal, and certain fungal diseases occur more frequently in diabetics. The hormonal changes that occur in females at the time of puberty are responsible for a thickening of the vaginal epithelium and for the production of more intracellular glycogen and lactic acid in the adult vagina. Therefore, the adult woman is more resistant than the young girl is to local vaginal infections. Pregnancy is associated with marked hormonal alterations and an increase in urinary tract infections.

## Naturally Occurring Microbiota Serve a Protective Role

Most animal and human surfaces that are exposed to the environment are inhabited by microorganisms, mostly bacteria and some fungi collectively known as the *normal microbiota*. Sites populated by the normal microbiota include the skin, and mucous membranes of the mouth, the upper respiratory tract, the urogential tract, and the gastrointestinal tract. The composition of the normal microbiota varies with the site. However, anaerobic bacteria are important components at all sites. The density of the normal microbiota also varies, greatly depending on the location. For example, the skin has low numbers ($10^3$–$10^4$/cm$^2$) bacteria, the eye has no normal microbiota, because of washing by lachrymal fluid and tears that contain lysozyme, even in the presence of the mechanical flushing action of salvia, the mouth has $10^8$ bacteria/ml of salvia (dental plaques contain $10^8$ bacteria/mg), the upper respiratory tract (nasal passage and nasophayarynx) maintains high numbers of bacteria, whereas the lower respiratory tract has no normal microbiota, the gastrointestinal tract at the stomach and proximal small bowel is virtually sterile, whereas the contents of the distal colon can contain $10^{11}$ bacteria/g of contents, comprising more than 400 species.

The normal microbiota clearly serves a protective role. For example, on the skin, the resident population of organisms can provide protection against the proliferation of unwanted microorganisms through the release of plasmid-encoded antibiotic peptides called *bacteriocins*. Gram-negative bacteria of the skin microbiota are the primary producers of bacteriocins. The bacteriocins produced by *E. coli* in the large intestine are called *colicins*; these can bind to receptors on sensitive bacteria to cause their lysis. Colicins can also alter ribosomes or disrupt energy production. Another example occurs when the anaerobic component of the gastrointestinal normal microbiota is eliminated by antimicrobial therapy. This therapy increases the susceptibility of patients to infection by enteric pathogens such as *Shigella* and *Salmonella*. However, the extent to which the normal microbiota participates in host defense and the mechanisms by which it prevents colonization or infection by pathogens are incompletely defined. Nonetheless, some mechanisms have been characterized using germ-free animals; they include competition for nutrients, for receptor sites on epithelial cells, and secrete inhibitory substances.

## MINI SUMMARY

Innate immunity serves as the first line of defense and includes both external and internal nonspecific responses. External defenses occur in those areas of the body exposed to the outside environment (the contact areas for pathogens). The unbroken skin and mucous membranes of the respiratory, alimentary, and urogenital tracts are important mechanical barriers to invasion by microorganisms. The human body also produces many antimicrobial chemical secretions, whose production is focused in these tracts. By competing with pathogens, the normal microbiota of a host provides protection.

# THE CELLULAR DEFENSES, THE LEUKOCYTES, ARE NUMEROUS AND HAVE KILLING AND REGULATORY ACTIVITIES

When microorganisms breach the external defense mechanisms of the host, they still have to contend with internal defense mechanisms—the second line of defense in innate immunity. Components of internal defense mechanisms constitute formidable barriers to infection. They include cellular mediators like phagocytic cells (neutrophils, macrophages, and dendritic cells) and cytotoxic natural killer (NK) cells, a wide variety of soluble factors that mediate how these cells respond, and the engulfment and destruction of pathogens by phagocytic cells (Figure 3-3). How these cells sense microbial invasion is discussed first, followed by discussion about the individual cells.

## Innate Immunity Relies on a Limited Number of Secreted and Cell-Based Receptors as the Key Sensors of Microbial Infection

The innate system, present in all multicellular organisms, is the oldest host defense system. Complex multicellular organisms arose in the presence of rapidly dividing single-cell microbes, to counteract this rapidity host recognition needed to be prompt. Thus, the innate immune system developed a variety of germline-encoded receptors that are secreted into the bloodstream and tissue fluids, or expressed on the cell surface or in intracellular compartments, or in the cytosol (Figure 3-4). These receptors, called *PRRs*, target conserved molecules (such as lipopolysaccharide [LPS], peptidoglycans, double-stranded RNA [dsRNA], and zymosan) that are shared by bacteria, viruses, fungi, and protozoa, called *PAMPs*; the secreted receptors include *mannose-binding lectin (MBL), C-reactive protein (CRP), serum amyloid protein (SAP), and LPS-binding protein (LBP)*; the cell-based receptors include *scavenger receptors, mannose receptor, Toll-like receptors (TLRs), nucleotide-binding oligomerization domain (NOD) proteins, retinoic-acid-inducible gene 1 (RIG-1)-like receptors (RLRs)*. Pattern recognition receptors are involved in recognition, opsonization, activation of complement, phagocytosis, and type I

|  | **INNATE IMMUNITY** | | **ADAPTIVE IMMUNITY** | |
|---|---|---|---|---|
|  | Recognition | Effectors | Recognition | Effectors |
| **Humoral** | LBP, CD14, collectins, complement C3b, pentraxins | Lysozyme, antimicrobial peptides, cytokines, complement, lactoferrin, acute phase proteins | Antibodies | Antibodies, complement components |
| **Cellular** | TLRs, Dectin-1, CD14, fMet receptor, NOD1, NOD2 | Proteases, antimicrobial peptides, CAMs, respiratory burst products, neutrophils, macrophages, dendritic cells, NK cells, others | BCR, TCR, MHC molecules | Plasma cells, helper T cells, cytotoxic T cells |

Abbreviations: LPS-binding protein, LBP; complement component 3b, C3b; Toll-like receptors, TLRs; N-formyl-methionyl receptor, fMet receptor; nucleotide-binding oligomerization domain-1 and -2, NOD1 & NOD2 proteins; cell-adhesion molecules, CAMs; natural killer cells, NK cells; B cell receptor, BCR; T cell receptor, TCR; major histocompatibility complex, MHC

**FIGURE 3-3** Effectors of innate and adaptive immunity.

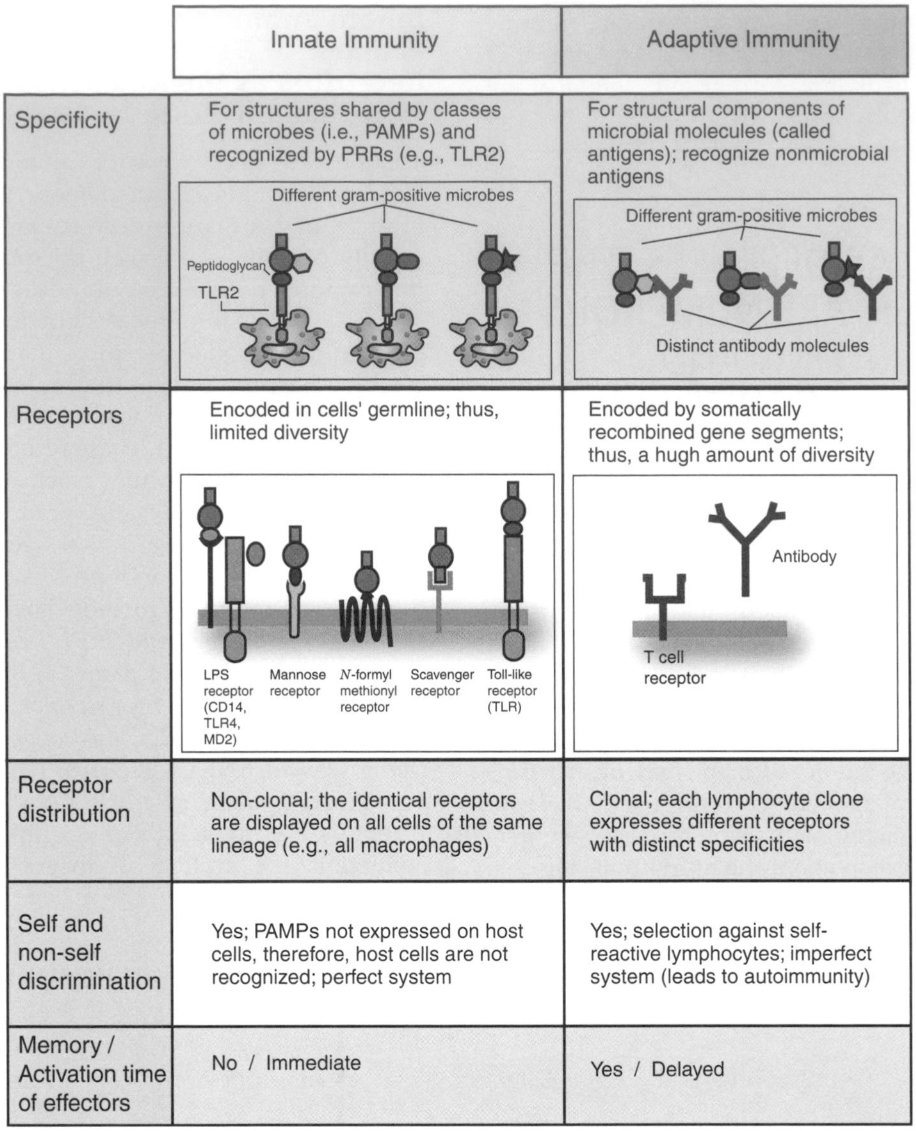
Innate Immunity
Adaptive Immunity
Specificity
For structures shared by classes of microbes (i.e., PAMPs) and recognized by PRRs (e.g., TLR2)
Different gram-positive microbes
Peptidoglycan
TLR2
For structural components of microbial molecules (called antigens); recognize nonmicrobial antigens
Different gram-positive microbes
Distinct antibody molecules
Receptors
Encoded in cells' germline; thus, limited diversity
LPS receptor (CD14, TLR4, MD2)
Mannose receptor
N-formyl methionyl receptor
Scavenger receptor
Toll-like receptor (TLR)
Encoded by somatically recombined gene segments; thus, a hugh amount of diversity
Antibody
T cell receptor
Receptor distribution
Non-clonal; the identical receptors are displayed on all cells of the same lineage (e.g., all macrophages)
Clonal; each lymphocyte clone expresses different receptors with distinct specificities
Self and non-self discrimination
Yes; PAMPs not expressed on host cells, therefore, host cells are not recognized; perfect system
Yes; selection against self-reactive lymphocytes; imperfect system (leads to autoimmunity)
Memory / Activation time of effectors
No / Immediate
Yes / Delayed

**FIGURE 3-4 Innate and adaptive immune recognition**. The integrity of the body is maintained by multiple defense systems. Protection against infection can be innate (inborn and unchanging) or acquired (developed during the lifetime of the host). Innate immune system recognition molecules are germline-encoded receptors called *pattern recognition receptors* (*PRRs*), which recognize conserved structures shared by classes of microbes called *pathogen-associated molecular patterns* (*PAMPs*).

interferon (IFN) activation of proinflammatory signaling pathways.

Secreted pattern-recognition molecules, or PRRs, bind to microbial cell walls, targeting them for recognition by the complement system and phagocytes; the PRRs act as opsonins. **Mannose-binding lectin, CRP**, and **SAP** are synthesized in the liver and are secreted into the serum as components of the acute-phase response (discussed later) during the early stages of infection. Mannose-binding lectin along with surfactant proteins A and D form a structurally related family of molecules called *collectins*, so named because they consist of a N-terminus collagenous domain (responsible for effector functions) and a carbohydrate-recognizing, calcium-dependent lectin C-terminus domain (responsible for ligand recognition). Mannose-binding lectin binds specifically to terminal mannose residues, which are abundant on the surface of many Gram-positive and Gram-negative bacteria and yeast, as well as some viruses and parasites. Mannose-binding lectin associates with MBL-associated serine proteases

(MASP), which are related to the serum proteases, C1r and C1s, of the classical complement system (see Chapter 11). MASP1 and MASP2 are activated by MBL and initiate the lectin pathway of complement by cleaving C2 and C4 proteins. Unlike the C1 proteases of the classical complement pathway, which required antigen-antibody complexes for their activation, MASPs are activated by MBL binding to microbial ligands. Surfactant proteins A and D, found on the mucosal surfaces of the lung and gastrointestinal tract, recognize similar microbial ligands as MBL and act as opsonins. The other two members of secreted PRRs are CRP and SAP. They are structurally related members of the pentraxin family that like MBL are rapidly produced in the liver in response to proinflammatory cytokines, such as interleukin-6 (IL-6), and function as opsonins on binding to bacterial surface phosphorylcholine. CRP and SAP can also bind to C1q component of the classical complement pathway and thus activate it in the absence of antigen-antibody complexes.

Another secreted PRR is **LPS-binding protein (LBP)**. A circulating lipid transfer protein produced by the liver that delivers monomeric LPS to the high-affinity LPS receptor CD14 expressed on macrophages, neutrophils, and dendritic cells, permitting the quick detection of a Gram-negative infection. The LPS-sensing pathway involves more than LBP or CD14, because they do not directly alert cells; CD14 does not have a transmembrane region, so accessory molecules are needed for signal transduction. The accessory molecule is Toll-like receptor 4 (TLR4; see below); however, TLR4 recognition of LPS requires the co-receptor MD2, a lipid-binding protein—the LBP-bound LPS is transferred to CD14, and then to MD2, thereby activating TLR4-signaling pathways (discussed shortly).

**Scavenger receptors**, originally defined in macrophages and endothelial cells and now dendritic cells and others, are a family of cell-surface transmembrane glycoprotein PRRs that are defined by their ability to recognize modified low-density lipoproteins. They can also bind either microbial ligands that include microbial surface constituents (LPS and lipoteichoic acid) or intact Gram-negative and Gram-positive bacteria, plus damaged host cells and tissues, and apoptotic and senescent host cells; they exhibit broad ligand-binding specificities, a typical feature of PRRs. The cell-surface expression of unique molecular structures associated with microbes or altered self-constituents not found on normal host tissues and cells provides a perfect target. Scavenger receptors are divided into at least six classes of structurally unrelated receptors; the prototype molecule is SR-A. Their importance in host defense is suggested by increased susceptibility to bacterial, viral, and protozoan infections in scavenger receptor-deficient mice. Nonetheless, as their name, and role in LPS clearance and in host apoptotic cell engulfment, implies, scavenger receptors are PRRs devoted to mopping up ligands.

**Mannose receptor** (CD206), expressed by primarily macrophage populations, recognizes mannose, fucose, and N-acetylglucosamine. Even though mannose receptors mediate the clearance of endogenous glycoproteins, such as lysosomal hydrolases, the main function is thought to be binding and leading to phagocytosis of bacterial, viral, fungal, and protozoan pathogens. Also, mannose receptor uptake of mannosylated antigen facilitates its presentation to T cells; thus, in addition to its homeostatic function mannose receptor doubles up as a means to enhance antigen acquisition for presentation to the adaptive immune system. In addition to mannose receptor, the C-type lectin DC-SIGN (CD209; unique to dendritic cells and binds to ICAM-3 on naïve T cells), Dectin-1 (yeast β-glucan receptor; found on dendritic cells, macrophages, and neutrophils), and Dectin-2 (yeast zymosan receptor) are also implicated in pattern recognition.

Another family of PRRs is the plasma membrane-associated and intracellular (vesicle) membrane-associated **Toll-like receptors** (**TLRs**). How a host senses the invasion of pathogen microbes relies to a great extend on TLRs, which recognize specific molecular patterns inherent in microbes, the PAMPs, and signals the first alarm that an infection is present. Stimulation of different members of the TLR family induces distinct gene expression patterns, which not only leads to the activation of innate immunity but also leads to the initiation and determination of effector functions of antigen-specific adaptive immunity. The discovery of the TLR family began with the identification of *Drosophila* Toll, a receptor expressed by insects and was required for dorso-ventral polarity during fly embryogenesis. Later studies on *Drosophila* carrying a loss-of-function mutation in the *Toll* gene revealed that Toll also has importance in insect innate immune responses against fungal infections. Homologues of Toll were identified, and so far, 10 TLR family members have been identified in humans (Table 3-1) and 13 in mice.

Toll-like receptors are transmembrane glycoproteins with a single α-helix that spans the cell membrane (Figure 3-5). They share a conserved structure in their extracellular domains (ectodomains), which consists of blocks of 24–29 amino-acid motif repeats (XLXXLXLXX; where X is any amino acid and

**TABLE 3-1 Toll-like Receptors (TLRs) and Their Ligands**

| TLRs* | TLR location/Subcellular localization | Ligands | Ligand origin |
|---|---|---|---|
| TLR1 | Ubiquitious/Cell membrane | Triacyl lipopeptides | Mycobacteria |
| TLR2 | Myeloid cells, mast cells, NK cells, mDCs, αβ & γδ T cells/Cell membrane | Envelope protein<br>GPI-linked proteins<br>Lipoproteins<br>Lipoteichoic acid<br>Peptidoglycans<br>Zymosan | Virus<br>Trypanosomes<br>Mycobacteria<br>Gram-positive bacteria<br>Gram-positive bacteria<br>Fungi |
| TLR3 | mDCs, NK cells/Intracellular | Double-stranded RNA | Viruses |
| TLR4 | Monocytes, mast cells, neutrophils, γδ regulatory T cells; golgi in gut epithelial cells/Cell membrane; Golgi | Fusion protein<br>Glycoinositolphospholipids<br>LPS<br>Mannan | Respiratory syncytial virus<br>Fungi<br>Gram-negative bacteria<br>Fungi |
| TLR5 | Epithelial cells, NK cells, monocytes, mDCs/Cell membrane | Flagellin | Bacteria |
| TLR6 | Myeloid cells, mast cells, B cells/Cell membrane | Diacyl lipopeptides<br>Lipoteichoic acid<br>Zymosan | Mycobacteria<br>Gram-positive bacteria<br>Fungi |
| TLR7 | pDCs, B cells, eosinophils/Intracellular (endosomal) | Single-stranded RNA | Viruses |
| TLR8 | NK cells, T cells, myeloid cells/Intracellular (endosomal) | Single-stranded RNA | Viruses |
| TLR9 | pDCs, B cells, NK cells; surface of tonsillar cells/Intracellular (endosomal) | CpG-containing DNA<br>Herpesvirus DNA | Bacteria, protozoa, virus<br>Viruses |
| TLR10 | B cells, pDCs/Cell membrane | Unknown | Unknown |
| TLR11 | Murine uroepithelium/Cell membrane | Unknown<br>Profilin | Uropathogenic bacteria;<br>*Toxoplasma gondii* |
| TLR12 | Murine uroepithelium/Cell membrane | Unknown | Unknown |
| TRL13 | Cell membrane | Unknown | Unknown |

*Some TLRs form dimers: TLRs 1 & 2, TLRs 2 & 6, and TLR4 with itself. (Humans express ten TLRs, enumerated 1 through 10. Mice do not express TLR10, but do express TLRs 1 through 9, and have three additional paralogs [11, 12, and 13] that are not represented in humans.)

L is leucine), called **leucine-rich repeats** (**LRRs**). Each TLR can contain up to 42 blocks of LRRs, and a subset of LRRs forms the TLR ligand-binding portion. The 135–160 amino-acid-long cytoplasmic tail of TLRs is called the *Toll/IL-1R (TIR) domain* so named for its homology to the intracellular domain of interleukin-1 receptor family members. The TIR domain couples downstream signal transduction to receptor engagement. Three highly homologous regions called *boxes 1, 2,* and *3* characterize the TIR domain and serve as binding sites for intracellular signaling molecules that also contain TIR domains; they are called *adaptor proteins* and are associated with TLR-ligand engagement. Four TIR-containing adaptor proteins mediate the TLR signaling pathway. The adaptor protein-TLR association is through homophilic TIR domain interactions and each TLR induces distinct responses with different adapter combinations. TLR signaling is initiated by ligand-induced dimerization of TLRs, which can form heterodimers (such as TLR2 and TLR1) or homodimers (such as TLR4 with itself).

All TLRs, except TLR3, signal using the adaptor protein *myeloid differentiation primary-response protein 88 (MyD88)*. After ligand binding, MyD88 is recruited to the receptor complex, which is then joined by *IL-1R-associated kinases (IRAKs)*, ultimately ending in the activation of the NF-κB pathway and MAP-kinase pathways (Figure 3-6). Nuclear factor-κB activation instigates the transcription of many genes influential in innate immune effector functions, such as the production of proinflammatory cytokines and costimulatory molecules. It also augments adaptive immunity by mediating signaling pathways of B and T cells.

The preceding TLR signaling pathway is called the *MyD88-dependent pathway*. Even though TLR2 and TLR4 signaling pathways require activation of the MyD88-dependent pathway, the adapter protein TIR domain-containing adaptor protein (TIRAP) is also needed. Some TLR family members trigger the induction of type I IFN production in a MyD88-independent manner; thus, it is called the *MyD88-independent pathway*. TLR3 and TLR4 use

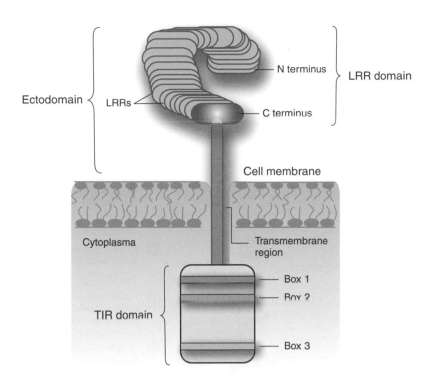

**FIGURE 3-5 Toll-like receptor structure.** The schematic diagram shows the extracellular, transmembrane, and cytoplasmic domains of the Toll-like receptors. The extracellular domain, or ectodomain, is composed of tandem repeats of leucine-rich regions called *leucine-rich repeats (LRRs)*. LRRs contain the ligand-bind sites, how they recognize their ligands is unknown. A single transmembrane α-helix connects the LRRs to the cytoplasmic domain. The conserved cytoplasmic domain that is called *Toll/IL-1 receptor (TIR) domain*, which contains three highly homologous regions known as *boxes 1, 2,* and *3.* See text for further description.

this pathway to induce IFN-β and IFN-inducible genes, substituting TIR domain-containing adaptor inducing IFN-β (TRIF) for MyD88. In addition, TRIF is essential for the induction of proinflammatory cytokines in the TLR4 signaling pathway. The remaining adaptor, TRIF-related adaptor molecule (TRAM), is necessary for the TLR4-mediated MyD88-independent pathway because it acts as a bridge between TLR4 and TRIF.

TLR3 and TLR4 mediated activation of the transcription factor IFN-regulatory factor 3 (IRF3), which induces IFN-β and IFN-inducible genes and leads to the production of type I IFNs IFN-α and IFN-β. TLR7 and TRL9 also induce IFN-α and IFN-β production, but through different signaling pathways. Even though type I IFNs are most closely associated with their antiviral activities, thus their major role in innate antiviral immunity, they have diverse antiviral-devoid functions in the development of adaptive immunity. They promote memory T cell proliferation, prevent T cell apoptosis, and induce CD4+ and CD8+ T cell IFN-γ production. The largest amounts of type I IFN are produced by specialized dendritic cells (DCs) called *plasmacytoid DCs (pDCs)*, which express high levels of TLR7 and TLR9. Ligand engagement of these TLRs induces pDCs to produce IFN-α.

In mammals, at least 13 TLRs have been identified and functions have been ascribed to 12 of them. This set of TLRs can detect a broad array of bacteria, viruses, fungi, and protozoa (see Table 3-1). TLRs are crucial components of the innate immune system because they recognize conserved motifs on pathogens, which are referred to as PAMPs that are biologic patterns/structures unique to, and necessary for, the survival of microorganisms but not generated by the host. For example, one such pattern is the conserved bacterial lipid-A pattern in LPS, a component of the Gram-negative bacterial cell wall. LPS is necessary for microbial survival; thus, bacteria

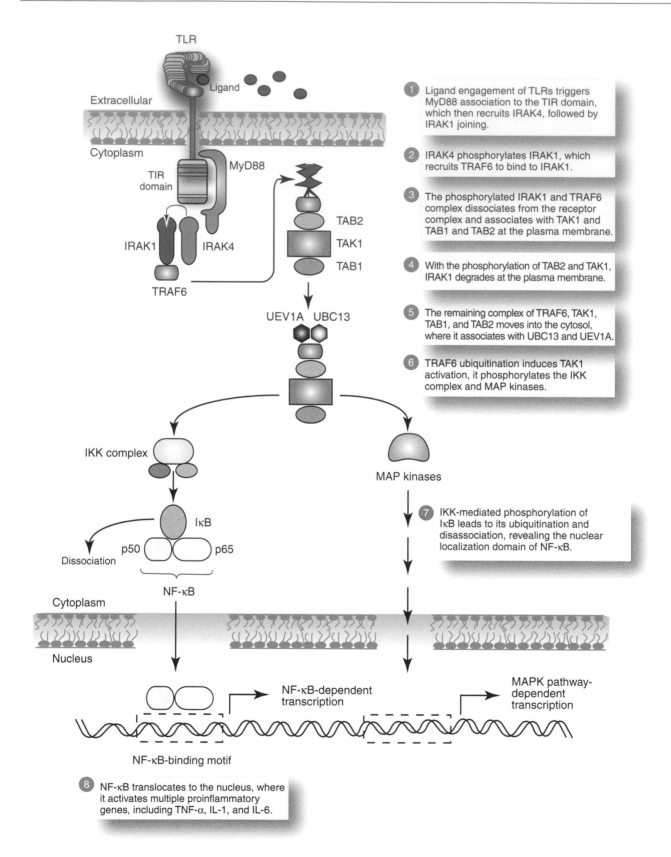

**FIGURE 3-6 TLR signaling pathway.** Abbreviations: MyD88, myeloid differentiation primary-response protein 88; IRAK, IL-1R-associated kinase; TRAF6, tumor-necrosis-factor-receptor-associated factor 6; TAK1, transforming-growth-factor-β-activated kinase 1; UBC13, ubiquitin-conjugating enzyme 13; UEV1A, ubiquitin-conjugating enzyme E2 variant 1; IKK, inhibitor of nuclear factor-κB [IκB]-kinase complex; MAP, mitogen-activating protein kinases; NF-κB, nuclear factor-κB.

always express this marker (if they shed or alter their LPS in order to evade innate immunity, they are no longer viable). The same can be said for the loss of viruses' nucleic acid or fungi's cell wall component zymosan. So universal are PAMPs that the ability to identify them is encoded into the germline DNA of multicellular organisms—pattern-recognition receptors (PRRs), such as TLRs, are evolutionary conserved germline-encoded transmembrane proteins; our body's innate immune system has the inherent capacity to identify any organism that displays these patterns and to mount a rapid response to eliminate it. The TLRs differ from one another in their expression pattern, their ligand specificities, and depending on the cell type and molecule, the localization of TLRs is restricted to the cell surface or cell organelles, particularly the endolysosomal compartment. Some TLRs form dimers: TLRs 1 and 2, TLRs 2 and 6, and TLR4 with itself, TLR5 also may dimerize with itself. Toll-like receptor pairing influences their ligand specificity. TLR2 and TLR1 or TLR6 form heterodimers, TLR1/2 and TRL2/6, which discriminate between the molecular structure of diacyl and triacyl lipopeptides, respectively. TLR2 recognizes lipoproteins/lipopeptides and peptidoglycans from Gram-positive and Gram-negative bacteria, and lipoteichoic acid from Gram-positive bacteria, a phenol-soluble modulin from *Staphylococcus aureus*, glycolipids from *Treponema maltophilum*, and atypical LPS from nonenterobacteria, whose structures are different from typical LPS of Gram-negative bacteria. During viral replication by RNA viruses, dsRNA is generated, which is recognized by TLR3. The best-characterized TLR is TLR-4, the major receptor for most bacterial LPS, which is expressed on neutrophils, macrophages, and dendritic cells. It recognizes lipid A of LPS; this occurs through the TLR4/MD2/CD14 complex (mentioned earlier). TLR5 recognizes flagellin, the major portion of bacterial flagella. TLR5, expressed on the basolateral surface of intestinal epithelial cells, but not their apical side, may serve as a sensor for pathogenic bacteria that invade across the epithelium. TLR7 and TLR8 recognize ssRNA from viruses such as human immunodeficiency virus, vesicular stomatitis virus (VSV), and influenza virus. TLR9 detects unmethylated CpG DNA motifs found most commonly in prokaryotic genomes and DNA viruses. TLR9 induces antiviral responses by sensing DNA virus CpG DNA.

The recognition of microbes at the cell-surface or in vesicles is covered by the TLR system, but what about in the cytosol (Figure 3-7)? There is a Toll-like receptor (TLR)-independent system in the cytosol represented by the **nucleotide-binding** **oligomerization domain (NOD) proteins NOD1** and **NOD2**—NOD1 and NOD2 act as intracellular PRRs. The NODs are part of another innate immunity microbial-recognition system called the *nucleotide-binding domain LRR-containing family (NLRs)* of more than 20 proteins in humans that recognizes microbial components derived from bacterial peptidoglycans in the cytoplasm and also sense endogenous products released by dying cells. NOD1 binds tripeptide peptidoglycan breakdown products; NOD2 binds to muramyl dipeptide derived from peptidoglycan degradation of Gram-positive bacterial cell walls. The TLRs and NOD receptor structure is similar (see Figure 3-7); they rely on pathogen recognition by an LRR domain, albeit in the cytosol rather than at the cell surface or in vesicles. Moving to the N-terminus of the NOD receptor structure, the LRR domain is followed by a NOD domain, which as an ATP-dependent dimerization domain, and the last domain caspase-recruitment domain (CARD) is a protein-protein interaction cassette. The downstream signaling pathways in the TLR and NOD systems are different. The NOD proteins are expressed in antigen-presenting cells (such as macrophages and dendritic cells) and epithelial cells. The importance of these proteins is underscored by the fact that NOD1 participates in host defense against *H. pylori* infections and 10-15% of Crohn's disease patients have mutations in the gene encoding NOD2. Other members of the NLR family form molecular machines called *inflammasomes*, which are involved in the activation of proinflammatory cytokines such as IL-1 and IL-18.

What about the recognition of viral components that are present in the cytosol? The TLRs and NODs cannot recognize them. Two members of the cytoplasmic proteins of the retinoic-acid-inducible gene I (RIG-I)-like receptor (RLR) family, **RID-I** and **melanoma differentiation-associated gene 5 (MDA5)**, can recognize viral proteins in the cell's cytosol (see Figure 3-7). RIG-I and MDA5 are composed of two N-terminal CARDs and a C-terminal DEXD/H-box RNA-helicase domain.[2] They are intracellular sensors of dsRNA, which induce the production of type I IFNs. RIG-I can recognize RNA viruses such as Newcastle disease virus, vesicular stomatitis virus, Sendai virus, paramyxoviruses, influenza virus, and Japanese encephalitis virus. MDA5 is required for picornavirus detection

---

[2]The DEXD/H box RNA helicases can unwind dsRNA with their intrinsic ATPase activity. They are found in almost all organisms from viruses to mammals and mediate many important processes, including RNA interference.

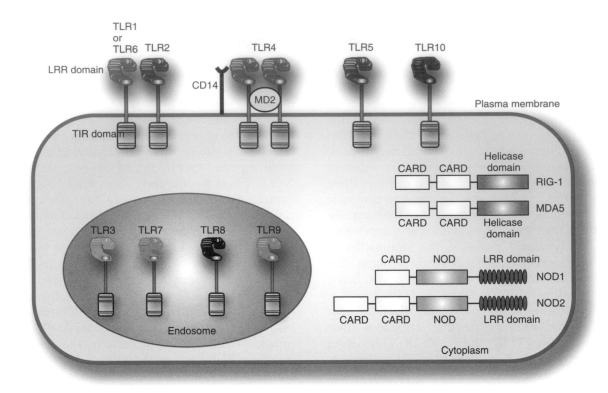

**FIGURE 3-7 Cellular location of TLRs, NOD1 and NOD2, RIG-1 and MDA5.** The NOD (nucleotide-binding oligomerization domain) proteins NOD1 and NOD2 are cytosolic proteins composed of three domains: a carboxyl-terminal LRR domain (binds ligand); a central NOD (a region with ATPase activity that facilitates self-oligomerization; and an amino-terminal domain composed of protein-protein interaction domains called *caspase-recruitment domain* (*CARD*). Like NODs, RLRs are cytosolic proteins but are only composed of two types of domains: two N-terminal CARD domains and a C-terminal Helicase domain (binds dsRNA). Both TRLs and NODs use their LRRs to recognize microbial components, whereas RLRs use their Helicase domain.

and polyinosine polycytidylic acid-induced IFN-α production.

The innate immune system, through specialized host-cell receptors (PRRs) recognize molecules (PAMPs) expressed exclusively by microorganisms, rapidly deciphers the type of infection, provides first line protection, and instigates the appropriate effector class of adaptive immune responses. The interrelationship between innate recognition of microorganisms by TLRs, NODs, and others, which leads to immediate protection and eventual long-term adaptive immunity is illustrated in Figure 3-8.

### Killing Microbes by Either Internalizing Them (Phagocytosis) Using Scavenger and Specialized Cells or Killing Them Outright by Contact, and the Production of Inflammatory Molecules

Unlike the receptors used in adaptive immunity that are expressed only on lymphocytes, the innate immune system's diverse array of pathogen-specific receptors, we discussed above, are distributed by, and expressed on, many different immune and nonimmune cell types. Nonetheless, once the innate immune system recognizes the pathogens, it depends mainly on four cell types to kill these pathogens: neutrophils, macrophages, dendritic cells, and natural killer (NK) cells. Each of these cells mediates its activity at different stages of infection and targets different types of pathogens. Other cells that release inflammatory mediators (basophils, mast cells, and eosinophils) will be discussed in later chapters.

Metchnikoff first recognized the importance of phagocytosis as a general defense mechanism against infection. He called human amoeboid, particulate-eating cells *phagocytes* (from the Greek words *phagein*, "to eat," and *kytos*, "cell"). **Phagocytosis** is a quintessential means by which cells in the body resist infection by pathogenic microorganisms.

Phagocytes internalize extracellular macromolecules by endocytosis and particulate matter by phagocytosis. Virtually all cells are capable of **endocytosis**, whereas only specialized cells like

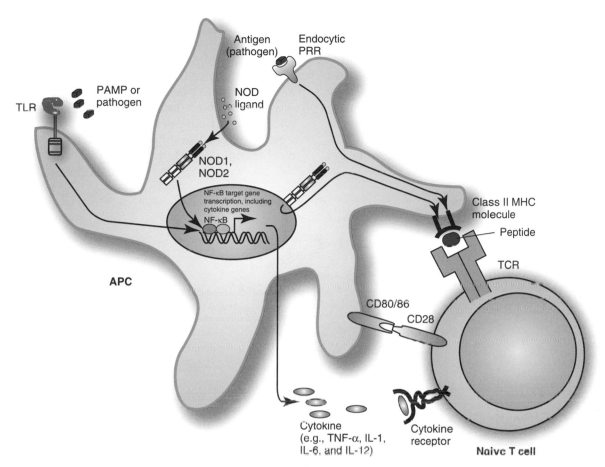

**FIGURE 3-8 Role of TLRs and NODs in innate and adaptive immunity**. Pattern-recognition receptors (PRRs), such as Toll-like receptors (TLRs) and nucleotide-binding oligomerization domain (NOD) proteins sense the presence of infection through recognition of pathogen-associated molecular patterns (PAMPs). Recognition of PAMPs by TLRs expressed on (or in) antigen-presenting cells (APCs) and intracellular ligands by NOD proteins, upregulates cell-surface expression of costimulatory (CD80 and CD86) molecules and class II major histocompatibility complex (class II MHC) molecules. TLRs and NODs also mediate the activation of signaling pathways including those downstream of nuclear factor-κB (NF-κB), which induce expression of cytokines, such as tumor necrosis factor-α (TNF-α), interleukin-1 (IL-1), IL-6, IL-12, and chemokines and their receptors, and trigger events associated with APC maturation. Induction of CD80/86 on APCs leads to the activation of T cells specific for pathogens that triggered the TLR and NOD signaling. IL-12 contributes to the differentiation of activated T cells into T helper (T_{H})1 effector cells. It is unknown whether TLRs and NODs can induce T_{H}2 cell responses. The mechanism by which NOD proteins enhance transcriptional activity of MHC class II transactivator (CIITA), which leads to class II MHC molecule synthesis, is unclear (see Chapter 7).

neutrophils, macrophages, and dendritic cells are capable of phagocytosis. In endocytosis, macromolecules are internalized by invagination and pinching off of small regions of the plasma membrane, to form small vesicles. Endocytosis occurs either by nonspecific pinocytosis (the internalization of fluids or solutes) or receptor-mediated endocytosis (the selective internalization of macromolecules after binding to specific receptors). Either process leads to the fusion of the resultant vesicles with each other and their delivery to endosomes, which

are intracellular acidic sorting compartments. In phagocytosis, particulate material, including whole pathogens, is internalized when the plasma membrane expands around the material forming large vesicles (10–20 times larger than endocytic vesicles) called *phagosomes*.

The two major types of phagocytes are neutrophils and macrophages; dendritic cells are specialized phagocytic cells. When infection occurs, neutrophils are recruited from the blood to the infected area. In contrast, for macrophage precursor cells, circulating monocytes move from the blood into the tissues and become tissue-resident macrophages. Monocytes and macrophages constitute the functional network of cells generally called the *mononuclear phagocyte system*. The neutrophils and macrophages not only carry out phagocytosis; they are also equipped with a potent arsenal of antimicrobial substances. Even though immature dendritic cells are phagocytic, they are not efficient in bacterial clearance, but they are proficient at antigen processing and

antigen loading of MHC molecules for presentation to antigen-specific T cells. Macrophages can also present antigen-derived peptides to specific T cells.

The fourth major cell in innate immunity is the nonphagocytic cell, the natural killer (NK) cell. It is a lymphocyte-like cell that functions as an important mediator of innate immune defense against viruses. NK cells contribute to the host immune response to viral infections through direct and indirect cytolytic mechanisms or cytokine production.

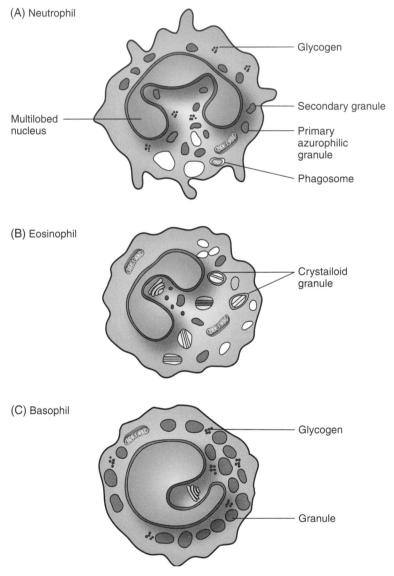

(A) Neutrophil

Glycogen

Multilobed nucleus

Secondary granule

Primary azurophilic granule

Phagosome

(B) Eosinophil

Crystailoid granule

(C) Basophil

Glycogen

Granule

**FIGURE 3-9 Typical morphology of granulocytes.** The differences in the shape of the nucleus and in the shape and number of cytoplasmic granules distinguish the cells. Eosinophils, for instance, have an affinity for acidic dyes such as eosin; basic methylene blue reacts to granules in the basophil; and granules of the neutrophil stain with both. The most numerous immune cells in the blood are the neutrophils. See Table 2-1 for cell percentages in the blood.

## Neutrophils Are Short-Lived, Highly Motile Phagocytic Killers; They Do Not Present Antigen

As 70% of all blood leukocytes, **neutrophils** are the most common leukocyte found in the blood of most mammals. Neutrophils are short-lived. Unlike the other phagocytic cells we will discuss, neutrophils do not reside in the tissues before infections, after spending roughly 12 hr in the blood, they are recruited by resident macrophages that have encountered pathogens and enter the tissues, where they live only 1 to 3 days. They have an irregular nucleus, shaped like a segmented sausage (Figure 3-9); therefore, they also are called *polymorphonuclear leukocytes*. Neutrophils are the first leukocytes to appear at an infection site; they arrive with a significant antimicrobial arsenal—their main weapon is phagocytosis. They are highly phagocytic, respond to chemotaxis, and undergo diapedesis (migration of cells across the blood vessel lining and into tissues) as a result of local inflammation (discussed later). These activities are mediated through the interaction of many different neutrophil receptors with their targets. In addition to (1) lectin receptors, (2) scavenger receptors, (3) TLRs, (4) receptors for antibody molecules, (5) complement receptors, (6) chemokine receptors, and (7) molecules that mediate rolling and sticking at sites of inflammation, neutrophils contain receptors for N-formyl methionyl peptides (fMet). fMet is derived from bacterial protein and mitochondrial protein breakdown—a chemotactic warning sign of bacteria.

The recognition of invariant and widely distributed microbial molecules by lectin receptors, scavenger receptors, TLRs particularly TLR2 and TLR4, and complement component receptors on neutrophils makes it difficult for pathogens to escape detection by neutrophils. The direct receptor engagement of neutrophils with invaders and their engulfment (phagocytosis) is enhanced when invaders are coated (*opsonized*) with antibodies (humoral arm of adaptive immunity) or complement or both. Some serum complement components opsonize pathogens in the absence of antibodies. Microbe-engaged neutrophils spread pseudopodia around organisms and internalize them into a saclike structure called a *phagosome*. Organism-killing granules are emptied into these sacks. Neutrophils contain two types of granules: lysosomes (also called primary granules) and secondary granules. The contents of primary granules are: myeloperoxidase (involved in respiratory burst), lysozyme (destroys cell walls), cationic proteins called *defensins* and *cathelicidins* (antibacterial peptides), and hydrolases (degrade proteins). The contents of secondary granules are: lysozyme, lactoferrin (antibacterial, binds iron), and collagenase (degrades collagen). Neutrophils can be considered "suicide cells" because they are killed in the process of killing. These killed neutrophils are the major component of pus in infections. Nonetheless, they are the principals in ridding the body of the continual tide of invading microorganisms.

The process of phagocytosis first requires adherence of the microbe to the phagocytic cell. Electrostatic forces are involved in initial attachment, since divalent cations such as $Ca^{2+}$ and $Mg^{2+}$ are required. Serum substances called *opsonins* facilitate firm attachment and ingestion. Opsonins include acquired or naturally occurring antibodies and a component of the complement system (C3b). Neutrophils have specific receptors on their surfaces for such antibodies, as well as for the C3b complement fragments. The opsonins first become attached to the surface of microbes, thus making them more "palatable" to phagocytes (Figure 3-10).

After the phagocyte attaches a microbe to its surface, it sends out projections called *pseudopodia* that surround the microbe during ingestion (Figure 3-11). These pseudopodia fuse and form a phagocytic vacuole called a *phagosome* that contains the microbe. The phagosome then pinches off from the membrane and enters the cytoplasm. Subsequent events depend on the activity of cytoplasmic granules called *lysosomes*, which contain digestive enzymes and microbicidal substances. The lysosomes move toward the phagosome, fuse with its membrane, and form a digestive vacuole called a *phagolysosome*. The lysosomes discharge their toxic contents into the phagolysosome, thus initiating the intracellular killing and digestion of the microorganism. The digested contents are then eliminated in a process called **exocytosis**.

Within the phagolysosome, immediately after fusion with the lysosome, there is a brief rise in pH and neutral proteases and cationic proteins are active. Subsequently, the pH becomes acidic (pH 3.5 to 4.0) and acid proteases become active, both killing many bacteria. The lysosomal enzymes emptied into the digestive vacuole include lysozyme and a variety of other hydrolytic enzymes that break down the macromolecular components of microorganisms. Over 60 different enzymes have been found within lysosomes; they include: acid proteases, which are active at acid pH and include enzymes such as glycosidase, lipase, nuclease, and acid phosphatase; cationic proteins, which are found in neutrophil granules and in some macrophages and damage the lipid bilayer of Gram-negative organisms under alkaline conditions; defensins and cathelicidins, families of

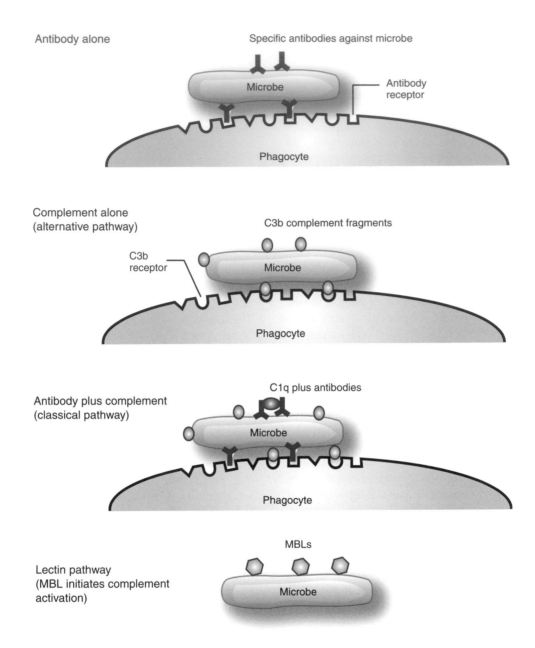

**FIGURE 3-10 Mechanisms of microbial opsonization**. It is a process whereby phagocytosis is enhanced by the deposition of opsonins on the antigen. Adherence of microbes to phagocytes is enhanced by receptors on the phagocyte surface. Receptors are specific for both antibodies (generated only during the adaptive immune response) and complement fragments on the microbes. Mannose-binding lectin (MBL) coats target microbes and initiates the complement cascade directly, which in turn leads to production of complement components such as C3b. Whether antibodies, complement components, or acute phase reactants like MBL, they all can act as opsonins.

wide-spectrum cationic antimicrobial and cytotoxic peptides present in neutrophil granules; lactoferrin, which is found in neutrophil granules and binds tightly to iron, therefore depriving bacteria of this essential element; lysozyme, a muramidase enzyme that hydrolyzes peptidoglycan in bacterial cell walls; and neutral proteases, which are active near pH 7 and include enzymes such as collagenase, elastase, and some cathepsins.

The preceding list indicates that activated phagocytes in the process of killing internalized microbes produce a number of antimicrobial and cytotoxic

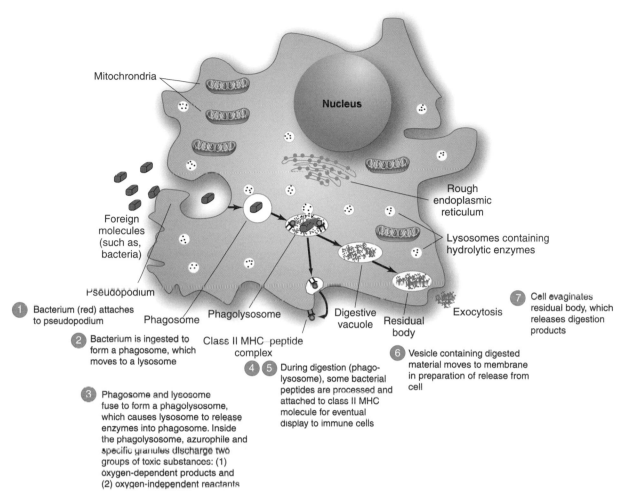

Mitochrondria

**Nucleus**

Rough
endoplasmic
reticulum

Foreign
molecules
(such as,
bacteria)

Lysosomes containing
hydrolytic enzymes

Pseudopodium

**7** Cell evaginates
residual body, which
releases digestion
products

**1** Bacterium (red) attaches
to pseudopodium

Phagosome

Phagolysosome

Digestive
vacuole

Residual
body

Exocytosis

**2** Bacterium is ingested to
form a phagosome, which
moves to a lysosome

Class II MHC–peptide
complex

**6** Vesicle containing digested
material moves to membrane
in preparation of release from
cell

**4** **5** During digestion (phagolysosome), some bacterial
peptides are processed and
attached to class II MHC
molecule for eventual
display to immune cells

**3** Phagosome and lysosome
fuse to form a phagolysosome,
which causes lysosome to release
enzymes into phagosome. Inside
the phagolysosome, azurophile and
specific granules discharge two
groups of toxic substances: (1)
oxygen-dependent products and
(2) oxygen-independent reactants

**FIGURE 3-11 Phagocytosis.** Cells of the mononuclear phagocyte system are attracted to the site of infection by factors released by pathogens, damaged host cells, and other blood components. The phagocytes engulf the pathogens, using pseudopodia, and internalize them as membrane-bound organelles (*phagosomes*) within the phagocyte. The phagosomes fuse with other organelles (*lysosomes*) containing hydrolytic enzymes. These organelles are then called *phagolysosomes*. Inside the phagolysosome, azurophile and specific granules discharge two groups of toxic substances into the organelle: (1) oxygen-dependent products formed by reactive oxygen metabolites and (2) oxygen-independent reactants, such as proteases, lactoferrin, and phospholipase $A_2$. Organisms killed by the action of superoxide ions, hypochlorite, and hydrogen peroxide. The phagocyte's activity is enhanced by other parts of the immune system.

substances. The toxic effects of these substances involve oxygen-dependent and -independent killing mechanisms (Table 3-2). The major microbicidal mechanism of activated phagocytes is produced by the "respiratory burst." Shortly after phago-cytosing a microbe, the activated phagocytic cell increases its oxygen consumption to support the increased metabolic activity of phagocytosis. This is associated with increased activity of the hexose monophosphate shunt, which generates highly toxic oxygen metabolites, including singlet oxygen, superoxide, hydrogen peroxide, hydroxyl radicals,

and hypochlorite. Neutrophils also synthesize lysozyme, various enzymes, and defensins and cathelicidins whose activity is not dependent on oxygen. Within the phagolysosome, enzymes, low pH, or oxygen metabolites kill most microbes within 10 to 30 minutes, although complete destruction can take a few hours.

The combined actions of the lysosomal enzymes and toxic oxygen metabolites are usually sufficient to destroy all invading microorganisms. However, microbes vary their response to phagocytic activity. Gram-positive bacteria are rapidly destroyed.

**TABLE 3-2** Neutrophil and Macrophage Mediators of Antimicrobial and Cytotoxic Activity

| Oxygen-dependent killing | Oxygen-independent killing | |
|---|---|---|
| Reactive oxygen intermediates | Reactive nitrogen intermediates | |
| $O_2^{\cdot-}$ (superoxide) | NO (nitric oxide) | Defensins and cathelicidins |
| $OH\cdot$ (hydroxyl radicals) | $NO_2$ (nitrogen dioxide) | Lysozyme |
| $H_2O_2$ (hydrogen peroxide) | $HNO_2$ (nitrous acid) | Hydrolytic enzymes |
| HOCl (hypochlorous acid) | | TNF-$\alpha$ (macrophages only) |
| $NH_2Cl$ (monochloramine) | | |

Gram-negative bacteria are somewhat more persistent because their cell wall is relatively resistant to digestion.

## Macrophages Are Long-Lived, Highly Motile Phagocytic Sentinels with an Overwhelming Array of Biological Activities

Along with neutrophils, **macrophages** are phagocytic cells but are considered the central player in innate immunity because of their essential role in innate immune functions and multiple roles in host defense. Macrophages are the "big eaters" of the immune system. The first cell type that biologists identified as protecting the host from a microorganism intrusion, macrophages were once derided as the "garbage collectors" of the immune system. During the 110 years since the Russian zoologist Elie Metchnikoff (1845–1916) discovered macrophages (also called *mononuclear phagocytes*), scientists have realized that they are also important regulators of adaptive immunity (see Chapter 2). *Tissue macrophages* and their blood precursors, *monocytes* (Figure 3-12), are

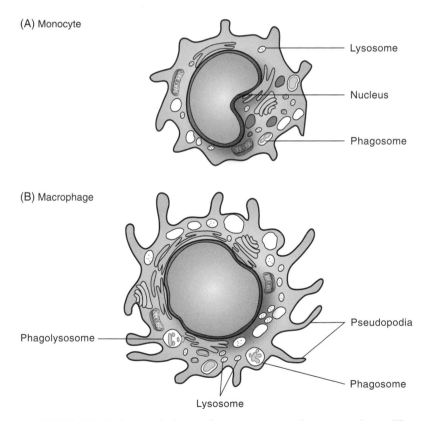

(A) Monocyte

Lysosome

Nucleus

Phagosome

(B) Macrophage

Phagolysosome

Pseudopodia

Phagosome

Lysosome

**FIGURE 3-12 Typical morphology of a monocyte and a macrophage.** The blood precursors of macrophages are monocytes. Monocytes are five- to tenfold smaller than macrophages and contain fewer organelles, particularly lysosomes. (Cells are not drawn to the same scale).

part of the mononuclear phagocyte system because they share a common lineage and because their primary function is phagocytosis.

Circulating monocytes give rise to a variety of mature tissue-resident macrophages (and dendritic cells) that are distributed in peripheral tissues and organs throughout the body where they are most likely to encounter pathogens early in an infection. Tissue macrophages are seeded in a variety of guises throughout the body, where they stay for 2 to 3 months. They are named according to their residency in the many tissues they inhabit (see Figure 2-7). Macrophages measure 10 to 50 μm in diameter and their morphology varies, depending on their state of activity. Resting macrophages on encounter with pathogens or other stimuli become activated, that is, they become fully competent to mediate a broad array of antimicrobial activities, including enhanced phagocytosis and killing of pathogens, enhanced production of inflammatory mediators, and increased expression of class II MHC molecules. The latter augments their ability to present antigen to helper T cells—connecting innate and adaptive immunity.

The processes of adherence, ingestion, and digestion of microbes in macrophages are generally similar to those of neutrophils, although there are some important differences. Macrophages have the ability to change their surface shape—forming ruffles—and to differentiate. They also secrete at least 100 different metabolic products, ranging from lysozyme to collagenase to complement components, which contribute to antimicrobial defense. They do not move in response to the same chemotactic chemicals (chemokines) as neutrophils. The lysosomal enzymes of macrophages also differ from those of neutrophils. Macrophages do not have the same cationic proteins

found in neutrophil cell granules, nor do they produce highly toxic oxygen metabolites as efficiently. These differences are reflected in their ability to deal with ingested microorganisms. For example, macrophages are much less effective than neutrophils in killing the yeast *Candida albicans* or the bacterium *M. tuberculosis*. However, macrophages activated by IFN-γ can kill these microorganisms. Activated macrophages also kill pathogens with defensins, cathelicidins, nitric oxide, lysozyme, and molecules that compete with essential nutrients.

Macrophages express receptors that are directly involved in mechanisms of innate resistance: the macrophage mannose receptors, scavenger receptors, complement receptors, receptors for antibodies, lectin receptors, CD14, and TLRs. The fact that the ligands for these receptors are almost universally expressed in bacteria allows macrophages to rapidly recognize and respond to bacterial invaders.

As discussed in Chapter 2, macrophages are versatile cells that can play four roles: accessory, secretory, effector (a response to eliminate or neutralize an organism), and regulatory.

## Dendritic Cells Are Immature Microbe-Capturing Sentinels That Shift to Mature T Cell-Activating Cells

**Dendritic cells (DCs)** have important and unique immune functions (Figure 3-13). These bone marrow-derived cells have a characteristic star-like morphology, caused by finger-like processes radiating from a central hub. Dendritic cells are better known for their orchestration of adaptive immunity—different mature DC subsets activate helper T cell and cytotoxic T cell adaptive immune

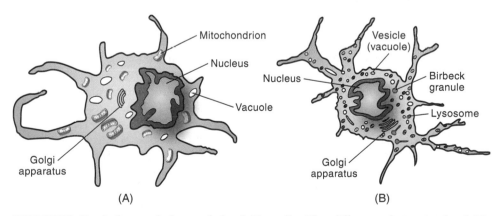

**FIGURE 3-13 Typical morphology of dendritic cells.** The difference between dendritic (A) and Langerhans (B) cells is mainly their area of residence in the body, which is the lymph nodes and skin, respectively. The Birbeck granule is unique to Langerhans cells. The Birbeck granule's function is unknown.

responses. Before DCs can activate antigen-naïve T cells, they must complete a maturation program that is instigated by interaction with invading pathogens or other immune cells. The key to initiating an immune response to pathogens is the recognition of their PAMPs, which is mediated by TLR family members, several of which are expressed by immature DCs. After pathogen encounter, recognition, internalization, migration to lymphoid tissues, now mature, DCs become efficient at stimulating naïve T cells, a process that is coincident with increased expression of antigen-presenting class I and class II MHC molecules and costimulatory molecules. Because of the latter characteristics, mature DCs, along with B lymphocytes and macrophages are considered APCs.

Nonetheless, immature DCs also have a crucial direct defense against pathogens. Tissue-residing immature DCs, such as DCs in the epidermis of the skin, where they are known as *Langerhans cells*, are phagocytic cells constantly sampling the surrounding milieu. These DCs express a number of PRRs, including mannose receptors, scavenger receptors, and several TLRs, used to recognize pathogens. Much like phagocytosis by macrophages, the binding and engulfment of pathogens by DCs can also lead to direct antimicrobial responses, such as, the killing of pathogens by the production of reactive oxygen species, nitric oxide, and defensins. Langerhans cells also can produce IL-6, IL-12, and tumor necrosis factor-α (TNF-α), cytokines that induce inflammation. Another DC subset called *plasmacytoid DCs*, which expresses TLR7 and TLR9, corresponds to a specialized cell population that produces significant amounts of type I IFNs (IFN-α and -β) in response to TLR-virus engagement. These IFNs block viral replication. Taken together, DCs provide bridge between innate and adaptive immunity, they continuously sample their surrounding environment for invading pathogens, killing them, and carrying a snapshot of the them to lymphoid tissues, where they induce the activation of effectors of adaptive immunity (see Chapter 10).

## Natural Killer Cells Are Antiviral Hunter-Killers and Conveyers of Activating Signals to the Immune System

**Natural killer (NK) cells** are large (12 to 15 μm in diameter) granule-containing lymphocytes (Figure 3-14), distinct from B and T lymphocytes, that protect in the absence of any known immunization; thus, they are associated with innate immunity. NK cells are a type of lymphocyte, and as their name

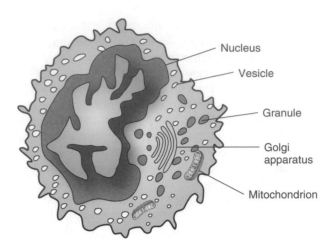

**FIGURE 3-14 NK cell.** (A) the typical morphology of a NK cell. In the peripheral blood, NK cells are histologically identified as large granular lymphocytes because they are larger than small lymphocytes and they contain many azurophilic granules.

implies, they kill various target cells without a need for additional activation—they are poised as effector cells for an immediate response. When NK cells bind to potential target cells, there are interactions between inhibitory (class I MHC molecule-binding) and activating (carbohydrate-binding) receptors with counterparts available on the virus-infected target cells, and the integration of signals transmitted by these receptors determines whether the NK cell detaches and moves on or stays and kills the target (see Chapter 10). For example, if the target cell self-class I MHC molecule levels are too low or absent for binding of NK cell inhibitory receptors, but binding of carbohydrate by lectin-like activating receptors occurs, the NK cell cannot inhibit the activation signal to kill—the virally infected target is killed.

NK cells are not phagocytic and do not have the conventional surface markers of other lymphoid cells of the adaptive immune system. They are instrumental in innate immune responses because they provide the first line defense against viruses—they lyse virus-infected cells. This early lysis either clears the viral infection or curbs its increase until days later when the adaptive immune system's virus-specific, cytotoxic T cells engage the infection. (Unlike NK cells, cytotoxic T cells need to be activated before they differentiate into cells with the ability to kill virally infected cells.) NK cells, once considered to be primitive nonspecific executioners, are now known to be sophisticated assassins that not only directly execute innate immune responses but also regulate the outcome of adaptive immunity through complex interplay with DCs. For example, NK cells provide for the early production of IFN-γ and TNF-α, which drive the maturation of DCs. Also, IFN-γ is major activator of macrophages and coercer of helper T cell development. NK cells also are considered important cytotoxic cells in adaptive immune responses because they express membrane receptors for the tail portion of antibody molecules (see Chapter 15).

## MINI SUMMARY

Innate immunity uses germline-encoded PRRs to target PAMPs that are shared by bacteria, viruses, fungi, and protozoa. The secreted receptors include mannose-binding lectin (MBL), C-reactive protein (CRP), serum amyloid protein (SAP), and LPS-binding protein (LBP); the cell-based receptors include scavenger receptors, mannose receptors, Toll-like receptors (TLRs), and nucleotide-binding oligomerization domain (NOD) proteins. Pattern recognition receptors are involved in opsonization, activation of complement, phagocytosis, and activation of proinflammatory signaling pathways. The three general groups of cellular mediators of non-specific internal innate defense are phagocytic cells—neutrophils, macrophages, and dendritic cells; a fourth cell is nonphagocytic, the NK cells, which can directly kill virally infected target host cells without internalizing them.

# THE CHEMICAL DEFENSES, THE AUGMENTERS OF CELLULAR DEFENSES, LEAD TO PROMOTION OF INFLAMMATION AND INDUCTION OF ADAPTIVE IMMUNITY

In addition to the cellular mediators of the body's internal defense, soluble mediators contribute to host resistance. Earlier, we mentioned fibronectin and β-lysin. Another mechanism of innate resistance is the production of products of the lectin complement pathway and the alternative pathway of complement activation. The complement pathways are activated by a cascade of enzymatic events in which the first molecule becomes activated, it in turn

activates the next in the series, and so-forth until all the complement components of the pathways are used. The advantages to a cascade system are that (1) it lends itself to multiple targets of control, which is necessary here because the complement system is nonspecific and thus capable of attacking host cells as well as microorganisms, and (2) the sequential development at each step of potent biological mediators that amplify protection. Other products, known as proinflammatory cytokines, greatly amplify innate immunity by acting on other immune and nonimmune cells without directly affecting the invading microbes themselves. In a systemic manner, these cytokines mediate the clearance of pathogens from the host; clearance is accomplished by attracting cells to the site of infection, diverting blood flow to the affected tissue so as to favor the influx of cells capable of killing microbes, and enhance the cells' antimicrobial activity once they arrived. The pathogenic insult, and the host's innate response to it, lead to tissue injury—a double-edged sword. Another example of a stepwise resolution, the elimination of pathogen, leads to inflammation.

## Complement, an Interlocking Set of Proteins, Rapidly Activated by Innate Recognition Proteins or Later Activation by Secreted Antibody, Which Kill Blood-Borne Pathogens

**Complement**, as one of the serum enzyme systems, mediates inflammation, opsonization of microbes, and causes membrane damage to pathogens. The complement system consists of almost 30 serum proteins that can be activated by: the classical pathway (discussed in Chapter 11), which is activated by certain antibodies bound to antigens (that is, it works in concert with adaptive humoral immunity); the alternative pathway, which is activated on microbial cell surfaces in the absence of antibody; or the lectin pathway, which is activated by the binding of plasma mannose-binding lectin (MBL) to mannose residues in microbial proteins and polysaccharides but not in mammalian molecules (Figure 3-15).

The names classical pathway and alternative pathway arose because the classical pathway was discovered and characterized first, but the alternative pathway is phylogenetically older. Many of the lectin pathway components are shared with the classical pathway. Although the complement activation pathways differ in how they are started, all of them lead to the generation of enzyme complexes capable of cleaving the third complement (C) protein C3. Once they

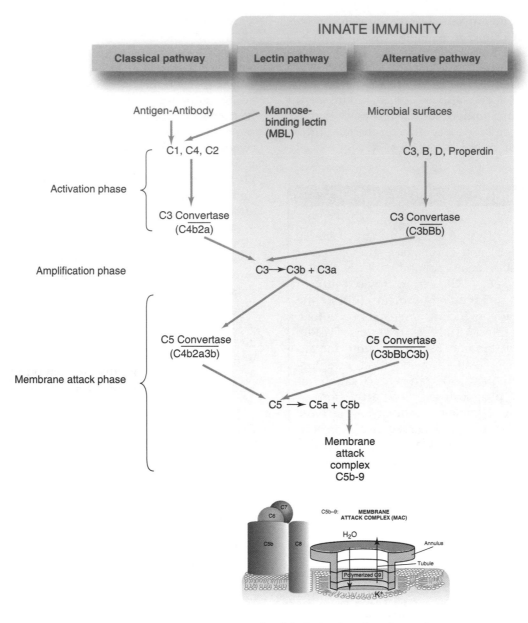

**FIGURE 3-15 Three complement activation pathways.** All three pathways generate C3 convertase, which leads to C5 convertase and C5b and the remaining complement components (C6, C7, C8, and C9) forming the membrane-attack complex. Innate immune system complement activation (lectin and alternative pathways of complement activation) is in the absence of specific antibodies (classical pathway [see Chapter 11]), which are generated during adaptive immune responses.

converge, if the cascades go to completion, it forms a channel called the *membrane-attack complex* across the outer membrane of Gram-negative bacteria, killing the bacteria.

The **alternative pathway** constitutes the component of natural defense against infections that can operate without antibody participation (see Chapter 11). Activation of the alternative complement pathway is considered a nonspecific activation of the complement cascade. The alternative pathway is triggered by microbial polysaccharides or endotoxin contained in the cell membranes of Gram-negative bacteria, protozoa, or yeasts and teichoic acid from cell-wall compartments of Gram-positive bacteria. This pathway can occur in body fluids rather than on a cell surface and does not require the presence of the antigen-antibody complex. It can crudely discriminate between microbial cells and self-tissues and activate a number of powerful antimicrobial responses.

In addition to activating lytic mechanism that can directly kill pathogens, breakdown components of complement are recognized by receptors on macrophages and neutrophils that augment phagocytosis of bacteria. For example, bacteria that have C3b bound to their surface are said to have undergone **opsonization** (see Figure 3-10). Two other complement receptors found on neutrophils, mast cells, and NK cells bind to inactive C3b (iC3b). C3b and iC3b receptor-dependent phagocytosis of microorganisms is an important defense mechanism against systemic bacterial and fungal infections.

The process of complement activation during an infection produces intermediates, the **anaphylatoxins** C3a and C5a, which can induce or enhance inflammation. C3a receptors are expressed on basophils, mast cells, smooth muscle cells, and lymphocytes. C5a receptors are expressed on mast cells, basophils, neutrophils, monocytes/macrophages, and endothelial cells. When soluble complement intermediate molecules bind to their receptor on a particular cell, they invoke a response. For example, C3a and C5a can cause the release of mediators (such as histamines) from tissue-resident mast cells that increase vascular permeability, which enhances inflammation. C5a causes neutrophil activation and acts as a chemoattractant.

As in the alternative pathway, the binding of microbial polysaccharides to circulating plasma lectins MBL triggers the **lectin pathway** of complement activation in the absence of antibody (see Chapter 11). MBL binds to mannose residues on polysaccharides, and because it is structurally similar to a subunit of the first complement component C1, C1q, it triggers the complement system either by activating the C1 serine esterase complex (like C1q) that cleaves C4 or by associating with another serine esterase, called *mannose-binding protein-associated serine esterase (MASP)*, which also cleaves C4. Apart from being activated without antibody (like the alternative pathway), the reminder of the lectin pathway is the same as the classical pathway.

In sum, the complement system is protective in three general ways:

- Its early steps stimulate the inflammatory response. (In fact, the intimacy is extraordinary. The DNA consensus elements binding transcription factors activated by some proinflammatory cytokines are also found in the promoters of several complement genes—you "turn on" one, you "turn on" on the other.)
- Its intermediate steps release substances that attract phagocytic cells and render them highly active.
- Once activated, the complement system leads to the assembly of lytic complexes that cause lysis of invading microorganisms.

## Cytokines, Signaling Proteins That Recruit, Coordinate, Activate, Control Defensive Cells, Induce Inflammation, and Then Turn Off These Responses or Prod the Adaptive Immune System for a Specific Attack

**Cytokines**, a class of molecules functionally similar to hormones that mediate signaling between cells; they have a vital role in communication between different immune system cells. Cytokines are regulatory and effector molecules that act at picomolar concentrations usually at close range on cytokine receptors expressed by target cells. Cytokines are involved in signal transduction; they activate genes for growth, differentiation, and cell activity. They play a primary role in mediating the host's defense against internal and external antigenic insults. Cytokines can be derived from any cell, immune or nonimmune. Only Type I IFNs α and β and the proinflammatory cytokines TNF-α, interleukin-1 (IL-1), IL-6, CXC-chemokine ligand 8 (CXCL8; formerly called *IL-8*), and IL-12 are discussed below; cytokines are detailed in Chapter 9.

**TABLE 3-3** Classification of Interferons

| Interferon | Cellular source | Inducer | Other name |
|---|---|---|---|
| IFN-α | B and T lymphocytes and macrophages | Viruses, polyribonucleotides, tumors, chemicals | Type I, viral |
| IFN-β | Fibroblasts | Viruses, polyribonucleotides, chemicals | Type I, fibroblast |
| IFN-γ | T lymphocytes and NK cells | Antigens, T-cell mitogens | Type II, immune |

### Interferons Are Cytokines That Mediate Antiviral Effects

In 1957, Alick Isaacs and Jean Lindenmann found an interesting substance produced by cells that had been infected with virus. This substance, which they called **interferon** (IFN; because it interferes with viral replication), protected other cells from infection with the same or unrelated viruses. According to present research, IFNs are still the only natural substance with the distinctive ability to inhibit intracellular viral replication.

There are several kinds of IFN (Table 3-3), each made by a different cell type. Interferon-α (IFN-α) is produced by leukocytes; interferon-β (IFN-β) is produced by fibroblasts (a type of cell in tissues); and interferon-γ (IFN-γ), which also is called *immune interferon*, is produced by antigen-sensitized T cells.

Interferons are small proteins produced by eukaryotic cells in response to viral infection or dsRNAs, RNAs (viral or synthetic). The infected cell produces IFN for a few hours, even for a day, but

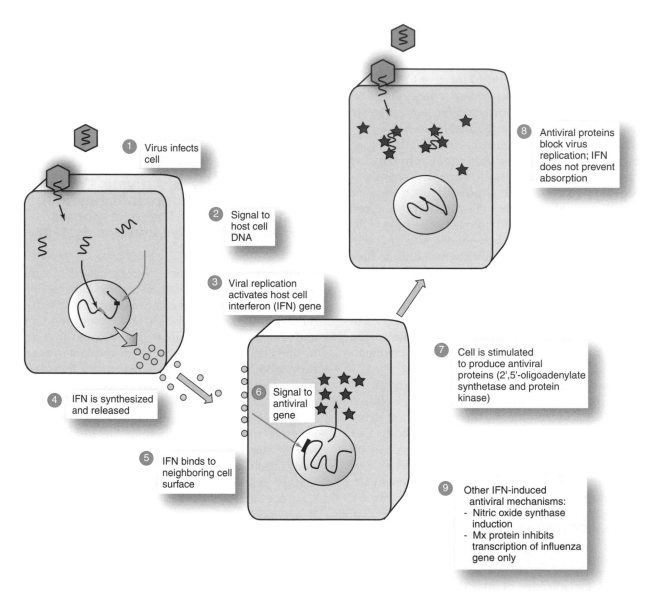

**FIGURE 3-16 The molecular basis of interferon's antiviral activity.** Virus infection-induced IFN-α and -β synthesis activates antiviral mechanisms in neighboring uninfected cells, which enables them to resist viral infection. IFNs activate two genes with direct antiviral activity: a 2′5′-oligoadenylate synthetase that activates a latent endoribonuclease capable of degrading viral RNA, and a protein kinase that inhibits the phosphorylation of e1F-2 and blocks translation of proteins.

the IFN production does not save the cell producing it. Interferon is excreted and used by other cells. When these cells become infected with virus, the IFN causes the cells to produce molecules that prevent replication of the infecting virus (Figure 3-16) (see Chapter 9).

Interferons prime cells to respond to viruses. Interferons α and β act on an uninfected cell by binding to receptors on the cell surface, causing the cell to synthesize another protein that remains in the cell and protects it from infection by all other viruses. The overall effect is the inhibition of viral gene transcription by degradation of mRNA and the induction of RNA-dependent protein kinase production that inactivates protein synthesis. In this way, the cycle of virus replication is interrupted, and either the infection is halted or the process is slowed down sufficiently to enable the specific immune response to eliminate the infecting virus. Specifically, IFN first induces the production of a molecule called *2,5-oligoadenylate synthetase*. If a cell that has interacted with IFN, and is producing 2,5-oligoadenylate synthetase, becomes infected with virus, the virus activates the enzyme to produce 2,5-linked oligoriboadenylate. The presence of this compound in turn activates a preexisting, inactive molecule called *endoribonuclease L* that degrades viral mRNA and thus inhibits viral protein synthesis. Interferon-γ stimulates macrophages to produce antimicrobial agents such as nitric oxide, a molecule with antiviral activity in IFN-activated macrophages. Two other antiviral proteins are induced by IFN: a protein kinase and a molecule called *Mx*. The protein kinase phosphorylates an initiation factor called $e1F_2$, and its phosphorylation inhibits viral protein synthesis by blocking elongation of dsRNA. The Mx protein acts on influenza virus mRNA by inhibiting its transcription and translation.

Interferons lack virus specificity because they do not react directly with the virion but instead induce a general antiviral state in host cells. Conversely, IFNs are species-specific with respect to the species of cells that produced them; that is, they induce little or no resistance in cells from other species. Thus, human IFN is most effective in protecting human cells and poorly protective for mouse or chicken cells. Similarly, mouse IFN has no action on chicken or human cells.

Interferon is also capable of promoting the natural cytotoxic activity of NK cells and activates macrophages and dendritic cells. However, the primary protective role of IFNs is against naturally acquired viral infections, because IFNs are produced locally and more promptly than specific antibodies.

## Proinflammatory, or Inflammation-Promoting, Cytokines Orchestrate Inflammation

**Tumor necrosis factor-α (TNF-α)** is the primary cytokine that mediates inflammation. TNF-α is mainly produced by activated macrophages at the site of infection. TNF-α produces two types of changes in the cells lining the blood vessels. One effect is a vascular swelling, or increase in the diameter of the venules. This leads to increased blood flow, hence the heat and redness (erythema) associated with inflammation. Associated with vascular swelling is an increase in vascular permeability leading to a leakage (edema) of fluids and macromolecules into the extravascular space. The increased leakage leads to an increase in antibodies, complement, and other important serum molecules. A second effect is the induction of vascular endothelium to express adhesion molecules (such as E-selectin) that can lead to extravasation (cells actively move out of the blood vessels) of monocytes and leukocytes (discussed below). In combination with the chemokine CXCL8 (discussed shortly), TNF-α induces neutrophils to be more cytotoxic.

TNF-α also has systemic effects. It causes fever by interacting with the regulator mechanism in the hypothalamus of the brain. If systemic bacterial infection induces TNF-α, the local effects are spread throughout the blood vascular system. The result is a loss of plasma volume due to increased vascular permeability. This leads to shock, disseminated-intravascular coagulation with depletion of clotting factors and consequent bleeding, multiple organ failure (from loss of clotting factors), and death. Along with IL-1 and IL-6, TNF-α promotes the acute phase response leading to the production of acute phase proteins (discussed shortly).

Many cytokines are now designated as **interleukins** (between leukocytes). **Interleukin-1 (IL-1)**, produced mainly by activated macrophages, acts locally to activate vascular endothelium, and to stimulate chemokine production by endothelial cells and macrophages. Like TNF-α and IL-6, IL-1 acts systemically to induce the production of acute phase proteins by the liver, and on the hypothalamus to increase body temperature.

**Interleukin-6 (IL-6)**, produced mainly by macrophages, acts locally to increase adaptive humoral immunity, and it has a large number of systemic effects. It is produced in response to microbes and to IL-1 and TNF-α, and it causes hepatocytes to produce and mobilize acute phase proteins (see discussion of acute phase response below) into the blood circulation.

**TABLE 3-4** Major Proinflammatory Cytokines TNF-$\alpha$, IL-1, and IL-6 and Their Effects

| Effect | TNF-$\alpha$ | IL-1 | IL-6 |
|---|---|---|---|
| Increased vascular permeability | + | + | + |
| Increased adhesion molecules on vascular endothelium | + | + | − |
| Synthesis of acute phase proteins by liver | + | + | + |
| Induction of IL-6 | + | + | − |
| Induction of CXCL8 | + | + | − |
| Fibroblast growth | + | + | − |
| Platelet production | − | + | + |
| Fever induction (endogenous pyrogen) | + | + | + |

The combination of IL-1 and IL-6 causes, in addition to fever and an acute phase response, neutrophil mobilization from the bone marrow and changes in fat and muscle metabolism to help increase body temperature. Most of these effects contribute to antipathogen immunity: Increased body temperature does little to decrease bacterial and viral replication; activation of macrophages causes more cytokine production (increasing inflammatory responses) and increased antigen-presenting activity; increased numbers of neutrophils aid in combating bacteria; and the acute phase proteins along with complement components are antibacterial. The activities of TNF-$\alpha$, IL-1, and IL-6 are summarized and compared in Table 3-4.

**Interleukin-12 (IL-12)**, a monocyte/macrophage-dendritic cell-derived cytokine, is induced by bacteria, bacterial products, bacterial DNA, and intracellular parasites. It directs the generation of a subset of helper T cells to produce IFN-$\gamma$, which enhances the cytotoxicity of NK cells. It is also considered a proinflammatory cytokine because it augments TNF-$\alpha$ activity and induces nitric oxide production. Because of these activities, it can be considered the jump-starter of inflammatory (and adaptive cell-mediated immune) responses.

Another group of cytokines contribute to antimicrobial activity; they are called **chemokines**. Chemokines are small, secreted proteins that are synthesized by T cells, macrophages, vascular endothelial cells, and other cells and are mainly involved in leukocyte chemoattraction but also induce changes in leukocyte adhesion molecules enabling firm attachment of leukocytes to endothelial cells at an infection site. **CXC-chemokine ligand 8 (CXCL8)** is a member of the chemokine family of cytokines (see Chapter 9). CXCL8 contributes to extravasation (escape of cells from the blood into tissues) by binding to CXC-chemokine receptor 1 (CXCR1)- or CXCR2-expressing neutrophils and activating them to express adhesion molecules. There are many human chemokines, which are produced in response to bacterial products and viruses.

## MINI SUMMARY

Internal defense mechanisms include chemical barriers that consist of soluble mediators. These mediators, which play important roles in the internal defense mechanisms of a host, include complement and cytokines. Complement plays an important role in resistance against infection and is a principal soluble mediator of antimicrobial inflammatory responses. There are three overall pathways of complement activation, two are involved in innate immunity, the alternate pathway and the lectin pathway. Cytokines are soluble proteins produced and secreted by sensitized cells. These include interferons, small proteins that inhibit intracellular viral replication. Their primary role is to protect against naturally acquired viral infections. Other cytokines such as TNF-$\alpha$, IL-1, IL-6, IL-12, and CXCL8 mediate nonspecific protection through the induction of microbicidal activities associated with inflammation (next topic of discussion).

# THE BIOLOGICAL DEFENSES, RECRUITMENT AND PROMOTION OF PROFESSIONAL PHAGOCYTES, RECOGNIZE AND KILL PATHOGENS BUT DO NOT SPARE SELF-TISSUES

If a pathogen has survived the preceding barrage of innate immune elements, particularly the professional "eating cells" with broad specificity for different classes of microbes, it now faces its strongest challenges: the inflammatory response, a complex group of reactions that is initiated by chemical mediators whenever phagocytic cells are attempting to prevent infection.

## Guided Leukocyte Migration and Resulting Inflammation, the Seek-and-Destroy Mission of the Immune System

Leukocytes circulate continually throughout the body using the blood and lymph systems, and they actively migrate into tissues at the site of infection. This continual movement (recirculation) assures that the maximum number of antigen-naïve cells will be activated by antigen (such as pathogens) irrespective of what part of the body an infection occurs, and these antigen-activated cells will migrate to sites to remove pathogens aggressively. Billions of motile leukocytes continually recirculate from the blood to tissues and then into lymph to the lymphoid organs. A versatile, coherently functioning system of intercellular soluble and cell-based communication molecules navigates these cells along their pathways. This pattern of movement is critical to the development of an inflammatory response. Inflammation is another component of the internal innate defenses, which consists of a complex group of reactions initiated by chemical mediators whenever phagocytosis alone fails to prevent infection. The process of inflammation is summarized in Figure 3-17.

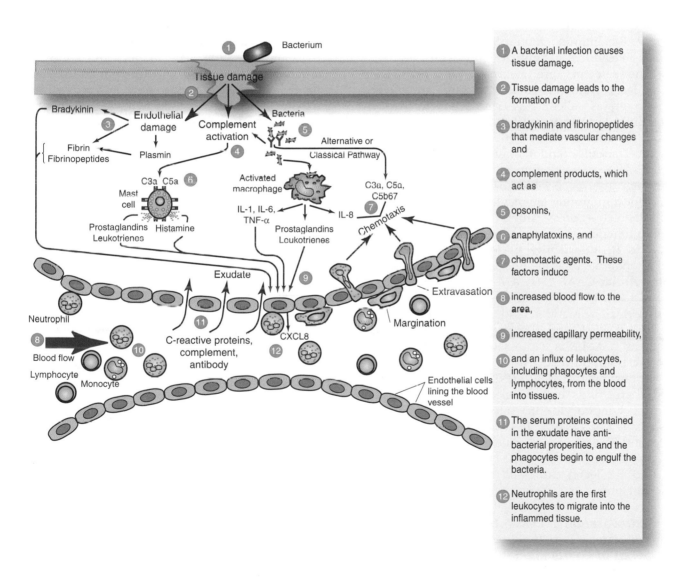

**FIGURE 3-17 Overview of a local acute inflammatory response**. Inflammation is the response of tissues to injury, with the function of bringing serum molecules and immune system cells to the site of infection damage.

### The Guideposts, Cell-Adhesion Molecules, Inform Innate Immune Cells Where to Exit into Extralymphoid Tissues and Sites of Inflammation

In order that circulating leukocytes enter inflamed tissue or peripheral lymphoid organs, they must adhere to, and pass through, the endothelial cells lining the walls of blood venules. This process is called **extravasation** (or *diapedesis*). Leukocyte-specific **cell-adhesion molecules (CAMs)** expressed on the vascular endothelium control leukocyte trafficking from the blood into the surrounding tissues. Some CAMs are express constitutively; others are induced by localized concentrations of inflammatory cytokines or activated cells. Recirculating leukocytes display CAM receptors, thereby allowing them to extravasate into the tissues. Most CAMs fall into four families: the selectin family, integrin family, the immunoglobulin (Ig) superfamily, and mucin-like addressin family (Figure 3-18).

The **selectins** are a group of three CAMs with lectin domains that can bind to specific carbohydrates called *sialyl-Lewis$^X$*, which are usually linked to **mucin-like molecules**. *P-selectin* (*CD62P*) and *E-selectin* (*CD62E*) are expressed on the vascular endothelium, whereas *L-selectin* (*CD62L*) is expressed on most circulating leukocytes. Selectins are responsible for the early stickiness that slows migrating leukocytes. Different leukocyte populations express **integrins**, α- and β-chain heterodimeric proteins, allowing these cells to bind to **Ig-superfamily CAMs** displayed by vascular endothelium. Ig-superfamily CAMs include **intercellular-CAM 1** (**ICAM-1**), *ICAM-2, ICAM-3, vascular-CAM (VCAM)*, and *mucosal adhesion CAM-1* (*MAdCAM-1*). ICAM-1 and VCAM are induced by TNF-α, IL-1, and IFN-γ at inflammatory sites, whereas ICAM-2 is expressed constitutively. With the exception of MAdCAM-1, the other CAMs bind to various integrin molecules. MAdCAM-1, a mucin addressin, binds both L-selectin and integrins. It controls lymphocyte entry into mucosa. The mucins, also called *vascular addressins*, display ligands to selectins. The neutrophil mucin-like CAM *P-selectin glycoprotein ligand 1* (*PSGL1*) molecule binds to E- and P-selectin expressed on inflamed vascular endothelium.

### Extravasation of Cells into Tissues Is a Regulated Multistep Process Involving a Series of Coordinated Interactions Between Leukocytes and Endothelial Cells

The production of inflammatory cytokines and other mediators at the site of inflammation instigates the appearance of CAMs on the local blood venules. This vascular endothelium, said to be *inflamed* or *activated*, is one form of the specialized endothelium that allows cells to undergo extravasation, the process by which cells migrate across the endothelium into tissues. The other specialized endothelium, directing lymphocyte extravasation, is the postcapillary high-endothelial venules (HEVs) of the lymph nodes and Peyer's patches of the gut; as discussed in Chapter 2. As such, the inflammatory response and normal lymphoid recirculation are related events that involve a regulated interaction between neutrophils or lymphocytes, and the vascular endothelium.

The leukocyte/lymphocyte-vascular endothelium interactions and subsequent extravasation involve a series of sequential, overlapping steps, each of which confers specificity to the process and determines whether a particular cell will be targeted for the tissue in question. Neutrophils are usually the first cells to be activated by an inflammatory response, causing them to attach to inflamed endothelium, penetrate it, and migrate into the extravascular tissue. Monocytes and eosinophils undergo a similar process. Neutrophil extravasation can be divided into four steps: (1) attachment and rolling, (2) activation, (3) arrest and adhesion, and (4) extravasation (Figure 3-19). The steps begin with E-selectin-dependent primary adhesion to vascular endothelium through neutrophil expressed mucin-like CAMs. This loose adhesion leads to brief tethering, detachment, and retethering, the neutrophil tumbles end-over-end along the endothelium, thus called *rolling*. During rolling, neutrophils are activated by chemoattractive molecules called *chemokines* such as CXCL8. The chemokine binds to neutrophil receptors triggering an integrin-mediated firm adhesion to Ig-superfamily endothelium CAMs and the neutrophils' *arrest*. Now firmly attached to endothelial cells, the neutrophils penetrate the vessel wall.

### Microbe Internalization by Phagocytic Cells Triggers Proinflammatory Signals Initiating a Salutary but Tissue-Damaging Acute Inflammatory Response

Inflammation consists of localized and systemic responses. The mechanisms of innate immunity are summarized in Table 3-5. Inflammation of a particular body region is indicated by the suffix *-itis*; for example, inflammation of the tonsils is called *tonsillitis*, and inflammation of the appendix is called *appendicitis*. The five cardinal signs of inflammation were first described roughly 2000 years ago. The five distinct symptoms that accompany **acute**, or

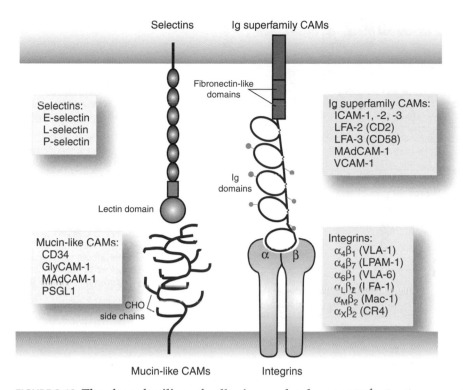

**FIGURE 3-18 The four families of adhesion molecules, general structures, and selected members**. Cell adhesion molecules (CAMs) drive the movement of circulating leukocytes to peripheral lymphoid tissues and inflamed tissues, a process called *extravasation*. Selectins are a group of three separate but closely related CAMs present on leukocytes (L-selectin [CD62L]), activated endothelium (E-selectin [CD62E]), and on platelets and activated endothelium (P-selectin [CD62P]) that bind to mucin-like CAMs, a group of heavily glycosylated serine- or threonine-rich proteins (e.g., CD34, GlyCAM-1, and PSGL-1 [P-selectin glycoprotein ligand; CD162])—the binding between leukocytes and endothelium directs leukocyte recirculation and promotes leukocyte activation. The selectins are a single-chain glycoprotein with a similar modular structure that includes an extracellular calcium-dependent lectin domain. Integrins are a family of cell surface receptors that are transmembrane glycoproteins consisting of noncovalent heterodimers (two subunits, α and β). They are physiologically important because they participate in cell-cell and cell-matrix adhesion. Integrins are activated by chemokines to bind with high affinity to ligands. There are two main integrin subfamilies; members of each family express a conserved β chain ($\beta_1$, or CD29, and $\beta_2$, or CD18) associated with different α chains. Leukocytes usually expressed the $\beta_2$ subfamily of integrins, which bind to cell-surface ligands called *intercellular CAMs (ICAMs)*, e.g., ICAM-1 (CD54), -2 (CD102), -3 (CD50), and VCAM (CD106) expressed on vascular endothelial cells. ICAMs are members of the immunoglobulin (Ig) superfamily so they are also called *Ig-superfamily CAMs*. MAdCAM-1 contains both mucin- and Ig-like domains, is expressed on mucosal endothelium, and directs lymphocyte movement into mucosa.

short-term, **inflammation** are redness, swelling, heat, pain, and following severe episodes the loss of function. Inflammation collectively involves a series of vascular events that serve as a defense mechanism. Inflammation includes (1) clotting mechanism activation, (2) increased blood flow, (3) increased capillary permeability, and (4) enhanced influx of phagocytic cells. Initiated within minutes of physical trauma or bacterial infection, this process leads to increase in vascular diameter (vasodilation), thereby increase of blood volume to the area—the cause of heat and tissue redness. Vascular permeability also increases and leads to leakage of fluids into the extravascular space (edema), particularly at postcapillary venules. In some instances, this causes extravasation of leukocytes, which contributes to the swelling and redness

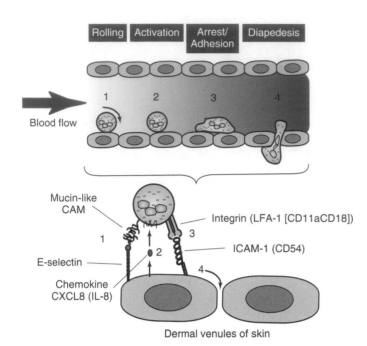

**FIGURE 3-19 The movement of cells out of the blood vessels and into the tissues (extravasation).** Usually, neutrophils are the first cells to appear at the site of a local acute inflammatory response, followed by monocytes (convert to macrophages in tissues) and lymphocytes. There are four sequential, overlapping steps in neutrophil extravasation. Cell-adhesion molecules and chemokines are involved in the first three steps of neutrophil extravasation.

in the area. The leakage of fluid from the bloodstream activates the kinin, clotting, and fibrinolytic systems (Figure 3-20). Many of the early-localized vascular changes are due to direct and indirect effects. Plasma enzyme mediators like bradykinin and fibrinopeptides induce vasodilation and increased vascular permeability directly, whereas complement anaphylatoxins (C3a and C5a) mediate vascular changes indirectly. The anaphylatoxins induce local mast cell degranulation with release of histamine, which is a potent mediator of inflammation, causing vasodilation and smooth-muscle contraction. Following cell damage or vascular endothelial damage, membrane phospholipid metabolism also leads to the generation of other mediators like prostaglandins and leukotrienes, which can also contribute to the vasodilation and increased vascular permeability.

A fundamental activity of the inflammatory response is the activation of neutrophils, causing them to migrate from the blood vasculature to the extravascular tissues. They are recruited by tissue-resident macrophages that have been sampling their surrounding environment. Neutrophils are the most abundant of the leukocytes. Even though they have a half-life of only hours, their high numbers and phagocytic ability make them essential in combating

the constant barrage of infectious organisms. Therefore, within hours of the onset of vascular changes, neutrophils adhere to the endothelial cells of the postcapillary venules, migrating out of the blood into the extravascular spaces (see Figure 3-19). Here they phagocytose the invading pathogens and release mediators that amplify the inflammatory response. The mediators recruit monocytes that are converted to activated macrophages in the inflammatory site. The activated macrophages arrive roughly 6 hours after an inflammatory response begins. As activated cells, they exhibit increased phagocytosis and an increased release of mediators and cytokines that continue to amplify the inflammatory response. The cytokines include TNF-$\alpha$, IL-1, and IL-6; they induce many of the localized and systemic changes observed in the acute inflammatory response (see Table 3-4). Locally, all three cytokines induce coagulation and an increase in vascular permeability, by generating increased expression of adhesion molecules on vascular endothelial cells. TNF-$\alpha$ stimulates expression of E-selectin, an endothelial adhesion molecule that selectively binds neutrophils; IL-1 induces increased expression of ICAM-1 and VCAM-1, which bind to integrins on lymphocytes and monocytes. Circulating neutrophils, monocytes, and lymphocytes adhere to a blood vessel wall by recognizing these adhesion

**TABLE 3-5 Summary of Innate Immunity Mechanisms**

| Barriers | Mechanism |
|---|---|
| *Mechanical* | |
| Skin | A mechanical barrier that restricts microbial entry |
| | Acidic environments that retard microbial growth |
| Mucous membrane | Mucus entraps microbes |
| | Cilia propels microbes out of body |
| | Normal microbiota competes with pathogens for binding sites and nutrients |
| *Physiologic* | |
| Temperature | Normal body temperature inhibits the growth of some pathogens |
| | Increased body temperature (fever) inhibits the growth of some pathogens |
| Oxygen tension | Host areas that have high oxygen content inhibit the growth of some pathogens |
| pH | The stomach's acidic pH kills most ingested microbes |
| Chemical mediators | Lysozyme degrades bacterial cell wall |
| | Complement components lyse microbes or facilitates their phagocytosis |
| | Interferon induces antiviral protection in uninfected cells |
| | Cytokines that amplify cytotoxic, phagocytic, and inflammatory barriers; and induce fever |
| *Cytotoxic* | |
| | Natural killer (NK) cells can directly kill virally infected cells, and release cytokines that amplify phagocytic and inflammatory barriers |
| *Phagocytic* | |
| Neutrophils | Chief early phagocytic cells that internalize, kill, and digest microbes but die in the process |
| Macrophages | Chief late phagocytic cells that act as neutrophils but unlike them they do not die and have important functions in specific immunity |
| Dendritic cells | Specialized phagocytic cells with limited microbe-clearing ability but highly efficient APCs |
| *Inflammatory* | |
| | Vascular leakage allows antibacterial serum proteins into infected tissue |
| | Mediators that attract phagocytes and enhance their activity in affected areas |

molecules and then move through the vessel wall (extravasation) into the tissue spaces.

TNF-α and IL-1 also act on macrophages and endothelial cells, inducing production of the chemokine CXCL8. CXCL8 contributes to the neutrophil influx by increasing their adhesion to vascular endothelial cells and by acting as a chemotactic factor. Other cytokines, such as IFN-γ, serve as chemotactic factors for macrophages, thereby bringing increased numbers of phagocytic cells to the site of antigen deposition. In addition, IFN-γ and TNF-α activate macrophages and neutrophils, promoting increased phagocytic activity and increased release of lytic enzymes into the tissue spaces. The result is an influx of cells that participate in clearance of the organism and healing of the tissue.

During clearance of the pathogen, an **acute phase response (APR)** can occur, which involves a shift in the levels of various proteins secreted by the liver into blood. In APR, levels of some plasma proteins decrease, while levels of others increase. This response—to infection, burns, trauma, and neoplasia—alters the blood sedimentation rate, which was once the common measure of whether a patient was sick.

TNF-α, IL-1, and IL-6 are produced by activated macrophages, that is, macrophages that have been stimulated by LPS, C5a, or chemokines. TNF-α and IL-1 induce heptocytes to produce one set of **acute phase proteins** including serum amyloid protein, whereas IL-6 induces another set including fibrinogen, C-reactive protein, and mannose-binding protein. TNF-α and IL-1 activate the coagulation system by altering the balance of the procoagulant and anticoagulant activities of vascular endothelium.

IL-6 causes hepatocytes to produce and mobilize two important acute phase proteins into the blood circulation. These two acute phase proteins are important because they mimic the action of antibodies (see Chapter 4). The acute phase protein, *C-reactive protein* (mentioned earlier), is a member of the *pentraxin* protein family, which binds to phosphorylcholine on microbial surfaces (but not mammalian cells) to opsonize the microbe and initiate the complement cascade. A second protein, *mannan-binding protein* (also mentioned earlier), is a member of a structurally related family of proteins, called *collectins* (lectins with collagen domains). This calcium-dependent lectin binds to mannose moieties on bacterial surfaces. It can act as an opsonin for

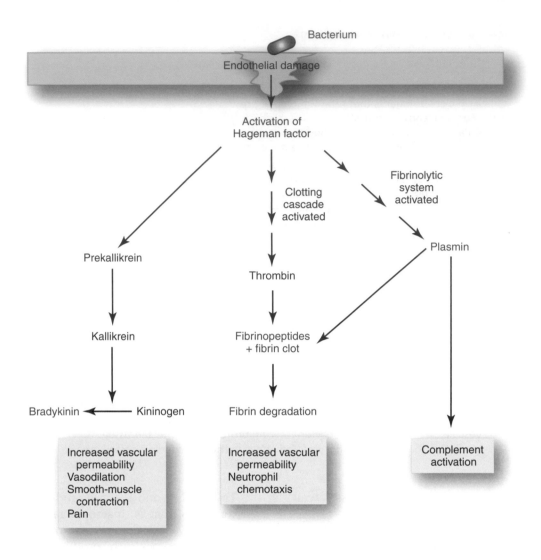

**FIGURE 3-20 Induction of plasma enzyme mediators.** Inflamed tissue activates the kinin, clotting, and fibrinolytic systems, leading to the production of plasma enzyme mediators. These mediators cause vascular changes that augment inflammation directly or indirectly (the latter situation arises when plasmin not only degrades fibrin clots but also activates the classical complement system).

monocytes (but not macrophages) and can initiate the complement cascade. These two acute-phase proteins mimic some of the properties of antibodies before an antibody response has a chance to become established. Within a day or two, these two proteins provide a primitive yet effective recognition system for the immune system to distinguish a broad range of microbes from mammalian cells and to effectively deal with them. Additionally, C-reactive protein or IL-6 concentration is used as an indicator of illness.

The final stage of inflammation is tissue repair, when all harmful agents or substances removed or neutralized at the inflammation site. The ability of a tissue to repair itself depends in part on the tissue involved. Skin, being a relatively simple tissue, has a high capacity for regeneration. But nerve tissue in the brain, which is highly specialized and complex, appears to regenerate very slowly. Taken together, inflammatory barriers are innate immunity's most effective means to prevent the entrance and establishment of infectious agents.

## MINI SUMMARY

Phagocytic cells destroy invading microorganisms. They need to migrate from the blood into the site microbe infection. The innate immune response relies on a precise temporal and spatial positioning of neutrophils within infected tissues. Tissue-resident macrophages that have sampled the invading microbes, and the organisms themselves, release chemotactic molecules called *chemokines*, thereby recruiting and positioning the neutrophils at the site of infection and shaping their functional properties. Precision and specificity in this process are achieved by varying patterns of chemokine receptors and cell adhesion molecules expressed on the cell surface of neutrophils and endothelial cells. Chemokine-recruited and positioned neutrophils are a key component of inflammatory activity during the clearing of pathogens—phagocytosis can trigger inflammation. Inflammation and fever are complex responses by a host against microbial infection. It is a response that results from tissue injury and involves increased blood supply to the site of injury, increased capillary permeability, movement of leukocytes from the capillaries into the surrounding site, and finally repair of the infected tissue.

# SUMMARY

The immune system is classified into two subsystems: the innate and adaptive immune systems. Innate immunity is considered a nonspecific response but is immediate, whereas the adaptive immunity is a specific response but takes time. The *innate immune system* (or *innate immunity*) is the most ancient and most common form of host defense against infection. As "innate" implies, it is immunity that preexists and functions independently of a microbial invader. The reactions to foreign invaders, *immune responses*, of the innate and adaptive systems lead to protection that is called *immunity*. They are tightly interwoven systems; vertebrates cannot survival without either.

Constitutive host factors such as nutrition, age of the host, physical and emotional stresses, and genetic factors influence host resistance to infection by pathogens.

Innate immune system can be divided into external and internal defenses. The external first-line defenses, exposed to the outside environment, are mechanical barriers, which include skin and mucous membranes. Unbroken skin is impervious to most microorganisms, but it also produces sebum that maintains the skin pH levels low enough to be inhibitory to most microbes. Skin-resident microorganisms produce *bacteriocins*. The mucous membrane covers most areas throughout the body, such as, the respiratory, alimentary, and urogenital tracts with a sticky substance (traps microbes) that contains antimicrobial agents. These agents include *lysozyme*, *defensins* and *cathelicidins*, *lactoferrin*, *fibronectin*, and *β-lysin*. Respiratory tract cilia sweep mucus-entrapped microbes upward to the throat. Normal microbiota usually out-compete pathogens.

Immune system, whether innate or adaptive, revolves around some core elements, which includes recognition of the pathogenic invader, killing the recognized pathogen, and ignoring host tissues and cells. This recognition relies on a limited number of germline-encoded (hard-wired) receptors called *pattern recognition receptors* (*PRRs*), which recognize conserved microbial-associated products expressed by microbial pathogens, called *pathogen-associated molecular patterns* (*PAMPs*), but not by the host. Thus, innate immune system sensors can only target microbes; this inability is not the case with adaptive immunity. PAMPs are the microbes' "molecular signatures" that are essential for their survival; therefore, if a pathogen tries to lose or mutate its PAMPs it would be lethal to the microorganism. PRRs can be extracellular (secreted or cell surface-associated) or intracellular (vesicle membrane-associated or in the cytosol) molecules such as soluble *mannose-binding lectin* (*MBL*), *C-reactive protein* (*CRP*), *serum amyloid protein* (*SAP*), and *LPS-binding protein* (*LBP*); the cell-based receptors include *scavenger receptors*, *mannose receptors*, *Toll-like receptors* (*TLRs*; they can be extracellular or intracellular molecules), *nucleotide-binding oligomerization domain* (*NOD*) *proteins*, and the retinoic-acid-inducible gene I (RIG-I)-like receptor (RLR) family, *RID-I* and *melanoma differentiation-associated gene 5 (MDA5)* (intracellular molecules found in the cytosol of the cell).

The TLRs are the most important sensors of the innate immune system because they initiate inflammatory and immune responses. The extracellular portions of TLRs, *leucine-rich repeats* (*LRRs*), recognize PAMPs. The ligand match ups for TLRs are, TLR1 + lipopeptides, TRL2 + lipopeptides and peptidoglycan, TLR3 + dsRNA, TLR4 + LPS, TLR5 + flagellin, TLR6 + lipopeptides and zymosan, TLR7 + single-stranded RNA, TLR8 + single-stranded RNA, and TLR9 + CpG-containing DNA. Each TLR is endowed with a *Toll/IL-1 receptor* (*TIR*) *domain* motif that serves as signaling adapter when TLR are engaged with ligand. This engagement leads to the activation of signaling pathways that induce antimicrobial genes and inflammatory cytokines. For signaling to occur, there must be dimerization of TLRs. Stimulation of dendritic cell TLRs triggers their maturation and leads to increased antigen-presenting capacity and the induction of costimulatory molecules. Thus, microbial recognition by TLRs activates innate immune killing mechanisms and helps to direct adaptive immune responses to pathogen-derived antigens.

Once pathogens breach external defenses, the host's internal defense is largely dependent on professional phagocytic cells that engulf and destroy pathogens; they include *neutrophils, macrophages, dendritic cells (DCs)*, and *natural killer (NK) cells*. The two major groupings of phagocytic cells are called *polymorphonuclear phagocytes* and *mononuclear phagocytes*. NK cells fall into neither of these groups. All of these cells express PRRs.

Neutrophils, macrophages, and DCs mediate microbial killing by *phagocytosis* (cell-eating), which is the receptor-dependent engulfment of large particles and microorganisms, internalization into large intracellular vesicles, and subsequent killing by multiple mechanisms. *Endocytosis* is mediated by all cells and involves the vesicular uptake of fluid and macromolecules. *Exocytosis* is the process by which cells release unused molecules contained in membrane-bound vesicles when the vesicle fuses with the plasma membrane. Neutrophils and macrophages are considered the professional phagocytes; DCs are considered paraprofessional phagocytes, that is, they are not as efficient at clearing pathogens but more efficient at processing antigen for presentation to T cells.

The *polymorphonuclear phagocytes*, the *neutrophils*, are of key importance in the containment of infection. They are short-lived, specialized killers, endowed with a broad array of weapons with which to destroy their microbial prey. Even though they are stand-alone phagocytic cells, they function better in the presence of proteins made by the humoral arm of the adaptive immune response, that is, bacteria coated (*opsonization*) with bacteria-specific antibodies.

The *mononuclear phagocytes* are the blood *monocyte-derived* **macrophages**, and the closely related *dendritic cells (DCs)*, some of which are also of monocyte origin. Macrophages are distributed throughout the host's body so that macrophages will rarely be far away from the invasive microorganism. Macrophages are a heterogenous population of cells; they are morphologically diverse cells that need to be activated to mediate their primary functions, which include enhanced phagocytosis and killing of pathogens, enhanced production of inflammatory mediators, and increased expression of class II MHC molecules (they are antigen-presenting cells [APCs]). Even though macrophages are important scavenger cells capable of phagocytosis and killing of microbes, their most important functions may be supervisory. Through the elaboration of chemotactic cytokines, they recruit neutrophils to the site of infection. Like macrophages, DCs exhibit a variety of guises (such as the *Langerhans cells* of the skin and the *plasmacytoid dendritic cells* of the blood). Even though DCs are in the minority among the phagocytes, they are the most efficient at presenting antigen to naïve T lymphocytes by class II MHC molecules—they are the premier APCs. Macrophages also are APCs. Thus, macrophages and DCs, using TLRs to recognize microbes, can direct adaptive immune responses to antigens derived from microbial pathogens.

Another important cell of the innate immune system is the nonphagocytic NK cell. NK cells are specialized lymphocytes that provide a first line of defense through their ability to kill virus-infected host cells. Unlike cytotoxic T cells of adaptive immunity, NK cells cannot mount a memory response when re-exposed to the same viral antigen; however, because they are constitutively or "naturally" present cells their response is immediate. NK cell function is tightly controlled by a fine balance of inhibitory and activating receptor signals as well as mediated by proinflammatory cytokines. NK-cell inhibitory receptors bind self-MHC class I molecules, which blocks activating signals leading to killing; however, the absence of self-MHC class I molecules removes the block thereby leading to killing. This feature enables them to limit the spread of viruses that subvert innate and adaptive immune defenses by selectively down-regulating the expression class I MHC molecules.

The innate immune system continues its protection using chemical mediators that boost and regulate cellular defenses and induce inflammation. The principal mediators are *complement* and *cytokines*. Microbes or their products can induce the *alternative* and *lectin pathway of complement activation*, which leads to a cascade reaction producing complement components that opsonize microorganisms, are chemotactic for neutrophils, induce inflammation, and cause lysis of microorganisms. Cytokines are the major group of chemical messengers of host defense, in that they regulate communication between innate immune system cells, between adaptive immune system cells, and immune cells between the two systems. Cytokine production is not limited to immune cells; nonimmune cells can make them and response to them. The primary groups of cytokines associated with innate immune responses include *interferons* (IFN-α and -β), which inhibit viral replication, activated NK cells, macrophages and DCs, and augment APC activity and cytokines that clearly promote inflammation are called *proinflammatory cytokines* and *chemokines*. The proinflammatory cytokines include *TNF-α, IL-1, IL-6, and IL-12*, if administered to humans, they produce augmented cell activity, tissue destruction, inflammation, and fever. Some cytokines, such as IL-12, augment not only innate immunity but also drive adaptive immunity by the production of IFN-γ. An example of a proinflammatory chemokine, small chemotactic cell-activating cytokines, is *CXCL8* (formerly called *IL-8*).

The causal relationship between innate immunity and inflammation is widely accepted—it is the price of innate immune responses. The description of inflammation's sequential development follows. Pathogenic microbe insult into the body leads to tissue damage, which instigates a multifactorial network of chemical signals that initiate and maintain a host response designed to "heal" the injured tissue. In turn, the immune response attempting to clear the pathogen furthers tissue damage, the combine effect is known as *acute inflammation*. It involves activation and directed migration of first neutrophils, followed by monocytes from the venous system to sites of pathogen deposition. Chemotactic cytokines, named *chemokines*, recruit neutrophils and dictate the natural progression of the inflammatory response. For neutrophils, a four-step mechanism of recruitment to sites of infection is initiated by tissue-resident activated macrophages and microbe-released products, the overall process involves (1) attachment and rolling, (2) activation, (3) arrest and adhesion, and (4) *extravasation* (migration of cells across the endothelium into tissues). These steps include: activation of a sequential series of *cellular adhesion molecules* (*CAMs*), particularly *selectins* (*L−*, *E−*, and *P-selectin*), integrins (such as, *intercellular adhesion molecule 1* [*ICAM1*]), and *addressins* (such as, *P-selectin glycoprotein ligand 1* [*PSGL1*]), which eventually leads to neutrophil transmigration through the endothelium to sites of infection. To expedite pathogen elimination, during inflammation, an *acute phase response* occurs, which entails the production of *acute phase proteins* (such as *C-reactive protein* and *mannose-binding lectin*) by the liver. These molecules act as opsonins by activating the complement system. Pathogen clearance leads to tissue repair and resolution of inflammation.

# SELF-EVALUATION

## RECALLING KEY TERMS

Acute Inflammation
Acute phase proteins
  C-reactive protein (CRP)
Acute phase response (APR)
Cell-adhesion molecules (CAMs)
Chemokines
  CXCL8 (formerly IL-8)
Complement
  Alternative pathway
  Lectin pathway
Cytokines
Dendritic cells
Endocytosis
Exocytosis
Extravasation
Immunity
Immune response
Leucine-rich repeats (LPPs)
Lipopolysaccharide (LPS)-binding protein (LBP)
Lysozyme
Macrophages
Mannose-binding lectin (MBL)
Mannose receptors
Natural killer (NK) cell
Neutrophils
Nucleotide-binding oligomerization domain (NOD)
  proteins
Opsonization
Pathogen-associated molecular patterns (PAMPs)
Pattern recognition receptors (PRRs)
Phagocytosis
Proinflammatory cytokines
  Interferons (IFN-α, -β, and -γ)
  Interleukin-1 (IL-1)
  Interleukin-6 (IL-6)
  Interlukin-12 (IL-12)
  Tumor necrosis factor-α (TNF-α)
Scavenger receptors
Serum amyloid protein (SAP)
Toll-like receptors (TLRs)

## MULTIPLE-CHOICE QUESTIONS

1. Innate immunity mediates its activities directly through all of the following except (a) natural killer cells, (b) chemical barriers, (c) tears, (d) T lymphocytes, (e) inflammation (f) phagocytosis, (g) none of these. (*See pages 63 to 65*)

2. All of the following are characteristics of innate immunity, except it is (a) nonspecific, (b) rapid,

(c) inducible, (d) absent of immunologic memory, (e) constitutive, (f) none of these. *(See pages 63 to 65)*

3. Phagocytosis is preceded by (a) a respiratory burst, (b) extravasation, (c) antigen (such as a pathogen) binding to phagocyte, (d) integrin binding to ICAMs, (e) chemotaxis, (f) none of these. *(See pages 81 to 83.)*

4. Differences between innate and adaptive immunity include (a) innate immunity is specific, whereas adaptive immunity is nonspecific, (b) adaptive immunity includes the ability to distinguish self from non-self, whereas innate immunity does not, (c) innate immunity does not possess immunologic memory, whereas adaptive immunity does, (d) adaptive immunity does not include an antibody response, whereas innate immunity does include this response, (e) none of these. *(See pages 71 and 72.)*

5. The following are all mechanisms used by the innate immune system that prevent the penetration of pathogens into the host's tissues, except (a) the skin, (b) physiological barriers (pH, temperature), (c) alternative complement pathway, (d) cilia of the respiratory tract, (e) normal flora of digestive tract, (f) a and b, (g) a and c, (h) b and c, (i) none of these. *(See pages 66 to 70.)*

6. Natural killer (NK) cells (a) kill target cells that express low levels of class II MHC molecules, (b) are induced to kill virus-infected cells through carbohydrate-bind receptors, (c) kill target cells that express high levels of class I MHC molecules, (d) need to interact with antigen-presenting dendritic cells to kill target cells, (e) are none of these. *(See pages 86 and 87.)*

7. Selectins (a) are used by neutrophils to kill Gram-negative bacteria, (b) are expressed on neutrophils and vascular endothelium, (c) are integrins that can bind ICAMs, (d) include ICAM1, ICAM2, and ICAM3, but not VCAM, (e) are all of these, (f) are none of these. *(See pages 94 and 95.)*

8. Inflammation, caused by pathogens crossing epithelial barriers and establishing infection, is presented as the following symptoms. (a) an increase in cell flow to the site of infection, (b) an increased vascular permeability at the site of infection, (c) redness at the site of infection, (d) swelling at the site of infection, (e) a and b, (f) c and d, (g) all of the above, (h) none of these. *(See pages 93 to 98.)*

9. The process of neutrophils leaving the blood to enter a site of infection is called (a) trafficking, (b) opsonization, (c) chemotaxis, (d) migration, (e) none of these. *(See pages 95 and 96.)*

10. Pathogen-associated molecular patterns (PAMPs) are/can be (a) molecules shared by a certain class of microbes, (b) flagellin, (c) lipopolysaccharides (LPS), (d) molecules necessary for survival of microorganisms, (e) all of these, (f) none of these. *(See pages 63 and 71.)*

## SHORT-ANSWER ESSAY QUESTIONS

1. Why do you think some scientists consider innate immunity more important than adaptive immunity?

2. Why do you think humans are resistant to canine distemper and dogs are not?

3. What is meant by predisposing factors of host resistance?

4. Discuss external and internal innate defenses. How do the skin and the mucous membrane form effective barriers to infectious agents?

5. Why would you think that the defense mechanisms in the urogenital tract are unable to protect an individual from a sexually transmitted disease like gonorrhea?

6. What are some of the specific chemical substances secreted by the body that are unfavorable for microbial growth or even killing invading microorganisms?

7. Describe the activation of the alternative and lectin complement system.

8. What is the mechanism of phagocytosis in neutrophils? In macrophages? Why might the body have two phagocytic cell systems?

9. What do you predict would be the consequence of an individual with a neutrophil deficiency, or a C5a deficiency?

10. What is the function of NK cells? Why are they important?

11. Briefly describe the major events in the acute inflammatory response.

12. The cardinal signs/lesions of inflammation are redness, swelling, heat, pain, and loss of function. What are the benefits of these lesions?

13. Give reasons for the symptoms manifested by the inflammatory response.

14. What do you think the benefits of an acute phase response are? Disadvantages to this response?

15. If fever is induced to provide protection, why do we usually try to reduce it when we are sick?

# FURTHER READINGS

Akira, S. and K. Takeda. 2004. Toll-like receptor signaling. *Nat. Rev. Immunol.* 4:499–511.

Akira, S. and K. Takeda. 2004. Toll-like receptor signaling. *Nature Rev. Immunol.* 4:499–511.

Akira, S., S. Uematsu and O. Takeuchi. 2006. Pathogen recognition and pathogen immunity. *Cell* 124:781–801.

Beutler, B. 2004. Innate immunity: An overview. *Molecular Immunol.* 40:845–859.

Brown, E.J., and H.D. Gresham. 2003. Phagocytosis. In *Fundamental Immunology*, 5th ed. W.E. Paul, ed. Philadelphia: Lippincott Williams & Wilkins. p. 1105–1126.

Carroll, M.C. 1998. The role of complement and complement receptors in induction and regulation of immunity. *Ann. Rev. Immunol.* 16:545–568.

Colonna, M., G. Trinchieri, and Y-J. Liu. 2004. Plasmacytoid dendritic cells in immunity. *Nat. Immunol.* 5:1219–1226.

Imhof, B.A. and M. Aurrand-Lions. 2004. Adhesion mechanisms regulating the migration of monocytes. *Nat. Rev. Immunol.* 4:432–444.

Iwasaki, A. and R. Medzhitov. 2004. Toll-like receptor control of the adaptive immune responses. *Nat. Immunol.* 5:987–995.

Kawai, T. and S. Akira. 2006. Innate immune recognition of viral infection. *Nat. Immunol.* 7:131–137.

Kiyoshi, T., T. Kaisho, and S. Akira. 2003. Toll-like receptors. *Annu. Rev. Immunol.* 21:335–376.

Kumagai, Y., O. Takeuchi, and S. Akira. 2008. Pathogen recognition by innate receptors. *J. Infect. Chemother.* 14.86–92.

Lanier, L.L. 2005. NK cell recognition. *Annu. Rev. Immunol.* 23:225–274.

Lemaitre, B. 2004. The road to toll. *Nat. Rev. Immunol.* 4:521–527.

Levy, O. 2007. Innate immunity of the newborn: Basic mechanisms and clinical correlates. *Nat. Rev. Immunol.* 7:379–390.

Medzhitov, R. 2003. Innate immune system. In *Fundamental Immunology*, 5th ed. W.E. Paul, ed. Philadelphia: Lippincott Williams & Wilkins. p. 497–518.

Medzhitov, R., and C. Janeway, Jr. 2000. Innate immunity. *New Engl. J. Med.* 343:338–344.

Nathan, C. 2006. Neutrophils and immunity: Challenges and opportunities. *Nat. Rev. Immunol.* 6:173–182.

O'Neill, A.J. 2005. Immunity's early warning system. *Sci. Amer.* 38–45.

O'Neill, L.A.J. and A.G. Bowie. 2007. The family of five: TIR-domain containing adaptors in Toll-like receptor signaling. *Nat. Rev. Immunol.* 7:353–364.

Pisetsky, D.S. 1996. Immune activation by bacterial DNA: A new genetic code. *Immunity* 5:303–310.

Rosenberg, H.F., and J.I. Gallin. 2003. Inflammation. In *Fundamental Immunology*, 5th ed. W.E. Paul, ed. Philadelphia: Lippincott Williams & Wilkins. p. 1151–1170.

Shortman, K. and S.H. Naik. 2007. Steady-state and inflammatory dendritic-cell development. *Nat. Rev. Immunol.* 7:19–30.

Strober, W., P.J. Murray, A. Kitani, and T. Watanabe. 2006. Signaling pathways and molecular interactions of NOD1 and NOD2. *Nat. Rev. Immunol.* 6:9–20.

Taylor, P.R., L. Martinez-Pomares, M. Stacey, H-H. Lin, G.D. Brown, and S. Gordon. 2005. Macrophage receptors and immune recognition. *Annu. Rev. Immunol.* 23:901–944.

Uematsu, S. and S. Akira. 2006. Toll-like receptors and innate immunity. *J. Mol. Med.* 84:712–725.

Ulevitch, R.J. 2004. Therapeutics targeting the innate immune system. *Nat. Rev. Immunol.* 4:512–520.

Zhang, X., and D.M. Mosser. 2008. Macrophage activation by endogenous danger signals. *J. Pathol.* 214:161–178.

# CHAPTER FOUR

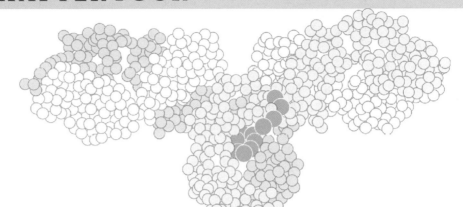

# ANTIGENS AND ANTIBODIES

*Immunology: Understanding the Immune System, Second Edition*, by Klaus D. Elgert
Copyright © 2009 John Wiley & Sons, Inc.

a. All antibody classes have either λ or κ light chains.
b. IgG is the major antibody in the blood, but it is able to enter tissue spaces and coat antigens, speeding antigen uptake.
c. IgA concentrates in body fluids to guard the entrances of the body.
d. IgM is the largest antibody; it tends to remain in the blood, where it can lead to efficient killing of bacteria.
e. IgD remains membrane-bound and somehow regulates the cell's activation.
f. IgE is found in trace amounts in the blood, but it still triggers allergies.

**9.** The C domains mediate the biological effector functions of antibodies.

## OBJECTIVES

The reader should be able to:

**1.** Differentiate between an antigen's inductive and reactive abilities.
**2.** Explain the factors that bestow immunogenicity on molecules.
**3.** Describe the discrete and distinctive sites on an antigen that is recognized by the immune system.
**4.** Understand what haptens are and how they can be used to test the specificity of antibodies.
**5.** Explain how antigenic determinants can be studied; describe their size; and discuss some important characteristics of protein antigenic determinants.
**6.** Understand how the characterization of antibody structure led to the comprehension of antibody function.
**7.** Distinguish between the overall structure and the fine structure of antibodies.
**8.** Describe the variable and constant regions of an antibody's light and heavy chains.
**9.** Explain the organization of the variable regions of an antibody's light and heavy chains; define complementarity-determining regions and domains.
**10.** Name and compare the biological and chemical characteristics of the five classes of antibodies.
**11.** Discuss the differences in the biological effector functions of antibodies.

An overview of immunity, in Chapter 1, of the major players in immunity, in Chapter 2, and of the conserved antigen recognition, in Chapter 3, set the stage for an exploration of immunology and how the immune system can prevent disease or, alternatively, how it can cause or aggravate disease. The immune system recognizes many different "foreign" substances (or *antigens*) and can distinguish them from those substances native to the body. The ability to recognize a specific foreign antigen and distinguish self from nonself is the essence of the immune response. The immune system specifically recognizes antigen through receptors on B and T cells. These cells recognize different kinds of antigens, and they recognize antigens in very different ways. This chapter emphasizes the properties and characteristics of antigens

needed to induce an antibody response and the structure and function of molecules, the antibodies, which are induced. The T cell's interaction with antigen is detailed in Chapters 8 and 10.

An **antigen** (Gr. *anti-*, against; and *gen*, of *gignomai*, to generate), *when introduced into a host, induces the formation of specific antibodies and T lymphocytes that are reactive against the antigen.* The definition for antigen is *operational*; a substance is called an *antigen* only when it induces a particular response, whether positive induction (formation of an antibody or sensitized T cell) or negative induction (no formation of an antibody or sensitized T cell). Irrespective of positive or negative induction, many substances that are introduced into the body, such as foods and drugs, do not cause antibodies or sensitized T cells to form and thus are not antigens. An antigen can be a bacterium, a fungus, a parasite, or a virus. Most tissue or cells from other individuals act as antigens. Antigens are usually proteins or polysaccharides or combinations of the two; lipids and nucleic acids usually do not induce formation of antibodies or sensitized T cells. Antigens can be introduced into the body through many routes: intradermal, subcutaneous, intramuscular, intravenous, intraperitoneal, and orally.

## ANTIGENS MAY EXHIBIT IMMUNOGENICITY AND ANTIGENICITY

The immune system protects against pathogens but cannot distinguish between good and bad invaders; all invaders are recognized as foreign or nonself. Antigens can be distinguished by two properties: (1) they *induce* an immune response and (2) they *react specifically* with the elements of the immune system they induce. The only exceptions are small molecules called *haptens*. They are a special kind of antigen that will be discussed later in the chapter.

*The ability of a substance (the antigen) to induce humoral (antibodies) or cell-mediated (activated T cells) immunity is called* **immunogenicity**. The inducing substance is called an **immunogen**. However, a given substance may or may not elicit an immune response, depending on the status of the immune system. Soluble proteins or polysaccharides can elicit humoral immunity. In contrast, only proteins (and some lipids or glycolipids) elicit cell-mediated immunity because they are not recognized directly but must be broken down to small peptides that are displayed together with MHC molecules on a cell's membrane.

*The ability of a substance to react with the specific antibodies (or activated T cells) that it induces is called* **antigenicity**. In this context, the substance is more appropriately called an *antigen*. An antigen also is immunogenic if it can induce the formation of antibodies and activated T cells. Although not every biologic molecule is immunogenic, almost every kind can be antigenic, whether small or large or polysaccharide, protein, lipid, or nucleic acid. Therefore, all immunogens are antigens but not all antigens are immunogens. Customarily, the term antigen is used to describe either the two properties (immunogenicity and antigenicity) or the reactivity (binding to immune system elements).

## AN ANTIGEN HAS FOUR SPECIFIC FEATURES

Antigens capable of stimulating an immune (antibody) response have at least four common characteristics: (1) high molecular weight, (2) chemical complexity, (3) solubility (biodegradability), and (4) foreignness.

1. *Usually, only macromolecules are immunogenic. The larger the molecule, the more immunogenic it is likely to be.* A general rule is that molecules with a molecular weight of 5000 or greater are immunogenic. Some substances with low molecular weights are antigens (such as insulin, with a molecular weight of 5700), but no minimum threshold molecular weight exists that leads to lack of immunogenicity. Substances weighing less than 1 kD (such as L-tyrosine-p-azobenzene arsonate, 400 molecular weight) are weakly immunogenic. Even though macromolecules can be immunogenic, their building blocks (amino acids, nucleotides, fatty acids, lipids, and monosaccharides) are normally not immunogenic. Later in the chapter, we will address the conundrum of how these building-block molecules can react with specific antibodies yet not be immunogenic.

2. *Immunogenic molecules require some degree of chemical complexity and heterogenicity.* Large substances lacking chemical complexity, such as nylon, polyacrylamide, and Teflon, are not immunogens. Regardless of their size, polypeptides that are homopolymers with repeating units of a single amino acid are not immunogenic. Immunogenicity increases with amino acid residue diversity. Globular proteins consisting of the 20 different amino acid residues have a complex composition and demonstrate multiple levels of organization (primary, secondary, tertiary, and quaternary). The complexity of these molecules is caused by their chemical composition and by the spatial arrangements of the amino acids because amino acid order determines three-dimensional folding. Aromatic amino acids contribute to immunogenicity significantly more than do nonaromatic residues. The chemical composition and spatial arrangements of globular proteins make them the most potent immunogens, followed by polysaccharides. The immunogenicity of polysaccharide antigens also depends on the three-dimensional conformation of their epitopes, but their conformation is affected by the extensive side-chain branching through glycosidic bonds.

3. *Intact antigens are broken down into immunogenic pieces.* Cells must interact with antigens before humoral or cell-mediated immunity can be induced. T cells cannot react directly with antigen yet they are required to help B cells produce antibodies to most antigens; therefore, antigen must be processed and presented associated with MHC molecules. Antigen-presenting cells degrade the substances in a manner that enhances the immunogenicity of the antigenic substance; this is called *antigen processing* (see Chapter 7).

4. *Immunogens must be recognized as foreign.* Immunogenicity is an operationally dependent property; the immune system must recognize a molecule as foreign, or nonself to mount an immune response. Generally, the greater the phylogenetic distance between the species being immunized and the source of the molecule used for immunization, the more immunogenic the molecule. There are exceptions; highly conserved molecules such as collagen and cytochrome c are poorly immunogenic across species. On the flipside, there are also exceptions with self-antigens, such as, corneal tissue and sperm, which are considered antigens sequestered from the immune system. If these antigens are inoculated into the host of origin, they can be immunogenic. The host is normally unresponsive to self-antigen. This inability to react, or tolerate, self-antigens occurs during lymphocyte development (it will be discussed in Chapter 8).

Whether an antibody response, or an immune response in general, develops, the type of immune response that develops, and the magnitude of an immune response is dictated by additional parameters (Table 4-1). The chemical and physical nature of an antigen has profound effects on the immunogenicity of an antigen. For example, the chemical complexity of a protein antigen will dictate the concentration and the class of antibody produced. Polysaccharide and lipid antigens induced humoral immunity; antibodies of the IgM class predominate (these types of antigens are unable to associated with MHC

**TABLE 4-1 Factors That Affect Primary Antibody Response Development**

| |
|---|
| Chemical and physical nature of the antigen |
| Dosages of antigen |
| Frequency of antigen exposure |
| Route of antigen exposure |
| Use of adjuvants |
| Genetic makeup of the host receiving the antigen |

molecules; therefore, T cells are not involved). In contrast, protein antigens induced both humoral and cell-mediated immune responses. If it is a humoral response, it leads to antibody class switching, affinity maturation, and memory cell development (discussed later and detailed in Chapter 6). Responses against antigens with low immunogenic potency (such as proteins rich in D-amino acids) can be amplified if the antigen persists in the host's tissues. The dosage of antigen can affect the development of the primary antibody response, and the smallest effective dose depends on the method of administration. Minute or excessive doses can cause specific unresponsiveness (tolerance). The frequency of antigen exposure and the routes of administration (environmental exposure versus injection) also affect the development of the primary antibody response. Repeated small injections of a toxoid evoke a greater antibody response than does one injection of the same total amount. The route of antigen exposure influences immune responses, intradermal (i.d.; into the skin)/subcutaneous (s.c.; beneath the skin) or intramuscular (i.m.; into the muscle) administration of antigens is collected by draining lymph nodes and leads to immunogenic responses. Antigen administered intravenously (i.v.) (into a vein) are collected in the spleen, where the beginnings of a humoral response occur; however, i.v. and orally administered antigens can induce tolerance and allergic reactions.

The immune response can be modified to enhance the antibody or cell-mediated immune response against antigens. **Adjuvants** (L. *adjuvere*, to help) are substances mixed with antigen before injection, which nonspecifically enhance or modify the immune response to that antigen. Adjuvants are a heterogeneous group of substances. In general, they enhance the immunogenicity of protein antigens by converting soluble proteins into particulate forms, which enhances phagocytosis and by administering a bacteria or bacterial product with the antigen, which enhances local inflammation reactions. Adjuvants can consist of cell-wall constituents (the active constituent is muramyl dipeptide) from acid-fast bacteria (*Mycobacterium tuberculosis*), Gram-negative bacteria such as *Bordetella pertussis*, and bacteria of the *Brucellae* group. Other adjuvants can consist of alum (aluminum sulfate), mineral oil, lanolin, detergents (surface active agents), acrylic particles, and polynucleotides such as polyinosinic-polycytidilic (poly IC).

The most popular adjuvant is Freund's adjuvant. **Complete Freund's adjuvant** is prepared by mixing mineral oil, lanolin (a detergent to disperse the oil into small droplets), and heat-killed *M. tuberculosis*

**TABLE 4-2 Mechanisms of Action of Adjuvants**

1. Increased phagocytic uptake, become better APCs (increased class II MHC and costimulatory molecule expression), and local delayed release of antigen (depot effect)
2. Delayed destruction and elimination of antigen
3. Lengthened contact of antigen with immunocompetent cells
4. Local granuloma formation
   a. Migration of leukocytes to site of antigen localization
   b. Increase in the number of leukocytes involved

**MINI SUMMARY**

For an antigen to induce an immune response (immunogenicity), it must usually be a nonself, complex molecule of high molecular weight that can be degraded by certain types of immune cells. Once the antigen has induced an immune response, it can react with the immune elements it induced (antigenicity). There are additional biologic parameters such as the dose and route of antigen exposure, the inclusion of adjuvants, which enhance immunogenicity, with antigen, and the genotype of the host, all can affect immunogenicity.

(to induce strong granuloma formation), then adding a saline solution of test antigen and emulsifying the mixture. The result is a viscous milky-white emulsion consisting of droplets of antigen surrounded by oil. **Incomplete Freund's adjuvant** is prepared in the same manner as complete adjuvant but *M. tuberculosis* is left out. Adjuvants are given subcutaneously or intradermally to avoid systemic granuloma formation. The mechanisms of action of adjuvants are summarized in Table 4-2. The major difference between complete and incomplete Freund's adjuvant seems to be the population of CD4$^+$ T cells it activates. Complete Freund's adjuvant activates $T_H1$ (inflammatory) cells, probably through the bacterial components invoking macrophage production of IL-12. Incomplete Freund's adjuvant induces activation of $T_H2$ (helper) cells.

Granuloma formation, a by-product of muramyl dipeptide activity, occurs at the site of adjuvant inoculation after several days. First, fibroblasts, monocytes, macrophages, lymphocytes, and giant cells are seen. Within a few days, the cellularity and vascularity are diminished and fibrous tissue thickens because of more collagen deposits. Granuloma formation causes (1) the migration of leukocytes to this area; (2) an increase in the number of cells involved in the immune response; (3) induction of adenylate cyclase activity (which increases cell permeability and stimulates lymphocytes); and (4) delayed antigen destruction and prolonged antigen retention. The use of adjuvants blends the primary and secondary responses, with a resulting increase in the immune response.

Lastly, a host's genetic constitution plays a major role. If the host does not have the "immune-response" genes, the genes that encode MHC molecules for the antigen's particular antigenic determinants to interact with, a primary antibody response will not occur, even if the substance meets the requirements for immunogenicity (see Chapters 7 and 8).

# ANTIGENIC DETERMINANTS (EPITOPES) ARE THE CONTACT POINTS FOR THE IMMUNE SYSTEM'S ELEMENTS

*A whole antigen does not induce an immune response.* Instead, the cells of the immune system recognize discrete and distinctive sites on an antigen. Antigens can be considered to have two functional regions called the *hapten* and the *carrier*. The haptenic portion of the antigen is made up of sites called **antigenic determinants** (also called **epitopes**). If an epitope is purified in the laboratory and introduced into a host, it alone is not immunogenic; but as part of the rest of the antigen (which acts as a carrier), the epitope becomes immunogenic. *Epitopes are the immunologically active portions of an antigen that can react with antibodies (free and surface-associated) and T-cell antigen receptors (after antigen processing).* Epitopes come into direct contact with the binding sites of antibodies. For complex antigens such as proteins, the interaction between an epitope and an immune element probably involves all four (primary, secondary, tertiary, and quaternary) levels of protein organization. Table 4-3 compares B-cell and T-cell antigen recognition (T-cell recognized epitopes are discussed in Chapters 7, 8, and 10). The presence of at least one epitope makes a molecule an antigen. Interaction of epitopes with elements of the immune system determines the specificity of antigen-receptor reactions. Furthermore, many antigens contain distinct overlapping epitopes. Most amino acid residues on an antigen are not part of the epitopes but rather constitute the carrier portion of the molecule.

The ability of a host to mount an immune response to each determinant is genetically controlled

**TABLE 4-3 Recognition of Antigen by B Cells and T Cells**

| Parameter | B cells | T cells |
|---|---|---|
| Type of antigen recognized | | |
|     Lipids | + | − |
|     Polysaccharides | + | − |
|     Proteins | + | + |
| Properties of the epitope | | |
|     Accessible | + | −(internal) |
|     Shape | Usually conformational | Denatured linear peptides |
|     Amino acids | Hydrophilic | Amphipathic |
|     Mobility | + | −(bound by MHC molecules)* |
| Recognition unit | Ag-Ab complex | TCR-Ag-MHC molecule complex |
| Binding to soluble antigen | + | −(binds to cell surface-associated antigen |
| MHC restriction | − | + (recognizes fragmented antigen presented by MHC molecules) |

*Abbreviations: MHC, major histocompatibility complex; Ag, antigen; Ab, antibody; TCR, T-cell receptor.

(see Chapters 7 and 8). The MHC genes decide a host's ability to respond to an epitope. Although a host may possess the structural genes to produce the right immune response molecules (such as synthesis of a specific antibody), it may not have the necessary MHC genes (such as those to allow the synthesis of the specific antibody). The more antigenic determinants an antigen possess, the greater the probability that the individual will have the "immune response" genes to permit an immune response against some of the determinants.

---

### MINI SUMMARY

An entire antigen molecule does not induce an immune response; instead, antigenic determinants, or epitopes, induce immunity. The more antigenic determinants possessed by an antigen, the more likely and the more diverse the immune response. How and what epitopes a B and T cell recognize are fundamentally different.

---

# HAPTENS, ANTIGENIC BUT NOT IMMUNOGENIC MOLECULES, CAN BE USED TO TEST THE SPECIFICITY OF ANTIBODIES

Antigenic determinants interact first with membrane antibody and induce immunity and then with the cell-free form of the antibody. The specificity of these interactions can be tested by using a small substituent, or *hapten*, on the antigen that induced

the antibody response. In 1921, Karl Landsteiner observed that an alcohol extract of horse kidney failed to induce antibodies when inoculated into rabbits, but antibodies did form against a homogenate of the kidney tissue combined with the extract. However, if he covalently coupled the alcohol kidney extract to a larger carrier, it induced antibody formation. Landsteiner called the small molecules (those that induced antibody formation only when coupled to a larger molecule) *haptens* (Gr. *hapto*, to bind, to fasten). Landsteiner's elegant pioneering studies with haptens clarified our understanding of the specificity of antigen-antibody interactions.

Landsteiner's work also suggested that one could develop adaptive immunity to many biological haptens (such as small organic molecules, small peptides, and steroid hormones) not meeting the standard criteria for immunogenicity. **Haptens** *are defined as molecules that are not immunogenic in themselves but that can react (antigenicity) with preformed antibodies of the right specificity*. Haptens are classified according to how many determinants they have. *Simple haptens* have only one antigenic determinant, whereas *complex haptens* have two or more different antigenic determinants.

How do preformed antibodies originate if haptens are not immunogenic? The answer is that immunity to a hapten is developed by coupling the hapten to a *carrier molecule*, and this hapten-carrier complex is immunogenic. The complex induces immunity that is hapten-specific. Carriers themselves may or may not be immunogenic. If the carrier is immunogenic, the hapten usually modifies the carrier so that the hapten becomes an antigenic determinant. The carrier has its native antigenic determinants as well as the new determinants introduced by the coupled hapten (*pure antigenic determinants are functionally equivalent to haptens)*. A carrier can also be nonimmunogenic if it lacks some of the criteria for immunogenicity. Conjugation of hapten to this carrier confers immunogenicity by making the molecule more complex.

The use of haptens allowed immunologists to test how the immune system recognizes antigens in a specific manner. Karl Landsteiner performed a series of experiments in the 1920s that explained the specificity of antigen-antibody reactions. He prepared antibodies specific for a hapten of known chemical structure. Then he tested whether other haptens of defined structure would cross-react with the original antibodies. From the cross-reactions observed, he concluded that the chemical groups in a hapten and their positions were important in determining how antibodies recognize a haptenic group.

While this text cannot include a detailed description of all of Landsteiner's work, Table 4-4 lists his conclusions after many years of work. In brief, the main way antigenic determinants are recognized is by their chemical structure. The chemical structure of a molecule determines its specificity and its degree of cross-reaction.

## MINI SUMMARY

Landsteiner discovered substances called haptens that are functionally equivalent to antigenic determinants. Haptens can combine with the antibody but cannot induce an immune response unless they are bound to larger "carrier" molecules. A hapten is antigenic but not immunogenic by itself. Landsteiner analyzed antibody specificity using haptens and determined that the level of cross-reactivity suggested the degree of specificity.

**TABLE 4-4** **Landsteiner's Conclusions on Antibody Specificity**

1. Antibodies react most strongly with the homologous hapten (antigen).
2. Cross-reactions show definite patterns that can be related to chemical structure.
   a. The **chemical nature** of the groups on haptens is critical in cross-reactions.
   b. **Position**: when substitutions are made in the same position, cross-reactions occur.
   c. **Size**: when substitutions are made with groups of equal size, cross-reactions are more likely.
   d. **Charge**: if substitutions maintain their electrical charge, cross-reactions are more likely.
   e. **Stereoisomerism**: The immune system can distinguish between the D and L forms of a molecule.

# ANTIGENIC DETERMINANTS OF MACROMOLECULES ACT AS THEIR FINGERPRINTS

Although haptens seem to be equivalent to antigenic determinants, determinants on polysaccharide and protein macromolecules are not seen in the same immunologic fashion. A series of experiments done in the 1960s and 1970s and continuing today with crystallographic studies molecularly defined how antibodies specifically recognize and interact with antigen through antigenic determinants.

## An Antibody-Recognized Epitope Is About 6 Sugar, or 15 to 22 Amino Acid, Residues in Size

One of the simplest polysaccharide antigens is a homopolymer of glucose called *dextran* ($10^4$–$10^5$ kD). It is produced by the bacterial (*Leuconostoc mesenteroides*) degradation of sucrose. Dextran's predominant linkages are α-1,6 glycosidic bonds. Dextran was used to determine the size of polysaccharide antigenic determinants recognized by the immune system. First, rabbits were immunized to get anti-dextran antibodies. Second, dextran was fragmented by acid hydrolysis to get fragments ranging from monosaccharides to the larger oligosaccharides. After hydrolysis, the fragments were separated into monosaccharides, disaccharides, trisaccharides, and so on. Third, the reactivity of anti-dextran antibodies to the purified sugar fragments of defined length was tested. *Thus, the size of the epitope was determined by determining the size of the antibody's antigen-binding site.*

The quantitative inhibition of the dextran-antidextran reaction by the sugar fragments (haptens) revealed the size of the dextran antigenic determinants. Antigenic determinants of dextran consist of six glucose residues (hexasaccharide was the best ligand with antidextran antibodies) in an α-1,6 linkage. The epitope is small (about $34 \times 12 \times 7$ Å), and represents a segment less than 1 kD in a molecule having a molecular weight in the millions. Further studies also concluded that the determinants were repeated (many copies of the same determinant in each dextran molecule). *The epitopes of carbohydrates (or phospholipids) are completely a function of the covalent structure of the molecule caused by extensive side-chain branching, while the epitopes of proteins are a function of both covalent structure and noncovalent folding of the molecule.*

Using homopolymers of amino acids or polymer-protein conjugates as antigens yielded antigenic determinant sizes similar to those for dextran.

When antibodies specific for peptides consisting of 1 to 4 alanine residues and one glycine residue coupled to RNase were reacted with tetrapeptides, the greatest reactivity occurred. Similar kinds of experiments with other polymer-protein complexes showed that antigenic determinants of proteins were made up of 4 to 6 to 8 amino acids. If, however, a structural analysis (x-ray crystallography of antigen-antibody complexes) is used to characterize a protein epitope, it leads to the view that an epitope consists of 15 to 22 residues assembled from residues from several different discontinuous portions of the polypeptide chain. Thus, small protein epitopes and large globular protein antigens bind differently to antibodies. Nonetheless, whether antibodies bind small peptides or larger epitopes on antigens, the antibody's antigen-binding regions are not different.

## Antibody-Recognized Protein Antigenic Determinants Have Four Important Characteristics

Synthetic polypeptides can be used to characterize antigenic determinants because one can vary amino acid composition, spatial arrangement, molecular weight, charge, or molecular conformation; one can then evaluate the significance of these parameters for antigen specificity. Protein fragments obtained by enzymatic digestion also can be used to characterize epitopes.

### Antigenic Determinants Must Be Accessible to Antibodies

Synthetic copolymers were used to characterize antigenic determinants; both their immunogenicity and cross-reactivity of specific copolymers were tested. One of the synthetic multichain copolymers was called *(T,G)-A-L* because it contained L-tyrosine and L-glutamic acid residues attached to multi-poly-DL-alanines that were in turn coupled to a polylysine backbone. This molecule and a similar molecule, A-(T,G)-L, are shown schematically in Figure 4-1. Results from these experiments showed that antigenic determinants must be at the surface to come into contact with immune cells or antibodies. Surface regions of an immunogen induce immunity and can react with specific antibodies. Thus, a cardinal feature of immunogenicity is **accessibility**. *Accessibility implies that antigenic determinants usually consist of hydrophilic amino acid structures on the surface of proteins. These determinants are called topographic determinants.* Along with charge, accessibility may decide why a particular region of an antigen molecule acts as a determinant. This ability to serve as an antigenic determinant is called *immunopotency*.

### Antigenic Determinants May Be Continuous or Discontinuous

The remainder of our discussion on antigens in this chapter will examine the characterization of antigenic determinants on two globular proteins, myoglobin and lysozyme. The oxygen-binding protein sperm whale molecule myoglobin consists of one polypeptide chain with 153 amino acid residues (16.7 kD), and 75% of the residues are rearranged in $\alpha$ helices (Figure 4-2). Anti-myoglobin antibodies were prepared by immunizing rabbits with the native molecule. To identify the antigenic determinants, myoglobin was cleaved into several fragments, the fragments representing the entire molecule were purified, and the reactivity of individual fragments with anti-myoglobin antibodies specific for the intact protein was tested. The results suggested that myoglobin contains five determinants separated by immunosilent regions. Each epitope is small, with a molecular weight between 600 and 1000, and consists of 6 to 10 amino acid residues. Epitope sequences are rich in basic amino acid residues, suggesting that antibody binding with these antigenic determinants is through polar (hydrophilic) interactions and that nonpolar amino acids just stabilize binding by hydrophobic interactions. The epitopes are located on the surface of the molecule in the nonhelical corners (residues 15–21, 56–62, 94–100, 111–120, and 146–153). Five antigenic sites were described for the myoglobin molecule. Each antigenic determinant has a unique amino acid sequence. *Epitopes of this type are called* **continuous**, *or* **linear, determinants** *because the amino acid residues that make up the determinants comprise part of the primary sequence of the polypeptide. These epitopes were located in the flexible regions of the immunogen.* Continuous antigenic determinants are often preserved when an antigen is fragmented. However, this conclusion can lead to confusion because what is called a "continuous" epitope of a protein, in fact, usually is only a portion of a larger discontinuous epitope.

The latest view of the antigenic structure of myoglobin proposed that instead of restricted, single segments (the proposed five sites) of a peptide chain containing sequential residues, the antigenic sites are assembled from several different segments throughout the chain. Thus, the antigenic determinants are topographic; furthermore, any part of the myoglobin's surface may be antigenic, not just the five proposed sites. Furthermore, epitopes immunogenic for antibody production are not the same as those for T-cell responses. For example, residue 109 of myoglobin seems to be a pivotal site recognized by T cells. No antibodies have been identified that bind to this site.

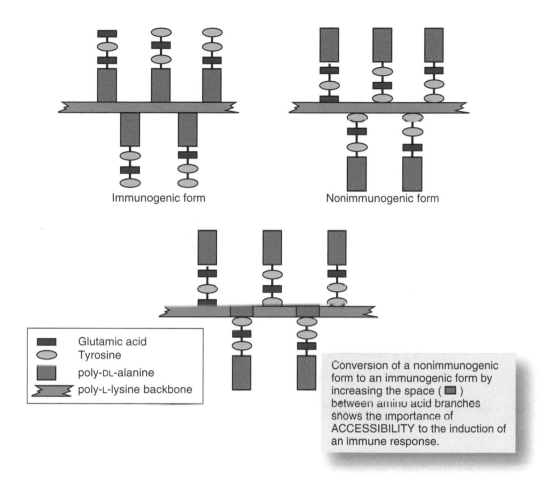

Immunogenic form    Nonimmunogenic form

Glutamic acid
Tyrosine
poly-DL-alanine
poly-L-lysine backbone

Conversion of a nonimmunogenic form to an immunogenic form by increasing the space ( ■ ) between amino acid branches shows the importance of ACCESSIBILITY to the induction of an immune response.

**FIGURE 4-1 Chemical structure of the synthetic multichain copolymer (T,G)-A-L and variant A-(T,G)-L.** Anti-(T,G)-A-L antibodies recognize the tyrosine-glutamic acid portion. Sela constructed a variant with the same composition as (T,G)-A-L but with the chemical formulation A-(T,G)-L. The only difference between the two is that the positions of alanine chains and the tyrosine-glutamic acid copolymer are reversed. In contrast to (T,G)-A-L, A-(T,G)-L is not an immunogen and anti-(T,G)-A-L antibodies do not cross-react with A-(T,G)-L. If A-(T,G)-L has wider spacing among the side chains, this molecule is immunogenic and cross-reacts with anti-(T,G)-A-L antibodies. The A-(T,G)-L molecule has close side-chain spacing; thus, tyrosine-glutamic acids are hidden or masked determinants. (Adapted from M. Sela, 1969. *Science* 166:1365.)

Studies using hen egg-white lysozyme showed that discontinuous antigenic determinants exist. Lysozyme is an enzyme that consists of one polypeptide chain comprising 129 amino acid residues with a molecular weight of 14,500. The determinants of lysozyme are **discontinuous** or **conformational** or, in more contemporary terminology, **assembled topographic determinants**. *These epitopes are made up of amino acids spaced distantly from one another on the polypeptide backbone. The separated regions are brought close together when the molecule folds* (Figure 4-3). Amino acid residues 1 to 12 and 122 to 129 combine to form one of the main surface epitopes of lysozyme. The two distant regions are

brought together when the molecule folds and are held together by a disulfide bridge between cysteines at positions 6 and 127. If the disulfide bonds are broken, the regions separate and the epitope is destroyed. All antigenic determinants of lysozyme are discontinuous because antibodies prepared against the native molecule fail to react with denatured lysozyme.

The first difficulties with earlier interpretations arose when investigators realized that the set of antigenic specificities produced after immunization with the native protein did not represent the entire potential antigenic repertoire—any part of a globular antigen surface has the potential to be antigenic.

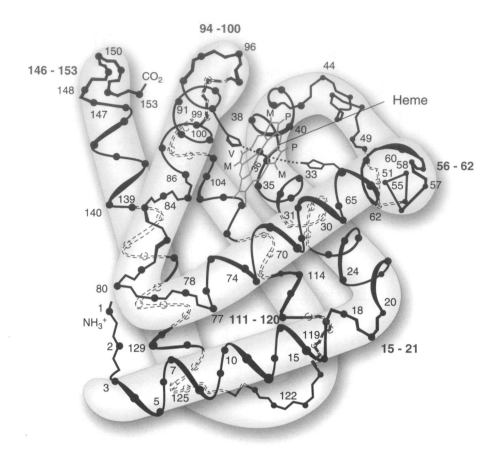

**FIGURE 4-2 Model of the myoglobin chain**. The three-dimensional structure of the myoglobin molecule was determined by crystallographic and amino acid sequence studies. (Adapted from Atassi, M.Z. and A.L. Kazim. 1978. *Adv. Exp. Med. Biol.* 98:9.)

An individual's immune response is directed toward immunodominant sites. This bias can be shown by using monoclonal antibodies. In fact, using monoclonal antibodies suggested that most, if not all, of the hen egg lysozyme surface could be antigenic, *consisting of multiple overlapping determinants*. Other studies using inbred strains of immunized mice suggest that the immune response is biased in any host because the predominant antibodies recognize only a few antigenic sites (*immunodominant epitopes*) on the surface of lysozyme. The immune response depends on the genetic constitution of the recipient and the regulatory interactions occurring during that immune response. Nonetheless, the repertoire of specificities is more diverse than the actual specificity repertoire expressed in a host's serum following immunization. Such results are succinctly summarized in the following statement:

Immunogenicity of an intact protein is less than the sum of the immunogenicity of its pieces. (R.A. Lerner. 1984. *Adv. Immunol.* 36:9.)

### Antigenic Determinants Have Some Amino Acid Residues That Are More Important Than Others

An important antigenic determinant of lysozyme is in the "loop peptide" (amino acid residues 60 to 83) (see Figure 4-3). This determinant establishes that some amino acid residues within a determinant are more important than others. Antibodies were prepared that recognized the loop peptide and several constructed synthetic loops with alanine substituted for different amino acids of the loop. The reactivity of these loops with antibodies specific for native lysozyme revealed the phenomenon called **immunodominance** (Figure 4-4)—some elements of an epitope contribute more to antigenicity than others.

### Antigenic Determinants Are Mobile

Besides *intrinsic* (structural characteristics of antigenic determinants) and *immunoregulatory* (tolerance, immune gene response, and specificity of T-cell help) *mechanisms*, **antigenic site mobility** also has

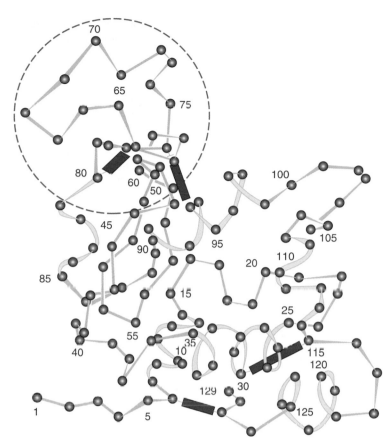

**FIGURE 4 3** **Model of the lysozyme chain** The three-dimensional structure of the lysozyme molecule was determined by crystallographic and amino acid sequence. The dotted circle indicates the loop region. (Adapted from C.C.F. Blake *et. al*. 1965. *Nature* 206:757.)

importance in the immunogenicity and antigenicity of proteins, such as cytochrome c, hemoglobin, insulin, and myoglobin. Antigen site mobility suggests that antigen recognition is a multistep process, which facilitates complementarity between an antibody's binding site and the epitope; it involves side-chain movements of the antigen. Binding can be divided into two phases: (1) precollision orientation of a determinant and an antibody-combining site by electrostatic forces, and (2) the induced fit accomplished by site-specific rearrangement of a determinant and an antibody-combining site structure. Characteristics of determinants recognized by B cell membrane-bound or free antibody are summarized in Table 4-5.

# ANTIGENS INDUCE ANTIBODY FORMATION

In the preceding part of the chapter, antigens as recognized by B-cell immunoglobulin receptors or free

antibody were described.[1] The remainder of the chapter describes the antigen-specific receptors present on B cells and secreted by plasma cells that bind antigens and mark them for destruction by the immune system. Interaction of membrane-bound antibody with cognate antigen induces antigen-specific B-cell proliferation, leading to plasma cells secreting an identical but soluble form of the membrane antibody—antibodies bind antigens in the recognition phase (membrane molecules [B-cell receptors]) and the effector phase (soluble effector molecules) of humoral immunity. Antibody characteristics as soluble molecules will be emphasized. Most antigens are complex macromolecules with numerous epitopes; therefore, they elicit a heterogeneous production of antibodies.

---

[1]We use the term *antigen*, even though *immunogen* may be more accurate at times, as explained earlier in chapter.

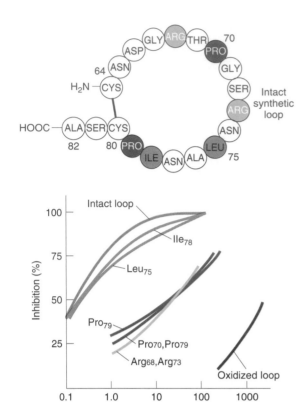

**FIGURE 4-4 Alteration of immune reactivity of the loop peptide of lysozyme.** Replacement of certain amino acid residues by alanine in the synthetic loop peptide reduced immune reactivity of the antibody directed against the native molecule. The synthetic loop similar to native lysozyme reacts most strongly with specific antibodies. Loops containing alanine instead of leucine at position 75, and isoleucine at position 78, reacted almost as well as the correct loop. Leucine and isoleucine residues were of little importance in reactivity with specific antibodies. However, the change of arginine at position 68 or of proline at position 79 profoundly affected the reactivity of the loop with antibodies. When the amino acids in these positions were substituted, they caused changes in the conformation (the manner in which the loop is folded). A change from arginine to alanine (from a positive charge to nonpolar) or from proline to alanine led to a more flexible molecule. Thus, some amino acid residues in an epitope are more important in immunological activity than others. (Synthetic loop adapted from R. Arnon, E. Maron, M. Sala, and C.B. Anfinsen. 1971. *Proc. Natl. Acad. Sci. USA.* 68:1450. Anti-loop inhibition curve adapted from E. Teicher, E. Maron, and R. Arnon. 1973. *Immunochemistry* 10:265.)

*The secreted recognition proteins found in the serum[2] and other body fluids of vertebrates that react specifically*

---

[2]Antibody-containing serum is called *antiserum*, in contrast to *normal serum* (the clear yellowish fluid collected when

## TABLE 4-5 Mini Summary: Characteristics of Antigenic Determinants

1. Antigenic determinants are **small**.
2. *All* of the surface of a protein may be immunogenic and antigenic.
3. Antigenic determinants must be **accessible** and are composed of **assembled topographic determinants**.
4. **Charge** and **polarity** add to antigenic determinant immunogenicity.
5. Antigenic determinants are **conformation-dependent**.
6. Antigenic determinants have **immunodominant building blocks**. Factors such as *conformation* and *accessibility* are important in determining immunodominance.
7. **Antigen site mobility** contributes to protein antigenicity.
8. An individual's immune response to a protein antigen (1) is dictated by its genetic makeup, (2) depends on the structural differences between the antigen and the recipient's self-proteins, and (3) depends on the immunoregulatory mechanisms operating in that individual's immune system.

---

*with the antigens that induced their formation are called* **antibodies**. Antibodies belong to a family of globular proteins called **immunoglobulins**. The terms *antibody* and *immunoglobulin* are used interchangeably throughout this text. *Immunoglobulins, however, are defined as a family of globular proteins that comprise antibody molecules and molecules having patterns of molecular structure (antigenic determinants) in common with antibodies.* The term *immunoglobulin* can be used to refer to any antibody-like molecule, regardless of its antigen-binding specificity.[3]

# THE STRUCTURE OF AN ANTIBODY IS RELATED TO ITS FUNCTION

The function of an antibody is to bind foreign or nonself molecules—antigens, neutralizing them or signing them up for removal. The host can produce a vast array of antibodies that are structurally similar (all are Y-shaped molecules) yet unique. This

---

whole blood is separated into its solid and liquid parts) that does not contain antibody to a specific antigen.

[3]MHC molecules and T-cell antigen receptors are the other two kinds of molecules used by the immune system to recognize antigen. Their role in antigen recognition is discussed in Chapters 7 and 8, and 10, respectively.

variability was a startling finding, because all other protein molecules made by an individual are identical; they all have the same amino acid sequence. However, antibodies come in millions of different amino acid sequences and are the most diverse proteins known (see Chapter 6).

*The chemical structure of antibodies explains three functions of antibodies: (1) binding versatility, (2) binding specificity, and (3) biological activity.* A mammal is capable of responding to more than 100 million antigenic determinants and can even respond to artificial antigens that do not exist in nature. Because the amino acid sequence differs in the arms of various antibody molecules, each different antibody can bind specifically to one unique epitope. Thus, the arms of an antibody molecule confer the versatility and specificity of responses that a host can mount against antigens. The stem region of an antibody molecule decides its biological activity and defines whether the response against a particular antigen will lead to complement-mediated lysis, enhanced phagocytosis, or (in some cases) allergy. These activities start once antibodies bind to antigen.

## Isolation and Biochemical Characterization Studies Determined the Basic Structural Components of Antibodies

### Initially, Antibodies Were Identified Only by Their Electrical Charge

Since the 1890s, immunologists have known that the molecules of humoral immunity are present in serum. In 1939, Tiselius and Kabat performed electrophoretic studies with rabbit antiserum specific for ovalbumin.[4] They found that electrophoresis of serum from unimmunized rabbits resolved serum proteins into four dominant families of differing mobility. The albumins were the fastest-migrating (most negatively charged) fraction, followed by the alpha- ($\alpha$), beta- ($\beta$), and gamma- ($\gamma$) globulins (Figure 4-5). Tiselius and Kabat then hyperimmunized rabbits with hen ovalbumin to get a strong antibody response. When they electrophoresed the immune serum, they observed a large increase in the $\gamma$-globulin fraction and concluded that antibodies were $\gamma$-globulins. After they absorbed out the anti-ovalbumin antibodies with the antigen ovalbumin, they observed that the electrophoretic pattern was the same as the pattern for the preimmune serum. This observation thus supported their conclusion that *antibodies are $\gamma$-globulins*,

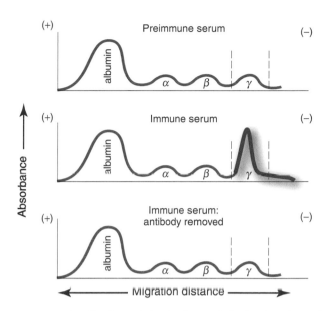

**FIGURE 4-5 Antibody activity in the $\gamma$-globulin fraction of serum**. The electrophoretic pattern of rabbit serum before immunization (top), after immunization (middle), and after absorption (bottom) of the antibody with specific antigen is illustrated.

which were called *immunoglobulins*. We now know that immunoglobulin G (IgG) is mostly found in the $\gamma$-globulin fraction but significant amounts of IgG and other classes of antibodies are found in the $\alpha$ and the $\beta$ fractions of serum. Antibodies can be separated further by ultracentrifugation. Studies performed in the 1940s and 1950s revealed that antibody molecules are heterogeneous in size. They range in molecular weight from 150 to roughly 1000 kD.

### Fragmentation Studies Showed That Antibodies Are Made Up of Two Identical Light Chains and Two Identical Heavy Chains

In the late 1950s and early 1960s, Rodney Porter of Great Britain and Gerald Edelman of the United States elucidated the chemical structure of antibodies.[5] Edelman structurally studied $\gamma$-globulins and myeloma proteins, while Porter's experiments focused on a specific antibody from the $\gamma$-globulin fraction of rabbit serum called *Immunoglobulin G* or *IgG*. Edelman and Porter's approaches to the characterization of the IgG molecule were different. Edelman characterized IgG molecules using chemical solvents, whereas Porter used protein-degrading enzymes. Our understanding of antibody structure draws from the two scientists' results.

---

[4]Electrophoresis is the migration of charged molecules after the introduction of an electric current.

[5]Porter and Edelman shared the 1972 Nobel Prize in Medicine for their structural studies of antibodies.

To generate subunits of IgG, Edelman treated rabbit IgG with dithiothreitol (a reducing agent that disrupts disulfide bonds), iodoacetamide (an alkylating agent that prevents reassociation of the disrupted disulfide bonds), and a denaturing agent (a substance that disrupts noncovalent interactions). When the treated antibodies were passed through sizing columns, he identified two subunits in equimolar ratios. He designated the larger subunit (50 kD) as the **heavy, or H, chain** and the smaller subunit (23 kD) as the **light, or L, chain**. Because the molecular weight of the original IgG molecule is 150 kD, he concluded that the IgG molecule consisted of two heavy and two light chains linked by disulfide bonds and noncovalent interactions.

Porter fragmented rabbit IgG with the proteolytic enzyme *papain* in the presence of the reducing agent cysteine. Papain hydrolyzed peptide bonds in IgG

and produced three fragments (I, II, and III). The three fragments had similar molecular weights (50 kD) but different charges. Two of the three fragments were identical and retained the ability to bind antigen. These two fragments were called the **Fab fragments** (for *fragments of antigen-binding*). Because the intact IgG is bivalent and the two Fab fragments each could bind antigen, Porter concluded that the Fab fragments must be univalent. The third fragment produced by papain digestion did not bind with antigen and crystallized during cold storage. Porter called this piece the **Fc fragment** (for *fragment crystallizable*). Thus the ratio of Fab to Fc is 2 to 1. Edelman confirmed Porter's results by cleaving and electrophoresing human IgG into two antigenically different fractions equivalent to the two fragments from rabbit IgG (Figure 4-6).

In similar studies, Alfred Nisonoff used *pepsin*, which hydrolyzes different sites on the IgG molecule

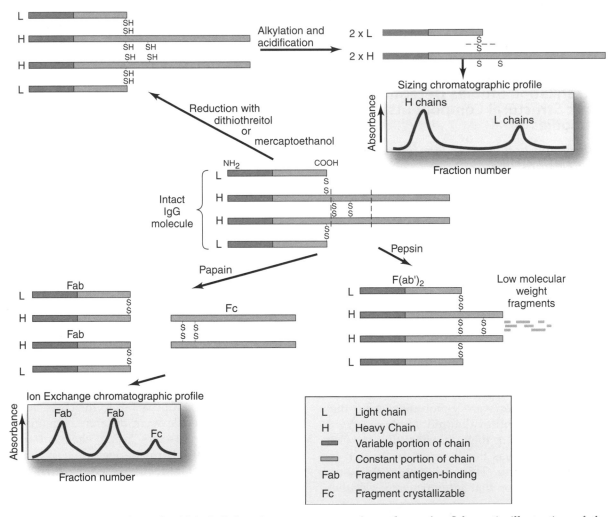

**FIGURE 4-6 Fragmentation of rabbit IgG by the enzymes papain and pepsin.** Schematic illustration of the chromatography of reduced and papain-digested (also pepsin-digested) rabbit IgG. The results show the basic structure of all antibodies. See text for further explanation.

than does papain. IgG treated with pepsin yielded one large fragment with a molecular weight (100 kD) double that of one Fab fragment, and many small fragments. Nisonoff called the large fragment **F(ab′)₂**. This fragment also could bind antigen, but unlike the Fab fragment, it led to a visible serological reaction. It had both of the antigen-binding sites of IgG (the chains remained linked) and could be treated further with reducing agents to yield two Fab-like fragments called **Fab′**. Collectively, the two enzymes cleave at about the same region of the IgG molecule. Papain splits the molecule on one side, and pepsin on the other side, of the bond that holds Fab fragments together (see Figure 4-2).

Following these studies, Porter showed that either Fab or Fab′ fragments compose the entire light chain and part of the heavy chain. These data led to the formulation of the structure of an antibody and are summarized in Table 4-6. IgG is used as the prototype antibody to explain the basic structure of all antibodies.

## Sequencing Studies Explained the Fine Structure of Antibodies—the Variable and the Constant Regions on the Chains

The primary structure of antibodies was determined by amino acid sequencing of myeloma proteins.

---

**TABLE 4-6** Mini Summary: Characteristics of the IgG Molecule*

1. IgG (150 kD) consists of two light chains and two heavy chains; each light chain pairs with a heavy chain and each heavy chain pairs with another heavy chain.
   a. Covalent interchain disulfide bonds and noncovalent interactions link the chains.
   b. The two light chains (23 kD each) and two heavy chains (50 kD each) are identical.
2. Papain digestion produces two Fab fragments and one Fc fragment.
   a. Fab fragments (50 kD) consist of the entire light chain and part of the heavy chain.
   b. Fab fragments contain the antigen-binding sites.
   c. The Fc fragment (50 kD) crystallizes in cold and does not bind antigen.
3. Pepsin digestion produces one large fragment (100 kD) called F(ab′)₂ and degrades the remainder of the heavy chains into small pieces.
   a. When the large fragment is treated with reducing agents, the disulfide bridges are disrupted, giving two Fab-like fragments, Fab′.
   b. Each of the Fab′ fragments is made up of the entire light chain and a slightly longer part of the heavy chain.

---

*Even though characteristics are given for the IgG antibody molecule, we will see that all antibody molecules have similar overall structures and some common properties.

*Myeloma proteins* are molecules that have the characteristic structure of antibodies but originate from a disease state rather than from an immune response to a specific antigen. These pathologic immunoglobulins are formed by individuals with **multiple myeloma**, a cancer of antibody-forming (plasma) B cells. Myeloma proteins were invaluable in the resolution of antibody structure because they are produced in large quantities (up to 95% of patient immunoglobulins) and are usually homogeneous in a patient, whereas in a normal immune response the antibodies are heterogeneous in composition. Serum antibodies are *polyclonal antibodies*, because they are produced by the descendants of several B cells that recognize different epitopes on the same antigen. The resulting heterogeneity of serum antibodies makes them unsuitable for sequence studies. The main work involved a light-chain myeloma protein, called the *Bence-Jones protein* (first described in 1847 by Henry Bence-Jones). Bence-Jones proteins are immunoglobulin light chains excreted in the urine of myeloma patients. Amino acid sequence comparisons of Bence-Jones chains led to a startling finding. Each chain consisted of a large region that was constant in different types of antibodies (even from unrelated species) and a similar sized region that was highly variable among different Bence-Jones proteins. This large region, called the **constant (C) region**, has amino acid sequences in the carboxyl terminal end (residues 109 to 214) of the light chains that are almost identical. The opposite end of the light chain, the amino terminal end (residues 1 to 108), shows great variability in amino acid sequence among the chains and is called the **variable (V) region**. These studies also showed that most species have two types of light chains (discussed later): **kappa (κ)** and **lambda (λ)**.

The amino acid sequence of antibody heavy chains showed similar regions. The first 113 amino acid residues of the heavy chain[6] again showed great variability among myeloma heavy chains, while the remaining part of the heavy chain consisted of amino acids that were almost identical (the constant regions). This implies that molecules binding different determinants have different V light ($V_L$) and V heavy ($V_H$) regions. A group of words can illustrate the concept:

---

[6]The length of the heavy-chain V region varies. The V heavy-chain region is somewhat larger (about 123 amino acid residues) than the V light-chain region (about 108 amino acid residues). V-region length depends on CDR length. The CDRs (discussed shortly), especially CDR3s of IgMs, can be quite large.

*P-S-Y-C-H-O-L-O-G-Y, P-H-Y-S-I-O-L-O-G-Y,* and *I-M-M-U-N-O-L-O-G-Y*. All have a constant region ("*O-L-O-G-Y*") and a variable region, the first five letters of each word. Because the primary structure, the amino acid sequence, accounted for variable and constant light and heavy chain regions and causes the antiparallel β-pleated sheet secondary structure characteristic of antibody molecules, which dictates the three-dimensional structure, the unique sequence of amino acid residues and shape for each V region leads to the large diversity of structure, which accounts for antibody specificity.

Although antibodies are complex globular proteins, they do possess some structural repetitiveness. *Each antibody chain has a tandem series of repeating homology units roughly 110 amino acid residues in length called* **immunoglobulin domains,** *which fold independently into a compact globular structure* (Figure 4-7). Within each domain, an intrachain disulfide bond forms a "sphere-like" structure of roughly 60 amino acids.

All proteins that exhibit this structural motif belong to the **immunoglobulin superfamily** (see Chapters 7 and 8). The term *superfamily* designates genes that encode proteins with redundant characteristic structures that may have arose from a common primordial gene. Domains are separated by less ordered regions of the peptide chains. The light chain of IgG has two domains called $V_L$ and $C_L$. The heavy chain of IgG has four domains: one $V_H$ and three in the $C_H$ region ($C_H1$, $C_H2$, and $C_H3$ or $C_\gamma1$, $C_\gamma2$, and $C_\gamma3$). The heavy-chain V unit shows similarity to the V part of the light chain, while the three C-region units show strong homology to each other and to the C region of the light chain. X-ray crystallographic analysis revealed that each domain has a characteristic tertiary structure consisting of two β-pleated sheet structures called an **immunoglobulin fold**. Each domain has a sandwich-like structure with a hydrophobic amino acid interior. A disulfide bridge near the center of the domain covalently links layers. When the $V_L$ chain

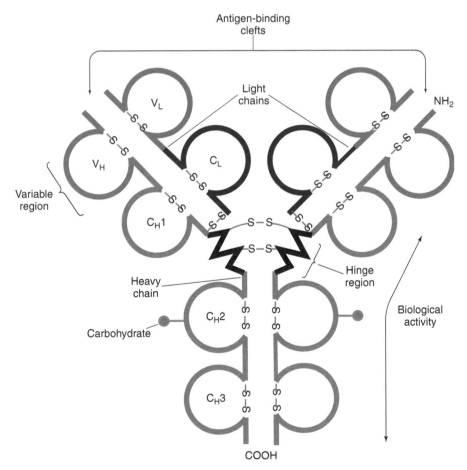

**FIGURE 4-7 Schematic representation of IgG domains**. Areas of variability and constancy, divided into segments of 110 amino acid residues, within an IgG molecule (and for all antibodies) are known as *domains*. The IgG molecule has a V and C domain for each light chain and one V and three C domains for each heavy chain.

framework residues assume this three-dimensional arrangement, hydrophilic amino acid "loops" are held out from the sandwich. These loops represent the complementarity-determining regions, which we will discuss shortly. Their amino acid residues define the size and shape of the loops. When heavy and light chains are brought together to form an IgG molecule, extensive noncovalent interactions occur between $V_L$ and $V_H$, $C_L$ and $C_H1$, $C_H2$ and $C_H2$, and $C_H3$ and $C_H3$. These regions of interaction are shown by the "three-dimensional" model in Figure 4-8.

Variability of the amino acid sequences in the V regions is not random but precisely organized. It is concentrated within certain sections of the V region of a chain, and these sections have substantial sequence variation from protein to protein. The greatest variability in the light- and heavy-chain V regions are roughly in the same position, around residues 30, 55, and 95. These areas are called **hypervariable regions** or **complementarity-determining regions** (**CDRs**). Moving from the amino-terminal end of either an antibody light or heavy chain, the three regions are called *CDR1*, *CDR2*, and *CDR3*—three in the light-chain V region and three in the heavy-chain V region. Each CDR is about 10 amino acid residues in length. Hypervariable regions are called *CDRs* because these segments line the antigen-binding site. Intervening sequences between the CDRs have restricted variability and show little difference in amino acid sequence between chains. These invariant segments make up

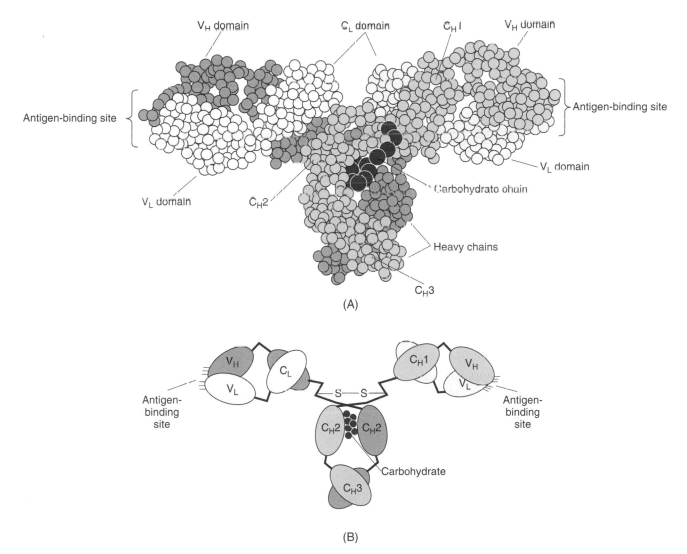

(A)

(B)

**FIGURE 4-8 Three-dimensional model of IgG.** From studies by X-ray crystallography and electron microscopy, (a) the three-dimensional structure of IgG can be depicted as a Y-shaped molecule. Each sphere represents an amino acid residue. The two light chains are shades of yellow and the heavy chains are shades of orange. (b) The schematic cartoon shows how domains interact. (Adapted from E.W. Silverton, M.A. Navia, and D.R. Davies. 1977. *Proc. Natl. Acad. Sci. USA* 74:5140.)

the **framework residues**, which compose about 85% of the V region. Framework residues define the positioning of the CDRs. The V region folds so that the CDRs are exposed on the surface of the chain. When the light and heavy chains are joined, the CDRs of the chains form a cleft that serves as the antigen-binding site of an immunoglobulin. Because the amino acid sequences of the CDRs determine the shape and ionic properties of the antigen-binding site, the CDRs define *the specificity of the antibody*. A schematic representation of heavy and light chains is shown in Figure 4-9 and detailed in Figure 4-10.

The association of the CDRs and the antigen-binding site of an antibody was confirmed by crystallographic studies. An example of such a study is the binding of antibody specific for the hapten phosphorylcholine (Figure 4-11). X-ray diffraction studies of antigen-antibody complexes suggest that several CDRs make bind to an antigen and in some cases all

six CDRs contact the antigen. The $V_H$ domain seems to contribute more to antigen binding than the $V_L$ domain. Not only is the variability and amino acid composition of CDRs important in antigen binding but also the ability of CDRs to change their conformation during antigen binding, this change in antibody shape allows for a better complementary fit with the epitope.

Antibody constant domains do not bind antigen but are responsible for biologic effector functions (detailed later in chapter), which are dictated by each domain's amino acid sequence. Antibodies also demonstrate **segmental flexibility**, which means that the two Fab portions can move relative to one another on antigen binding. The angle varies from 60 to 180 degrees. This flexible region where the arms meet the stem of the Y contains an extended peptide sequence rich in proline residues called the **hinge region** and is located between the $C_H1$ and $C_H2$ domains. Only

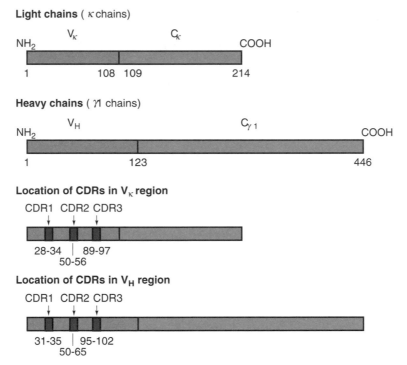

**FIGURE 4-9 Amino acid sequence of light and heavy chains: Localization of variability.** Antibodies have two identical light and heavy chains. Each chain is divided into two regions, the variable (V) and constant (C) regions. The amino-terminal end contains the V region, while the carboxyl-terminal end contains the C region. In the V region are areas of increased variability called *hypervariable regions* or *complementarity-determining regions* (*CDRs*, marked by arrows); while the numbers below the arrows give the amino acid residue positions. The CDRs of the light and heavy chains form the antigen-binding sites. The more conserved amino acids between the CDRs are called *framework residues*; they hold the CDRs in place. See text for further explanation.

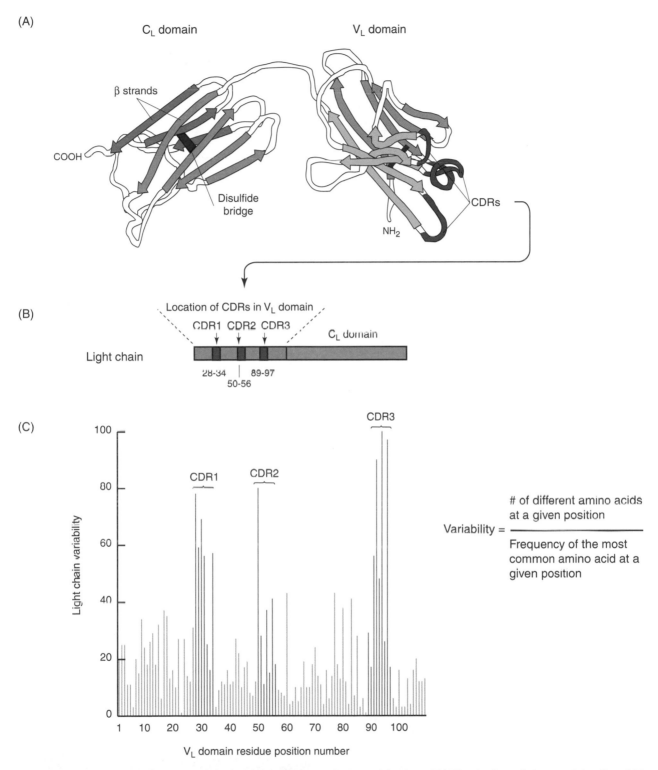

**FIGURE 4-10 Light-chain immunoglobulin-fold structure: CDR positioning.** (A) The β-pleated sheets of the C and V domains are held together by the disulfide bond and hydrophobic interactions. The β-sheet strands are shown in different colors. The regions with increased amino acid variability, hypervariable regions or complementarity-determining regions (CDRs), are shown in red. The heavy-chain domains (not shown) have the same overall structure. (B) A linear map of CDR locations. (C) The variability plot (also called *Wu and Kabat plots*) of a human $V_L$ domain is shown. It shows the presence and location of the hypervariable regions/CDRs within the V regions. (D) Continued on the next page.

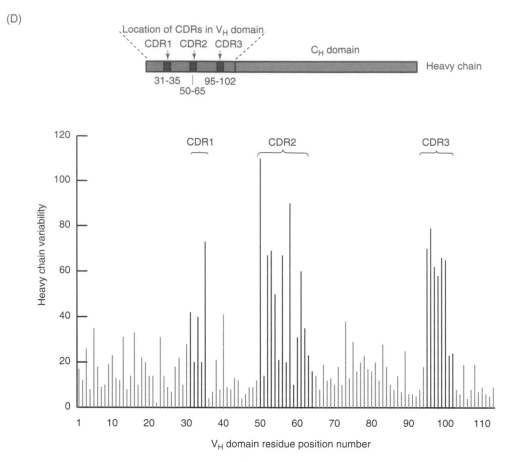

(D)

**FIGURE 4-10** (*Continued*).

IgG, IgA, and IgD antibody molecules[7] have hinge regions. Even though IgM and IgE do not have hinge regions, they have additional 110-amino acid domain ($C_H2/C_H2$) with hinge-like characteristics. IgG, IgA, and IgD have three C-region domains and a hinge region, whereas IgM and IgE have four C-region domains and no hinge region. The heavy chains of IgM and IgA antibody molecules possess additional amino acid residues on the carboxyl terminal end of the last $C_H$ domain. These areas, called **tailpieces**, permit IgM and IgA to interact with like antibodies and form multimeric molecules. Multimeric IgM and IgA also have a polypeptide called the **joining (J) chain**, which is disulfide-linked to the tailpieces and stabilizes the multimeric structure. All antibody molecules can be expressed either as a **membrane-bound immunoglobulin** or a **secreted immunoglobulin**. In its membrane-bound form, the heavy chain $C_H3/C_H3$ domains of IgG, IgA, and

IgD and the $C_H4/C_H4$ domains of IgM and IgE antibody molecules possess additional amino acid residues on the carboxyl terminal end of the last $C_H$ domain, which is divided into a hydrophilic, extracellular 26-amino-acid-spacer sequence, a hydrophobic transmembrane sequence, and a cytoplasmic tail. The amino acid length of the spacer and cytoplasmic tail vary among antibody class, whereas the transmembrane sequence is constant. In its secreted form, antibodies have additional hydrophilic amino acids that contribute to their effector functions. Antibodies also contain carbohydrates; the percentage and location of the carbohydrate molecules differ according to the class of antibody.

**MINI SUMMARY**

Amino acid sequencing of light chains shows that variability is localized at the amino terminal end of the chains in the V regions. The other, carboxyl ends are identical and are called the constant, or C, regions. This variability arrangement is the

---

[7]The five antibody classes—IgG, IgA, IgM, IgD, and IgE—will be discussed shortly.

Phosphorylcholine

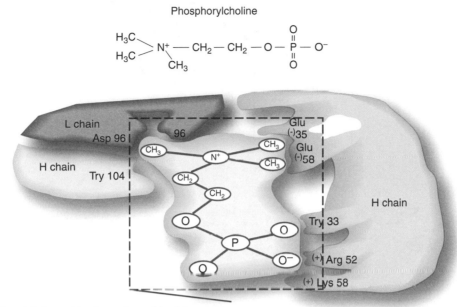

The cleft formed by the amino acids of the heavy (H) and light (L) chain complementary determining region (CDR) "holds" the antigenic determinant, in this case the hapten phoshorylcholine.

**FIGURE 4-11** Antigen-combining site of an antibody for the hapten phosphorylcholine showing the complementarity between an epitope and an antibody-combining site. The amino acids lining the CDRs bind to the epitope through weak, noncovalent interactions. The three CDRs of the heavy chain and one CDR of the light chain contribute to the combining site.

same for heavy chains. Light chains also possess two repeated homology units (domains), and heavy chains possess four to five domains. The three-dimensional structure of antibodies shows that domains are folded in similar configurations, with the V-light and V-heavy units lying together to form the V domains of the complete antibody molecule. V-domain variability is concentrated in segments called complementarity-determining regions (CDRs) or hypervariable regions. The CDRs line the walls of the antigen-binding sites in antibody molecules. Segments between the CDRs are highly conserved regions called framework residues. The light- and heavy-chain V domains shape the antigen-binding cleft, which are formed by the three CDRs from each chain. Changes in amino acid residues at the position of this cavity change its shape and thus its specificity. The amino acid sequencing of antibody light and heavy chains divides them into V regions for antigen recognition and C regions for biological effector functions.

## The Antibody's Antigenic Determinants—Called Isotypes, Allotypes, and Idiotypes—Determine the Variability in Antibody Structure

*Humans express five groups of antibodies, called* **immunoglobulin (Ig)**, *or* **antibody, classes**. The five classes of antibodies, designated *IgG, IgA, IgM, IgD,* and *IgE,* differ in their physicochemical (charge, size, and solubility) and serologic (*in vitro* reactions with antigens) properties, and *in their behavior as antigens.* The latter characteristic usually is the one used to divide immunoglobulins into the five classes.

Antibodies are divided into classes by the antigenic determinants on their heavy chains. Antibodies themselves can be immunogenic. For example, if one immunizes a rabbit with human antibodies, the rabbit's immune system does not see an antibody molecule but rather a foreign complex glycoprotein. The rabbit responds by making antibodies to the human antibodies, and this antiserum can be used to distinguish at least three types of determinants or epitopes (*isotypic, allotypic,* and *idiotypic*) that can then

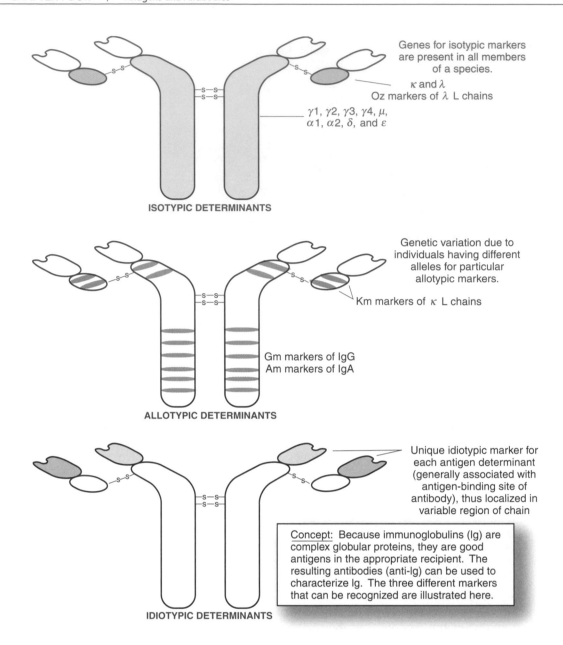

Genes for isotypic markers
are present in all members
of a species.

κ and λ
Oz markers of λ L chains

γ1, γ2, γ3, γ4, μ,
α1, α2, δ, and ε

**ISOTYPIC DETERMINANTS**

Genetic variation due to
individuals having different
alleles for particular
allotypic markers.

Km markers of κ L chains

Gm markers of IgG
Am markers of IgA

**ALLOTYPIC DETERMINANTS**

Unique idiotypic marker for
each antigen determinant
(generally associated with
antigen-binding site of
antibody), thus localized in
variable region of chain

Concept: Because immunoglobulins (Ig) are
complex globular proteins, they are good
antigens in the appropriate recipient. The
resulting antibodies (anti-Ig) can be used to
characterize Ig. The three different markers
that can be recognized are illustrated here.

**IDIOTYPIC DETERMINANTS**

**FIGURE 4-12 Nomenclature of antibody variability.** Three overall variants of antibody exist.
Going from general to specific variation, the first, known as *isotypic variation*, refers to the different
heavy (H) and light (L) chain classes (IgG, IgA, IgM, IgD, and IgE) and subclasses (such as human
IgG1 through IgG4). Most *allotypic variation* occurs in the C region of H and L chains, but some has
been found in the framework residues of V regions. The last variation, called *idiotypic*, is found
only in the V regions of the heavy and light chains.

be used to classify antibodies into *isotypes, allotypes,*
and *idiotypes* (Figure 4-12).

### Isotypes Are Variants Present in All Members of a Species

*The heavy-chain antigenic determinants that define the
antibody class are called* **isotypic determinants**. *The antibody molecule is an* **isotype** (G. *iso,* the same). *Isotypic*

*determinants distinguish constant-region sites.* Thus, an
antibody specific for the heavy chain of IgG reacts
with only IgG molecules. Antigenic determinants
that define the heavy chain of IgG, IgA, IgM, IgD,
and IgE are given the Greek letters gamma (γ), alpha
(α), mu (μ), delta (δ), and epsilon (ε), respectively.
Other isotypic heavy-chain determinants define differences within a class and thus are called **antibody**

**subclasses**. IgG has four subclasses, called $\gamma1$, $\gamma2$, $\gamma3$, and $\gamma4$ or IgG1, IgG2, IgG3, and IgG4. In humans, IgG1, IgG2, IgG3, and IgG4 are found in normal serum in the approximate proportions of 65, 25, 5, and 5%, respectively. Two subclasses have also been found in IgA, designated $\alpha1$ and $\alpha2$ or IgA1 and IgA2.

Antigenic determinants on the constant regions of light chains classify them as either $\kappa$ or $\lambda$ types. Humans have only one gene for the $\kappa$ C region, but the $\lambda$ chain has at least four functional C-region genes. The four $\lambda$ chain isosubtypes are designated $\lambda1$, $\lambda2$, $\lambda3$, and $\lambda6$. Light-chain antigenic determinants are *not* useful in determining antibody class or subclass because $\kappa$ and $\lambda$ chains are associated with all classes and subclasses. Within an antibody molecule, both heavy chains and both light chains are identical. All of the genes for isotypic determinants are expressed in a normal individual; therefore, all isotypic determinants are present on some antibodies of all members of a species.

### Allotypes Are Variants Caused by Intraspecies Genetic Differences

**Allotypic determinants** *are encoded by one allele (variation) of a given antibody gene and are present on the antibodies of some members of a species. These antibodies are called* **allotypes** (G. *allos*, other). Alternate alleles encode antigenically distinct allotypic markers; they differ by one to four amino acids. The genes encoding allotypic determinants are inherited in a Mendelian fashion and illustrate the genetic diversity within a species (*polymorphism*). Allotypic nomenclature consists of the right class and subclass marker followed by each allele in parentheses—for example, G2m(23), G4m(4a), A2m(1), or Km(3). The $\gamma$, $\alpha$, and $\kappa$ chains have allotypic determinants called **Gm, Am**, and **Km**. All four $\gamma$ chain isotypes have allotypes (humans have at least 25 Gm markers). Only IgA2 has allotypes designated A2m(1) and A2m(2). The $\kappa$-light chain allotypes are called Km(1), Km(2), and Km(3). No allotypes have been described for IgM, IgA1, IgD, IgE, or the $\lambda$ chain.

### Idiotypes Are Variants Caused by Structural Heterogeneity in the Antibody V Regions

**Idiotypic determinants** (also called **idiotopes**) *are found in the V region in or near the antigen-binding site of the antibody molecule. These determinants classify antibodies into* **idiotypes** (G. *idios*, one's own) *and are common to antibodies having specificity for the same foreign antigenic determinant.* Each individual has as many different idiotypes as it has different antigen-specific antibodies. These determinants are individual-specific. Idiotypic determinants reflect the antibody-combining site's structure and usually depend on the arrangement of heavy and light chains.

---

**MINI SUMMARY**

The antigenic determinants of antibodies show three levels of variability. The determinants (from general to specific) are called isotypic, allotypic, or idiotypic and classify antibody molecules into isotypes, allotypes, and idiotypes, respectively. Isotypic determinants, found on the C-region part of heavy chains, divide antibodies into five classes (or isotypes) called IgG, IgA, IgM, IgD, and IgE. Isotypic determinants also can be used to classify antibody light chains into $\kappa$ and $\lambda$ types. Isotypic differences can be used to partition classes into subclasses or subtypes. Allotypic determinants, found on the C-region part of heavy chains, are carried by only some individuals within a given species and are inherited in a Mendelian fashion. Idiotypic determinants are individual-specific and represent the antigen-combining site of an antibody.

---

# THERE ARE FIVE CLASSES OF ANTIBODIES BASED ON THE STRUCTURE OF THEIR HEAVY-CHAIN C DOMAINS

## All Antibody Classes Have Either $\lambda$ or $\kappa$ Light Chains

As mentioned earlier, the two determinants used to define antibody light chains are called kappa ($\kappa$) and lambda ($\lambda$). Each chain has a molecular weight of about 23 kD and exists as one polypeptide chain of about 214 amino acid residues. The first 108 amino acids make up the V region, followed by roughly 110 amino acids that make up the C region. These two regions compose the $V_L$ and $C_L$ chain domains. $\lambda$-light chains exhibit minor differences in amino acid sequences that are used to classify $\lambda$ chains into four subtypes. The ratios of $\kappa$ to $\lambda$ light chains vary greatly within mammalian species. In mice, it is 95 to 5; in humans, it is about 60 to 40, and in cats it is 95 to 5 $\lambda$. The $\kappa$ to $\lambda$ ration reflects the numbers of V-region gene segments in each isotype and their recombination efficiency into functional light-chain genes. However, there is no difference in either chain's ability to pair with a heavy chain.

## IgG Is the Major Antibody in the Blood, but It Is Able to Enter Tissue Spaces and Coat Antigens, Speeding Antigen Uptake

IgG, primarily induced by protein antigens, constitutes about 80% (12.5 mg/ml) of the antibody in serum. The IgG (150 kD) is composed of two light chains (either κ or λ) and two heavy chains (γ). Disulfide bonds covalently hold the four polypeptide chains together. Human IgG consists of four subclasses (isotypes), which are numbered in order of their decreasing serum concentrations (IgG1, IgG2, IgG3, and IgG4). The four subclasses have 90 to 95% identity with each other in the C-region domains. The γ chain is made up of four domains, one in the V portion and three in the C portion of the chain. The γ1 chain is the shortest heavy chain, with 446 amino acid residues. On the $C_H2$ domain (at position 297) of all γ chains is attached one carbohydrate group that controls the quaternary structure of this domain. The chief distinguishing characteristic among the four IgG subclasses is the pattern of interchain linkages in the hinge region. The four IgG subclasses also have distinguishing biologic activities: IgG1, IgG3, and IgG4 can cross the placenta; in increasing efficiency of complement activation IgG2 > IgG1 > IgG3, IgG4 cannot activate complement; and IgG1 and IgG3 bind to phagocytic cells through high-affinity Fc receptors mediating opsonization, IgG4 has intermediate affinity, and IgG2 has low affinity. Table 4-7 summarizes the biological, chemical, and physical properties of the five classes of antibodies and Figure 4-13 shows their structures.

## IgA Concentrates in Body Fluids to Guard the Entrances of the Body

Human IgA constitutes only 13% (2.1 mg/ml) of the antibody in human serum, but it is the predominant class of antibody in extravascular secretions. In the serum, IgA is a mainly a 160-kD monomer. The IgA is present in secretions (tears, saliva, nasal secretions, bronchial and digestive tract mucus, and mammary gland secretions) as a dimer or tetramer and called **secretory IgA**. It is composed of a J chain and a secretory component. The organization of monomeric and secretory IgA is depicted in Figure 4-14.

The *J chain* is a 16-kD polypeptide consisting of 129 amino acid residues and one carbohydrate group. It is synthesized by plasma cells and attaches to IgA (or IgM) at the time of plasma cell secretion. The J chain attaches to the carboxyl terminal penultimate cysteine of both monomeric IgA α3 domain tailpieces, the C-terminal 18 amino acid extensions present on IgA heavy chains but lacking from the heavy chains of immunoglobulin classes, which do not polymerize (such as IgG). J chains facilitate IgA polymerization. (The J chain is also present in polymeric IgM.) The remaining peptide, a 70-kD polypeptide of five immunoglobulin-like domains, called *secretory component*, is produced by epithelial cells and attaches to the Fc region domains of dimeric IgA. IgA-producing plasma cells home to subepithelial tissue, where their secreted dimeric IgA binds to receptors for polymeric immunoglobulin (Ig) molecules called **poly-Ig receptors** (Figure 4-15; and see Figures 4-16 and 4-17). These receptors are found on the basolaterial surface of most mucosal epithelia. Once dimeric IgA binds to the epithelial cells through poly-Ig receptors, it is internalized by receptor-mediated endocytosis. The vesicle containing the dimeric IgA–poly-Ig receptor complex moves through the cytoplasm to the luminal membrane of epithelial cells, where the vesicle fuses with the plasma membrane, the poly-Ig receptors are cleaved from the membrane and bind to dimeric IgAs, and are released as secretory IgA into the mucous secretions. (Polymeric IgM is also transported into mucous secretions in a similar manner; however, it accounts for a much smaller percentage than IgA.) The secretory component provides resistance to enzymatic cleavage of IgA while in mucosal secretions. Secretory IgA affords a first-line defense at main entry sites for many pathogens.

The α chain is made up of one V domain and three C domains. IgA1 is the most prevalent form in serum, but IgA2 is slightly more prevalent in secretions. Only IgA2 has allotypic determinants, and only the A2m(1) uniquely lacks interchain disulfide bridges between light and heavy chains. Instead, chains are linked to their own counterparts (one light chain to the other light chain). Another difference between IgA allotypes is the size of their hinge regions.

## IgM Is the Largest Antibody; It Tends to Remain in the Blood, Where It Can Lead to Efficient Killing of Bacteria

IgM is secreted by plasma cells, primarily induced by polysaccharide antigens, as a 950-kD pentamer that makes up about 8% (1.25 mg/ml) of the antibody in the serum. The five monomeric IgM molecules are arranged radially, the Fab fragments pointing outward and the Fc fragments pointing to the center

**TABLE 4-7  Biological, Chemical, and Physical Properties of Human Antibodies**

| Property | IgG1 | IgG2 | IgG3 | IgG4 | IgA1 | IgA2 | IgM | IgD | IgE |
|---|---|---|---|---|---|---|---|---|---|
| Molecular weight (kD) | 150 | 150 | 160 | 150 | 160 (m), 300 (d) | | 950 (p) | 175 | 190 |
| Heavy chain | γ1 | γ2 | γ3 | γ4 | α1 | α2 | μ | δ | ε |
| Other chains | −[a] | − | − | − | J chain (16 kD), secretory component (70 kD) | J chain (16 kD), secretory component (70 kD) | J chain (16 kD) | − | − |
| Concentration range in serum (mg/ml) | 5–12 | 2–6 | 0.5–1 | 0.2–1 | 1.4–4.2 | 0.2–0.5 | 0.25–3.1 | 0.03–0.4 | 0.0001–0.0002 |
| Percent of total Ig | 45–53 | 11–15 | 3–6 | 1–4 | 11–14 | 1–4 | 10 | 0.2 | 0.004 |
| Biologic half-life in serum (days) | 21–24 | 21–24 | 7–8 | 21–24 | 5–7 | 4–6 | 5–10 | 2–8 | 1–5 |
| Carbohydrate content (%) | 2–3 | 2–3 | 2–3 | 2–3 | 7–11 | 7–11 | 10–12 | 9–14 | 12–13 |
| Classical complement pathway activation | + | +/− | ++ | − | −(activates alternative pathway) | − | +++ | − | − |
| Placental transfer | + | +/− | + | + | − | − | − | − | − |
| Binding to phagocytes via Fc receptor | ++ | +/− | ++ | + | − | − | − | − | − |
| Induction of allergic activity | − | − | − | − | − | − | − | − | ++ |
| Mucosal transport | − | − | − | − | ++ | ++ | + | − | − |
| Naïve mature B cells expression | − | − | − | − | − | − | + | + | − |

[a]Presence of absence of component; activity levels: high = ++; medium = +; low = +/−; none = −.
[b]d = dimer; m = monomer; p = pentamer.

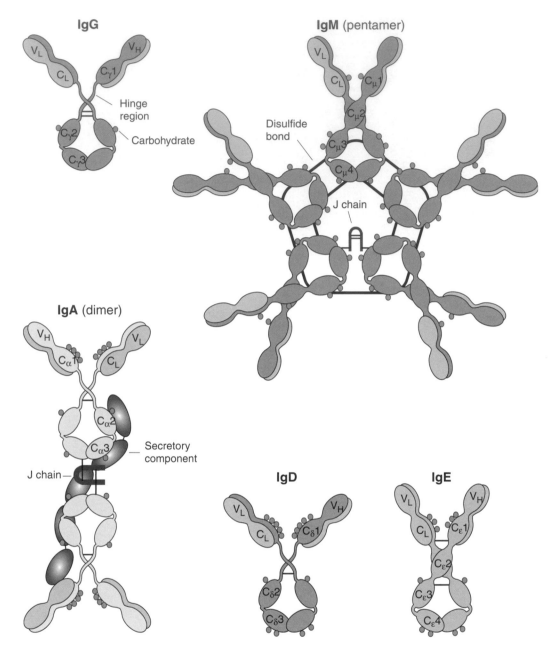

**FIGURE 4-13 Structures of the five major classes of secreted antibodies.**

of the circle (see Figure 4-13). The five monomeric molecules are held together by disulfide bonds that linked their constant-region domains (Cμ3/Cμ3) and their Cμ4/Cμ4 domains. Each pentameric IgM contains a J chain, which is disulfide-linked to two of the 10 μ chains. IgM is the first antibody to appear during an immune response and the first formed by a developing fetus. Because of its many antigen-binding sites, IgM can quickly clump antigen and efficiently activate complement. IgM acts as one of the main receptors on the surface of mature B cells, along with IgD.

When IgM is a surface receptor, it is in its monomeric form.

The IgM μ chain consists of 576 amino acid residues, with 452 making up the C region. Unlike γ and α chains, which have three C-region domains, the μ chain has four. The five carbohydrate groups are in the $C_H1$ and $C_H3$ domains and in the part of the μ chain where the J chain binds. The $C_H2$ domain of the μ chain is equivalent to the hinge regions of the γ and α chains. The μ chain has two interchain disulfide bonds.

**IgA** (monomer)

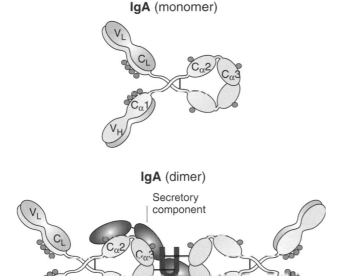

**IgA** (dimer)

Secretory
component

J chain

**FIGURE 4-14 Human secretory IgA.** This is made up of two monomeric IgA molecules, a joining (J) molecule and a secretory component (SC), with molecular weights of 160,000 (each monomer), 15,000, and 75,000, respectively. Intact secretory IgA has a molecular weight of 390,000. The two monomers of IgA are joined by their Fc ends by the J chain. The secretory piece is probably wrapped around the two IgA monomers.

## IgD Remains Membrane-Bound and Somehow Regulates the Cell's Activation

IgD (175 kD) constitutes roughly 0.2% (40 μg/ml) of the antibody in human serum. IgD is an antibody whose function remains unknown, even though, along with IgM, it is one of the main receptors on mature B cells. As naïve mature B cells interact with cognate antigen, other antibodies replace IgD. There is no known effector function associated with IgD. The δ-chain C region is divided into three domains and consists of 383 amino acid residues (see Figure 4-13). The hinge region of IgD consists of 64 amino acid residues, longer than any other antibody class.

## IgE Is Found in Trace Amounts in the Blood, but It Still Triggers Allergies

Human IgE (190 kD) makes up less than 0.003% (0.4 μg/ml) of the antibody in serum. IgE binds through its Fc part to mast cells or basophils. On later exposure to the same antigen, mast cells and basophils bind antigen with membrane-bound IgE, causing degranulation of granule content into the

extracellular regions, which trigger allergic reactions. IgE protects against parasites by releasing mediators that attract eosinophils. Like the μ chain, the ε chain contains four C-region domains. IgE is made up of about 13% carbohydrate. The ε chains are similar in size to μ chains, except that ε chains lack the 18 amino acid residues for J-chain binding (see Figure 4-13). For further discussion of IgE, see Chapter 12.

# THE C DOMAINS MEDIATE THE BIOLOGICAL EFFECTOR FUNCTIONS OF ANTIBODIES

Whereas a small part of the V region on an antibody determines the antigen specificity, single domains in the C region of heavy chains determine the effector functions. *Biologic activities of antibodies divide into three general areas: (1) protection, (2) placental transfer, and (3) cytophilic (literally, "cell-loving") properties.* (The biologic function of membrane antibody as the B cell receptor for antigen is discussed in Chapter 6.) Although antibody binding blocks the attachment of toxins or viruses (called *neutralization*), antibodies alone cannot directly destroy a foreign organism. Instead, antibodies mark them for destruction by other defense systems. When IgM or IgG (except IgG4) binds to antigen, the complement system is activated and promotes bacterial lysis or accelerated phagocytic uptake. IgM or IgG molecules that have not reacted with antigen do not activate complement. IgM also mediates agglutination reactions. The coating (*opsonization*) of organisms with primarily IgG antibodies leads to enhanced phagocytosis by macrophages and neutrophils. Antibodies allow for the interaction of several cell types with antigen-antibody complexes through the cells' Fc receptors. Several examples of human Fc receptors are illustrated in Figure 4-16 and Fc receptors for IgG are detailed in Table 4-8. Multiple biologic functions can be triggered through the cross-linking of any of the Fc receptor classes. Macrophages have enhanced engulfment of antigen-antibody complexes through Fc receptors. B-cell Fc receptor engagement by antigen-antibody complexes regulates B-cell activation. Other cell types expressing Fc receptors (CD16) can use ADCC, to lyse target cells coated with IgG. Certain antibodies, like IgA, can be localized to the lumens of mucosa-lined organs to provide mucosal immunity. Because of their characteristic immunoglobulin-like extracellular domains (share the Ig fold domain structure), Fc receptors belong to

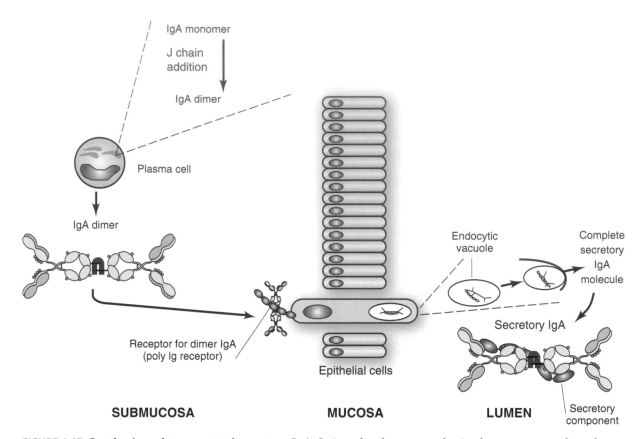

**FIGURE 4-15 Synthesis and transport of secretory IgA.** IgA molecules are synthesized as monomers, but plasma cells secrete them as dimers linked by the J chain. These IgA molecules bind to the poly immunoglobulin receptor on the interior surface of the epithelial cells. The complex is endocytosed and passed through the epithelial cells lining the lumens of the body, where the complex acquires the secretory component by cleavage of the receptor and finally enters the lumen as secretory IgA.

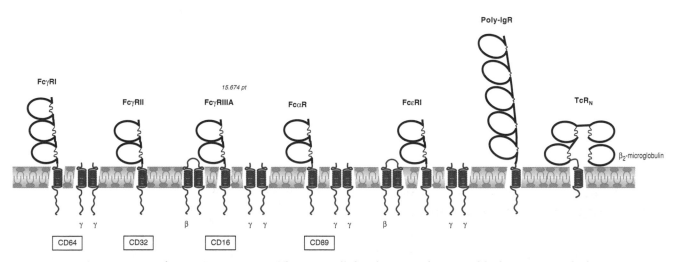

**FIGURE 4-16 The structure of some Fc receptors.** The extracellular domains shown in black interact with the Fc portions of antibody molecules. These domains have the characteristic β-pleated sheet/Ig fold structure that places them in the Ig superfamily. Where present, the accessory signaling molecules are shown in violet. The CD names are include were assigned.

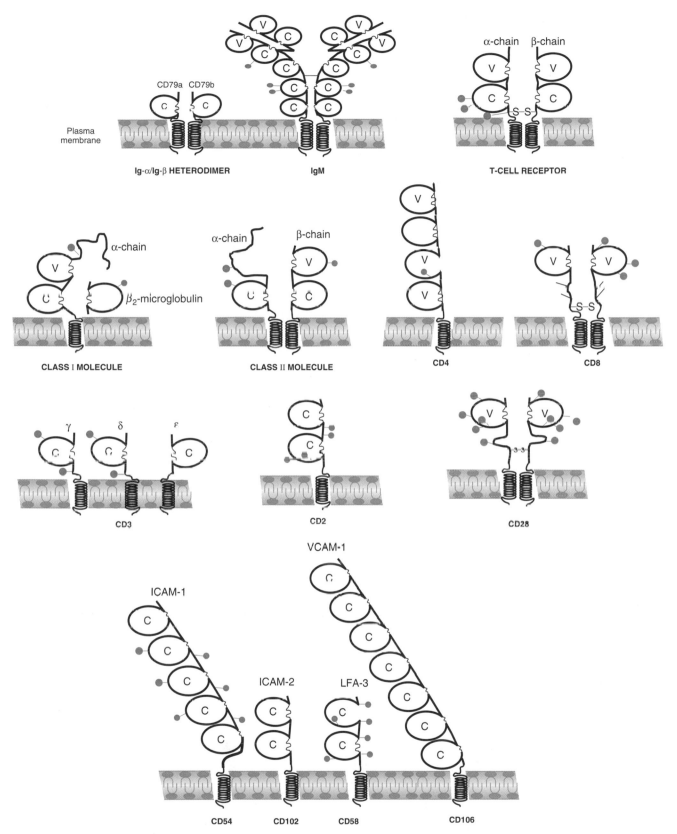

**FIGURE 4-17 Some members of the Ig superfamily of surface glycoproteins**. The carboxyl-terminal ends of all members except β2-microglobulin are anchored into the plasma membrane. Members of this family that are not pictured are CD121a (IL-1R), CD80 (B7-1), CD86 (B7-2), the Fc receptors, neural cell adhesion molecule, and platelet-derived growth factor receptor.

**TABLE 4-8** Human IgG Fc Receptors

| CD Name | Common name | Molecular weight (kD) | Affinity ($K_d$) | Distribution |
|---------|-------------|----------------------|------------------|--------------|
| CD16 | FcRIIIA | 50–65 | $2 \times 10^{-6}$ M | Granulocytes, macrophages, NK cells, neutrophils |
| CD32 | FcRII | 40 | $5 \times 10^{-7}$ M | B cells, eosinophils, granulocytes, macrophages |
| CD64 | FcRI | 75 | $1 \times 10^{-8}$ M | Monocytes, macrophages, cytokine-activated neutrophils |

*Note*: Three classes of human Fc receptor for IgG have been defined. The high-affinity FcRI is constitutively expressed on monocytes, macrophages, and cytokine-activated neutrophils, while the lower-affinity FcRII is widely distributed (found on immune and nonimmune cells). FcRIIIA has the lowest affinity of the three Fc receptors and is the main Fc receptor on neutrophils.

the immunoglobulin superfamily. There are many other immunoglobulin superfamily members that are critical to the development of immune responses (Figure 4-17). Many of these members will be discussed in other chapters.

The second area of biologic activity associated with the antibodies is the movement of maternal antibody across the placenta to the fetus. The human fetus and newborns have limited immune responses. Mechanisms of adaptive immunity are not at full strength until some time after birth. Most of the protection for a fetus or newborn comes from maternal IgG that crosses the placenta during pregnancy. The **neonatal Fc receptor (FcR$_N$)** for IgG is important for the transplacental transfer of maternal IgG (see Figure 4-16). Only IgG can cross the placenta because only the γ-chain $C_H1$ and $C_H3$ domains can bind to placental cells expressing FcR$_N$. Maternal IgA, secreted in breast milk, neutralizes pathogens in the infant's gut.

The third area of biologic activity is the binding of IgE to mast cell and basophil receptors through their Fc regions. Because of this "stickiness," IgE antibodies are called *cytophilic antibodies*. The reaction following the second exposure of specific antigen with IgE molecules bound to mast cells triggers allergic responses. The IgE molecule and allergic responses are detailed in Chapter 12.

**MINI SUMMARY**

Antibodies are divided, based on their heavy chain structure, into five chemically distinct classes—four kinds of IgG and two kinds of IgA, plus IgM, IgD, and IgE. Each class plays a different role in the immune system's defense strategy. IgG, the major antibody in the blood, coats microorganisms to speed up their uptake by phagocytic cells. The dimeric IgA concentrates in body fluids to guard the entrances of the body. IgM, a pentamer, is the most effective activator

of complement (and therefore is the best indirect killer of blood-borne bacteria). IgD is found almost exclusively on the surface of B cells, where it may regulate the cell's activation. IgE, found in trace amounts in the blood, attaches itself to specialized cells, where it triggers the symptoms of allergies.

Antibodies have many biologic activities. They can prevent toxins and viruses from entering cells, whereas other antibodies coat bacteria or target cells to make them more palatable or vulnerable to attack by certain immune cells. Antigen-antibody complexes also can activate complement. Some antibodies, like IgG, cross the placenta and provide protection to the fetus. IgE can promote allergies, attach to Fc receptors on B cells, and inhibit B-cell activation.

# SUMMARY

*Antigens* are considered nonself as measured by specific responses of the humoral (antibody-making) or cell-mediated (T lymphocyte) immune system. *Immunogenicity* is the ability of a substance (*immunogen*) to trigger the immune system in a naïve (previously unexposed) host. *Antigenicity* is the ability of a substance (*antigen*) to react with lymphocyte receptors or antibody once they have been induced. Antigens capable of inducing an immune response have four common characteristics: (1) high molecular weight, (2) chemical complexity, (3) biodegradability, and (4) foreignness. These characteristics are affected by the dose and route of antigen exposure, the inclusion of adjuvants, which enhance immunogenicity, with antigen, and the genotype of the host.

The entire antigenic structure is not involved in the immune response. *Antigenic determinants*, or *epitopes*, are small regions of the antigen that interact with the cells or antibodies of the immune system. Small antigens called *haptens* must be conjugated to larger *carrier molecules* before they can induce an immune response. Once the immune response has been induced, the hapten alone can interact with antibody. Hapten-carrier conjugates were used to assess the specificity of antigen-antibody reactions. Studies of antibody specificity using haptens led to the conclusions that the (1) chemical nature, (2) position, (3) size, (4) charge, and (5) stereoisomerism of chemically defined antigenic determinants are important in the specificity of antigen-antibody interactions. Antigenic determinants that contact the antibody molecule are small (6 sugar residues or 15 to 22 amino acid residues) and must be *accessible*. Antigenic determinants can consist of *continuous* or *discontinuous* amino acid sequences. The latter determinants depend on the native (unaltered) spatial conformation and are called *assembled topographic determinants*. Within a given protein's (or carbohydrate's) antigenic site, certain amino acid (or sugar) residues are more immunologically important than others (*immunodominance*). Antigen site mobility also contributes to protein antigenicity.

Humoral immunity involves a class of *immunoglobulins* called *antibodies*. The electrophoretic mobility of antibodies usually places them in the *γ-globulin fraction* of serum. Antibodies can directly inactivate antigens and indirectly lead to their destruction through enhanced phagocytosis and complement activation. Antibody classes differ in antigenicity, charge, function, and size. These differences explain antibody functions such as (1) versatility in antigen binding, (2) binding specificity, and (3) biologic activities.

A typical antibody molecule (the prototype class of immunoglobulin is IgG) is made up of four polypeptide chains with a molecular weight of about 150 kD. The four chains are divided into two identical *light chains* and two identical *heavy chains*. An antibody molecule is Y-shaped, with two identical *antigen-binding sites* at the ends of the arms of the Y. The light and heavy chains contribute to the antigen-binding sites. Each antibody molecule can bind to two identical antigenic determinants. Where the arms meet, the stem of the Y is known as the *hinge region*. The hinge region allows *segmental flexibility* of the antibody molecule. The two antigen-binding ends (or amino-terminal ends) of the antibody molecule are called the *Fab fragments* (for fragment antigen binding), whereas the stem (or carboxyl-terminal end) of the Y is considered to be the *Fc fragment* (for fragment crystallizable). The Fc

region of the antibody molecule is responsible for its biologic properties, which include activation of the complement system (leading to enhanced phagocytosis), placental transfer, and binding to cell-surface receptors. Myeloma proteins were important in early characterization studies on antibodies.

The amino-terminal end of an antibody is called the *variable*, or *V*, *region* and the carboxyl-terminal end is called the *constant*, or *C*, *region*. The C region is the about the same size as the V region in the light chain and three or four times larger than the V region in the heavy chain. The V regions of light and heavy chains form the antigen-binding sites. Light and heavy chains consist of repeating, similarly folded homology units or *domains*. The light chain has one V-region ($V_L$) domain and one C-region ($C_L$) domain, whereas the heavy chain has one V region ($V_H$) and three or four C-region ($C_H$) domains. The most variable parts of the V regions are limited to several small *hypervariable regions* or *complementarity-determining regions* (*CDRs*). The light- and heavy-chain V regions contain three CDRs. The CDRs come together at the amino-terminal end of the antibody molecule to form the antigen-binding site, which determines *specificity*. The invariant regions of amino acids, between the CDRs, make up about 85% of the V regions and are designated *framework residues*.

Antigenic determinants that define antibody classes are called *isotypic determinants*, and the classes are referred to as *isotypes*. Isotypic determinants also define *subclasses of antibodies*. The IgG class consists of four subclasses, while the IgA class has two subclasses. Light chains are made up of two classes, κ and λ. Either κ or λ chains can be associated with any class of heavy chain. A κλ chain combination never occurs on the same antibody molecule. Only one isotype of the κ chain exists, while there are four isotypes of λ chains. *Allotypic determinants* define antibodies called *allotypes* and are encoded by genes that have several alleles. Allotypes have been characterized for all four subclass chains of IgG, the IgA2 subclass chain, and the κ chain. They are called *Gm, Am*, and *Km*, respectively. *Idiotypic determinants* define antibody molecules called *idiotypes*. These determinants are located at the antigen-binding site.

The five different *classes of immunoglobulins* are called *IgG, IgA, IgM, IgD*, and *IgE*, each with a distinctive heavy chain designated γ, α, μ, δ, and ε, respectively. IgG is the major antibody in the blood, but it is capable of entering tissue spaces, where it coats antigens, speeding their uptake. IgA concentrates in body fluids to guard the entrances of the body. The extracirculatory dimeric IgA and the circulating IgM are polymerized by a glycopeptide *J chain*. A glycoprotein *secretory component* is added to dimeric IgA by mucosal epithelial cells. This antibody molecule is called *secretory IgA*. IgM is the largest antibody; it tends to remain in the blood, where it can efficiently kill bacteria. IgD remains membrane-bound and somehow regulates the cell's activation. IgE is found in trace amounts in the blood and triggers allergies.

# SELF-EVALUATION

## RECALLING KEY TERMS

Accessibility
Allotypes
Allotypic determinants
  Am
  Gm
  Km
Antibodies
Antibody subclasses
Antigen
Antigenic determinants
Antigenic site mobility
Antigenicity
Constant (C) region
Continuous (linear) determinants
Discontinuous (conformational or assembled
  topographic) determinants
Epitopes
Fab fragment
Fab' fragment
F(ab')₂ fragment
Fc fragment
Framework residues
Gm markers
Haptens
Heavy (H) chain
Hinge region
Hypervariable regions (complementarity-determining
  regions [CDRs])
Idiotypes
Idiotypic determinants (or Idiotopes)
Immunodominance
Immunogen
Immunogenicity
Immunoglobulin (or antibody) classes
Immunoglobulin domains
Immunoglobulin superfamily
Immunoglobulins
  Membrane-bound immunoglobulins
  Secreted immunoglobulins
Isotype

Isotypic determinants
Joining (J) chain
Km markers
Light (L) chain
Multiple myeloma
Neonatal Fc receptor (FcR$_N$)
Secretory IgA
Segmental flexibility
Tailpieces
Variable (V) region

## MULTIPLE-CHOICE QUESTIONS

*(An answer key is not provided, but the page[s] location of the answer is.)*

1. Which of the following is unlikely to induce an antibody response? (a) polysaccharides, (b) lipids, (c) proteins, (d) proteins to which carbohydrate side chains are attached, that is, glycoproteins, (e) none of these. *(See page 107.)*

2. Haptens (a) are not antigenic by themselves, (b) are macromolecules, (c) are usually protein-like, (d) cannot bind to an antibody molecule unless coupled to a carrier, (e) are none of these. *(See pages 110 and 111.)*

3. The following characteristics may make an antigen immunogenic: (a) high molecular weight, (b) chemical complexity, (c) biodegradability, (d) all of these are needed but not sufficient, (e) none of these. *(See pages 107 and 108.)*

4. Consider two protein antigens, *X* and *Y*. Antigen *X* has a molecular weight of 150,000 and is made up of a single repeating epitope. Antigen *Y* has a molecular weight of 100,000 and is made up of 10 different types of epitopes. Which antigen is more immunogenic? (a) antigen *X*, (b) antigen *Y*, (c) of equal immunogenicity, (d) neither is immunogenic, (e) cannot be determined from data given, (f) none of these. *(See pages 107 and 108.)*

5. All amino acid residues within a determinant contribute equally to immunologic reactivity. (a) true, (b) false. *(See pages 114 and 116.)*

6. A human myeloma protein (IgM-κ) is used to immunize a rabbit. The resulting antiserum is then absorbed with a large pool of IgM purified from normal human serum. Following this absorption, the antiserum is found to react only with the particular IgM myeloma protein used for immunization; it is now defined as an anti-idiotypic antiserum. With what specific portion(s) of the IgM myeloma protein would

the antiserum react? (a) constant region of the κ chain, (b) variable regions of the μ and κ chains, (c) constant region of the μ chain, (d) J chain, (e) none of these. *(See pages 125 to 127.)*

7. Which of the following statements, concerning papain cleavage of IgG is incorrect? (a) the Fc fragment contains part of the heavy chain, (b) the Fab fragment contains both heavy-chain and light-chain determinants, (c) the Fc fragment interacts specifically with certain lymphoid cell receptors, (d) the Fab fragment is divalent, (e) antisera prepared against the Fc fragment are specific for the IgG class of immunoglobulins, (f) none of these. *(See pages 117 to 119.)*

8. The antigen-binding sites of an antibody molecule are located in the (a) C region of light chains, (b) V region of light chains, (c) C region of heavy chains, (d) V region of heavy chains, (e) V regions of both light and heavy chains, (f) none of these. *(See pages 120 to 122, and 125 to 127.)*

9. The class-specific antigenic determinants of immunoglobulins are associated with the (a) light chain, (b) heavy chain, (c) J chain, (d) secretory component, (e) none of these. *(See pages 126 and 127.)*

10. The greater resistance of secretory IgA to proteolytic enzymes is assumed to be a consequence of the (a) binding of the secretory component, (b) predominantly dimeric nature of secretory IgA, (c) antiprotease activity of heavy chain, (d) presence of the J chain, (e) none of these. *(See page 128.)*

11. IgG is not (a) the major antibody that confers passive immunity on the fetus, (b) divided into five subclasses, (c) made up of two antigen-binding sites, (d) any of these. *(See pages 128 and 129.)*

12. IgM is (a) not involved in agglutination (clumping) reactions, (b) found as a pentamer on the B lymphocyte's surface, (c) the predominant antibody in the serum, (d) a pentamer in the blood, (e) none of these. *(See pages 128 and 129.)*

13. IgA (a) is the predominant antibody in colostrum, (b) is present on the surface of all naïve mature B cells, (c) has a molecular weight of 150,000, (d) mediates precipitation reactions, (e) is none of these. *(See pages 128 and 129.)*

14. Which of the following represent allotypes? (a) λ light chains, (b) IgA2, (c) Gm, (d) Km, (e) *c* and *d*, (f) none of these. *(See pages 126 and 127.)*

15. Idiotypes are (a) located in the C region of the light chain, (b) located in the C region of the heavy chain, (c) are located in and around the antigen-binding region of an antibody molecule, (d) none of these. *(See page 127.)*

## SHORT-ANSWER ESSAY QUESTIONS

1. Explain the difference between immunogenicity and antigenicity.
2. An entire antigen molecule does not induce an immune response. Explain.
3. List and briefly explain any three characteristics of antigenic determinants.
4. Haptens can be used to test the specificity of antibodies. Why and how?
5. Describe the two opposing views of what constitutes a protein's antigenic determinant. What role did monoclonal antibodies play in initiating the new views of antigenic determinants?
6. The structure of an antibody molecule is related to its function. Explain.
7. The analysis of antibody molecules by papain and pepsin fragmentation led to similar yet different results. Explain.
8. What is the difference between an immunoglobulin and a myeloma protein? Why were myeloma proteins critical to the early studies on antibody structure?
9. What are antibody domains?
10. The variability of the amino acid sequence in the antibody's V region was not random but precisely organized. Explain. Differentiate between complementarity-determining regions and framework regions.
11. Explain the statements "antibodies can be antigens" or "antibodies are used to characterize antibodies."
12. Briefly discuss immunoglobulin isotypic, allotypic, and idiotypic determinants. Give examples of each.
13. Why can't light chains be used to classify antibodies?
14. List the five classes of antibodies and give a key biologic property of each.

## FURTHER READINGS

Amit, A.G., R.A. Mariuzza, S.E.V. Phillips, and R.J. Poljak. 1986. Three-dimensional structure of an antigen-antibody complex at 2.8 AA resolution. *Science* 233:747–753.

Benjamin, D.C., J.A. Berzofsky, I.J. East, F.R.N. Gurd, C. Hannum, S.J. Leach, E. Margoliash, J.G. Michael, A. Miller, E.M. Prager, M. Reichlin, E.E. Sercarz, S.J. Smith-Gill, P.E. Todd, and A.C. Wilson. 1984. The antigenic structure of proteins: A reappraisal. *Annu. Rev. Immunol.* 2:51–101.

Berzofsky, J.A. 2003. Immunogenicity and antigen structure. In *Fundamental Immunology*, 5th ed. W.E. Paul, ed. Philadelphia: Lippincot Williams & Wilkins. p. 631–684.

Kelly, D., S. Conway, and R. Aminov. 2005. Commensal gut bacteria: Mechanisms of immune modulation. *Trends Immunol.* 26:326–333.

Kindt, T.J., and J.D. Capra. 1984. *The Antibody Enigma*. New York: Plenum Press.

Landsteiner, K. 1962. *The Specificity of Serological Reactions*, rev. ed. New York: Dover Publications.

Laver, W.G., G.M. Air, R.G. Webster, and S.J. Smith-Gill. 1990. Epitopes on protein antigens: Misconceptions and realities. *Cell* 61:553–556.

Mazumdar, P.M.H. 2003. Immunoglobulins: Structure & function. In *Fundamental Immunology*, 5th ed. W.E. Paul, ed. Philadelphia: Lippincot Williams & Wilkins. p. 47–68.

Novotny, J., M. Handschumacher, E. Haber, R.E. Bruccoleri, W.B. Carlson, D.W. Fanning, J.A. Smith, and G.D. Rose. 1985. Antigenic determinants in proteins coincide with surface regions accessible to large probes (antibody domains). *Proc. Natl. Acad. Sci. U.S.A.* 83:226–230.

Ravetch, J.V. 2003. Fc receptors. In *Fundamental Immunology*, 5th ed. W.E. Paul, ed. Philadelphia: Lippincot Williams & Wilkins. p. 685–700.

Rojas, R., and G. Apodaca. 2002. Immunoglobulin transport across polarized epithelial cells. *Nat. Rev. Immunol.* 3:1–12.

Tainer, J.A., E.D. Getzoff, Y. Paterson, A.J. Olson, and R.A. Lerner. 1985. The atomic mobility component of protein antigenicity. *Annu. Rev. Immunol.* 3:501–535.

Woof, J.M., and D.R. Burton. 2004. Human antibody–Fc receptor interactions illuminated by crystal structures. *Nat. Rev. Immunol.* 4:1–11.

Woof, J.M., and M.A. Kerr. 2006. The function of immunoglobulin A in immunity. *J. Pathol.* 208:270–282.

Wu, T.T., and E.A. Kabat. 1970. An analysis of the sequences of the variable regions of Bence-Jones proteins and myeloma light chains and their implications for antibody complementarity. *J. Exp. Med.* 132:211–250.

# CHAPTER FIVE

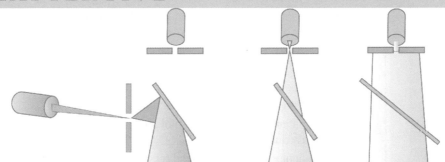

# ANTIGEN-ANTIBODY INTERACTIONS AND SOME EXPERIMENTAL SYSTEMS

2. Secondary antigen-antibody interactions occur when primary antigen-antibody complexes aggregate to form large visible lattices.

   a. Precipitation is the combination of soluble antigen with specific antibody, which leads to the formation of an insoluble aggregation.

      1) The zone phenomenon shows the reversibility of precipitation reactions.

      2) Precipitation reactions can be tested in many ways.

         a) Precipitation reactions can occur in fluids.

         b) Precipitation reactions can occur in gels.

   b. Agglutination is the combination of a particulate (insoluble) antigen with specific antibody, which leads to a clumping of particles.

      1) The agglutination of red blood cells is called hemagglutination.

      2) The naturally occurring antibodies that react with RBC antigens and cause hemagglutination can be used to distinguish human blood groups.

         a) The best-known human blood group system is the ABO system.

         b) Another important human blood group system is the Rh system.

3. Monoclonal antibodies are pure antibodies with single epitope specificities.

   a. Monoclonal antibody development improves on nature.

   b. Monoclonal antibodies have many applications.

4. The transfer of cloned genes provides information on the *in vivo* activity of immune genes.

5. Immune system characterization using gene expression patterns from microarrays.

## OBJECTIVES

The reader should be able to:

1. Explain a primary antigen-antibody interaction; list three important characteristics.

2. Name and understand the forces that foster primary antigen-antibody interactions.

3. Distinguish between antibody affinity and avidity.

4. Give an account of the strength of primary antigen-antibody interactions using equilibrium dialysis and define K and $K_0$.

5. Compare and contrast the RIA and ELISA; discuss the advantages and disadvantages of each procedure.

6. Describe the direct and indirect fluorescent antibody methods; comment on confocal microscopy and flow cytometry.

7. Convey the basics of Western blotting.

8. Explain a secondary antigen-antibody interaction; discuss how a lattice forms.

9. Define a precipitation reaction; understand the physical basis for immunoprecipitate formation; understand why appropriate soluble antigens and antibodies become insoluble when they react.

10. Explain the zone phenomenon.

11. List and distinguish between various procedures used to determine the presence and quantity of soluble antigen and antibody in a fluid and in a gel.

12. Assess the reasons for using the different gel precipitation reactions.

13. Distinguish between an agglutination reaction and a precipitation reaction; give the advantages of each.

14. Discriminate between a direct agglutination and an indirect agglutination reaction.

15. Comment on the three varieties of hemagglutination testing.

16. Understand the connection between naturally occurring antibodies and red blood cell antigens in classifying human blood groups.

17. Describe the ABO blood group; comment on the antigen on the cell, the antibody in serum, the percentage of the U.S. population possessing the antigen, and the respective genotypes and phenotypes of each group.

18. Appreciate the importance of the Rh system; realize that antibodies against Rh antigens are different from antibodies against ABO antigens.

19. Assess the role of Rh antigens in hemolytic disease of the newborn; comment on the fact that passive antibody administration prevents immunization in the recipient and thereby prevents hemolytic disease of the newborn.

20. Contrast conventional antibody and monoclonal antibody development; discuss hybrid monoclonal antibodies.

21. Describe the general procedure for developing transgenic mice; comment on transgenic knockout mice.

22. Tell how microarray analysis changes the "one-gene-one-experiment" paradigm.

In the previous chapters, we have hinted at immunologic techniques used to characterize innate and adaptive immune responses. Many of these immunologic assays depend on a bimolecular association between antigen and antibody, much like the association between an enzyme and its substrate but unlike enzyme-substrate interactions there is no alteration in either antigen or antibody. The antigen and antibody interaction revolves around the highly specific, noncovalent association between an epitope and complementarity-determining regions in antibody light and heavy chain variable domains. The specificity of these interactions is the crux of immunologic tests that detect, characterize, and quantify antigens, antibodies, immune complexes, and cells involved in the humoral immune response. Most of the immunologic techniques we will mention depend on the fundamental properties of antigen-antibody interactions; others involved molecular biologic methods, genetic engineering, cell culturing, and animal models. The chapter starts with a discussion on the nature of the antigen-antibody interaction, describes immune assays that measure or exploit this interaction, and ends with descriptions of other assay systems that have contributed to our understanding of the immune system.

As you read in the preceding chapter, antibodies react specifically with the epitopes of the antigen that stimulated their formation. Antibodies are found in blood serum, the fluid left after blood has clotted.

**Serology** *is the science dealing with the in vitro interactions of antibodies with antigens.* Antibodies can be used to discriminate and identify an infinite number of substances or pathogens. *The interaction of an antigenic determinant and an antibody molecule is called a* **primary antigen-antibody interaction**, and the cardinal characteristic of primary antigen-antibody interactions is that they are *invisible*. Methods that use primary antigen-antibody interactions are some of the most sensitive tests known. The conversion of invisible primary interactions to macroscopically visible ones leads to *secondary antigen-antibody interactions* such as precipitation and agglutination.

*In vitro* antigen-antibody interactions are indispensable in: (1) clinical applications, (2) assessment of the basics of the immune response, and (3) research applications. The earliest clinical application of antibodies was in the diagnosis of infectious disease. Pathogens cultivated from the patient can be identified using an antibody of known specificity. Alternatively, antibody specific for the pathogen can be detected in a patient's bloodstream. The latter method is used for pathogens not easily cultivated. An additional clinical application of antibodies is their use in the identification of cell surface antigens. This application can determine blood group and organ transplant incompatibilities. Antibodies have been used to characterize immune cells and follow their maturation. Applications of these techniques have been used throughout the biologic sciences. Methods using antibodies range from measuring drugs and hormones to developing taxonomic schemes. These varied and important applications began with the understanding of antigen-antibody interactions.

# PRIMARY ANTIGEN-ANTIBODY INTERACTIONS OCCUR WHEN INDIVIDUAL ANTIGENIC DETERMINANTS BIND TO THEIR APPROPRIATE ANTIBODY-COMBINING SITES

## Antibody Interlocks with Antigen Much as a Key Matches a Lock

The primary antigen-antibody interaction is dependent solely on the interaction of an epitope with the antigen-binding site of an antibody. An antigenic determinant is precisely complementary to the cleft or groove of the antibody's binding site (Figure 5-1). The amino acids lining the antigen-binding site bind tonobreak thenobreak epitope by weak noncovalent interactions, and the hypervariable regions of the heavy and light chains participate in antigen binding. The engagement of an antigen determinant at the binding site of an antibody mirrors both a key

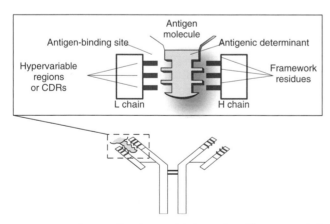

**FIGURE 5-1 The antibody-combining site.** This is a cleft formed by the hypervariable, or complementarity determining regions (CDRs), of antibody heavy and light chains. The antigenic determinant (epitope) rests within this complementarity cleft. The CDRs provide the 10 to 12 amino acids that contact the epitope. Framework residues do not directly contact the epitope but produce the folding of the variable regions (thus present CDRs) and maintain the integrity of the antibody-combining site.

matching a lock (because of specificity) and a hand fitting into a glove (because of antigen-site mobility).

## The Antigen-Antibody Interaction Is Precise; This Precision Is Called Specificity

The precise fit of an antibody with an antigenic determinant indicates a high degree of specificity. Limitations to antibody specificity are recognized but usually antibodies directed against one epitope are not complementary to epitopes of another antigen. For example, antibodies made against influenza virus do not react with or protect against polio virus. However, if two different antigens share some epitopes, then an antiserum will recognize and bind these shared antigenic determinants. The result is called **cross-reactivity**. Antiserum is made up of a population of antibodies reacting specifically with the homologous antigens but cross-reacting with heterologous antigens because of shared epitopes. Antibodies recognize the total configuration of antigens rather than just their chemical composition. This mechanism of specific recognition allows antibodies to distinguish among slight changes in primary structure, charge, optical configuration, and steric conformation of an antigen. Specific recognition of antigens is the hallmark of antibodies and the reason for their almost unlimited use as quantitative reagents.

## Primary Antigen-Antibody Interactions Have Three Important Characteristics

*A primary antigen-antibody interaction is a reaction dependent only on the interaction of an antigenic determinant and the combining site of an antibody.* Three important characteristics of primary antigen-antibody interactions are recognized: (1) they are rapid interactions (occurring in seconds), (2) they are *not* dependent on electrolytes (such as salts or buffered solutions), and (3) they are *not* visible in the classical sense (because the binding involves an individual epitope and its correct antibody-combining site). Methods that measure primary antigen-antibody interactions are used (1) to quantify antigen or antibody, (2) to detect or localize antigen, and (3) to convert them to visible, measurable reactions.

## Four Types of Noncovalent Interactions Hold Antigenic Determinants Within the Antibody-Combining Site

An antigen binds to an antibody by multiple noncovalent bonds. These interactions are weak (about 5 kcal/mol) compared to covalent bonds

(90–100 kcal/mol) and are effective only over short distances. Bonds are effective only when groups of atoms on one molecule fit complementary recesses on the other molecule. The kinds of noncovalent interactions important in antigen-antibody interactions are presented in Figure 5-2.

*Coulombic* (also termed *electrostatic* or *ionic*) interactions are attractive forces between oppositely charged groups in antigenic determinant and the antigen-binding sites of an antibody. These charged groups are dependent on the pH of their environment. Coulombic interactions also are affected by the salt concentration of the reaction because ions can compete for the sites. For strong charge-charge interactions to take place, molecules must be close. This closeness means that the antigen-binding cleft must be highly complementary to the epitope in shape if this interaction is to play a role in antigen binding.

*Van der Waals forces* are interactions among the electron clouds of all molecules when they are brought close to each other. Attractive forces result from the interactions between the charge fluctuation from electron movement in one molecule and the fluctuating charge distribution in another molecule. When the two molecules approach one another, oscillating dipoles are induced in the electron cloud of each, and a net attractive force results. The closer the complementarity among the electron clouds, the stronger the attractive force.

*Hydrogen bonding* results from the interaction between a hydrogen atom linked to an electronegative atom in one molecule and an unshared electron pair of an electronegative atom of another molecule. This hydrogen bonding forms hydrogen bridges between molecules. In proteins, this bonding can take the form of the carboxyl group of peptide bonds interacting with (1) the amide nitrogen of peptide bonds,

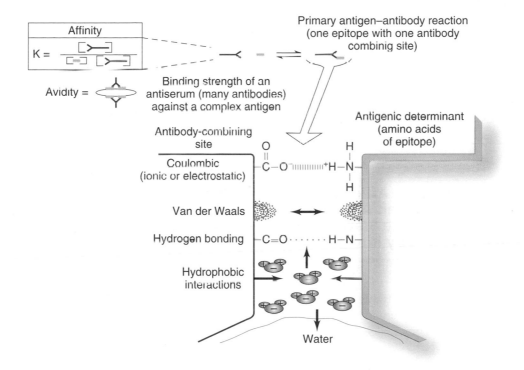

**FIGURE 5-2 The intermolecular noncovalent associations between antigens and antibodies.** Four types of forces hold antigens (epitopes) within the antibody-combining site. For these forces to work, the interacting groups must closely approach each other. *Coulombic (ionic or electrostatic) forces* are caused by attractive forces between oppositely charged groups of proteins in an epitope and antibody-combining site. *Van der Waals forces* are interactions among the electron clouds of molecules brought close to each other. *Hydrogen bonding* is caused by hydrogen bridges between electronegative atoms of close molecules. *Hydrophobic interactions* are caused by the association of nonpolar, hydrophobic groups in an aqueous environment. The important point in all these interaction forces is the distance between the interacting molecules. Any change from optimal distances leads to ineffective binding.

(2) the hydroxyl groups of the amino acid residues threonine and serine, or (3) the hydroxyl groups of carbohydrates. Hydrogen bonds are sensitive to heat.

*Hydrophobic bonds* result from the association of nonpolar (hydrophobic) groups (such as the amino acids leucine and phenylalanine) in an aqueous environment. In globular proteins, the nonpolar amino acid residues are in the interior of the molecule and polar amino acids (such as lysine and aspartic acid) are at the exterior. Large, complementary, hydrophobic regions exist, and the attraction between antigen and antibody molecules is significant. Fifty percent of the binding ability between an antigenic determinant and amino acids at an antigen-binding site may be caused by hydrophobic bonds. Changes in pH and salt concentrations of the reaction medium have minimal effects on the strength of hydrophobic interactions.

---

### MINI SUMMARY

Interaction between antigen and antibody leads to the formation of an immune complex. Noncovalent interactions between antigens and antibodies involve weak chemical forces. No covalent bonds are formed. Antigen-antibody interactions result from (1) coulombic forces, (2) Van der Waals forces, (2) hydrogen bonding, and (4) hydrophobic interactions.

---

## The Strength of Attraction (Affinity) Between an Antibody and an Antigenic Determinant Determines the Stability of a Primary Antigen-Antibody Interaction

The preceding sections suggest the importance of complementarity in determining the strength of antigen-antibody interactions; the tighter the fit, the stronger the interaction. Complementarity allows several noncovalent forces to be created. *The strength of antigen-antibody bonds between one epitope and an individual antibody's antigen-binding site is called* **antibody affinity**. *It differs from* **avidity**, *which is the binding strength between a multivalent antibody and a multivalent antigen.*

The affinity between an antibody's antigen-binding site and an epitope can be analyzed thermodynamically[1] because the noncovalent bonds

between antibody and epitope are dissociable (or reversible). *The reaction of an epitope with an antigen-binding site can be expressed by the following equation, called the* **intrinsic binding reaction**:

$$Ag + Ab \Leftrightarrow [Ag - Ab] \qquad (1)$$

Analyzing Ag-Ab systems by the law of mass action gives the affinity constant, $K$. The right ($\rightarrow$) and left ($\leftarrow$) arrows represent the reaction directions for association and dissociation constants, respectively. Thus, the **equilibrium constant** expressed as an **association constant** ($K$: antibody affinity) would be

$$K = \frac{[Ag - Ab]}{[Ag][Ab]} \qquad (2)$$

where *[Ag-Ab]* is the concentration of complexed antigen, *[Ag]* is the concentration of free antigen, and *[Ab]* is the concentration of free binding sites of antibody at equilibrium. Another way of describing these reactants is: *[Ag-Ab]* is the concentration, at equilibrium, of the occupied antibody sites, *[Ag]* is the concentration of the free (unbound) antigen molecules, and *[Ab]* is the concentration of vacant antibody sites. $K$ is a thermodynamic expression of the tendency of an antibody to bind an antigenic determinant (expressed in liters per mole). $K$ expresses the affinity of the antibody for an antigen: the higher the value of $K$, the more affinity an antibody has for an antigen. How $K$ is studied experimentally is presented in the following section on equilibrium dialysis.

## Equilibrium Dialysis, a Primary Antigen-Antibody Interaction, Can Be Used to Measure Affinity

**Equilibrium dialysis** is an important procedure for measuring the affinity of small molecules (such as haptens) for antibodies. It provides a thermodynamically sound method for obtaining association constants because measurements are performed at equilibrium. Because equilibrium dialysis easily distinguishes free antigen from antigen-antibody complexes, free antigen concentration is measured to determine affinity.

---

[1]Panic may set in at the mere mention of the word *thermodynamics*. The following quotation by the physicist

Arnold Summerfield will not make the discussion easier, but perhaps it will place the next section in perspective. "Thermodynamics is a funny subject. The first time you go through the subject, you don't understand it at all. The second time you go through it, you think you understand it . . . except for one or two small points. The third time you go through it, you *know* you don't understand it, but by that time you are so used to the subject that it doesn't bother you any more."

Equilibrium dialysis has some limitations. For example, (1) it must be performed with haptens because only they are small enough to be dialyzed; (2) purified hapten and antibody are required because the molar concentrations of each must be known; (3) hapten concentration must be measured by coloring or radioactively labeling the hapten; and (4) it assumes that all antibody-combining sites are identical and bind hapten independently of one another. The latter assumption cannot be made when a heterogeneous preparation of antibodies (whole antiserum) is used.

Because known amounts of hapten and antibody are used, equilibrium dialysis is essentially a method that measures the diffusion of haptens across a semipermeable membrane (Figure 5-3). Hapten is placed only on one side of the membrane, but at equilibrium the hapten concentration ($[H]$) on both sides is equal. If the experiment is repeated with hapten placed on one side and antibody placed on the other side, at equilibrium the $[H]$ is again the same on both sides. Taking a closer look at the solution at equilibrium (reaction II in Figure 5-3), the *free [H]*

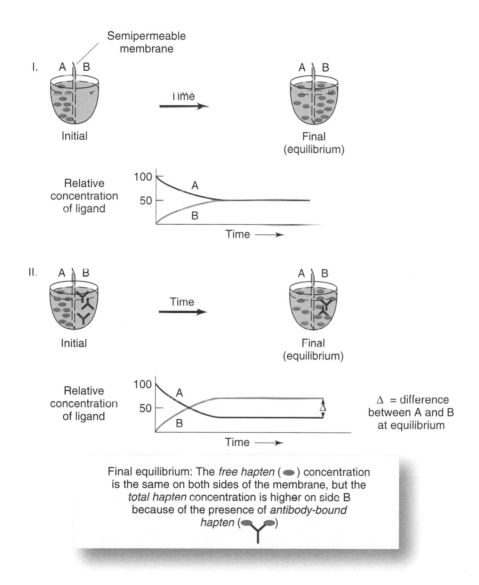

FIGURE 5-3 **Equilibrium dialysis.** *I.* In chamber A, the solid gray ovals represent univalent haptens that can freely diffuse between the two chambers. With time, the hapten concentration becomes equal on both sides of the membrane. *II.* If antibodies are added to chamber B (antibodies cannot cross the membrane), the final equilibrium state changes. The *free hapten concentration* is the same on both sides of the membrane, but chamber B contains more *total hapten* than chamber A.

is the same on both sides of the membrane in both chambers *but* the total *[H]* is higher in chamber B because some hapten is bound to antibody. Because the membrane is semipermeable—permeable to hapten but impermeable to antibody—the *H-Ab complex* cannot cross the membrane. These results can be used to determine affinity and are described below. The reaction will also work if hapten and antibody are placed on the same side of the membrane and a buffer solution on the other side.

Because volumes and the free *[H]* (at equilibrium) are the same on both sides of the membrane, the bound hapten ($[H_{Ab}]$) equals the total hapten ($[H_{Total}]$) minus twice the free hapten ($[H_{Free}]$). The $[H_{Ab}]$ can be calculated using the following formula:

$$[H_{Ab}] = [H_{Total}] - 2[H_{Free}] \qquad (3)$$

Next, measurements are carried out in which the *[Ab]* is held constant and the initial *[H]* is varied. The $[H_{Ab}]$ is determined in each experiment. Because these reactions can be expressed on a molar basis, it is possible to calculate the ratio of moles of hapten bound per mole of antibody (designated *r*) at the concentration of free hapten measured (designated *c*). These calculations assume that the binding of hapten at one site does not influence the reaction at another site, and that all sites have the same association constant. As a result, Equation 2 can be transformed into a new equation:

$$\frac{r}{c} = nK - rK \qquad (4)$$

where *r* equals the moles of hapten bound per mole of antibody, *c* equals free hapten concentration ($[H_{Free}]$) at equilibrium, *n* equals antibody valence (number of combining sites), and *K* equals the association constant. Equation 4 is mathematically determined from Equation 2 by dividing the numerator *[H-Ab]* and the denominator *[Ab]* by the *[Ab]*. Equation 4 states that the curve that represents *r/c* values as a function of *r* is a straight line. Thus, the data are usually plotted according to Scatchard[2] as *r/c* against *r* (Figure 5-4). Because this equation leads to a straight line, the intercept of the line on the abscissa (the point where *r/c = 0*) is equal to *n* (*n* corresponds to the number of antibody-combining sites, that is, antibody valence). The intercept of the line with the ordinate is equal to *nK*. The slope of the equation equals the reciprocal of the association constant (-*K*). In fact, in haptenic excess (high *[H_{Free}]*) close to saturation of the antibody-combining site, represented in Equation 4 as

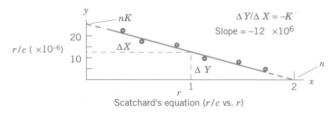

**FIGURE 5-4 Scatchard analysis of specific binding of haptens to antibodies.** The plot of *r/c* versus *r* gives a straight line of slope −*K*.

*c*, the *r/c*. Ratio approaches zero. Therefore *r* is almost equal to *n* because in the equation *r/c = nK − rK*.

Aside from showing the affinity of antibody for antigen, equilibrium dialysis was the first experimental method to define antibody valence (for IgG, *n* = 2; for IgM, *n* = 10). Scatchard analysis also allows an estimate of antibody homogeneity in a given experiment. If the antibody preparation is heterogeneous (antiserum collected after immunization) or if the interaction of hapten with one antibody-combining site influences another site, a straight line is not obtained because the antibody molecules have different association constants (*K*). The next few paragraphs describe how to determine the *K* of antiserum.

Because antibodies produced by conventional immunization are heterogeneous, Scatchard's analyses usually do not produce a straight line (Figure 5-5). Because antibodies differ in affinity, Equation 4 is not linear; therefore, *K* cannot be read off the graph because there is a combination of affinities resulting from the different clones that are responding to antigen. The question then is: "How do you determine affinity of antibody produced by immunization?"

If Equation 4 leads to nonlinearity, it is useful to determine an average value called $K_0$ rather than *K*. $K_0$ is defined by the *[H_{Free}]* required to occupy

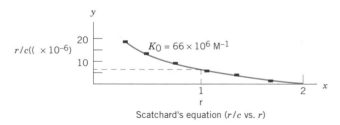

Scatchard's equation (*r/c* vs. *r*)

**FIGURE 5-5 Scatchard plot of a heterogeneous solution of antibodies.** Antibodies produced by conventional immunization are heterogeneous; thus, a Scatchard analysis is difficult. The fact that antibody-epitope pairs have diverse binding constants leads to nonlinearity in *r/c* compared with *r*. Therefore, it is useful to determine an average value, $K_0$.

half the antibody-combining sites. Thus, if $r = n/2$ is substituted in Equation 4, the results are:

$$\frac{1}{c} = 2K - 1K \qquad (5)$$

or

$$K_0 = \frac{1}{c} \qquad (6)$$

where $K_0$ equals the reciprocal of the $[H_{Free}]$ when half the antibody-combining sites are filled; for example, if the antibody is IgG, when $r = 1$, half the combining sites are bound. $K_0$ is called the **average intrinsic association constant** and is a measure of the **average affinity**. For example, if $K_0 = 10^8$ liters/mole, half of the antibody-combining sites are bound to hapten when $[H_{Free}]$ is $1 \times 10^{-8}$ M. $K_0$ for antisera range from $10^4$ to $10^9$ M$^{-1}$. Thus, Equation 1 would be expressed as

$$Ag + Ab \longleftrightarrow \longrightarrow [Ag - Ab] \qquad (7)$$

At equilibrium, the concentration of the Ag-Ab complex is high compared to that of free Ag or Ab.

The affinity information derived from equilibrium dialysis is important because it shows that $K_0$ or antibody affinity increases in an animal repeatedly challenged with antigen. The biologic significance of this selection is that low-affinity antibody production is shut off, while high-affinity antibody production is selected. High-affinity antibodies are more likely to bind pathogens and activate the effector mechanisms of humoral immunity.

---

### MINI SUMMARY

The affinity of antigen and antibody interactions can be tested by equilibrium dialysis. It measures the concentration of free and bound hapten. Scatchard plots of the data can be used to calculate the affinity ($K$) and antibody valence ($n$). Because antigens and antibodies are not homogeneous, the curves are not linear. An average affinity ($K_0$) can be determined. $K_0$ increases with time after antigen exposure and with the number of exposures.

---

## Other Methods Detect Primary Antigen-Antibody Interactions

Primary interaction methods have some common features. They all (1) require the use of purified antigen or antibody, (2) must be quantitative and sensitive, (3) usually use isotopic or fluorescent labeling, and (4) involve the separation of free antigen or antibody molecules from antigen-antibody complexes. A description of four such methods follows.

### *Fluorescence Quenching, in Which an Antigenic Determinant Fits into an Antibody-Combining Site to Block Fluorescence, Can Be Used to Detect Primary Antigen-Antibody Interactions*

Because antibodies are proteins, they emit fluorescent energy in the ultraviolet spectrum. The amino acids phenylalanine, tryptophan, and tyrosine absorb ultraviolet light at 280 nm. This absorption excites electrons from the ground state, leading to energy emitted as visible light (350 nm), called *fluorescence* (Figure 5-6). If antibody specific for hapten is exposed to ultraviolet light, the amount of fluorescence can be measured. By varying the amount of hapten added to the antibody, the amount of fluorescence can be determined as a function of hapten added. As more hapten is added, the fluorescence drops. The hapten *quenches fluorescence* when it is bound to antibody because it may cover aromatic amino acid residues at the antibody-combining site or it may absorb emitted

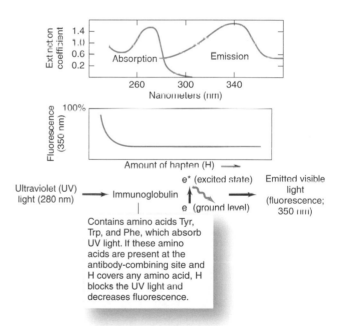

**FIGURE 5-6 Principle of fluorescence quenching and plotting of fluorescence quenching.** The top graph shows the absorption and emission spectra of a purified antibody (for example, antibody against the hapten dinitrophenyl). The middle graph shows the decline in fluorescence (fluorescence quenching) of the antibody as it binds increasing amounts of hapten. The mechanism behind fluorescence quenching is depicted at the bottom of the figure.

light when bound to antibody. Thus, the quenching of fluorescence is related to the amount of hapten bound. Measurements similar to $K_0$ can then be made (see Figure 5-6). A more basic aspect of the method is that it will detect the absence or presence of a hapten-antibody interaction.

### Radioimmunoassay (RIA), in Which Radioactively Labeled and Unlabeled Substances Compete, Can Be Used to Detect Primary Antigen-Antibody Interactions

RIA was popularized by Yalow and Berson in 1960.[3] Since its introduction, RIA has become one of the most widely used assays because of its sensitivity in detecting biologic molecules. RIAs can detect picogram amounts ($10^{-12}$ g). Most classic immunologic reactions before RIA could not detect such small amounts of antigen or antibody (they detected microgram amounts) because the mass of the individual antigen-antibody reaction is too small for them to measure. *RIAs involve the binding of low concentrations of highly radioactively labeled antigen to low concentrations of specific antibody that are sensitive to competition of unlabeled antigen. One antibody reacts with either labeled or unlabeled antigen.*

---

[3]Rosalyn Yalow received the Nobel Prize in 1977 for her work.

Yalow and Berson set out to measure the amount of insulin in the blood. They incorporated radioactive isotopes into antigen molecules, so that their Equation 1 became

$$Ag^* + Ab \Leftrightarrow [Ag^* - Ab] \qquad (8)$$

where * represents the radiolabel (the Ag*-Ab complex is at equilibrium). Antigen molecules are so radioactive that even picogram amounts can easily be detected. The Ag*-Ab complex, therefore, is detected by its radioactivity, not by its mass. Yalow and Berson proposed that there would be *competition* between radioactively labeled insulin and known amounts of unlabeled blood insulin, both trying to bind to a limited number of antibody molecules specific for insulin (Figure 5-7). As they added more unlabeled antigen, the amount of radioactive antigen bound to antibody dropped because some labeled antigen was displaced from the binding sites. Thus, by measuring the amount of free-labeled antigen in solution, they could determine the concentration of unlabeled antigen. They used the results from this assay system to set up a standard curve to measure insulin in the blood (Figure 5-8). Thus, by reduction of labeled insulin bound to antibody, they could determine the insulin concentration in the blood—a method elegant in its simplicity.

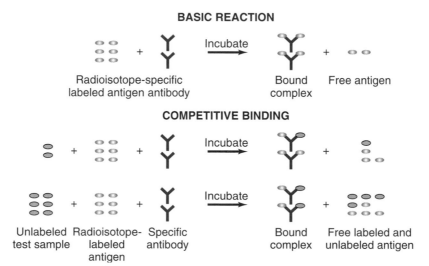

**BASIC REACTION**

Radioisotope-specific labeled antigen antibody    Incubate    Bound complex    Free antigen

**COMPETITIVE BINDING**

Unlabeled test sample   Radioisotope-labeled antigen   Specific antibody    Incubate    Bound complex   Free labeled and unlabeled antigen

**FIGURE 5-7 Principle of RIA in testing for insulin.** Competition for antibody binding occurs between known amounts of labeled insulin (darkened circles) and unknown amounts of unlabeled blood insulin. As more unlabeled antigen is added, the amount of radioactive antigen bound to antibody drops because some unlabeled antigen binds to antibody. The result is less radioactivity associated with antibody. The amount of radioactive insulin bound to antibody is measured as a function of unlabeled insulin added.

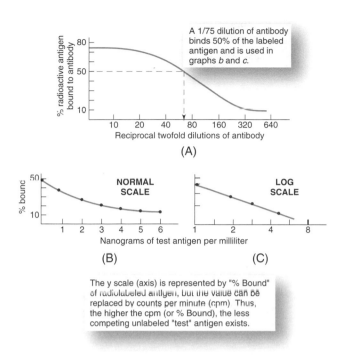

A 1/75 dilution of antibody binds 50% of the labeled antigen and is used in graphs *b* and *c*.

(A)

NORMAL SCALE

LOG SCALE

Nanograms of test antigen per milliliter

(B)                    (C)

The y scale (axis) is represented by "% Bound" of radiolabeled antigen, but the value can be replaced by counts per minute (cpm). Thus, the higher the cpm (or % Bound), the less competing unlabeled "test" antigen exists.

**FIGURE 5-8** Standard curve for RIA.

### Enzyme-Linked Immunosorbent Assay (ELISA), in Which Enzyme-Labeled Antibody Binds an Antigen, Leading to Substrate Breakdown and Color Change, Can Be Used to Detect Primary Antigen-Antibody Interactions

A group of primary antigen-antibody interactions analogous to RIA are called *enzyme immunoassays*; the most widely used form of these assays is the **enzyme-linked immunosorbent assay** (**ELISA**). ELISA uses an enzyme for labeling rather than a radioisotope. Like the radioisotope, the enzyme is covalently coupled to the antibody; in principle, this is the only difference between ELISA and RIA. ELISA measures bound enzyme activity rather than bound counts per minute. Quantification requires measuring the color intensity of the colored products generated by the enzyme and added substrate. The intensity of the color is equivalent to the amount of labeled antibody bound to antigen. Enzymes used in ELISA include β-galactosidase, glucose oxidase, peroxidase, and alkaline phosphatase. ELISA has replaced RIA in many clinical and basic science laboratories. RIAs are potentially hazardous and tedious, require bookkeeping, and involve radioisotopes. These reasons, combined with the commercial availability of plate readers that can measure the absorbance of 96 wells in less than a minute, accounts for the ELISA's growing popularity. ELISA and RIA are similar in sensitivity. Theoretically, ELISA can be more sensitive than RIA

because each enzyme molecule can generate hundreds of thousands of colored product molecules that can be measured. In contrast, $^{125}$I molecule decays only once.

***There are three variants of the ELISA.*** Three basic ELISA techniques have clinical value: the indirect ELISA, for the detection and measurement of antibody, the sandwich ELISA, and the competitive ELISA, the latter two for the detection and measurement of antigen. The various ELISA tests are shown diagrammatically in Figure 5-9.

The *indirect ELISA* is used as a qualitative or quantitative assay for antibodies, which is used to detect, among other things, antibodies against the human immunodeficiency virus, the cause of AIDS (see Figure 5-9). The initial step involves coating the well wall with antigen by adsorption. Test antiserum is added and allowed to incubate. If any antibodies in the test antiserum have bound to the immobilized antigen, their presence is detected by adding an enzyme-conjugated secondary antibody (enzyme-tagged anti-antibody, or antibody made against the isotype of the primary specific antibody). Enzyme substrate is then added; the rate of its hydrolysis is associated with a color change proportional to the concentration of antibody present in the test sample. This color change can be monitored visually or by a spectrophotometer.

As already noted, ELISA is used to assay for antibody. But the method also can be used as a qualitative or quantitative assay for antigens, such as, by the *sandwich ELISA*. Antiserum samples are added to the wells in a plate, and the antibodies in the antiserum adhere to the inner surface of each well (see Figure 5-9). The test antigen is added; if the antigen is homologous or specific for the antibody, it attaches to the antibody immobilized on the well surface. An enzyme-conjugated secondary antibody is then added. It will bind to the antigen already fixed by the first antibody, creating an antibody (with enzyme)-antigen-antibody "sandwich." Finally, an enzyme substrate is added to react with the enzyme. The rate of enzyme action is directly proportional to the quantity of enzyme-linked antibody present, which, in turn, is proportional to the amount of test antigen. Enzyme hydrolysis of the substrate causes a color change in the solution that can be seen visually or measured with a spectrophotometer, an instrument used to analyze color changes in a solution.

Another type of ELISA, the *competitive ELISA*, is used to detect or quantify soluble antigens, particularly if both a specific antibody and preparations of pure or semi-pure antigen are available (see

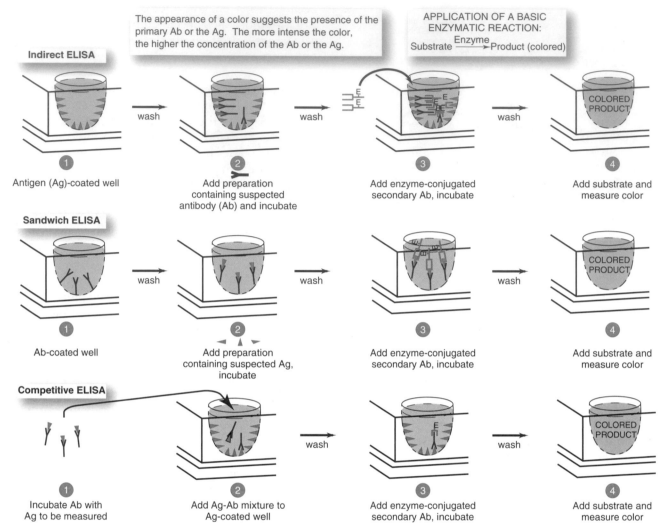

**FIGURE 5-9 ELISA variants**.

Figure 5-9). The test antigen and specific antibody are preincubated, and then the antigen-antibody test mixture is added to an antigen-coated well. The more antigen present in the mixture, the less antibody available to bind to the well-associated antigen. As in the other ELISAs, enzyme-conjugated secondary antibody is added and can be used to determine the amount of primary antibody bound to well-associated antigen as in the indirect ELISA.

The ELISA has been used for the detection of many infectious viruses, bacteria, fungi, and parasites such as protozoa. For example, one antiserum sample from a pregnant woman can be screened simultaneously for infections caused by rubella virus (the agent for German measles, which can cause congenital malformations or fetal death) and by type 2 herpesvirus (which can cause severe congenital nervous system malformations and smallness of the head in the offspring).

*The ELISPOT detects single antibody-secreting cells specific for a given antigen.* Assays analogous to ELISAs, used to quantify antigen-specific cells, are called *enzyme-linked immunospot (ELISPOT) assays.* Antibody-forming cells are detected by overlaying lymphocytes on a plate coated with the specific antigen. The specific antibody binds to the antigen surrounding the cells that secrete it. ELISPOT assays can visualize this type of antibody binding, that is, enzyme-conjugated secondary antibody is added, followed by substrate, which produces a colored spot around the antibody-secreting cells. The technique also is used to identify cells secreting a particular cytokine. For example, cytokine-secreting subsets of T cells can be uncovered by overlaying them on plates coated with anti-interferon-γ (IFN-γ) antibody to capture the IFN-γ. The spot of cytokine is detected by using another antibody to a different epitope of the IFN-γ.

### Fluorescent Antibody Technique, in Which Fluorescently Tagged Antibodies Bind to the Appropriate Antigen, Causing the Antigen to Fluoresce, Can Be Used to Detect Primary Antigen-Antibody Interactions

Another widely used method to detect primary antigen-antibody interactions is **immunofluorescence**. It is a cytochemical or histochemical technique used for the detection and localization of antigens. Its uses generally include (1) detection of antigen on the surface of intact cells or internal antigen within tissue and cell sections and (2) diagnostic detection of antibody specific for pathogens in a patient's serum. The technique uses antibody coupled to fluorescent dyes. The originator of immunofluorescence, A.H. Coons, developed the technique to show the presence of bacteria in tissue sections. When antibody is coupled to a fluorescent dye, the antibody binds to antigen and preparations that are placed in a fluorescent microscope fluoresce.

Fluorescence is the emission of visible light of a characteristic wavelength when irradiated with light of a different color (or shorter wavelength). Incident or absorbed light is at a higher energy level than the emitted wavelength. Organic dyes that emit absorbed light at characteristic wavelengths are called **fluorochromes**. The two most commonly used fluorochromes in immunofluorescence, **fluorescein** and **rhodamine**, have characteristic absorption and emission spectra. Fluorescein's absorption maximum is at 490–495 nm; its characteristic green color is emitted at 517 nm. Rhodamine's absorption maximum is at 550 nm; it emits its characteristic red color at 580 nm. Thus, different excitation and barrier filters must be used in the fluorescence microscope to visualize the characteristic colors of these two fluorochromes.

To conjugate fluorochromes with antibodies, fluorochromes with chemically reactive groups are mixed with purified antibody of the desired specificity. The chemical forms of fluorescein and rhodamine used to react with antibody are *fluorescein isothiocyanate* and *tetramethylrhodamine isothiocyanate*, respectively. These compounds readily bind covalently to proteins at an alkaline pH. To optimize fluorescence, as many dye molecules as possible are attached to antibody molecules without changing the reactivity of the antibody with the antigen.

Two staining techniques are used in immunofluorescence: (1) the **direct fluorescent antibody method** and (2) the **indirect antibody method fluorescent antibody method**. *In the direct test, the fluorescently labeled antibody has specificity for the antigen to be detected. In the indirect test, antibody with specificity for the desired antigen is unlabeled and a second, fluorescently labeled, antibody with a specificity for the first antibody (an antibody to an antibody) is then added to the mixture.* The basic principle for direct and indirect immunofluorescence is shown diagrammatically in Figure 5-10 and Figure 5-11, respectively.

Indirect immunofluorescence methods are more widely used than direct ones because they have two advantages: (1) greater sensitivity and (2) greater versatility. *Direct* methods are less sensitive because only one or two labeled antibodies bind to each antigenic site. This level of binding leads to low fluorescence intensity. In *indirect* methods, many fluorescent (secondary) antibodies bind to each unlabeled (primary) antibody. As a result, more fluorescence occurs at each antigenic site. Primary antibodies with specificity for each antigen to be detected must be labeled in the direct method. In the indirect method, one labeled antibody can be used to detect any antigen when the primary antibody is made in the same species. Both methods have achieved widespread use in clinical applications because of their great usefulness as a sensitive and specific diagnostic tool. Table 5-1 gives a partial list of direct and indirect immunofluorescence applications in clinical immunology.

*Immunohistochemical specimen analysis using confocal scanning microscopy.* Ordinary fluorescence microscopy is not typically used for structural studies. A new approach using fluorescence, **confocal scanning microscopy**, allows imaging of complex three-dimensional objects. In light microscopy, the thinner the sample sections the crisper the image—specimen parts below or above the plane of focus are blurred. Sample sectioning destroys three-dimensional architecture, and some samples cannot be sliced into sections before viewing. Confocal scanning microscopy overcomes this problem (Figure 5-12). During confocal microscopy,

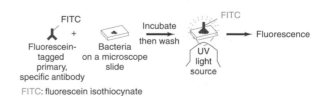

FITC: fluorescein isothiocynate

**FIGURE 5-10 Direct immunofluorescence.**

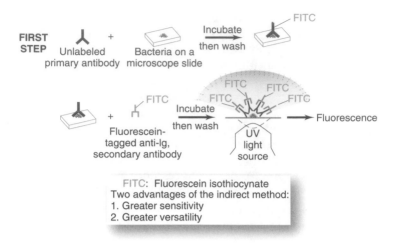

**FIGURE 5-11 Indirect immunofluorescence.**

**TABLE 5-1 Clinical Applications of Immunofluorescence**

1. Detection of complement components in tissues
2. Detection of antibodies in tissues
3. Detection of specific antibody in fixed tissue
4. Identification of microorganisms in culture or tissue
5. Identification of T and B cells in blood
6. Identification of transplantation antigens in different organs
7. Identification of tumor antigens on cancerous tissues

electronic imaging methods allow focusing on a chosen plane in a thick specimen while rejecting the light that is derived from out-of-focus regions. The result is a crisp, thin optical section. The microscope processes a series of optical sections taken at different depths of the specimen. The information is retrieved by a computer and reconstructed into a three-dimensional image.

In contrast to ordinary fluorescence microscopy, which illuminates the entire specimen at once, a confocal microscope's optical systems focus a spotlight onto a single point at a specific specimen depth (see Figure 5-12). Passing laser light through an illuminating pinhole generates a bright spotlight; the emitted specimen fluorescence is then collected and presented at the entry port of a light detector. The detector aperture is placed confocal to the illuminating pinhole—the point where the specimen's emitting illuminating point rays come to a focus. Thus, in-focus light reaches the detector, while out-of-focus is excluded from the detector. A two-dimensional image is produced by sequentially collecting the data from each point in the plane of focus by repeated horizontal line (raster) scanning of the specimen.

*Immunofluorescence staining of immune cells for detection of surface antigens.* The direct interaction of antibodies tagged with a fluorescence tracer and the target cells allows quantification of the amount of an antibody probe present on the target cells, and isolation of pure lymphoid cell populations, The use of a sophisticated instrument called a flow cytometer or fluorescence-activated cell sorter (FACS) can rapidly measure the fluorescence intensity on many lymphocytes and isolate the cells on the basis of their fluorescence intensity (Figure 5-13). The use of the FACS to identify and separate lymphoid cells or particles that can be tagged with a fluorescent dye is called **flow cytometry**. A detailed description of flow cytometry is beyond the scope of our discussion; however, Table 5-2 gives a partial list of applications of flow cytometry in different areas of biology and medicine.

Instruments of flow cytometry are capable of analyzing properties of single cells in suspension as they travel through a stream of fluid intersected by a beam of laser light. Cells flow through this stream of fluid sequentially as individual cells and allow the laser beam to intersect with each cell. By combining light scatter and volume or granularity measurements with fluorescently tagged secondary antibodies directed against a specific primary antibody, subpopulations of cells can be easily identified and analyzed. The analytical data allow the selection of properties by which to sort cells. The FACS combines this analytic ability with the ability to sort cells (see Figure 5-13).

### Western Blotting Identifies a Specific Protein Antigen in a Complex Mixture of Proteins

**Western blotting** (also called **immunoblotting**) is a technique used to identify a specific protein

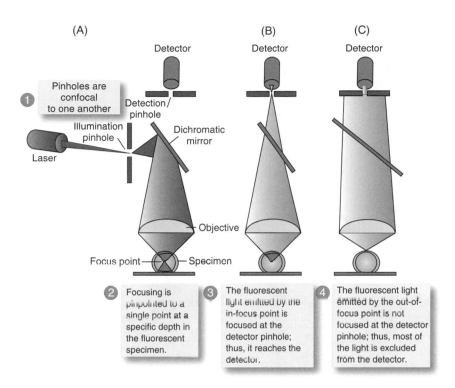

FIGURE 5-12 **The principle of confocal scanning microscopy.** (A) The arrangement of optical components is similar to that of the fluorescence microscope; the major exception is that a laser light passed through a pinhole illuminates the specimen at a point of focus. (B) The emitted fluorescence from this specimen focal point is focused at the second (confocal) pinhole (the detection pinhole). (C) The emitted fluorescence from out-of-focus points in the specimen is not focused and does not contribute to the final image. The light beam scanning across the specimen generates a sharp two-dimensional image of the exact plane of focus; therefore, the light from out-of-focus regions of the specimen does not degrade the displayed image.

in a complex mixture of proteins. It is named for its similarity to Northern blotting, which detects RNAs, and Southern blotting, which detects DNA fragments. In Western blotting, a protein mixture is separated by electrophoresis on a polyacrylamide slab gel that has been treated with sodium dodecyl sulfate, a dissociating agent. The protein bands are transferred to a nitrocellulose membrane by capillary blotting or electrophoresis (electro-blot), and the individual protein bands are identified by flooding the blot with antigen-specific primary antibody, followed by incubation and washing, and finally addition of radiolabeled or enzyme-labeled secondary antibody specific for the primary antibody. The antigen-antibody complexes (bands) that form are visualized by autoradiography or substrate addition, respectively (Figure 5-14). If labeled primary specific antibody is unavailable, antigen-antibody complexes can be detected by

adding a secondary anti-isotype antibody that is either radiolabeled or enzyme-labeled; the band is visualized by autoradiography or substrate addition, respectively. Western blotting can also be used to identify a specific antibody in a mixture; that is, the separated antibody bands are visualized with a labeled antigen. For example, HIV envelope and core proteins and the HIV-infected individual's antibodies to these components can be detected.

## MINI SUMMARY

Many methods have been developed to assess primary antigen-antibody reactions. They include (1) fluorescence quenching, (2) RIA, (3) various types of ELISAs, (4) various types of immunofluorescence, and (5) Western blotting.

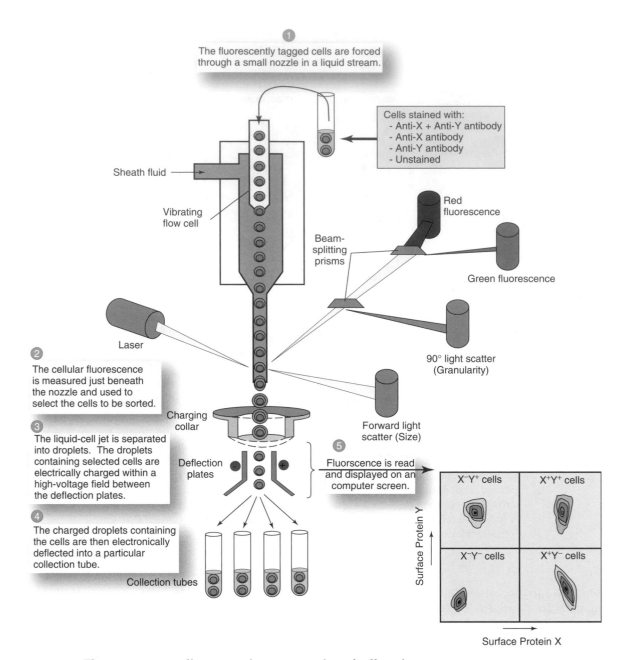

**FIGURE 5-13** Flow cytometry—diagrammatic representation of cell sorting.

# SECONDARY ANTIGEN-ANTIBODY INTERACTIONS OCCUR WHEN PRIMARY ANTIGEN-ANTIBODY COMPLEXES AGGREGATE TO FORM LARGE VISIBLE LATTICES

Whereas primary antigen-antibody interactions involve the binding of an antibody molecule with an individual antigenic determinant of an antigen, **secondary antigen-antibody interactions** involve the combination of an antigenic determinant and an antibody-combining site followed by aggregation of antigen-antibody complexes into macroscopically visible precipitates or clumps. The aggregate formed is a visible manifestation of the antigen-antibody interaction.

In contrast to the primary interaction of antigen and antibody, which is almost instantaneous, the aggregation phase may take hours to days to reach a maximum. The secondary reaction also requires

**TABLE 5-2 Applications of Flow Cytometry**

### General Applications

1. The cell cycle and cell growth: Analyze DNA and RNA content, cell size, bromodeoxyuridine incorporation to determine position in cell cycle and sorting cells in different cell cycles for studies in culture or biochemical analysis.
2. Cell differentiation: Detect and quantify variations in surface antigens, nucleic acids, enzymes, and functional characteristics during normal and abnormal cell differentiation.
3. Immunology: Any application used above but now applied to immune cells.
4. Microbiology: Measure the same parameters in prokaryotic cells as for eukaryotic cells.

### Clinical Applications

1. Hematology: Differential counting of peripheral blood cells.
2. Immunology: Determine the dysfunction in an immune response caused by changes of T and/or B cells by analyzing their surface markers.
3. Microbiology: Count bacteria in urine samples.
4. Oncology: Determine the nucleic acid content of malignant cells or expression of tumor-specific surface antigens.

electrolytes for maximum formation. More important, the secondary antigen-antibody reaction is visible.

The two visible reactions are called *precipitation* and *agglutination*. Precipitation is the combination of *soluble antigen* with specific antibody, which leads to the formation of an insoluble aggregation. In contrast, agglutination is the combination of a *particulate* (*insoluble*) *antigen* with specific antibody. This reaction leads to a clumping of particles.

The mechanism of aggregate formation was first proposed in 1934 by J.R. Marrack, who stated that aggregates are a lattice. The lattice is a network of alternating antigen and antibody molecules. The lattice theory is based on the fact that antigen and antibody molecules being *multivalent*. Each antigen molecule is linked to more than one antibody molecule, or, conversely, each antibody molecule binds more than one antigen molecule (Figure 5-15).

**Immune precipitation** *occurs when antigen and antibody combine in solution and form a visible aggregate*. The precipitation reaction was first described in 1897 by R. Kraus. This reaction provided the immunologist with an *in vitro* method for quantifying antigen-antibody interactions and analyzing the chemistry and mechanism of the interaction. Before this time, antibody activity was assessed only by the *in vivo* neutralization of toxins that had been

mixed *in vitro* with different doses of antibody. By the mid-1930s, precipitation reactions were shown to happen in different stages or zones. To date, the precipitation reaction and all its variations are one of the most widely used immunologic procedures. These procedures can be carried out in a fluid or gel medium.

## Precipitation Is the Combination of Soluble Antigen with Specific Antibody, Which Leads to the Formation of an Insoluble Aggregation

The mechanism of precipitation includes both the hydrophobicity and the size of the lattice. *Hydrophobicity* affects the inability of a molecule to dissolve in water because of the reduction or lack of polar groups. During lattice formation, the antibody molecules become tightly packed together and foster hydrophobic protein-protein interactions. The net result is that their interactions with water decrease. Maximum precipitation occurs in the presence of salts because salts (or electrolytes) foster hydrophobic interactions. The other characteristic of a lattice, important in the formation of a precipitate, is its size. Because antigen-antibody complexes dissociate and reassociate, the size of the complexes increases and, in turn, the lattice grows. The large complexes sediment to the bottom of the tube, becoming a precipitate.

### The Zone Phenomenon Shows the Reversibility of Precipitation Reactions

Originally, paradigms suggested that antigen-antibody complexes formed and precipitated irreversibly. However, J. Danysz reported important observations in 1902 about precipitation and other secondary antigen-antibody reactions. His observations of toxin-antitoxin interactions supported the reversibility of antigen-antibody interactions, called the *Danysz phenomenon*.

Another observation made in the early 20th century showed that a variation in the ratio of antibody to antigen leads to different levels of lattice formation, and thereby to different amounts of precipitate. This phenomenon, called the **zone phenomenon** (Figure 5-16), divides the precipitation reaction into three zones: (1) *antibody excess zone* (prozone), (2) *equivalence zone*, and (3) *antigen excess zone* (postzone).

In the first part of the precipitin curve, or **antibody excess zone**, the lattice has a high ratio of antibody molecules to antigen molecules. Not all antibody molecules, however, are able to interact

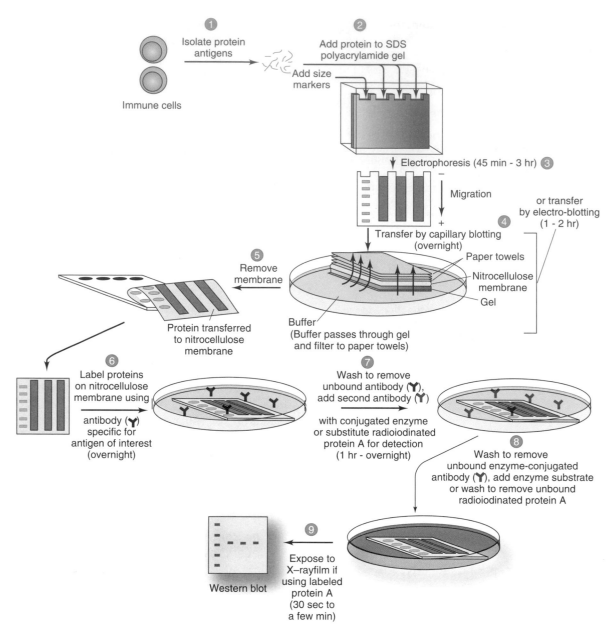

**FIGURE 5-14 Western blotting—analyzing protein by gel electrophoresis and blotting**. It is a process used to identify proteins that have been separated by gel electrophoresis and then transferred to a membrane (blot). The blot is incubated with a primary antibody that binds to antigens on the blot. The bound antibody can be detected by using either a secondary enzyme-conjugated antibody or protein A, both directed against the primary antibody. If the primary antibody is against a sequential epitope, denaturing gels can be used. If the primary antibody is against a structural epitope, nondenaturing gels must be used. (Protein A is a protein that specifically binds to IgG antibodies).

with antigen, so some antibody is free in the supernatant. If not all the antibody is bound, the precipitate formed is less than maximum.

In the middle of the precipitin curve, the **equivalence zone**, the ratio of antibody to antigen in the lattice is lower than in the antibody excess zone. All antigen and antibody molecules, however, are in the lattice. Supernatants are usually devoid of either detectable antigen or antibody. Thus, the immune precipitate is at its maximum.

In the last part of the precipitin curve, the **antigen excess zone**, the ratio of antibody to antigen in the lattice decreases still more. The antigen-antibody complexes that are formed are small. Once the ratio of

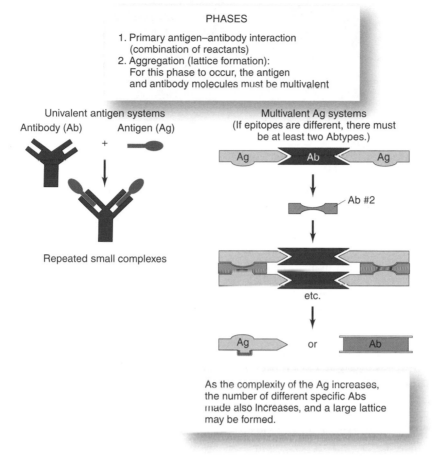

**FIGURE 5-15 Lattice formation.** This suggests a scenario for aggregate formation. Primary antigen-antibody reactions are almost instantaneous when antigen and antibody are mixed. Within a few seconds, small antigen-antibody complexes are formed. Because antigen-antibody reactions are reversible, antigen and antibody molecules dissociate and reassociate until large aggregates form, which may take hours to days. When the size of the aggregates exceeds a particular threshold, the aggregates spontaneously become insoluble and fall out of solution (precipitate)—the visible antigen-antibody reaction. The secondary antigen-antibody reaction of precipitation occurs in two distinct stages: (1) rapid formation of soluble antigen-antibody complexes that are invisible and (2) slow aggregation of these complexes to form a visible precipitate.

antibody to antigen in the lattice falls below a threshold, the lattice is soluble. Supernatants in antigen excess contain free antigen. Thus, the precipitation is less than maximum.

Other factors affect precipitation, such as (1) *temperature*, (2) *pH*, (3) *salt concentration*, and (4) *reaction volume*. The affinity constants ($K_0$) of antibody for antigen vary with changes in each of these conditions. For example, the affinity for hydrogen bonds and polar bonds is reduced as temperature increases. In contrast, many antigen-antibody interactions have a higher affinity in the cold than at room temperature

or at 37 °C. In contrast, temperature has little effect on the affinity of hydrophobic or nonpolar interactions. Maximum precipitation is observed in the physiologic pH range of 6 to 8. Outside this range, the amino acid residues in antibody-combining sites ionize. Physiologic salt concentrations (0.15 $M$ NaCl) lead to maximum precipitation. If the antigen-antibody interactions are dominated by ionic interactions, high salt concentrations will reduce the affinity. Because antigen-antibody aggregation depends on kinetic collisions to form a lattice, the reaction volume is important.

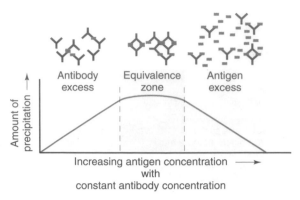

**FIGURE 5-16 Zone phenomenon—Lattice formation leading to a precipitate**. To demonstrate the zone phenomenon, a series of tubes are set up, each with an equal amount of antibody. To each of the tubes, an increasing amount of antigen is added; then the amount of precipitate formed is measured. Initially, as more and more antigen is added, more precipitate is formed, until a maximum is reached. If still more antigen is added, less precipitate is formed. If enough antigen is added, no more precipitate forms.

---

## MINI SUMMARY

The observable reaction (secondary antigen-antibody reaction) that can follow a primary antigen-antibody reaction depends on the nature and form of the antigen or on the precipitation of soluble antigen molecules. Exclusion of water from a lattice and a lattice's size dictate whether a precipitate forms. Formation of a precipitate is a reversible reaction (as demonstrated by the zone phenomenon). Factors such as temperature, pH, salt, and reaction volume also affect secondary antigen-antibody reactions.

---

### Precipitation Reactions Can Be Tested in Many Ways

Precipitation reactions can be tested in a number of different ways using either *fluids* or *gels*. When precipitation occurs in a fluid, the antigen and antibody react in solution. In a gel, antigen and antibody react in a porous, semisolid medium. Fluid precipitation reactions include the qualitative interfacial or ring test, the two semiquantitative precipitin tests and the quantitative precipitin reaction. Gel precipitation reactions include diffusion, electrophoresis, or a combination of the two.

### Precipitation Reactions Can Occur in Fluids.
In 1902, Ascoli demonstrated precipitation using the **interfacial** or **ring test**. Antiserum is placed in small

tubes, and an antigen solution is carefully laid over the antiserum. Antiserum is placed at the bottom of the tube because it is usually viscous. If it is carefully overlaid, mixing of the two reactants does not occur. Generally, the antigen concentration is increased from tube to tube, while the antiserum concentration remains constant. Antigen and antibody react at the interface of the two solutions, forming a visible band or ring with a cloudy (opaque) appearance. The ring test is a rapid, simple, qualitative way to detect antigen or antibody and can be used in forensic and public health medicine.

Two semiquantitative precipitin tests were developed in the 1920s. They are widely used in clinical laboratories to detect pathogens or antibody specific against pathogens. These tests had their origin in the assessment of toxin neutralization by antitoxins. Ramon developed a test in 1922 to titrate antitoxin, mixing varying amounts of antitoxin with a constant amount of toxin. He found that the mixture that precipitated was not toxic when injected into an animal. The procedure led to what is now called the *Ramon procedure*, or, more contemporarily, the *β procedure*, and to its counterpart, the *Dean-Webb procedure*, or *α procedure*.

The **Ramon** or **β, procedure** is carried out in a series of tubes, each containing the *same amount of antigen* (anywhere from 0.01 to 1.0% antigen concentration per tube). Serial dilutions of antibody are added to the tubes and mixed with the antigen; the tubes are then incubated. Within a few hours, the tubes can be observed for a precipitate. Results are expressed as a **titer**, which in the β procedure is the highest dilution (or smallest amount) of antibody that will cause precipitation with a given amount of antigen. Precipitation occurs in a narrow range. The zone phenomenon in the β procedure is reversed because the prozone is caused by antigen excess and the postzone by antibody excess.

If a fluid precipitation test is performed in the sequence described for the zone phenomenon, it is called a **Dean-Webb procedure**, or more contemporarily, the **α procedure**. In this test, tubes contain *constant amounts of antibody* to which varying dilutions of antigen are added. The *titer* for the α procedure is the highest dilution (or smallest amount) of antigen that will cause precipitation with a given amount of antibody.

Much more antibody is needed for the α procedure than for the β procedure. However, the α procedure precipitates over a broader range of dilutions because antigen is multivalent. Precipitation occurs in a narrower group of dilutions in the β procedure because the main precipitating antibody is bivalent. Thus, antibody is more easily diluted beyond its functional concentration. The α procedure is more extensively used because antisera will precipitate over a wide range of antigen dilutions. The α procedure allows us to compare antibody potencies under identical conditions.

The β and α procedures are semiquantitative. In both procedures, the higher the titer, the more specific the antibody that an antiserum contains. The titers can be used to diagnose disease states. These methods also allow comparisons of the antibody present in antisera but *do not* tell the absolute amount of specific antibody in an antiserum. Some of the precipitin reactions discussed in the next section do show this quantity.

*Precipitation Reactions Can Occur in Gels.* Antigen and antibody also can react in a gel matrix to give a visible precipitate, which is usually seen as an opaque band. Precipitation reactions in gels have many applications in immunology because they (1) are convenient and quick, (2) can quantify antigens, (3) can measure relationships among antigens, and (4) can give the number of antigen-antibody systems. The gels used are chemically and immunologically inert to avoid interference with the antigen-antibody interactions. Most commonly used gels are agar or agarose and cellulose acetate. A 0.5 to 1.0% agarose solution is commonly used because the resulting gel has large pores that permit passage of large antigen and antibody molecules. Because agarose forms a transparent gel, antigen-antibody interactions appear as an opaque white precipitate in a transparent background. In contrast to the agarose gel, cellulose acetate is an opaque white matrix. Thin layers of cellulose acetate are bound to plastic strips. When antigen and antibody interact in the cellulose acetate medium, the opaque precipitates can be visualized using a dye. Irrespective of the gel used, antigen and antibody either move naturally (*diffuse*), are forced to move (*electrophoresis*), or move by a combination of diffusion and electrophoresis.

The rate of diffusion of a protein in a liquid is proportional to the concentration gradient times the diffusion coefficient of the protein. Diffusion coefficients of antibodies are low because they are large molecules. A distance of 5 to 20 mm often takes antibodies 1 or more days to cover. To stabilize the liquid phase for such a long time, a gel matrix is added to provide support without hindering the diffusion. Antigens and antibodies are placed in wells cut into the matrix and diffuse toward one another by concentration differences. Either molecule

is small compared to the size of the gel pores. When antigen and antibody meet in equivalence zone proportions, a precipitate is formed. The pores of the gel, however, are not clogged. Antigen and antibody molecules may migrate through the precipitate and the pores.

Diffusion methods are characterized by the number of reagents that diffuse and the directions in which they diffuse. Two arrangements are used: (1) double diffusion in two dimensions (Ouchterlony method) and (2) single diffusion in two dimensions (Mancini method). As the geometry of the reactants entering the gel is adjusted, several characteristics such as the antigenic identity, partial cross-reactivity, purity of antigens, specificity of antibodies, and number of antigen-antibody systems present can be determined.

The **double immunodiffusion** (the **Ouchterlony method**) is performed in pure agarose gelled in a Petri dish or on a microscope slide; at least two, usually three, wells are cut in the pattern shown in Figure 5-17.

The Ouchterlony method can provide an estimation of the lowest number of antigen-antibody systems present. The number of precipitin bands formed is the *minimum* number of antigen-antibody systems present because the precipitin bands of different antigen-antibody systems may overlap due to similar diffusion rates. Diffusion rates of antigens are proportional to their concentration and to the intrinsic properties of the antigens (such as size and shape). The Ouchterlony method also provides qualitative comparisons of antigens, such as whether two antigens the same, somewhat related, or distinct (Figure 5-18). However, it cannot be used to determine antigen concentration.

A variation of the double immunodiffusion method called **radial immunodiffusion** (the **Mancini method**) can measure antigen concentration (Figure 5-19). A predetermined concentration of antibody is incorporated into a thin layer of agar on a rectangle-shaped slide, which contains a series of wells (see Figure 5-19B). Serial dilutions of known concentrations of pure antigen (the standard) are placed in successive wells; the remaining wells receive test samples of unknown antigen concentration. Antigen diffuses into the antibody-containing agar, a gradient forms, at a given radius of diffusion, the antigen concentration is equivalent to the antibody concentration in the gel (the equivalent zone), and a precipitin ring forms. The higher the antigen concentration, the farther the antigen diffuses and the larger the area (or diameter) of the ring. The diameter of the precipitin ring is proportional to the concentration of antigen (see Figure 5-19C).

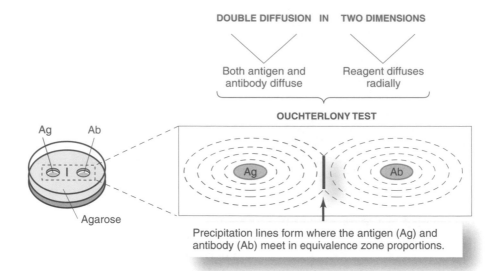

**FIGURE 5-17 Double Immunodiffusion—Ouchterlony method**. The antigen and antibody diffuse toward one another, and precipitin lines form where antigen and antibody meet in equivalence zone proportions.

The Mancini test can be used to determine the concentration of an antigen in a mixture of diverse antigens. It is widely used in clinical laboratories in the diagnosis of myelomas and agammaglobulinemias.

Most antigen-antibody systems are too complex for Ouchterlony immunodiffusion because the precipitate bands are too close together or too many bands are present. Grabar and Williams introduced **immunoelectrophoresis** to overcome these problems. Immunoelectrophoresis combines immunodiffusion (the ability to precipitate in a gel with specific antibody and antigen) with electrophoresis (the characteristic mobility in an electric field). Immunoelectrophoresis is used for (1) detecting and identifying individual components in multiple antigen-antibody systems, (2) determining the purity of an antigen-antibody system, (3) determining the efficacy of a fractionation procedure for isolating a given antigen, and (4) recognizing pathologic serum proteins. A diagram of immunoelectrophoresis is shown in Figure 5-20. Immunoelectrophoresis is a qualitative technique that can be modified to detect quantitative anomalies. As a quantitative technique, its variant is called *rocket electrophoresis*.

### MINI SUMMARY

Various procedures are used to determine the presence and quantity of soluble antigen and antibody. Fluid precipitin tests (such as the α

and β procedures) can be qualitative or quantitative. Precipitation reactions in a gel can be either the result of diffusion methods (Ouchterlony and Mancini) or electrophoresis methods (immunoelectrophoresis).

## Agglutination Is the Combination of a Particulate (Insoluble) Antigen with Specific Antibody, Which Leads to a Clumping of Particles

The preceding section discussed the study of interactions between antibodies and soluble antigens and presented some techniques used to assess these interactions. *This section deals with the clumping, or* **agglutination**, *of particulate antigens by specific antibodies. Clumping results from formation of a lattice in which antigen and antibody are cross-linked*. While precipitation reactions are quantifiable, agglutination methods are qualitative or semiquantitative at best. Nonetheless, agglutination reactions can be used in many applications, and they possess a high degree of sensitivity.

Agglutination reactions can be classified as either *direct* or *indirect. In the* **direct agglutination reaction**, *the antigenic determinant is a normal constituent of the particle surface*. For example, an antigen on a bacterial cell surface or the blood group substances (such as the ABO antigens) on human blood cells can be directly agglutinated by specific antibody. When the particle is a red blood cell (RBC), the reaction is called

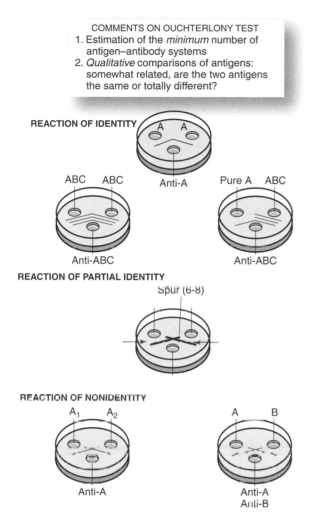

FIGURE 5-18 Ouchterlony method—Qualitative comparisons of antigens.

Two different agglutination testing methods are available for the direct and the indirect agglutination procedures. They are the *qualitative slide tests* and the *semiquantitative tube tests*. The qualitative slide test is quick and convenient. A suspension of particulate antigen is mixed with antiserum and incubated for several minutes on a microscope slide (or concavity slide). Clumping shows that the two reactants of the antigen-antibody system are present. The semiquantitative tube test is analogous to the β-precipitation procedure because antigen concentration is held constant and varying dilutions of antibodies are added to tubes or wells of a microtiter plate. The concentration of the last tube to give a positive reaction by clumping (that is, the highest dilution or the least amount of antibody at which agglutination occurs) is expressed as the antibody titer.

### The Agglutination of Red Blood Cells Is Called Hemagglutination

**Hemagglutination** reactions are read by the sedimentation patterns of the RBCs observed at the bottom of a tube or well. Because RBCs that react with antibody are sticky, they interact with the tube, and spread-out patterns (*agglutination*) result. If the RBCs do not react with antibody, they roll to the bottom of the tube and form a tight button.

Hemagglutination testing has **three** variations. (1) *reverse passive hemagglutination*, (2) *passive hemagglutination inhibition*, and (3) *nonimmune hemagglutination inhibition*. **Reverse passive hemagglutination** is so named because antibodies rather than antigens are absorbed to RBCs. Serial dilutions of antigens are added to each tube. The least amount of antigen that leads to agglutination is the titer of the antibody. **Passive hemagglutination inhibition** results from inhibition of agglutination of antigen-tagged RBCs. Inhibition occurs because free antigen competes with the bound antigen. The higher the concentration of free antigen, the greater the inhibition of agglutination.

*Nonimmune hemagglutination* results from the cross-linking of RBC by lectins or viruses. Lectins are plant or animal proteins or glycoproteins that specifically bind to certain monosaccharides. Many lectins have more than one sugar-binding site per molecule. The lectin phytohemagglutinin agglutinates human erythrocytes, and many of the myxoviruses (such as influenza virus and Newcastle disease virus) agglutinate the RBCs of certain species. The ability of viruses to agglutinate RBC leads to a method of detecting antibody specific for these viruses.

In the **nonimmune hemagglutination inhibition test**, a standard number of RBCs is chosen. Using

*hemagglutination. In the* **indirect agglutination reaction,** *a molecule that is ordinarily soluble is attached to a particle and rendered insoluble.* Attachment of a soluble antigen to a particle converts what would have been a precipitation reaction into an agglutination reaction. This conversion is advantageous because agglutination reactions are about 1000 times more sensitive than precipitation reactions. Figure 5-21 diagrammatically presents the reason for this increased sensitivity.

During indirect agglutination, soluble antigens are passively adsorbed or chemically coupled to particles or "carriers." Particles such as colored polystyrene latex particles or charcoal are often used. One of the most widely used particles is the RBC. This form of indirect agglutination is called **passive hemagglutination**. The advantages of using RBCs as carriers are their availability, ease of storage, and high visibility (because of the red color of the cells).

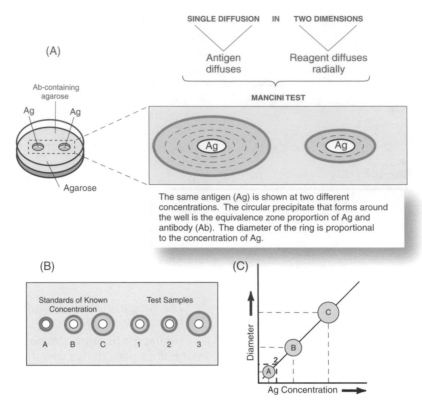

**FIGURE 5-19 Radial Immunodiffusion—Mancini method.** (A) If wells are filled with the preparations containing the same antigen but of different concentrations, the antigens diffuse into the antibody-containing agar forming circular precipitin rings around the wells. (B) The "standard" wells contain the serial dilutions of known concentrations of pure antigen. The test sample wells contain unknown concentrations of the antigen. (C) The diameter of the circular precipitin ring is used to plot a calibration curve of antigen concentration against diameter. The unknown antigen concentration is read of line.

this amount of RBCs, the amount of virus needed to agglutinate the RBCs can be determined. Serum is taken from an individual possibly infected by virus or one who has been immunized. Serial dilutions of antiserum are added to a constant amount of virus, and the mixture is incubated for 1 to 2 hr. After the incubation, the RBCs and tubes are observed for hemagglutination. Antibody specific for the virus combines with the virus and blocks its RBC receptors. Thus, virus can no longer agglutinate the RBCs. If the antibody becomes more dilute, eventually there are too few antibodies to prevent agglutination. The titer is reported as the highest dilution of antibody that inhibits hemagglutination.

## MINI SUMMARY

Agglutination is the aggregation of insoluble antigens by antibodies. Agglutination can be direct or indirect. Agglutination of red blood cells is called hemagglutination and can take three forms: (1) reverse passive hemagglutination, (2) passive hemagglutination inhibition, and (3) nonimmune hemagglutination inhibition.

### The Naturally Occurring Antibodies That React with RBC Antigens and Cause Hemagglutination Can Be Used to Distinguish Human Blood Groups

The RBCs of one individual are rarely, if ever, identical to the RBC of another. The difference lies in the chemical markers on the cell surfaces called **blood group antigens**. The function of blood group antigens is unknown. More than 15 blood group systems that contain more than 200 alloantigens have been identified, but only the *ABO* and *Rh blood groups* will be discussed. The principles of antigen-antibody relationships operating in these two blood cell antigen systems also can be applied and extended to many

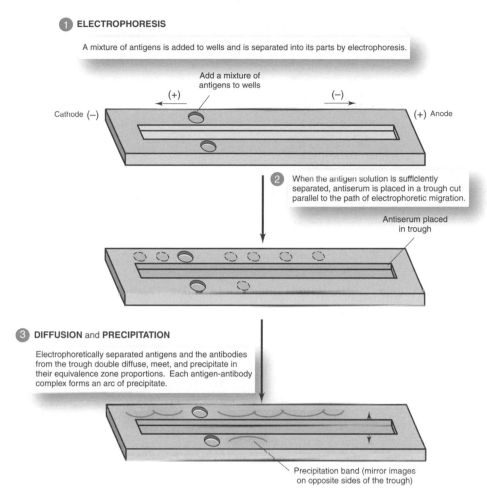

**1** **ELECTROPHORESIS**

A mixture of antigens is added to wells and is separated into its parts by electrophoresis.

Add a mixture of antigens to wells

(+)

(−)

Cathode (−)

(+) Anode

**2** When the antigen solution is sufficiently separated, antiserum is placed in a trough cut parallel to the path of electrophoretic migration.

Antiserum placed in trough

**3** **DIFFUSION** and **PRECIPITATION**

Electrophoretically separated antigens and the antibodies from the trough double diffuse, meet, and precipitate in their equivalence zone proportions. Each antigen-antibody complex forms an arc of precipitate.

Precipitation band (mirror images on opposite sides of the trough)

**FIGURE 5-20 Immunoelectrophoresis.** In the first step, a mixture of antigens is separated into its parts by electrophoresis. Then the antigen solution is placed in a small well in the gel layer (2 to 3 mm in thickness) on a microscope slide prepared in an alkaline buffer solution of about pH 8.5, and an electric field is established. At pH 8.5 most proteins become negatively charged and move through the gel to the anode, though antibodies are mostly neutral or slightly negatively charged and move only slightly toward the anode. Because proteins have different charges, they have different electrophoretic mobilities and so move to different positions in the gel. At the end of the electrophoretic separation, each protein has moved to its characteristic position according to its isoelectric point at the pH conditions used. At the end of 1 to 2 hr, when the antigen solution is sufficiently separated, antiserum is placed in a trough cut parallel to the path of electrophoretic migration. Electrophoretically separated antigens and the antibodies from the trough double diffuse, meet, and precipitate in their equivalence zone proportions. Each antigen-antibody complex forms an arc of precipitate.

other blood group systems that have lesser degrees of immunologic significance. Some blood group antigens are listed in Table 5-3.

***The Best-Known Human Blood Group System Is the ABO System.*** Karl Landsteiner described the ABO blood group antigens in 1900.[4] He performed

simple experiments in which RBCs and sera from many individuals were mixed in all possible combinations. The RBCs of some individuals were agglutinated by the serum of others. Because of the agglutination patterns he observed, he determined that all human RBCs could be classified as one of four blood groups by the presence or absence of two alloantigens, *A* and *B*. These antigens represent the *A* and *B blood group substances*. Individuals who lack the blood group antigens have antibodies specific for these antigens in their serum. These antibodies

---

[4]He received the 1930 Nobel Prize in Medicine for this work.

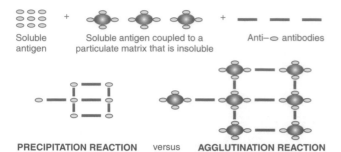

Soluble antigen | Soluble antigen coupled to a particulate matrix that is insoluble | Anti–○ antibodies

PRECIPITATION REACTION   versus   AGGLUTINATION REACTION

**FIGURE 5-21 Conversion of a precipitation reaction to an agglutination reaction.** When a small (soluble) antigen is coupled to larger (insoluble) particles, the lattice that is formed is larger, thus making it more visible using the same amount of antibody. That is, a precipitation reaction is converted to an agglutination reaction.

are responsible for hemagglutination reactions. Because individuals who have not been transfused with ABO-incompatible blood have these antibodies, where do the antibodies specific for blood group antigens come from? Because the chemical structure of certain blood group antigens is duplicated in many foodstuffs and bacteria, ingestion of these natural substances or infection by bacteria may be enough to cause antibody production if no similar material has been inherited. Some indirect evidence for this theory is that germ-free animals do not develop anti-blood group antibodies. The blood group antigens are *heterophile* antigens. Because of exposure to these heterophile antigens, virtually everyone over the age of 6 months who lacks either of these antigens produces antibody. *Humans form antibodies against the blood group antigens they do not express. These antibodies are called* **naturally occurring antibodies** *or* **isoagglutinins**. Isoagglutinins (also called *isohemagglutinins*) may be of the IgM, IgG, or IgA class. Most individuals have a mixture of IgM and IgG, but virtually any combination may be seen. Their production starts at 3 months of age, reaches its highest level during adolescence, and decreases with advancing age. In the adult population, great variation in the titer of these antibodies occurs. Usually, anti-A titers are higher than anti-B titers.

When RBCs are tested with serum known to contain a specific antibody and agglutination does not occur, the cells are assumed to lack the antigen against which the antibody is directed. Conversely, clumping implies that the cells possess the antigen. Two common antibodies, anti-A and anti-B, are used to show this reaction. Using these two antibodies, the U.S. population is divided into the *A, B, O,* and *AB blood groups.* Table 5-4 shows the results of such testing and the inheritance pattern for these antigens.

**TABLE 5-3 Partial List of Human Blood Groups**

| Discovery date | System | Phenotype | Percentage of population |
|---|---|---|---|
| 1900 | ABO | A | 41 |
| | | B | 9 |
| | | O | 46 |
| | | AB | 4 |
| 1927 | MN | MN | 50 |
| | | MM | 25 |
| | | NN | 25 |
| 1927 | P | $P_1$ | 75 |
| | | $P_2$ | |
| 1939 | Rh | $Rh^+$ | 85 |
| | | $Rh^-$ | 15 |
| 1945 | Lutheran | $Lu(a^- b^+)$ | 92 |
| | | $Lu(a^+ b^+)$ | 7.9 |
| | | $Lu(a^+ b^-)$ | 0.1 |
| 1946 | Lewis | $Le(a^- b^-)$ | 70 |
| | | $Le(a^+ b^-)$ | 25 |
| | | $Le(a^- b^-)$ | 5 |
| 1946 | Kell | k | 90 |
| | | Kk | 9.8 |
| | | K | 0.2 |
| 1950 | Duffy | $Fy(a^- b^+)$ | 50 |
| | | $Fy(a^+ b^+)$ | 35 |
| | | $Fy(a^+ b^-)$ | 15 |
| 1951 | Kidd | $Jk(a^+ b^+)$ | 50 |
| | | $Jk(a^+ b^-)$ | 25 |
| | | $Jk(a^- b^+)$ | 25 |
| 1954 | Diego | $Di(a^+)$ | 36,[1] 8 to 12[2] |
| 1962 | Xg | $Xg(a^-)$ | 85,[3] 65[4] |
| | | $Xg(a^+)$ | 15,[3] 35[4] |

[1]South-American Indians
[2]Japanese
[3]Women
[4]Men

### MINI SUMMARY

Landsteiner discovered the ABO blood group in 1900. The ABO system is characterized by RBC antigens identified with naturally occurring antibodies (isoagglutinins) found in individuals lacking the corresponding antigen. The origin of these antibodies is uncertain. Blood group antigens are important in transfusion and forensic medicine.

***Another Important Human Blood Group System Is the Rh System.*** In 1939, a report by Levine and Stetson discussed findings on serum of a type O patient who had suffered a transfusion reaction after

**TABLE 5-4** The ABO Blood Groups

| Blood group | Antigen on cell | Antibody in serum | Percentage of U.S. population possessing antigen | Inheritance of blood group antigens | |
|---|---|---|---|---|---|
| | | | | Genotype | Phenotype |
| A | A | anti-B | 41 | AA, AO | A |
| B | B | anti-A | 9 | BB, BO | B |
| O | — | anti-A, anti-B | 46 | OO | O |
| AB | A, B | — | 4 | AB | AB |

receiving type O blood from her husband. The patient had received no previous transfusion, but her second pregnancy ended in the delivery of a macerated fetus. After the transfusion reaction, the patient's serum agglutinated not only her husband's group O RBCs but also 80 of 104 group O RBC samples. Levine and Stetson suggested that the woman made antibodies against a fetal antigen genetically transmitted from her husband. No name was given to the antibody or antigen.

At the same time, Landsteiner and Wiener immunized rabbits and guinea pigs with RBCs from *Macacus rhesus* monkeys and studied the resultant antibodies. In 1940, they reported that the rabbit and guinea pig anti-rhesus antibodies agglutinated not only monkey RBCs but also the RBCs of 85% of humans. Also in 1940, Wiener and Peters reported the similarity between human antibodies following transfusion reactions and the anti-rhesus antibodies and suggested that the human and animal antibodies agglutinated the same RBCs. The names **Rh** (from *rh*esus monkey) for the antigen and anti-Rh for the antibody were then accepted because the antibody described by Levine and Stetson was indistinguishable from the anti-Rh antibody described by Landsteiner and Wiener.

Human RBCs are classified as $Rh^+$ if the Rh antigen is on their membrane or $Rh^-$ if the Rh antigen is absent. The presence or absence of Rh antigen (also called *D antigen*) is determined by testing the RBCs with anti-$Rh_0$ (also called *anti-D*) antibodies. A positive reaction (agglutination of erythrocytes by anti-D) suggests that the cells have D antigen. If anti-D antibodies do not agglutinate the cells, they lack the D antigen. About 85% of the U.S. population is $Rh^+$ and 15% is $Rh^-$. The sera of $Rh^-$ individuals do not contain anti-D antibodies. The absence of anti-D antibodies suggests that there are no natural substances chemically similar to the D antigen and therefore no naturally occurring antibodies. If an $Rh^-$ person is found to have anti-D antibodies, that person has been exposed to $Rh^+$ RBCs. The two ways for $Rh^+$

RBCs to enter the circulation of an $Rh^-$ person are through (1) transfusion of blood from an $Rh^+$ donor or (2) the passage of fetal $Rh^+$ RBC through the placenta to the $Rh^-$ mother.

Reagents used to test for the presence or absence of Rh antigens are prepared from the serum of $Rh^-$ individuals who have produced anti-D antibodies. Even though these antibodies are needed to prepare test reagents and are harmless to the RBCs of the individual who produced them, one goal of blood transfusion is to prevent antibody formation. However, this antibody does cause problems in transfusion or pregnancy. Antibody of an immunized recipient may destroy the donor's cells. During pregnancy, maternal antibody may destroy the RBCs of the fetus.

There is no way to prevent fetal RBCs from reaching the mother during delivery, but the formation of anti-D antibodies can be suppressed by treatment immediately postpartum. For transfusions, the formation of anti-D is prevented by accurate typing of recipients and donors and the selection of $Rh^-$ blood for all $Rh^-$ recipients.

Following Landsteiner and Levine's description of the Rh antigen and antibodies, Levine demonstrated anti-Rh antibodies in the sera of several women who delivered babies suffering from the disease erythroblastosis fetalis. In 1941, Levine and his associates described the importance of isoimmunization in the pathogenesis of this disease. This disease is now called **hemolytic disease of the newborn**.

Hemolytic disease of the newborn has largely been eliminated by immunologic treatment. The disease is usually observed in the later pregnancies of an $Rh^-$ woman who has delivered $Rh^+$ children. In earlier pregnancies when the woman carries an $Rh^+$ fetus, fetal RBCs leak into the maternal circulation and serve as the immunogenic stimulus to produce anti-Rh antibodies. Mixing of fetal RBCs usually happens during delivery (parturition) when the placenta separates from the uterus. Anti-Rh antibodies are primarily of the IgG class and cross the placenta during later pregnancies to attack $Rh^+$ fetal RBCs, unlike anti-ABO antibodies that are of the IgM class and do not cross the placenta.

Symptoms of hemolytic disease of the newborn begin when the maternal antibodies attack and destroy the fetal RBCs. The fetus attempts to replace the RBCs (erythrocytes) by pouring immature RBCs, or **erythroblasts**, into the bloodstream. Presence of the erythroblasts in hemolytic disease of the newborn has led to the term **erythroblastosis fetalis**. At birth the child appears blue because of anemia. In severe cases the child is stillborn. After birth the child appears jaundiced because the hemoglobin from the ruptured RBCs breaks down into different end products, one of which is a yellow pigment called *bilirubin*. A newborn's liver has little or no glucuronyl transferase, which is needed for the conversion of bilirubin to the nontoxic bilirubin glucuronide. Therefore, it cannot remove excessive amounts of bilirubin. High amounts of bilirubin are dangerous because bilirubin is extremely toxic if deposited in tissue.

Hemolytic disease of the newborn can be treated before or after delivery. The most widely used treatment is exchange transfusion performed within a few hours of birth. A complete blood transfusion removes the damaged RBCs and circulating maternal antibodies. However, if amniocentesis shows that the fetus is not likely to survive to be delivered at term, early induction of labor may be tried. In the most severe cases, in which it is predicted that the fetus will die before it has matured enough for premature delivery, intrauterine transfusions have been successful.

Prevention of antibody production following Rh-incompatible pregnancy is possible because of research based on two classic observations: (1) ABO incompatibility of the fetus and mother partly prevents the Rh$^-$ mother from producing anti-Rh$_0$ (anti-D) antibodies, and (2) passive antibody administered in adequate doses along with its corresponding antigen prevents immunization in the recipient.

Investigators observed that Rh$^-$ women who bore Rh$^+$ children who were ABO incompatible seldom became sensitized to the Rh$^+$ antigen (D antigen). If the fetal cells are ABO incompatible, the mother has isoagglutinins that rapidly remove the fetal cells from the maternal circulation and prevent sensitization to the Rh antigen. This observation has led to a novel immunologic method to prevent hemolytic disease of the newborn. Shortly after delivery of an Rh$^+$ child, the mother is given passively transferred anti-Rh antibodies. These antibodies are prepared in male Rh$^-$ volunteers by immunization with Rh$^+$ RBCs.

The commercial material designed to suppress maternal antibody production on exposure to Rh$_0$ (D)

positive incompatible fetal RBC is called **RhoGAM**.[5] The principle of RhoGAM action is that passive anti-D antibodies given to the Rh$^-$ mother at delivery prevent her from responding to the immunogenic stimulus of incompatible fetal RBC entering her circulation at parturition. By preventing anti-D antibody production at delivery of the first infant, the later Rh$^+$ infant of this mother is protected from hemolytic disease of the newborn. Even though the exact mechanism of suppression is not known, there are three related concepts: (1) correct doses are required because too low a dose of antibody will enhance antibody production rather than suppress it; (2) IgG and IgM will prevent sensitization; and (3) there is no need to give RhoGAM during pregnancy. Protection is accomplished if it is administered within 72 hr of delivery. To date this is the only clinical situation that requires specific immunosuppression.

---

**MINI SUMMARY**

Human RBCs can be divided into two groups based on their expression of Rh antigen (also called D antigen). Roughly 85% of the population express Rh antigen and are considered Rh$^+$, while the remaining 15% do not express Rh antigen and are considered Rh$^-$. The discovery of the Rh system lead to the eventual solution to the problem of hemolytic diseases of the newborn called erythroblastosis fetalis. This disease can be prevented with the use of RhoGAM.

---

# MONOCLONAL ANTIBODIES ARE PURE ANTIBODIES WITH SINGLE EPITOPE SPECIFICITIES

Normal serum contains $10^{16}$ antibody molecules per milliliter. These antibodies can be collected from experimental animals and have long been an important tool of investigators, who have used them to identify or label molecules or cells and to separate molecules or cells from mixtures. A concern,

---

[5]RhoGAM is taken from *Rh$_0$* (D) Immune Globulin (Human) or more specifically *Rh$_0$ Gam*ma G immunoglobulin. The concentrated IgG is prepared by alcohol fractionation so that the risk of transmitting hepatitis is low.

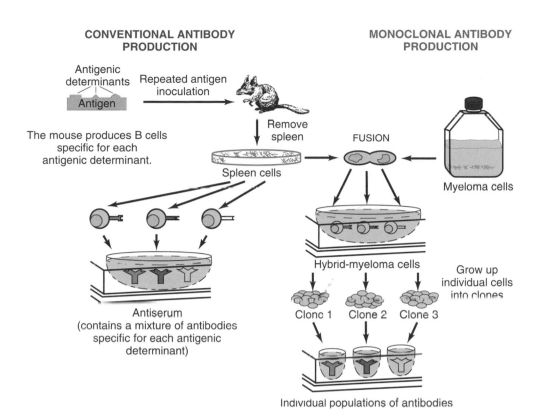

**CONVENTIONAL ANTIBODY PRODUCTION**

Antigenic determinants

Antigen

Repeated antigen inoculation

The mouse produces B cells specific for each antigenic determinant.

Remove spleen

Spleen cells

Antiserum
(contains a mixture of antibodies specific for each antigenic determinant)

**MONOCLONAL ANTIBODY PRODUCTION**

FUSION

Myeloma cells

Hybrid-myeloma cells

Grow up individual cells into clones

Clone 1   Clone 2   Clone 3

Individual populations of antibodies

**FIGURE 5-22 Conventional antisera compared with monoclonal antibody production.** The main difference between the two ways of producing antibodies is the resulting preparations; one is heterogeneous, while the other is homogeneous. B-cell-derived hybridomas can be separated into individual clones and grown indefinitely. One clone gives rise to identical daughter cells, all producing one antibody idiotype (a monoclonal antibody) directed against a specific antigenic determinant. See text for further explanation.

however, has always been the variability of antisera (Figure 5-22). The development of hybridization techniques allowed for the production of one kind of *specific* antibody by immortalized antibody-producing cells. Methods were then developed to screen for and produce large numbers of these antibodies for use in many applications.

Antibodies of a single idiotype produced by immortalized B cells are called **monoclonal antibodies**. Regrettably, normal antibody-secreting cells are end cells of a differentiation series; thus they cannot be maintained in culture. In contrast, myeloma cells are immortal. Therefore: "Why not use immunoglobulins produced by myeloma cells?" The reason myeloma immunoglobulins cannot be used is twofold: (1) their antigen specificity is usually unknown and (2) it is difficult to tailor-make antigen-specific myelomas. The second problem is overshadowed by the question "Is the combining site of the myeloma protein an accurate representation of the antibody produced during an immune response?" What would happen if one combined

the characteristics of each cell into one? Georges Kohler and Cesar Milstein fused cells secreting antibody of a single specificity with myeloma cells. The resulting clone of cells is a *hybrid*-myeloma or a **hybridoma**. The hybridoma cells inherit the lymphocyte's property of specific-antibody production and the immortality of the myeloma cell. In 1975, Kohler and Milstein published a short paper in *Nature* detailing how continuous cultures of fused cells secreting a monoclonal antibody of predefined specificity were produced. They were awarded the 1984 Nobel Prize in Medicine for their work.

## Monoclonal Antibody Development Improves on Nature

How are hybridomas produced? Mice are immunized with specific antigen (Figure 5-23), and spleens from hosts with the highest titers are collected. The separated spleen cells are mixed with myeloma cells that cannot produce immunoglobulins of their own; thus,

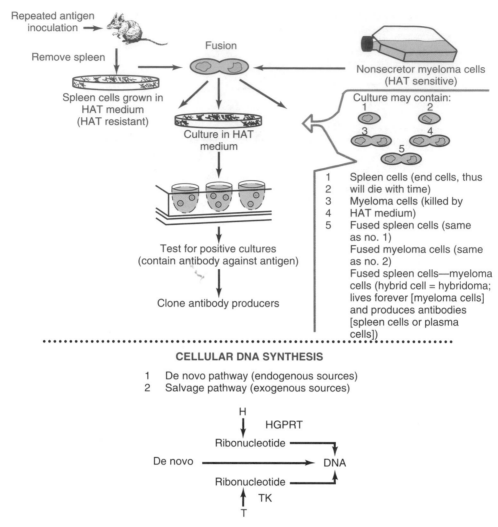

**FIGURE 5-23 Standard procedure for the development of monoclonal antibodies.** Hypoxanthine (H) and thymidine (T) are required for the salvage pathway. Aminopterin (A) blocks *de novo* DNA synthesis; thus, myeloma cells deficient in HGPRT enzyme *cannot* grow in HAT medium. However, B-cell-myeloma cell hybrids have the HGPRT enzyme; thus, they can grow because they use the salvage pathway for DNA synthesis. TK, thymidine kinase. See text for further explanation.

the myeloma cells do not interfere with the production of normal antibody by the fused B cells. Mouse spleen cells are mixed with the myeloma cell line in a ratio of roughly 10 to 1 in the presence of polyethylene glycol to change membrane permeability and allow cell fusion.

Because cell fusion is random, the cell culture contains a mixture of myeloma-spleen cell fusions, myeloma-myeloma fusions, spleen-spleen cell fusions, single myeloma cells, and single spleen cells. *Selection for only myeloma-spleen cell fusions is accomplished by culturing the cell mixture in* **hypoxanthine-aminopterin-thymidine (HAT) medium** (see Figure 5-23). Aminopterin is a folic

acid analog that blocks the *de novo* biosynthesis of purines and pyrimidines vital for DNA synthesis. Myeloma cells used in hybridoma production lack the enzyme hypoxanthine-guanine phosphoribosyl transferase (HGPRT⁻), so they cannot use the exogenous hypoxanthine to synthesize purines by the salvage pathway. Aminopterin also blocks their endogenous synthesis of purines and pyrimidines. In HAT medium, the myeloma-myeloma cells and free myeloma cells die in the first week. Although single spleen cells and spleen-spleen cell fusions express HGPRT and therefore are not selected against by HAT medium, these cells have limited growth in culture and die in 2 weeks. Myeloma cells (HGPRT⁻)

**TABLE 5-5** Applications of Hybridoma Technology

1. Generation of routine serologic reagents
2. Monoclonal antibodies against viruses
3. Monoclonal antibodies against parasites
4. Monoclonal antibodies to define mouse and human differentiation and tumor antigens
5. Monoclonal antibodies to the human MHC encoded antigens
6. In clinical pharmacology, immunosuppressants in transplantation and autoimmune reactions and a targeting vehicle for treatment of cancers
7. In cell biology studies, such as anti-tubulin and anti-actin antibodies
8. In plant physiology studies

that have fused with HGPRT$^+$ spleen cells now have the enzyme and can grow in HAT medium. About 500 hybrids are formed per mouse spleen, and 20 to 30 of them produce specific antibody. The correct antibody-producing hybridomas are then identified.

## Monoclonal Antibodies Have Many Applications

Monoclonal antibodies ushered in a new era in immunologic research and in the application of immunologic assays to basic and clinical questions. The impact of hybridoma technology is obvious when we begin to look at the many situations in which it has been successfully used (Table 5-5).

Monoclonal antibodies are not without problems: (1) the affinity for antigen may be low, (2) individual species of monoclonal antibodies do not readily activate complement or precipitate or agglutinate antigens *in vitro*, and (3) monoclonals are difficult to use *in vivo* in humans because of the difficulty of producing human, as opposed to mouse, hybridomas. To avoid these problems, antibody-gene DNA that has been manipulated *in vitro* is introduced into myeloma cells. The process is called **transfection**, and the resulting transfected cells are called **transfectomas**. *Transfection is the integration of donor DNA into a cell's chromosomes* (Figure 5-24). *If the recipient cell lacks the genetic trait encoded by the donor DNA, the recipient cell acquires that trait.*[6] Transfection uses several recombinant DNA techniques to produce an entire new family of novel, tailor-made monoclonal antibodies called either **hybrid, chimeric,** or **recombinant, monoclonal antibodies**. The goal is to *humanize* antibody.

---

[6]Transfection is the mammalian counterpart to bacterial transformation.

Custom-made antibodies can be molecules with variable regions joined to different isotypic constant regions. These antibodies could enhance the binding of antigen-specific antibodies to protein A (a cell wall component of staphylococci that binds specifically to the Fc portion of IgG) by changing the Fc part, or could change the antibody's ability to bind complement (keep same antigen reactivity but change effector function). Custom-made antibodies also can be generated that have unique heavy- and light-chain combinations. This situation would allow for one antibody molecule to bind two different antigenic determinants. Furthermore, molecules with Fab antibody sequences can be fused with nonantibody sequences (such as enzyme or toxin sequences). This approach could make chimeric antibodies that are part antibody and part enzyme (which has use in immunoassays) or part toxin (antibody directs toxin to specific a site). The applications of these recombinant antibodies seem limitless.

Why not bypass hybridoma technology and even immunization? You can. Lymphocyte V-region gene repertoires are harvested or assembled *in vitro* and cloned for display of heavy- and light-chain Fab fragments on the surface of bacteriophage, thus the name *phage display antibodies*. Rare phage display antibody is selected by binding to antigen, and soluble Fab fragments are expressed from infected bacteria. Ironically, we are using the bacteria that our immune system is designed to defend against to make antibodies.

# THE TRANSFER OF CLONED GENES PROVIDES INFORMATION ON THE *IN VIVO* ACTIVITY OF IMMUNE GENES

In 1980, scientists randomly inserted foreign DNA into the mouse genome by microinjection of fertilized eggs, reimplanted the embryos into foster mothers, and analyzed the resultant progeny. The general method for producing transgenic mice is depicted in Figure 5-25. In about 10–25% of the offspring, called **transgenic mice** *(part of their germline genes come from a genetically distinct host; they gain a gene)*, the injected DNA, or transfected DNA—the cloned foreign genes are called **transgenes**. Because a transgene is introduced into the chromosomal DNA of a single cell embryo, the DNA will integrated into germline cells and somatic cells; thus, it is transmitted to progeny in a Mendelian fashion. This

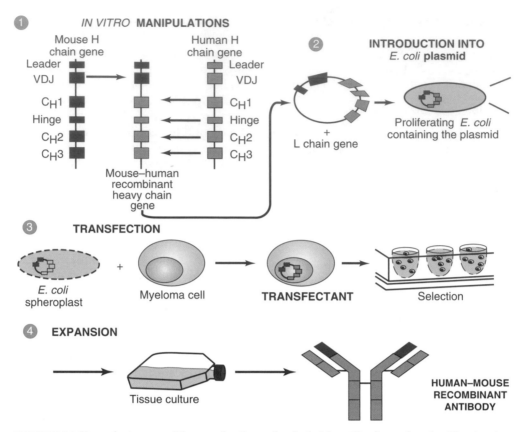

**FIGURE 5-24 Transfectomas—The production of a hybrid antibody molecule**. The *in vitro* manipulations include ligating the gene containing the sequence of interest (for an antibody, enzyme, toxin, and so on; in this case, combining mouse and human antibody genes into one molecule) into an expression vector such as a eukaryotic cell plasmid. The plasmid is introduced into *E. coli*, the bacteria are grown, and the *E. coli* containing the plasmid with integrated DNA is selected for. These cells are treated with lysozyme to remove the bacterial cell walls, and the resulting spheroplasts are fused (*transfection*) with myeloma cells. After fusion, the stable cells (*transfectants*) are identified and selected. These cells represent the *transfectomas*. Last, the transfectomas are amplified by growing them as ascites or in tissue culture, and the resulting recombinant antibodies are isolated.

allows for the production of transgenic mouse lines, whose members all contain the transgene thereby providing an important model for studying the immune system—affords a means to observe the expression of a given immune system-associated gene *in vivo*. The greatest benefit of using transgenic mice may be the discovery of gene therapy treatments against congenital and genetic dysfunctional diseases.

The limitation of transgenic mice is that transgenes are rarely inserted into their normal positions; they are integrated randomly within the mouse genome. If inserted into the wrong site, a needed gene may be transcriptionally inactive, and consequently it is not expressed. Targeted gene transfer avoids these problems and places transferred genes in specific germline sites. Targeted gene transfer is used to

develop transgenic mice with mutant genes—*these mice lose the function of a gene*. The mutant gene is generated by insertion of a construct, usually containing the selection marker *neo*, into an exon of the target gene, rendering the gene nonfunctional. The nonfunctional gene construct is introduced into embryoic stem (ES), which are grown up in culture. The targeted ES cells are selected and microinjected into a blastocyst, which is implanted into the uterus of a foster mother. The chimeric offspring contain cells from the host blastocyst and from the donor stem cells. The mutation disrupts the desired gene, leading to no functional gene product expression. These gene **knockout mice** are used to test the lack of a particular gene product to immune reactivity (e.g., mice lacking particular MHC molecules, cytokines, or receptors).

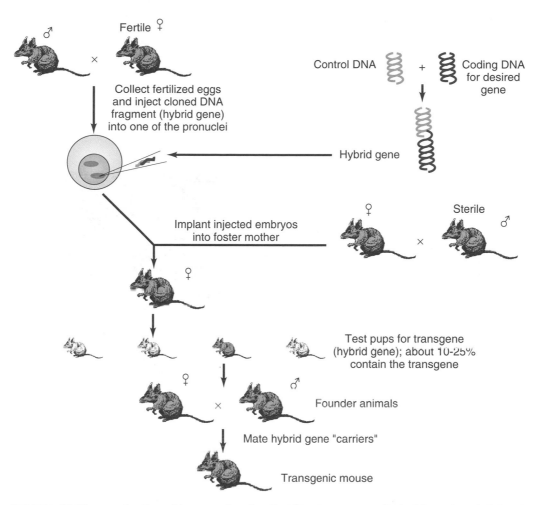

**FIGURE 5-25 The production of transgenic mice.** Fertilized eggs are collected from female inbred mice that have been hormonally superovulated and then mated. About 12 hr after fertilization one-cell embryos are flushed from the oviduct, injected with cloned DNA by insertion of a thin glass needle into the male pronucleus, reimplanted in the oviduct of a pseudopregnant foster mother, and allowed to come to term. The pseudopregnant foster mother is prepared for pregnancy by mating with a sterile male. Two weeks after birth, the pups' genomic DNA is extracted from small pieces of the tails and analyzed for the transfected gene using Southern blotting. When the transgenic mice (containing the gene question) are sexually mature, they each can serve as founders of a line.

# IMMUNE SYSTEM CHARACTERIZATION USING GENE EXPRESSION PATTERNS FROM MICROARRAYS

It is estimated that there are roughly 20,500 genes in the human genome, a smaller but significant portion of these genes are associated with the immune system. A functional organism (or immune system) needs to turn this genetic blueprint into expressing each of these genes in a specific temporal and spatial context. New technologies allow the study of gene expression on a large scale—new methods get past the "one-gene-one-experiment" paradigm. A biologically based way to characterize the immune system has arisen from the science of genomics. One genomics method uses **microarrays** to measure the expression of thousands of genes simultaneously (called *gene profiling*).

Gene profiling requires the availability of large collections of cDNAs immobilized on glass (called *DNA microarrays*) or sets of synthetic oligonucleotides immobilized on silica wafers or chips (called *oligo microarrays*). The target (free nucleic acid sample

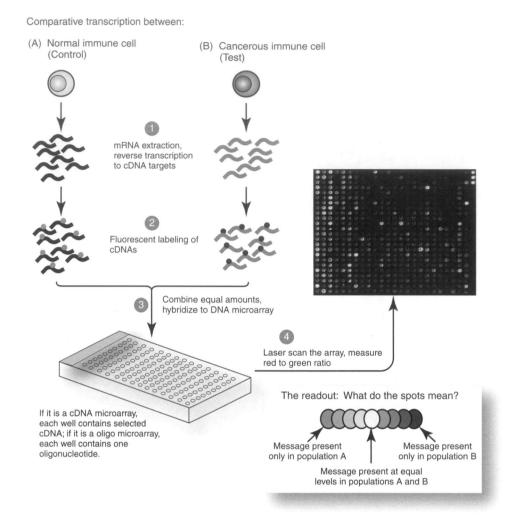

**FIGURE 5-26 DNA microarray analysis comparing samples from normal immune cell and cancerous immune cell**. The analysis using cDNA microarrays is illustrated. mRNA is isolated from cells or tissues, reverse-transcribed to cDNA, fluorescently labeled during target preparation, and labeled-targets hybridized to cDNA microarray. (See text).

whose identity/abundance is being detected) source for cDNA and oligo microarrays are the same, but the target preparation differs depending on the microarray. The example illustrated in Figure 5-26 shows the comparative transcription of two different cell types using DNA microarrays. In DNA microarrays, distinct fluorochromes are used to label the different sources of cDNAs targets. A green fluorochrome is used to label normal immune cell cDNA, and a red fluorochrome is used to label cancerous immune cell cDNA (see Figure 5-26). RNA is extracted from the cells (or tissues) to be studied and used to make fluorescently labeled cDNA from mRNA in the extract (mRNA is reverse-transcribed to cDNA). The first strand synthesis from population A cell mRNA is done using one nucleotide conjugated to a green

fluorescent dye. This process is repeated with population B cell mRNA but using a nucleotide conjugated to a red fluorescent dye. Both tagged target cDNAs are then hybridized to a DNA microarray, that is, the microarray is overlayed with the labeled cDNAs targets, which hybridize by base pairing with matching probe fragments (tethered nucleic acid with known sequence), leading to a green or red fluorescence emission. The array is then scanned at two different wavelengths to distinguish between the green and red fluorescence, signal strengths of each fluorescence emission signal are determined and compared, and the resulting data are presented as a ratio. If a single target hybridizes from a particular cell cDNA (see Figure 5-26), the cDNA will fluoresce either green or red. If both targets hybridize to the cDNA, an intermediate yellow fluorescent (the combination of the green and red fluorescent dyes) is detected.

If one uses the oligo microarray, the initial preparation of mRNA isolation and cDNA production from the two cell populations is similar but the target cDNA is usually labeled with a biotin-tagged nucleotide during first-strand synthesis of the mRNA. The biotin-labeled cDNA is hybridized to the oligo microarray and detected using fluorescently tagged streptavidin. The process is repeated with the other cell's cDNA but on a second oligo microarray; this can be done because of the increased accuracy of oligonucleotide placement in replicate microarrays.

## MINI SUMMARY

Antigen-specific B cells from an immunized mouse can be fused with immortal B-cell myeloma cells to form hybridomas. Hybridomas have both the specific antibody-producing ability of the B cell and the immortality of the tumor cell. Transfectomas (cells resulting from the integration of donor DNA into the recipient cell's chromosomes) can be generated to produce tailor-made antibodies, called hybrid, chimeric, or recombinant monoclonals.

Cloned genes (transgenes) can be inserted into germline DNA of mouse embryos, leading to progeny (transgenic mice) that express the chosen gene. Knockout transgenic mice represent transgenic mice where a target gene has been replaced ("knockout") by its nonfunctional counterpart.

Gene profiling using microarrays allows for simultaneous comparative transcriptional examination of many genes from different tissues and cells.

# SUMMARY

The function of antibody is to combine with antigen. This combination *in vivo* may be enough to neutralize toxins and some viruses, but a secondary interaction of the antigen-bound antibody with another effector agent, such as complement or phagocytic cells, is usually required for disposal of larger antigens such as bacteria. The *in vitro* interaction of antibody with antigen, however, has led to the development of many techniques that form the basis of *serology*.

Interaction of antigen with antibody can be divided into two stages. The first interaction of an antigenic determinant (or epitope) with its corresponding antigen-binding site on an antibody is called a *primary antigen-antibody reaction*. If the primary antigen-antibody reaction is followed by the aggregation of antigen-antibody complexes into macroscopically visible clumps, the aggregate is called the *secondary antigen-antibody reaction*. The *lattice hypothesis* offers a satisfactory explanation of aggregation of antigen-antibody.

The ability of an antibody molecule to combine with one antigen is referred to as its *specificity*. This specificity resides in the part of the antibody molecule, called the *Fab* portion, that contains the *combining site*. Antigen-antibody binding depends on a close three-dimensional fit. The closer the fit between the combining site and a given antigenic determinant of the antigen, the stronger the noncovalent forces between antigen and antibody. These forces are represented by (1) coulombic (ionic or electrostatic) forces, (2) Van der Waals forces, (3) hydrogen bonding, and (4) hydrophobic interactions. The strength of these forces between an epitope and an antibody-combining site is called *antibody affinity*. In contrast, *avidity* is the binding strength between a multivalent antibody and a multivalent antigen.

*Equilibrium dialysis* can be used to determine association constants by measuring the interaction of haptens and antibodies. A *Scatchard equation* can be used to determine antibody affinity. Using equilibrium dialysis, one can show that the *average intrinsic association constant* increases in animals or individuals with time and with repeated antigenic challenge.

Primary antigen-antibody reactions can be measured using *fluorescence quenching, radioimmunoassay (RIA)*, various forms of *enzyme-linked immunosorbent assays (ELISAs)* and related assays (such as *ELISPOT*, which can detect the production of antibodies and antigens at the single-cell level), and *immunofluorescence* (such as *direct* and *indirect immunofluorescence, confocal scanning microscopy*, and *flow cytometry*), and *Western blotting*.

The combination of a soluble antigen with its appropriate antibody can lead to an aggregate that falls out of solution (*precipitation*) and is called a *precipitate*. Formation of a precipitate is caused by the hydrophobicity and size of the lattice. Lattices form in different stages or zones is called the (1) *antibody excess zone*, (2) *equivalence zone*, and (3) *antigen excess zone*.

Precipitation reactions are performed in fluids and gels. Precipitation in a liquid medium can be shown by a *ring test*. The two important fluid, semi-quantitative precipitation tests are (1) the *Ramon* or *β procedure* and (2) its counterpart, the *Dean-Webb* or *α procedure*. These precipitation tests are qualitative or, at best, semiquantitative. Precipitation also can be demonstrated in a semisolid medium such as agar. The most common immunodiffusion precipitation test in a gel is called the *Ouchterlony method* (also called *double immunodiffusion*). Three different patterns or reactions can be observed using the Ouchterlony method: (1) *reaction of identity*, (2) *reaction of partial identity*, and (3) *reaction of nonidentity*. A variation of the Ouchterlony method, the *Mancini method* (also called *radial immunodiffusion*) can quantify antigen.

Complex mixtures of antigens can be separated by application of an electric current, and then the electrophoresed antigens are allowed to diffuse and react with antibody in another well or within the agar; this process is called *immunoelectrophoresis*.

The combination of an *insoluble* (particulate or cellular) antigen with its appropriate antibody can lead to clumping and is called *agglutination*. An important difference between the precipitation and agglutination methods is that the first are quantifiable, while the second are qualitative or semiquantitative at best. However, agglutination methods have wide applications and a high degree of sensitivity. Agglutination reactions are divided into two general types: (1) *direct* and (2) *indirect*.

Direct agglutination of RBCs is called *hemagglutination*. Hemagglutination can be modified to *indirect hemagglutination* by attaching antigens to RBCs. Three forms of hemagglutination testing are done: (1) *reverse passive hemagglutination*, (2) *passive hemagglutination inhibition*, and (3) *nonimmune hemagglutination inhibition*.

The natural agglutination of RBCs that may follow transfusion of blood is due to the occurrence of *blood group antigens* on RBCs. At least 200 different known blood group antigens are used to separate cells into more than 15 blood groups. The most well-characterized blood group antigens are the human alloantigens of the *ABO* and *Rh blood groups*. Antibodies *residing* in individuals that react with blood group antigens they do not express are called *naturally occurring antibodies* or *isoagglutinins*. The use of these antibodies separates the U.S. population into four blood groups: *A, B, O,* and *AB*.

Forty years after Landsteiner discovered the ABO antigens, he and Wiener discovered another RBC antigen system called the *rhesus*, or *Rh, antigens*. The presence or absence of the Rh (or D) antigen on RBCs indicates whether one is Rh$^+$ or Rh$^-$, respectively. No naturally occurring antibodies to the D antigen have been found. Rh$^-$ individuals develop antibodies to the D antigen only on exposure to Rh$^+$ red blood cells.

Development of antibodies to Rh antigens is important in the pathogenesis of the disorder *hemolytic disease of the newborn*, also called *erythroblastosis fetalis*. During the disorder, an Rh$^-$ mother produces anti-Rh (or D) antibodies, which cross the placenta and destroy the fetus's Rh$^+$ RBCs. At birth the child appears blue because of anemia. In severe cases the child is stillborn. This disease in Rh-incompatible pregnancies is avoided by passively administering anti-Rh IgG antibodies to the mother at the time of birth. These antibodies, called *RhoGAM*, block immunization against the D antigen.

When antibody-forming cells are fused with myeloma cells, the resulting clone of cells is a *hybridoma*. Hybridoma cultures are the source of *monoclonal antibodies* of predefined antigen specificity. Use of monoclonal antibodies has revolutionized modern biology. *Transfectomas* (transfected cells) have led to the creation of novel, tailor-made monoclonal antibodies called either *hybrid, chimeric,* or *recombinant monoclonal antibodies*.

*Transgenes* can be incorporated into mouse embryonic cell germline DNA, leading to *transgenic mice* expressing the transgene. Transgenic knockout mice result from targeted gene replacement by a nonfunctional form of the gene, so the gene of interest is not expressed.

Modern genomic analysis tools, such as *microarrays*, give us a systematic way to simultaneously observe and characterize thousands of gene expression profiles comparing different tissues and cells.

# SELF-EVALUATION

## RECALLING KEY TERMS

**ABO blood groups**
**Agglutination**
  **Direct agglutination reaction**
  **Indirect agglutination reaction**
**Antibody affinity**
**Association constant (K)**
**Average affinity**
**Average intrinsic association constant (K$_0$)**
**Avidity**
**Blood group antigens**
**Cross-reactivity**
**Dean-Webb (or α) procedure**
**Direct fluorescent antibody method**
**Enzyme-linked immunosorbent assay (ELISA)**
**Equilibrium constant**
**Equilibrium dialysis**
**Erythroblastosis fetalis**

Erythroblasts
Fluorescein
Fluorochromes
Hemagglutination
  Nonimmune hemagglutination inhibition
  Passive hemagglutination
  Passive hemagglutination inhibition
  Reverse passive hemagglutination
Hemolytic disease of the newborn
Hybrid, chimeric, or recombinant, monoclonal
  antibodies
Hybridoma
Hypoxanthine-aminopterin-thymidine (HAT)
  medium
Immune precipitation
Immunoelectrophoresis
Immunofluorescence
Indirect fluorescent antibody method
Interfacial (or ring) test
Intrinsic binding reaction
Mancini method (Radial immunodiffusion)
Microarrays
Monoclonal antibodies
Naturally occurring antibodies (or isoagglutinins)
Ouchterlony method (Double immunodiffusion)
Primary antigen-antibody reactions
Radioimmunoassay (RIA)
Ramon (or β) procedure
Rh blood groups
Rhodamine
RhoGAM
Secondary antigen-antibody reactions
Serology
Titer
Transfection
Transfectomas
Transgenes
Transgenic mice
Zone phenomenon
  Antibody excess zone
  Antigen excess zone
  Equivalence zone

## MULTIPLE-CHOICE QUESTIONS

*(An answer key is not provided, but the page[s] location of the answer is.)*

1. Direct fluorescent antibody methods are more sensitive and versatile in antigen detection than indirect fluorescent antibody methods. (a) true, (b) false. *(See pages 151 and 152.)*

2. A procedure widely used in clinical laboratories to visually detect antigens in cell sections or on the cell surface is (a) the hemolytic test, (b) the Ouchterlony test, (c) RIA, (d) the fluorescent antibody test, (e) all of these. *(See pages 151 and 152.)*

3. The $r/c$ versus $r$ plots (Scatchard plots) of equilibrium dialysis data are usually linear when the antibody is produced by immunization. (a) true, (b) false. *(See pages 146 and 147.)*

4. The affinity of specific antibody increases during an immune response. (a) true, (b) false. *(See page 147.)*

5. Equilibrium dialysis (a) is useful with macromolecular antigens, (b) does not require known concentrations of antibody and hapten, (c) yields estimates of antigen valence, (d) is most easily performed with colored or radioactively labeled haptens, (e) is none of these. *(See pages 144–147.)*

6. The type of interaction that does not play a role in antigen-antibody reactions is (a) covalent bonds, (b) Van der Waals forces, (c) disulfide bridges, (d) electrostatic forces, (e) hydrophobic interactions, (f) none of these. *(See pages 142 and 143.)*

7. Primary antigen-antibody reactions require long incubation periods to occur. (a) true, (b) false. *(See page 142.)*

8. Which of the following assays directly measures the primary interaction between antibody and antigen and is not dependent on secondary interactions? (a) quantitative precipitation tests, (b) agglutination tests, (c) precipitation tests, (d) fluorescence quenching tests, (e) none of these. *(See pages 147 and 148.)*

9. RIA depends on the antibody binding to labeled or unlabeled antigen with equal effectiveness. (a) true, (b) false. *(See pages 148 and 149.)*

10. In the $r/c$ versus $r$ plot obtained from an equilibrium dialysis experiment, using monoclonal IgM antibody against DNP, the $x$ intercept would be (a) 1, (b) 2, (c) 4, (d) 10, (e) cannot be determined with the information given, (f) none of these. *(See page 146.)*

11. Fluorescent antibody methods (a) are less sensitive when indirect methods are used, (b) use fluorescein to yield an apple green fluorescence, (c) are more versatile when direct methods are used, (d) are useful in the ultrastructural localization of antigens, (e) are none of theses. *(See pages 151 and 152.)*

12. Interactions important in the combination of an antibody's antigen-binding site with an epitope include (a) covalent bonds, (b) Van der Waals forces, (c) disulfide bridges, (d) electrostatic forces, (e) *b* and *d* are correct, (f) none of these. *(See pages 143 and 144.)*

13. In a precipitin reaction (a) the gel diffusion method of Ramon cannot be used, (b) the nature

of the antigen is not important, (c) the test is usually carried out by adding increasing amounts of antiserum to constant amounts of antigen, (d) the reaction may occur with haptens, (e) none of these. (*See pages 155 to 159.*)

14. If a solution of pure antigen is placed in two adjacent wells and the homologous antibody is placed in the center well, the two precipitin bands join at their contiguous ends and fuse. The pattern is known as (a) the reaction of identity, (b) the reaction of nonidentity, (c) the reaction of partial identity, (d) the cross-reaction, (e) none of these. (*See pages 159 and 161.*)

15. In the α procedure, the titer is the highest dilution of antibody to give a positive test. (a) true, (b) false. (*See pages 158 and 159.*)

16. Immunoelectrophoresis combines the principles of (a) electrophoresis, (b) precipitation, (c) agglutination, (d) *a* and *b* are correct, (e) *a* and *c* are correct. (*See pages 160 and 163.*)

17. Equivalence zone precipitates form when equal numbers of antigen and antibody molecules form a lattice. (a) true, (b) false. (*See pages 156 to 158.*)

18. The Ouchterlony technique can be used to determine whether two antigens share some but not all determinants. (a) true, (b) false. (*See page 159.*)

19. Factors that affect the amount of immune precipitate formed include (a) pH of the reaction medium, (b) molar ratio of antibody to antigen, (c) salt concentration, (d) reaction volume, (e) all of the above, (f) none of these. (*See page 157.*)

20. Antigen and antibody do not combine in the region of antigen excess. (a) true, (b) false. (*See pages 156 to 158.*)

21. The reaction that occurs when antibody and soluble antigen are mixed is demonstrated by the (a) agglutination test, (b) adsorption test, (c) precipitation test, (d) hemagglutination test, (e) none of these. (*See page 155.*)

22. In the prevention of hemolytic disease of the newborn (a) mothers are given complete blood transfusions after delivering Rh$^+$ children, (b) marriages between Rh-incompatible couples are discouraged, (c) Rh$^-$ mothers delivering Rh$^+$ children are given anti-Rh antibodies, (d) Rh$^+$ mothers delivering Rh$^-$ children are given anti-Rh antibodies, (e) none of the above, (f) none of these. (*See pages 165 and 166.*)

23. Passive hemagglutination reactions (a) are more sensitive than indirect agglutination, (b) use antigens that are normal constituents of the particle surface, (c) can be used to estimate the number of epitopes, (d) are widely use in ABO blood typing, (e) none of these. (*See page 164.*)

24. Agglutination is (a) more sensitive than a precipitation reaction, (b) the reaction of a soluble antigen with antibodies, (c) the reaction of an insoluble antigen with an antibodies, (d) *a* and *b* are correct, (e) *a* and *c* are correct. (*See page 161.*)

25. Maternal sensitization to a baby's Rh antigen may be prevented by ABO incompatibility between them. (a) true, (b) false. (*See page 166.*)

26. The fusion of what cells leads to a hybridoma cell line that secretes monoclonal antibodies? (a) plasma cells and myeloma cells, (b) monocytes and lymphocytes, (c) lymphocytes and lymphoma cells, (d) plasma cells and activated T cells, (e) none of these. (*See pages 167 and 168.*)

## SHORT-ANSWER ESSAY QUESTIONS

1. Differentiate between a primary and a secondary antigen-antibody reaction. What are three important characteristics that distinguish the two reactions?

2. The cross-reactivity of antibodies presents problems for the science of serology. Explain.

3. What kinds of noncovalent interactions are important in antigen-antibody interactions? What aspect of these interactions is probably most important and why?

4. How is equilibrium dialysis used to measure primary antigen-antibody reactions?

5. Distinguish between antibody affinity (or **K**) and average antibody affinity (or **K$_0$**).

6. How is fluorescence quenching used to measure primary antigen-antibody reactions?

7. Briefly discuss the RIA, and suggest its pros and cons.

8. RIAs are being replaced by ELISAs. Why? Describe the different variants of the ELISA test.

9. Describe the two types of immunofluorescence tests. What is the advantage of the indirect procedure over the direct procedure? What are some commonly used fluorochromes, and what colors do they emit? How are fluorscent dyes used in flow cytometry?

10. When describing secondary antigen-antibody reactions, what do we mean by a lattice formation?

11. What makes precipitation reactions visible reactions? What two factors are important in the development of precipitation reactions?

12. Discuss how the zone phenomenon shows the reversibility of precipitation reactions. What factors other than the proportion of antigen and antibody affect precipitation?

13. Compare and contrast the Ramon or β procedure and the Dean-Webb or α procedure. The antibody titers of these two procedures are defined differently; why?

14. The Ouchterlony test is an example of double diffusion in a two-dimension test. Explain.

15. Three patterns can be observed using the Ouchterlony test. What are they, and what do they show?

16. What is the major advantage of immunoelectrophoresis tests over immunodiffusion tests?

17. Briefly discuss how agglutination differs from precipitation.

18. Why are agglutination tests more sensitive than precipitation tests?

19. Differentiate between direct and indirect agglutination reactions. What is a major advantage of indirect agglutination reactions?

20. What is hemagglutination? Briefly describe three types.

21. The first blood group system to be described was what? By whom? What type of antigens are blood group antigens? What are the antibodies called that react against blood group antigens?

22. What are the four divisions of the ABO blood system? What antigens are expressed on the RBCs of individuals of each group, and what antibodies against these antigens are found in their blood?

23. If an Rh⁻ person has anti-D antibodies, what are the two ways in which these antibodies could have developed?

24. What causes hemolytic disease of the newborn, and how can it be prevented?

25. Compare conventional antibody production with monoclonal antibody production.

26. The use of transfectomas to create novel, tailor-made monoclonal antibodies has reduced some of the limitations of monoclonal antibodies. Explain.

27. AIDS is a difficult disease to study because it is difficult to reproduce the process by which the human immune system responds to HIV. How could transgenic mice lessen this problem?

28. How has micrroarray-based gene analysis changed the way we diagnosis diseases?

## FURTHER READINGS

Alkan, S.S. 2004. Monoclonal antibodies: the story of a discovery that revolutionized science and medicine. *Nat. Rev. Immunol.* 4:53–56.

Berzofsky, J.A., I.J. Berkower, and S.L. Epstein. 2003. Antigen-antibody interactions and monoclonal antibodies. In *Fundamental Immunology*, 5th ed. W.E. Paul, ed. Philadelphia: Lippincott Williams & Wilkins. p. 69–106.

Coligan, J.E., B.E. Bierer, D.H. Margulies, E.M. Shevach, and W. Strober, ed. 2005. *Short Protocols in Immunology.* Hoboken, NJ: John Wiley & Sons, Inc.

Kohler, G. 1986. Derivation and diversification of monoclonal antibodies. *Science* 233:1281–1286.

Kohler, G., and C. Milstein. 1975. Continuous cultures of fused cells secreting antibody of predefined specificity. *Nature* 256:495–497.

Milstein, C. 1980. Monoclonal antibodies. *Sci. Am.* 243:66–74.

Milstein, C. 1986. From antibody structure to immunological diversification of immune response. *Science* 231:1261–1268.

Chase, M.W., and C.A. Williams. 1971. *Methods in Immunology III*. New York: Academic Press.

Davies, D.R., E.A. Padlan, and S. Sheriff. 1990. Antigen-antibody complexes. *Annu. Rev. Biochem.* 59:439–473.

Garvey, J.S., N.E. Cremer, and D.H. Sussdorf. 1977. *Methods in Immunology*, 2nd ed. Reading, MA: W.A. Benjamin.

Hughes-Jones, N.S., and C.A. Clark. 1982. Haemolytic disease of the newborn. In *Clinical Aspects of Immunology*, 4th ed. ed. P.J. Lachmann, and D.K. Peters. Oxford: Blackwell Scientific.

Johnstone, A., and R. Thorpe. 1987. *Immunochemistry in Practice*, 2nd ed. Oxford: Blackwell Scientific.

Kabat, E.A. 1976. *Structural Concepts in Immunology and Immunochemistry*, 2nd ed. New York: Holt, Rinehart and Winston.

Kabat, E.A. 1978. The structural basis of antibody complementarity. *Adv. Protein Chem.* 32:1–76.

Marcus, D.M., ed. 1981. Blood group immunochemistry and genetics. *Semin. Hematol.* 18:1–3.

Nowotny, A. 1979. *Basic Exercises in Immunochemistry*, 2nd ed. New York: Springer-Verlag.

Price, T.H., ed. 2008. *Technical Standards for Blood Banks and Transfusion Services*, 25th ed. Bethesda, MD: Amer. Assoc. Blood Banks.

Rose, N.R., et al. 1997. *Manual of Clinical Laboratory Immunology.* Washington, DC: American Society of Microbiology.

Steensgaard, J. 1984. The mechanism of immune precipitation. *Immunol. Today* 5:7–10.

Sturgeon, P. 1983. *Erythrocyte Antigens and Antibodies*, ed. W.J. Williams, J. Bentler, A. Erslev, and W. Rundles. New York: McGraw Hill.

Weir, D.M., ed. 1986. *Handbook of Experimental Immunology, Vol. I: Immunochemistry*, 4th ed. Oxford: Blackwell Scientific.

Wilson, I.A., and R.L. Stanfield. 1994. Antigen-antibody interactions: New structures and new conformational changes. *Opin. Chem. Biol.* 8:857–867.

Yalow, R.S., and S.A. Berson. 1960. Immunoassay of endogenous plasma insulin in man. *J. Clin. Invest.* 39:1157–1175.

Yalow, R.S. 1980. Radioimmunoassay. *Rev. Biophys. Bioeng.* 9:327–345.

# CHAPTER SIX

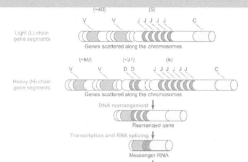

# THE GENETICS OF ANTIBODY FORMATION AND STRUCTURE

## OBJECTIVES

The reader should be able to:

1. Understand how the number and organization of immunoglobulin gene segments contribute to the generation of antibody diversity.
2. Outline Tonegawa's experiment to prove the hypothesis of two genes—one polypeptide; understand why comparing the immunoglobulin genes (DNA) of embryonic (germline) and adult (somatic) cells was the crux of his experiment; realize that Tonegawa's results suggested that immunoglobulin

germline genes rearranged to form a functional immunoglobulin gene and a joining (J) region follows the variable (V) region.

3. Draw the organization of immunoglobulin light-chain and heavy-chain genes.

4. Give an account, in the context of the heptamer-nonamer and 12/23 rule, of V-J joining for light-chain genes and D-J joining and V-(D-J) joining for heavy-chain genes.

5. Understand how allelic exclusion leads to antibody molecules of single antigen specificity.

6. Explain how transcription controls immunoglobulin gene expression.

7. List and discuss the mechanisms that contribute to antibody diversity; give some possible numbers of immunoglobulin genes resulting from these mechanisms.

8. Appreciate the connection between RNA processing and the coexpression of IgM and IgD and the progression of membrane to secreted IgM.

9. Comment on site-specific DNA recombination as a mechanism for class switching.

10. Describe the physiology of immunoglobulin express.

The previous chapters suggest that vertebrate immune systems can respond to millions of antigens, even newly synthesized molecules not present in nature, by producing specific antibodies against each. Antibody diversity is possible because a host has millions of B cells that each produce a unique antigen-binding antibody molecule. An individual must have an *antibody* (or T-cell receptor) *repertoire*, or total population of antibody specificities, large enough to ensure that there will be an antibody with an antigen-binding site to fit any antigenic determinant (estimated to be higher than 100 million different antibody molecules). Because antibodies are proteins, and genes encode proteins, such a large number of antibodies would call for 100 million immunoglobulin genes. However, the genome of a body cell accounts for perhaps 25,000 genes, and immunoglobulin genes make up only a small proportion of them. Nonetheless, *the information to encode all these antibodies must be present in the DNA.* How can a few genes encode an unlimited number of antibodies? The surprising answer is that intact immunoglobulin genes are assembled from a limited number of bits and pieces of DNA scattered on a chromosome. The resulting unusual immunoglobulin organization of unique variable regions and a limited number of constant regions on the same polypeptide chain directly relates to the DNA's organization. How this happens is the subject of this chapter. In short, the body uses (1) mechanisms that are unique to the immune system: DNA rearrangement for generation of antibody diversity (and control thereof) and allelic exclusion and (2) mechanisms that are just the normal processes of cell biology: RNA splicing to remove introns and biosynthesis of a cell-surface or secreted glycoprotein.

# THE GENETIC BASIS OF ANTIBODY DIVERSITY IS EXPLAINED BY THE RANDOM RECOMBINATION OF INHERITED VARIABLE-REGION GENE SEGMENTS

The human genome is not large enough to have all the genes necessary for such a limitless diversity in antibody structure. Two groups of theories emerged to explain the presence of so many immunoglobulin genes. *The **germline theories** stated that all genes encoding immunoglobulins are present in the germinal cells (that is, the egg and sperm).* The opposite hypotheses, the **somatic theories**, *stated that the genome had a limited number of immunoglobulin genes and antibody diversity is generated later by some sort of somatic genetic change (mutation or recombination) of a few germline variable- (V) region genes during differentiation of B-cell precursors to mature (somatic) B cells.*

The germline theories postulate that each immunoglobulin polypeptide chain is synthesized from a cistron[1] present in the germ cell (gamete). The genes encoding antibody specificity against the entire repertoire of antigenic determinants are inscribed in the genome of the person and inherited from the parents. The fusion of sperm and ovum

---

[1] The term *cistron* is used to describe a tandem gene that is jointly transcribed and is used when specifying a hereditary unit of function.

(parental germline cells) leads to an individual with a genome containing genetic information to respond to any antigenic determinant from the moment of conception. This scenario implies that immunoglobulin genes are passed from generation to generation through germline cells—no special genetic mechanisms are needed to generate antibody diversity. The concept seemed simple enough, and even logical, but one simple fact, not known at that time, but realized once immunoglobulins amino acid sequences were determined, destroyed its credibility: the undifferentiated (embryonic) cells have more immunoglobulin genes than do their immunologically mature progeny (somatic) cells.

The somatic theories postulated that an individual inherits a few immunoglobulin genes from germline cells. Somatic theories use two hypotheses to explain the mechanisms used to generate antibody diversity. The *somatic recombination hypotheses* suggest that antibody diversity results from germline DNA having many V-region segments that are each able to join to a single constant- (C) region gene segment. The *somatic mutation hypotheses* suggest that antibody diversity results from a single germline gene undergoing extensive mutation, but only in its V region. This mutation leads to an immunoglobulin chain with a unique V-region amino acid sequence, although all immunoglobulin chains have the same C region. Thus, immunoglobulins diversify by somatic recombinations and mutations that occur during differentiation of stem cells into naïve mature B lymphocytes. Consequently, immature immune cells destined to become B cells must have a high rate of somatic recombinations or random mutations among the few germline immunoglobulin V-region gene segments they inherited. The result is a host with many different genes encoding antibodies capable of responding to an infinite variety of antigens. As will be seen, *some mechanisms proposed by both theories contribute to antibody diversity.*

## B Cells Have Multiple Copies of Separate V-Region Gene Segments

Irrespective of the theories proposed to explain antibody diversity, they could not explain the diversity and constancy within each antibody molecule and the fact that identical V regions used different C regions. To resolve the contradictions between the germline and somatic theories, immunologists tried to determine the number and the organization of immunoglobulin genes present in germline cells. Immunoglobulin structure was difficult to explain using traditional genetics. Because classic molecular

biology holds that one gene encodes one polypeptide chain, an immunoglobulin would need two genes: one for the heavy chain and one for the light chain. It made sense to assume that one gene encoded the entire light or heavy chain because the V and C regions of either chain were seamlessly connected to one another in the molecule. However, this assumption turned out to be incorrect. In 1965, Dreyer and Bennett proposed that two separate genes encode *each* immunoglobulin chain—one encodes the V region, the other the C region. The *hypothesis of two genes, one polypeptide* was based on the presence of V and C regions in each chain. When the amino acid sequences of many kappa (κ) light chains were compared, some segments of the chains always differed in sequence (V regions), and other segments were always the same on all chains (C regions). Furthermore, sequence studies of myeloma heavy (H) chains showed that the *same* $V_H$ region can associate with *different* $C_H$ regions. This phenomenon is called *class*, or *isotype, switching* and will be discussed shortly. If one genetic element encodes the entire heavy chain, the same half of the $V_H$ gene must be linked to different halves of $C_H$-region genes (a great deal of redundant information). Dreyer and Bennett proposed that there were only single copies of class and subclass C-region genes encoded in the germline separately from the hundreds of V-region genes. They felt that immunoglobulin chains were specified in two discontinuous stretches of DNA. They asked: If one gene encoded V and C regions, why was variability limited to the amino-terminal end of the chain and not found in the C region? If distinct genes encoded each region, the lack of carboxyl-terminal end variability could be explained. They proposed that the V region was connected by a normal peptide link to the C region. For this kind of linking, a mechanism must exist to synthesize one molecule by joining two different segments together. They advanced the notion that this happens at the level of DNA. Incorporation of Dreyer and Bennett's hypothesis into selective theories of immunoglobulin formation would mean that during differentiation of cells, culminating in mature B cells, events occur that lead to the joining of $V_L$ and $C_L$ genes and $V_H$ and $C_H$ genes—that DNA rearranges to produce a functional immunoglobulin gene. If different V- and C-region genes were linked, each progeny B cell would be committed to express receptors of unique antigen specificity while maintaining the biologic effectiveness of their few C regions.

Dreyer and Bennett's novel and controversial notion was correct, but more complex than they envisioned and the molecular biologic methods to test their hypothesis were unavailable at the time. After many years, in 1976 Tonegawa and his colleagues provided definitive experimental evidence for Dreyer and Bennett's hypothesis. Using a technique called *Southern blotting*, they showed DNA rearrangements (the genes for the V and C regions are separated and then joined during the course of B-cell differentiation), leading to a *complete*, or *functional*, *gene* that the cell then expressed as its antibody product. Tonegawa's group did this experiment by comparing the structure of a κ light-chain gene (DNA) from myeloma cells[2] (analogous to all adult immune cells), which produce this immunoglobulin chain, and embryonic mouse cells (analogous to all adult nonimmune cells), which do not. The experiment began with the isolation of full-length radioactive messenger RNA (mRNA) encoding the V and C regions of a κ chain secreted by a myeloma cell line—the probe for both V and C regions. Some of this radioactive mRNA was broken in half and the 3' half was used as a probe for the C region. Because the labeled mRNA is complementary to the gene that encodes the light chain, it can be used as a probe in hybridization experiments with DNA from mouse embryo cells and myeloma cells.

Tonegawa's experiment showed that the sizes of DNA fragments of immunoglobulin-containing genes differs in embryonic and somatic DNA; the results of the experiment are schematically depicted in Figure 6-1. It showed that immunoglobulin germline gene segments rearranged to form a functional immunoglobulin gene. The nucleotide sequence data, however, still showed a physical separation of the genes. Genes were close together but not contiguous. The genes are separated by noncoding **inter**vening sequences (also called **introns**) of about 1200 nucleotides.[3] Genes used for coding, or the sequences that are *ex*pressed, are called **exons**. Two genes–one polypeptide, plus the rearrangement of germline DNA, leads to a commitment to express a receptor. Functional genes for lambda (λ) and κ light chains and heavy chains (and T-cell receptors) are generated in the same manner.

Tonegawa and his associates got another surprise when they compared the nucleotide sequence of the embryonic DNA containing the light-chain V-region gene to the number of amino acids in the light-chain V region. The V-region gene stopped after the codon for amino acid 98, yet there were about 110 amino acid residues in the V region of the light chain. The V-gene segment was too short to encode the entire V region. The missing DNA segment, encoding the remaining 13 amino acids, was in the embryonic DNA about 1200 base pairs downstream before the start of the C-region gene. The 1200 base pairs are the exact size of the intron found in the V-region gene of the mature B cell. The gene segment was called J for *joining*.

The research of Tonegawa and colleagues showed that the V, J, and C segments (exons) of embryonic (germline) DNA were widely separated; *but during the maturation of a B cell, the V and J segments become joined and form the **composite coding sequence** (or **functional gene**)[4] for a light-chain V region*. Voila! Antibody diversity results from somatic recombination, or gene shuffling. The VJ-region coding sequence remains separated from the C-region coding sequence by an intron. The intron is not excised until after the entire stretch of DNA is transcribed into RNA (this process is discussed later). mRNA is then translated into an immunoglobulin light chain. (The joining scenario is similar for immunoglobulin heavy chains, except for the presence of a third unique V-region gene segment.) For this and related experiments, Susumu Tonegawa received the 1987 Nobel Prize in Medicine.

## Immunoglobulin Gene Segment Organization Allows for a Precise Sequence of Random Recombination of These Segments

Subsequent immunoglobulin DNA cloning and sequencing suggested even greater complexity than Dreyer and Bennett imagined. Mice and humans have three multigene families found on different chromosomes that encode immunoglobulin chains (Table 6-1). Each family contains coding sequences called **gene segments** that are arranged in groups of variable (V), diversity (D), and joining (J) segments, and constant (C) exons. *The light chain is encoded by three distinctive gene segments,* **variable- (V) gene segments** *(roughly 300 base-pairs long),* **joining-(J) gene segments** *(roughly 50 base-pairs long), and* **constant (C) gene segments** *(roughly 300 base-pairs long)—all separated by variable lengths of noncoding DNA. The embryonic form of κ- and λ-chain (and heavy-chain) genes also includes a short DNA sequence (an exon) encoding a 19 amino acid-long* **leader (L)**, *or* **signal, peptide**, *preceding each V-gene segment. This exon*

---

[2]Remember, from Chapter 4, that myeloma cells are malignant plasma cells secreting homogeneous immunoglobulin.
[3]Introns were first described in adenovirus, β-globin, and ovalbumin genes shortly before Tonegawa's work was done.

---

[4]When describing immunoglobulin genes, the term *genes* takes on added meaning: it refers either to the segments, or exons, of the DNA encoding only the V and C regions or to the DNA encoding the complete light or heavy chain.

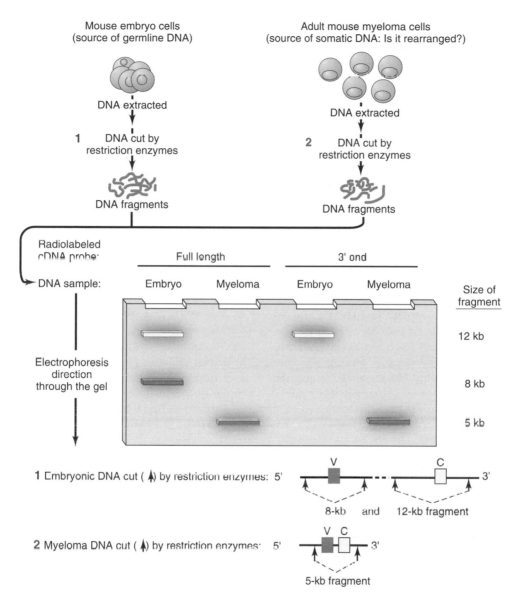

**FIGURE 6-1 Arrangement of V- and C-gene segments during B-cell maturation.** Tonegawa showed that V and C genes have different arrangements in embryonic (germline) and adult (somatic) DNA. Both DNAs were digested to completion with restriction enzymes and separated by gel electrophoresis. The gel was cut into slices, the fragments were eluted from the slices and denatured to single-stranded fragments, and the fragments were hybridized with mRNA encoding the κ chain. By using a V-region probe combined with a C region (full-length mRNA) or a C-region probe alone (3′ half of the mRNA), the κ mRNA hybridized by its C-region portion to one DNA fragment, while its V-region portion hybridized to a separate DNA fragment when DNA from the embryo was used. Because the mRNA hybridized to two different embryonic DNA fragments, the genes encoding the $V_\kappa$ and $C_k$ are physically separated. In the somatic DNA, one restriction fragment hybridized to the full-length mRNA probe and the 3′-end mRNA probe (both probes reacted with DNA fragments of the same size). V and C genes are closer together in myeloma cells than in embryonic cells. Thus, the germline immunoglobulin genes rearranged. The results proved Dreyer and Bennett's hypothesis.

**TABLE 6-1 The Chromosomal Location of Immunoglobulin Genes**

| Gene | Chromosome | |
|---|---|---|
| | Mouse | Human |
| κ light chain | 6 | 2 |
| λ light chain | 16 | 22 |
| Heavy chain | 12 | 14 |

encodes the hydrophobic part of the polypeptide chains. The signal peptides are found in secretory and transmembrane proteins and are important for the transport of immunoglobulin molecules from the ribosomes into the lumen of the endoplasmic reticulum, where they are cleaved off.

Light-chain V-gene segments encode amino acid residues 1 to 95 (including the first two complementarity-determinig regions [CDRs; see Chapter 4]), J-gene segments encode amino acid residues 96 to 108 (including the last CDR), and C genes encode the remainder of the chain (Figure 6-2). These light-chain CDRs are encoded on a noncontiguous piece of DNA. The gene segments for the first two CDR regions, however, are contiguous; therefore, they are not free to assort on their own. The V-segment group is next to but not contiguous to

the DNA segment (J region) encoding the remaining 13 amino acids of the light-chain V-region protein sequence. The V- and J-gene segment groups are separated by a large intron (for λ-chain DNA roughly 70 kb; for κ-chain DNA roughly 23 kb). J-gene segments within the J group lie next to, but separated from, each other by short introns. The J-segment group is separated by an intervening sequence of about 1.2 kb from the C-region gene. The joining of different V-gene segments with different J-gene segments leads to sequence variability.

Vκ segments each encode the first two CDRs and three framework regions of the κ chain V region, plus a few CDR3 amino acid residues. Jκ segments each encode the remainder of CDR3 and the fourth framework region. The Cκ exon encodes the complete κ-light chain C-region. DNA encoding the human κ chain includes roughly 40 functional Vκ segments, five Jκ segments, and one Cκ gene segment, as well as some pseudogenes (in mouse segments) that contain frameshrift and/or stop codons. Human λ-chain DNA contains roughly 30 functional Vλ segments and four functional sets of Jλ and Cλ segments. As κ-chain DNA, λ-chain DNA also contains some pseudogenes. An individual Jλ segment always pairs with its corresponding Cλ exon, unlike Jκ segments which

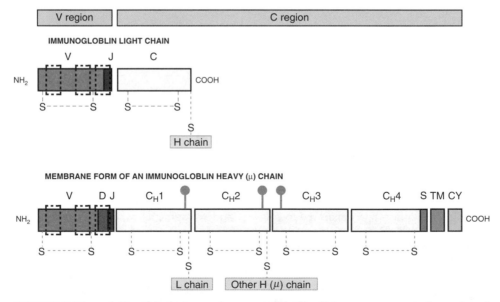

**FIGURE 6-2 The relationship between immunoglobulin (Ig) gene segments (exons) and light and heavy (μ) chain domains.** The Ig light chain is encoded by two incomplete, or segmented, exons (V and J) and one complete exon (C). The Ig heavy chain, here the membrane form of the μ chain, is encoded by three incomplete, or segmented, exons (V, D, and J) and six complete exons (C$_H$1–4, and the transmembrane [TM] and cytoplasmic [CY] exons). The approximate locations of intrachain and interchain disulfide bridges (S–S), of carbohydrates (●) and of CDR regions (dashed boxes) are given.

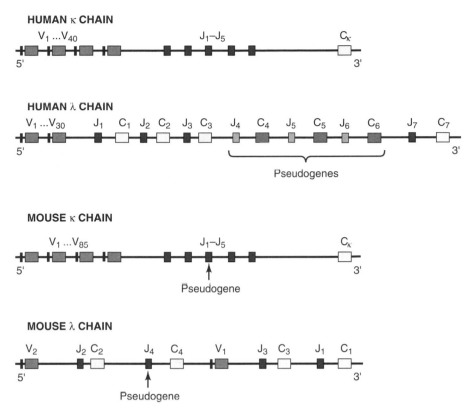

**FIGURE 6-3** Organization of germline immunoglobulin genes for mouse and human κ **and** λ **chains**. The human κ chains have 40 $V_L$ genes, five $J_L$ genes, and single copies of $C_L$ genes. The human λ chain has a gene arrangement similar to that of its mouse counterpart, but has more V, J, and $C_L$ genes (30 $V_L$ genes, 4 $J_L$ genes). The mouse κ chains have 85 $V_L$ genes and 4 $J_L$ genes. Only four of the five mouse $J_κ$ segment genes are expressed. The $J_3$-segment gene encodes a protein sequence never found in mouse κ chains—a pseudogene (↑). In contrast, the mouse λ-chain V region has only three germline V genes, three $J_L$ genes, and four $C_L$ genes, each flanked on the 5′ side with $J_L$ genes. All V genes are preceded by a leader sequence.

all pair with the same Cκ exon. The arrangement of genetic elements in human and mouse germline DNA for κ and λ chains is schematically represented in Figure 6-3; in the mouse, the genes for λ chains are simpler than those for κ chains, at least in the number of total gene segments and resulting combinations.

*The organization of heavy-chain gene segments is similar to the organization of light-chain gene segments, but heavy-chain gene segments also contain* **diversity-(D) gene segments** *(roughly 50 base pairs long), and each C-region gene segment has one or more associated coding segments called* **membrane (M) exons**, *represented by a transmembrane (TM) exon and a cytoplasmic (CY) tail exon* (Figure 6-4). As for light chains, each heavy-chain V-gene segment is preceded by a leader exon. *Heavy chains are encoded by four different gene segments,* $V_H$, $D_H$, $J_H$, *and* $C_H$ (see Figure 6-2). V-gene segments encode amino acid residues 1 to 94

(including the first two CDRs and three framework regions), D-gene segments encode amino acid residues 95 to 97, J-gene segments encode amino acid residues 98 to 113, and C-gene segments encode the remainder of the chain. CDR3 is encoded by the last few nucleotides of $V_H$, all of $D_H$, and the first part of $J_H$, while the remainder of the $J_H$ gene segment encodes framework region 4. Heavy-chain CDR3 is a component of the region created by the joining of $V_H$, D, and $J_H$ segments, thereby contributing significantly to receptor diversity (discussed shortly). The end of the J-gene segment group and $C_μ$ segment are separated by roughly 7 kb. The separation between C-gene segments ranges from 4.5 to 55 kb. *The heavy-chain C region is encoded by multiple C exons.* Structural studies of immunoglobulin heavy chains show four C-region structural domains in the μ and ε chains and three structural domains and a hinge

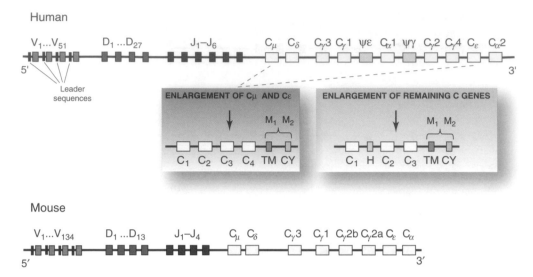

**FIGURE 6-4 Organization of germline immunoglobulin gene segments for human and mouse heavy chains.** The $C_1$-$C_4$-$M_1$-$M_2$ is the exon sequence for the four structural constant (C) domains and membrane (M) exons (represented by transmembrane [TM] and cytoplasmic [CY] exons) for $\mu$ and $\varepsilon$ chains. $C_1$-$H$-$C_2$-$C_3$-$M_1$-$M_2$ is the exon sequence for the structural C, hinge (H), C domains, and M exons for $C_\delta$, $C_{\gamma3}$, $C_{\gamma1}$, $C_{\gamma2b}$, $C_{\gamma2}$, and $C_\alpha$ chains. The $M_1$ (TM) and $M_2$ (CY) exons encode the transmembrane and cytoplasmic segments of the membrane form of the chain, respectively. The organization of human germline immunoglobulin-gene segments is similar to that of the mouse; however, there are fewer V-gene segments (51), roughly 27 D-gene segments, 6 functional J-gene segments (and three pseudogenes not shown), and C-gene sequence is $C_\mu$, $C_\delta$, $C_{\gamma3}$, $C_{\gamma1}$, $C_\varepsilon2$, $C_\alpha1$, $C_{\gamma2}$, $C_{\gamma4}$, $C_\varepsilon1$, and $C_\alpha$. All V-gene segments are preceded by a leader sequence.

region in the $\delta$, $\gamma$, and $\alpha$ chains. The overall sequence of heavy-chain C-region gene segments is $C_\mu$, $C_\delta$, $C_\gamma$, $C_\varepsilon$, and $C_\alpha$; this sequence seems to correlate with the sequence of antibody expression during B-cell differentiation and IgM production during the first exposure to all antigens. Sequencing of the genes for these heavy chains shows that separate DNA exons encode each of the domains and the hinge regions. Furthermore, all C genes have one or more M exons 3' to their last C-domain gene segment. These exons encode a roughly 40-amino-acid sequence that constitutes the TM and CY domains at the carboxyl-terminal end of the membrane-bound forms of heavy chains. This hydrophobic tail participates in the attachment of immunoglobulins destined for the membrane of B cells. The introns and noncoding DNA, separating light and heavy chain exons, are not without importance; the introns contain nucleotide sequences that affect transcription and RNA splicing, while the noncoding DNA sequences contain nucleotide sequences that control DNA rearrangements. These activities will be discussed shortly.

The immunoglobulin gene organization of naïve mature B cells contrasts sharply with the arrangement of all other cells. In fact, all cells except B cells contain immunoglobulin genes in their germline configuration. The generation of receptor (immunoglobulins or T cell receptors) diversity depends on the ability of B cells (and T cells) to somatically alter this germline configuration. Embryonic cells inherit the immunoglobulin light-chain genes as four segments (L, V, J, and C). The L and C segments are exons; the V and J segments are incomplete exons that are joined by recombinational events at the DNA level to complete the third exon, V-J. The heavy-chain gene locus in germline DNA is more complex. This locus is inherited as five segments (L, V, D, J, and C). The L and C segments are exons (but remember that heavy-chain C regions are encoded by multiple exons; see Figure 6-4) and the V, D, and J segments are incomplete exons that are joined through a two-step recombinational event at the DNA level to complete the third exon, V-(D-J). These antigen-independent recombination events are instigated by sequence-specific endonucleases that cut the DNA flanking the gene segments and followed by joining of the DNA ends by nonhomologous end-joining (NHEJ) proteins. Both heavy-chain and light-chain V-region gene rearrangements occur in an ordered sequence during

B-cell maturation in the bone marrow (see also Chapter 10). Heavy-chain V-region gene rearrangements occur first, followed by light-chain V-region gene rearrangements. Even though rearrangements occur in an ordered sequence, they are random events that lead to random determination of B-cell antigen specificity. These rearrangements lead to functionally rearranged genes capable of encoding functional light and heavy chains in naïve mature B cells. How this occurs is detailed in the next few sections.

## Conserved Signals for Recombination Flank V-Region Gene Segments

In differentiating B cells, a rearrangement of genomic DNA leads to V-gene segments joining with J-gene segments for light chain production and D-gene segments joining with J-gene segments followed by DJ joining with V-gene segments for heavy chain production. This rearrangement leads to either *deletion* of the DNA separating these gene segments in the embryonic DNA or *inversion* (in rare cases), depending on the orientation of the V and J segments. *Germline DNA sequences at the immediate 3′ ends of each $V_L$ or $V_H$ gene segments, 5′ and 3′ to each $D_H$ gene segments, and at the immediate 5′ ends of each $J_L$ or $J_H$ gene segments serve as DNA* **recombination signal sequences (RSSs)** *that help to control all of the DNA rearrangements.* Figure 6-5 illustrates the location and organization of these sequences in the germline immunoglobulin DNA. RSSs are composed of a conserved palindromic heptamer and a conserved AT-rich nonamer separated by nonconserved 12- or 23-nucleotide-long spacers. These 12- or 23-nucleotide-long spacer sequences correspond to one and two turns of the DNA helix; thus, they are called **one-turn RSSs** and **two-turn RSSs**, respectively. The $V_\kappa$ segment is flanked on its 3′ side by a one-turn RSS and the $J_\kappa$ segment on its 5′ side is flanked by a two-turn RSS. The order is reversed in λ light-chain DNA. In heavy-chain DNA, the $V_H$ and $J_H$ segments have two-turn RSSs, the $D_H$ segments are flanked on both sides by one-turn RSSs (see Figure 6-5). Whether light or heavy chains are synthesized, *the joining of separate V-J or D-J and V to D-J gene segments on the DNA strand is governed by the* **heptamer-nonamer** *and* **spacer 12/23 rule**. *These joinings occur only if their heptamer-nonamers are oriented in opposite directions and are separated by 12 or 23 nucleotides.* This ensures that light chains only make V-J recombinations and heavy chains V-(D-J) recombinations.

During deletional V(D)J recombination in light-chain (and heavy-chain) genes, these short,

highly conserved (identical in all V-, D-, and J-gene segments) RSSs are the complementary sequences that come together to form a stem-loop structure containing V- and J-gene segments and introns to be deleted (Figure 6-6). These stem-loop configurations—V(D)J recombination sites, the junctions between RSSs (signal sequences for short) and coding sequences—are catalyzed by immunoglobulin gene enzymes collectively called **V(D)J recombinase**. The two genes, adjacent to one another on Chromosome 11p13, which induce immunoglobulin gene recombination, are called **recombination activation genes 1** and **2** (**RAG1** and **RAG2**). They encode the proteins (RAG-1 and RAG-2), which comprise the lymphocyte-specific components of the recombinase that act synergistically and are required to mediate V-(D-J) recombination; without them, humans make no immunoglobulins or T-cell receptor proteins and they have no mature B or T cells. These enzymes, along with **terminal deoxynucleotidyl transferase** (**TdT**), are the only known immune cell-specific gene products that mediated V-(D)-J recombination and they act only in the early developmental stages of B cells (and T cells) and only during assemble of their antigen receptors. They are active in pre-B (and pre-T) cell lines but not in antibody-secreting myeloma cells. RAG genes are expressed in the $G_0$ and $G_1$ phases of the cell cycle and are quiescent in proliferating B (and T) cells. During early B-cell differentiation, immunoglobulin gene rearrangement also is controlled by recombinase accessibility to DNA. Proteins that condense into a structure called *chromatin*, which prevents uncontrolled DNA expression, cover most regions of eukaryotic DNA. However, the chromatin structure of immunoglobulin gene segments opens as the B cell starts to develop, exposing the segments to the recombinases that mediate DNA rearrangement. The activation and regulation of RAG1 and RAG2 recombinase correlates with specific transcription factor expression that drives early B cell differentiation. For example, the generation of the earliest B cell progenitors depends on the transcription factors early B cell factor (EBF) and the E box proteins E2A, which coordinately activate the B cell gene expression program that initiates immunoglobulin heavy-chain gene rearrangements by opening immunoglobulin loci and inducing expression of recombination-related proteins (RAG1, RAG2, and TdT) at the onset of B-cell lymphopoiesis.

A more detailed view of the configuration required for deletional V-J joining is presented in Figure 6-7. The first RSS consists of seven nucleotides (a CACAGTG heptamer) arranged as a consensus

## NUCLEOTIDE SEQUENCE OF DNA RSSs

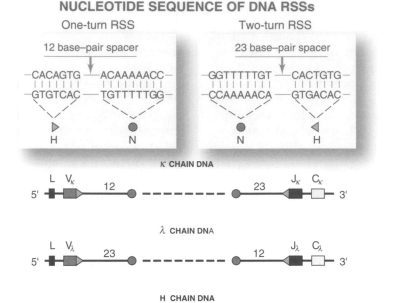

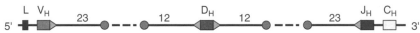

**FIGURE 6-5 Location and organization of DNA RSSs of germline immunoglobulin DNA**. Recombination of V-, D-, and J-gene segments occurs by the joining of specific sequences flanking $V_L$ and $J_L$ segments of light-chain germline DNA and $V_H$, $D_H$, and $J_H$ segments of heavy-chain germline DNA. The organization of these RSSs is as follows: a 7-base-pair sequence (heptamer [H]) identical in all V-, D-, and J-gene segments, followed by a 12-base-pair or 23-base-pair random sequence, and then a 9-base-pair (nonamer [N]), also identical in all V-, D-, and J-gene segments. Recombination occurs only between an element with a 12-base-pair spacer and an element with a 23-base-pair spacer and their H-N are oriented in opposite directions. This rule ensures that a V-gene segment is always joined to a J-gene segment but never to another V-gene segment. For example, the H and N sequences, 3′ to a V-gene segment and separated by nonconserved 12- or 23-base-pair spacers, recognize complementary N and H sequences of opposite orientation 5′ to a J-gene segment. This interaction brings light-chain V- and J-gene segments together, forming loops of noncoding intervening DNA that are excised. In heavy-chain germline DNA, the V- and J-gene segments are flanked by 23-base-pair spacer elements, and the D-gene segments, which can recombine at both ends, are flanked on both sides by 12 base-pair spacer elements. The direction of the triangles gives the orientation of the H and N sequences.

sequence 3′ to the V-gene segments with its oppositely oriented, complementary heptamer (CACTGTG) 5′ to the J-gene segments. The palindromic heptamer is followed by an AT-rich nonamer (ACAAAAACC) that appears 12 nucleotides 3′ of the V heptamer and then by its complement nonamer (GGTTTTTGT), also oriented in the opposite direction, which appears 23 nucleotides 5′ of the J heptamer. (The RSS arrangement in heavy chains is similar to that in light chains, except for D-gene segments, which are flanked on both sides by the abutting heptamer of the RSSs [see Figure 6-5].) Although the sequences

of the 12- and 23-nucleotide-long spacers are not important, the lengths are. The lengths correspond to one and two turns of the double helix. The recognition sequences have a directional reading sense to them.[5] These RSSs are the site-specific substrates for *RAG1* and *RAG2* gene-encoded V(D)J

[5]The complementary strands of DNA are read from 5′ → 3′; because each strand is of opposite polarity $\frac{5'\rightarrow 3'}{3'\leftarrow 5'}$, the directional reading sense leads to heptamers and nonamers of opposite orientation.

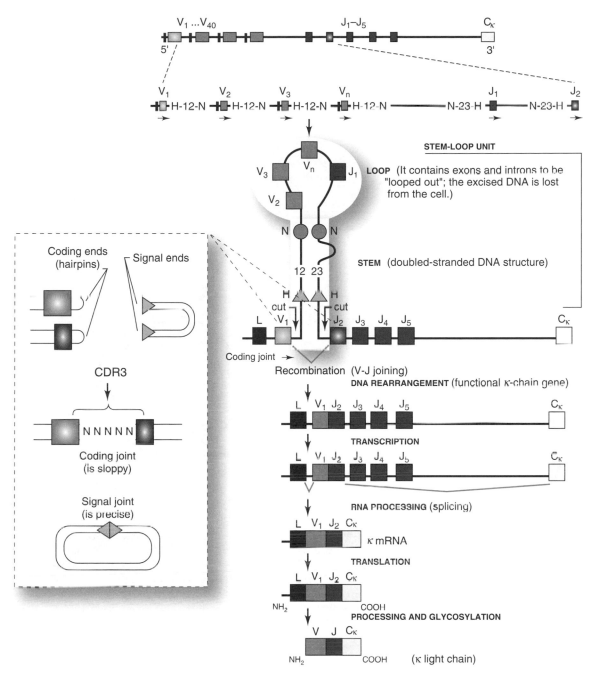

**FIGURE 6-6 Deletional joining of V-J DNA segments leads to a complete V-region exon that generates a mature germline transcript.** This joining mechanism occurs when the V and J segments to be joined have the same transcriptional orientation (horizontal arrows [→]). The top of the figure shows a close-up of the germline nucleotide sequence (the leader [L] sequences 5′ to the V segments are shown as black bars). V-coding segments are flanked on their 3′ edge by a palindromic heptamer (H) and an AT-rich nonamer (N) separated by either a 12- or 23-base spacer. This combination (H-12-N or N-23-H) is the DNA *recombination signal sequence (RSS)*. J-coding segments have a similar arrangement on their 5′ edge but with an opposite orientation. The H-N and the 12–23 spacer sequences specify joining of $V_L$-$J_L$ (here $V_1$ to $J_2$) DNA segments in immunoglobulin genes. To bring $J_2$ next to $V_1$, the intervening introns and exons are pushed up into a stem-loop structure. This structure acts as a substrate for a V(D)J recombinase enzyme, induced by *RAG1* and *RAG2* genes, bringing the two gene segments together for recombination at the cut sites (they are precisely at the RSS's heptamer junction with the gene segment [for illustrative purposes are moved]). The now complete or functional V-region gene is transcribed to produce a primary, or nuclear, transcript that is spliced to remove unwanted sequences, butting the $C_\kappa$ exon to the 3′ side of the V-J exon. The spliced RNA is translated into a complete κ light chain. V-shaped blue lines indicate recombination.

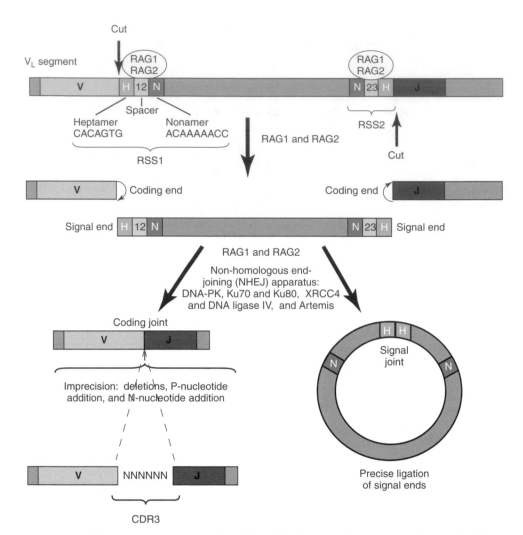

**FIGURE 6-7 RSSs offer a mechanism for V-J (or V-D-J) recombination—deletional joining.** This diagram illustrates the removal of intervening DNA (includes introns and exons) to form the contiguous coding V- and J-gene segments of κ chains. The V-J gene segments are flanked by inverted RSSs on the same DNA strand. The *RAG gene*-encoded recombinases are activated to *precisely* cut one strand of the double-stranded DNA at the heptamer-RSS border with their respective gene segments. The 3′-hydroxyl groups at the coding ends react with the 5′-phosphate groups on the complementary uncut strands to form hairpin structures and double-stranded breaks at the signal ends. Excision (← *CUT*) of the intervening DNA (circular extrachromosomal DNA) and subsequent repair activity by NHEJ protiens brings together (recombination) the respective V- and J-gene segments encoding the V region of an immunoglobulin light chain. The nucleotide sequence at the joining borders of the V and J segments encodes amino acids at positions 95 and 96 in the mature κ chain. The joining of coding ends is imprecise; this imprecision allows for further increases in diversity. (A similar scenario exists for heavy chains, but an additional D-gene segment is found between the V- and J-gene segments [see also Figure 6-14].) See text for further explanation. (Adapted from M.S. Schlissel. 2003. *Nat. Rev. Immunol.* 3:890).

recombinase (endonucleases). The RAG protein complexes bind to RSS1 and RSS2 and then to each other, which causes the segments to line-up with one another. A precise DNA double-strand cut at the heptamer-gene segment border generates intermediates with four DNA ends. The *coding ends* are DNA sealed-hairpin structures and the *signal ends*, excised from the chromosome, are blunt and 5′ phosphorylated. The rejoining steps require DNA-repair proteins DNA-dependent protein kinase

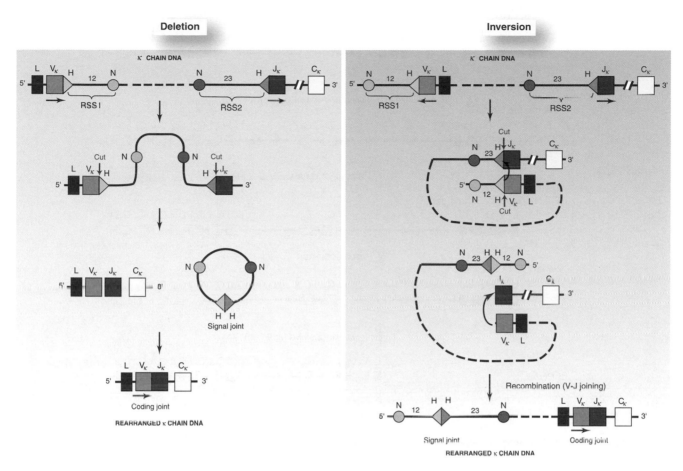

**FIGURE 6-8 Deletional and inversional joining of V-J DNA segments leads to a complete V-region exon that generates a mature germline transcript.** Deletional joining (left side of illustration) occurs when the intervening DNA between V- and J-gene segments are deleted ("looped out"), followed by ligation of segments. Inversional joining (right side of illustration) occurs when the V- and J-gene segments to be joined have opposite transcriptional orientations (indicated by horizontal arrows [ ← → ]). Following V- and J-gene segment recombination, transcription, RNA processing, and translation occur, as described in Figures 6-6 and 6-7.

(DNA-PK), Ku, X-ray repair cross complementing protein 4 (XRCC4), DNA ligase IV, and Artemis. The DNA-double-strand break is first identified by the DNA-PK complex composed of Ku70 (a DNA end-binding protein) and Ku80, the latter recruits DNA-PK. DNA-PK activates the nuclease activity of Artemis, which opens the coding-end hairpins. The DNA ligase IV-XRCC4 complex mediates the ligation of the V and J segments, which remain on the chromosome to form a coding joint. XRCC4 augments DNA ligase IV activity. The same complex precisely joins the heptamer sequences to form a signal joint, which is a circular piece of extrachromosomal DNA that is lost from the cell's genome as it divides. Coding joints are imprecise; they contain short deletions, palindromic nucleotide repairs (P-nucleotide addition), and nontemplated nucleotide additions

(N-regions) that are introduced by TdT. N-region additions only occur in heavy-chain gene segment recombinations. This imprecision leads to increased diversity in CDR3. These mechanisms associated with increased immunoglobulin diversity will be discussed shortly.

The mechanism we used to describe V(D)J recombination, to this point, involves deletion of intervening DNA between gene segments. If the V- and J-gene segments do not have the same transcriptional orientation, inversional deletion of DNA followed by ligation of adjacent gene segments can occur. It is illustrated in comparison with deletional recombination in Figure 6-8.

The mechanism for V-J recombination in light chains resembles that for heavy-chain V-D-J recombination. Whereas light-chain V-region recombination

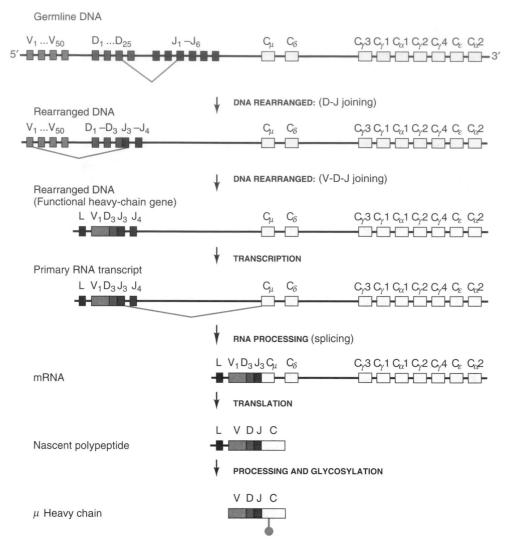

**FIGURE 6-9 Joining of D-J and V-D-J DNA segments leads to a complete V-region exon that generates a mature heavy-chain germline transcript, followed by transcription, and synthesis of a human μ heavy chain.** The functional heavy chain exon (V-D-J gene) results from a two-step combination of three gene segments: first, D and J are joined; second, one of the many V genes is joined to the D-J complex. In this example, $D_3$ and $J_3$ join and then $V_1$ joins the $D_3$-$J_3$ complex. The location of carbohydrate (●) is schematic, leader sequences (not shown) precede each V gene, and each C gene consists of multiple exons that are not shown. V-shaped blue lines indicate recombination.

is one event (random joining of a V segment to a J segment), heavy-chain V-region recombination involves two events (first the random joining of a D segment to a J segment, then the joining of a V segment to the D-J piece), which leads to a functional gene that encodes a μ heavy chain, as illustrated in Figure 6-9. Whether light or heavy chains are synthesized, only gene segments that are flanked by RSSs with dissimilar spacer lengths can combine with one another due to the limitation known as the heptamer-nonamer and spacer 12/23 rule. This ensures that light chains only

make V-J recombinations and heavy chains V-(D-J) recombinations.

## The Orderliness of Immunoglobulin Gene Rearrangements Yields Cells of a Single Antibody Specificity

Because individual B cells make antibody specific for only one antigenic determinant and both heavy- and light-chain alleles could lead to successful rearrangements, a mechanism must be used to limit B-cell expression to only one type of heavy chain and one type of light chain. If a B cell made λ and κ chains, each chain would have different V regions and bind more than one epitope. Furthermore, each cell has two copies of each immunoglobulin gene family (the maternal and the paternal λ, κ, and heavy-chain gene families). Each B cell makes two choices during development: (1) whether to express κ or λ chains (a given B-cell clone cannot produce some immunoglobulin molecules with κ chains and others with λ chains) and (2) whether to use maternal or paternal gene pools or genes from each. *This phenomenon of expressing either the maternal or paternal allele of an immunoglobulin gene in a given B cell is known as* **allelic exclusion** (Figure 6-10) *and is unique to immunoglobulin (and T-cell receptor) genes*. Pre-B-cell receptor signaling enforces allelic exclusion (see Chapter 10), which is accomplished by adherence to a strict sequence of rearrangement events and by regulatory mechanisms. Pre-B-cell receptor signaling regulates allelic exclusion by: (1) directly reducing *RAG1* and *RAG2* expression leading to a decline in V(D)J recombinase activity, (2) indirectly reducing *RAG2* expression through targeted protein degradation leading to further decline in V(D)J recombinase activity, and (3) reducing V(D)J recombinase access to the heavy-chain locus. These mechanisms lead to: (1) genes on one chromosome remaining in the germline configuration, which prevents their expression, and (2) the successful rearrangement of one gene family (light or heavy) suppressing rearrangement of the corresponding genes on the homologous chromosome. The ability and choice of allele to undergo recombination is controlled through targeted changes in chromatin accessibility, DNA methylation and histone modification—the developing lymphocyte senses successful gene rearrangement (some kind of feedback inhibition mechanism) that leads to signals that alter gene expression, enforce a period of proliferative growth, and cause chromatin structure changes that alter recombinase access to DNA. Even though RAG1 and RAG2 expression ceases for the heavy chain, they are reexpressed later in B-cell development to carry out light-chain locus rearrangement (see Chapter 10).

*Allelic exclusion involves an ordered sequence during gene rearrangement* (Figure 6-11). All stem cells contain the germline configuration of immunoglobulin genes, but once these cells are stimulated to become B cells, a strict sequence of rearrangement events starts in the immunoglobulin loci. Because both heavy-chain alleles are accessible to recombinase, heavy-chain (μ) gene rearrangement (V-D-J joining) begins with $D_H$-to-$J_H$ joining on both heavy-chain alleles that leads to efficient bi-allelic $D_H$-to-$J_H$ rearrangement.

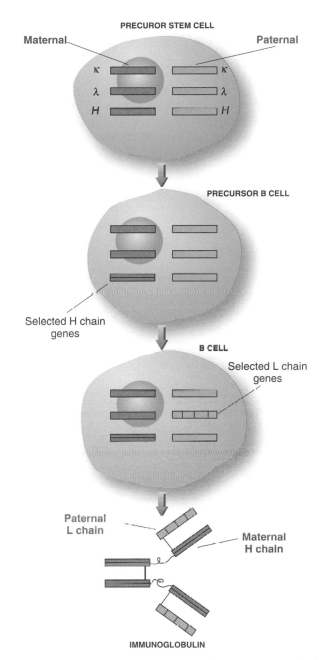

**FIGURE 6-10 Allelic exclusion**. B cells produce antibodies with only one kind of antigen-binding site. To do so, they must make strict sequential choices in immunoglobulin-gene activation. Each B cell must first choose among six gene pools; maternal and paternal κ-, λ-, and heavy-chain gene pools. The B cell can express only one light-chain gene and one heavy-chain gene.

Inefficient V-to-$DJ_H$ rearrangement decreases the likelihood of in-frame heavy-chain gene rearrangement in both alleles. If rearrangement is productive in one allele, a functional gene results that both inhibits rearrangement on other alleles (*allelic exclusion*) and stimulates κ-chain gene rearrangement. Nonproductive

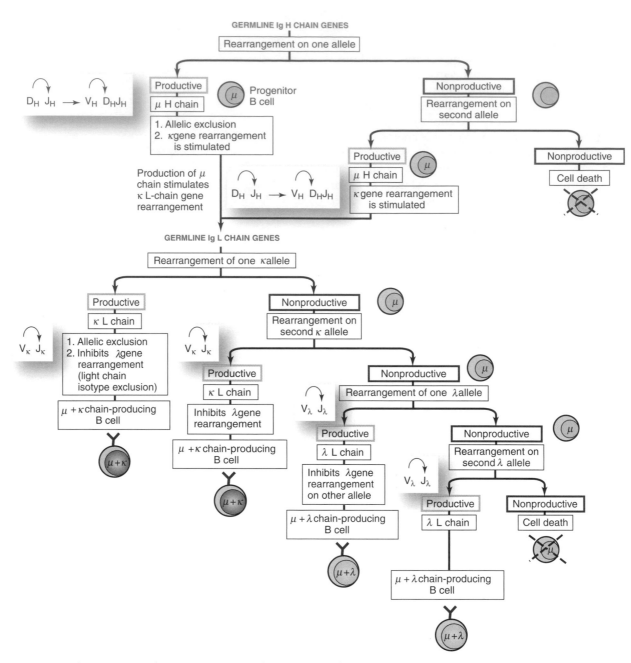

**FIGURE 6-11 The sequence of rearrangement and expression of immunoglobulin heavy ($\mu$) and light chains.** Allelic exclusion is accomplished by following an ordered sequence of DNA rearrangements that stops further rearrangements when the desired ones have been reached.

rearrangements may result from deletions, frame shifts, or mutations that lead to stop codons. The consequences of a nonproductive $\mu$-gene rearrangement lead to rearrangement on the second allelic chromosome, which can be either productive or nonproductive. A second nonproductive heavy-chain gene rearrangement leads to cell death. As with heavy-chain genes, successful light-chain gene rearrangement has to occur at one allele at a time; however, unlike

heavy-chain genes, light-chain genes can undergo successive rearrangement events. The $\kappa$ light-chain locus tends to undergo rearrangement before the $\lambda$ light-chain locus. If the $\kappa$ light-chain locus V-J rearrangement fails to produce a functional light chain, the rerrangements can be repeated with the unused V and J gene segments up to five times (humans have five $J_\kappa$ gene segments) on each chromosome before moving on to the other chromosome and attempting

$\lambda$ light-chain gene rearrangement. This enhances the changes of producing a successful intact light chain. Nonetheless, successful rearrangement in $\kappa$ genes prevents rearrangement on the other allele (called *light chain isotype exclusion*) and prevents $\lambda$-gene rearrangement. (Unlike B-cell immunoglobulin heavy chains, light chains do not undergo class switching [once they make $\kappa$ chains they do not switch to making $\lambda$ chains on antigen contact].) If all the $\kappa$-gene segment rearrangements are nonproductive, rearrangement on the second allele occurs and leads to either a productive or nonproductive rearrangement. A productive rearrangement results in a $\kappa$-chain-producing B cell, while nonproductive rearrangements in all $\kappa$-gene segments lead to rearrangement on one $\lambda$ allele. This productive or nonproductive cycle repeats itself for the $\lambda$-chain-producing B cell. After these recombinations occur, further DNA rearrangements are inhibited. The result is the expression of only one type of heavy and one type of light chain in a given B cell. This expression leads to IgM ($\mu$) and IgD ($\delta$) antibody receptors and phenotypically establishes a $B_{\mu+\delta}$ cell (considered a mature B cell).

## Cell-Specific Transcription Controls Immunoglobulin Gene Expression

In the preceding sections, functional immunoglobulin gene assembly was discussed, but not how its expression is controlled. Two types of regulatory elements affect transcription: *cis*-regulators and *trans*-regulators. *Cis*-regulators are DNA sequences on a given chromosome and act only on adjacent genes; *trans*-regulators are soluble molecules that are made by one gene and interact with genes on the same or different chromosomes. Three types of *cis*-regulatory DNA sequences are found in eukaryotic genes: **promoters, enhancers**, and **silencers**. Promoters, about 100 base-pairs long, are usually located roughly 200-base pairs upstream from the site where transcription begins. The promoter site is where RNA polymerase binds DNA and is the start site for transcription of DNA. The enhancer element, located upstream or downstream of promoter and associated with silencers, controls the rate of transcription from that particular promoter. Silencers are nucleotide sequences that operate in both directions over a distance to dowregulate transcription. The *trans*-regulators, called **DNA-binding proteins** or **nuclear factors** (**NF**), can inhibit or stimulate the activities of promoters and enhancers. *Trans*-regulators provide a link between external signals and gene expression.

Immunoglobulin gene expression is one of the best-characterized examples of transcriptional gene regulation (Figure 6-12). The promoters for immunoglobulin gene transcription are associated with each $V_H$- and $V_L$-segment coding sequences and located just upstream from the leader sequence, the $D_H$ segment and the $J_\kappa$ clusters are preceded with promoters, while the heavy-chain enhancer is located in the intron between the last J segment (but 5' of the $S_\mu$ switch site) and the first C-region gene segment, $C_\mu$. Because of its location, the heavy-chain enhancer can continue to act after class switching. The other heavy-chain enhancer is located 3' of the $C_\alpha$-gene segment. The $\kappa$-light chain has two enhancers, one ($E_\kappa$) located between $J_\kappa$-gene segment and the $C_\kappa$-gene segment; the other ($3'_\kappa$ E) is located 3' of the $C_\kappa$-gene segment. The $\lambda$-light chain also has two enhancers, which are located 3' of $C_\lambda 4$ ($\lambda 2$-4E) and 3' $C_\lambda 1$ ($\lambda 3$-1E). Silencers are found adjacent to some heavy-chain and $\kappa$-chain enhancers but not $\lambda$-chain enhancers. Each V region is preceded by its own promoter. Enhancers influence promoters, but in the germline DNA for immunoglobulin genes, enhancers are too widely separated from promoters to affect their activity.

Interestingly, transcriptional promoter sequences are not efficient enough to promote transcription, and the enhancer element is roughly 250 kb pairs away from the promoter. This separation ensures that unrearranged V segments are not influenced by the enhancer and that all rearranged genes are influenced by the same enhancer 5' of the $C_\mu$ switch site thereby continuing to work after class switching has occurred. The promoter and enhancer are brought to within roughly 2 kb pairs of each other (close enough for transcription to be activated) only after DNA rearrangement. However, activation of transcription occurs only in the presence of *trans*-regulatory factors.

In short, once light- or heavy-chain germline DNA is rearranged, the gene segment sequence for a light chain is

*leader exon | intron | V-J exon | intron | C exon*

and the gene segment sequence for a heavy chain is

*leader exon | intron | V-D-J exon | intron | C exons.*

These rearrangements bring light-chain promoters (upstream from the leader exons of all V-gene segments) into proximity with potent, complex enhancers (usually located in the intron between J- and C-gene segments and the 3' end of the locus). The heavy-chain promoters precede all V-gene segments, the D-gene segment cluster, and a number

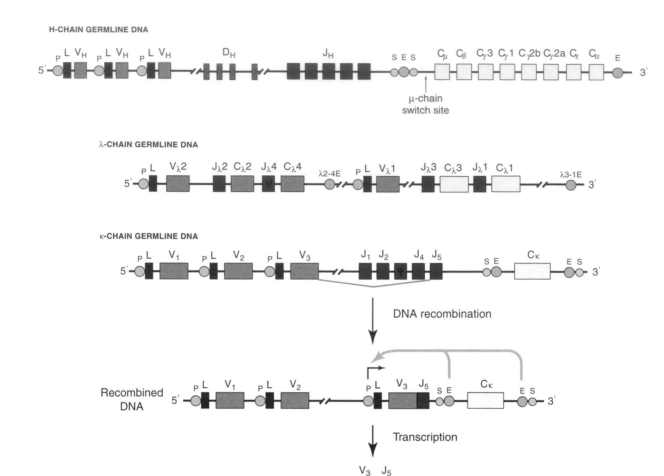

**FIGURE 6-12 Transcriptional regulation of mouse immunoglobulin genes by promoters, enhancers, and silencers.** DNA rearrangement (V-[D]-J joining) brings the appropriate promoter (P; colored light red) close to the enhancer (E; colored light green), leading to transcription of a functional gene ($V_3J_5$). To complete activation of transcription, the nuclear factors bind to the promoter and enhancer sequences, respectively (not shown). Silencers (S; colored beige). Promoters not shown are located before the $J_H$ cluster, some $C_H$-region genes, and $J_\kappa$ cluster. V-shaped blue lines indicate recombination.

of C genes (see Figure 6-12). This arrangement enables the enhancer to activate transcription from the promoter. RNA polymerase transcribes from the leader segment through the C-gene segment to generate a primary RNA transcript. RNA processing enzymes remove the introns and yield mRNA. The mRNA is translated and the leader sequence is cleaved, leading to an immunoglobulin light or heavy chain (see Figure 6-19). The rates of RNA turnover and RNA translation influence antibody production.

## Numerous Mechanisms Contribute to Antibody Diversity

B cells can use various strategies to generate antibody diversity. As described earlier, explanations for the source of antibody diversity revolved around

the germline theory, which suggested that variability in immunoglobulin chains was encoded by genes found in the host's germline DNA and inherited by offspring through germline cells—existing genes are transmitted to your offspring. In contrast, somatic theories suggested that germline genes are altered by mutation and recombination during maturation of somatic cells—roughly 160 germline gene segments are transmitted to our offspring and are subject to change during the life of the immune cell. Experimental results supported contributions from both models.

Several mechanisms (Table 6-2) control the diversity of immunoglobulin structure; they include: the **multiplicity of V, D, and J germline gene segments**, the **combinatorial joining freedom of these gene segments**, and **combinatorial association freedom of light and heavy chains**. Additional mechanisms

**TABLE 6-2** Germline Immunoglobulin Gene Inventory

| | Light chains | | | | Heavy chains | |
| | Mouse | | Human | | Mouse | Human |
| Segments | κ | λ | κ | λ | H | H |
| --- | --- | --- | --- | --- | --- | --- |
| V | 85 | 3 | 40 | 30 | 134 | 51 |
| D | 0 | 0 | 0 | 0 | 13 | 27 |
| J | 4 | 3 | 5 | 4 | 4 | 6 |

add further antibody diversity by generating different amino acid sequences at the junctions of V-, D-, and J-gene segments, typically associated with CDR3—the region that has the most contacts with antigen; they include: **junctional flexibility**, which arises from both *imprecise DNA rearrangement*, and **P-region nucleotide addition** and **insertion of random N** (nucleotide) **regions** between regions D- and J-derived segments in D-J or V-(D-J) recombination. Diversity also arises from **somatic hypermutation**.

Diversity is increased incrementally by the inventory of gene segments in the germline repertoire that encode certain segments of the immunoglobulin polypeptide chain (see Table 6-2). The inherited germline V-region gene segments contribute to antibody diversification. Furthermore, the combination of these gene segments in the building of somatic light-chain and heavy-chain genes that can again be used in many combinations contributes to diversity. V-J joining in light-chain genes or V-D-J joining in heavy-chain genes is completely random during differentiation from immature to mature B lymphocytes. An almost infinite number of gene permutations, encoding the V region, caused by different combinations of V and J (light C) and V, D, and J (heavy C) explains why antibody diversity is so great. The result of this random joining is a population of B cells expressing different light and heavy chains, but each cell expresses only one antigen-binding site. Once V-J and V-D-J recombination are accomplished, any light chain can associate with any heavy chain to form a complete $L_2H_2$ immunoglobulin molecule. Random association of light and heavy chains leads to further antibody diversity.

The V-(D)-J joining required to form functional V-region genes should be precise; otherwise, the joining will lead to a frame-shift mutation. However, because of junctional flexibility or imprecision or short deletions, more antibody diversity is achieved because of the imprecise joining of V with J, D with J, or V with D. An example is the joining of $V_\kappa$ to $J_\kappa$ (see Figures 6-6 and 6-9). In the example shown in Figure 6-13, at least three new genes could be generated, leading to three different

amino acids at position 96 in the mature κ chain. The fact that there are 40 V-gene segments that can join with each of the five J-gene segments shows that junctional flexibility is an important contributor to antibody diversity. Furthermore, this coding-joint junctional flexibility occurs within CDR3 of light- and heavy-chain DNA—the greater the diversity in CDR3, the more unique contacts with antigens. The cellular enzymes that catalyze these rearrangements would not know the final reading frame of the gene; therefore, two-thirds of these joints lead to a nonfunctional gene in which the translational reading frame is lost. Junctional flexibility, therefore, is not without cost to the organism because it also causes generation of missense genes.

The other mechanisms for junctional diversity are by the random addition of nucleotides in light and heavy-chain genes or only heavy-chain genes (Figure 6-14)—repairing the single-stranded DNA cut at a junction of a V-(D)J gene segment and attached signal sequence (RSS). The result of this cleavage is that the nucleotides at the end of the coding sequences form closed DNA hairpins. The hairpins are opened by the nuclease activity of Artemis, which leaves a short single-strand at the end of the coding sequence; repair enzymes (DNA ligase IV) add complementary nucleotides to this strand (called *P-region nucleotide addition*) leading to a coding joint with a palindromic sequence (hence the name *P-nucleotides*). The hairpin cut position leads to sequence variation in the coding joint—the coding joint is in the midst of CDR3.

Another similar process that does not occur in light-chain genes is called *insertion of random N (nucleotide) regions*. Joining of $V_H$ and $D_H$ or $D_H$ and $J_H$ gene segments leads to insertion of nucleotides at the junctions of V or J with D segments. These extra portions, called **N regions** (nontemplated nucleotide additions), are inserted between $V_H$ and $D_H$ or $D_H$ and $J_H$ segments as part of the joining process. The random nucleotide addition is catalyzed by a terminal deoxynucleotidyl transferase (TdT). No genetic template has been is found for these extra nucleotides. These sequences offer an enormous additional element of antibody diversity because the addition of up to 15 (perhaps more) nucleotides at each junction (D to J and V to DJ) could generate $1.42 \times 10^9$ different possible combinations at each junction. The diversity is localized in the CDR3 of heavy-chain genes.

Because the exact amino acid sequence of many immunoglobulins does not precisely match with what would be predicted by their prototype germline nucleotide sequences, somatic mutations must be

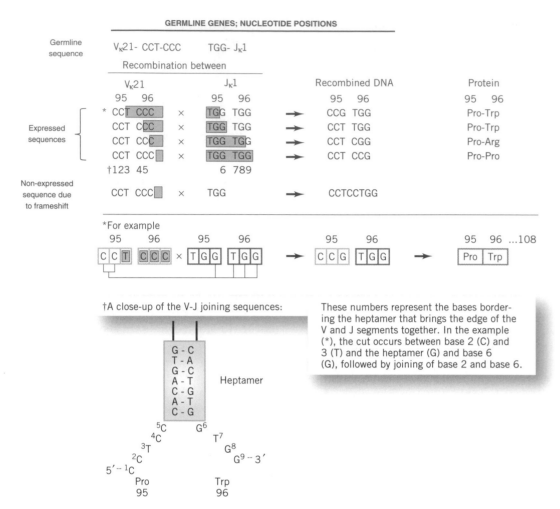

**FIGURE 6-13 Increased antibody diversity due to joining flexibility at the V-J recombination site**. This recombination is flexible at the exact nucleotide position of the joining site if it is in phase with the coding sequence. Joining between $V_\kappa$ and $J_\kappa$ always occurs at the same position (a codon-generating amino acid residue at position 96 of the mature $\kappa$ chain), but there is some variation in the precise site of the cut. Joining variation can result from adjustment of the point of recombination in the three nucleotides at the beginning of the J-gene segments (encode amino acid residue 96). The result is the generation of different triplet codons at the recombination site and therefore the insertion of a different amino acid at position 96 in immunoglobulin $\kappa$ chains. This imprecise joining accounts for some of the variability in the third CDR of light chains (V-J joining) and of heavy chains (V-D and D-J joining). The third CDR is considered to be the most variable part of both light and heavy chains and forms part of the antigen-binding site. Bases enclosed in red boxes indicate deletions.

important for further diversification of antibodies. The somatic mutations, replacement (not deletions or insertions) of individual nucleotides, which cause amino acid replacements are detectable mainly in the regions encoding the three CDRs of both heavy and light chains, in particular the first and second CDRs (Figure 6-15). This localization of mutations suggests a specific antibody **hypermutation somatic**[6]

mechanism that recognizes the DNA primarily of immunoglobulin heavy- and light-chain V-gene segments. Somatic hypermutation occurs mainly in non-IgM antibodies. Somatic hypermutation of immunoglobulin heavy- and light-chain V-region genes is activated by exposure to antigen and occurs only at the centroblast stage of B-cell differentiation in germinal centers, structures that develop in

[6]The spontaneous rate of mutation in mammalian genes other than immunoglobulin V genes is roughly $1 \times 10^{-7}$; the mutation rate is estimated to be $1 \times 10^{-3}$ per V-gene base pair per cell division—hence the *hyper* in *hypermutation*.

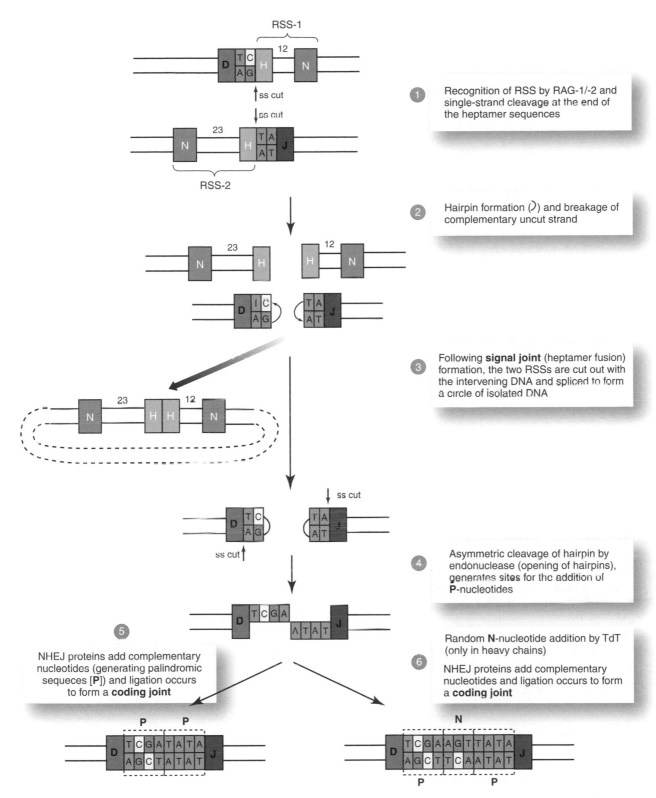

**FIGURE 6-14 Junctional diversification through P- and N-nucleotide addition at D-J or V-DJ joints.** The random insertion of nucleotides occurs by P-nucleotide and N-nucleotide addition. All four strands are cut (indicated by small up and down arrows [↑↓]) by doubled-stranded endonuclease at junctions of RSSs and coding sequences. The two heptamers (H; green boxes) join end to end surrounded by their nonamers (N; purple boxes). The coding sequences do not join but are held close to one another by joining proteins. Doubled-stranded endonucleases remove some nucleotides from the D and J ends, which generate sites for the addition of P-nucleotides. Terminal deoxynucleotidyl transferase (TdT) randomly adds nucleotides. DNA polymerase copies the added nucleotides, and a ligase seals the structure.

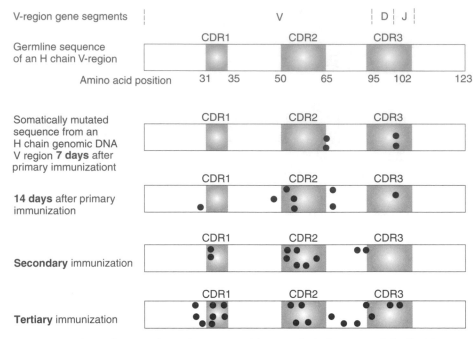

**FIGURE 6-15 Somatic mutation of rearranged heavy-chain immunoglobulin V genes.** This involves the replacement of individual nucleotides in a completed V-D-J segment with alternative nucleotides, leading to random variation mainly around CDR1 and CDR2. In light chains, most of the mutations also cluster around CDR1 and CDR2 (not shown). The black dots and their positions indicate where mutations causing amino acid differences have occurred at different times after immunization. The transition mutations of C to T or G to A occur more frequently than would be expected if the mutations occurred randomly. These point mutations occur in hotspots; the C in the WRC motif and G in the complementary GYW are the preferred sites for C deamination by activation-induced cytidine deaminase (AID). In fact, mutation rates seem to correlate with the frequency of these sequence motifs.

secondary lymphoid organs due to antigen exposure that induces T cell-dependent B cell responses (see Chapter 2). Somatic hypermutation increases with time after the first exposure of the antigen, and the frequency of mutations increases after additional exposures to the same antigen. The combination of somatic hypermutation, generating many new B cells with slightly changed antigen-binding specificities, and the preferential selection of these cells by ever decreasing concentrations of antigen with increasing time after exposure, account for the increases in antibody affinity during an immune response. This phenomenon is called **affinity maturation**— preferential selection of B cells with higher affinity receptors. Somatic mutation, therefore, is thought to be restricted to B cells differentiating into memory cells, which explains the increased antibody affinity in the secondary response. The secondary response is faster and greater, in part, because the memory B cells' antibody receptors have a higher affinity for antigen. Thus, somatic mutation increases

antibody diversity and fine-tunes the antibody response.

Table 6-3 lists the mechanisms contributing to the diversification of antibodies and shows how they can be used in the calculation of diversity. The importance of immunoglobulin-gene rearrangements is that enormous diversity can be generated with relatively few germline genes. The contribution of junctional flexibility is three different amino acids at each junction ($V_L$-$J_L$, $D_H$-$J_H$, and $V_H$-$D_H J_H$); therefore, for the light chain there are three new genes and for the heavy chain there are nine new genes. For example, the rearrangements of only 163 germline genes (adding up the number of gene segments that may be used by the first three mechanisms in Table 6-3) can lead to roughly 2.64 million different antibody molecules, each with unique antigen specificity. This number is a conservative estimate because the contributions of junction imprecision, P- and N-region insertions and somatic hypermutation to antibody diversity are not figured in but do occur under normal conditions.

**TABLE 6-3 Mechanisms Contributing to Human Antibody Diversity: Some Calculations**

1. Multiplicity of V, D, and J genes (Germline repertoire)
2. Combinatorial freedom
   a) Combinatorial joining (V-J or V-D-J gene segment joining)
   b) Combinatorial association (light & heavy chains)
3. Junctional diversity (associated with CDR3 junctions)
   a) Junctional flexibility — imprecise DNA recombination
   b) P-nucleotide addition — repair leads to palindromes
   c) N-nucleotide addition — insertion of random N (nucleotides) regions
4. Somatic hypermutation

**Estimated Light-Chain Gene Segments**

$V\kappa$ = 40        $V\lambda$ = 30        1. Germline repertoire
        x                x                        x
$J\kappa$ = 5         $J\lambda$ = 4         2a. Combinatorial joining

        200              120  Total light-chain
                              gene segments

**Estimated Heavy-Chain Gene Segments**

$V_H$ = 51        1. Germline repertoire
        x                x
$V_D$ = 27        2a. Combinatorial joining
        x                x
$V_J$ = 6         2a. Combinatorial joining

        8,262            Total heavy chain gene segments

        (200 + 120)      Total light-chain gene segments

        x                2b. Combinatorial association

        8,262            Total heavy-chain gene segments

        $\approx 2.64 \times 10^6$    Baseline diversity*

*This number does not consider the contribution of #3a junctional imprecision, #3b P nucleotide addition, #3c N nucleotide addition, or #4 somatic hypermutation to antibody receptor diversity; therefore, the actual diversity would be significantly higher.

**MINI SUMMARY**

Amino acid sequencing led to the discovery of variable (V) and constant (C) regions in immunoglobulin chains. Neither the germline nor the somatic theory alone could completely account for the incredible diversity necessary in the V segment of an immunoglobulin chain while retaining constancy of sequences in the remainder of the molecule. In 1976, direct evidence showed how the gene segments were brought together. An experiment comparing κ-chain gene structure in embryonic cells and in adult myeloma cells showed that embryonic DNA has separated gene segments for the V and C regions, while adult DNA has adjacent gene segments. Three unlinked gene families encode the λ, κ, and heavy chains; however, at each locus, V-region genes are linked to their respective C-region genes. V-J joining is needed to assemble a functional light-chain gene. To assemble a heavy-chain V-region gene, D-J joining and V-(D-J) joining are required. At the borders of V-, D-, and J-gene segments and near the recombination sites are special conserved sequences called *RSSs* and are composed of heptamers and nonamers separated by either a 12- or 23-bp spacer. Heptamers and nonamers and the 12–23 spacer rule govern V-J and V-D-J joining. The DNA, encoding V regions, is moved closer to the C-region DNA to create the functional immunoglobulin genes found in B cells.

Each B cell produces only one kind of light chain and one kind of heavy chain. This phenomenon is called *allelic exclusion* and is unique to immunoglobulin (and T-cell receptor) genes. Use of maternal or paternal immunoglobulin genes allows an ordered sequence that helps define B-cell differentiation. Once the cell has assembled a composite, functional immunoglobulin gene, further DNA rearrangements are inhibited. These antigen-specific surface antibodies are expressed (their heavy-chain class may change during antigen-dependent B-cell differentiation, their antigen specificity does not).

Immunoglobulin gene transcription is controlled by *cis*-regulators (promoters and enhancers) and by DNA-binding proteins that bind to these *cis*-regulators.

The diverse repertoire of antibody specificities is generated by multiple germline gene segments, V, D, and J genes, for variable regions, random combinatorial joining of these gene segments and chain association, junctional diversity (composed of imprecision and short deletions, and P- and N-nucleotide addition) and somatic hypermutation.

# SEVERAL PHYSIOLOGIC PROCESSES AFFECT IMMUNOGLOBULIN GENE EXPRESSION

Immunoglobulin primary gene expression involves V-(D)-J rearrangement, which leaves intervening DNA sequences, noncoding introns, and J gene segments; in the heavy-chain gene segments each domain corresponds to an exon, the noncoding introns need to be excised and the remaining exons connected by RNA splicing. Mechanisms in the nucleus, involving posttranscriptional processing of immunoglobulin light- and heavy-chain primary transcripts, delete the intervening DNA sequences, create different functional mRNAs, and ship the mRNAs out of the nucleus to be translated by ribosomes into light and heavy chains. These mechanisms allow individual B cells to simultaneously express IgM and IgD and produce secreted or membrane forms of immunoglobulins.

Another change occurs post V-D-J recombination, which involves an additional recombination but of C-region exons called *class switching* or *class-switch recombination*. Because antibodies initially function as recognition molecules, how does the immune system combine antibody specificity with each of its protection effector functions? As we saw in Chapter 4, the immunoglobulin's stem portion (heavy-chain C regions) mediates protection effector functions, such as activation of complement components, binding to macrophages, opsonization, and localization of antibodies to different areas of the body. The immune system has evolved mechanisms to join fully assembled, functional V-D-J exons to different heavy-chain C-region exons, which allows B cells to use antibodies with different functions but the same antigenic specificity. These mechanisms are discussed below.

## The Coexpression of IgM and IgD by a Single B Cell Involves Alternative RNA Processing, Not DNA Rearrangement

Dual expression of IgM and IgD signifies an immunocompetent and mature B cell. Even though both immunoglobulins have different heavy-chain isotypes, they both have the same V regions and thus the same antigen specificity. Simultaneous expression of $\mu$ and $\delta$ chains is difficult to understand because expression of a $\delta$ chain would require deletion of the $\mu$-gene segments. In fact, experiments show that in cells expressing $\mu$ and $\delta$ receptors, the $\mu$ and $\delta$ genes remain in a germline configuration. The simplest explanation is that the $\mu$ and $\delta$ mRNA are derived from the same gene transcript pathways regions by *alternative RNA processing/splicing pathways*.[7] Figure 6-16 illustrates such a mechanism. Two different species of mRNA are produced from a long primary RNA transcript containing both $C_\mu$ and $C_\delta$ genes, yet they have the same heavy-chain V sequence (the V-D-J complex). The close proximity (4.5 kb) of

---

[7]Alternative RNA splicing is a common process in gene regulation whereby alterations in splice site choices establishes the segments of coding sequence that are retained in the final mRNA transcript. This process permits one gene to create different forms of the same protein that differ in the final amino acid sequence and thus in their biological function.

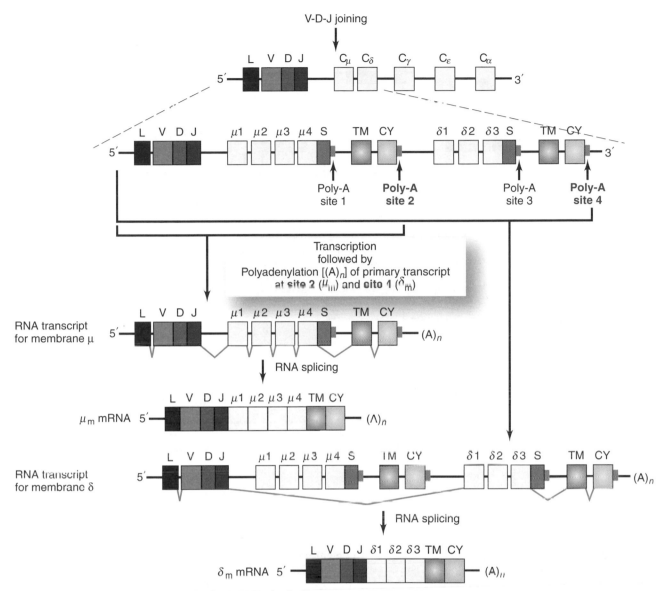

**FIGURE 6-16 Mechanism for the simultaneous expression of μ and δ chains.** During the mature antigen-naïve stage of their development, B cells express IgM and IgD. Even though the membrane immunoglobulins are of different classes, they have the same antigen-binding sites. For this to happen the cells produce long primary RNA transcripts containing Cμ and Cδ sequences. At the intron/exon boundaries of a primary transcript are splice sequences, that signal the position where splicing occurs. The polyadenylation at site 2 or 4, the splicing of introns, and the placement of two different C-region sequences contiguous to the same V-region sequence (V-D-J complex) lead to coexpression of IgM and IgD. V-shaped blue lines indicate splicing. Both processing pathways occur simultaneously. (See Figure 6-17 for description of S site.)

Cμ and Cδ and the lack of a switch site (discussed shortly) between them allow transcription of the entire VDJCμCδ region. The primary transcript contains four polyadenylation signal sequences, or poly-A sites. A μ heavy-chain is expressed if polyadenylation occurs at poly-A site 2 and the introns between the VDJ complex and the Cμ mRNA are spliced, butting the Cμ mRNA next to the VDJ complex. In contrast, a δ heavy chain is expressed if polyadenylation occurs at poly-A site 4 and the introns between the VDJ complex and the Cδ mRNA are spliced, butting the Cδ mRNA next to the VDJ complex. These alternative RNA splicing pathways must occur simultaneously because mature B cells display both IgM and IgD on their membrane.

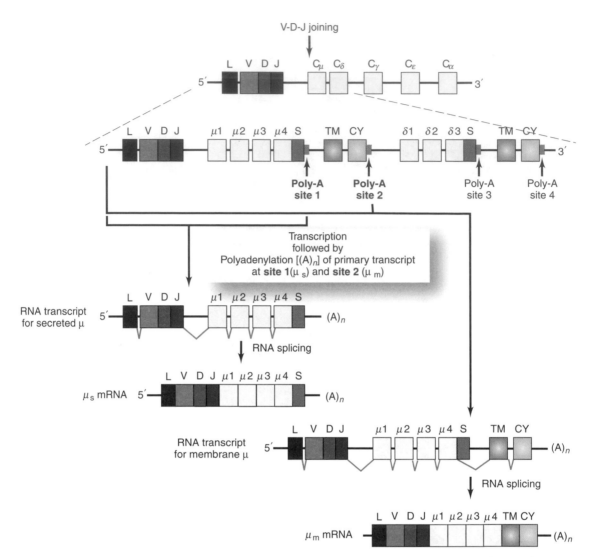

**FIGURE 6-17** **Model for generation of secreted and membranous forms of IgM**. The two forms of IgM are created from one Cμ-gene segment. The $C_\mu 4$ exon of the DNA Cμ exon cluster is bordered on its 3′ end by the S site, which encodes the hydrophilic sequence of the $C_H 4$ domain of secreted IgM. Either the secreted or the membranous mRNA transcript is formed, depending on whether site 1 or 2 of the primary DNA transcript undergoes polyadenylation. V-shaped blue lines indicate splicing.

## The Progression of Membrane to Secreted IgM Also Involves Alternative RNA Processing

Once the B cell chooses a particular DNA exon encoding the antigen-binding site of an immunoglobulin, it is a commitment for the life of the B cell and its progeny to produce only that site (how tightly it binds to that antigen can change but the specificity remains the same; see the earlier discussion about somatic hypermutation). As mentioned already, the first B cells to appear express a membrane-associated IgM molecule complexed with either κ or λ light chains. The transition from membrane to secreted IgM occurs at the level of mRNA processing and converts the B cell from a recognition cell to an effector cell. B cells expressing surface IgM synthesize two structurally different μ chains, one adapted for membrane incorporation ($\mu_M$) and the other adapted for secretion ($\mu_S$). The quantity of each chain expressed is affected by antigenic stimulation and reflects the stage of B-cell differentiation. The $\mu_M$ chain is 20 amino acids longer that the $\mu_S$ chain. The two forms arise by *alternative RNA processing of a primary transcript* (Figure 6-17). The mRNA encoding the two forms of μ chains is derived from one $C_\mu$ gene locus that consists of the four separated exons. The 3′ end of $C_\mu 4$ exon contains a nucleotide sequence called *S*, which encodes the hydrophilic portion of the $C_H4$ domain of secreted IgM. The two RNA differ in their 3′ regions, following the coding sequence for the fourth domain of the μ C region. Mature mRNA species contain either the information for the 20-amino-acid-long tail of the secreted form or that for the 40-amino-acid-long membrane-binding peptide encoded by two M exons located 1.8 kilobases to the 3′ side of the μ C4 domain segment. The two M exons encode the transmembrane (TM) and cytoplasmic (CY) portions of the μ chain, respectively. These two μ-chain mRNAs are generated from the transcripts of one μ gene by a developmentally regulated poly-A addition either at the 3′-untranslated region of the $\mu_S$ (poly-A site 1) or at the 3′-untranslated region of the $\mu_M$ (poly-A site 2). Poly-A addition to one of the two splicing sites determines whether a $\mu_S$ or a $\mu_M$ is created. If polyadenylation occurs immediately 3′ to the end of the μ C4 exon, RNA splicing leads to $\mu_S$ mRNA. If transcription proceeds to the second polyadenylation site 3′ to the $\mu_M$ exon, the $\mu_M$ mRNA is produced. The splicing site for $\mu_M$ is conserved at the end of the final domain of immunoglobulin heavy chains, suggesting that this method of posttranslational processing is used to produce either secreted or membrane-bound forms of other immunoglobulin heavy chains. *Thus, two functionally distinct polypeptides can be created from a single heavy-chain C-gene locus, depending on which way RNA processing occurs.*

---

**MINI SUMMARY**

RNA transcripts often contain noncoding intervening sequences and introns, which are copied from the corresponding regions of a gene. RNA splicing removes introns and joins the RNA exons that were on opposite ends of the introns.

Immature B cells express only IgM molecules. Mature B cells have membrane-bound IgM and IgD. RNA processing allows these individual plasma cells to express both and secrete IgM antibodies. Because the $C_\delta$ gene lies closer to the $C_\mu$ gene than the other C-region genes do, RNA processing may extend past the $C_\mu$ gene through the $C_\delta$ gene, forming a transcript containing both genes.

RNA processing is also important in the progression from the membrane-bound form to the secreted form of immunoglobulin. The change from the membrane form to the soluble form of IgM is caused by RNA splicing.

---

## Site-Specific DNA Recombination in Heavy-Chain C-Region Genes Leads to Class Switching

*Besides the changes that switch immunoglobulin production from a membrane form to a secreted form, B cells can undergo changes that promote antibody isotype (class) switching.* Class switching occurs in two stages: (1) initially mature naïve B cells simultaneously express IgM and IgD, and (2) within a clone, B cells can progress from synthesizing a μ heavy chain (IgM) to γ, ε, or α heavy-chain C-region isotypes. As discussed earlier, the mechanisms for the first stage involves alternative RNA splicing. The second stage involves *class switch recombination*, a complex and incompletely understood process; it occurs roughly one week after T cell-dependent antigen immunization when mature B cells have migrated to secondary lymphoid organs, are proliferating in germinal centers, and about the same time are undergoing somatic hypermutation.

Class switching occurs when a B cell that is simultaneously producing the membrane forms of IgM and IgD is stimulated by antigen to produce immunoglobulin of the non-IgM class. For the B cell to accomplish this switch, segments of $C_H$-region DNA must be deleted; *the entire V-D-J segment, including the promoter and enhancer, must be transferred to a downstream C gene, with deletion of the intervening DNA.* Class switching allows for expression of antibodies that have the same antigen specificity but are of a different isotype (IgG, IgE, or IgA) and thereby still react with the same antigen but mediate different effector functions—the $C_\mu$ region of the immunoglobulin is irreversibly replaced by another $C_H$ region, while the $V_H$ region remains the same.

Antigen- and cytokine-induced differentiation of B cells triggers **class switching** or **heavy-chain switching** and is mediated by another kind of DNA rearrangement called **class switch recombination** (**CSR**). As V(D)J recombination, CSR is a cut and paste mechanism in which breaks are initiated in two participating DNA regions followed by their fusion. This deletional-recombination reaction, i.e., CSR, requires the deamination of deoxycytosine residues in both strands of DNA by the enzyme activation-induced cytidine deaminase (AID). AID deaminates cytidine residues, generating uridines. The resulting uridine/guanine mismatches are recognized by uracil-N-glycosylase, which removes the uridine leaving sites without a base. These abasic sites may be cleaved by a specific endonuclease, leading to DNA nicks, which in turn lead to staggered double-stranded DNA breaks that occur in intervening sequences between the $V_H$ and $C_H$ genes, deletion of the intervening sequences, followed by DNA repair, and transcription. The DNA breaks occur in specific regions in the introns that contain highly repetitive tandem 1–10 Kb in length sequences with G-rich nontemplate strands. The nucleotide sequences of these regions, called **switch**, or **S, regions**, can be represented by GAGCT, GGGGT, or GGGCT. The S regions, in the 5′ intronic regions, are located 1–5 kb immediately upstream of each $C_H$ gene except for the $C_\delta$ gene. Class switch recombination leads to the placement of the complete $V_H$ gene (the V-D-J complex) next to another $C_H$ gene, leading to a rearranged $C_H$ locus and deletion of the intervening sequence as an episomal circle. The DNA ends are modified by nucleases and/or polymerases, creating blunt ends that are joined by NHEJ mechanisms.

An unusual characteristic is that CSR in the S regions is preceded by transcription through a particular S region to the corresponding $C_H$ gene. In response to specific cytokines (such as interleukin-4 [IL-4]) and CD40-CD40L interaction, transcription is initiated from a cytokine responsive promoter upstream of an exon (known as the I exon) that precedes all $C_H$ genes that undergo CSR. Transcription progresses through the S region and terminates downstream of the switching $C_H$ gene, this leads to a germline transcript containing the I and $C_H$ exon sequences. The primary transcript is spliced by unknown factors to eliminate the intronic S region and to join the I exon to the $C_H$ exons, producing mature germline transcripts that do not encode protein. Why germline transcription occurs in CSR is speculative. Nonetheless, because germline transcription always precedes CSR, transcription is postulated to render S-region chromatin structures accessible to CSR recombinases and to produce DNA structures that act as substrates for CSR recombinases.

An example of the classic pathway to IgE switching, illustrated in Figure 6-18, involves the $T_H2$–type cytokines IL-4 and IL-13 and the interaction of the B-cell surface molecule CD40 with T cell CD40L (CD154). These three reactants or "switch factors" induce sequential class switching, which leads to the sequential deletion of intervening DNA sequences. The two switch regions are brought into close proximity and cleaved by an unknown enzyme(s). The intervening DNA sequences are looped out from the chromosome between S recombination sites, deleting the DNA as an excised circle, and bringing a new C-region gene close to the rearranged V-D-J gene segments. Because this process is accompanied by deletion of genes 5′ to the $C_H$ gene being expressed,

the cell no longer can switch back to an isotype encoded 5′ to the isotype being expressed by the B cell.

T cell-derived cytokines such as IL-4, IL-5, transforming growth factor-beta (TGF-β), and interferon-γ (IFN-γ) activate and direct the switching process in B cells (see Chapter 10). For instance, IL-4 causes B cells to switch from IgM to IgE (IgG1 in mice) synthesis, IL-5 and TGF-β cause a switch to IgA synthesis, and IFN-γ causes a switch to IgG2a synthesis. These cytokines probably expose the S sites to regulators of DNA recombination and transcription.

## Biosynthesis of Membrane or Secreted Antibodies Involves the Presentation of Antibodies as Vesicle Membrane-Attached Antibodies or the Release of Antibodies from Vesicles

Membrane-associated and secreted antibody production progresses through similar pathways. The RNA polymerase II enzyme copies the assembled gene (DNA) into a nuclear RNA transcript. RNA splicing removes introns and joins exons. The resulting functional mRNA leaves the nucleus and binds to a ribosome. The leader sequence is translated and binds to a signal recognition protein, which stops further translation. This complex moves to the surface of the endoplasmic reticulum, where it docks, using the signal recognition protein, and starts the assemblage of immunoglobulins. The mRNAs are translated at the surface of the endoplasmic reticulum, and the translated chains subsequently enter the lumen of the endoplasmic reticulum. Within the lumen, the leader sequence is removed by enzymatic cleavage. At this stage in the process, the pathway splits. Immunoglobulins destined for the cell membrane do not pass completely through the endoplasmic reticulum membrane. The hydrophobic carboxyl-terminal segment of surface-bound immunoglobulins, which is encoded by an M exon(s), inhibits passage of the heavy chain and facilitates its anchoring to the membrane. Membrane-bound antibody remains attached to the endoplasmic reticulum membrane, with the antigen-binding sites pointing into the lumen. Enzymes add carbohydrates in N-glycosidic linkages to specific amino acids in the heavy chains as the endoplasmic reticulum moves into the Golgi apparatus. More sugars are added while the antibody molecules are in the lumen of the Golgi body. Immunoglobulins then move to the cell surface by vesicles. When they reach the plasma membrane, the vesicles fuse and either release the secreted form of immunoglobulins or present the vesicle membrane-attached

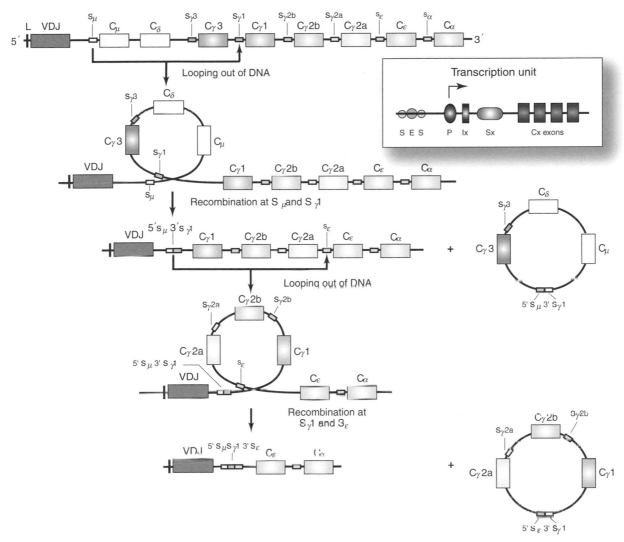

**FIGURE 6-18 A possible molecular mechanism for IL-4-induced sequential antibody class switching from IgM to IgG1 to IgE.** Each C exon except $C_\delta$ is preceded by a promoter, and I exon (I), and a switch (S) site. A looping-out mechanism has been proposed to explain the molecular excision of genes during class switching. During the first looping-out reaction, a DNA segment between $S_\mu$ and $S_\gamma 1$ recombination sites (yellow and green boxes, respectively) is excised as an episomal circle and the new $C_\gamma 1$-region gene is spliced to the V-D-J gene, leading to the IgM to IgG1 switch. During the second looping out reaction, the DNA segment between $S_\mu$ and $S_\varepsilon$ or $S_\mu S_\gamma 1$ and $S_\varepsilon$ recombination sites is excised as a circle and the new $C_\varepsilon$-region gene is spliced to the V-D-J gene, leading to the IgG1 to IgE switch. The inset (yellow box) generically represents the $C_H$ genes ($C_X$ exons) as transcription units, which are transcribed from cytokine-inducible I-promoters (P) upstream of the I-exon ($I_X$) through S regions and the corresponding $C_H$ exons. The resulting primary transcript is processed leading to a mature germline non-coding transcripts.

immunoglobulins to the outside of the cell. These events are summarized in Figure 6-19.

## MINI SUMMARY

The mechanism for heavy-chain class (isotype) switching involves a DNA class switch recombination, that is, from IgM to a class other than IgD. This kind of DNA rearrangement includes special segments, called switch, or S, regions. These regions lie 5′ to the heavy-chain C-region genes, except for $C\delta$. The S region before the $C_\mu$ gene is used to bring the other C-region genes contiguous to the V-D-J segment by cutting out the intervening genes and splicing the C-region genes to the S region.

The synthesis of membrane or secreted immunoglobulin is determined at the level of

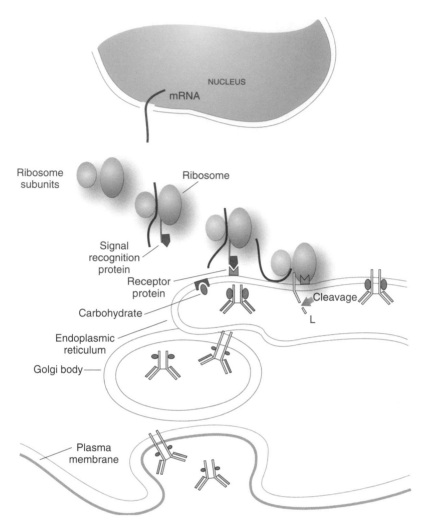

**FIGURE 6-19 Biosynthesis of membrane and secreted immunoglobulin.** Following transcription, the primary RNA transcript immediately associates with proteins, joins the pool of heterogeneous nuclear RNA, is chemically modified, is spliced to remove any introns, and is transported as mature mRNA across the nuclear membrane into the cytoplasm. In the cytoplasm, the mRNA is translated with the help of a ribosome. Leader peptides pull the developing polypeptides (the immunoglobulins) into the lumen of the endoplasmic reticulum and partially glycosylate the polypeptides. They are delivered by transport vesicles to the Golgi, where they are glycosylated further. The fully glycosylated polypeptides are then transported in vesicles to the plasma membrane. The presence of a hydrophobic transmembrane region determines whether the polypeptides remain anchored in the membrane of the vesicles for insertion into the plasma membrane or remain free in the vesicles for release to the exterior when the vesicles fuse with the plasma membrane.

mRNA processing. The inclusion of the membrane (M) or cytoplasm exons in the mature mRNA leads to immunoglobulins either as receptors or as soluble molecules. Also determined by mRNA processing.

# SUMMARY

How is the seemingly limitless antibody diversity generated using a few genes?

Amino acid sequencing indicates that antibody diversity and specificity are achieved by the joining of a large number of different V regions to a few C regions for light and heavy chains. Genetic studies showed that κ and λ light-chain and heavy-chain genes are on different chromosomes (three separate gene pools); however, the V-region genes are near the C-region genes. Immunoglobulin genes increase by expanding the number of V-region genes that associate with one set of C-region genes. For this process to work, the gene segments encoding different parts of the V regions of light and heavy chains must be brought together by normal peptide linkage at the level of DNA. A comparison of the immunoglobulin genes of embryos (germline configuration) and plasma cells (germline configuration or a somatic contribution) confirmed the two gene–one polypeptide hypothesis. Two things were learned: (1) there was rearrangement of germline immunoglobulin genes and (2) the genes were separated by *noncoding intervening sequences*. Germline DNA is rearranged and assembled in somatic cells, generating functional immunoglobulin genes.

Light-chain gene families contain one or more *C-region genes* and sets of *V-* and *J-gene segments*; the heavy-chain gene families contain these *gene segments* and also *D-gene segments*. To make an immunoglobulin molecule, light- and heavy-chain gene segments must be assembled. Assembly is catalyzed by immunoglobulin gene enzymes collectively called *V(D)J recombinase*. The two genes that induce immunoglobulin gene segment recombination are called *recombination activation genes 1 and 2 (RAG1 and RAG2)*. They encode the proteins (RAG-1 and RAG-2) that act synergistically and are required to mediate V-(D-J) recombination. To make the light-chain gene, V-gene segments are assembled by one DNA recombination event that joins a $V_L$ segment to a $J_L$ segment. After (V-J) gene segment joining, the V-J exon (*functional gene*) and the C exon are joined at the level of RNA by RNA splicing. Because the V-region gene segments in heavy-chain genes contain an additional D-gene segment, two DNA recombination events occur for heavy-chain V-region gene assembly. In the first step, the $D_H$ gene segment is joined to a $J_H$ gene segment. In the second step, a $V_H$ gene segment is joined to the rearranged D-J exon. Each of the assembled gene segments (V-J or V-D-J) is then co-transcribed with the right C-region exon to produce an mRNA molecule that encodes the complete polypeptide chain.

Light-chain V-J exons and heavy-chain V-D-J exons join at specific *recombination signal sequences (RSSs)*. The RSSs are composed of a conserved palindromic sequence of seven bases (heptamer) and of AT-rich nine bases (nonamer), separated by either 12 (*one-turn RSS*) or 23 (*two-turn RSS*) nucleotides whose sequences are varied and unimportant. The joining event is governed by the *heptamer-nonamer and 12/23 rule*. The V-J or D-J and V-(D-J) joinings happen only if their heptamer-nonamers are separated by 12 or 23 nucleotides.

Before exposure to antigen, B cells choose whether to express λ or κ chains and whether to use maternal or paternal gene pools—*allelic exclusion*. Allelic exclusion is part of an ordered sequence in the development of rearrangement: (1) heavy-chain gene rearrangements, (2) κ-chain gene rearrangement, and (3) λ-chain gene rearrangement (successful κ-gene rearrangement prevents λ-chain gene rearrangement), (4) immunoglobulin receptors; then antigen exposure leads to (5) class switching and finally to (6) antibody secretion. Cell-specific transcription controls the expression of functional immunoglobulin genes.

Humans inherit roughly 160 germline gene segments, the *germline repertoire* contribution to diversity. In humans, the random association of 40 V-gene segments with 5 J-gene segments at the κ locus or 30 V-gene segments and 4 J-gene segments at the λ locus generates a great deal of antibody diversity. When this random association is combined with the association of roughly 51 $V_H$-gene segments, about 25 D-gene segments, and 6 $J_H$-gene segments, antibody diversity is increased even more. This random association of gene segments is called *combinatorial joining*. Because it takes a light and a heavy chain to form an antibody's antigen-binding sites, diversity increases by the number of different light chains multiplied by the number of different heavy chains—*combinatorial association*. The V-J, D-J, or J-D joining does not always occur at the same base pair next to the heptamer of RSSs. The imprecise joining leads to different amino acid sequences and different polypeptide chains. This imprecise joining is called *junctional flexibility* or *junctional imprecision*. Junctional flexibility introduces extra diversity into the third CDR. Further junctional diversity can occur by *P-nucleotide addition* in light- and heavy-chain gene segment joining and by a template-free insertion of *N* (nucleotides) *regions* by *terminal deoxyribonucleotidyl transferase (TdT)* between D- and J-derived segments in D-J or V-(D-J) recombination for heavy-chain genes. The different antibodies generated from fully assembled immunoglobulin genes are further increased 10- to 100-fold by *somatic hypermutation* when exposed to antigen. Somatic hypermutation leads to *affinity maturation*. These numerous sources of antibody diversity lead to more than $10^{10}$ different immunoglobulin molecules.

RNA processing determines how single B cells coexpress membrane IgM and IgD and whether B-cell immunoglobulin genes encode either membrane or soluble forms of immunoglobulins. All B cells at first secrete immunoglobulins with the μ heavy chain (IgM). These cells coexpress μ and δ heavy chains, but after antigen stimulation in the presence of helper T cells and antigen-presenting cells, they undergo proliferation and differentiation into plasma cells that secrete IgM immunoglobulins. Some of these cells also become memory cells. During the immune response, however, some B cells will convert to make antibodies of other classes but keep the same antigen specificity as the original IgM immunoglobulin molecules. This *class switching* or *class switch recombination* is the result of $B_{\mu+\delta}$ cells replacing their heavy-chain V regions with γ, α, and ε C regions. Thus, antibodies are produced with different biologic properties but retain their original antigen specificity. Light-chain class switching does not occur.

# SELF-EVALUATION

## RECALLING KEY TERMS

Affinity maturation
Allelic exclusion
Class switching (or class switch recombination)
Combinatorial association freedom of light and heavy chains
Combinatorial joining freedom of gene segments
Composite coding sequence (functional gene)
Constant- (C) gene segments
Diversity- (D) gene segments
DNA-binding proteins (or nuclear factors [NF])
Enhancers
Exons
Gene segments
Germline theory
Heptamer-nonamer & spacer 12/23 rule
Imprecise DNA rearrangement
Insertion of random N regions
Introns (intervening sequences)
Joining- (J) gene segments
Junctional flexibility
Leader (or signal peptide) sequence
Membrane (M) exons
Multiplicity of V, D, and J germline gene segments
N regions
P-region nucleotide addition
Promoters
Recombination activating genes 1 & 2 (RAG-1 & RAG-2)
Recombination signal sequences (RSSs)

One-turn RSSs
Two-turn RSSs
Silencers
Somatic hypermutation
Somatic theories
Switch (S) regions
Terminal dexyncleotidyl transferase (TdT)
Variable- (V) gene segments
V(D)J recombinase

## MULTIPLE-CHOICE QUESTIONS

*(An answer key is not provided, but the page[s] location of the answer is.)*

1. The sequence in which antibody gene rearrangements occur when murine stem cells differentiate into B lymphocytes is (a) κ chains or λ chains first, then heavy chains, (b) κ chains, then λ chains, then heavy chains, (c) λ chains, then heavy chains, then κ chains, (d) heavy chains, then κ chains, then λ chains, (e) the sequence is totally random, (f) none of these. *(See pages 192 and 193.)*

2. Synthesis of a complete, soluble IgG heavy chain requires the action of (a) 2 gene segments, (b) 5 gene segments, (c) 7 gene segments, (d) 9 gene segments, (e) 12 gene segments, (f) none of these. *(See page 186.)*

3. A commitment by a B cell to make a single light chain is (a) triggered by V-J joining, (b) known as *class switching*, (c) triggered by V-D-J joining, (d) caused by deletion of forbidden clones, (e) none of these. *(See pages 193 and 194.)*

4. Somatic hypermutation accounts for some degree of antibody diversity. These mutations (a) account for the C-gene switch during differentiation, (b) occur at random in the different loci that control immunoglobulin synthesis, (c) tend to involve only the V genes, (d) predominantly affect the κ genes, (e) scramble the order of genes and gene fragments, (f) none of these. *(See pages 199 and 200.)*

5. Nucleotide sequences 3′ to each V gene and 5′ to each J gene for light chains that aid in the deletion of intervening V and J genes during B-cell maturation are (a) leader sequences, (b) switching sites, (c) recombination signal sequences, (d) excluded alleles, (e) the splice sites, (f) none of these. *(See page 187.)*

6. The generation of antibody diversity is best explained by (a) germline diversity, (b) somatic mutation, (c) adaptation to the environment,

(d) a combination of germline gene numbers, recombination events, and somatic mutations, (e) combinatorial association of germline genes, (f) none of these. *(See pages 180 and 181.)*

7. A clone of antibody-forming cells can switch from synthesizing one class of antibody to synthesizing another class. Such switches involve changes in (a) V regions of heavy and light chains, (b) C region of heavy chains, (c) C region of light chain, (d) C and V regions of heavy chains, (e) C and V regions of heavy and light chains, (f) none of these. *(See pages 205–207.)*

8. Allelic exclusion may be explained by (a) one chromosome having nonsense rearrangements, (b) one chromosome remaining in the germline configuration, (c) *a* and *b*, (d) neither *a* nor *b*, (e) none of these. *(See pages 192–194.)*

9. Which of the following correctly describes immunoglobulin genes? (a) they exist as several discrete segments in the germline DNA, (b) they do not require several somatic translocation events before transcription into mRNA, (c) they do not use a combinatorial association scheme to achieve greater diversity, (d) the light- and heavy-chain gene segments are on the same chromosomes, (e) none of these. *(See pages 182, 184, 185, and 197.)*

10. At the molecular level, when a plasma cells is making IgA antibody, you would find (a) mRNA specific for neither λ nor κ light chains, (b) a DNA sequence for V-D-J genes translocated near the μ DNA exon, (c) mRNA specific for both λ and κ light chains, (d) *a* and *b*, (e) none of these. *(See pages 206 and 207.)*

11. If all mechanisms that generate antibody diversity are used and you had 300 V- and 5 J-region gene segments for a light chain and 300 V-, 10 D-, and 5 J-region gene segments for a heavy chain, you could encode (a) exactly 1500 specificities, (b) exactly 22,500 specificities, (c) exactly 22,500,000 specificities, (d) a few more than 22,500,000 specificities, (e) none of these. *(See pages 201.)*

12. The switch mechanism for changing IgM to IgG does not involve (a) recombination at the DNA level at certain points in the introns, (b) use of gene segments encoding V, D, and J regions, (c) selection of a new light chain, (d) loss of exons between the V region of the heavy chain and the gene to which the switch occurs, (e) none of these. *(See page 207.)*

## SHORT-ANSWER ESSAY QUESTIONS

1. Why is it important to have antibody diversity?
2. Differentiate between the germline theory and the somatic theory of antibody diversity.
3. How are both the germline and somatic mechanisms sources of antibody diversity?
4. Why did the amino acid sequencing of antibody light chains lead Dreyer and Bennett to buck the dogma of *one gene-one polypeptide* and propose that two genes code for each antibody chain?
5. Briefly discuss Tonegawa's approach to answering Dreyer and Bennett's hypothesis.
6. In addition to showing that DNA segments come together to form a functional antibody gene, Tonegawa's experiments showed two other things. What were they?
7. Draw the organization of germline DNA for a k light chain and heavy chain. What is the V-region gene segment difference between light and heavy chains?
8. The words *race car* and *sex at noon taxes* represent palindromes. What are palindromes, and what is their importance in V-region gene construction?
9. What are the two DNA recombination events required to assemble a functional heavy-chain V-region gene?
10. The events in the preceding process are governed by the heptamer-nonamer and spacer 12/23 rule. Explain.
11. Briefly discuss the four mechanisms that contribute to antibody diversity.
12. The progression of membrane to secreted IgM involves differential RNA splicing. Explain.
13. How do you explain the fact that a particular B cell can display and secrete different antibody isotypes, yet each B cell is specific for only one antigenic determinant?
14. Class switching occurs in two stages. What are they?
15. Discuss allelic exclusion; what is it, and how is it regulated?

## FURTHER READINGS

Bergman, Y., and H. Cedar. 2004. A stepwise epigenetic process controls immunoglobulin allelic exclusion. *Nat. Rev. Immunol.* 4:753–761.

Casali, P., Z. Pal, Z. Xu, and H. Zan. 2006. DNA repair in antibody somatic hypermutation. *Trends Immunol.* 27:314–321.

Chaudhuri, J., and F.W. Alt. 2004. Class-switch recombination: Interplay of transcription, DNA deamination and DNA repair. *Nature Rev. Immunol.* 4:541–552.

Dreyer, W.J., and J.C. Bennett. 1965. The molecular basis of antibody formation: A paradox. *Proc. Natl. Acad. Sci. U.S.A.* 54:864–869.

Geha, R.S., H.H. Jabara, and S.R. Brodeur. 2003. The regulation of Immunoglobulin E class-switch recombination. *Nat. Rev. Immunol.* 3:721–732.

Hozumi, N., and S. Tonegawa. 1976. Evidence for somatic rearrangement of immunoglobulin genes coding for variable and constant regions. *Proc. Natl. Acad. Sci. U.S.A.* 73:3628–3632.

Jung D., C. Giallourakis, R. Mostoslavsky, and F.W. Alt. 2006. Mechanism and control of V(D)J recombination at the immunoglobulin heavy chain locus. *Annu. Rev Immunol.* 24:541–570.

Longerich S., U. Basu, F. Alt, and U. Stord. 2006. AID in somatic hypermutation and class switch recombination. *Curr. Opin Immunol.* 18:164–174.

Max, E.E. 2003. Immunoglobulins: Molecular genetics. In *Fundamental Immunology*, 5th ed. W.E. Paul, ed. Philadelphia: Lippincott Williams & Wilkins. p. 107–158.

Roth, D.B. 2003. Restraining the V(D)J recombinase. *Nat. Rev. Immunol.* 3:656–666.

Selsing, E. 2006. Ig class switching: Targeting the recombinational mechanism. *Cur. Opin. Immunol.* 18:249–254.

Stavnezer, J. J.E.J. Guikema, and C.E. Schrader. 2008. Mechanism and regulation of class switch recombination. *Annu. Rev. Immunol.* 26:261–292.

Tonegawa, S. 1983. Somatic generation of antibody diversity. *Nature* 302:575–581.

# CHAPTER SEVEN

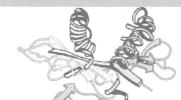

# THE MAJOR HISTOCOMPATIBILITY COMPLEX AND DEVELOPMENT OF IMMUNITY

## CHAPTER OUTLINE

1. The discovery of the MHC exposes the connection between genes and the immune response.
   a. The discovery of the mouse MHC establishes the foundation for the immunogenetics of the immune response.
   b. The discovery of the human MHC revolved around serologic and genetic analyses of linkage.
2. The MHC is a cluster of genes responsible for molecules that are essential to T-cell function.
   a. Class I region genes encode class I molecules that present intracellular antigenic peptides to CD8+ T cells.
   b. Class II region genes encode class II molecules that present extracellular antigenic peptides to CD4+ T cells.
   c. Class III region genes encode class III molecules, some complement proteins, cytokines, and other proteins unrelated to MHC class I and class II molecules.
3. The immune response is MHC-linked; the genes encode structures that allow immune functions.
4. MHC restriction means that T cells are programmed to interact with foreign peptides on cells only in association with class I or class II MHC molecules.
5. MHC molecules are promiscuous antigen receptors.
6. Control of MHC molecule expression is critical to T-cell responsiveness.
7. Antigen recognition requires antigen processing and preferential presentation of peptides by either class I or class II MHC molecules.
8. Antigen recognition requires antigen processing and preferential presentation of nonpeptides by non-MHC-encoded class I-like CD1 molecules.

## OBJECTIVES

The reader should be able to:

1. Understand the connection between a trait and a gene; realize that MHC genes encode molecules that allow immune responses (the trait).

---

2. Appreciate the use of inbred mice for studying the genetics of the immune response; distinguish between inbred and congenic mice.

3. Comprehend that the MHC is a cluster of genes encoding molecules that are needed for T cells to recognize antigen.

4. Draw maps of the H-2 and HLA complexes.

5. Identify the H-2 and HLA complex regions that encode class I molecules; describe and draw class I molecules; list the traits associated with the class I loci.

6. Identify the H-2 and HLA complex regions that encode class II molecules; describe and draw class II molecules; list the traits associated with the class II loci.

7. Comment on the function of class III genes.

8. Understand how class II genes ("Ir" genes) are MHC-linked and encode structures that allow immune functions; realize that the collection of class II genes, or haplotype, dictates an animal's ability or inability to respond to a particular antigen; appreciate how these genes might affect the immune response.

9. Define MHC restriction.

10. Describe an experiment that shows MHC restriction between T and B cells, between T cells and macrophages, and between cytotoxic T cells and virally infected cells; explain the difference between CD4$^+$ T-cell and CD8$^+$ T-cell MHC restriction.

11. Discuss what is recognizing what in the MHC molecule complex.

12. Explain why cytokines are important to MHC molecule expression.

13. Outline antigen processing and presentation.

14. Describe the molecules that can recognize lipid antigens.

Genetics affects the immune response through three systems: (1) the genes that encode antibody chains, (2) the genes that encode the T-cell antigen receptors (TCRs), and (3) the genes in the **major histocompatibility complex** (**MHC**) that control the responses to T-cell-dependent antigens and the ability to distinguish between self and nonself. Because T cells are responsible for the full expression of immunity—humoral and cell-mediated immunity, they use MHC molecules to discriminate between different types of antigens. In fact, unlike B cells whose receptors, antibodies, can recognize antigens alone, most T cells cannot recognize antigen alone, antigen must be associated with MHC molecules; peptide-MHC complexes are the ligands for TCRs. MHC-encoded molecules are antigen-presenting molecules—they display antigen-derived peptides—therefore, the host's MHC molecule repertoire influences resistance to infections but conversely they are implicated in susceptibility to autoimmune diseases. Because the mechanisms for the development of antibody and of TCR diversity are discussed in Chapters 6 and 8, only the immunogenetics of the human and murine MHC and its role in the development of immunity is presented here. The term MHC suggests some association between tissue acceptance and rejection; the importance of MHC molecules in clinical transplantation is discussed in Chapter 14.

*The defining characteristic of MHC genes is that they encode polymorphic molecules that allow immune responses.* Two groups of MHC genes, called *class I* and *class II MHC genes*, control the expression of two classes of surface molecules called *class I* and *class II MHC molecules*, respectively. The class I molecules were initially described because of immune responses to transplanted tissue, and the class II molecules were important in the regulation of the immune response. We now know that these surface glycoproteins are the molecules that allow cellular interactions through antigen presentation to T cells. Thus, these molecules are critical to T cells because most T cells cannot recognize free or soluble antigens; they only recognize parts of proteins (peptides) bound to these MHC molecules. The T cell's antigen receptor exhibits dual specificities, one for antigenic peptide and the other for the class I or class II MHC molecule. A CD4$^+$, helper T (T$_H$), cell's TCR recognizes antigen bound to a class II MHC molecule. In contrast, a CD8$^+$, cytotoxic T (T$_C$), cell's TCR recognizes antigen bound to a class I MHC molecule. This focusing of T-cell antigen recognition through class I and II MHC molecules is known as *MHC restriction*. The controlled restriction between CD4$^+$ T$_H$ cells and APC class II MHC molecules, and between CD8$^+$ T$_C$ cells and target-cell class I MHC molecules, is the genetic basis for the functional specificity of T lymphocytes. Class I molecules are also important in the recognition of host cells by natural killer (NK) cells. Although B cells can recognize and react with free antigen by their surface-bound antibodies, T cells cannot recognize antigen in its natural state. Protein antigen must first be broken down and the peptides of the antigen bound to an MHC molecule by an antigen-presenting cell (APC); this is called *antigen processing and presentation*. Genes within the MHC also encode certain complement components, enzymes, molecules involved in antigen processing, and cytokines. Immunity is the ability to respond to, and be protected against, foreign infectious agents. MHC genes orchestrate these protective activities.

# THE DISCOVERY OF THE MHC EXPOSES THE CONNECTION BETWEEN GENES AND THE IMMUNE RESPONSE

In the mid-1930s in England, Peter Gorer was attempting to characterize blood group antigens in the mouse. He found that strains of mice could be distinguished because of three genes that encoded cell-surface antigens. Two antigens (called *antigen I* and *III*) were common to all strains and varied only in amount, while the other (*antigen II*), found in some strains, correlated with tumor graft rejection. In the late 1940s, Gorer joined Snell at the Jackson Laboratories in Bar Harbor, Maine. George Snell realized that for genetic or immunologic analyses to proceed required that "transplantation" genes be studied on an individual basis—he introduced the notion of histocompatibility genes and how to develop inbred mice that differed by a single histocompatibility (H) gene. The use of inbred mice led to the description of the genes controlling graft rejection. Gorer and Snell found that the genetic locus encoding *antigen II* and the locus important for graft rejection were one and the same. Snell coined the term **histocompatibility** (*histo* means tissue) to denote cell-surface antigens that determine whether one tissue is compatible with another. In

reference to Gorer's **antigen II**, the locus was designated **H-2**. As described below, the H-2 was not one gene but a complex of closely linked genes. This gene complex is the MHC of the mouse.

In the early 1950s in France, Jean Dausset observed that patients who had multiple blood transfusions had antibodies to the lymphocytes from other, or *allogeneic*, individuals but not to their own lymphocytes. Thus, the antibodies were called *alloantibodies* and their target antigens were called **alloantigens**. These antibodies were the first antibodies to define human histocompatibility antigens, now termed **human leukocyte antigens** (**HLA**). In 1958 Dausset defined the first HLA determinant. The **HLA complex** is the human MHC and is the analog of the murine H-2 complex.

Because most individuals will never need transplants, the question arises: "What do these genes and the molecules they encode do in everyday life?" Research by Baruj Benacerraf in the 1960s and 1970s answered this question by showing that the MHC genes control cellular interactions among immune cells. Snell, Daussett, and Benacerraf received the 1980 Nobel Prize in Medicine, but because Nobel Prizes are not awarded posthumously, Peter Gorer did not share in the Prize.

Because of Snell's work, today there are over 200 *inbred* lines of mice and of their fine-tuned partners, the *congenics*. Others now include transgenic, knockout, and conditional knockout mice with directed and conditional mutations of revelvant genetic loci. Without these animals, genetic analysis of the immune response would have been difficult, if not impossible, because the equivalent of inbred mice would be human identical twins.

## The Discovery of the Mouse MHC Establishes the Foundation for the Immunogenetics of the Immune Response

The mouse MHC (the H-2 complex) was discovered as the genetic locus that encoded molecules responsible for tissue acceptance and rejection when swapped between inbred strains of mice. It was found that the MHC was a cluster of genes (locus) on a single chromosome, in the mouse on chromosome 17. The loci within the MHC are highly **polymorphic**, that is, there are many gene versions, or **alleles**, which exist at each locus in different members of the population. Not only are there different alleles of each gene in a host but also duplicated genes with similar functions. The MHC is highly **polygenic**, that is, there are several genes for MHC products.

The tools of immunogenetics—identifying relevant genes—involved the breeding of mice followed by the analysis of the progeny. The repetitive breeding of siblings through 20 generations leads to all members of an *inbred strain* being identical (**syngeneic**) at all genetic loci. Except for the sex chromosomes, all other chromosomes of an inbred strain are homozygous, producing identical homozygous progeny. The progeny loci must be of either parental homozygous genotype, with no heterozygous loci; the resulting progeny are then defined as *inbred*. Certain inbred strains such as A, CBA, DBA/2, and C57BL/10 have been designated prototype stains. Mice that have inherited the same MHC alleles as the prototype strain have the same haplotype but differ in the genes outside the MHC complex. Table 7-1 shows some well-characterized and commonly used inbred strains of mice.

The crossing of different inbred strains can, on rare occasions, lead to $F_1$ progeny in which a genetic crossover has occurred at a defined chromosomal location, so that the affected chromosome has different collections of genes, or haplotypes, at each end. These $F_1$ progeny are called *recombinant mice* and can be used to characterize segments of a chromosome. An MHC **region** is a segment of a chromosome serving as the site for at least one defined gene. For example, the comparable regions in the H-2 complex are called $K, I, S, D,$ and $L$, and in the HLA complex they are called $D, B, C,$ and $A$. Regions are further divided into areas of related loci called **subregions**. Within the MHC region, a genetic **locus** is the position of a gene encoding a single polypeptide chain, separated by recombination from flanking genes (such as the H-2 K region = H-$2^k$ locus).

In the strictest sense, **alleles** are alternate forms of genes that occupy corresponding positions (loci) on paired chromosomes; only one allele is expressed per haploid genome. In the MHC, however, alleles may represent alternate forms of individual loci and regions. The allele representing MHC genes of an inbred strain is designated by italicized superscript lowercase letters (see Table 7-1). For example, the

prototype DBA/2 strain has the allelic name of H-$2^d$ whereas H-$2^k$ is the name for the prototype CBA strain. The superscripts *d* and *k* are arbitrary designations used to refer to a collection of alleles in a strain. For nonrecombinant strains, the allelic name represents individual regions (genes) and the entire MHC. In contrast, the allelic name for recombinant strains stands for regions of the MHC or individual genes within the region, according to the original inbred strain from which the region was derived. For example, the designation is H-$2^{bq1}$ for a recombinant interval between the H-2 K region and the H-2 I-A subregion.

An MHC **haplotype** is the particular collection of alleles of MHC genes present on a single chromosome that encodes a specific characteristic or function, such as the immune system's MHC markers. Because inbred mice are homozygous, they have a single haplotype. The haplotype of the inbred strain BALB/c would consist of *d* alleles at all H-2 complex regions and subregions ($K^d I$-$A^d I$-$E^d S^d D^d$). Recombinant H-2 haplotypes involving neighboring regions have different allelic designations. For example, the A.TL strain has undergone two recombinant events, leading to three different allelic designations ($K^s I$-$A^k I$-$E^k S^k D^d$), receiving the K and D regions from the H-$2^s$ and H-$2^d$ haplotypes, respectively, and intervening regions from the H-$2^k$ haplotype. The problem with this type of scheme for defining haplotypes is that there are not enough lowercase letters in the alphabet to describe all the possible recombinant haplotypes. This problem has been alleviated by assigning compound letters (H-$2^{bq1}$). In humans, the HLA haplotype is written HLA-A*0101, -B*0701, -C*0101, -DP*0101, and so forth, where each HLA allele is given a number. HLA molecules encoded by the class I and class II loci are identified by four-digit numbers, such as A*0101, with the letter of the locus as a prefix and separated from the number by an asterisk. The four-digit number represents the alleles of the individual loci, with the first two digits indicating the allelic group (type) and the last two digits indicating the subtype. The HLA molecule designations are the same as the designations of alleles at the individual loci. MHC molecules for which "good" antisera are unavailable have an extra prefix, "w," (taken from HLA *w*orkshops). Remember that humans are usually heterozygous; thus, they have a haplotype from each parent. However, for immunogenetic studies, animals that are entirely homozygous at every genetic locus are required. Inbred mice are an example of a homogeneous population of animals. Inbreeding changes the allelic and genotypic frequencies of a population and increases the frequency of homozygotes for

**TABLE 7-1 Some Commonly Used Inbred Mouse Strains**

| Some prototype strains | Strains with the same haplotype | Haplotype |
|---|---|---|
| A | A/He, A/Sn, B10.A | a (H-$2^a$) |
| CBA | AKR, B10.BR, C3H | k (H-$2^k$) |
| C57BL/10 | C57BL/6, C57L, C3H.Sw | b (H-$2^b$) |
| DBA/2 | BALB/c, SEA, NZB | d (H-$2^d$) |

individual genes. As mentioned above, *inbred mice* are produced by sequential pedigreed brother-sister matings for at least 20 generations; they are *all genetically identical*.

The genetic analysis of the H-2 complex was made possible with the development of **congenic mouse strains**; mice which are identical throughout their entire genomes except for a selected locus or closely linked loci that prevent the exchange of a graft. Thus, the background genes remain constant against a differing MHC, combinations of MHC loci, or an individual MHC locus. These animals make it possible to follow the effects of one gene against a constant genetic background. H-2 congenic strains are most easily produced by the *intercross-backcross breeding scheme*. Figure 7-1 illustrates the intercross-backcross breeding scheme used to produce congenic mice. The availability of inbred and congenic mouse strains led to mapping of the position and function of H-2 complex genes. These studies identified different MHC gene products and determined whether they are encoded by separate loci.

## The Discovery of the Human MHC Revolved Around Serologic and Genetic Analyses of Linkage

The understanding of human MHC immunogenetics developed much more slowly than for mice. Immunogenetics of mice took advantage of inbred and congenic strains and the ability to transplant tissue at will. In humans the genetic analysis of the MHC deals with the definition of serologic specificities and analysis of family and population genetics.

In the early 1950s, evidence for the human counterpart to the mouse H-2 complex was beginning to accumulate. The evidence came from the analysis of sera from patients who had received multiple transfusions. These patients' sera often agglutinated leukocytes from unrelated donors, and the agglutination patterns suggested definable antigens in human populations. These sera were the first to define **human leukocyte antigens**, hence **HLA**, and in part led to the characterization of the **HLA complex**. HLA antigen-specific antisera are still used to characterize and define HLA antigens. Since the mid-1960s, workers have met in a series of international workshops and exchanged antisera in order to analyze the histocompatibility antigens on leukocytes; this work has led to some standardization of HLA specificities and a more uniform HLA nomenclature. By the early 1970s, these serologic specificities had been grouped into three series, designated *HLA-A, HLA-B,* and *HLA-C* (*HLA-X, -E, -J, -H, -G,* and *-F* have been

added since then). They are the cell-surface molecules that are the human counterpart of the mouse H-2 K, D, and L region molecules and, collectively are called *class I MHC molecules*. Another group of molecules, the *class II MHC molecules*, detected by their ability to induce proliferation of foreign T cells *in vitro* (called the *mixed leukocyte reaction [MLR]*; discussed in Chapter 14), were described shortly thereafter and were termed *HLA-D*. The first class II gene products detected by alloantibodies and MLRs mapped to the HLA-D region and were called *HLA-D region-related* or *HLA-DR*. The HLA-D region now is known to consist of several families of class II genes besides *DR*; therefore, another letter, near R in the alphabet, was added to the designation: *DP, DO, DM,* and *DQ*.

The other way of analyzing the human MHC involved genetic linkage analysis, which required the typing of segregation patterns in families. Genetic analysis was simplified because each HLA haplotype is transmitted as a single Mendelian codominant trait (for example, if maternal genes encode HLA-A 1, HLA-B 1, and HLA-C 1 class I MHC molecules and paternal genes encode HLA-A 2, HLA-B 2, and HLA-C 2, an offspring would codominantly express all six class I MHC molecules on all cells). In contrast, for class II genes, heterozygous individuals inherit six (DP, DQ, and DR from each parent) different polymorphic alleles, but more than six class II MHC molecules can be expressed per cell; usually 10–20 different class II MHC molecules are expressed per cell. This increase results because there may be two or three functional $\beta$-chain genes and one functional $\alpha$-chain gene for some class II loci (class II molecules consist of two chains called $\alpha$ and $\beta$; see Figure 7-7); therefore, additional class II MHC molecules are produced by the combination of one $\alpha$-chain gene with more than one $\beta$-chain gene within the same allelic locus or the combination of an $\alpha$-chain gene from one allelic locus and a $\beta$-chain gene from another. Genetic analysis was made more difficult because humans exhibit a great deal of polymorphism. The analysis of human class I genes currently indicates 303 A alleles, 559 B alleles, and 150 C alleles; the class II genes show similar polymorphism, 20 DP$\alpha$ and 108 DP$\beta$ chain alleles, 25 DQ$\alpha$ and 56 DQ$\beta$ chain alleles, and 3 DR$\alpha$ and 440 DR$\beta$ chain alleles. *Polymorphism* refers to the large number of multiple alleles in individuals (or animals) at the same chromosomal locus. For instance, if we analyzed chromosome 6, HLA locus A, of 303 individuals, each individual could have a different allele at that locus; thus, each locus would encode a different MHC protein. The same situation can occur on the other chromosome of the pair. Polymorphism is one of the most striking features of the MHC. This

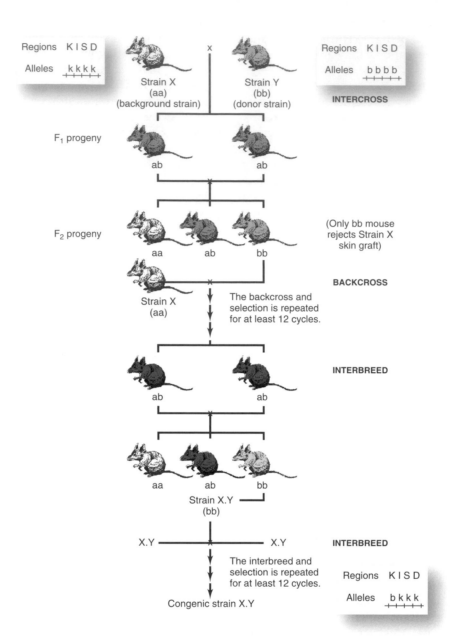

**FIGURE 7-1 Production of a hypothetical congenic strain X.Y.** To start the process, two different inbred strains that differ at the K locus are crossed. The background strain X (H-2$^a$, possessing the k allele at the K locus) must be a homozygote, and the donor strain Y (H-2$^b$, possessing the b allele at the K locus) may or may not be a homozygote (here a *bb* homozygote). To study the effect of the b allele, we must create a line genetically identical to strain X, but carrying the b allele. Production starts with the first intercross of two inbred strains, leading to an F$_1$ generation that is heterozygous at all loci (*ab*). F$_1$ progeny are interbred producing an F$_2$ generation. The homozygous *bb* F$_2$ progeny that reject a strain X skin graft are backcrossed to strain X (*aa*) and yield *ab* heterozygotes. (Any F$_2$ progeny that do not reject a strain X graft are eliminated from future breeding.) The heterozygous *ab* donor, who vigorously rejects a strain X skin graft, is now backcrossed to a background strain X (*aa*). For selected loci, all the progeny will again be heterozygotes (*ab*); that is, all the offspring will accept strain X's skin graft. These *ab* heterozygotes are again backcrossed to strain X (aa). This procedure is usually repeated for 12 consecutive generations, each time selecting the *ab* heterozygotes for mating to the *aa* background strain X. At each backcross the progeny become more and more like strain X except at strain Y's K locus, which is selected for on strain Y's ability to reject strain X skin grafts. The *ab* heterozygous progeny from the 12th generation have more than 99% of their genes derived from strain X. These mice are heterozygous for one histocompatibility locus contributed by strain Y. The result of interbreeding the ab heterozygotes would yield 25% *aa* homozygotes, 50% *ab* heterozygotes, and 25% *bb* homozygotes. By interbreeding of the *bb* mice, we get a line X.Y that is congenic to (similar to) strain X but carries the b rather than the k allele at the K locus on an X background.

feature is at the root of transplant failures and the success of antigen presentation. Familial studies showed variation in the prevalence and frequency of HLA antigens from one population to another. The other caveat was that the frequencies of certain haplotypes were higher than would be predicted by random association. The reason for this *linkage disequilibrium* is unknown. Nonetheless, humans are heterozygotes for most, if not all, HLA loci. Most leukocyte antigens belong to the *HLA complex*. The gene clusters and the molecules they encode will be detailed next.

## MINI SUMMARY

Expression of histocompatibility molecules is controlled by genes or groups of genes (loci) located close together (linked) on the same chromosomal strand. This segment of the chromosome is called the major histocompatibility complex, or MHC. In mice and humans the respective MHCs are called H-2 and HLA complexes.

Antigens responsible for provoking graft rejection are classically called transplantation antigens. Because rejection seemed to be an inherited phenomenon, studies to isolate and identify the responsible genes were begun using inbred and congenic mice.

Evidence for the human MHC arose from serologic and genetic linkage analyses. Serologic results suggested definable antigens in human populations called human leukocyte antigens, or HLA. Description of these antigens led, in part, to the characterization of the HLA complex. According to serologic specificities, these antigens were first grouped into three series, designated HLA-A, HLA-B, and HLA-C, followed later by HLA-D (and three subregions). Like mice, humans show a great deal of polymorphism.

# THE MHC IS A CLUSTER OF GENES RESPONSIBLE FOR MOLECULES THAT ARE ESSENTIAL TO T-CELL FUNCTION

*A group of closely linked genes determines tissue compatibility (graft survival). These genes are called the* **major histocompatibility complex** *or* **MHC**. *Antigens provoking a transplantation reaction are called major histocompatibility antigens. The MHC is a large, complex*

**TABLE 7-2 Partial List of Traits Under the Control of the MHC**

1. *Class I MHC molecules/region*
   a. Transplantation antigens
   b. Serologically detected membrane antigens
   c. Cellular target antigens for cell-mediated lympholysis
2. *Class II MHC molecules/region*
   a. Class II-region leukocyte antigens
   b. T cell and APC interactions
   c. Immune response regulation
   d. Mixed leukocyte reaction
   e. Graft-versus-host reaction
   f. Tumor virus susceptibility
   g. Peptide transport (TAP1, TAP2)
   h. Generation of peptides from cytosolic proteins (LMP2, LMP7)
3. *Class III MHC molecules/region*
   a. Complement levels
   b. Cytokines (TNF-$\alpha$, -$\beta$)
   c. Enzymes
   d. Heat-shock proteins

genetic region that controls not only the exchange of tissue but also the myriad cellular interactions of immune cells, the production of certain serum proteins, and the production of some cytokines and enzymes (Table 7-2). The MHC of mice and humans are called the *H-2 complex* and the *HLA complex*, respectively. *The H-2 and HLA complexes encode at least three major families of molecules: classes I, II, and III* (Figure 7-2). The class I and class II molecules are membrane-bound glycoproteins that are involved in antigen presentation to T cells. In contrast, the class III MHC molecules show no structural or functional similarity to class I and class II molecules. All of the vertebrates that have been studied possess an MHC, and functions ascribed to the MHC also are found in invertebrates such as sponges and colonial tunicates.

Because there are many genes in the HLA and H-2 MHC that encode mostly nonpolymorphic MHC-like molecules, of which most functions are unknown, the classification can be divided into classical MHC class I gene-encoded molecules called **class Ia molecules**; the other group of nonclassical class I genes that encode MHC class I-like molecules called **class Ib molecules**. (I signifies the Roman numeral I [one] not the alphabetical designation Ia, which is an older name for the murine class II MHC region.) Some class Ib gene-encoded molecules that perform specific functions include: (1) H-2 M3 (unknown if there is a human equivalent) is a murine protein that binds tightly to *N*-formylmethionine (*N*-f-met) residues. With few exceptions, such proteins are produced by prokaryotes; thus, they may be expressed by invading bacteria ($T_C$ cells can

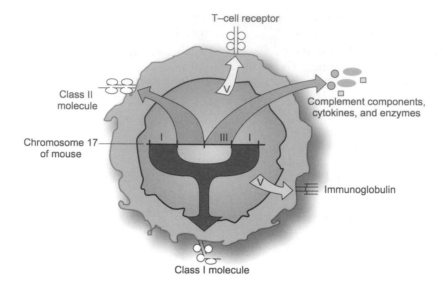

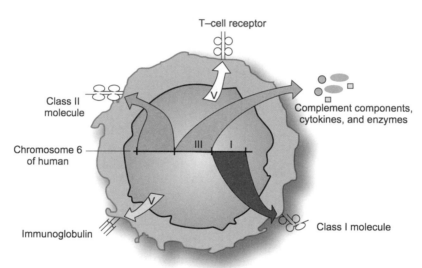

**FIGURE 7-2 The chromosomal location of the H-2 and HLA complex and the sites encoding class I and class II molecules.** The H-2 and HLA complex are organized differently; however, they encode for the same kinds of molecules. Two different groups of genes encode the V regions of Igs and T-cell receptors. All molecules are drawn in the same cell for illustrative purposes only.

recognize *N*-f-met-containing peptides presented by these class Ib molecules). (2) HLA-G, a human protein, which is the only MHC molecule expressed on trophoblast cells may protect the fetus from being recognized as foreign. It may also play a role in antigen recognition by NK cells. (3) Human MHC class I chain-related (MIC) molecules that are expressed at low levels in epithelial cells when under "stress" conditions that influence heat-shock proteins. MIC molecules are recognized by NK cells, $\gamma\delta$ T cells, and some CD8$^+$ T cells. There are also class II-like molecules, such as, HLA-DM, which encode

a heterodimer DM$\alpha$/DM$\beta$ that facilitates antigen loading by class II molecules.

The **H-2 complex**, a small segment located on chromosome 17, includes about 2000 kb of mouse DNA. The linear sequence of genes is called the **H-2 map** (Figure 7-3). The H-2 map can be divided into six regions because of the immunologic functions or molecules each region encodes. The six regions are **K, I, S, D, L,** and **Qa/Tla**, presented in linear sequence from left to right. These six regions contain genes encoding class I, II, and III molecules. In addition, within the class II regions of the H-2 and HLA

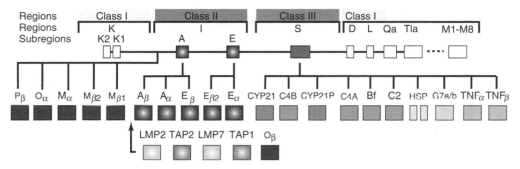

**FIGURE 7-3 H-2 complex map.** The H-2 complex contains the genes that encode three different classes of molecules involved in immune responses. These molecules are called *class I, II,* and *III MHC molecules.* Class I and II MHC molecules are cell-surface glycoproteins that present antigens, and class III MHC molecules are not antigen-presenting molecules. The class III region, between the S and D regions, contains genes that encode complement system components (C4, complement component 4; Bf, complement component factor B; C2, complement component 2), steroid 21-hydroxylases (CYP21, CYP21P), heat-stock proteins (HSP), valyl-tRNA synthetase (G7a/b), and tumor necrosis factors α and β (TNF-α, -β). Another set of genes, called *Qa* and *Tla genes,* encodes cell surface molecules on lymphocytes; these molecules are structurally similar to the molecules encoded by class I MHC genes. Their function is unknown. Genes considered to be associated with antigen processing (LMP2 and LMP7 [proteasome subunits]) and transport (TAP1 and TAP2 [peptide-transporter subunits]) are found between the M$_{\beta1}$ and A$_\beta$ loci (the location is designated by the up arrow [↑]; discussed later in chapter). (To ease descriptive comparisons between MHCs from different species, the generic term for regions should be used—class I, class II, or class III.)

complexes are genes for peptide transporters called *transporters associated with antigen processing-1 and 2 (TAP1, TAP2),* as well as the proteasome subunits called *low molecular weight proteins-2 and -7 (LMP2, LMP7).* The structures of these genes are involved in antigen processing.

The **HLA complex** is located on the short arm of chromosome 6 and spans roughly 4000 kb of human DNA (Figure 7-4). The HLA complex gene loci are organized differently (left to right: class II, III, and I regions) from the H-2 complex. Other than the mouse and probably the rat, all other mammals have the human type of MHC organization. The HLA complex consists of (reading from left to right): **DP, DN, DM, DO, DQ,** and **DR class II loci**; some **complement components,** steroid 21-hydroxylases, heat-stock proteins, valyl-tRNA synthease, and tumor necrosis factor-α and -β (TNF-α and -β) **class III loci**; and **B, C,** X, E, J, **A,** H, G, and F **class I loci.** As mentioned earlier, the genes of the H-2 and HLA complexes are highly polymorphic.

## Class I Region Genes Encode Class I Molecules That Present Intracellular Antigenic Peptides to CD8$^+$ T Cells

In humans, the **class I region** covers roughly 2000 kb of DNA and contains about 20 genes (see Figure 7-4). In mice, the class I region is separated into two

regions, which are at opposite ends of the H-2 complex (see Figure 7-3). The class I region genes encode **class I molecules** that are present on the surface of almost all nucleated cells of the body. Class I molecules are required for the recognition of antigen originating in the cytosol of cells; to be precise, they present antigenic peptide derived from intracellular antigen, such as, a virus, to T cells (see Chapter 10). They are codominantly expressed on nucleated cells; that is, class I alleles of both chromosomes of a pair are expressed. The class I region products were originally termed serologic defined antigens[1] because several antibodies could be raised against the products of their alleles. The human class I region genes encode the classical class I MHC molecules called *HLA-A, HLA-B,* and *HLA-C*; their murine counterparts are called *H-2K, H-2D,* and *H-2L*. Class I MHC molecules allow CD8$^+$ T cells, most of which are T$_C$ cells, to react with virally infected cells, chemically modified cells, allografts, and tumor cells. Class I MHC molecules are also recognized by NK cells. Many nonclassical class I genes have been identified in the human and mouse MHC. In humans, the nonclassical class I

---

[1]Older terminology referred to class I MHC molecules as the *classic transplantation antigens, H-2K* and *H-2D antigens,* or *serologically defined (SD) antigens.*

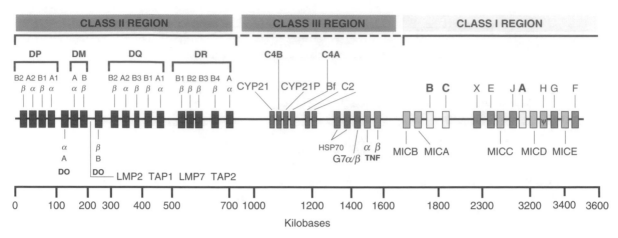

**FIGURE 7-4 HLA complex map.** HLA loci lie on the short arm of chromosome 6. The HLA complex consists of three regions called *class II, III,* and *I* (from left to right). The class II region contains the loci for HLA-DP to DR, the class III region contains the loci for proteins unrelated to MHC molecules, and the class I region contains the loci for HLA-B, -C, -X, -E, -A, -H, -G, and -F. The DP locus lies closest to the centromere, and the F locus is farthest. The class II region is subdivided into several loci, or families. The DP, DO, DM, DQ, and DR families have both α (A) and β (B) loci. Genes considered to be associated with antigen processing (LMP2 and LMP7) and transport (TAP1 and TAP2) are found within the class II region between the DM and DO loci. A group of genes unrelated to MHC genes, located between the DR and B loci (the class III region), encode cytochrome p450 21-hydroxylases (CYP21B and CYP21A), complement molecules (C2, C4A, C4B, and properdin factor B [Bf]), heat shock protein (HSP70), valyl-tRNA synthetase (G7a/b), and TNF-α and -β. (Kilobase distances are not to scale.)

genes include *HLA-E, HLA-F, HLA-G, HLA-J, HLA-X,* (*HLA-H* is a pseudogene [Ψ]), and a family of genes called *MHC class I chain-related (MIC) molecules,* which includes *MICA* through *MICE*; their murine counterparts include three regions downstream from the L region called *H-2Q, H-2T,* and *H-2M.*

The α chains of class I MHC molecules are transmembrane glycoproteins with a molecular weight of about 45 kD (Figure 7-5). They are noncovalently associated with a 12-kD glycoprotein termed $\beta_2$-*microglobulin*[2] that is encoded on human chromosome 15. The $\beta_2$-microglobulin chain is associated with the extracellular part of the class I molecule but is not bound to the cell membrane. The $\beta_2$-microglobulin maintains class I MHC molecules in their native conformation. The class I MHC molecule is about 345 amino acids long with the first 280 residues extracellular, about 25 hydrophobic residues embedded in the plasma membrane, a short stretch of hydrophilic residues, and the remaining 30 residues in the cell. It has three external domains ($\alpha_1, \alpha_2,$ and $\alpha_3$) of about 90 amino acid residues each, a transmembrane region, and a cytoplasmic region. Mouse α chains contain two N-linked oligosaccharides, while their human

counterparts contain one. The polymorphic $\alpha_1$ and $\alpha_2$ domains fold together to form an antigen-binding cleft with a floor consisting of eight-stranded antiparallel β-pleated sheets and the sides consisting of α-helices; the cleft is large enough (about 25 Å × 10 Å × 11 Å) to bind peptides of 8 to 10, usually 9, amino acids. The cleft is closed at its ends so it cannot accommodate larger peptides. The floor of the antigen-binding cleft contains conserved residues that bind the terminal residues of the peptides. It is the peptide-binding site for foreign peptides that are presented to $CD8^+$ $T_C$ cells. *Class I MHC molecules act as receptors for protein antigen-derived peptides.* The importance of class I (and II) MHC molecules as receptors is discussed shortly. The class I molecules not only bind and present peptide but also serve as recognition molecules for $CD8^+$ $T_C$ cells. The nonpolymorphic $\alpha_3$ domain is not involved in peptide binding and presentation, but it does interact with the T-cell coreceptor molecule, CD8 (see Chapters 8 and 10). The $\alpha_3$ domain is considered to be immunoglobulin (Ig)-like because it contains an Ig fold structure. The $\beta_2$-microglobulin molecule also exhibits the Ig fold structure; it is also invariant among all class I molecules. The Ig fold structure places class I molecules and $\beta_2$-microglobulin in the Ig superfamily (see Chapter 4). All three external domains play an important role in both positive (development of MHC

---

[2]The name $\beta_2$-*microglobulin* is derived from its electrophoretic mobility ($\beta_2$), size (*micro*), and solubility (*globulin*).

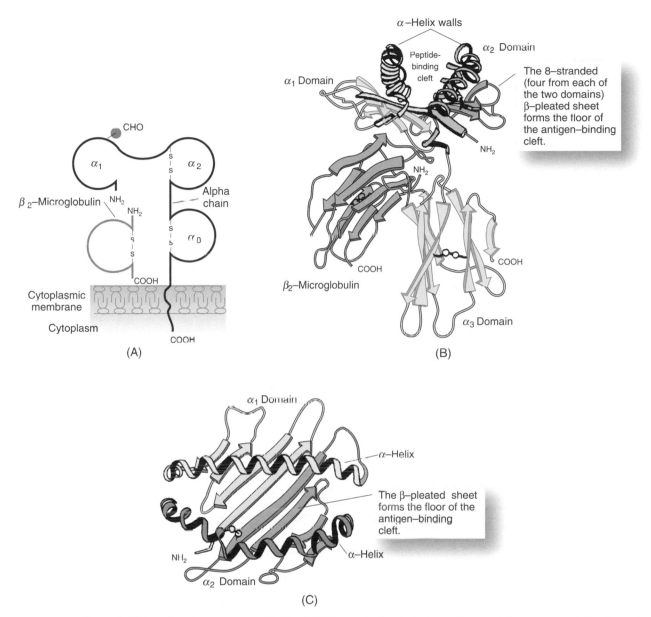

**FIGURE 7-5 Class I MHC molecule structure.** (*A*) The MHC-encoded α chain is made up of three extracellular domains (α₁, α₂, and α₃). The α₁ domain is at the NH-terminal end of the chain, the most distal from the membrane, and contains a carbohydrate (CHO) unit. The second domain (α₂), along with the α₁ domain, is polymorphic and contains the allogeneic determinants unique to each individual. The nonpolymorphic α₃ domain is noncovalently associated with the non-MHC-encoded chain, called β₂-*microglobulin*. The next domain is the 40 amino acid residue transmembrane section of the α chain. A short hydrophilic section followed by 30 amino acid residues of the α chain is found in the cytoplasm. (*B*) The side view of the class I molecule clearly shows its antigen-binding groove. As drawn, the top portion of the class I molecule is distal from the cell membrane while the bottom is proximal to the membrane. The transmembrane and cytoplasmic domains are not shown. (*C*) The view from the top, as the T-cell receptor would see it, shows a representation of the α₁ and α₂ that form the cleft consisting of a base of antiparallel β strands and sides of α helices.

restriction) and negative (development of immunologic tolerance) selection of the T-cell repertoire (see Chapter 13). The 30-amino-acid-long cytoplasmic tail has protein kinase A and *src* tyrosine kinase phosphorylation sites.

Class I molecules require the interaction of $\beta_2$-microglobulin and peptide with the class I molecule to be conformationally stable. In fact, the expression of cell surface class I molecules necessitates the presence of all three components. If a cell cannot produce $\beta_2$-microglobulin, it will not express class I molecules even though the cell is capable of making class I molecules. Furthermore, the associated peptide does not need to be a foreign antigenic peptide, uninfected/normal cells express self-peptides in their class I molecules. So a heterozygous individual codominantly expresses on every nucleated cell the class I molecule encoded by both alleles at each MHC locus (i.e., six different class I molecules, HLA-A, -B, and -C alleles from each parent). Similarly, an $F_1$ mouse inherits K, D, and L alleles from each parent and thus expresses six different class I molecules.

The representative structure for class I genes typical of HLA and H-2 complexes consists of a 5′ leader exon followed by six exons separated by introns (Figure 7-6), which encode the different domains of the class I molecule. Class I molecules are constitutively expressed on almost all nucleated cells, but their level of expression varies for different cell types. Lymphocytes exhibit the highest levels of class I molecule expression (roughly $5 \times 10^5$ molecules per cell), in contrast to cells such as fibroblasts, liver cells, muscle cells, and neural cells that express low levels. Some cells such as neurons and sperm cells do not express class I molecules.

*The $\alpha_1$ and $\alpha_2$ domains of the class I MHC molecule contribute to extreme polymorphism.* Estimates from serologic and functional analyses were mentioned earlier. Each allele is present in high frequency, and the products of these alleles may differ from each other by only a few amino acids. The variable sequences of class I molecules are not distributed throughout the chain, they are bunched in the $\alpha_1$ and $\alpha_2$ domains (Figure 7-7). The distribution pattern for polymorphic amino acid residues of class II MHC molecules is also concentrated in their membrane-distal $\alpha_1$ and $\beta_1$ domains. This polymorphism allows for the variation in the peptide-binding cleft needed to bind the many possible peptides and extends the range of antigens to which the immune system can respond. This polymorphism also

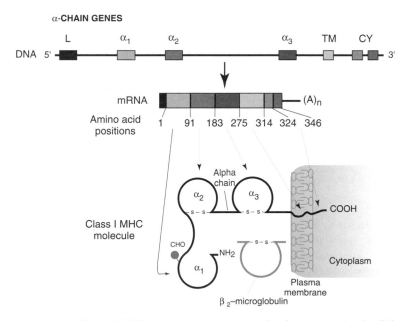

**FIGURE 7-6 Class I MHC gene organization.** The first exon (leader [L] sequence) encodes the signal peptide, which mediates insertion of the peptide into the endoplasmic reticulum during translation. The α chain's three external domains—$\alpha_1$, $\alpha_2$, and $\alpha_3$—are encoded by three exons. The transmembrane (TM) domain is encoded by the next exon. The remaining two exons encode the cytoplasmic (CY) domain(s). $\beta_2$-microglobulin is encode by a gene on a different chromosome.

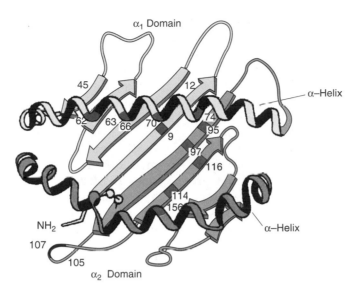

**FIGURE 7-7** The location of polymorphic amino acid residues in the $\alpha_1$ and $\alpha_2$ domains of a class I HLA molecule. (Adapted from P. Parham. 1989. *Nature* **342**:617.)

accounts for the immunogenic differences of class I MHC molecules in different individuals (the reason for graft rejection). Collectively, *class I MHC molecules (1) are highly polymorphic, (2) are found on virtually all nucleated cells, and (3) are targets for $CD8^+$ $T_C$ cells. Traits associated with the expression of class I MHC molecules include (1) graft rejection, (2) MHC restriction of $CD8^+T_C$ cell reactions against cell-surface antigens, (3) stimulation of antibody production, and (4) cell-mediated lysis reactions.*

Although class I MHC molecules are the primary target for $CD8^+$ $T_C$ cells, a host does not normally encounter these as foreign antigens, that is, as transplantation antigens. However, class I regions encode molecules involved in the generation of immunity against our virus-infected, chemically modified cells or tumor cells. The vigorous graft rejection that occurs against class I region-incompatible tissue is mimicked when endogenous "grafts" (such as virally infected cells or tumor cells) arise. $T_C$ cells are not preprogrammed to be occupied with class I MHC molecules on foreign tissue. Instead, they are preoccupied with detecting modified-self class I MHC molecules. Self-class I MHC molecules are required to distinguish between normal and altered self-cells, rather than to simply identify nonself cells.

### MINI SUMMARY

The mouse MHC, or H-2 complex, is located on chromosome 17. The class I—or K, D, and L—regions encode class I molecules. The characteristic combination of H-2 K and H-2 D class I molecules constitutes an H-2 haplotype. Genes encoding class I MHC molecules are extremely polymorphic; polymorphism is clustered in the $\alpha_1$ and $\alpha_2$ domains. The nonpolymorphic $\alpha_3$ domain provides a binding site for the $T_C$ cell's coreceptor CD8. Class I MHC molecules are integral membrane glycoproteins found on almost all nucleated cells. Structurally, they are made up of a polypeptide chain encoded by the MHC, noncovalently associated with another, smaller polypeptide called *$\beta_2$-microglobulin* not encoded by MHC genes.

Human genes of the MHC, or HLA, complex, are arranged close together on chromosome 6. Like the H-2 complex, the human counterpart can be divided into class I, II, and III regions. The class I, or B, C, and A, region, encodes class I cell-surface molecules. Their structures and functions are similar to their mouse equivalents.

### Class II Region Genes Encode Class II Molecules That Present Extracellular Antigenic Peptides to $CD4^+$ T Cells

The HLA complex class II (or D) region is roughly 1000 kilobases upstream from the nearest human class I loci (see Figure 7-4). Three (DP, DQ, and DR) of six subregions encode molecules resembling murine class II MHC molecules, which are designated H-2 I-A and H-2 I-E. DP, DQ, and DR loci contain at least one α- and β-chain pair of genes. The murine class II region, the I (here the letter, not the Roman numeral) region maps between the K and S regions, and is divided into two *subregions*; the linear sequence is I-A and I-E. These formerly called *immune response (Ir) genes* in the I-A and I-E subregions encode the class II MHC molecules. In addition to the genes encoding the classic MHC molecules, the HLA and H-2 class II regions have many genes that encode nonclassic MHC molecules. Pseudogenes also exist in some of these loci. Also, four non-class-II genes are found between the HLA-DM and HLA-DO genes and upstream of the mouse I-A subregion. Two (LMP2 and LMP7) of the four genes are involved with antigen processing and the other two (TAP1 and TAP2) with transport of peptides into the endoplasmic reticulum. Molecules encoded by the DQ locus are equivalent to the mouse I-A subregion-encoded molecules, while those encoded by the DR locus are similar to the I-E subregion-encoded molecules of the mouse.

Class II MHC molecules are assembled from a 32 to 34 kD α chain and a 29 to 32 kD β chain and associated with one another by noncovalent interactions (Figure 7-8). Unlike class I molecules, both class II molecule chains are encoded by MHC genes. Both chains are transmembrane proteins with a cytoplasmic, hydrophilic carboxyl terminus. As in the mouse, each chain consists of four domains. The two extracellular domains in each chain (the membrane-distal domains $\alpha_1$ and $\beta_1$, and the membrane-proximal domains $\alpha_2$ and $\beta_2$) are about 90 amino acids each. Both the α and β chains have a short (11–13 amino acids) hydrophilic peptide that connects the extracellular domains to a short (22 amino acids), membrane-binding, hydrophobic region and a short (15 amino acids), hydrophilic C-terminal domain located in the cytoplasm. The polymorphic class II molecule $\alpha_1$ and $\beta_1$ domains are analogous to the class I molecule $\alpha_1$ and $\alpha_2$ domains, they contain the antigen-binding site for processed antigenic peptides; they are the domains recognized by antigen receptor of CD4$^+$ T cells. Polymorphic amino acid residues concentrating in the α-helical sides and β-pleated sheet floor of the peptide-binding site provide the diversity for different peptide specificities and affinities. The overall antigen-binding cleft of the class II molecule is similar to its class I molecule counterpart, the $\alpha_1$ domain contributes four floor strands and one of the α helix walls and $\beta_1$ domain contributes the other four floor strands and the other α helix wall. Unlike the class I molecule, the class II molecule antigen-binding cleft has open ends, so it can accommodate larger peptides (range in size from 13–18 amino acid residues, perhaps larger). The class II molecule membrane-proximal domains $\alpha_2$ and $\beta_2$ are nonpolymorphic and folded into Ig-like domains, placing class II molecules in the Ig superfamily. The $\beta_2$ domain (perhaps also the $\alpha_2$ domain) provides the binding site for the coreceptor CD4 molecules of $T_H$ cells. X-ray crystallography shows that the three-dimensional structure of class II MHC molecules is similar to that of class I MHC molecules. However, unlike class I MHC molecules, class II MHC molecules occur as a dimer of αβ heterodimers with their antigen-binding clefts orientated in opposite directions that allows simultaneous interaction with two T-cell receptor complexes. The other major difference between class I and class II molecules is their difference in peptide-MHC molecule interactions (discussed in later). Class II MHC molecules bind and present extracellular peptides to CD4$^+$ T cells. The domains of human class II α and β chains have strong homology with the appropriate murine class II MHC molecules domains.

Like class I MHC molecules, class II MHC molecules are heterodimeric cell-surface glycoproteins but are expressed primarily on antigen-presenting cells (APCs; macrophages, dendritic cells, B cells, thymic epithelial cells, and some other cells, such as human endothelial cells that can be induced to express class II MHC molecules). Class II MHC molecules regulate the recognition of foreign antigenic peptides derived from extracellular antigens presented by APCs to CD4$^+$ T cells, most of which are helper T ($T_H$) cells.

Like class I MHC molecules, class II MHC molecules are highly polymorphic cell-surface proteins. This polymorphism in class II molecules leads to variation at the peptide-binding sites and TCR interaction sites. Although activated human and rat T cells express class II molecules, activated mouse T cells do not (the functional significance of class II expression on human T cells is uncertain but *in vitro* and *in vivo* evidence supports an APC function for T cells).[3] The specialized classes of dendritic cortical epithelial cells of the thymus and dendritic cells in the secondary lymphoid organs express high levels of class II MHC molecules. These cells are important in thymic selection of T cells and the presentation of

---

[3]In their guise as APCs, class II$^+$ human T cells downregulate the immune response by inducing anergy in T cells that have already been activated and cytotoxicity in resting T cells. This inhibitory mechanism may be important for T-cell homeostasis.

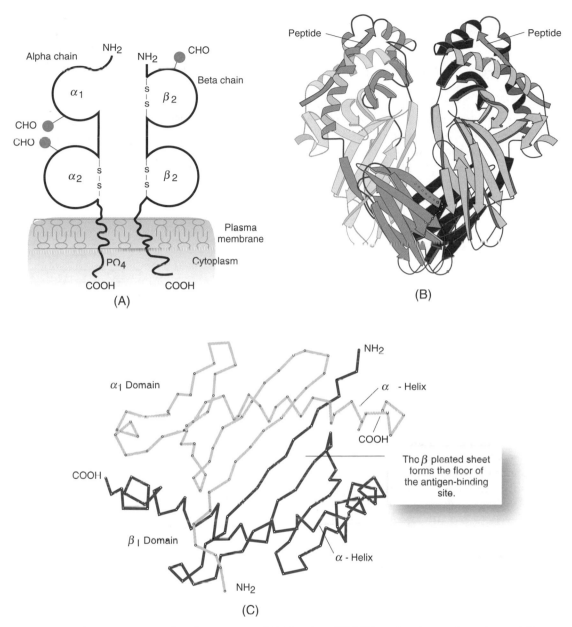

**FIGURE 7-8 Class II MHC molecule structure.** (A) The class II MHC molecule consists of two different chains (α and β) that are noncovalently linked. Each chain has four domains. Two domains for each chain are extracellular, one section of each chain is embedded within the plasma membrane, and each chain has a short tail in the cytoplasm. Both chains have carbohydrate (CHO) units attached, but more CHO is on the α chain. (B) The side view of the crystallized class II molecule, which cocrystallized as a dimer of the αβ heterodimer shown in A. One class II molecule is shaded in red and orange, the other in black and gray, and the peptides as blue arrows. The α chains are shaded lighter, while the β chains are shaded darker. (C) The crystalline structure of a class II MHC molecule (top view) as it might appear to a T-cell receptor. The overall structure is similar to that of the class I MHC molecule. The β-pleated sheet that forms the floor of antigen-binding groove is made up of the α1 (orange) and β1 (red) domains. (Adapted from J.H. Brown et al. 1993. *Nature* **364**:33.)

antigen to naïve T cells, respectively. *Class II MHC molecules are needed in the following interactions: (1) APCs presenting foreign peptide in association with class II MHC molecules to the right CD4⁺ T cells and (2) B-cell and T_H-cell cooperation requiring class II MHC marker recognition by CD4⁺ T cells.*

Both the α and β chains of the class II molecules are encoded within the class II region of the human and murine MHC. The class II chains also associate with a nonpolymorphic molecule that is encoded by a gene outside the MHC. This transiently connected chain is called the γ, or the *invariant, chain* (CD74) and associates with newly synthesized class II MHC molecules. The invariant chain makes the class II molecule peptide-binding sites inaccessible to antigenic peptides while in the endoplasmic reticulum. It also affects the cellular routing of the class II molecule-antigen complex during antigen processing.

Class II molecules require the interaction of an α chain, a β chain, and a bound antigenic peptide to make it conformationally stable. In fact, the expression of cell surface class II molecules necessitates the presence of all three components. In the absence of antigenic peptide, the APC will not express class II molecules. As class I molecules, the associated peptide does not need to be a foreign antigenic peptide, APCs not processing foreign antigen express self-peptides in their class II molecules. A heterozygous individual codominantly expresses on all APCs the class II molecule encoded by both alleles inherited from each parent (i.e., one set of HLA-DP, -DQ, and -DR alleles from each parent). Similarly, an F₁ mouse inherits I-A and I-E alleles from each parent. However, class II molecules are composed of two different chains encoded by two different genes; therefore heterozygous individuals will not only express the six parental class II molecule alleles but also molecules containing α and β chains from different chromosomes (i.e., six parental class II molecules and six class II molecules containing α and β chains from combinations from either parent). The number of class II molecules is further increased in humans and mice because they have multiple β-chain genes; humans also have multiple α-chain genes. These combinations lead to roughly 10 to 20 different class II molecules. Figure 7-9 illustrates this process for humans.

Structures of the genes encoding the α and β chains of class II MHC molecules of humans and mice are shown in Figure 7-10. The genes are organized with 5′ leader exon, followed by α₁ or β₁, α₂ or β₂, transmembrane exon, and ending with one or more cytoplasmic exons. The expression of class II MHC molecules is tightly regulated at the transcriptional

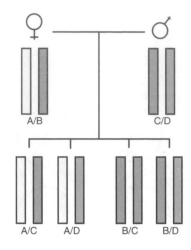

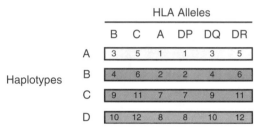

**FIGURE 7-9 A hypothetical example of the codominant expression of class I and class II MHC molecules on a human APC.** All APCs that express class I MHC molecules express two different alleles if the individual is heterozygous at a particular locus. For example, the macrophages of an individual heterozygous at the class I HLA -A, -B, and -C alleles will express six different class I α chains each with an identical β₂-microglobulin, which may be derived from either parent. At its simplest level, six different class II molecules (DP, DQ, and DR from each parent) would be expressed (shown here); however, the α chains of one class II allele can combine with β chains of the same or other allele for that locus, which leads to an increased number of different class II molecules expressed.

level by cell-specific transcriptional factors and by specific cytokines (discussed later). In contrast to class I MHC molecules, which are constitutively expressed on almost all nucleated cells, class II MHC molecules are normally expressed only on APCs, dendritic cells, macrophages, B cells, and a few other cell types (Table 7-3). As with class I MHC molecules, differences in class II MHC molecule expression exist among class II⁺ MHC–expressing cells. However, unlike class I molecules, class II molecule expression increases following exposure to certain cytokines (discussed later). Class II molecule expression is downregulated by agents such as corticosteroids, prostaglandins, and some viruses. These same viruses can downregulate class I molecule expression.

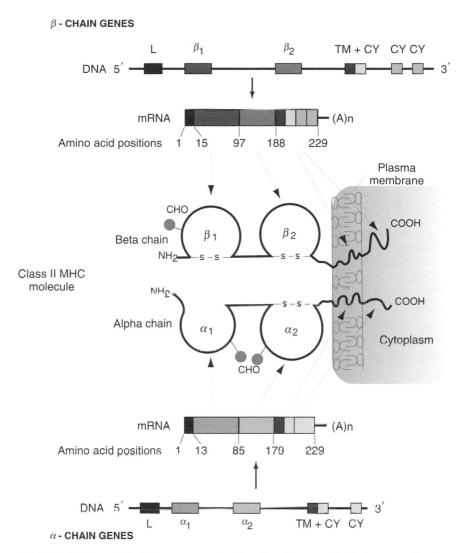

**FIGURE 7-10  Class II MHC gene organization.** For the α- and β-chain genes, the first exon encodes leader (L) signal peptide, which has the same function as described for the class I MHC molecule genes. The second and third exons encode the $\alpha_1$ and $\alpha_2$ or $\beta_1$ and $\beta_2$ domains. The fourth exon for the α-chain gene encodes the transmembrane (TM) domain, the short cytoplasmic (CY) domain, and the last exon encodes the remainder of the cytoplasmic portion. Exons four and five for the β genes encode slightly different regions than the α genes. The fourth, excluding L exon, β-gene exon encodes the TM domain and part of the CY domain. The next two exons encode the remainder of the CY domain. The regulatory sequences (not shown) are 5' to the leader sequences, which include (from the 5' terminus) W, $X_1$, $X_2$, Y, (SXY module; mentioned later in the chapter) and TATA.

To close our discussion on the class II MHC region, let us summarize by restating that *the class II MHC genes (formerly called Ir genes but a good functional description) from these regions encode class II MHC molecules that are found primarily on APCs, dendritic cells, macrophages, and B cells.* These molecules permit $CD4^+$ $T_H$ cells to "see" antigen and activate other specific immune cells.

## Class III Region Genes Encode Class III Molecules, Some Complement Proteins, Cytokines, and Other Proteins Unrelated to MHC Class I and Class II Molecules

The remaining MHC region of humans and mice is called the **class III region**. The human and mouse class III regions contain a heterogeneous assemblage

**TABLE 7-3** Cellular Distribution of Class II MHC Molecules

| Cells | Level of class II MHC molecule expression and expression following exposure to cytokines |
|---|---|
| Macrophages | Weak; increased by interferon-γ (IFN-γ) |
| B cells | Constitutive; decreased by IFN-γ, increased by IL-4 |
| T cells | During activation in humans and rats but not mice |
| Dendritic cells | Constitutive; increased by TNF-α |
| Langerhans cells | Constitutive; increased by IFN-γ |
| Endothelial cells | No expression; induced by high levels of IFN-γ |
| Epithelial cells/stromal cells | No expression; induced by high levels of IFN-γ |

of genes. The genes that encode class III molecules are located between the class I and class II regions of both the HLA (between HLA-DR and HLA-B subregions) (see Figure 7-4) and H-2 (sometimes called the *S region* and is situated between the I and D regions) complexes. Class III region genes encode the complement molecules C2, C4A, and C4B, and the associated complement molecule properdin factor B (Bf). Genes for two steroids cytochrome p450 21-hydroxylases (CYP21 and CYP21P), two heat-shock proteins (HSP70), valyl-tRNA synthetase (G7a/b), and the two cytokines TNF-α and -β are found in this region. Mouse class III genes have functions equivalent to those of their human counterparts.

---

**MINI SUMMARY**

The human and murine class II MHC regions are divided into subregions. The HLA D region is divided into many subregions; the best-characterized ones are called DP, DQ, and DR. The I region of the H-2 complex, situated between the K and S regions is divided into two subregions, called I-A and I-E. Unlike the class I genes, the class II genes encode membrane glycoproteins expressed mainly on APCs, dendritic cells, macrophages, and B cells. Structurally, class II MHC molecules consist of two noncovalently linked polypeptide chains, called α and β. MHC genes encode both chains. The $\alpha_1$ and $\beta_1$ domains of the respective chains contribute to their polymorphism; both domains form the antigen-binding cleft. The nonpolymorphic $\alpha_2$

and $\beta_2$ domains provide sites for the coreceptor CD4 to bind. The class II MHC molecules are critical in immune cell interactions.

The human class III genes are situated between the DR and B subregions; the murine S region is situated between the I and D regions. The class III region of both species contains genes that encode complement proteins, specific enzymes, heat-shock proteins, and the cytokines TNF-α and -β.

---

# THE IMMUNE RESPONSE IS MHC-LINKED; THE GENES ENCODE STRUCTURES THAT ALLOW IMMUNE FUNCTIONS

A hint of the function of MHC molecules came from early experiments by Benacerraf and his co-workers, who were attempting to produce a homogeneous preparation of antibodies by immunizing guinea pigs with simple synthetic polypeptides. Some animals produced antibodies, while others did not. Further investigations by Benacerraf, McDevitt, and Sela and their respective collaborators confirmed that the host's ability to respond to selected antigens is controlled by inherited genes. For example, an animal carrying a particular MHC gene might respond to a given antigen; another animal carrying a different MHC gene might not respond. In these *responder* and *nonresponder animals*, the MHC appeared to function as then called *immune response (Ir) genes*. The discovery by other researchers that these genes are located within the mouse MHC evoked the required investigations for decoding the complexity surrounding the control of immune responses.

Most of our understanding of the control of the immune response comes from observations that inbred animals develop different degrees of immunity (from high to low to no response) when exposed to antigens. Responsiveness to these antigens is transferred to offspring in a Mendelian fashion. Development of antibody and/or cellular immunity is controlled by MHC-linked autosomal dominant "Ir" genes. The following examples (experiments performed by Benacerraf and McDevitt) suggest that was the case.

When outbred Hartley guinea pigs were immunized with dinitrophenylated poly-L-lysine

(DNP-PLL), 30% of them produced anti-DNP antibodies and were called *responders* (strain 2). Others did not respond in a humoral fashion and were called *nonresponders* (strain 13). Breeding experiments suggested that the ability to respond to DNP-PLL by producing antibodies is controlled by a dominant autosomal gene.

Later breeding experiments used the strain 2 and strain 13 guinea pigs to determine if responsiveness was associated with one gene or a group of linked genes. The experiments consisted of immunizing strain 2 and 13 guinea pigs ($2\times13$)$F_1$ progeny, and ($2\times13$)$F_1 \times 2$ and ($2\times13$)$F_1 \times 13$ backcrossed guinea pigs with DNP-PLL, glutamic acid-alanine (GA) copolymer, or glutamic acid-tyrosine (GT) copolymer. The results, given in Table 7-4, show that immune responsiveness to these antigens (1) was limited to certain strains of guinea pigs, (2) was segregated to different genetic regions of different strains (that is, the ability to respond to the antigens was transmitted to the $F_1$ progeny as a dominant trait), and (3) was under MHC-gene control and

highly specific because the reverse responsive ability held true for the antigen GT.

The use of inbred mice by McDevitt allowed for fine-tuning of the contribution of MHC genes to immune response control. The "Ir" genes, which control the immune response to many antigens, were mapped to the class II region of the H-2 complex (Table 7-5). To summarize, *a direct relationship exists between an animal's MHC haplotype and its ability or inability to respond to a specific antigen.* The explanation for this variability in immune responsiveness is presented later in the chapter.

The localization of class II region genes in the same region of the chromosome as the "Ir" genes prompted the idea that the class II MHC molecules may be the products of these genes. Characterization of class II region gene function began with the production of antibody against MHC molecules (Figure 7-11). These antibodies blocked antigen-specific $T_H$ cells from interacting with the appropriate antigen on APCs. Thus, the $T_H$ cell recognized protein antigen only in association with one particular class II

**TABLE 7-4 Relationships Between Inheritance of Ir Genes and the MHC Loci of Strain 2 and 13, ($2\times13$)$F_1$, and Backcrossed Animals**

| Antigens | Immune responsiveness of different strains | | | | |
| --- | --- | --- | --- | --- | --- |
| | 2 | 13 | ($2 \times 13$)$F_1$ | ($2 \times 13$)$F_1 \times 2$ | ($2 \times 13$)$F_1 \times 13$ |
| DNP-PLL | + | − | + | + (100%)* <br> − (50%) | + (50%) |
| GA | + | − | + | + (100%) <br> − (50%) | + (50%) |
| GT | − | + | + | + (50%) <br> − (50%) | + (100%) |

*Numbers in parentheses represent the percentages of animals producing (+) or not producing (−) antibody to the immunizing antigen when $F_1$ progeny (heterozygotes) are backcrossed with either homozygous responders or nonresponders.

**TABLE 7-5 Immune Responsiveness of Various H-2 Haplotypes**

| H-2 haplotype | Representative strains | Immune response to the following antigens* | | | | |
| --- | --- | --- | --- | --- | --- | --- |
| | | BGG | OVA | GA | GLPhe | (T,G)-A-L |
| a | A | + | − | + | − | − |
| b | C57BL/6 <br> C57BL/10 | − | + | + | − | + |
| d | BALB/c <br> DBA/2 | − | + | + | + | ± |
| k | AKR <br> CBA <br> C3H | + | − | + | − | − |
| s | SLJ | ? | ± | + | − | − |

*The production of (+) or no production of (−) specific antibody following immunization with antigen. The antigen abbreviations are: BGG, bovine gamma globulin; OVA, ovalbumin; GA, glutamic acid-alanine copolymer; GLPhe, glutamic acid-lysine-phenylalanine; (T,G)-A-L, (tyrosine-glutamic acid)-alanine-lysine copolymer.

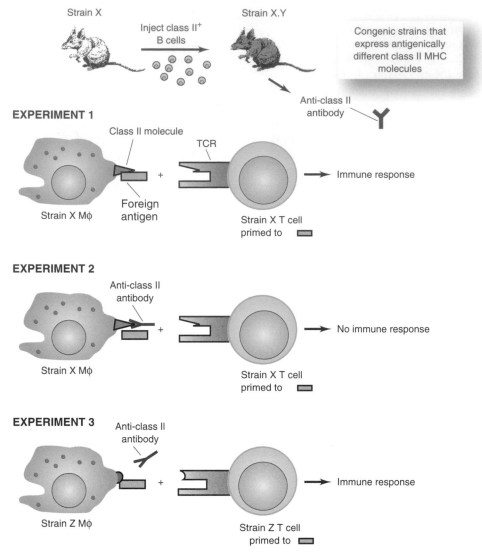

**FIGURE 7-11 Blocking class II MHC molecules inhibits cellular interaction**. Reciprocal immunization of different congenic H-2 recombinant mouse strains (or strain 2 and strain 13 guinea pigs) with each other's lymphoid cells evoked antibodies specific for antigenic determinants on class II (Ia) MHC molecules. Primed T cells need to interact with antigen presented in association with class II molecules on macrophages (Mφ) (Experiment 1). Masking of Mφ class II MHC molecules by these antibodies blocked the response of primed T cells to their respective priming antigen (Experiment 2). In Experiment 3 an immune response occurs because anti-X-Ia antibodies are specific for Strain X Ia molecules; therefore, they cannot block strain Z Ia molecules.

MHC molecule. This phenomenon is called **MHC restriction** (detailed in later in chapter); *the T cell simultaneously recognizes a protein antigen-derived peptide and a self class II (or I) MHC molecule displayed by an APC. Thus, T cells must recognize both self and nonself together. The formerly called Ir-gene products (now called class II MHC molecules) supply the vehicle for cellular interactions and permit specific regulation of the immune response.*

Two models have been proposed to explain how the MHC genes influence the immune response: (1) the **determinant-selection model**, *in which the failure of some MHC molecules to bind certain antigens underlies the genetic unresponsiveness of some hosts*; and, (2) the **holes-in-the-repertoire model**, *in which the MHC influences the immune response by shaping the repertoire of functional T cells*. The determinant-selection model accounts for the results shown in Tables 7-4 and 7-5 by proposing that immune response variabilities are caused by MHC polymorphism within a species, which generates differences in MHC molecule structure. These differences in structure affect the strength of MHC molecule interactions with a given processed antigen. Some of the most compelling evidence for the determinant-selection model is derived from competitive binding studies using various antigenic peptides and purified class II MHC molecules. Usually, the capacity of particular class II MHC molecules to bind an antigenic peptide parallels the responder status of that haplotype (Table 7-6); for example, BALB/c and DBA/2 mice are of the $H-2^d$ haplotype and are good

responders to ovalbumin (see Table 7-5). In contrast, the holes-in-the-repertoire model accounts for the results in Tables 7-4 and 7-5 by proposing the absence of T cells that can recognize a given antigen-MHC molecule complex. If a peptide binds to the appropriate MHC molecule in a certain inbred mouse strain but does not stimulate a response in that strain, the strain probably lacks (by clonal deletion or anergy) the responsive T cells (Table 7-7). *The melding of these two models suggests that the selectivity of MHC molecules binding antigens combines with holes-in-the-T-cell repertoire to set the boundaries of an individual's immune responsiveness.* The antigen specificity and class II

**TABLE 7-6  The Relationship Between MHC Restriction and Binding of Peptides to Class II MHC Molecules**

| Labeled peptide | Percentage of labeled peptide bound to | | | | Competitive Inhibition of OVA (323–339) binding to I-A$^d$ by unrelated peptides |
|---|---|---|---|---|---|
| | I-A$^d$ | I-E$^d$ | I-A$^k$ | I-E$^k$ | |
| Ovalbumin (323–339) | **11.8** | 0.1 | 0.2 | 0.1 | |
| Influenza hemagglutinin (130–142) | **18.9** | 0.6 | 7.1 | 0.3 | + + ++ |
| Hen-egg lysozyme (46–61) | 0.0 | 0.0 | **35.2** | 0.5 | |
| Hen-egg lysozyme (74–86) | 2.0 | 2.3 | **2.9** | 1.7 | ++ |
| Hen-egg lysozyme (81–96) | 0.4 | 0.2 | 0.7 | **1.1** | |
| Myoglobin (132–153) | 0.8 | **6.3** | 0.5 | 0.7 | |
| Pigeon Cytochrome (88–104) | 0.6 | 1.2 | 1.7 | **8.7** | ⊥ |
| Mouse Cytochrome (88–103) | 0.1 | 1.0 | 1.7 | **5.3** | |
| λ repressor protein (12–26) | 1.6 | **8.9** | 0.3 | 2.3 | ++ |

*Note:* The results show that different peptides can bind to the same purified class II MHC molecules. Also, the peptides that block (ranging from slightly [±] to highly inhibitory [+ + ++]) ovalbumin (OVA) (323–339) binding to the appropriate class II MHC molecule are also effective in competing with APC presentation of that peptide to OVA (323–339)-specific T cells (not shown). The boldface numbers represent significant binding and show known MHC restrictions of those peptides, that is, OVA is I-A$^d$-restricted, and so on. The numbers in parentheses indicate the amino acid residues included in each peptide.
Source: Adapted from S. Buus et. al. 1987. *Science* **235**:1353.

**TABLE 7-7  The Relationship Between MHC Binding of Processed Antigen and T-Cell Stimulation**

| Hen-egg lysozyme peptide | | | | | | | | | | | |
|---|---|---|---|---|---|---|---|---|---|---|---|
| (Amino acid residue position numbers) | | | | | | | | | | | |
| 52 | 53 | 54 | 55 | 56 | 57 | 58 | 59 | 60 | 61 | Binding to I-A$^k$ | Stimulation of specific T cells |
| 1. Asp | Tyr | Gly | Ile | Leu | Gln | Ile | Asn | Ser | Arg | + | + |
| 2. Asp | Tyr | Gly | Ile | **Phe** | Gln | Ile | Asn | Ser | Arg | + | − |
| 3. Asp | **Ala** | Gly | Ile | Phe | Gln | Ile | Asn | Ser | Arg | + | − |
| 4. Asp | Tyr | Gly | Ile | Leu | Gln | Ile | Asn | Ser | **Ala** | − | − |
| 5. Asp | Ala | Gly | **Ala** | Phe | Gln | Ile | Asn | Ser | Ala | + | + |

*Note:* Peptide 1 is the native hen-egg lysosome (fragment 52–61) that binds to the murine MHC class II I-A$^k$ molecule and stimulates a panel of T-cell hybridomas. Peptides 2 through 5 are synthetic versions of peptide 1 that differed by single amino acid substitutions (boldface numbers). Peptides 2 and 3 bind to the class II MHC molecule but do not stimulate T cells, suggesting that residues 56 and 53 are not critical for binding but are critical for contacting the TCR. Peptide 4 neither binds to the MHC molecule nor stimulates T cells, suggesting that Arg 61 may be involved in contacting the class II MHC molecule. Peptide 5 binds to the MHC molecule and stimulates T cells, suggesting that Ile at position 55 is not critical for binding to the MHC molecule or to the TCR. Asp 52, Ile 58, and Arg 61 contact the MHC molecule, while Try 53, Leu 56, and Gln 57 contact the TCR. The remaining four residues are not involved in either function and may serve as spacer residues.
Source: Adapted from E.R. Unanue and P.M. Allen. 1987. *Science* **236**:551.

**IMMUNE RESPONSE**

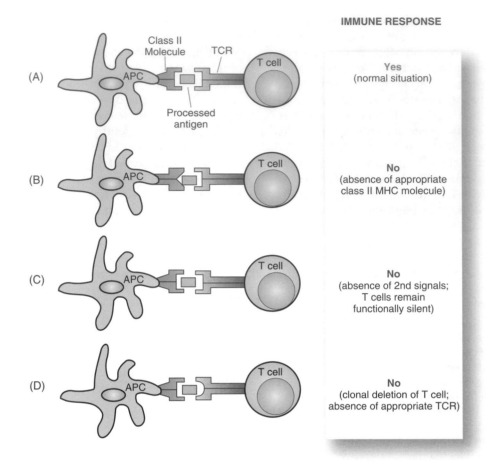

**FIGURE 7-12 The MHC can influence immune responsiveness.** (*A*) This scenario represents the typical interaction required between an APC and a T cell for a normal immune response to occur. (*B*) The host does not have the appropriate MHC genes to encode the required MHC molecule. (*C*) The host has the right MHC molecule and TCR for interaction to occur, but the T cell does not receive a second signal (surface activation molecules and cytokines). (*D*) The reactive T cell has been deleted during maturation.

gene- (Ir-gene) regulation of immune responsiveness to the antigen are explained in three ways in Figure 7-12.

## MINI SUMMARY

''Ir'' genes (now called class II genes) are associated with the MHC and control immune responsiveness. An animal's haplotype dictates its ability or inability to respond to a specific antigen.

For T cells to control an immune response, they must recognize foreign antigen in association with one particular class II MHC molecule. Specific class II MHC molecules provide the vehicles for cellular interactions and the basis for the specific regulation of the immune response.

# MHC RESTRICTION MEANS THAT T CELLS ARE PROGRAMMED TO INTERACT WITH FOREIGN PEPTIDES ON CELLS ONLY IN ASSOCIATION WITH CLASS I OR CLASS II MHC MOLECULES

Unlike B cells, which can bind free antigen, T cells cannot. T-cell receptors recognize complexes composed of antigen-derived peptides and self-MHC molecules. Thus, MHC-restricted recognition prevents the activation of T cells by circulating free antigen. T cells mediating cell-cell interactions are activated and deliver signals only when they interact with target cells displaying foreign peptides. These activated T cells are either class II MHC-restricted CD4$^+$ T cells, which as T$_H$ cells mediate cooperative functions, or class I MHC-restricted CD8$^+$ T cells, which as T$_C$ cells mediate cytotoxic functions (Figure 7-13). The target cells can be APCs but are generally thought of as cells bearing foreign antigen (such as virally infected cells or tumor cells).

MHC-restricted interplay between activated T cells and APCs or target cells occurs when MHC-restricted T cells simultaneously recognize foreign epitopes on presented peptides and MHC molecules (how MHC molecules bind peptides will be discussed later). Class II genes control restriction between CD4$^+$ T$_H$ cells and APCs. Class I MHC molecules act as antigen-presenting structures and restriction elements directing the attack of CD8$^+$ T$_C$ cells against virally infected cells, chemically modified cells, cells of transplanted tissues, and tumor cells. For a T$_C$ cell to react to cell-bound antigen, the T$_C$ cell must simultaneously recognize antigenic peptide and self-class I MHC molecules. Class I MHC restriction molecules are expressed on nearly all nucleated cells because all cells can be parasitized. Class I MHC molecules associated with foreign peptides alert CD8$^+$ T$_C$ cells to the presence of body cells that have been changed for the worse and need to be eliminated. Class II-restriction molecules are expressed primarily on cooperative cells (the APCs macrophages, dendritic cells, and B cells).[4] Class II MHC molecules combine with peptides derived from foreign antigen in a way that showcases the antigen and captures the attention of the CD4$^+$ T$_H$ cell. *This controlled restriction is the basis for the functional specificity of T lymphocytes.* Thus, T cells react to peptide-derived protein antigen only in association with self-class I or -class II MHC molecules.

The following experiments dramatize the fact that immune cells must concurrently recognize self and nonself for an immune response to occur. Results from experiments dealing with MHC-restricted recognition between (1) T and B cells, (2) macrophages and T cells, and (3) T cells and virally infected target cells will be briefly summarized.

For antigen-specific antibodies to be produced, T$_H$ cells and B cells must interact. Figure 7-14 shows

that T$_H$-B-cell interactions are dependent on only H-2 I region (class II MHC region) commonality. When the class II MHC region is the same, cooperation occurs that leads to antibody production (see Chapter 10 for further details).

Macrophages are front-line defenders that seize and display antigen interaction pieces on their surfaces to CD4$^+$ T cells. To test the "immunologic literacy" between macrophages and T cells (MHC restriction), antigen-pulsed macrophages are mixed with T cells of the same or different MHC haplotype. Figure 7-15 shows that macrophages can present antigen in a successful manner only to T cells that share the same MHC haplotype. A successful T-cell proliferative response to antigen occurs when the T cells and macrophages come from hosts of the same strain.

The self-MHC restriction of CD8$^+$ T$_C$ cells is presented in Figure 7-16. Comparative assessment of the cytotoxic ability of mouse T$_C$ cells mixed with virally infected target cells from the same or different haplotype mice suggested that class I MHC restriction controls T$_C$-cell activity. T$_C$ cells kill only syngeneic infected targets. Studies using congenic strains of mice showed that T$_C$ cells and target cells must share class I MHC molecules encoded by either the K or D MHC regions. Thus, T$_C$ cells are class I MHC restricted. Zinkernagel and Doherty received the 1996 Nobel Prize for this and other work that contributed to the understanding of cell-mediated immunity.

---

> **MINI SUMMARY**
>
> CD4$^+$ T$_H$ cells recognize antigen only when antigenic peptide is presented with class II MHC region-encoded molecules on APCs. In contrast, virally infected target cells and their specific CD8$^+$ T$_C$ cells can interact only when proper class I MHC region-encoded molecules on target cells plus associated foreign peptide are there to bind with TCRs on T$_C$ cells. This controlled MHC restriction is the genetic basis for the functional specificity of T lymphocytes. T cells react to foreign antigen only when it is associated with self-class I or II MHC molecules.

# MHC MOLECULES ARE PROMISCUOUS ANTIGEN RECEPTORS

The realization that the immune system did not develop MHC molecules to protect us against

---

[4]The further importance of class II MHC restriction is seen by making nonimmune class II$^-$ cells competent APCs, that is, transfecting fibroblasts with genes encoding the α and β chains of class II MHC molecules. The fibroblasts now can present antigen to CD4$^+$ T cells. (See Chapter 5 for a description of transfection.)

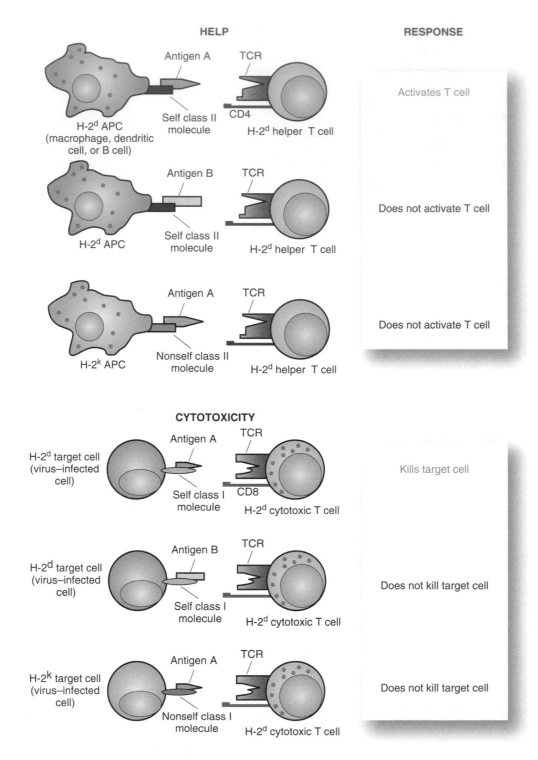

**FIGURE 7-13 MHC restriction of helper and cytotoxic T cells.** CD4$^+$ T$_H$ cells are activated by antigen presented in association with class II MHC molecules on APCs (such as dendritic cells, macrophages, or B cells). In contrast, CD8$^+$ T$_C$ cells are activated by antigen presented in association with class I MHC molecules on APCs, better known as *target cells* (such as virally infected cells.)

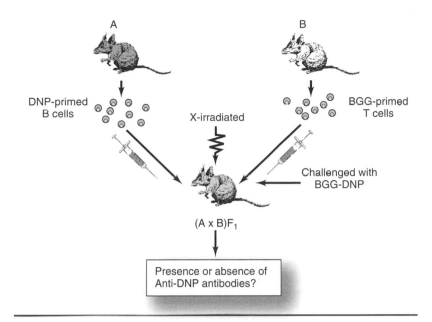

| H-2 haplotype (K I S D) | | H-2 region differences | Cooperation |
|---|---|---|---|
| B cells | T cells | | |
| skkd | kkkk | K + D | + |
| skkd | kkdd | K + S | + |
| kkdd | skkd | K + S | + |
| kkkd | skkd | K | + |
| kkkd | kkdd | S | + |
| sssd | skkd | I + S | − |
| sssd | kkdd | K + I + S | − |
| ssss | skkd | I + S + D | − |
| ssss | kkdd | K + I + S + D | − |

**FIGURE 7-14 MHC restriction of T- and B-lymphocyte cooperation in antibody production.** Congenic mice differing at various H-2 loci were immunized with bovine gamma globulin (BGG) or dinitrophenyl (DNP), and T and B cells, respectively, were collected. The harvested cells were adoptively transferred into irradiated $F_1$ recipients, challenged with BGG-DNP, and the anti-DNP antibody response measured. A successful (+) cooperative interaction led to anti-DNP antibody formation. Further proof for the class II-region restriction of this interaction can be provided by blocking studies; that is, the response can be blocked by preincubating the B cells with anti-class II MHC molecule (anti-I-A or -I-E) antibodies (see Figure 7-11.)

attacking transplants even though self-cells altered by infection were "rejected" like transplanted cells suggested that MHC molecules were displaying antigen. The antigenic universe is large, to say the least, yet we express a limited number of MHC molecules. Furthermore, every antigenic peptide that an immune response is directed against must be able to associate with an MHC molecule—class I and class II MHC molecules bind and present antigen to $CD8^+$ T cells and $CD4^+$ T cells, respectively. The fine specificity associated with Ig and TCRs does not carry over into MHC molecules. Each MHC

molecule shows a broad specificity for peptide binding; therefore, MHC molecule-peptide binding is considered promiscuous.

In 1987, the crystallographic structure of a human class I MHC molecule was described. The molecular structure clearly showed the presence of an antigen-binding cleft composed of a β-pleated sheet floor bordered on its sides by two long α-helices, separated by an 11-Å-deep groove 25 Å long and 10 Å wide located on the top surface of the molecule (see Figure 7-5). In fact, the cleft contained a piece of processed antigen, which suggested that class I, and

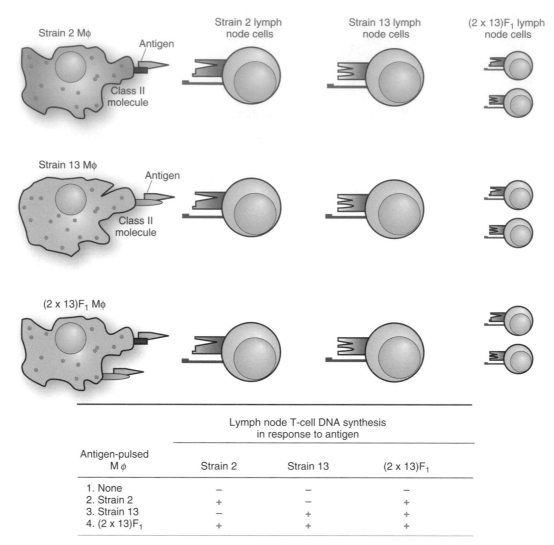

| Antigen-pulsed Mφ | Lymph node T-cell DNA synthesis in response to antigen | | |
|---|---|---|---|
| | Strain 2 | Strain 13 | (2 × 13)F₁ |
| 1. None | – | – | – |
| 2. Strain 2 | + | – | + |
| 3. Strain 13 | – | + | + |
| 4. (2 × 13)F₁ | + | + | + |

**FIGURE 7-15  MHC restriction of T-lymphocyte and macrophage (Mφ) cooperation in T-cell activation.** Lymph node T cells from either strain 2, strain 13, or (2×13)F₁ antigen-immunized guinea pigs were cocultured with no Mφs or antigen-pulsed Mφs from either strain 2, strain 13, or (2 × 13)F₁ guinea pigs. The pulsed Mφs present antigen in association with class II MHC molecules. The mixture is incubated for 72 hr, and cellular division is measured by the uptake of a radiolabel into the proliferating T cells. Proliferation is indicated by a + sign and no proliferation by a – sign. Even though Mφs are required for induction of T-cell proliferation, T cells respond only when antigen is presented by Mφs with the same haplotype (syngeneic Mφs.)

probably class II, MHC molecules behave like receptors that have one binding site for peptides from the original intact foreign protein. *MHC molecules are peptide receptors*—self-MHC molecules are cell-surface receptors, which present noncovalently attached peptides derived from foreign proteins to T cells. In addition to their structure, the polymorphism of MHC molecules supports their receptor role. In fact, most of the known polymorphic amino acids of the class I MHC molecule are in the antigen-binding groove (see Figure 7-7), as are the residues important for T-cell recognition. Despite their extreme polymorphism, MHC molecules have only one binding site

for many different peptides. Because each individual expresses six different class I molecules and up to 12 different class II MHC molecules, each MHC molecule must display many different peptides. Furthermore, MHC molecules bind peptides tightly ($K_d \cong 10^{-6}M$), and when proteins bind tightly, the fit is very specific. How can a single MHC molecule, which binds with high affinity to peptides, act as a specific receptor when it must bind a sizable part of the antigenic universe? As will be shown, MHC molecules recognize the amino acid side chains and do not bother as much with the peptide's backbone structure that differ from peptide to peptide. These features allow an

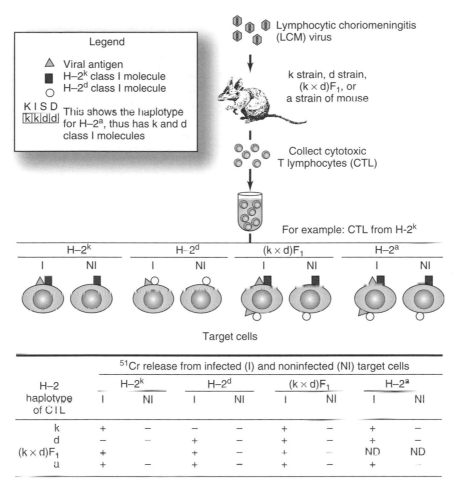

| | H-2ᵏ | | H-2ᵈ | | (k × d)F₁ | | H-2ᵃ | |
|---|---|---|---|---|---|---|---|---|
| | I | NI | I | NI | I | NI | I | NI |

Target cells

| H-2 haplotype of CTL | ⁵¹Cr release from infected (I) and noninfected (NI) target cells | | | | | | | |
|---|---|---|---|---|---|---|---|---|
| | H-2ᵏ | | H-2ᵈ | | (k × d)F₁ | | H-2ᵃ | |
| | I | NI | I | NI | I | NI | I | NI |
| k | + | − | − | − | + | − | + | − |
| d | − | − | + | − | + | − | + | − |
| (k × d)F₁ | + | | + | − | + | − | ND | ND |
| a | + | − | + | − | + | − | + | − |

**FIGURE 7-16 MHC restriction of cell-mediated cytotoxicity.** The schematic illustration gives only the example of H-2ᵏ mice exposed to LCM virus, but the protocol is the same for H-2ᵈ, (k × d)F₁, and H-2ᵃ mice. Cytotoxic T lymphocytes (CTL) are collected from H-2ᵏ-primed mice and tested for their ability to kill (+) either H-2ᵏ, H-2ᵈ, (k × d)F₁, or H-2ᵃ virally infected target cells. Killing is haplotype-restricted. CTL recognize viral antigen only in association with self-class I MHC molecules. Because class I MHC molecules are codominantly expressed, F₁ animals have both H-2ᵈ and H-2ᵏ class I MHC molecules and, therefore, are good targets for either haplotype of CTL. ND represents experiments that were not done. (The parental H-2 haplotypes are k/d for the H-2ᵃ recombinant that has a crossover between the I and S region. They are H-2ᵏ at the K and I loci but H-2ᵈ at the S and D loci.)

MHC molecule to bind many different peptides at the same site. The relationship between receptor activity and the extreme polymorphism of class I MHC genes is reflected in the different peptide-accommodating specificities of the respective peptide-binding sites, that is, each type of class I MHC molecule (A, B, and C in humans or K, D, and L in mice) and allelic variant (such as, HLA-A*0201 and HLA-A3) binds a unique set of antigenic peptides. As mentioned earlier, most nucleated cells express roughly $10^5$ copies of class I MHC molecules on their surface; therefore, each cell can simultaneously express many different peptides.

Crystal structures and elution studies show that the class I MHC molecule recognition site accommodates antigenic peptides that are eight to 10 amino acids long, usually nine, and that they contain specific amino acids at their amino and carboxyl termini that bind to invariant sites at each end of all class I MHC molecule antigen-binding clefts. The peptides exist in a flexible, extended chain in conformation with most of their surfaces buried in the binding groove. Class I MHC molecules restrict peptide size by blocking the peptide-binding grooves at either end, causing the longer peptides to simply bulge out of the groove

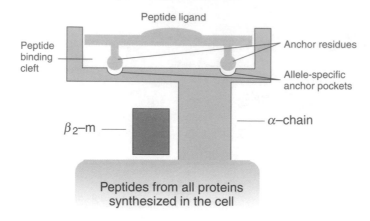

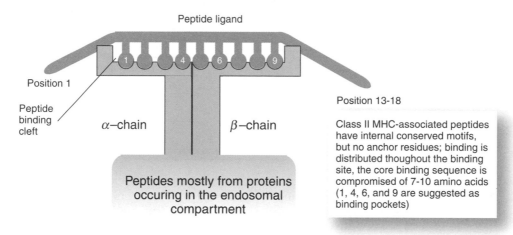

**FIGURE 7-17 Class I and class II MHC molecules interacting with peptides.**

in the middle—the peptide contact point for T cells (Figure 7-17).

Higher-resolution structures show a distribution of pockets at both ends of the antigen-binding cleft that are formed by polymorphic residues in the floor and walls of the class I groove. The pockets tether the amino and carboxyl ends of a peptide called **anchor residues** through hydrogen bonding and help dictate the peptide's orientation. The complementarities between these pockets and anchor residues seem to be the molecular basis of peptide-binding specificity for class I MHC molecules. Peptide uniformity is governed by motifs that are defined by conserved amino acids at certain positions. Typically, the second and nine positions are anchors that are occupied by a single amino acid residue of the antigenic peptide. The location of these anchors varies with class I alleles

(Figure 7-18). The carboxyl terminus anchor residues are usually hydrophobic or basic amino acids. The limited number of anchors accommodates conserved amino acids and forms the basis for allele-specific peptide binding. The amino acid residues that line the groove of the polymorphic MHC molecule form pockets that accommodate the amino acid side chains of an antigenic peptide. The location and shape of these pockets vary with the allelic form of the molecule. *The specific interactions are between amino acid side chains ("pockets") of the MHC molecule and the peptide chain's anchor residues. The broad specificity of MHC molecules occurs because they interact with the common backbone structures of peptides.*

In contrast to class I MHC molecule antigen-binding clefts, the ends of the class II antigen-binding grooves are open-ended, enabling peptides to

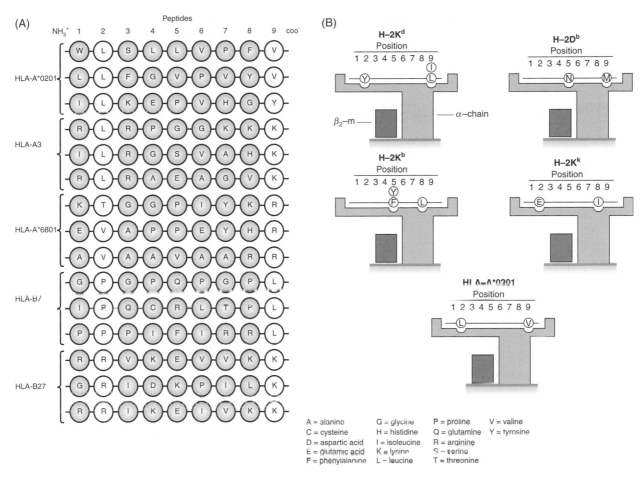

**FIGURE 7-18 MHC allele-specific, peptide-binding motifs of peptides eluted from class I MHC molecules.** (A) Examples of HLA anchor residues (yellow) in nonameric peptides eluded from several human class I molecules. (Adapted from J. Klein and A. Sato. 2000. *N. Engl. J. Med.* **343**:702.) (B) The cartoon version of class I MHC molecules is represented by $\beta_2$-microglobulin ($\beta_2$-m) and the MHC-encoded α chain. The distal $\alpha_1$ and $\alpha_2$ domains make up the receptor for peptide, while the $\alpha_3$ domain is adjacent to the cell membrane. The restriction elements are enclosed in boxes, the amino acid residue positions are numbered from 1 to 9, and the anchor residues (one-letter amino acid codes) are enclosed in circles. For example, the 9-amino-acid-long peptides presented by H-2 K$^d$. MHC molecules have the following characteristics: position 2 is almost always occupied by tyrosine, while position 9 is occupied by amino acids with hydrophobic aliphatic side chains, mainly leucine or isoleucine.

protrude from them (see Figure 7-17). This open-endedness allows longer (an average of 15–18 residues) peptides to bind. Similarly to class I molecules, class II MHC molecules can accommodate many different peptides. Elution of bound peptides and X-ray crystallography studies show that class II MHC molecule–peptide binding differs from that of class I molecules. The peptides are longer, do not have the conserved anchor residues at their ends as class I MHC-bound peptides, and the ends of the peptide are not bound. Class II-associated peptides may share allele-specific motifs. The mode of peptide binding to class II molecules is different from class I peptide binding. The class II-bound peptides are

in an extended conformation, binding to class II molecules by interactions along the length of the antigen-binding cleft. Peptides that bind to class II MHC molecules are at least 13 amino acids in length. The peptides are held by their side chains that extend into pockets lined by polymorphic residues and by interactions between their backbone and the binding cleft's conserved amino acid side-chains that line the cleft. Some structural studies suggest that peptide residues 1, 4, 6, and 9 are held by class II MHC molecule binding pockets. These pockets are more accommodating of different amino acid side chains than their class I molecule counterparts, which makes it more difficult define anchor residues and predict which peptides will bind to certain class II MHC molecules. Further experimentation, analyzing the molecular interactions between peptides and class II molecules, is needed to complete the description.

---

**MINI SUMMARY**

Class I and II MHC molecules are broadly specific, high-affinity cell-surface receptors for self and foreign peptides. The bimolecular complex of MHC molecule and peptide fragment is the specific ligand for TCRs.

---

# CONTROL OF MHC MOLECULE EXPRESSION IS CRITICAL TO T-CELL RESPONSIVENESS

MHC molecule expression determines whether T cells will recognize foreign antigen thereby leading to an adaptive immune response. Given their importance in adaptive immunity, the MHC genes are tightly regulated. In contrast to class I MHC molecules, which are expressed on almost all nucleated cells, constitutive expression of class II MHC molecules is confined to APCs, such as dendritic cells, macrophages, B lymphocytes, and thymic epithelial cells. Nonetheless, class I and class II MHC molecule expression can be induced by immune regulators and on cell activation. For example, class II MHC molecule expression can be induced by inflammatory cytokines (of which interferon-$\gamma$ [IFN-$\gamma$] is the most potent) or on activation of human T cells. *Cis*-acting regulatory promoter elements mediate the transcription of class I MHC (and $\beta_2$-microglobulin) genes. Of these regulatory elements, the class II MHC gene promoters also have the SXY module. The MHC class II transactivator (CIITA), synthesized in response to IFN-$\gamma$, contributes to the activation of class I MHC molecule promoters but it is essential for class II MHC promoter activation. MHC class II transactivator functions through interactions with regulatory factors bound to the SXY module.

Cytokines (discussed in Chapter 9) play a major role in MHC molecule expression. Type I (IFN-$\alpha$ and IFN-$\beta$) and type II (IFN-$\gamma$) IFNs and TNF-$\alpha$ and -$\beta$ increase the rate of constitutive transcription of class I genes. IFN-$\gamma$ and TNF-$\alpha$ induce the formation of the transcription factor interferon regulatory factor-1 and enhancer A, respectively, which in turn bind to IFN-stimulated response element and nuclear transcription factor $\kappa$B of class I MHC gene promoters.

These events lead to upregulation of gene transcription for the class I $\alpha$-chain, $\beta_2$-microglobulin, LMP proteasome subunits, and TAP peptide transporters. Because IFNs are produced in early innate responses to many viral infections and TNF-$\alpha$ in response to many microbial infections, it provides a connection of the innate response to the adaptive response by increased antigen presentation to specific T cells. In contrast, adenoviruses and malignant tumor cells can downregulate class I MHC molecule expression.

IFN-$\gamma$ also is important in the regulation of class II MHC molecules. As indicated above, IFN-$\gamma$ is essential for the induction of CIITA, which leads to increased class II MHC molecule expression not only on APCs but also non-APCs, such as intestinal epithelial cells, vascular endothelial cells, and pancreatic cells. Innate immune system NK cells produce IFN-$\gamma$ during viral infections, thereby stimulating the adaptive immune response. Activated T cells also produce IFN-$\gamma$, thereby augmenting the adaptive immune response. TNF-$\alpha$ increases the expression class II MHC molecules by maturing dendritic cells. The cytokine interleukin-4 can increase the expression of class II MHC molecules by resting of B cells, whereas IFN-$\gamma$ downregulates their expression on B cells. Corticosteroids and prostaglandin also downregulate expression of class II MHC molecules.

---

**MINI SUMMARY**

Molecular components tightly regulate the genes that encode MHC molecules. The expression of MHC molecules is influenced particularly by cytokines such as IFNs and TNF-$\alpha$, which stimulate the transcription of MHC genes.

---

# ANTIGEN RECOGNITION REQUIRES ANTIGEN PROCESSING AND PREFERENTIAL PRESENTATION OF PEPTIDES BY EITHER CLASS I OR CLASS II MHC MOLECULES

An antibody can recognize proteins, lipids, polysaccharides, nucleic acids, and small molecules, whereas *most T cells can recognize only protein antigens*. Only antigen-derived peptides can form stable complexes with class I and class II MHC molecules; lipids and polysaccharides cannot be recognized by classical MHC-restricted T cells and fail to induce cell-mediated immunity.

Although similar types of gene segments and DNA rearrangement events generate the receptors used by both B and T cells, these cells recognize antigen in different ways (Table 7-8). Antibody receptors bind conformational epitopes thus they can recognize the difference between native and denatured antigens, while TCRs bind to linear peptide epitopes derived from native antigens thus they cannot recognize the difference between native and denatured antigens. Because T cells by themselves are blind to antigen, native antigen is internalized and processed by APCs. *The conversion of a native, nonstimulatory protein to an immunogenic, MHC-associated peptide for T cells is called* **antigen processing** *and* **presentation**. *As a result, the most immunodominant epitope of the native antigen is displayed to the T cell.*

$T_H$ and $T_C$ cells use the same TCR genes and recognize a peptide of the processed native protein antigen, but the $CD4^+$ $T_H$ cell recognizes peptide in association with class II MHC molecules, and the $CD8^+$ $T_C$ cell recognizes peptide in association with class I MHC molecules. The remaining paragraphs of this section present an example of how class I MHC-restricted $T_C$ cells and class II MHC-restricted $T_H$ cells recognize antigen molecules. The differences lie in the pathways of antigen processing and presentation, which are usually determined by the route by which antigen enters a cell.

Early experiments using agents that impermeabilized APC membranes or altered the pH APC endosomes suggested that APCs, namely macrophages, processed bacterial antigen for presentation to $T_H$ cells. Also studies on the specificity of $T_C$ cells generated by immunization with influenza virus produced an unexpected finding. $T_C$ cell clones were generated that were specific for the internal nucleoprotein (a viral component not expressed on the membrane of the target cell) rather than for the membrane-expressed hemagglutinin molecule. To further confirm these results, short synthetic peptides

corresponding to certain regions of the nucleoprotein molecule were pulsed on target cells. The *in vitro* exposure of nucleoprotein-specific $T_C$ cells to these target cell-presented synthetic fragments led to target cell killing. Thus, it is unnecessary for the intact nucleoprotein to be on the cell surface; a degraded or fragmented form serves as the target antigen. These results suggested that antigen processing was an active metabolic process, which lead to antigenic peptide displayed with class I or class II MHC molecules on the cell surface.

Because class I MHC- and class II MHC-restricted T cells recognize similar forms of degraded antigen, antigen processing and presentation is a generalized activity of all cells, so all cells could be called *antigen-presenting cells*. However, by convention, cells that display class I MHC molecule-associated peptide to $CD8^+$ $T_C$ cells are called *target cells*. In contrast to class I MHC molecules which are expressed on the cell surface of all nucleated cells, only specialized cells display class II MHC molecule-associated peptide to $CD4^+$ $T_H$ cells; they are called **antigen-presenting cells** (**APCs**).

There are three types of APCs that are called *professional APCs* because they express class II MHC molecules and costimulatory molecules; they include dendritic cells, macrophages, and B cells (Table 7-9). Nonprofessional APCs include fibroblasts, glial cells, pancreatic beta cells, thymic and thyroid epithelial cells, and vascular endothelial cells, which can be induced by IFN-$\gamma$ to express class II MHC molecules or costimulatory molecules.

Antigen presentation divides the world of antigens into two categories that can be presented to T cells by class I and class II MHC molecules—endogenous, or intracellular, antigens and exogenous, or extracellular, antigens. Endogenous pathogens grow in host cell cytosol; they include viruses, intracellular bacteria, and protozoan parasites. These cytosolic antigens are either synthesized or degraded in the cytoplasm, delivered to the endoplasmic reticulum (ER) after being degraded, and complexed with class I MHC molecules in

**TABLE 7-8  B and T Cells Distinguish Between Different Forms of Antigen**

| | | Secondary immune response* | |
| Primary immunizing antigen exposure | Secondary antigen exposure | B cells | T cells |
|---|---|---|---|
| Native protein | Native protein | + | + |
| Native protein | Denatured protein | − | + |
| Denatured protein | Native protein | − | + |
| Denatured protein | Denatured protein | + | + |

*B-cell-mediated antibody production (+) or no production (−); T-cell-mediated, delayed-type hypersensitivity (+) or no reaction (−).

**TABLE 7-9 Properties and Functions of Professional APCs**

| | Dendritic cells | Macrophages | B cells |
|---|---|---|---|
| Ag uptake | Phagocytosis, Endocytosis | Phagocytosis | Receptor (Ig)-specific endocytosis |
| Class II MHC expression | Constitutive; increases with maturation; increased by IFN-γ | Induced by IFN-γ | Constitutive; increased by IL-4 |
| Costimulatory activity | Constitutive; increases with maturation; inducible by CD40-CD40L interactions, by IFN-γ | Induced by LPS, IFN-γ, CD40-CD40L interactions | Induced by antigen receptor cross-linking, B cell CD40-T cell CD40L interactions |
| Function | Activate naïve T cells | Activated to kill in effector phase of cell-mediated immunity | Antigen presentation to T$_H$ cells, leads to antibody production |

the ER—*the cytosolic pathway of antigen processing.* Exogenous pathogens include bacteria, their toxins, extracellular protozoan parasites, and fungi. Endosomal antigens (such as protein antigens internalized by phagocytosis) are taken up into acidified endosomal compartments where they are processed for binding with class II MHC molecules—*the endocytic pathway of antigen processing* (see Figure 7-20). Each pathway leads to the appropriate T-cell response.

The cytosolic processing pathway (Figure 7-19) is used when the antigen originates from the inside of the target cell, such as when a cell has been infected by a virus and synthesizes distinctive, virus-specific proteins on ribosomes in its cytoplasm. To associate with class I MHC molecules, these proteins must be degraded into peptides and transported into the ER. All nucleated cells in the body can present such internally synthesized proteins to CD8$^+$ T$_C$ cells and trigger cytotoxic activity. A large cytoplasmic enzyme structure, or **proteasome**, which consists of cylindrical arrays of proteolytic enzymes with their active sites towards the cylinder center, degrades cytoplasm protein and is primarily responsible for processing of endogenous antigens. Endogenous antigens can be either pathogen proteins or self-cell proteins that are covalently linked to *ubiquitin*, which drives them to the proteasome for processing. Two class II MHC region-encoded proteases called *low molecular weight protein 2* and 7 (*LMP2, LMP7*) and a third non-MHC-encoded subunit *LMP10* are induced by interferon in response to virus infections. The induced proteases replace constitutive proteasome proteases and preferentially degrade proteins to peptides with basic and/or hydrophobic amino acid residues at their carboxyl termini. This peptide structure facilitates their transport from the cytosol to the ER and provides the anchor residues for class I binding cleft pockets. Two additional class II

MHC region-encoded proteins called *transporter associated with antigen processing 1 and 2 (TAP1, TAP2)* reside in the ER membrane with each containing an ATP-binding site in their cytosolic domain followed by hydrophobic transmembrane domains. The transport of peptides containing 8–10 amino acids by the TAP1/TAP2 complex into the ER lumen requires hydrolysis of ATP. In the ER lumen, following a series of steps that involve protein-folding *chaperones*, the antigenic peptides bind with newly synthesized class I MHC molecules. The first chaperone, *calnexin*, associates with partly folded class I molecules and prevents misfolding of class I molecules in the absence of antigenic peptide. The subsequent binding of β$_2$-microglobulin to class I α chains releases calnexin and the complete class I molecules form complexes with the chaperone *calreticulin* and with *tapasin*. Another enzyme called *ERp57*, stabilizes the complex by forming a disulfide bond with TAP-associated protein (tapasin) and noncovalently associates with calreticulin, and conveys the TAP transporter close to the antigenic peptide, which promotes peptide binding to class I molecules. Once peptides bind, the peptide-class I molecule complexes are release from TAP transporters, they exit the ER, and move through the Golgi to the plasma membrane.

The interaction of naïve CD8$^+$ T$_C$ cells with target cells, such as virally infected cells or tumor cells, is not enough to activate, induce proliferation, and drive them to differentiate into effector T cells. They not only need TCR–peptide-loaded class I molecule ligation but also must encounter APC costimulatory molecules or T$_H$ cell-derived cytokine signals. APCs can participate in the immune response to intracellular microbes that do not directly infect them. APCs can capture virally infected cells or tumor cells as *exogenous* antigens—the exogenous protein antigens are internalized, processed in the cytosolic pathway

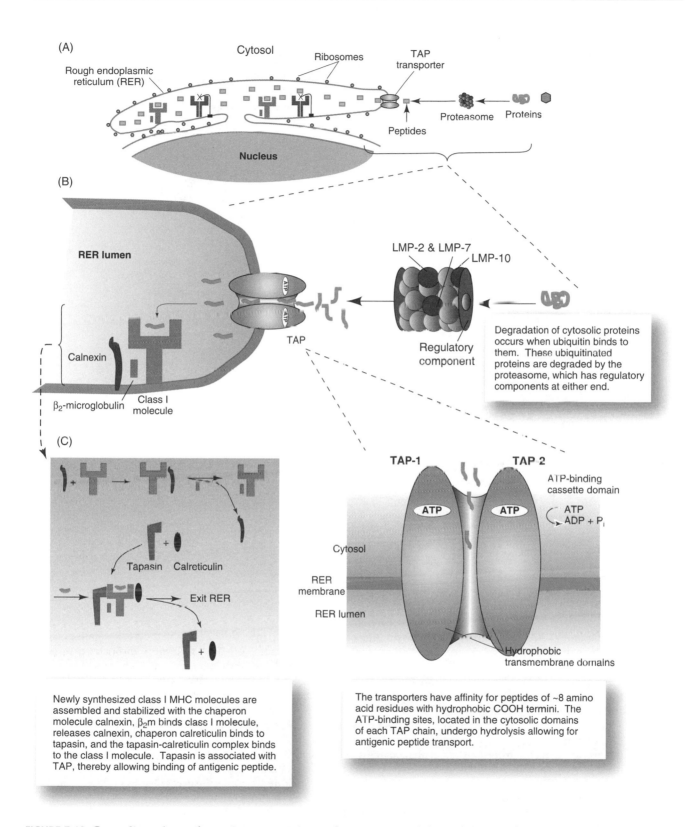

**FIGURE 7-19** Cytosolic pathway for antigen processing and presentation. (A) Degradation of antigenic peptides by proteasome, (B) transport of peptides from cytosol by transporter associated with antigen processing (TAP) to rough endoplasmic reticulum (RER), and (C) assemble and stabilization of class I MHC molecule followed by antigenic peptide binding. See text for more detail.

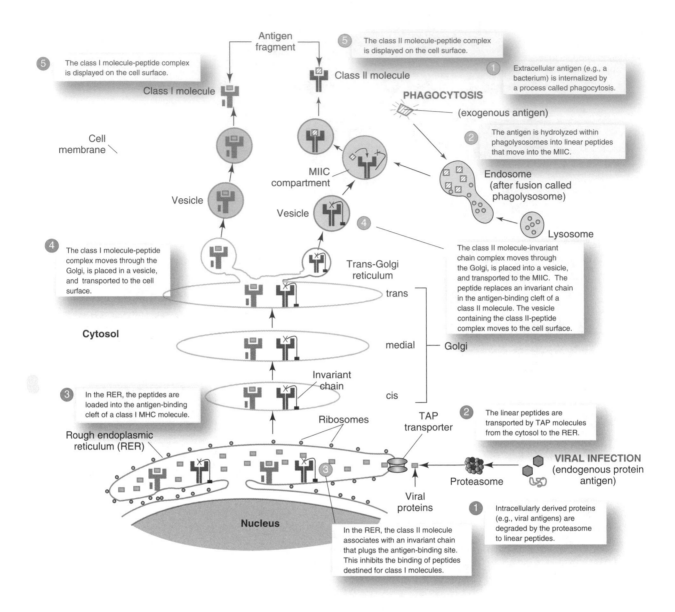

**FIGURE 7-20 Pathways for antigen processing and presentation—viral infection and phagocytosis.** Endogenous antigens, such as those derived from virus-directed synthesis of viral surface proteins or nucleoproteins, are processed in the ER and with the help of chaperone molecules the peptide associated with the class I molecule, and transported to the Golgi. Association of processed cytosolic antigen is a prerequisite for transport of class I MHC molecules to the cell surface, as is the binding with $\beta_2$-microglobulin ($\beta_2$m). Without peptide, the association of class I $\alpha$ chain and $\beta_2$m leads to an unstable complex that is inefficiently transported out of the ER. The antigen reaches the cell surface by forming a stable class I $\alpha$-chain-$\beta_2$m-peptide complex. Peptides in the cytoplasm, degraded by the proteasome, access the ER by specific TAP transporters.

Exogenous antigens are internalized by phagocytosis using a coated pit, which then enters endosomes. While the antigen resides in these acidified endocytic vesicles, partial proteolysis occurs. Once proteolysis of the antigen occurs and the invariant chain (Ii) is shed from the class II MHC molecule, making the molecule accessible to peptide binding, the immunogenic peptide becomes associated with class II MHC molecules moving to the cell surface. The two chains of the class II MHC molecule are assembled in the ER with the Ii to form a stable trimolecular complex and help in the routing of class II MHC molecules to endosomes containing exogenous processed antigen. The Ii inhibits the binding of peptides to the trimolecular complex in the ER. This complex is efficiently transported out of the ER, is directed to a post-Golgi compartment, and then is routed to an endosome called the *MIIC* where the Ii is proteolytically cleaved to CLIP, HLA-DM removes CLIP and loads peptide, and moves the vesicle containing the class II MHC—peptide-loaded complex to the cell surface.

(and in the endocytic pathway), and presented in association with class I MHC molecules to naïve CD8$^+$ T$_C$ cells initiating a primary response. This process is called **cross-presentation**, or **cross-priming**, because the APC presents antigenic peptide derived from exogenous antigen (the virus-infected cell or tumor cell) onto class I MHC molecules and activates the antigen-specific T$_c$ cells (see Chapter 10).

In contrast, the endocytic processing pathway is used when antigen is taken in from the surrounding medium by APCs by endocytosis or phagocytosis. The antigen is degraded in acidified endosomes, and its association with class II MHC molecules elicits T-cell help. Endosomes are increasingly acidic as they move further into the cytoplasm; this increased acidity activates proteases that degrade the antigens into peptides. Because antigens internalized through endocytosis or phagocytosis do not reach the ER, they do not associate with class I MHC molecules. However, some mechanism must exist to prevent peptides in the lumen of the ER from binding to newly synthesized class II MHC molecules. As class I α chains, class II α and β chains are synthesized on the rough ER and carried into the ER lumen but unlike class I molecules, they are assemble with another nonpolymorphic protein called the *invariant chain (Ii)*. Ii is a trimeric molecule composed of three 30-kD subunits, each subunit occupies a class II molecule-binding cleft. This "plugging" allows class II molecules to assemble in the absence of foreign or self-peptides present in the ER. In addition to preventing premature peptide binding, the Ii targets the class II molecules through the Golgi to a specialized low-pH peptide-containing vesicle called the *MHC class II compartment (MIIC)*, where the Ii is degraded. A fragment of the invariant chain, called *class II-associated invariant chain peptide (CLIP)*, remains bound to the class II molecules and prevents peptide binding. A class II-like molecule HLA-DM, not expressed on the cell-surface, catalyses the removal of CLIP, which leads to the loading of class II molecules with peptides. The peptide-loaded class II molecule then moves to the plasma membrane. Class II molecules without peptide are structurally unstable and are rapidly degraded. In the absence of infection, APCs present self-peptides. To summarize, Figure 7-20 shows schematic views for antigen processing and presentation to T cells during a viral infection or after phagocytosis.

The importance of antigen processing is evident in light of MHC restriction. Antigen processing explains how the few MHC molecules expressed by an individual interact with the many antigens against which immune responses are made. First, the conformational complexity of protein antigens is reduced by proteolytic processing and presentation of short peptides—the immunodominant determinants of the native protein. Second, the MHC site accommodates and binds a wide array of peptides with differing sequence. The practical consequence is that the combination patterns of MHC molecules and antigen decide whether T$_C$ or T$_H$ cells are activated—a choice that leads to the best immune response. These patterns are important because neither T$_C$ nor T$_H$ cell receptors nor class I or class II MHC molecules themselves can pick out intracellular or extracellular protein determinants. Intracellular antigen determinants lead to cytotoxic responses against parsitized cells (such as virus-infected cells), whereas extracellular antigen determinants lead to antibody responses against bacteria, their toxins, extracellular protozoan parasites, and fungi. Some cells, such as dendritic cells and macrophages, can simultaneously act as target cells and APCs.

## MINI SUMMARY

Antigen-derived peptides are presented to T cells with either class I or class II MHC molecules. Unexpected results suggest that class I- and II-restricted T cells recognize similar forms of antigen. The differences in antigen for the two types of T cells lie in the possible pathways of antigen processing and presentation. Assembly of the peptide-MHC molecule complexes occurs in two different intracellular compartments. Peptides derived from the degradation of cytosolic proteins and transported into the ER are found in complexes with class I MHC molecules. In contrast, peptides derived from exogenous proteins that enter the cell by phagocytosis or endocytosis are processed in acidic endosomes and become associated with class II MHC molecules.

# ANTIGEN RECOGNITION REQUIRES ANTIGEN PROCESSING AND PREFERENTIAL PRESENTATION OF NONPEPTIDES BY NON-MHC-ENCODED CLASS I-LIKE CD1 MOLECULES

Despite the overwhelming evidence for antigenic peptide-induced T cell activation, there are lipid and

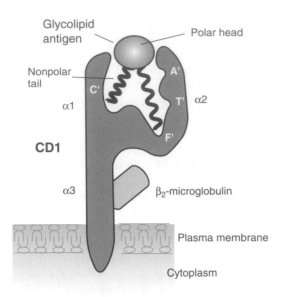

**FIGURE 7-21 CD1 molecule presentation of glycolipid antigen**. The human CD1B molecule consists of three extracellular domains ($\alpha_1, \alpha_2,$ and $\alpha_3$), a transmembrane domain, and a cytoplasmic domain. The $\alpha_1$ and $\alpha_2$ domains form the antigen-binding cleft that is composed of up to four pockets (A', C', F' and T') (not drawn to molecular scale or location) and two antigen portals (C' and F') (not shown), which were named because of their side-by-side locations and similar locations to the A, C and F pockets of MHC class I molecules. T' stands for tunnel. The antigen-binding cleft is lined by hydrophobic amino acids, which interact with the lipid's alkyl chains (nonpolar tail) allowing the variable components (polar head) of the antigen to protrude from the cleft, thereby available for direct interaction with antigen-specific TCRs.

glycolipid antigens, which begs the question: how are they recognized? The short of it is that members of the CD1 family of nonclassical class I molecules called **CD1 molecules** can present an array of lipids and glycolipids that comprise the membranes of mammalian cells and microbial pathogens to form antigen complexes that contact TCRs specifically and activate T cells.

There are five nonpolymorphic *CD1* genes on human chromosome 1 (*CD1A-E*), four (CD1A-D) of the five encoded proteins bind and present lipid antigens to T cells. All mammalian species studied have *CD1 genes*. The CD1 family is divided into two protein groups by amino acid homology: group 1 includes CD1A-C, whereas CD1D is the sole member of group 2. Like class I MHC molecules, CD1 molecules are transmembrane proteins that contain three extracellular domains ($\alpha_1, \alpha_2,$ and $\alpha_3$) (Figure 7-21). Similar to class I MHC $\alpha$ chains, the CD1 $\alpha$ chains form

complexes in the ER that consist of one $\alpha$ chain noncovalently paired with one $\beta_2$-microglobulin chain; they are expressed at the surface of many immune cells, including thymocytes, B cells, and dendritic cells. X-ray crystallography studies of CD1B show that the $\alpha_1$ and $\alpha_2$ domains form a large, deep hydrophobic antigen-binding cleft composed of up to four pockets (A', C', F', and T') and two antigen entrances, or portals (C' and F'), from the outer surface. The opening to the binding groove is narrower and the cavity volume is greater than their MHC counterparts. Nonetheless, the overall domain organization resembles class I MHC molecules with the hydrophobic antigen-binding site, forming channels or pockets that can accommodate lipid hydrocarbon chains. The narrow opening between the $\alpha$-helices permits the display of the lipid's polar moieties for recognition by TCRs; therefore, allowing the binding of different lipids linked to diverse polar head groups leading to an huge pool of possible CD1-presented glycolipid antigens. The different antigen classes presented by CD1 molecules include mycobacterial mycolates, phosphatidylinositols, sphingolipids and polyisoprenoid lipids. The group 1 CD1 molecules present glycolipid antigens to a wide variety of T cells including $\gamma\delta^+$ T cells (see Chapter 2) and a subset of $\alpha\beta^+$ CD8$^+$ T cells, whereas the group 2 CD1D molecules present their exogenous and endogenous glycolipid antigens mostly to an $\alpha\beta^+$ T cell subpopulation of limited TCR diversity called *NKT cells* (see Chapter 2). NKT cells also are known to bind CD1D-presented autologous antigens, reason unknown.

### MINI SUMMARY

Like the MHC molecules, the CD1 molecules mediate specific T-cell responses to various lipid antigens. Similar to the MHC system, CD1 molecules selectively obtain certain antigens by trafficking in different endosomal compartments. CD1A is found only in early endosomes, CD1B and CD1D internalize in late endosomes and lysosomes, and CD1C is found throughout early endosomes and late endosomes and lysosomes.

# SUMMARY

The large multigene locus called the ***major histocompatibility complex***, or ***MHC***, consists of several thousand kilobase pairs of DNA on a single chromosome.

The highly polymorphic genes within this segment of DNA encode a wide range of cell-surface structures that T cells must recognize in association with foreign antigen for a successful immune response.

Immunogenetics has its roots in the genetics of *histocompatibility* (sharing of transplantation antigens between two individuals or animals). Transplant rejection was first recognized in mice. Mouse models (inbred and congenic) are invaluable to research on the genetics of the immune response.

The two most thoroughly studied MHCs are the *histocompatibility antigen 2*, or *H-2*, and the *human leukocyte antigen*, or *HLA, complexes* of mice and humans, respectively. Genes of the H-2 and HLA complexes encode three classes of products, designated *class I, II*, and *III*. The H-2 complex was characterized using specially bred mice. Evidence for the human counterpart to the mouse H-2 complex arose from the analysis of sera from patients who had multiple transfusions. Their sera often agglutinated leukocytes from unrelated donors, and the agglutination patterns suggested definable antigens in human populations. These antigens were called *human leukocyte antigens*, or *HLA*. Description of these antigens led, in part, to the characterization of the *HLA complex*. According to serologic specificities, these antigens were first grouped into three series, designated *HLA-A, HLA-B*, and *HLA C*, and followed later by *HLA-D*. The first three cell-surface molecules are the human match to the mouse H-2-K, -D, and -L region molecules; thus, they are class I molecules. Class II molecules are termed *HLA-D* and are equivalent to the mouse class II MHC molecules. Like the mouse, the human, with as many as 3 to more than 550 alleles per loci, shows a great deal of polymorphism. Familial studies showed variation in the prevalence and frequency of HLA antigens from one population to another.

In order from left to right, the **HLA complex** consists of class II, III, and I regions. The HLA loci lie on chromosome 6. A group of genes located between the DR and B loci encodes class III region molecules including complement molecules (C2, C4, and factor B), enzymes, heat-shock proteins, and the cytokines TNF-$\alpha$ and -$\beta$. In order from left to right the regions are *DP, DO, DM, DQ, DR, class III region, B, C, X, E, J, A, H, G*, and *F*. The class II region is divided into several subregions: *DP, DO, DM, DQ*, and *DR*. The *B, C*, and *A* regions contain the genes encoding class I molecules expressed on all nucleated somatic cells and act in the presentation of viral antigens to CD8$^+$ T$_C$ cells. They also are the antigens recognized on grafted tissue by CD8$^+$ T$_C$ cells, leading to graft rejection. Class I molecules consist of two protein chains: a variant chain called $\alpha$, which is noncovalently associated with an invariant chain called $\beta_2$-*microglobulin*. The $\alpha$ chain is anchored by a short segment extending into the cell interior, while the remainder of the chain protrudes to the outside. The *DP, DQ*, and *DR* regions contain the genes encoding class II molecules. These molecules are expressed on APCs, such as, dendritic cells, macrophages, B cells, and on some epithelial cells and T cells. Class II MHC molecules are recognized in association with foreign antigenic peptide by CD4$^+$ T cells. Class II MHC molecules are made up of two noncovalently linked variant protein chains, called $\alpha$ and $\beta$. Both chains are encoded by MHC genes.

The *H-2 complex* is located on chromosome 17 of the mouse. The H-2 map is divided into at least six *regions*. It consists of (moving from left to right) the *K, I, S, D, L*, and *Tla;Qa regions*. The I region is further divided into the *I-A* and *I-E subregions*.

The murine class I region includes *K-, D-*, and *L-region genes* (or class I genes) encode *class I molecules*. The class II region contains *I region genes* (or class II genes), situated between the K and S regions, encode *class II molecules*. Because the class II MHC genes control the level of immune response to certain antigens, they are also called *immune response*, or *Ir, genes* in mice. The murine class III region contains class III genes (or *S region genes*), situated between the I and D regions, which encode components as described for their human counterpart.

Most T cells see foreign antigen only when antigen is on cell surfaces and in association with self MHC-encoded cell-surface molecules. This phenomenon is called **MHC restriction**. The TCR must simultaneously see foreign-antigen-derived peptides and self-MHC molecules for a successful immune response. T$_C$ cells can destroy only targets that have the right foreign antigenic peptide in association with its class I MHC molecules. T$_H$ cells must concurrently see foreign antigenic peptide in association with self-class II MHC molecules on APCs.

MHC molecules bind single peptides but their specificity is not restricted to a unique peptide; class I MHC molecules can bind various peptides because of their common structural features called *anchor residues*. Class I MHC molecule antigen-binding clefts have closed ends so they can accommodate peptides that are only 8–10 amino acid residues in length, whereas class II MHC molecules have open-ended clefts so they can bind 13–18 amino acid residues in length. Class II MHC molecules recognize peptides along the length of the binding cleft.

The level of innate and adaptive immunity is influenced largely by the interaction of T cells with peptide-loaded MHC molecules. Thus, the regulation of MHC molecule expression is tightly controlled during immune responses, particularly by cytokines like IFN-$\gamma$.

T cells by themselves are blind to antigen. They recognize only antigen that has been processed and presented by target cells or APCs. The antigen fragment is presented in association with class I or class II MHC molecules. Antigen that associates with class I molecules has been processed through the nonendosomal, or cytosolic, pathway, and antigen that associates with class II MHC molecules has been processed through the endocytic pathway. This conversion of a native, nonimmunogenic protein to an immunogenic peptide is called *antigen processing*.

Bacterial-derived nonpeptide (lipid and glycolipid) antigens are presented by non-MHC, nonpolymorphic class I-like *CD1 molecules*.

# SELF-EVALUATION

## RECALLING KEY TERMS

Alleles
Alloantigens
Altered-self model
Anchor residues
Antigen II
Antigen processing and presentation
CD1 molecules
Class I molecules
Class I region
Class II molecules
Class II region
Class III region
Congenic mice
Cross-presentation (or cross-priming)
Determinant-selection model
H-2
H-2 congenic mice
H-2 map
Haplotype
Histocompatibility
Histocompatibility antigen-2 (H-2) complex
  D region
  I region
    I-A subregion
    I-E subregion
  K region
  L region
  S region
  TIa;Qa region
HLA complex
  A region
  B region
  C region
  C2/C4 region
  DP region
  DQ region
  DR region
Holes-in-the-repertoire model
Human leukocyte antigens (HLA)
Inbred mice
Locus
Major histocompatibility complex (MHC)
MHC restriction
Proteasome
Region
Subregions

## MULTIPLE-CHOICE QUESTIONS

*(An answer key is not provided, but the page[s] location of the answer is.)*

1. Which of the following is true concerning the MHC in mammals? (a) in the mouse it is located on chromosome 18, (b) transplant rejection is determined by major histocompatibility antigens, (c) its primary function is the rejection of foreign transplants, (d) none of these. *(See pages 219 and 220.)*

2. The HLA-C region of the human MHC appears to be the functional equivalent of the H-2 I region of the mouse MHC. (a) true, (b) false. *(See pages 221 and 225.)*

3. On the HLA complex, the D/DR region (a) codes for cytokines, (b) codes for class I antigens, (c) codes for class III antigens, (d) codes for molecules found mainly on antigen-presenting cells, (e) none of these. *(See pages 225 and 226.)*

4. Molecules encoded by the K and D regions are characterized by (a) expression on immune cells only, (b) a requirement for interaction between T and B cells, (c) their affect on $T_C$ lymphocytes, (d) the presence of an $\alpha$ and a $\gamma$ chain, (e) none of these. *(See page 221.)*

5. Regions and subregions of the H-2 complex are defined by recombination (or crossover) events among distinct genes. (a) true, (b) false. *(See page 216.)*

6. The H-2 complex (a) is located on chromosome 6, (b) regulates T-independent antigen immune response, (c) was discovered by Dausset, (d) codes for transplantation antigens, (e) *a* and *d* are correct, (f) none of these. *(See pages 215, 219, and 220.)*

7. MHC molecules are highly polymorphic because (a) it helps the exchange of tissues or organs

among the various vertebrate species, (b) it decreases the possible interactions among the cells of the immune system, (c) it helps the spleen to perform a variety of regulatory functions, (d) it ensures that all members of a species are not equally susceptible to a pathogen, (e) none of these. *(See pages 224 and 225.)*

8. An MHC region is a segment of chromosome that serves as the locus for at least one marker gene. (a) true, (b) false. *(See page 216.)*

9. Class I molecules of the H-2 complex (a) are encoded by the I region, (b) are found mainly on lymphocytes, (c) are found in the same region that codes for complement components, (d) are highly polymorphic and unique for each strain, (e) none of these. *(See pages 221–225.)*

10. Concerning the structure of HLA-encoded class I MHC molecules, which of the following is true? (a) they comprise three polypeptides, (b) they contain a $\beta_2$-microglobulin, (c) they contain a heavy chain that traverses the lipid cellular bilayer, (d) *a, b,* and *c* are correct, (e) *b* and *c* are correct, (f) none of these. *(See pages 222–225.)*

11. Class I molecules are found on the following cells: (a) T cells, (b) kidney cells, (c) gametes, (d) all of the above, (e) none of these. *(See page 221.)*

12. Class II molecules (a) allow interaction between dendritic cells and T cells, (b) require interaction between T and B cells, (c) are located on immune cells, (d) all of the above, (e) none of these. *(See page 226.)*

13. In the HLA complex, class II molecules are encoded by the (a) I region, (b) K region, (c) D region, (d) the A, B, and C regions, (e) none of theses. *(See page 226.)*

14. Class III molecules are concerned with which of the following? (a) C4, C2, and factor B, (b) transplant rejection, (c) B cell idiotypes, (d) T cells, (e) none of these. *(See page 230.)*

15. The ability to respond to an antigen is transmitted to the offspring as a dominant trait. (a) true, (b) false. *(See page 231.)*

16. Unlike B cell antibody receptors or TCRs, each class I and II MHC molecule can bind many different peptides. (a) true, (b) false. *(See pages 240 and 241.)*

## SHORT-ANSWER ESSAY QUESTIONS

1. Even though the immune system rejects transplanted kidneys and hearts, its function is not to protect us against grafts. Why do people need histocompatibility antigens?

2. What is the connection between immunity and genes from the MHC?

3. Why are inbred/congenic mice so important to immunogenetic studies?

4. Compare and contrast the terms *region* and *locus* in the context of immunogenetics.

5. Briefly describe the structures of class I MHC and class II MHC proteins.

6. If we do not need protection against attack from foreign organs and tissues, why are class I MHC molecules so polymorphic? This polymorphism, or diversity, is different from the generation of diversity for antibodies. How?

7. Briefly describe how class II MHC molecules allow immune cells to communicate with one another. Why is this communication important? What is the relationship between class II MHC molecules and Ir genes?

8. Class III MHC molecules are not cell-surface proteins. What are they, and what do they do?

9. Explain the following statement: there is a direct relationship between an animal's MHC haplotype and its ability or inability to respond to a specific antigen.

10. Most T cells can react only with protein fragments. What is this process called, and how does it occur? Which pathway leads to antigen interaction with class I molecules and which leads to antigen interaction with class II molecules? Briefly describe each pathway. How are lipids and glycolipids accounted for?

## FURTHER READINGS

Barral, D.C., and M.B. Brenner. 2007. CD1 presentation: How it works. *Nat. Rev. Immunol.* 7:929–941.

Benacerraf, B. 1981. Role of major histocompatibility gene products in immune regulation. *Science* 212:1229–1238.

Bevan, M. 2006. Cross-priming. *Nat. Immunol.* 7:363–365.

Brown, J.H., et al. 1993. Three-dimensional structure of the human class II histocompatibility antigen HLA-DR1. *Nature* 364:33–39.

Cresswell, P. 2003. The biochemistry and cell biology of antigen processing. In *Fundamental Immunology,* 5th ed. W.E. Paul, ed. Philadelphia: Lippincott Williams & Wilkins. p. 613–630.

Dausset, J. 1981. The major histocompatibility complex in man. *Science* 213:1469–1474.

De Libero, G., and L. Mori. 2006. Mechanisms of lipid-antigen generation and presentation to T cells. *Trends Immunol.* 27:485–492.

Eisenlohr, L.C., L. Huang, and T.N. Golovina. 2007. Rethinking peptide supply to MHC class I molecules. *Nat. Rev. Immunol.* 7:403–410.

Horton, R., et al. 2004. Gene map of the extended human MHC. *Nat. Rev. Genetics* 5:889–899.

Jones, E.Y., L. Fugger, J.L. Strominger, and C. Siebold. 2006. MHC class II proteins and disease: A structural perspective. *Nat. Rev. Immunol.* 6:271–282.

Kelly, J., et al. 2005. Comparative genomics of major histocompatibility complexes. *Immunogenetics* 56:683–695.

Margulies, D.H., and J. McCluskey. 2003. The major histocompatibility complex and its encoded proteins. In *Fundamental Immunology*, 5th ed. W.E. Paul, ed. Philadelphia: Lippincott Williams & Wilkins. p. 571–612.

Parham, P. 2005. MHC class I molecules and KIRS in human history, health and survival. *Nat. Rev. Immunol.* 5:201–214.

Reith, W., S. LeibundGut-Landmann, and J-M. Waldburger. 2005. Regulation of MHC class II gene expression by the class II transactivator. *Nat. Rev. Immunol.* 5: 793–806.

Rock, K.L., I.A. York, and A.L. Goldberg. 2004. Post-proteasomal antigen processing for major histocompatibility complex class I presentation. *Nat. Immunol.* 5:670–677.

Rock, K.L., and L. Shen. 2005. Cross-presentation: Underlying mechanisms and role in immune surveillance. *Immunol. Rev.* 207:166–183.

Rodgers, J.R., and R.G. Cook. 2005. MHC class Ib molecules bridge innate and acquired immunity. *Nat. Rev. Immunol.* 5:459–471.

Snell, G.D. 1981. Studies in histocompatibility. *Science* 213:172–178.

Trombetta, E.S., and I. Mellman. 2005. Cell biology of antigen processing *in vitro* and *in vivo. Annu. Rev. Immunol.* 23:975–1028.

Vyas, J.M., A.G. Van derVeen, and H.L. Ploegh. 2008. The known unknowns of antigen processing and presentation. *Nat. Rev. Immunol.* 8:607–618.

Watts, C. 2004. The exogenous pathway for antigen presentation on major histocompatibility complex class II and CD1 molecules. *Nat. Immunol.* 5:685–692.

# CHAPTER EIGHT

# THE T-CELL RECEPTOR COMPLEX: CHARACTERIZATION, DIVERSIFICATION, COSTIMULATORY MOLECULES, THYMIC SELECTION, AND T-CELL ACTIVATION

## CHAPTER OUTLINE

1. Characterization of the TCR was difficult.
2. The structure of the TCR resembles in some ways the Fab portion of immunoglobulin.
3. The gene organization and diversification of the TCR resemble the immunoglobulin molecule's gene organization and diversification.
4. TCR association with the invariant proteins of the CD3 complex is required for TCR expression and T-cell activation.
5. Antigen recognition requires accessory molecules (or coreceptors).
   a. Accessory molecules for T cells function as adhesion molecules, signal transduction molecules, or both.
      1) CD4 and CD8 interactions with their counterreceptor, class II and class I MHC molecules, mediate adhesion and transduce signals.
      2) CD2 (LFA-2) interaction with its counterreceptor, CD58 (LFA-3), is tipped toward adhesion by T-cell activation.
      3) CD11aCD18 (LFA-1) interaction with its counterreceptors, CD54 (ICAM-1) and CD102 (ICAM-2), is needed for many immune cell functions.
   b. Other T-cell accessory molecules, costimulators, which regulate the response of antigen-activated T cells.
6. T cells specific for foreign peptides bound to self-MHC molecules are selected for maturation in the thymus.
7. The molecular basis of T-cell activation entails the formation of the immunological synapse, which initiates multiple signaling pathways.

## OBJECTIVES

The reader should be able to:

1. Outline the characterization of the TCR for antigen.

2. Draw the structure of the TCR and compare and contrast its structure with that of an antibody molecule.

3. Appreciate TCR-gene organization and the strategies for TCR diversification.

4. Realize that for the TCR to work, it needs the help of an associated set of cell surface molecules called CD3.

5. Appreciate that antigen recognition requires accessory molecules; discuss some examples of accessory molecules.

6. Discuss how T cells are selected in the thymus; define positive and negative thymic selection; comment on why these selection processes during the development of MHC restriction are difficult to understand.

7. Describe the molecular pathways for T-cell activation.

To identify and respond to their specific antigenic targets, T cells express roughly $10^5$ **T-cell receptors** (**TCRs**) on their surface. Although the TCR is structurally similar to an antibody, it cannot recognize antigen in its natural state, as a B-cell antigen receptor can. *Unlike the B-cell receptor, the TCR exists only at the cell surface. All T-cell interactions with antigens occur on the T-cell surface, and antigens for T cells are cell-bound molecules.* Furthermore, the antigens are recognized only when presented as antigen-derived peptide fragments by cells bearing specific class I or class II MHC molecules. The TCR is a heterodimer composed of either α and β or γ and δ chains. The generation of TCR diversity is similar to that of B cell receptors. Also as B cell receptors, TCRs have signal-transducing complexes associated with them. TCR structure, gene organization, molecular arrangement, and diversification are discussed first. Some cell-surface cosignaling molecules, many identified as crucial components of the immunological synapse, which cooperate with the TCR during recognition of antigen are discussed next. It is followed by a distillation of the complex steps required in T-cell development in the thymus. Engagement of the TCR and the resulting intracellular activation events that culminate in biologic function are described last.

# CHARACTERIZATION OF THE TCR WAS DIFFICULT

The observation that T cells were MHC restricted—need to recognize antigen and self-MHC molecules simultaneously—led to the formulation of two models: (1) the *dual-receptor model* and (2) the **altered-self model**. The dual-receptor model postulated the existence of two TCRs, one with complementarity for the antigenic determinant and a second with complementarity for class I or class II MHC molecules. The altered-self model postulated that the TCR recognized two individual units by distinct combining sites on the same receptor. The latter model suggested that the TCR recognized self-MHC molecules that were altered by the interaction with foreign antigenic peptide. This recognition model postulates a *single-receptor model* (as opposed to the *dual receptor model*) in which the TCR recognizes the antigenic determinant and the MHC gene product as a unit (Figure 8-1).

Current data favor the altered-self model. Anti-idiotypic antibodies raised against antigen-specific, MHC-restricted T cells of one clone recognized only the αβ TCR and only the αβ TCR of that clone. Other experiments by Kappler and Marrack (Figure 8-2) showed that recognition of antigen plus class II MHC molecules is determined solely by the αβ-containing TCR. Thus, the α and β chains of the TCR define both antigen and MHC specificity. These results also suggest that foreign antigen recognition and MHC restriction of the parent TCR are linked. Much data since these experiments continues to support the altered-self model of TCR recognition of antigen. *Thus, the TCR for antigen is also the receptor for MHC gene products. In the trimolecular complex that consists of TCR, antigen, and MHC molecule, two antigenic determinants are recognized by the TCR and the MHC molecule. Specific MHC molecule determinants also are recognized by the TCR.*

Despite the preceding data, unraveling the nature and structure of TCRs was much more difficult than figuring out the structure of B-cell receptors and antibodies. Initially, TCRs were presumed to be antibodies. The T-cell antibody model, however, was discarded when probes of immunoglobulin (Ig) genes

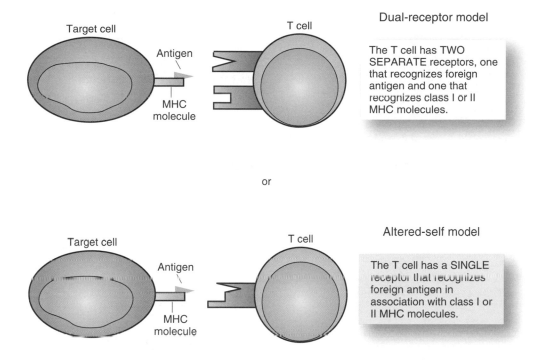

**FIGURE 8-1 The dual-receptor model versus the altered-self model for MHC-restricted antigen recognition by T cells.** The altered-self model opposes the counterpart incorrect dual- receptor model (of two independent TCRs: one for the antigen, the other for the MHC molecule).

in T cells showed that light-chain and heavy chain genes do not rearrange and that mRNAs for Ig chains are not present.

Until 1983, no direct data showed whether TCRs existed as physical entities and whether the isolated TCRs were the actual receptors. The enormous heterogeneity of T cells, with their corresponding structurally different antigen-specific receptors, further complicated the search. Two breakthroughs finally permitted TCR characterization: the development of monoclonal antibodies and T-cell hybridomas. The first glimpse of the TCR structure came when monoclonal antibodies specific for individual T-cell clones precipitated protein dimers essential for T-cell activation by antigen. This characterization was accomplished using T-cell hybridomas. T-cell hybridoma use allowed for the production of many T cells specific for one antigenic determinant. The resulting hybridomas were screened to find clones that had receptors for the desired antigen.

$T_H$ cell hybridomas, *used as immunogens*, were produced with specificity for several different antigenic determinants, such as cytochrome *c* and ovalbumin. Spleen cells from animals immunized with antigen-specific $T_H$ cell hybridomas were fused with myeloma cells, leading to hybrids that produced monoclonal antibodies against surface markers on the T-cell hybridomas. Several monoclonal antibodies were obtained that were directed against the TCR for various antigens. The antibodies met all the criteria for specificity against $T_H$ cell TCRs; their use lead to isolation of the receptor, its characterization as a two-chain structure with constant and variable domains.

Molecular biology approaches also were used to characterize the TCR. Rather than purifying the TCR proteins, the TCR genes were cloned to determine whether rearrangement between germline and mature T-cell DNA occurred. The strategy involved looking for mRNA that encoded the TCR. The approach was based on three assumptions: (1) the TCR gene is expressed only in T cells, (2) the mRNA is associated with the endoplasmic reticulum because receptor synthesis occurs on membrane-associated polysomes, and (3) the gene is rearranged in mature T cells. The last assumption was based on the known need for Ig-gene rearrangement to generate antibody specificity. Furthermore, B and T cells are exposed to the same antigenic universe; like Ig DNA rearrangement, some DNA rearrangement may determine the specificity of the TCR. To isolate TCR mRNA from all other mRNAs in the T cell, **subtractive hybridization** was used (Figure 8-3). In fact, the TCR structure was predicted

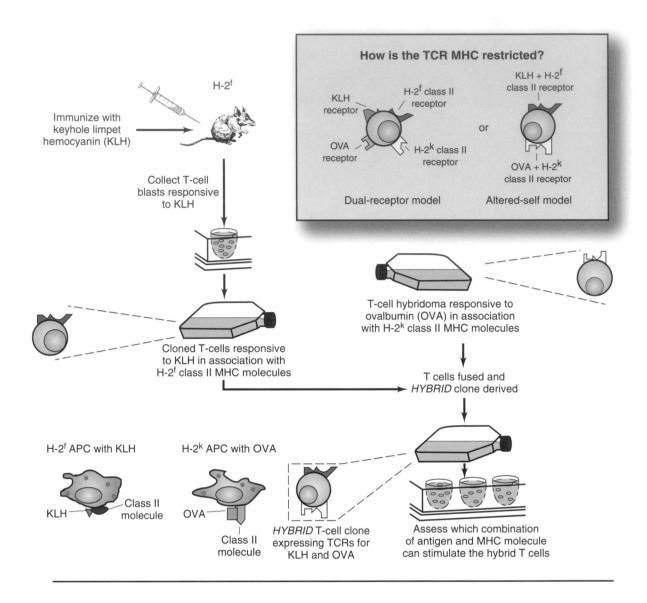

| | Antigen-MHC combination on APCs | | | |
|---|---|---|---|---|
| Responder cells | OVA/H-2$^k$ | OVA/H-2$^f$ | KLH/H-2$^k$ | KLH/H-2$^f$ |
| 1. OVA-responsive T-cell clone | + | – | – | – |
| 2. KLH-responsive T-cell clone | – | – | – | + |
| 3. Hybrid of fusion partners 1 & 2 | + | – | – | + |

**FIGURE 8-2  T-cell recognition of an antigen-MHC molecule combination; the TCR is also the receptor for MHC molecules.** The hybrid T cells react only to the two antigen-MHC combinations that stimulate the fusion partners. They do not respond to antigen recognized by one partner in association with the MHC molecule recognized by the other (OVA on H−2$^f$ cells or KLH on H−2$^k$ cells). The F$_1$ T cells' antigen receptors recognize the combination, not antigen or MHC molecules alone. The altered-self model represents the TCR's simultaneous recognition of antigen and MHC epitopes.

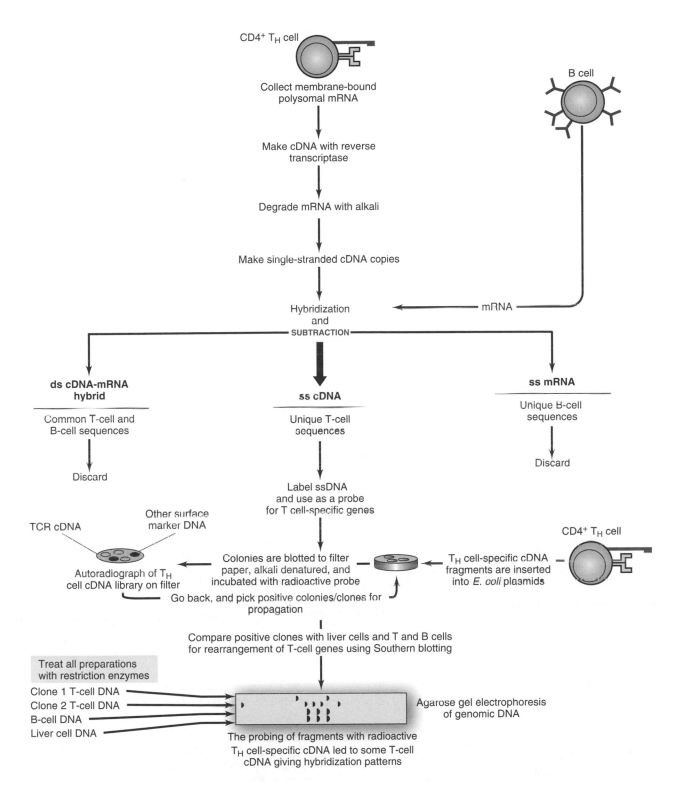

**FIGURE 8-3 Subtractive hybridization.** This method involves the isolation of membrane-associated mRNA from $T_H$ cell hybridomas specific for a particular antigen and the production of cDNA copies that hybridized with B-cell mRNA, leaving unique T-cell cDNA. The remaining cDNA is labeled and used to screen clones of a $T_H$ cell hybridoma cDNA library (these genes are constructed from cytoplasmic RNA also absorbed with B-cell mRNA; therefore, the clones that hybridize with the probe should contain a gene specific for the T cell). Finally, the clones are tested for genes which became rearranged in T cells. (Adapted from S. Hedrick et al. 1984. *Nature* **308**:149.)

mostly from the nucleotide sequence of the cloned genes.

The premise of subtractive hybridization was that B and T cells share about 98% of their mRNAs but *not* the mRNAs for the TCR. T-cell membrane-bound, polysomal mRNA first was converted into cDNA and subsequently hybridized with mRNA from B cells. Once the hybridized cDNA strands were discarded (*subtracted*), the remaining cDNA represented T-cell-specific mRNAs (including those for the TCR chains). This remaining nonhybridized cDNA then was labeled and used to probe a second $T_H$ cell cDNA clone library. Hybridization with the T-cell-specific, radioactive DNA probe identified the clones of interest in a cDNA library. The library consisted of *E. coli*–containing plasmids with T-cell-specific DNA fragments. Culture dishes containing the growing *E. coli* colonies were blotted to filter paper, to which some bacteria of each colony adhere. The blotted colonies, known as *replicas*, are denatured with alkali and incubated with the radioactive T cell-specific probe. Several cDNA clones were identified as $T_H$ cell specific. However, were these $T_H$ cell genes the rearranged TCR genes? This question was answered by comparing restriction-enzyme-treated genomic DNA from cells such as liver cells and B cells (TCR gene is in the germline configuration) and T cells—*the specific breakpoints in DNA, generated by restriction enzymes, are dependent on the nucleotide sequence. Thus, if the DNA is rearranged the nucleotide sequence would change. The enzymes would cut at different points, leading to fragments of different size.* The different fragments were separated by Southern blotting and probed with the labeled T-cell-specific cDNA. The Southern blot patterns suggested that the T-cell DNA rearranged, while the liver-cell and B-cell DNA did not. When the isolated rearranged T-cell genes were sequenced, and their amino acid sequence was derived, the β-chain gene of the TCR had been isolated. Subsequent experiments isolated the cDNA clones that encoded the α chain, the γ chain and lastly the δ chain. The doors were open for structural and functional studies on the TCR.

# THE STRUCTURE OF THE TCR RESEMBLES IN SOME WAYS THE FAB PORTION OF IMMUNOGLOBULIN

On either a resting or an activated T cell, the density of TCRs is about $10^5$ receptors. Individual T cells express only one type of functional TCR that consists of two polypeptide chains, which are encoded by separate genes. The chains, either α and β or γ and δ, are held together by disulfide bonds; they are built with the Ig fold as their backbone structure. The **αβ** and **γδ TCRs** are always found in close association with the CD3 complex. The αβ TCR molecules are expressed mainly on $CD4^+CD8^-$ $T_H$ cells and on $CD4^-CD8^+$ $T_C$ cells and permit specific recognition of antigenic peptides in association with MHC molecules. Roughly 95% of peripheral blood T cells express αβ TCRs. In contrast, the γδ TCR molecules are expressed on roughly 60% of double-negative ($CD4^-CD8^-$), $CD3^+$+hymic immature T cells, which are found in low numbers ($1\frac{1}{N}10\%$) in the peripheral blood and target microbial phospholipid antigens. $γδ$ $TCR^+$ T cells account for most of the T cells in the early stages of thymus ontogeny and in the epithelia. The localization of γδ T cells in notably epithelial layers of the intestines, which form a first line of defense between host and pathogen, suggests that they could perform a critical surveillance function at this portal of entry for many pathogens (see Chapter 2). The $γδ^+$-$CD3^+$ cells are a separate T-cell lineage distinct from $αβ^+$-$CD3^+$ cells. The physiologic importance of γδ TCR remains an enigma, even though the ligands for γδ TCR are primarily MHC class-I-like proteins, phospholipids (see Chapter 7), and heat shock proteins.[1] Class Ib molecules may be a target for γδ T cells. Also, some γδ T cells recognize "simple" rather than "compound" ligands such as MHC-peptide, but instead may bind to "surfaces" or epitopes the same way antibodies do. A group of nonMHC-encoded MHC-like molecules called *CD1 molecules* can present bacteria-derived lipid and glycolipid to γδ T cells; γδ T cells are not MHC-restricted (see Chapter 7).

The human heterodimeric glycoprotein αβ TCR consists of a 40- to 50-kD α chain linked by disulfide bonds to a 35- to 44-kD β chain. The γδ TCR consists of a 40- to 55-kD γ chain and a 38- to 42-kD δ chain. The structure of the TCR is similar to that of the Fab portion of an Ig or to that of two Ig light chains (Figure 8-4). Each chain has loops made of about 70 amino acids and, like Ig molecules, the α and γ chains of the TCR have V, J, and C regions. The β and δ chains also have a fourth region, called *diversity* (D). Each such region is

---

[1] Heat shock proteins (HSPs), or stress proteins, are found in many prokaryotic and eukaryotic cells. HSPs are induced by a variety of stresses and serve as important antigens of infectious agents.

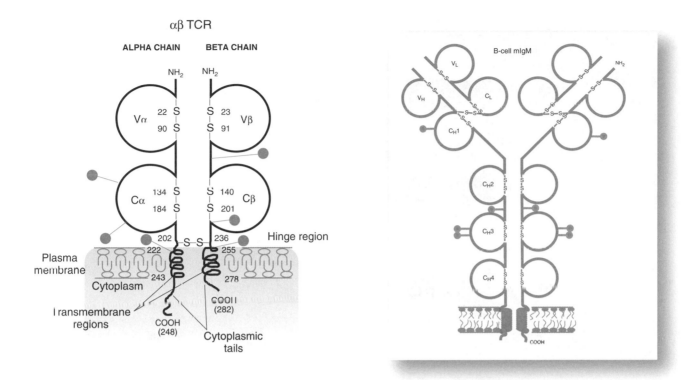

**FIGURE 8-4 Molecular structure of the TCR.** The TCR consists of two chains, α and β. Each has two extracellular domains, an amino-terminal V domain and a carboxyl-terminal C domain. Domains are stabilized by intrachain disulfide bonds between cysteine residues. The α and β chains are linked by an interchain disulfide bridge near the cell membrane (hinge region). Each chain is anchored on the membrane by a hydrophobic transmembrane segment and ends in the cytoplasm with a carboxyl-terminal segment rich in cationic residues. Both chains are glycosylated (•). A second TCR consists of γ and δ chains and is arranged like the αβ TCR. (For comparison, the yellow inset box includes the structure of B-cell membrane-bound IgM.)

encoded by distinct and separate segments of DNA. The analyses of crystallized TCR chains show CDR loops that are arranged the same as their Ig counterparts. The three CDRs (Figure 8-5), which appear equivalent to Ig CDRs, are found in both αβ and γδ chains. The first two CDRs are encoded by the V-gene segments; the third CDR is generated by junctional flexibility, P-nucleotide addition, and N-region nucleotide addition at the junctions between V and J segments in the α and γ chains or V, D, and J segments in the δ and β chains. TCR diversity is focused in the CDR3. Models of interaction between the TCR and MHC-peptide ligand complexes suggest that the TCR CDR3 is the primary contact point with the peptide epitope and that the other TCR V-region sites, particularly the CDR2 of α- and β-chain V regions, contribute to the specificity and stability of that interaction through direct contact with MHC determinants. Just as Ig heavy chains are encoded by C-gene segments with multiple exons, so are the

C regions of each TCR chain. The four exons that encode the C region, from amino to carboxyl termini, are: C, which encodes the largest part (including an intrachain disulfide bond); H, which encodes the hinge region (including a cysteine residue disulfide linking the α and β or γ and δ chains); TM, which encodes a hydrophobic transmembrane region of 21 or 22 amino acids (anchoring the TCR to the plasma membrane); and lastly, CY, which encodes a short cytoplasmic tail of 5–12 amino acids. The shortness of the cytoplasmic tails suggests that TCR chains do not transduce signals to the cytoplasm. The closely linked CD3 molecule (discussed later) carries out this function. Because the TCR is not secreted, differential RNA processing of TCR primary transcripts does not occur.

Although the genes encoding the V, J, D, and C segments of the TCR are expressed only in T cells, TCR genes are structurally related to Ig genes. These genes are part of the *Ig-gene superfamily* (see Chapter 4).

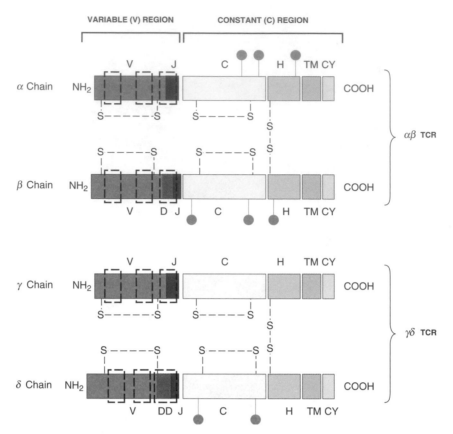

**FIGURE 8-5 The relationship between TCR gene segments and chain domains.** The α and γ chains are encoded by two incomplete, or segmented, exons (V and J) and four complete exons for the C region (C domain, hinge [H], transmembrane [TM], and cytoplasmic [CY] exons). The β and δ chains are encoded by three incomplete, or segmented, exons (V, D, and J) and four complete C-region exons like the α and γ chains. The approximate locations of intrachain and interchain disulfide bridges (S--S), of carbohydrates (•), and of complementarity-determining regions (CDRs; shown by dashed boxes) are given. (Adapted from M. Kronenberg, G. Siu, L.E. Hood, and N. Shastri. 1986. *Annu. Rev. Immunol.* **4**:529 and from M.M. Davis and P.J. Bjorkman. 1988. *Nature* **334**:395.)

# THE GENE ORGANIZATION AND DIVERSIFICATION OF THE TCR RESEMBLE THE IMMUNOGLOBULIN MOLECULE'S GENE ORGANIZATION AND DIVERSIFICATION

Mice and humans have four multigene families found on different chromosomes that encode TCR chains (Table 8-1). The TCR multigene family consists of α-, β-, γ-, and δ-gene segments. The germline gene and rearranged gene organization for the α, β, γ, and δ chains of the mouse TCR are shown in Figure 8-6. The organization of the human TCR gene families

is similar to that of the mouse but the number of segments differ.

The gene encoding the α TCR chain is localized to chromosome 14 in humans and mice. The human α chain consists of V, J, and C regions, which are encoded by 54 V-gene segments, 61 J-gene segments, and one C gene. The $J_\alpha$ locus is unusual because of its large repertoire (more J-gene segments than any other T- or B-cell receptor gene families). The TCR α-chain gene locus is analogous to Ig light-chain gene loci; they do not contain D gene segments and are rearranged only after their partner chain is expressed.

The β-chain gene segments are located on chromosome 7 in humans and chromosome 6 in mice. The β-chain V regions are encoded by three distinct gene segments, $V_\beta$, $D_\beta$, and $J_\beta$. Two C-region genes exist—$C_\beta 1$ and $C_\beta 2$—and a cluster of multiple J-gene

**TABLE 8-1** The Chromosomal Location and Number of TCR Gene Segments

| | Chromosome | | Number of gene segments | | | | | | | |
| | | | Mouse | | | | Human | | | |
| Gene | Mouse | Human | V | D | J | C | V | D | J | C |
|---|---|---|---|---|---|---|---|---|---|---|
| α chain | 14 | 14 | 100 | | 50 | 1 | 50 | | 70 | 1 |
| β chain | 6 | 7 | 20–30 | 2* | 2* | 2* | 57 | 2 | 13 | 2 |
| γ chain | 13 | 7 | 7 | | 3 | 3 | 14 | | 5 | 2 |
| δ chain | 14 | 14 | 10 | 2 | 2 | 1 | 3 | 3 | 3 | 1 |

*The β-gene family has two identical repeats of D (1 $D_\beta$), J (6 $J_\beta$), and C (1 $C_\beta$) segments.

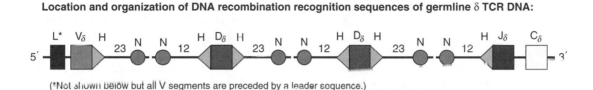

**Location and organization of DNA recombination recognition sequences of germline δ TCR DNA:**

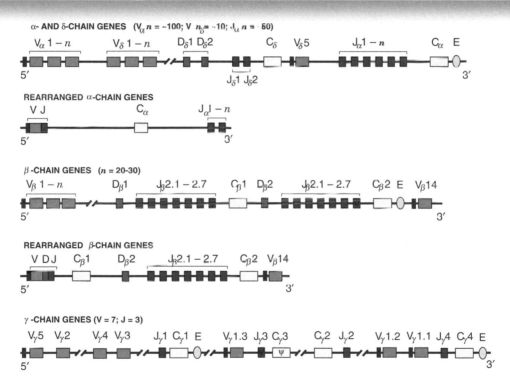

**FIGURE 8-6 Organization of mouse germline and rearranged TCR genes.** TCR germline DNA undergoes rearrangement by mechanisms similar to Ig-gene rearrangement: conserved heptamer (H) and nonamer (N) recognition sequences, with 12- or 23-base-pair spacers, flank each V, D, and J segment. Using the 12–23 joining rule, intervening DNA is removed by deletional or inversion mechanisms. The common feature of these four TCR multigene families is that they contain separate gene segments encoding V and C regions of the TCR, even though the δ-chain gene segments are in the midst of the α-chain gene segments. Leader sequences (not shown) precede each V-gene segment, and each C-gene segment consists of multiple exons that are not shown. A V-gene segment is brought together with a J-gene segment during lymphocyte ontogeny by DNA rearrangements to form a complete V-region gene. D-gene segments are involved where applicable, leading to a contiguous V-(D)-J exon. This exon is spliced together with the C-region segments at the level of RNA. The organization of mouse germline and rearranged TCR genes is similar (not shown). (0 = Enhancer) See text for further explanation.

segments are located uniquely 5′ to each of the $C_\beta$ genes and each J-gene cluster is preceded by a single D-gene segment. The β-chain locus rearranges before the α-chain locus. DNA joining of V, D, and J segments with the C gene forms a functional gene; this step occurs in mRNA when the unnecessary sequences are spliced out. In humans, there are 67 V-gene segments, 2 D-gene segments, and 14 J-gene segments that can rearrange to form the β-chain gene.

The γ-chain gene segments were uncovered during the search for the gene segments encoding the α and β proteins. The human and mouse γ-gene segments are found on chromosomes 7 and 13, respectively. The human γ gene locus consists of 14 V-gene segments and five functional repeats of J-gene segments and two C genes that rearrange during T-cell development in the thymus. Both the human and mouse γ genes encode a disulfide-linked chain with a molecular weight of 40- to 55-kD (depending on the extent of glycosylation). The γ chain is associated with a 38- to 42-kD δ chain. The human δ-chain gene segments are located between the $V_\alpha$ and $J_\alpha$ clusters on Chromosome 14. The δ chain is assembled from three V-gene segments, three D-gene segments, four J-gene segments, and one C gene.

*The TCR multigene family uses at least seven strategies* (Table 8-2) *for TCR diversification, which are similar to that used by Ig-gene rearrangements (there are exceptions): (1)* **multiple germline gene segments**, *(2)* **combinatorial joining of these segments**, *(3)* **junctional flexibility**, *(4)* **P-region addition**, *(5)* **random N-region addition**, *(6)* **alternative D-segment joining**, *and (7)* **combinatorial association of the α and β** or γ and δ **polypeptide subunits**. Even though TCR genes have fewer V-gene segments than does Ig, TCR diversity greatly exceeds Ig diversity. The greater TCR diversity is caused by some unique features of junctional diversification surrounding the coding sequences at junctional regions. Three phenomena contribute to the greater TCR junctional diversity: (1) as with Ig genes, but with four V-region junctions instead of three (V-J, V-D, D-D, and D-J), joining of TCR genes can be imprecise yet can lead to functionally rearranged genes, (2) P-region addition can occur in all TCR gene-segment joining (as for Ig gene rearrangement), and (3) N-region addition of up to 15–20 nucleotides can occur at the four different junctions in all four TCR chain genes (occurs only in Ig heavy-chain genes), and (4) unique to TCR genes, the arrangement of *recombination signal sequences* (*RSSs*) flanking $D_\beta$- and $D_\delta$-chain gene segments permits D segments to join to other D segments yet maintaining the 12–23 rule—leading to $(VDDJ)_\delta$ in mice and in humans $(VDDDJ)_\delta$. Alternative D-segment joining does not occur in Ig heavy-chain genes.

As in B cells, each V, D, J TCR germline segment is flanked by either heptamer (one-turn) RSSs or nonamer (two-turn) RSSs. The heptamer-nonamer or 12–23 rule, described for Ig-gene joining, also governs TCR-gene joining. Pre-T cells express recombination-activating genes-1 and -2 (*RAG-1* and *RAG-2*), which encode recombinase enzymes that recognize RSS1 and RSS2 to catalyze V-J and V-D-J joining through deletional or inversional mechanisms. As for Ig-gene rearrangement, RAG-1 and RAG-2 enzymes nick one strand of DNA between

**TABLE 8-2 Generation of Human TCR Diversity**

| | Potential combinations | | | |
|---|---|---|---|---|
| | αβ TCR | | γδ TCR | |
| 1. Multiple germline gene segments for variable regions | | | | |
| V | 50 | 57 | 14 | 3 |
| D | 0 | 2 | 0 | 3 |
| J | 70 | 13 | 5 | 3 |
| 2. Combinatorial joining of V-J or V-D-J segments | 50×70 = 3500 | 57 × 2 X 13 = 1482 | 14 × 5 = 60 | 3 × 3 X 3 = 27 |
| 3. Junctional flexibility | + | + | + | + |
| 4. P-region addition | + | + | + | + |
| 5 N-region nucleotide addition | V-J | V-D, D-J | V-J | V-D, D-D, D-J |
| 6. D-D segment joining | − | + (seldom) | − | + (often) |
| 7. Combinatorial association of chains | + | + | + | + |
| TOTAL DIVERSITY | | ≈ $10^{15}$ | | ≈ $10^{18}$ |

*Note:* + indicates that the mechanism contributes significantly to diversity. − indicates that the mechanism does not contribute to diversity. The contribution of junctional flexibility is due to the possible development of different amino acids at each junction (V-J, D-D, D-J, and V-[DJ]) due to four different contributing mechanisms. The contribution of N-region addition of 15–20 nucleotides at each junction could generate a huge number of different possible combinations at each junction. Like Ig light and heavy chains, any TCR α chain can associate with any β chain and any TCR γ chain can associate with any δ chain. So, combinatorial association of chains is another major contributor of diversity.

coding and signal sequences, coding end forms a hairpin structure whereas the signal end forms a 5′ double-strand break, and repair enzymes join the coding ends and join the signal ends and excise it as circular DNA. As in Ig genes, allelic exclusion allows only one of the two inherited α- (or γ-) chain loci and one of the two inherited β- (or δ-) chain loci to be functionally rearranged and expressed but exceptions exist. Because δ-chain gene segments are located within the α-chain gene cluster, once α gene segments are rearranged, δ gene segments are deleted excluding γδ-chain expression. β-chain gene segments are organized in two clusters; therefore, if rearrangement is nonproductive on the first attempt, it attempts to use the remaining cluster for a second try at rearrangement. Successful rearrangement at either attempt excludes rearrangement by the other β allele. The α-chain gene rearrangement can rarely occur in both α alleles simultaneously, because unlike Ig assembly that leads to termination of gene rearrangement and induces further B-cell differentiation, $V_\alpha$ TCR gene-segments continue to rearrange unless the receptor is positively selected (discussed later). Even though two different α chains can be expressed; this dual antigen specificity does not survive positive selection thereby ensuring that each T cell has only a single antigen specificity. The combination of these strategies could lead to $10^{18}$

different TCRs. *Somatic mutation does not occur in TCR genes.* Unlike a functional Ig, TCR affinity does not increase during a secondary T-cell immune response and isotypic switching does not occur.

To summarize, during intrathymic development, the TCR V regions are assembled from $V_\alpha$- and $J_\alpha$-gene segments for the α chain, $V_\beta$-, $D_\beta$-, and $J_\beta$-gene segments for the β chain, $V_\gamma$- and $J_\gamma$-gene segments for the γ chain, and $V_\delta$-, $D_\delta$-, and $J_\delta$-gene segments for the δ chain. At the joining site of each of these segments, nucleotides also are removed and added during recombination. This leads to tremendous TCR diversity. All these gene segments, acting together, determine TCR antigen specificity and MHC restriction.

# TCR ASSOCIATION WITH THE INVARIANT PROTEINS OF THE CD3 COMPLEX IS REQUIRED FOR TCR EXPRESSION AND T-CELL ACTIVATION

As B-cell Ig is associated with the Igα and Igβ signal transduction complex, the TCR is expressed on the T-cell membrane with a signal transduction complex called **the CD3 complex.** *The CD3 complex closely*

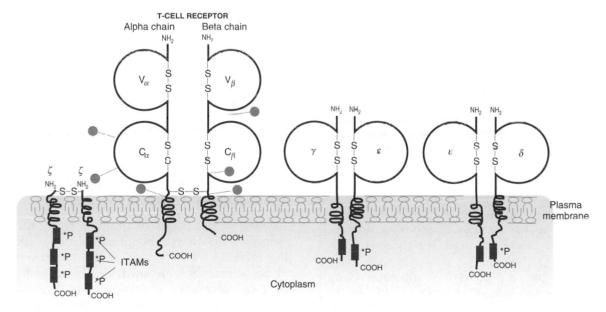

**FIGURE 8-7 The TCR-CD3 complex.** Shown is a seven-chain (δ, α, ε, γ, β, ζ, and η) model of the complex described in the text. The CD3 complex consists of three invariant peptide chains with individual molecular weights of 20 to 28 kD (δ = 20 kD, ε = 20 kD, γ = 25–28 kD molecular weigh). The disulfide-linked ζ-ζ (ζ = 16 kD) homodimers and the disulfide-linked ζ-η (η = 21 kD) heterodimer appear to be subunits that can associate with the TCR complex or other CD3 molecules; either form of the dimer can be found. The α and β TCR chains and the δ and γ CD3 chains are glycosylated (●), while the CD3 ε chain and the ζ and η chains are not. Phosphorylation (*P) can be elicited in the δ, γ, and ζ chains.

*associates with the human αβ and γδ TCR and plays a role in signal transduction after antigen binding* (Figure 8-7). The three invariant transmembrane proteins (γ, δ, and ε chains) that form the CD3 complex are noncovalently associated with the αβ TCR chains. A disulfide-linked ζ-ζ homodimer or a disulfide-linked ζ-η heterodimer independently associates with the TCR. Roughly 90% of ζ exists as a ζ-ζ homodimer, while 10% exists as a ζ-η heterodimer. The TCR complex consists of the αβ TCR noncovalently linked to the CD3 and ζ proteins. The CD3 complex regulates the assembly and expression of the TCR, and the TCR is not expressed if the CD3 complex is absent. The CD3 complex, along with the ζ/η chains, also controls signal transduction after ligand binding to the TCR. The γ, δ, and ε chains of CD3 have cytoplasmic domains that range from 44 to 81 amino acid residues in length. Each one of these domains contains a single copy of the signaling motif called **immunoreceptor tyrosine-based activation motif (ITAM)**. The ζ and η chains contain three copies of ITAM in their cytoplasmic domains. ITAMs are conserved segments, composed of (D/E)XXYXX(L/I)X6–8YXX(L/I), where X denotes any amino acid, found in the intracytoplasmic tails of CD3 and ζ proteins, Igα–Igβ (CD79a–CD79b), NK cell receptors and in several Ig Fc receptors that are targets for phosphorylation by tyrosine kinases, allowing them to interact with cytosolic enzymes. When the ITAM-containing receptors bind their ligands, the ITAMs' tyrosine residues become phosphorylated and form docking sites for other molecules mediating cell-activating signal transduction pathways, triggering a cascade of intracellular events that leads to T-cell activation. The process of T-cell activation is discussed later in the chapter.

---

**MINI SUMMARY**

The TCR differs from the B-cell receptor. TCRs exist only on the T cell's surface and recognize antigen fragments only when they are associated with MHC molecules. However, the TCRs and B-cell receptors belong to the Ig-gene superfamily. The TCR is made up of a heterodimer with an α and a β chain or a γ and a δ chain, and each chain has a V and a C domain. Gene segments for the V portion (antigen binding) of the TCR are generated in a scenario similar to that of Ig gene recombinations of V-, D-, and J-gene segments. These rearrangements occur during T-cell maturation but before antigen exposure. V-region rearrangements could lead to a diversity of $10^{18}$ different TCRs. The TCR gene

segments are not shared by B cells. A second kind of TCR exists that is derived from γ- and δ-gene rearrangements. The αβ TCR or γδ TCR is associated with the CD3 complex, which plays a role in signal transduction following TCR-antigen interaction, eventually leading to T-cell activation. The TCR also is associated with a disulfide-linked ζ-ζ homodimer or a disulfide-linked ζ-η heterodimer.

# ANTIGEN RECOGNITION REQUIRES ACCESSORY MOLECULES (OR CORECEPTORS)

Cell-surface molecules other than the TCR complex (αβ-CD3-ζη) affect the triggering and functional activity of T cells. *These molecules, called* **accessory molecules**, *are involved in lymphocyte adhesion and T-cell activation.* The accessory molecules can be further divided into those that ease physical interaction between antigen-presenting cells (APCs) and T cells (the adhesion molecules) and those needed for T-cell activation and proliferation (the *costimulator molecules*). Because some accessory molecules are intimately associated with TCR function, they are also called *coreceptors*. APCs provide costimulatory signals for T-cell activation. The cytokines *IL-1, IL-6,* and *TNF-α* or *-β* and chemokines *CCL19* and *CCL21* exhibit costimulator activity. When costimulators are absent during antigen presentation, tolerance to the displayed antigen occurs. (Cytokines are discussed in Chapter 9.) Some of the adhesion molecules are discussed below.

## Accessory Molecules for T Cells Function as Adhesion Molecules, Signal Transduction Molecules, or Both

Adhesive interactions of immune cells with other immune cells or with nonimmune cells is central to the successful functioning of the immune system. These interactions are mediated by different types of T-cell accessory molecules, which share some common properties; they (1) are invariant and nonpolymorphic, (2) bind ligands on APCs and target cells, vascular endothelial cells, and cells in extracellular matrix, (3) stabilize attachment between T cells and APCs or target cells by strengthening the bonds between them, (4) transduce signals, (5) can be used as identification markers, and (6) can be grouped into families. Four families of accessory/adhesion cell-surface molecules have been categorized (see Figure 3-18). Members of the Ig-gene superfamily, which include CD2, CD58, CD54, CD102, CD4, CD8, are important in regulating activated T-cell interactions during an immune response. Another group of adhesion molecules, the *integrin family*, accounts for antigen-independent adhesion and include CD11aCD18, CD11bCD18, CD11cCD18, and VLA molecules. Adhesion molecules, particularly the integrins, coordinate T-cell trafficking and serve directly as signaling molecules activating cell functions. Naïve T cells are programmed to recirculate through the seconday lymphoid tissues. In contrast, effector T cells must identify specific sites of antigen deposition in non-lymphoid tissues to exert targeted effector activity. Some members of these two families and other accessory molecules are discussed below.

### CD4 and CD8 Interactions with Their Counterreceptor, Class II and Class I MHC Molecules, Mediate Adhesion and Transduce Signals

*Unlike antibody effector functions mediated by $C_H$-chain regions, TCR C-region gene segments do not correlate with differences in T-cell function. Thus, the TCR is not enough to define T-cell functional responses.* The coreceptor molecules **CD4** and **CD8** define T-cell functional responses. CD4 and CD8 are members of the Ig-gene superfamily (see Figure 4-16). The 55-kD, single-chained CD4 molecule has four extracellular Ig V-like domains, a hydrophobic transmembrane region, and a long cytoplasmic domain that can be phosphorylated. In contrast, the CD8 molecule is a disulfide-linked heterodimer, consisting of an α chain and a β chain (30- to 38-kD each), or a homodimer of α chains. In either form of the molecule, both chains have a single N-terminal Ig V-like domain but a similar hydrophobic transmembrane region and a long (25–27 residues) cytoplasmic domain that can be phosphorylated. *The cellular distribution of CD4 and CD8 is mutually exclusive; either CD4 or CD8 molecules are found on mature T cells.* In humans, CD4 is also found in low numbers on monocytes and macrophages. CD4 and CD8 are two of the many accessory molecules on the surface of human T cells that enhance antigen-specific functions by acting as cell adhesion molecules—they are part of the *immunological synapse* (Figure 8-8), which will be discuss later in the chapter. *CD4 and CD8 molecules, which are transmembrane proteins with extracellular binding domains, transmembrane segments, and tyrosine kinase cytoplasmic domains, act as receptors for nonpolymorphic regions of class II and class I*

*MHC elements, respectively, and thereby contribute to adhesion and early signal transduction.* CD4, using its N-terminal, membrane-distal domain, binds to a site on the nonpolymorphic $\beta_2$ domain of the class II molecule. CD8, probably using the domains of both chains, binds to a site at the base of the class I molecule $\alpha_3$ domain. CD4 or CD8 and the TCR diffuse independently in the plane of the T-cell plasma membrane until they are brought together by corecognition of the foreign peptide-class I or -class II MHC molecule complex. The interactions between MHC products and accessory molecules do not just stabilize cell-cell interactions but also help T-cell activation. This idea is reinforced by the fact that CD4 and the α chain of the heterodimer CD8 are associated through their cytoplasmic tail to Lck, a protein-tyrosine kinase. In fact, CD4 and CD8 initiate T-cell activation through cytoplasmically associated Lck. Because of these kinds of links to TCR functions, CD4 and CD8 are also called *coreceptors*.

### CD2 (LFA-2) Interaction with Its Counterreceptor, CD58 (LFA-3), Is Tipped Toward Adhesion by T-Cell Activation

**CD2** (also called **lymphocyte function-associated antigen-2 [LFA-2]**) enhances antigen-specific functions by acting as a cell adhesion molecule. Roughly $5 \times 10^4$ CD2 molecules are found on most mature naive T cells (also found on human NK cells and thymocytes). CD2, a 45- to 50-kD glycoprotein and its ligand, **CD58 (LFA-3)**, a 55- to 70-kD glycoprotein, are members of the Ig-gene superfamily. CD58 is found on many different types of immune and nonimmune cells. The interaction between CD2 and CD58 promotes cell-cell adhesion as part of the immunologic synapse; this seems to promote and stabilize TCR searching for antigenic peptide-MHC complexes (see Figure 8-8). Once TCR binds to peptide-MHC complexes and signaling increase, the avidity of CD2 for CD58 increases.

### CD11aCD18 (LFA-1) Interaction with Its Counterreceptors, CD54 (ICAM-1) and CD102 (ICAM-2), Is Needed for Many Immune Cell Functions

Another group of important T-cell adhesion molecules, which mediates cell-cell, cell-extracellular matrix, and cell-pathogen interactions, are members of the integrin family (see Chapter 3). The immune system relies in part on integrins for leukocyte trafficking, migration, attachment to endothelial cells, and extravasation of cells into tissues, immunological synapse formation (T cell-attachment to APCs) and costimulation, and cytotoxic killing. During

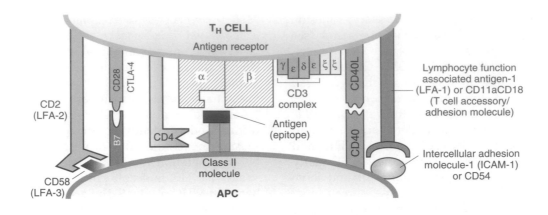

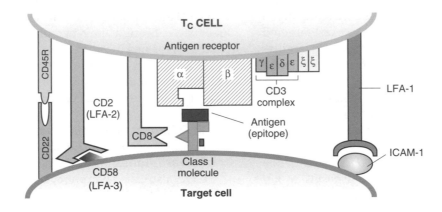

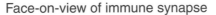

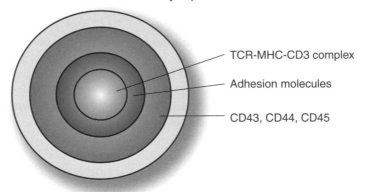

Face-on-view of immune synapse

**FIGURE 8-8 Model for accessory molecule-antigen receptor recognition by T cells—the immunologic synapse**. CD8 (or CD4) and the TCR-CD3 complex cooperate in the recognition of antigen. Each of these components recognizes different products of the MHC, leading to the formation of a quaternary complex during the process of antigen presentation. The CD8 and CD4 structures recognize invariant regions of class I and II MHC molecules, respectively, while the TCR-CD3 complex recognizes foreign peptides in the context of the same molecules. The other molecules, CD2 and CD11aCD18, play a key role in cell adhesion among leukocytes and between leukocytes and nonimmune cells. For example, the cytolytic response may proceed from low-affinity interactions between CD11aCD18 and CD54 (ICAM-1/2), causing initial cell contact between a T$_C$ cell and a target cell that eases antigen recognition to high-affinity ligand binding, resulting from ligated TCR-CD3-mediated signaling that activates CD11aCD18 through phosphorylation of its β chain. This strengthening of adhesion facilitates efficient delivery of the lethal hit. Dephosphorylation of CD11aCD18 to its low-affinity (inactive) state allows the T$_C$ cell to detach from the target cell.

an infection, effector T cells need to be guided to the infection sites. Antigen-naïve T cells, expressing L-selectin (CD62L), are enable to enter lymph nodes by binding to CD34 on high endothelial cells. Once activated, effector T cells loose L-selectin, increase expression of integrins (discussed below), exit the lymph nodes, and traffic to tissues contaminated with antigen.

**Lymphocyte function-associated antigen-1 (LFA-1)** is needed for many leukocyte functions, including B-cell responses, T-cell-mediated killing, $T_H$-cell responses, natural killing, ADCC by macrophages and neutrophils, and adherence of leukocytes to endothelial cells (see Figure 8.8). LFA-1 is a member of the integrin family of adhesion receptors. Each integrin molecule is made up of an α- and a β-subunit. There are three forms of the β-subunit called $\beta_1$ (CD29), $\beta_2$ (CD18), and $\beta_3$ (CD61) integrins. LFA-1 belongs to the $\beta_2$ subfamily and therefore can be called **CD11aCD18**. CD11aCD18 molecules are found on mature/activated T cells. During an inflammatory reaction, the vascular endothelium at the inflammation site releases cytokines and chemokines, together with TCR ligation by recruited T cells, rapidly increase CD11aCD18 expression and avidity for its ligand.[2] One ligand for CD11aCD18 is **intercellular adhesion molecule-1 (ICAM-1 [CD54])**, a molecule that is expressed on lymphocytes, monocytes, dendritic cells, endothelial cells, and fibroblasts. CD54, an 80- to 114-kD glycoprotein, is a member of the Ig-gene superfamily with five extracellular Ig-like domains. Its expression on APCs and endothelial cells is increased by a variety of inflammatory cytokines such as interferon-γ, IL-1, and TNF. The second CD11aCD18 ligand, **ICAM-2 (CD102)**, differs in tissue distribution from ICAM-1. ICAM-2 is found mainly on endothelial cells and is constitutively expressed. ICAM-2 expression is not increased by cytokines. In contrast to ICAM-1, ICAM-2 has only two extracellular Ig-like domains.

Another group of integrins, called **very late activation (VLA)** molecules, are important in cell-cell adhesion. VLA-1 through -6 are members of the $\beta_1$ subfamily of integrins. They share a common β chain, CD29, which is noncovalently associated with

VLA α chains (CD49a to CD49f). The conversion of antigen-naïve T cells to effector T cells leads to an increased expression of VLA-4 and LFA-1. VLA-4 binds to vascular cell adhesion molecule 1 (VCAM-1 [CD106]), a molecule expressed on cytokine- and chemokine-activated vascular endothelial cells in inflamed tissues, which facilitates tight adhesion and extravasation into inflamed tissues by chemokine-recruited effector T cells.

Collectively, T-cell activation, a 4 to 5 day process, is a sequential series of events moving from cellular interaction to effector function. T cells recognize and are activated by only a few APC-displayed peptide-MHC complexes. Because TCRs have low affinity ($K_d$ of $4 \times 10^{-4}$ to $6 \times 10^{-7}$ M) and high off-rate for their peptide-MHC complexes, antigen-independent adhesion probably occurs simultaneously with TCR engagement. That is, when the TCR is turned on, various adhesion molecules rapidly but temporarily upregulate their adhesion. Thus, the conjugate formation (*adhesion*) between a T cell and an APC may not be totally antigen-specific and involves the interaction of CD2 and CD11aCD18 with their respective ligands, integrins and their ligands, and CD4 and CD8 also may participate. TCR engagement with peptide and class I or II MHC molecules may be eased or stabilized by the interaction of CD4 or CD8 molecules with MHC molecules. How many TCRs need to be engaged by peptide-MHC complexes to initiate T-cell activation? The most recent evidence, as measured by $Ca^{2+}$ release, suggests even a single TCR-MHC complex causes $Ca^{2+}$ release and maximal $Ca^{2+}$ release is achieved in $CD4^+$ and $CD8^+$ T cells with the formation of as few as 10 TCR-MHC complexes.

## Other T-Cell Accessory Molecules, Costimulators, Which Regulate the Response of Antigen-Activated T Cells

Although antigen-specific T-cell activation is started through the TCR, TCRs do not stimulate proliferation if they engage *only* with peptide-MHC complexes. T cells require *costimulation*, a "second signal" (a concept introduced in Chapter 1) from APCs primarily through CD28–B7 family of interactions, respectively. Costimulation receptor function is completely dependent on TCR signals, and the role of costimulatory receptors is to modulate the TCR signal, the combined strength of these two signals determines whether naïve T cells will proliferate and differentiate into effector cells. The engagement of additional T-cell accessory molecules, including some of the tumor necrosis factor (TNF)/TNF receptor (TNFR) family

---

[2]This is an example of how integrin adhesiveness is uniquely regulated by a process called *inside-out signaling*. Stimuli received through chemokine, cytokine, and antigen receptors initiate intracellular signals that act on cytoplasmic domains of integrins and alter their adhesiveness for extracellular ligands.

and others (CD44 and CD45), provide the essential costimulatory signals needed for the full activation of T cells. The most prominent costimulatory receptor is CD28. Even though the term *costimulator* is used more often, they are *cosignaling molecules* and depending on their functional outcome are grouped into costimulators or positive costimulatory molecules that enhance TCR activity and coinhibitors or negative costimulatory molecules that inhibit TCR activity. Figure 8-9 illustrates some of these costimulators and the results of their interactions.

**CD28**, a 44-kD homodimeric glycoprotein receptor, is constitutively expressed on 90% and 50% of human peripheral blood CD4$^+$ and CD8$^+$ T cells, respectively, and is stimulated during engagement of T cells with APCs or target cells. CD28 is expressed by naïve and activated T cells. The CD28 family of receptors includes *cytotoxic T lymphocyte-associated protein 4 (CTLA-4 [CD152]), inducible costimulator (ICOS), programmed death 1 (PD-1 [CD279]), and B and T lymphocyte attenuator (BTLA)*. CD28, a member of the Ig-gene superfamily, is a transmembrane protein of 202 amino acids. The best-defined ligands for CD28 are the costimulatory molecules B7-1 (CD80) and B7-2 (CD86) (expressed on professional APCs, B cells, dendritic cells, and macrophages). B7 is also a member of Ig-gene superfamily; the B7 family of molecules includes B7-1, B7-2, ICOS ligand (also called *B7H*), B7-H1, B7-DC, B7-H3, and B7-H4. The interaction between CD28 and its counterreceptor, B7, is needed for APC-T cell cooperation and T-B-cell cooperation (see Chapter 10). CD28 serves as the top hierarchical surface component of a signal transduction pathway that not only stimulates cytokine (particularly IL-2) production, antiapoptotic protein (BCL-X$_L$) production, and T-cell growth and differentiation but also drives in cascade-like fashion subsequent costimulator interactions. For example, CD28 signals upregulate CD40 ligand expression, which leads to APC CD40 signaling, which in turn upregulates B7-1 and B7-2 expression—amplifies the T cell–APC interaction. Unlike CD28, only activated T cells express ICOS. T-cell ICOS binding to APC ICOS-L enhances the production of IL-4 and IL-10, Ig class switching, and the formation of germinal centers. A structurally homologous molecule to CD28, *CTLA-4*, despite its name, it is not restricted to cytotoxic T cells; it is expressed on activated and memory CD4$^+$ and CD8$^+$ T cells (as is ICOS). CTLA-4, PD-1, and BTLA are inhibitory receptors that bind to the negative constimulatory B7 family molecules. CTLA-4 inhibits T-cell activation by out competing CD28 for B7 binding, which leads to the termination of the T-cell response.

CTLA-4 has a higher affinity for B7 molecules than does CD28. The APC ligands for T-cell PD-1 receptor are B7-H1 and B7-DC, the ligand for BTLA is unknown. The receptors for B7-H3 and B7-H4 are unknown.

The TNF/TNFR superfamily include members, such as the 4-1BB (CD137), CD27, CD30, OX-40 (CD134) receptors and their ligands 4-1BBL, CD27L (CD70), CD30L (CD153), and OX-40L, respectively, also serve an important function in the costimulatory cross-talk between cells. One of the principals is the TNFR family member CD40, which is a 48 kD transmembrane glycoprotein cell-surface receptor constitutively expressed on B cells. Its ligand, CD40L, is a 34–39 kD membrane protein expressed on activated but not naive T cells. CD40L interaction with APC CD40 governs the magnitude and quality of humoral- and cell-mediated immunity. B cell CD40–T cell CD40L interaction in the presence of cytokines leads to intense clonal expansion, differentiation to Ig secretion, and enhancement of B-cell APC capacity. Dendritic cell CD40–T cell CD40L interaction in the presence of signals by toll-like receptors (TLRs), drives the maturation of dendritic cells to increased proficiency in antigen presentation, cytokine and chemokine production, and extended survival.

**CD44**, an acidic sulfated membrane glycoprotein, also is involved in cell-cell adhesion and T-cell activation. CD44 is expressed on mature T cells, thymocytes, B cells, erythrocytes, fibroblasts, monocytes and macrophages, and granulocytes. CD44 binds hyaluronate; therefore, it is important in binding endothelial cells and extracellular matrix. It affords easy binding for activated and memory T cells to endothelial cells associated with inflammation sites.

**CD45** (formerly called *leukocyte-common antigen*), a cell-surface glycoprotein with a cytoplasmic tyrosine phosphatase domain, is present on T and B cells, thymocytes, granulocytes, and monocytes. CD45 exists in many different isoforms; the ones expressed on a restricted group of cells are called *CD45R*. Naïve T cells expressed CD45RA, whereas memory T cells express CD45RO; however, there is no evidence to associated a particular function with expressed isoforms. CD45 is the most abundant cytoplasmic tyrosine phosphatase found associated with T cells; it catalyzes dephosphorylation of tyrosine residues in several substrates, such as Lck, the tyrosine kinase associated with CD4 and CD8 molecules. This kinase activation can trigger the next steps in T-cell activation. The ligand for the extracellular portion of CD45 remains unknown.

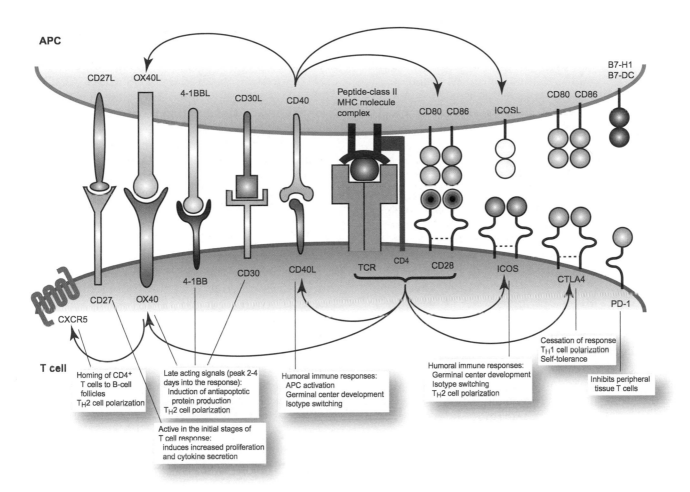

**FIGURE 8-9** The immunoglobulin-like CD28-B7 family and TNF receptor family of costimulators and their activities. CD28 plays the key role in promoting the full activation of naïve T cells after TCR stimulation. Only the costimulator molecules that are members of immunoglobulin superfamily (CD28 receptors and their B7 ligands) and tumor necrosis factor (TNF) superfamily are mentioned here. Both costimulators (molecule that promote TCR-mediated responses) and coinhibitors (molecules that demote TCR-mediated responses) are written as costimulators and the terms receptor and ligand are used to distinguish the signal transmission direction. The arrows suggest that the binding of CD28 and B7 molecules have direct effects, such as, cell proliferation, antiapoptotic molecule production, cytokine gene expression, and a second-wave of costimulator receptor expression. For example, the induction of CD40L expression and its ligation to APC CD40 instigates a cascade of activities from clonal expansion to augmented humoral responses to $T_H$ cell polarization to the expression of other receptors. (Adapted from O. Acuto and F. Michel. 2003. *Nat. Rev. Immunol.* 3:939.)

# T CELLS SPECIFIC FOR FOREIGN PEPTIDES BOUND TO SELF-MHC MOLECULES ARE SELECTED FOR MATURATION IN THE THYMUS

Bone marrow-derived progenitor T cells enter the thymus devoid of any surface molecules or antigen receptors characteristic of mature T cells. These progenitor cells will give rise to a major $\alpha\beta^+$, and a minor $\gamma\delta^+$, T cell population. The $\alpha\beta^+$ T cell population will eventually become CD4$^+$ T and CD8$^+$ T cells with a specificity repertoire that is large, self MHC-restricted, and self-tolerant. The thymus serves as the major site of T-cell repertoire development. The development process involves migration and proliferation, differentiation, and selection. All of these processes are the result of sequential interactions of thymocytes with cortical/medullary epithelial cells and thymic macrophages and dendritic cells. As the T cells develop in the thymus, different surface markers that regulate differentiation and selection appear and disappear in their membranes. By tracking the expression of these markers, we can follow the T cell's journey to maturity.

The overall scheme for human T-cell differentiation in the thymus can be monitored by the surface expression of coreceptors CD4 and CD8 (Figure 8-10). In the eighth or ninth week of gestation in humans (we now know that this is a 24-7 process that occurs throughout life), progenitor T (pro-T) cells migrate from the bone marrow and enter the thymus expressing neither CD4 nor CD8; they are called immature **double-negative (DN)** T cells and represent roughly 60% of CD4$^-$ CD8$^-$ thymocytes. These DN (CD4$^-$CD8$^-$CD3-$\zeta^-$TCR$^-$) T cells, which comprise 1–2% of thymocytes, enter the thymus at the cortico-medullary junction, progressively migrate to the subcapsular zone of the outer cortex, return through the cortex, move into the medulla, and exit into the periphery. This cellular migration is characterized by distinct stages: double-negative (DN; CD4$^-$CD8$^-$), double-positive (DP; CD4$^+$CD8$^+$), and finally single-positive (SP; CD4$^+$CD8$^-$ or CD4$^-$CD8$^+$) cells. All stages are associated with separate localizations in the thymus. The DN stage T cells can be further divided into four subsets: DN1—DN4 dependent on the differential expression of c-kit (receptor for stem cell factor), CD44 (an adhesion molecule), and CD25 (the $\alpha$ chain of the IL-2 receptor). The most immature thymocyte precursors, DN1 cells, are c-kit$^+$CD4$^-$CD8$^-$CD44$^+$CD25$^-$, which have multi-lineage potential, including myeloid-cell, NK cell, dendritic cell, B-cell, and T-cell potential. c-kit$^+$CD4$^-$CD8$^-$CD44$^+$CD25$^+$ DN2 cells lack B-cell potential but still have NK cell, dendritic cell, and T-cell potential. During the DN2 stage, the cells express recombination-activating genes (RAG-1 and -2) and simultaneous rearrangement of the TCR $\beta$-chain, TCR $\gamma$-chain, and TCR $\delta$-chain loci begins; rearrangement of TCR $\alpha$-chain genes does not occur, perhaps due to recombinase inaccessibility.

Which TCR chain loci win the rearrangement competition? The transduction of signals through the $\gamma\delta$ TCR or pre-TCR determines whether thymocytes become $\gamma\delta^+$ or $\alpha\beta^+$ T cells. If a $\gamma\delta$ TCR is completed before successful $\beta$-chain gene-segment rearrangement, it cannot lead to pre-TCR production, the thymocyte receives signals through the $\gamma\delta$ TCR, which terminates further $\beta$-chain gene-segment rearrangement and commits the cell to a $\gamma\delta$ lineage. If a successful $\beta$-chain is completed first and pairs with pre-TCR $\alpha$-chain to form a pre-TCR, signals are transduced through the pre-TCR, which terminates $\gamma$- and $\delta$-chain gene-segment rearrangement and commits the cell to an $\alpha\beta$ lineage. At the transition from the DN2 to DN3 stage, $\gamma\delta$ T cells begin their development; they represent less than 5% of mature thymocytes. Most DN2 thymocytes are destined to become $\alpha\beta$ T cells. In the DN3 stage, final T-cell lineage commitment occurs; the cells turn off c-kit and CD44 expression (c-kit$^-$CD4$^-$CD8$^-$CD44$^-$CD25$^+$). At this stage, cells stop proliferating, the TCR $\beta$-chain locus chromatin configuration is accessible to RAG-1 and -2-encode proteins thereby permitting TCR $\beta$-chain gene rearrangements, if a productive TCR $\beta$-chain is produced, it pairs with the invariant **pre-TCR $\alpha$-chain** and CD3 and $\zeta$ proteins forming a **pre-TCR** that signals for further differentiation toward the DN4 and DP stages. During the transition from DN3 to DN4, CD25 expression is halted (c-kit$^-$CD4$^-$CD8$^-$CD44$^-$CD25$^-$), the TCR $\beta$-chain locus becomes inaccessible (suppresses further gene rearrangement, which leads to allelic exclusion), and the cells experience several rounds of division during which RAG-1 and -2 are inactive. As the cell progresses to the DP stage, RAG-1 and -2 are reactivated; the cell converts to a TCR $\alpha$-chain locus rearrangement tolerant cell (TCR $\alpha$-chain locus chromatin configuration is now accessible), and the cell progresses to the *double-positive stage—cells express both CD4 and CD8 coreceptors.* The CD4$^+$CD8$^+$ **double-positive** (DP) cells (constitute 75–88% of thymocytes) are short-lived, rapidly dividing cells, once the cells stop proliferating and RAG-2 protein levels increase, TCR $\alpha$-chain locus rearrangement starts. The rapidly proliferation of thymocytes with productive $\beta$-chain gene rearrangements provides a larger clone of cells, where each cell can rearrange a different $\alpha$-chain gene that leads to unique antigen-specific $\alpha\beta$ TCRs. These DP CD3$^+$, $\alpha\beta$ TCR$^+$ thymocytes are now ready for the gauntlet of positive and negative selection (discussed next) into **single-positive (SP;** CD4$^+$CD8$^-$ or CD4$^-$CD8$^+$) cells. In the cortex, the DP cells, which represent the vast majority cells in the thymus, will undergo positive and negative selection, mature into SP cells, move into the medulla for another round of negative selection, and then they exit the thymus. Although only 1 to 3% of the cells are selected for entry to the periphery, *three main T-cell lineages are generated during T-cell development* (see Figure 8-10). (Four, if you include naturally occurring CD4$^+$CD25$^+$ T regulator cells [mentioned shortly; also see Chapter 10].)

How does the thymus limit TCR diversity so that mature T cells express only receptors for a foreign antigenic peptide-self-MHC molecule complex? *The labyrinthine process of acquiring MHC-restriction is called* **thymic selection.** *MHC-restriction is not preprogrammed into T cells, but is acquired by contact with humoral factors and by physical interaction of TCR-expressing cells with MHC molecule- and*

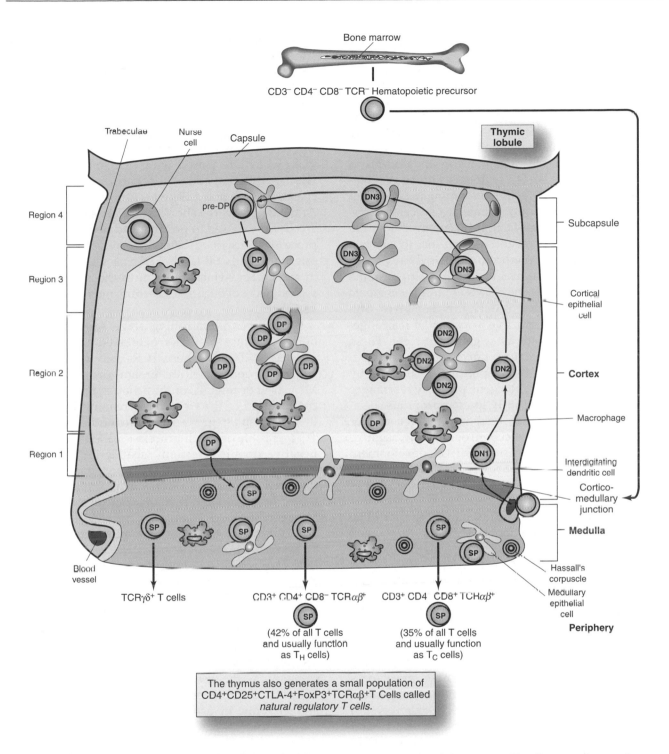

**FIGURE 8-10 Intrathymic human T-cell differentiation.** The development of the mature T cell repertoire can be followed by analyzing the expression of CD4 and CD8 molecules on thymocytes. CD25 and CD44 and CD3 and TCR molecules change along with CD4 and CD8 expression. In fact, CD25 and CD44 are used to divide CD4$^-$CD8$^-$ double-negative (DN) thymocytes into four subsets, DN1: c-kit$^+$CD44$^+$CD25$^-$; DN2: c-kit$^+$CD44$^+$CD25$^+$; DN3: c-kit$^-$CD44$^-$CD25$^+$; and DN4: c-kit$^-$CD44$^-$CD25$^-$. Cells expressing TCR$\gamma\delta$ (derived at the transition between DN2 and DN3 stages) and TCR$\alpha\beta$ are separate lineages that develop from common precursors. Subsets of thymocytes are divided into CD4$^-$CD8$^-$ double-negative cells, CD3$^-$CD4$^+$CD8$^-$ or CD3$^-$CD4$^-$CD8$^+$ transiently immature single-positive cells, CD4$^+$CD8$^+$ double-positive cells, and mature CD4$^+$CD8$^-$ or CD4$^-$CD8$^+$ single-positive cells. High levels of TCR expression start at the double-positive stage. The development of single-positive T cells is coincident with up-regulation of CCR7 and migration to the medulla. See text for more detail. (Adapted from C.C. Blackburn and N.R. Manley. 2004. *Nat. Rev. Immunol.* 4:278.)

*cytokine-expressing thymic cells during T-cell development in the thymus.*

TCR proteins tightly control T-cell development. The stages of α- and β-chain gene loci rearrangement progress through a similar sequence as seen in Ig heavy- and light-chain loci rearrangement during B-cell development (see Chapter 6). Just as Ig heavy-chain loci rearrangement occurs first in B cells, TCR β-chain loci rearrangement in thymocytes is always first, that is, D$_β$ segments join in V$_β$ segments, followed by V$_β$ segments joining to DJ$_β$-joined segments. If the rearrangements are successful, the cell can produce a pre-TCR, if all attempts fail, the cells must rearrange γ- and δ-chain loci to survive. Unlike B cells with nonproductive Ig heavy-chain gene-segment rearrangement, the β-chain germline gene-segment organization (two D$_β$ and J$_β$ segments upstream of C$_β$ genes; see Figure 8.6) gives thymocytes with nonproductive β-chain VDJ rearrangements four more attempts at getting it right. These additional attempts increase the chances for productive rearrangements. Developing αβ T cells die by apoptosis unless the TCR β gene properly rearranges and produces complete αβ TCRs of appropriate specificity. These T cells are then selected for further development (positive selection) or deletion (negative selection). Thus, the process of αβ T-cell development is controlled by the TCR at two separate stages: (1) by the TCR β chain and (2) by the V-region specificities of the complete αβ TCR (Figure 8-11).

As discussed earlier in the chapter, the germline genes used for construction of TCRs are rearranged and expressed in a random manner. This process generates immature TCRαβ$^+$ (and TCRγδ$^+$) thymocytes that express all the possible antigenic peptide and MHC specificities available for selection. At the beginning of the process, the DN1 c-kit$^+$CD44$^+$CD25$^-$ progenitor T cells, lacking CD3, ζ, or TCR, come in contact with the thymic environment and begin to proliferate and express CD25 becoming DN2 c-kit$^+$CD44$^+$CD25$^+$ pre-T cells. These pre-T cells undergo D$_β$-to-J$_β$ rearrangement (and rearrangement for γ- and δ-chain genes but not α-chain genes) followed by V$_β$-to-DJ$_β$ rearrangements, which lead to cytoplasmically detectable β-chain protein. DN2 pre-T cells also express CD3 and ζ molecules. The newly synthesized β-chain is expressed on the cell surface combined with the *pre-Tα chain*, and both chains are associated with the CD3 and ζ components to form the *pre-TCR*. The pre-TCR interacts with yet unknown ligands and halts β-gene rearrangements, induces proliferation, CD4 and CD8 coreceptor expression, and allows the now DP$^+$ cells to begin TCR α-chain locus rearrangements. While in the

subcapsular zone, a second wave of *RAG-1* and −2 gene expressions, the cells rapidly divide and rearrange their TCR genes. Although the γδ TCR is expressed first, the αβ TCR lineage represents the main developmental pathway (TCR γδ- and TCR αβ-expressing thymocytes are separate lineages with a common precursor). After α-gene rearrangement, the cells stop dividing and express increased complete TCR, which are paired with CD3 and ζ molecules. During differentiation, most cortical thymocytes coexpress CD4 and CD8 with higher levels of TCRs. At the DP stage, the short-lived (3 to 4 day life-span) T cells are exposed to positive and negative selection processes (described below). Positive and negative selection yields SP CD4$^+$CD8$^-$ or CD4$^-$CD8$^+$ cells in the cortex, which move into the medulla for a second wave of negative selection and finally into the periphery.

The second controlling stage screens the random repertoire of TCRs expressed on immature, unselected, T cells. These TCRs may recognize any antigenic peptide (self or foreign) displayed by any MHC (self or foreign) or they may not recognize any combination of the two. The screening is regulated by the variable-region specificities of the complete αβ TCR. This life or death process is called **positive** and **negative thymic selection**[3] (see Figure 8-11), which initially occurs in the cortex. *During positive selection, the T-cell repertoire is preferentially amplified for cells having low avidity αβ TCRs that recognize self- (future foreign) peptides only if presented by self-MHC molecules. During negative selection, T cells that have high-avidity TCRs reactive to abiquitous self-MHC molecules and associated self-peptides (and tissue-restricted self-antigens)[4] are eliminated.* Thymocytes unable to recognize any peptide–MHC molecules (no TCR signal) by default fail positive selection and die by apoptosis; that is, no TCR signal leads to death by neglect. Any positively selected T cells that are self-reactive are eliminated by a second wave of negative selection in the medulla. Therefore, positive and negative selections permit T-cell reactivity to foreign antigen only in association with the appropriate

---

[3]Positive selection means that the cells of interest are kept. In contrast, negative selection means that all cells but the ones of interest are kept, that is, positive selection for self-MHC restricted cells and negative selection of autoreactive T cells.

[4]Tissue-specific proteins would not be expected to be expressed in the thymus, yet some stromal cells in the thymic medulla express many tissue-specific proteins. Therefore, negative selection applies even to proteins restricted to tissues outside the thymus (see Chapter 13).

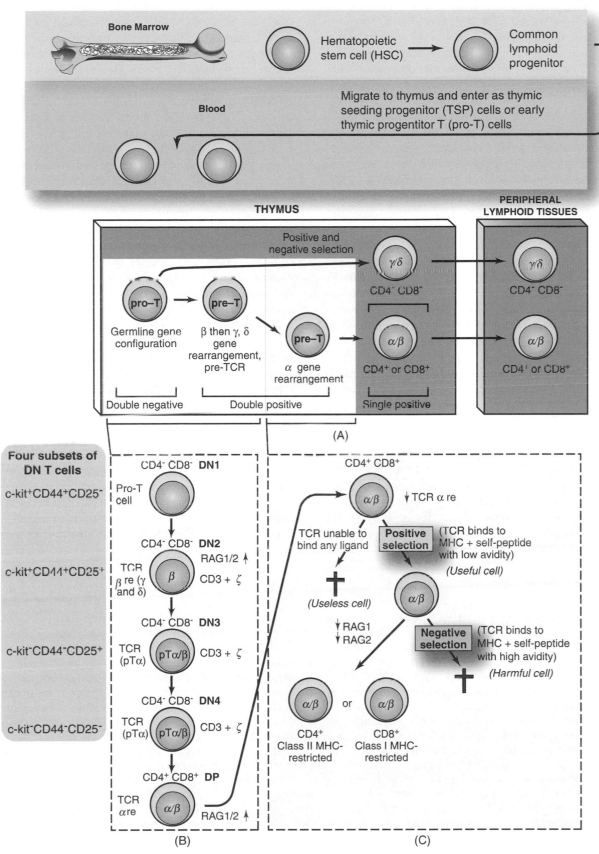

**FIGURE 8-11** *Continued*

self-MHC molecules and tolerance to self-antigens associated with self-MHC, respectively. Negative selection is often reached by clonal deletion or clonal anergy (see Chapter 13). Cortical epithelial cells that express class I and II MHC molecules associated with self-peptides determine the specificity of positive selection, while APCs (macrophages and dendritic cells) and to lesser extend medullary epithelial cells mediate negative selection. In either case, if the thymocyte TCR fits the MHC-peptide expressed by the respective cells, it will be positively (rescued from apoptosis) or negatively (induces apoptosis) selected. Because only thymocytes whose TCRs can bind foreign peptides and self-class I or II MHC molecules are left after thymic selection, *mature T cells are self-MHC-restricted and self-tolerant.* This intrathymic maturation process leads to at least three subsets of mature peripheral T cells: CD4$^+$CD8$^-$TCR$\alpha\beta^+$ class II-restricted T cells, CD4$^-$CD8$^+$TCR$\alpha\beta^+$ class I-restricted T cells, CD4$^-$CD8$^-$TCR$\gamma\delta^+$ T cells, and a small population of CD4$^+$ T cells that have regulatory properties; these T cells, called *natural regulatory T cells* (see Chapter 10), express high levels of cell-surface CD25 and CTLA-4 and the Forkhead transcription factor FOXP3. An alternative, extrathymic development pathway generates an additional group of T cells, CD4$^-$CD8$^-$TCR$\alpha\beta^+$, found in the periphery. They are abundant in some tissues, such as the gut (see Chapter 2). Their MHC restriction and antigen recognition characteristics are unknown. In the case of CD4$^+$ and CD8$^+$ mature T cells, positive selection has determined their cell-surface phenotype and functional potential, which leads to an appropriate roadmap for efficient effector T-cell development during an immune response.

Experimental use of knockout mice has provided evidence for some of the necessary components in thymic selection. For example, knockout mice unable to produce class I MHC molecules have normal distributions of DN, DP, and CD4$^+$ thymocytes but fail to produce CD8$^+$ thymocytes, whereas class II MHC molecule-deficient mice have normal distributions of DN, DP, and CD8$^+$ thymocytes but fail to produce CD4$^+$ thymocytes. The lymph nodes of class II MHC molecule-deficient mice lack CD4$^+$ T cells. These results provide direct evidence that positive selection of CD8$^+$ and CD4$^+$ T cells requires thymocyte binding of class I and class II MHC molecules. The human immunodeficiency diseases called *bare lymphocyte syndromes* (see Chapter 16) confirm the importance of MHC molecules in the development of CD4$^+$ and CD8$^+$ T cells; individuals that cannot express class II MHC molecules have CD8$^+$ T cells but few CD4$^+$ T cells, whereas individuals that cannot express class I MHC molecules have CD4$^+$ T cells but few CD8$^+$ T cells.

The thymic-selecting process sets up an MHC-restriction bias. Bias is equivalent to MHC restriction to the haplotype of the host thymus. Figure 8-12 schematically summarizes positive selection using bone marrow and thymus chimeras. The complexity of chimera experiments left their interpretation controversial. Other approaches have provided direct evidence supporting positive and negative selection as a necessary stage in T-cell development. These approaches include the creation of transgenic mice in which all the T cells had the same receptor or the exposure of normal mice to superantigens. (The development of transgenic mice is described in Chapter 5.)

---

**FIGURE 8-11 The development of αβ T cells.** Bone marrow-derived precursor T cells migrate to the thymus by the blood stream, undergo antigen-independent development to mature T cells, exit the thymus and seed periphery, where they experience antigen-dependent activation leading to the development of effector and memory cell. As thymocytes begin development, they express neither CD4 nor CD8, they are CD4$^-$CD8$^-$ cells; therefore, they called *double-negative (DN) cells.* They are subdivided into four subsets (DN1–DN4), which are characterized by their expression of surface molecules c-kit, CD44, and CD25.(*A*) This panel illustrates the overall sequence for the development of γδ$^+$ T cells (diverge at the transition between double-negative DN2 and DN3 stages) and αβ$^+$ T cells. Panels B and C detail the two stages of αβ T-cell development as controlled by the TCR. (*B*) The TCRβ-CD3 complex controls thymocyte growth, starts CD4 and CD8 expression and TCR α-gene transcription, and suppresses further TCR β-gene rearrangement (re). (*C*) The developmental control by the TCR β chain leads to the specificity of the complete αβ TCR. This TCR controls whether thymocytes die (†) when they are unable to bind any ligand, are rescued from programmed cell death when they bind the correct MHC-peptide complex (positive selection), or are deleted when they bind an MHC-self-peptide complex (negative selection). The consequences of positive selection are inhibition (↓) of the continuing TCR α rearrangement (re), increase in the density of TCR expression, and development of T cells into either class II-restricted CD4$^+$ cells or class I-restricted CD8$^+$ cells. Which MHC restriction path is followed depends on the specificity of their receptors. α-Chain rearrangement stops only when the αβ TCR has bound to the appropriate MHC-peptide ligands (positive selection), which terminates (↓) expression of the recombination activation genes (RAG1 and RAG2). See text for more detail.

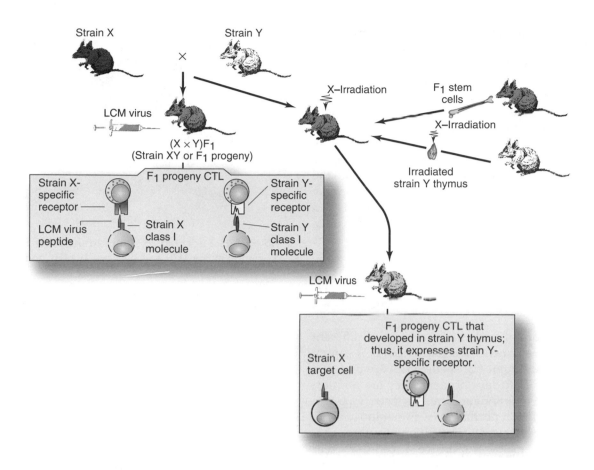

**FIGURE 8-12 Model for positive selection in the development of MHC restriction.** The $F_1$ progeny mouse is immunized with lymphocytic choriomeningitis (LCM) virus. $T_C$ lymphocytes (CTL) harvested from this mouse are able to kill cells from strain X and strain Y mice. To test the importance of the thymus in CTL MHC restriction, the $F_1$ progeny mouse is thymectomized and irradiated. This animal is reconstituted with stem cells from another $F_1$ mouse and the irradiated thymus from a strain Y mouse. Cells are allowed to develop in the $F_1$ mouse with a strain Y thymus. The experimental $F_1$ mouse is then immunized with LCM virus. The harvested CTL can kill virus-infected strain Y cells but not virus-infected strain X cells.

**TABLE 8-3 Demonstration of Positive and Negative Selection in SCID TCR Transgenic Mice**

| | | Selection | | | |
|---|---|---|---|---|---|
| **Experimental transgenic mice** | | **Positive** | **Negative** | **Transgenic TCR on mature T cells** | **Results if cells survive** |
| 1. | Male MHC $D^b$ H-Y$^+$ | Yes* | Yes | No | Harmful |
| 2. | Female MHC $D^b$ H-Y$^-$ | Yes | No | Yes (CD8$^+$ T cells)$^†$ | Useful |
| 3. | Female MHC $D^k$ H-Y$^-$ | No | No | No | Useless |

*If the male mouse's T cells react with foreign peptide associated with the appropriate MHC molecules, those cells are preserved (positive selection), mature, and populate the peripheral lymphoid tissue.
$^†$Only CD8$^+$ $T_C$ cells appear because the transgenic genes came from only cloned $T_C$ cells, suggesting that αβ TCR specificity for class I or class II MHC molecules determines whether a developing T cell becomes a $T_C$ cell or a $T_H$ cell, respectively.

Severe combined immune deficient (SCID) mice lack antigen-specific T- and B-cell immunity because their B and T cells cannot combine antigen-receptor gene segments. SCID mice were used to prove positive and negative selection (Table 8-3). In this experiment, specific α and β TCR genes were isolated from a cloned $T_C$ cell and introduced into SCID mice. The resulting TCR was specific for the intracellular H-Y peptide that is present in male mice (a self-antigen to them) but absent in females (a foreign antigen to them). Thus, these SCID mice displayed only the transgenic TCR on their developing lymphocytes. The TCR recognized the H-Y peptide only when associated with the class I MHC molecule $D^b$. In Table 8-3, line 1 shows that if a male mouse's T cells reacted with the self-H-Y peptide associated with the appropriate MHC molecule, those cells were deleted before they matured (negative selection). *Deletion occurred because the cells were harmful.* Line 2 shows that if a female mouse's T cells reacted with the foreign H-Y peptide associated with the appropriate MHC molecule, those cells were preserved and populated the peripheral lymphoid tissue (positive selection). *These cells were kept because they were useful.* Line 3 shows that in female mice lacking the appropriate MHC molecules, the transgenic TCRs were *useless* because they could not react with the $D^k$ MHC molecules. The cells did not mature and died by apoptosis.

Because normal hosts have millions of different TCRs, the development of a particular TCR cannot be followed. Although transgenic mice are useful in understanding TCR development, they are not normal animals. Superantigens can be used to prove negative selection in normal mice. Superantigens are molecules that are recognized differently from conventional antigens by responsive T cells, whereas conventional antigens bind within the polymorphic cleft on the top surface of class II MHC molecules and interact only with T cells bearing specific αβ TCRs. Superantigens bind to class II MHC molecules outside the antigen-binding cleft and stimulate T cells with distinct $V_β$-containing TCRs. **Superantigens** *are molecules that engage all TCRs containing a specific $V_β$ region irrespective of either the other components of the receptor or the MHC context of the antigen.* Although superantigens do not bind TCRs or MHC molecules at the same sites, as do antigenic peptides, they are presented by APC class II MHC molecules (Figure 8-13).

Superantigens are represented by two groups: exogenous bacterial enterotoxins and some infectious viruses and endogenous minor lymphocyte stimulating (*Mls*) antigens. The engagement of exogenous superantigens causes all T cells expressing a particular family of $V_β$ regions to proliferate, while the expression of endogenous self-superantigens in the developing mouse leads to a large deletion of self-reactive T cells during thymic maturation (these two activities put the *super* in *superantigens*). Superantigens illustrate negative selection because they selectively stimulate all T cells bearing particular $V_β$ regions (irrespective of $D_β$ $J_β$ gene segments or α chains) or lead to selective deletion of these same

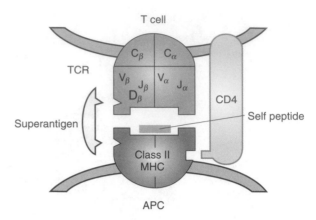

**FIGURE 8-13 Superantigens bind to the outer faces of the $V_β$ region of the TCR and the class II MHC molecule.**

**TABLE 8-4 Self-Superantigens Cause Negative Selection (Clonal Deletion) of $V_β 17a^+$ T Cells in Mice Expressing I-E$^+$ APCs**

| Mouse strains with or without I-E$^+$ APCs | Percentage range of peripheral T cells expressing TCRs using $V_β 17a$ |
|---|---|
| With | 0.0–0.1 |
| Without | 3.7–14.2 |

T cells *in vivo*. Table 8-4 shows that an endogenous superantigen, when presented in association with I-E class II MHC molecules, eliminated massive numbers of developing $V_β 17a^+$ T cells. $V_β 17a^+$ T cells were found only in the thymic cortex; they were missing from the thymic medulla and the peripheral lymphoid tissue. $V_β 17a^+$ T cells were not deleted in I-E$^-$ mice. These results suggest that in I-E$^+$ mice, developing $V_β 17a^+$ thymocytes encounter a self-peptide displayed by I-E class II molecules and are deleted. In their I-E$^-$ counterparts, there is no such complex to recognize; thus, no deletion occurs.

Even though thymic selection is drastic, 1–3% of T cells survive their travels through the thymus; the outcome of the selection modes suggests that no T cells should mature. What prevents this from happening? Furthermore, positive selection is driven by *self-antigens*, which produces mature peripheral T cells specific for *foreign antigens*. How? Current evidence offers two mutually nonexclusive models of thymic selection: the *avidity hypothesis* and the *differential-signal hypothesis*. In the avidity model, T cells with receptors of low avidity for self-MHC molecules are positively selected and leave the thymus, whereas all T cells with receptors of medium to high avidity for self-MHC molecules are negatively selected (clonally deleted). In the differential-signaling model, the TCR avidity

**TABLE 8-5 The Role of Peptides in Thymic Selection**

| Fetal thymus cultures* | Peptide presentation to DP thymocytes | Amount of peptide added[†] | Development of CD8[+] T cells |
|---|---|---|---|
| Normal host | Yes | None | Normal |
| TAP-1-deficient host | No | None | None |
| | No | Optimal | Normal |
| | No | High | None |

*Thymic lobules were collected from normal host (wild type) or TAP-1-deficient mice at 16 days of gestation and placed into fetal thymic organ culture. At this time, thymocytes have not undergone positive selection and their development can be follow *in vitro*. TAP-1-deficient mice express low levels MHC class I molecules on thymic epithelial cells, not enough to form peptide–MHC class I molecule complexes; therefore, there is little development of CD4$^-$CD8$^+$ thymic T cells because of the absence of class I-restricted thymocyte positive selection. When peptides are added to the cultures, class I molecules appear, peptides bind, and maturation of CD4$^-$CD8$^+$ T cells is restored.
[†]When low concentrations of peptide were added to the cultures, it induced low avidity TCR binding, leading to positive selection and normal levels of CD4$^-$CD8$^+$ T cells. In contrast, when high concentrations of peptide were added to the cultures, it induced high avidity TCR binding, leading to negative selection and very low levels of CD4$^-$CD8$^+$ T cells.

required for positive or negative selection is the same, and positive and negative selection are mediated by distinct signals from complexes of self-MHC molecules plus self-peptides presented by thymic stromal cells. When self-MHC–self-peptides convey weak or incomplete signals to the TCR positive selection occurs, whereas negative selection occurs if the signal is complete. Currently, our understanding thymic selection does not allow us to decide between the two models; there is experimental evidence for both.

To test the role of peptides in the avidity model of MHC-dependent positive T cell selection, TAP-1-deficient knockout mice were used (Table 8-5). These mice are unable to load the low numbers of class I molecules with cytosolic peptides; however, their cell-surface class I molecules, even though unstable, can be loaded with exogenously added peptides. Thymic lobules from TAP-1-deficient mice harvested at roughly the 16th day of gestation were used in fetal thymic organ cultures. These lobules contain DN thymocytes, which continue to develop in culture; however, CD4$^-$CD8$^+$ thymocyte development is blocked (the connection between MHC molecule expression and CD4 and CD8 expression were discussed earlier). However, peptide addition to the fetal thymic organ cultures derived from TAP-1-deficient mice, permits the formation of cell-surface peptide–MHC class I molecule complexes on thymic epithelial cells, which restores CD4$^-$CD8$^+$ T cell development. The results suggest that the positive and negative selection signals could be generated by the same peptide; the amount of peptide dictated which mode of selection occurred.

Positive selection interactions also determine the functional attributes (commitment to T$_H$ or T$_C$ cell lineages) of developing T cells, which are characterized by the respective downmodulation of CD4 or CD8 coreceptors. If the TCR is specific for a class II MHC molecule and its associated self-peptide, a thymocyte will corecognize a class II MHC molecule with its CD4 molecule. This corecognition somehow fixes the expression of CD4 and inhibits that of CD8. Likewise, a TCR specific for a class I MHC molecule and its associated self-peptide promotes a CD4$^-$ CD8$^+$ phenotype. Two models have been proposed to explain the mechanism of CD4 or CD8 lineage choice, which guarantees the correlation between TCR specificity and adoption of the T$_H$ or T$_C$ phenotype, respectively. The *instructive model* suggests that changes are signaled by the thymocyte "knowing" which MHC class its TCR, CD4, CD8 molecules recognized and instructing the cell to differentiate into CD4 or CD8 SP cells—one type of signal for class I MHC–TCR–CD8 coreceptor interactions, a different type of signal for class II MHC–TCR–CD4 coreceptor interactions. The *stochastic/selective model* suggests that CD4–CD8 lineage changes are the result of selected survival of cells that differentiated randomly into the appropriate SP subset—DP cell randomly downregulates CD4 or CD8, if remaining cell binds to the appropriate peptide-MHC class I or II molecule complex it survives (a CD8$^+$ or CD4$^+$ T cell, respectively), if it is unable to bind either complex it undergoes apoptosis. Irrespective of mechanism, SP cells downregulate one or the other coreceptors and completely changes their program of response to antigen.

## MINI SUMMARY

Markers such as CD3, CD4, CD8, and the TCR are used to follow the development of T cells in the thymus. Thymic selection bestows MHC restriction on T cells for recognition of antigen in association with self-MHC and for removal of autoreactive T cells during tolerance induction. Positive and negative selection hypotheses have been proposed to account for MHC restriction. Data from experiments using knockout, SCID TCR transgenic mice or superantigens support both modes of selection.

# THE MOLECULAR BASIS OF T-CELL ACTIVATION ENTAILS THE FORMATION OF THE IMMUNOLOGICAL SYNAPSE, WHICH INITIATES MULTIPLE SIGNALING PATHWAYS

Many adhesion molecules and the TCR-CD3 complex cooperate during antigen recognition. CD4 and CD8 also play an integral role in generating intracellular signals that lead to T-cell cytokine secretion and proliferation. Naïve mature T cells normally exist in a resting state and express all the structural elements of the TCR complex ($\alpha\beta$-CD3-$\zeta\eta$). In sum, for specific activation, T cells must bind physically to APCs or target cells. The interaction plane between the two cells (the **immunological synapse**) is a highly organized structure, consisting of a central cluster of signaling molecules (TCR-MHC, CD28-B7/[CTLA-4], CD40-CD40L) surrounded by a "glue" ring of adhesion molecules (CD11aCD18-CD54, CD2-CD58), followed by a peripheral ring containing CD44 and CD45 molecules—a bulls-eye zone pattern (see Figure 8-8).

Once the TCR engages the peptide-MHC complex, the ligated TCR moves into a lipid raft that contains adhesion molecules—forming the immunological synapse, and the T cells undergo a cascade of activation events that lead to proliferation and differentiation. Proliferation causes *clonal growth* of antigen-activated T cells, which expands the number of antigen-specific memory T cells. Differentiation causes secretion of cytokines and chemokines by $T_H$ cells and the lysis of target cells by $T_C$ cells. These cytokines and chemokines spur additional T-cell growth, attract other immune cells to the site of infection, and direct the activities of the cells once they arrive at the site. Some T cells become cytotoxic and set out to track down altered-self cells. T-cell activation and resulting effector functions, however,

are not simply on or off events. The TCR responds to minor changes in the peptide-MHC ligand with gradations in T-cell activation and effector functions.

On antigen exposure, a small number of immune cells proliferate to many and in doing so change their functional character—this process starts with ligand (antigen)-receptor (TCR) binding, which alters immune cell function. The signaling machinery engaged by TCRs is complex (Figure 8-14). This engagement is called *signal transduction*; it is the conversion of a signal from one form to another, that is, the process of conveying information from the outside of the cell to the inside. The receptor receives signals from its ligand; the antigenic peptide-MHC molecule is the ligand for TCRs (in the case of the BCR, it is antigen). All membrane receptors have a tripartite structure, extracellular domains that bind specific ligands, transmembrane domains that span the plasma membrane, and cytoplasmic domains that mediate signal transduction. The cytoplasmic domains of TCRs (and BCRs) are too short to contain the appropriate amino acid residues for signal transduction; therefore, TCRs are associated with other signaling molecules, such as, CD3.

The initial signal of antigen-binding to TCR leads to TCR movement into lipid rafts containing adhesion molecules, which cause receptor clustering into a characteristic bulls-eye structure called an *immunological synapse* (see Figure 8-8). This clustering signal is transduced into cytoplasmic chemical signals by the activation of receptor-associated protein kinases. Immune system protein kinases are enzymes that usually add phosphate groups to serine, threonine, and tyrosine residues on other enzymes; this process is called *phosphorylation* and can lead to activation or inactivation of the enzymes. Phosphorylation can also create binding sites on proteins, which facilitates the binding of cytoplasmically free proteins to phosphorylated membrane proteins; this concentrates the proteins and increases their chance to be phosphorylated. The flip side of this process is the removal of phosphate groups, *dephosphorylation*, by phosphatases, which leads to signal reversal.

As mentioned earlier, TCRs are intimately associated with the signal-transducing molecule CD3, which is composed of three dimers: $\gamma\varepsilon$, $\delta\varepsilon$, and either $\zeta\zeta$ or $\zeta\eta$. The transmembrane portions of the $\gamma$, $\delta$, and $\varepsilon$ chains are negatively charged, which allows close association with the positively charged transmembrane portions of the TCR $\alpha$ and $\beta$ chains. The $\zeta$ chains have few extracellular amino acid residues; most are associated with the transmembrane and cytoplasmic domains. The CD3 and $\zeta$ molecules' cytoplasmic domains are much longer than the TCR's and contain

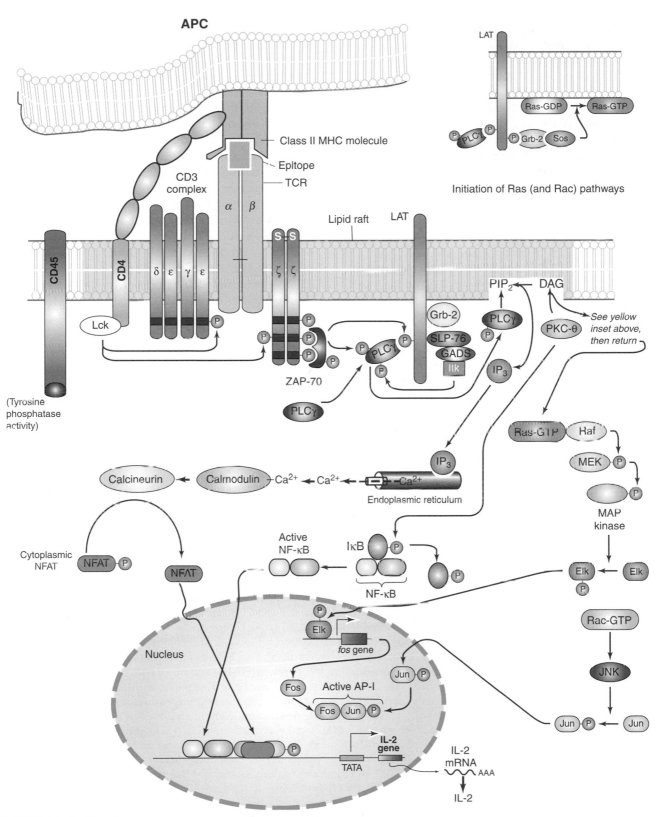

**FIGURE 8-14** *Continued*

specific amino acid sequences called *immunoreceptor tyrosine-based activation motifs (ITAMs)*, which can be phosphorylated by receptor-associated tyrosine kinases. After peptide-MHC molecule binding, TCRs cluster and the Src-family protein tyrosine kinase CD4/CD8-associated *lck* phosphorylate CD3 and ζ chain ITAMs; the CD3-associated *fyn* has similar activity as lck. This activation depends on CD45, a phosphatase that is required for receptor-mediated action of lymphocytes. Once both tyrosines of the ζ chain-associated ITAM regions are phosphorylated, they provide docking sites for the tyrosine kinase *ζ-associated protein of 70 kD (ZAP-70)*. ZAP-70 contains two internal domains with unique structures called *Src homology 2 domains (SH2)* and *Src homology 3 (SH3)* that permit noncovalent interactions with phosphotyrosines in other proteins (the "docking sites"). When ZAP-70 binds, it becomes active and phosphorylates a number of adapter proteins,[5] such as, linker of activated T cells (LAT), src-homology 2 (SH2)-domain-containing leukocyte protein of 76 kD (SLP-76), growth factor receptor-bound protein 2 (Grb2), and others. The adapter proteins become docking sites for cytoplasmic enzymes such as phospholipase Cγ (PLCγ) and proteins that activate ras and rac kinases, which in turn activate various cellular responses.

The active enzyme PLCγ hydrolyzes the membrane phospholipid phosphatidylinositol biphosphate

(PIP$_2$) into two second messenger molecules **diacylglycerol (DAG)** and **inositol 1,4,5-triphosphate (IP$_3$)**. DAG remains associated with the inner side of the plasma membrane and with Ca$^{2+}$ activates protein kinase C-θ (PKC-θ), which moves to the immunological synapse and activates the inhibitor of nuclear factor-κB [IκB]-kinase complex (IKK). IκB is complexed with the transcription factor *nuclear factor-κB (NF-κB)*, preventing its translocation to the nucleus. IKK phosphorylates IκB causing its removal from NF-κB and thereby allowing NF-κB translocation to the nucleus. As an activated transcription factor, NF-κB contributes to the expression of multiple cytokine and cytokine receptor genes. In contrast, IP$_3$ diffuses away from the membrane and releases Ca$^{2+}$ from the endoplasmic reticulum. The released Ca$^{2+}$ binds to calmodulin, this complex binds and activates the Ca$^{2+}$/calmodulin-dependent phosphatase calcineurin. The active calcineurin removes a phosphate group from the cytoplasmic inactive transcription factor *nuclear factor of activated T cells (NFAT)*, which permits NFAT to translocate into the nucleus. NFAT is required for the expression of IL-2, IL-4, TNF, and other cytokine genes.

The activation of PKC-θ is also important in the activation of the Ras pathway, which leads to the activation of mitogen-activated protein (MAP) kinases and ultimately contributes to the activation of the transcription factor *activated protein 1 (AP-1)*. Ras is a member of the family of 21-kD guanine nucleotide-binding proteins called *small G proteins* that link receptor phosphorylation to cytoplasmic kinases in many different cell types. Ras is loosely attached to the plasma membrane and is in an inactive form when bound to guanosine diphosphate

---

[5]The cell's cytoplasmic signaling molecules can interact with different receptors that send similar signals, however to bind different receptors adapter proteins are essential. Adapter proteins are not signaling molecules but connect signaling molecules with their targets.

---

**FIGURE 8-14 T-cell activation.** Following TCR–peptide-MHC molecule ligation, the CD4/CD8-associated Src-family protein tyrosine kinase (PTK), *Lck*, is activated, leading to phosphorylation of ζζ and CD3 module ITAMs of the TCR complex, which provides docking sites for ζ-chain-associated protein of 70-kD (ZAP-70). (CD3 also has an associated PTK called *Fyn* [not shown].) Activated ZAP-70 phosphorylates linker of activated T cells (LAT) and Src-homology 2 (SH2)-domain-containing leukocyte protein of 76 kD (SLP-76). Phosphorylated LAT then recruits several SH2-domain-containing proteins, including growth factor receptor-bound protein 2 (Grb2), Grb2-related adaptor protein (GADS) and phospholipase Cγ (PLCγ). Through its constitutive association with GADS, SLP76 is also recruited to LAT following TCR stimulation. SLP-76 also constitutively associates with the SH3 domain of PLCγ. Activation of PLCγ leads to the hydrolysis of phosphatidylinositol 4,5-bisphosphate to inositol 3,4,5-triphosphate (IP$_3$) and diacylglycerol (DAG). IP$_3$ production leads to increases of intracellular free Ca$^{2+}$ concentration—*leading to dephosphorylation of cytoplasmic nuclear factor of activated T cells (NAFT)*, whereas DAG can activate both protein kinase C-θ (PKC-θ)—*leading to phosphorylation, release of inhibitor of κB (IκB), and activation of nuclear factor κB (NF-κB)*, and Ras (yellow inset)—*leading through the MAP and JNK kinase pathway to activation of activation protein 1 (AP-1)*. Phosphorylated LAT recruits the SH2 domain of Grb2, and therefore, the Grb2-associated Ras guanosine nucleotide-exchange factor (GEF), son-of-sevenless (Sos), exchanging GTP for GDP forming active Ras-GTP. Ras-GTP activates a cascade of enzymes leading to the activation of MAP kinase, culminating in the formation of fos, one component of AP-1. Tyrosine phosphorylated SLP-76 also associates with Vav-1, a GEF protein that acts on another small G protein called *Rac*. Rac-GTP starts a Ras-parallel enzyme cascade leading to the activation of a MAP kinase called *Jun N-terminal kinase (JNK)*, leads to the formation of Jun, the second component of Ap-1, which dimerizes with fos to form AP-1. (See text for details.)

**TABLE 8-6 Expression of T$_H$ Cell Genes Following Antigen Interaction**

| Gene product | Function | Start of mRNA expression | Location | Fold increase after activation |
|---|---|---|---|---|
| | | IMMEDIATE* | | |
| c-fos | Cellular oncogene; nuclear-binding protein | 15 min | Nucleus | >100 |
| c-Jun | Cellular oncogene; transcription factor | 15–20 min | Nucleus | ? |
| NFAT | Transcription factor | 20 min | Nucleus | 50 |
| c-Myc | Cellular oncogene | 30 min | Nucleus | 20 |
| NF-κB | Transcription factor | 30 min | Nucleus | >10 |
| | | EARLY* | | |
| IFN-γ | Cytokine | 30 min | Secreted | >100 |
| IL-2 | Cytokine | 45 min | Secreted | >1000 |
| IL-3 | Cytokine | 1–2 hr | Secreted | >100 |
| TGF-β | Cytokine | <2 hr | Secreted | >10 |
| IL-2 receptor (p55) | Cytokine | 2 hr | Plasma membrane | >50 |
| TNF-β | Cytokine | 1–3 hr | Secreted | >100 |
| IL-4 | Cytokine | <6 hr | Secreted | >100 |
| IL-5 | Cytokine | <6 hr | Secreted | >100 |
| IL-6 | Cytokine | <6 hr | Secreted | >100 |
| c-Myb | Cellular oncogene | 16 hr | Nucleus | 100 |
| GM-CSF | Cytokine | 20 hr | Secreted | ? |
| | | LATE* | | |
| HLA-DR | Class II MHC molecule | 3–5 days | Plasma membrane | 10 |
| VLA-4 | Adhesion molecule | 4 days | Plasma membrane | >100 |
| VLA-1, -2, -3, -5 | Adhesion molecules | 7–14 days | Plasma membrane | >100, ?, ?, ? |

*These immediate, early, and late genes are named on the basis of their kinetics of activation: transcription within 15 min, 30 min to hours, and days for immediate, early, and late genes, respectively. Unlike early and late genes, transcription of immediate genes does not need protein synthesis. Immediate and early gene transcription occurs before mitosis, while late gene transcription occurs after mitosis.

(GDP) and active when it binds guanosine triphosphate (GTP). Ras activation involves two adapter proteins LAT and growth factor receptor-bound protein 2 (Grb2). ZAP-70-phosphorylated LAT serves as a docking site for Grb2, which recruits Ras guanosine nucleotide-exchange factor (GEF), son-of-sevenless (Sos), which exchanges GTP for GDP leading to Ras activation. Ras then activates a cascade of reactions that lead to the production of kinases called *MAP kinases*, which phosphorylate transcription factor Fos in the nucleus. Grb2 and Sos also recruit the GDP/GTP exchange protein Vav-1 that acts on a small G protein called *Rac*. Activated Rac initiates a Ras-parallel cascade of reactions that lead to the production of the MAP kinase called *c-Jun N-terminal kinase (JNK)*, which phosphorylates the transcription factor Jun. Once phosphorylated, Fos and Jun dimerize to form AP-1. AP-1 regulates IL-2 transcription.

As a result of NF-κB, NFAT, and AP-1 binding to DNA sequences, it starts transcription of 70 or more so-called *immediate, early,* and *late genes* that regulate activation (Table 8-6). Thus, multiple signal transduction cascades are activated within minutes by ligation of the TCR, which leads to proliferation and differentiation into effector cells.

**MINI SUMMARY**

The coreceptors CD4 and CD8 define the functional response of T cells. CD2 and CD11aCD18 contribute to cell-cell interactions that are essential for T-cell activation. The TCR–antigenic peptide-MHC molecule plus CD3 interaction provide the first signal to T-cell activation. T cell-expressed CD28, the pivotal molecule responsible for providing the second signal, is required for T-cell activation by interacting with members of the B7 family on APCs. Other T cell accessory molecules such as CD44, and CD45 also may play a role in cell-cell adhesion and T-cell activation. Occupancy of the TCR by its ligand leads to the initiation of multiple signaling pathways. CD4/CD8-associated tyrosine kinase p56[lck] initiates the pathways through the activation of ZAP-70, phosphorylates phospholipase Cγ (PLCγ). These pathways promote proliferation and differentiation of T cells into effector cells and production of cytokines.

# SUMMARY

In contrast to B cells, T cells do not bind free antigen. The *TCR* recognizes foreign antigen only in association with self-MHC molecules presented on a cell surface. The TCR was characterized using monoclonal antibodies and *subtractive hybridization*. The 90-kD antigen-specific, heterodimeric, glycoprotein TCR consists of two disulfide-linked polypeptides, either the α chain with the β chain or the γ chain with the δ chain. The TCR is encoded by several gene segments (V, D, J, and C) in a scenario similar to that of immunoglobulin gene rearrangements. Somatic hypermutation, however, does not occur in TCR V genes. V-region rearrangements could lead to a diversity of over 100 trillion different TCRs. TCR genes are structurally related to immunoglobulin genes and thus are part of the same supergene family called the *immunoglobulin (Ig) gene superfamily*. The *CD3 complex* associates with the TCR but is not part of the T-cell αβ or γδ heterodimer. The CD3 complex is involved in T-cell activation following antigen binding in association with MHC molecules by the αβ or γδ heterodimer.

The TCR does not define T-cell functional responses. Antigen recognition by T cells also requires *accessory molecules* that seem to define T-cell function. *CD4* and *CD8* coreceptor molecules correlate with the effector function of responding T cells. *Cell adhesion molecules*, such as *CD2*, *CD11aCD18 (LFA-1)*, *CD58 (LFA-3)*, and the *ICAMs*, also help T cell-antigen interactions. Other T-cell accessory molecules, including *CD28*, *CD44*, and *CD45*, also are important in cell-cell adhesion and T-cell activation.

Differentiation antigens such as CD3, CD4, CD8, and TCR are used to follow the maturation of T cells in the thymus. MHC-restricted antigen recognition is acquired as T cells mature in the thymus. This *thymic selection* is a process that creates a pool of T cells whose receptors recognize only an antigen–MHC complex rather than self or foreign molecules alone. T cells that fail this selection process die in the thymus. *Positive selection* is responsible for MHC restriction of antigen recognition, whereas *negative selection* is responsible for clonal deletion of autoreactive T cells (tolerance induction). The use of *transgenic mice* and *superantigens* has proved that positive and negative selection occur within the host.

On mature T cells, the occupancy of the TCR leads to activation of proliferation and differentiation into effector cells. This occupancy, TCR and coreceptors binding peptide-MHC molecule complexes, leads to phosphorylation of the ζ chain by tyrosine kinases p56[lck], binding, phosphorylation, and activation of ZAP-70 and the phosphorylation of adapter proteins, the activation of phospholipase Cγ (PLCγ), which converts PIP$_2$ to two second messengers IP$_3$ and DAG. The latter two molecules lead to increased cytoplasmic Ca$^{2+}$ production and PKCθ activation, Ca$^{2+}$ increase causes calcineurin and subsequent NFAT production, whereas PKCθ leads to NF-κB production. ZAP-70 incombination with PLCγ and adapter proteins lead to the activation of Ras and Rac forming Fos and Jun, which dimerize to form AP-1. Thus, multiple transduction cascades are induced by occupancy of the TCR that lead to cell proliferation, differentiation, and cytokine production.

# SELF-EVALUATION

## RECALLING KEY TERMS

**Accessory molecules**
 CD2 (LFA-2)
 CD4
 CD8
 CD11b/CD18 (LFA-1)
 CD28
 CD44
 CD45
 CD54 (ICAM-1)
 CD58 (LFA-3)
 CD102 (ICAM-2)
 VLA-1, -2, -3, -4, -5, -6
**Cell adhesion molecules**
**CD3 complex**
**DNA-binding proteins**
**Ig-gene superfamily**
 CD2 (LFA-2)
 CD4
 CD8
 CD28
 CD54 (ICAM-1)
 CD58 (LFA-3)
 CD102 (ICAM-2)

**Integrin family**
   CD11b/CD18 (LFA-1)
   VLA-1, -2, -3, -4, -5, -6
**Subtractive hybridization**
**Superantigens**
**T cell receptors (TCRs)**
   $\alpha\beta$ TCR
   $\gamma\delta$ TCR
**Thymic selection**
   Positive selection
   Negative selection
**Transcription factor**
   NF-$\kappa$B

## MULTIPLE-CHOICE QUESTIONS

*(An answer key is not provided, but the page[s] location of the answer is.)*

1. The TCR is composed of two polypeptide chains and is designed to recognize (a) a foreign antigenic determinant alone, (b) epitope plus an MHC molecule, (c) only an MHC molecule, (d) polysaccharide antigens, (e) none of these. *(See pages 258 and 259.)*

2. If T cells react with free soluble antigen, the interaction leads to a successful immune response. (a) true, (b) false. *(See pages 254 and 255.)*

3. Which combination of the following molecules is in the immunoglobulin gene superfamily? (a) class I, class II, and LFA-1, (b) CD2, CD58, and CD11aCD18, (c) CD4, CD8, and CD45, (d) CD54, TCR, and ICAM-2, (e) all of these are correct. *(See page 265–267.)*

4. As with antibodies, TCR affinity increases during a secondary immune response. (a) true, (b) false. *(See page 263.)*

5. The CD3 complex is made up of (a) $\gamma$, $\delta$, and $\varepsilon$ chains, (b) $\alpha$, $\delta$, and $\varepsilon$ chains, (c) $\zeta$, $\delta$, and $\varepsilon$ chains, (d) $\eta$, $\delta$, and $c$ chains, (e) none of these. *(See pages 263 and 264.)*

6. CD29 is the common $\beta$ chain on (a) LFA-1, (b) CD3, (c) VLA molecules, (d) CD2, (e) LFA-3, (f) none of these. *(See page 265–267.)*

7. CD45 marker can be used to distinguish between antigen naïve T cells and memory T cells. (a) true, (b) false. *(See page 269.)*

## SHORT-ANSWER ESSAY QUESTIONS

1. Briefly explain subtractive hybridization and state why this method was so important in the characterization of the TCR?

2. What does it mean to say that TCRs belong to the Ig supergene family? Briefly describe the heterodimeric structure of the TCR.

3. TCR genes use the same strategies as antibody genes to develop receptor diversity; however, TCR genes do not exhibit somatic hypermutation. Why?

4. The TCR is closely associated with another surface protein complex. What is its name and function?

5. T cells can react only with protein fragments. What is this process called, and how does it occur? Which pathway leads to antigen interaction with class I molecules and which leads to antigen interaction with class II molecules? Briefly describe each pathway.

6. What are accessory molecules? Give some examples and briefly discuss how they may be involved in antigen recognition by T cells.

7. Describe T-cell differentiation in the thymus using the CD4 and CD8 markers.

8. T cells do not recognize free antigen, as antibody receptors do. Speculate on why.

9. Briefly discuss the molecular events, collectively called *T-cell activation*, that lead to biologic function. What is the importance of diacylglycerol and IP$_3$ in T cell activation? What are key transcription factors in T-cell activation?

## FURTHER READINGS

Acuto, O., and F. Michel. 2003. CD28-mediated co-stimulation: A quantitative support for TCR signaling. *Nat. Rev. Immunol.* 3:939–951.

Bjorkman, P.J., M.A. Saper, B. Smarasoui, W.S. Bennet, J.L. Strominger, and D.C. Wiley. 1987. The foreign antigen binding site and T cell recognition regions of class I histocompatibility antigens. *Nature* 329:512–518.

Chen, L. 2004. Co-inhibitory molecules of the B7-CD28 family in the control of T-cell immunity. *Nat. Rev. Immunol.* 4:336–347.

Davis, D.M. 2006. Intrigue at the immune synapse. *Sci. Amer.* 294:48–58.

Davis, M.M., and Y-H. Chien. 2003. T-cell antigen receptors. In *Fundamental Immunology*, 5th ed. W.E. Paul, ed. Philadelphia: Lippincott Williams & Wilkins. p. 227–258.

Greenwald, R.J., G.J. Freeman, and A.H. Sharpe. 2005. The B7 family revisited. *Annu. Rev. Immunol.* 23:515–548.

Huppa, J.B., and M.M. Davis. 2003. T-cell-antigen recognition and the immunological synapse. *Nat. Rev. Immunol.* 3:973–983.

Kedzierska, K., N.L. La Gruta, J. Stambas, S.J. Turner, P.C. Doherty. 2008. Tracking phenotypically and functionally distinct T cell subsets via T cell repertoire diversity. *Mol. Immunol.* 45:607–618.

Luo, B-H., C.V. Carman, and T.A. Springer. 2007. Structural basis of integrin regulation and signaling. *Annu. Rev. Immunol.* 25:619–647.

Marrack, P., and J. Kappler. 1986. The T cell and its receptor. *Sci. Am.* 254:36–45.

Marrack, P., J.P. Scott-Browne, S. Dai, L. Gapin, and J.W. Kappler. 2008. Evolutionary conserved amino acids that control TCR-MHC interaction. *Annu. Rev. Immunol.* 26:171–203.

Rothenberg, A.V., and T. Taghon. 2005. Molecular genetics of T cell development. *Annu. Rev. Immunol.* 23:601–649.

Rothenberg, E.V., J.E. Moore, and M.A. Yui. 2008. Launching the T-cell-lineage development programme. *Nat. Rev. Immunol.* 8:9–21.

Rudd, C.E., and H. Schneider. 2003. Unifying concepts in CD28, ICOS, CTLA4 co-receptor signaling. *Nat. Rev. Immunol.* 3:544–556.

Rudolph, M.G., R.L. Stanfield, and I.A. Wilson. 2006. How TCRs bind MHCs, peptides, and coreceptors. *Annu. Rev. Immunol.* 24:419–466.

Sharpe, A.H., Y. Latchman, and R.J. Greenwald. 2003. Accessory molecules and costimulation. In *Fundamental Immunology*, 5th ed. W.E. Paul, ed. Philadelphia: Lippincott Williams & Wilkins. p. 393–418.

Hayday, A.C., and D.J. Pennington. 2007. Key factors in the organized chaos of early T cell development. *Nat. Immunol.* 8:137–144.

Takahama, Y. 2006. Journey through the thymus: Stromal guides for T-cell development and selection. *Nat. Rev. Immunol.* 6:127–135.

Teft, W.A., M.G. Kirchof, and J. Madrenas. 2006. A molecular perspective of CTLA-4 function. *Annu. Rev. Immunol.* 24:65–97.

Townsend, A., J. Rothbard, F. Gotch, B. Bahadur, D. Wraith, and A. McMichael. 1986. The epitopes of influenza nucleoprotein recognized by cytotoxic T lymphocytes can be defined with short synthetic peptides. *Cell* 44: 959–968.

Turner, S.J., P.C. Doherty, J. McCluskey, and J. Rossjohn. 2006. Structural determinants of T-cell receptor bias in immunity. *Nat. Rev. Immunol.* 6:883–894.

von Boehmer, H. 2005. Unique features of the pre-T-cell receptor α-chain: Not just a surrogate. *Nat. Rev. Immunol.* 5:571–577.

Weiss, A., and L.E. Samelson. 2003. T-lymphocyte activation. In *Fundamental Immunology*, 5th ed. W.E. Paul, ed. Philadelphia: Lippincott Williams & Wilkins. p. 321–364.

# CHAPTER NINE

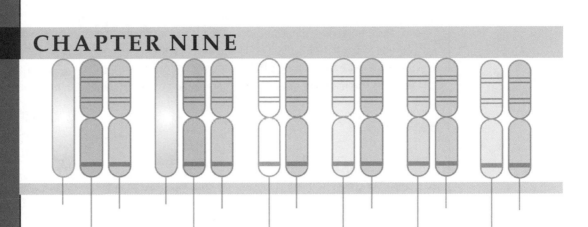

# CYTOKINES

## CHAPTER OUTLINE

1. The recognition of cytokines' importance originated with the realization that they maintain T-cell growth and activate lymphocytes.
2. Cytokines can be ascribed to numerous functional categories.
3. Nonspecific cytokines exhibit specificity by binding exact receptors on responsive target cells.
   a. Cytokine receptors are divided into five families and three subfamilies.
   b. Cytokine engagement of their counterpart receptors initiates signal transduction pathways that ultimately instruct the biologic activity of target cells.
4. Multiple cytokines influence innate immunity.
   a. IL-1, a pleiotropic proinflammatory molecule, is a major mediator of inflammatory responses to infection.
   b. Tumor necrosis factor is the major mediator of acute inflammatory responses to infection.
   c. IL-6 influences innate and adaptive immunity.
   d. IL-12, a proinflammatory cytokine that links innate and adaptive immunity.
   e. Type I interferons are antiviral molecules that mediate and regulate innate immunity.
   f. IL-10, an inhibitor of activated macrophages and dendritic cells, controls innate immunity.
5. Chemokines are small cytokines that selectively control adhesion, chemotaxis, and activation of leukocytes.
6. Multiple cytokines influence adaptive immunity.
   a. IL-2 is an autocrine T-cell growth factor.
   b. IL-4 is the signature cytokine of $T_H2$ cells.
   c. IL-5 is an eosinophil activation and differentiation factor that links T-cell activation with eosinophilic reactions.
   d. Interferon-$\gamma$ is a potent immunoregulatory molecule with additional antiviral and antiproliferative effects.

*Immunology: Understanding the Immune System, Second Edition*, by Klaus D. Elgert
Copyright © 2009 John Wiley & Sons, Inc.

e. Transforming growth factor-$\beta$, an inhibitor and a stimulator molecule, is important to the initiation, progression, and resolution of an immune response.

f. IL-13 is more than another $T_H2$ cell-derived cytokine.

7. Cytokines stimulate the growth and differentiation of hematopoietic stem cells.

## OBJECTIVES

The reader should be able to:

1. Comprehend how immune responses are controlled by cytokines.

2. Describe the role of cytokines in the development of immunity; define cytokines, lymphokines, interleukins, and chemokines; classify cytokines; discuss the characteristics of cytokines.

3. Tabulate the interleukins and their functions.

4. Gain historical perspective on cytokines' importance in maintaining T-cell growth.

5. Sequentially illustrate cytokine signal transduction.

6. Account for the origins of interleukin-1 (IL-1), its different forms, and its role in immune responses.

7. Describe tumor necrosis factor-$\alpha$'s contributions to inflammatory responses.

8. Understand how IL-12 links innate and adaptive immunity.

9. Convey how IL-10 controls innate immunity.

10. Distinguish between type I and type II interferons.

11. Broadly describe the four chemokine families.

12. Account for the origins of interleukin-2 (IL-2), its different receptor forms, and its role in immune responses; appreciate the autocrine nature of IL-2.

13. Describe the role of interferon-$\gamma$ in immunoregulation.

14. Describe the positive and negative immunoregulatory roles of transforming growth factor-$\beta$.

15. Name the hematopoietic cytokines and comment on each.

Development of immunity is a result of the antigen-dependent differentiation of antigen-reactive cells. This differentiation is regulated by cell-cell interactions and by soluble molecules called *cytokines*. These cytokines are not antigen-specific. The antigen-activated $T_H$ cell can be regarded as a signal transduction machine that receives an antigen-specific signal and converts it into antigen-nonspecific regulators of the immune response. Nonetheless, they are the mediators that stimulate inflammatory reactions associated with innate immunity, the activation and effector phases of adaptive immunity, and the development of hematopoietic cells.

**Cytokines**, *a class of low-molecular-weight molecules produced by many different cells in a highly regulated fashion, change the behavior and function of many different cells. Cytokines are* <u>regulatory</u> *and* <u>effector</u> *molecules that act at picomolar to nanomolar concentrations on cytokine receptors expressed by target cells.* Cytokines are involved in signal transduction; they activate genes for growth, differentiation, and cell activity. They play a cardinal role in mediating the host's defense against internal and external antigenic insults. *Cytokines are derived from any cell, immune or nonimmune.* **Lymphokines** *are cytokines derived from lymphocytes and* **monokines** *are cytokines derived from macrophages.* Thus all lymphokines or monokines are cytokines, but not all cytokines are lymphokines or monokines. A subset of cytokines, **chemokines**, is a group of low-molecular weight (8- to 12-kD) cytokines that play a major role in inflammation by mediating chemotaxis and activation of leukocytes. Table 9-1 presents a classification of cytokines. For simplicity's sake, we will usually refer to all cellular mediators as cytokines.

CD4$^+$ helper T ($T_H$) cells usually control proliferation and differentiation whereas CD8$^+$ cytotoxic T ($T_C$ cells) usually kill aberrant cells. Up

**TABLE 9-1 Possible Classification of Cytokines**

| Families of cytokines | Representative members |
|---|---|
| Hematopoietin (Interleukins; Colony-stimulating factors) | IL-1α, IL-1β, IL-2 to IL-34; G-CSF, GM-CSF, IL-3, IL-7, M-CSF |
| Interferon | IFN-α, IFN-β, IFN-γ |
| Chemokine | CXCL8 (IL-8), CCL2 (MPC-1), XCL1 (lymphotactin), CX3CL1 (fractalkine) |
| Tumor necrosis factor (Cytotoxic/ Immunomodulatory/Growth factors) | TNF-β, TNF-α, TGF-β |

to about 35 years ago, T-cell regulatory activity was credited primarily to cellular interactions mediated by antigen-specific receptors recognizing antigenic peptides associated with MHC molecules. However, cytokines are vital for successful immune responses, and distinct populations of $T_H$ cells (see Table 10-1) along with antigen-presenting cells (APCs) and non-lymphoid cells transmit growth and differentiation signals among immune cells by these molecules. These cytokine-mediated interactions occur in a cascade fashion, where a cytokine induces the target cell to produce one or more cytokines, which in turn may act on another target cell to synthesize other cytokines. Cytokines not only regulate lymphocyte activities but also influence the differentiation of hematopoietic cells, mast cells, fibroblasts, and osteoclasts. Cytokines also affect hematopoietic homeostasis, inflammation, immediate hypersensitivities, and wound healing. Table 9-2 presents some of the general characteristics of cytokines.

**TABLE 9-2 Characteristics of Cytokines and Their Receptors**

1. Cytokines are usually low molecular weight (usually <30 kD) glycoproteins that are biochemically distinct. They are divided into four groups: the hematopoietin family, the interferon family, the chemokine family, and the tumor necrosis family.

2. Cytokines are obtained from lymphoid and nonlymphoid tissues and cells.

3. Cytokines are *pleiotropic* (they can have multiple overlapping biological activities in disparate organ systems or cells); they are often *redundant* (different cytokines exhibit the same functions). For example, IL-2, IL-4, and IL-5 can induce proliferation of B cells (Figure 9-1)

4. Cytokines are involved in inflammation and immunity; they regulate the amplitude and duration of the response. Some cytokines act as regulators of cell division.

5. Cytokines are produced by lymphoid cells in response to:
   a. Nonspecific mitogenic stimulants and
   b. Specific antigenic stimulants (if previously sensitized).

6. Cytokines are compartmentalized. They are usually produced locally and transiently, acting in an **autocrine** (binding to the same cell that secreted the cytokine) or **paracrine** (binding to a nearby cell), rather than **endocrine** (binding to a distant cell), manner (see Figure 9-1). The cytokines produced during an immune response interact in a cascade fashion.

7. Cytokines are synthesized briefly, are secreted in nanomolar amounts, and are self-limiting; thus, they have high specific activity (great biological potency at low concentrations).

8. Cytokines are nonspecific and antigen-independent in mode of activity. They react directly with many different types of target cells (*pleiotropism*) through high-affinity ($K_d$ of $10^{-10}$ to $10^{-12}$ M) cell surface receptors specific for each cytokine or cytokine group. Many of these receptors have two polypeptide chains: a cytokine-specific α chain and a signal-transducing β chain. Some cytokines share chains (such as, the common γ chain), and some have three chains. Cytokine binding leads to a change in the pattern of cellular RNA and protein synthesis and to altered cell behavior. The target cells are as follows:
   a. Inflammatory cells: leukocytes (neutrophils, macrophages) and lymphocytes,
   b. Noninflammatory cells: endothelial cells, osteoclasts, and fibroblasts.

9. All cytokine receptors have the typical receptor structure: an extracellular domain, a single membrane-spanning domain, and a cytoplasmic domain. The conserved amino acid sequence motifs found in the extracellular domains are used to define the *cytokine-receptor families:* Ig superfamily receptors, class I cytokine receptors, class II cytokine receptors, TNF receptors, and chemokine receptors.

10. Cytokines interact in a network by:
    a. Inducing each other (cascade-like activity).
    b. Transmodulating cytokine cell surface receptors.
    c. Interacting synergistically or antagonistically on cell functions.

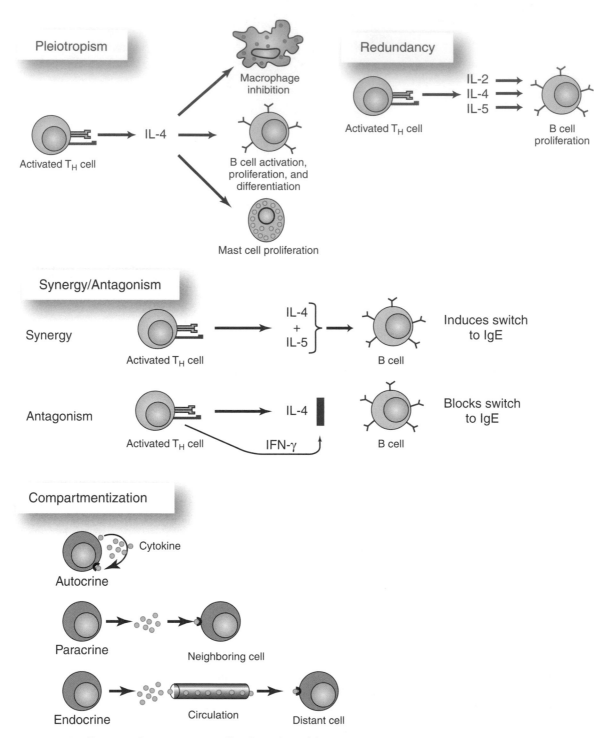

**FIGURE 9-1 Attributes and compartmentalization of cytokines.**

# THE RECOGNITION OF CYTOKINES' IMPORTANCE ORIGINATED WITH THE REALIZATION THAT THEY MAINTAIN T-CELL GROWTH AND ACTIVATE LYMPHOCYTES

The word *lymphokine* was first proposed by Dumonde and coworkers in 1969. However, the study of lymphokines began 9 years earlier with the discovery by Nowell that the plant lectin phytohemagglutinin caused lymphocytes to undergo mitosis. Within 5 years, reports described soluble mitogenic activities in the culture supernatants of lectin-stimulated human leukocytes. The initial conclusion was that the mitogenic factors were lymphocyte-derived. This conclusion was short-lived, since in 1970 it was reported that macrophages also produce mitogenic molecules. The name coined for the macrophage-derived mitogenic factor was *lymphocyte-activating factor (LAF)*. Differentiation between T-cell and macrophage mitogenic factors was difficult because the assay systems used to detect the molecules were similar.

The breakthrough that lessened these difficulties was a discovery by Gallo's group in 1976. They observed that culture supernatants from lectin-stimulated human peripheral blood lymphocytes promoted and maintained the long-term viability and proliferation of T cells in culture. The supernatants contained *T-cell growth factor (TCGF)*. Their discovery led to the long-term culture and clonal isolation of functional T cells. The culturing of cloned T cells allowed for a clear association of a T-cell- or macrophage-derived molecule with a particular biological assay. In 1978, Smith and colleagues used cloned T-cell lines for the development of a rapid, quantitative bioassay for mitogenic factor activities. Thus, in combination with more rigorous biochemical studies that isolated and characterized the cytokines, the wide array of mediators was shown to have fewer molecules than their many acronyms implied. This assay system resolved the enigma that factors derived from cells with different functional phenotypes (macrophages and T cells) produced identical biologic effects. From these studies, the interaction of immune cells with ligands (mitogens[1]

or antigens) was shown to be the signal that induced the production of soluble secondary signals.

---

**MINI SUMMARY**

Activation of immune cells leads to further regulation by soluble molecules called cytokines. These are a large group of low molecular weight, nonantigen-specific factors produced by lymphocytes, APCs, and nonlymphoid cells with different biologic effects, which change the behavior and function of many cells.

---

# CYTOKINES CAN BE ASCRIBED TO NUMEROUS FUNCTIONAL CATEGORIES

Cytokines can be functionally categorized by determining their direct or indirect involvement in immunity. Using this approach, cytokines can be divided, *but cautiously*, into three groups based on their participation in innate immunity versus adaptive immunity (but indirectly all of them work in adaptive immunity) and as stimulators of hematopoiesis. These activities also include control of cell growth and differentiation and wound healing. Irrespective of cytokine function, the principal cytokine producers are $T_H$ cells, dendritic cells, and macrophages. The produced cytokines only target cells with the appropriate receptors.

If the list of 100 activities published in 1979 (now more than 200) is a hint of the possibilities, the known and named members of the cytokine family surely will continue to grow. The application of recombinant DNA methods will see to that. The nomenclature is moving in the right direction to avoid confusion; a consensus was reached at the 6th International Congress of Immunology, 1986, that a factor should be given the name interleukin only after the nucleotide sequence encoding the factor is determined and effects on target cells demonstrated. To summarize cytokine-mediated regulation, Table 9-3 summarizes the present thinking on some cytokine

---

[1]Mitogens are substances such as concanavalin A (Con A) or phytohemagglutinin (PHA) and lipopolysaccharide (LPS) that induce cell division in a high percentage of T and

B cells, respectively. This occurs irrespective of the cells' antigen specificity. Thus, mitogens are *polyclonal activators* that if derived from plants are called *lectins* (Con A and PHA). Mitogens also are derived from bacterial cell wall components (such as lipopolysaccaride [LPS]).

**TABLE 9-3** Cytokine Abbreviations, Sources, and Functions

| Abbreviation | Sources | Functions |
|---|---|---|
| Interleukins | | |
| IL-1$\alpha$; IL-1$\beta$ | Monocytes, macrophages, endothelial cells, epithelial cells, and many others | Mediates host inflammatory responses: vasculature inflammation, fever, stimulates acute phase protein production, promotes $T_H2$ cell proliferation |
| IL-2 | $T_H0$, $T_H1$ | Stimulates T-cell growth or activation-induced cell death, costimulates B-cell proliferation, NK cell activation |
| IL-3 | $T_H$ cells, NK cells, mast cells | Stimulates hematopoietic cell growth (one of the CSFs); stimulates mast cell growth |
| IL-4 | $T_H2$ cells, mast cells | Promotes $T_H2$ cell growth; costimulates B-cell proliferation; enhances $IgG_1$ and IgE production; stimulates class II MHC molecule expression on B cells; inhibits $T_H1$ cells |
| IL-5 | $T_H2$ cells | Stimulates B-cell growth and antibody production; enhances IgA production by stimulated B cells; enhances eosinophil activation and differentiation |
| IL-6 | T cells, macrophages, endothelial cells, and others | Stimulates hematopoietic progenitors; induces production of acute phase proteins; stimulates T cell activation and IL-2 production; promotes B-cell proliferation and antibody secretion |
| IL-7 | Bone marrow cells, thymic stromal cells, and some T cells | Stimulates pre-B cells and pre-T cells (one of the CSFs) |
| IL-8 | (see Table 9-6) | |
| IL-9 | IL-2 activated $T_H$ cells | Stimulates T cell proliferation; mast cell activation |
| IL-10 | $T_H2$ cells, macrophages | Inhibits cytokine synthesis by $T_H1$ cells and activated macrophages; enhances B cell, thymocyte, and mast cell proliferation; in association with TGF-$\beta$, it stimulates IgA synthesis |
| IL-11 | Bone marrow stromal cells, fibroblasts | Stimulates megakaryocyte growth; growth factor for macrophage progenitors |
| IL-12 | Macrophages, dendritic cells | Induces IFN-$\gamma$ production from T and NK cells; enhance of NK cell cytotoxic activity; stimulates differentiation of $CD4^+$ T cells to $T_H1$ cells |
| IL-13 | Activated T cells, NK cells, and mast cells | Blocks inflammatory monokine production; shares activity with IL-4; growth factor for B cells |
| IL-14 | T cells | B-cell growth factor; inhibits antibody synthesis |
| IL-15 | Mainly dendritic cells and monocytic cell lineage, T cells, epithelial cells, and others | Shares IL-2 bioactivities: T cell and NK cell growth factor; augments NK cell activation |
| IL-16 | T cells | Chemotactic for $CD4^+$ T cells, $CD4^+$ macrophages, eosinophils; competes with HIV binding to CD4 molecule |
| IL-17 | Mainly $CD4^+$ T cells ($T_H17$ subset) | A family of six cytokines; proinflammatory activity; induces severe autoimmunity |
| IL-18 | Monocytic cell lineage, dendritic cells, and others | Promotes $T_H1$ cell differentiation; induces T cell IFN-$\gamma$ production; enhances NK cell activity |
| IL-19 | LPS-stimulated monocytes and B cells | Member of IL-10 family of cytokines that induces proinflammatory cytokines; alter $T_H1/T_H2$ balance by inhibiting IFN-$\gamma$ and enhancing IL-4 and IL-13 production |
| IL-20 | Monocytes and keratinocytes | IL-10 family member with similar activity as IL-19 |
| IL-21 | Activated T cells | Enhances NK cell and $T_C$ cell cytotoxicity and IFN-$\gamma$ production |
| IL-22 | Mainly $CD4^+$ T cells | IL-10 family member that inhibits epidermal differentiation and has activity similar to IL-19 and -20 |

**TABLE 9-3** *(Continued)*

| Abbreviation | Sources | Functions |
|---|---|---|
| IL-23 | Activated dendritic cells | IL-12 family member that stimulates CD4$^+$ T cells to produce IL-17 |
| IL-24 | B cells, fibroblasts, melanocytes, NK cells, and T cell subsets | IL-10 family member that induces IFN-$\gamma$ and TNF-$\alpha$ and low levels of IL-1$\beta$, IL-12, and GM-CSF |
| IL-25 | Bone marrow stromal cells, T cell subsets | IL-17 family member that induces production IL-4, IL-5, IL-13, and eotaxin; involved airway disease of the lung |
| IL-26 | T and NK cell subset | IL-10 family member with functions similar to IL-20 |
| IL-27 | Dendritic cells, macrophages, endothelial cells, and plasma cells | IL-12 family member that has pro- and anti-inflammatory activities |
| IL-28 A/B | Monocyte-derived dendritic cells | An IFN-like molecule that is coexpressed with IFN-$\beta$; exhibits antiviral activity and induces class I and II MHC molecule expression |
| IL-29 | Monocyte-derived dendritic cells | Activities similar to IL-28 A/B |
| IL-30 | Antigen-presenting cells | A subunit of IL-27 with functions similar to IL-27 |
| IL-31 | Primarily activated T$_H$2 cells, which can be induced by activated monocytes | Possible recruitment of monocytes, neutrophils, and T cells to areas of skin inflammation |
| IL-32 | Activated NK cells and peripheral blood mononuclear cells | IL-1 family member that is a proinflammatory cytokine; induces TNF-$\alpha$ |
| IL-33 | Smooth muscle cells, epithelial cells; levels by TNF-$\alpha$ and IL-1$\beta$-induced dendritic cells and macrophages | IL-1-like cytokine that induces T$_H$2 cell-associated cytokines |
| IL-34 | Unknown (binds to M-CSF receptor) | Unknown |
| IL-35 | CD4$^+$CD25$^+$FOXP3$^+$T$_{reg}$ cells | IL-12 family cytokine is required to mediate their suppressive activity |
| **Interferons** | | |
| IFN $\alpha$ | Lymphocytes, dendritic cells, and macrophages | Induces antiviral resistance; inhibits cellular proliferation; controls class I MHC molecule expression |
| IFN-$\beta$ | Fibroblasts, dendritic cells, and some epithelial cells | Same activity as IFN-$\alpha$ |
| IFN-$\gamma$ | CD4$^+$ and CD8$^+$ T cells, NK cells | Activates B cells, T cells, macrophages, and NK cells; induces class II MHC molecule expression on APCs; T$_H$1 cell signature cytokine; inhibits all activities of IL-4 on B cells; weakly inhibits viral replication |
| **Tumor necrosis factors** | | |
| TNF-$\alpha$ | Monocytes, macrophages, and others such as, activated T cells, fibroblasts, NK cells, and neutrophils | Vascular inflammation; regulates growth of many different cell types; causes apoptosis of target cells; induces acute phase proteins; promotes angiogenesis and cachexia; activates neutrophils and endothelial cells |
| TNF-$\beta$ | Activated T$_H$1 cells, B cells, astrocytes, fibroblasts, and endothelial and epithelial cells | Causes apoptosis of target cells; promotes fibroblast growth; inhibits osteoclasts and keratinocyte growth; induces terminal differentiation of monocytes; activates neutrophils, enhances adhesion |
| **Colony-stimulating factors** | | |
| CSF | Colony-stimulating factors *See pages 315–316 for other aliases* | Stimulate the growth of colonies of granulocytes and macrophages from bone marrow progenitor cells; some activate mature macrophages |
| **Others** | | |
| TGF-$\beta$ | Many different cell types | Inhibits and stimulates extracellular matrix formation; also inhibits B-, T-, and NK-cell activity; switches antibody production to IgA |

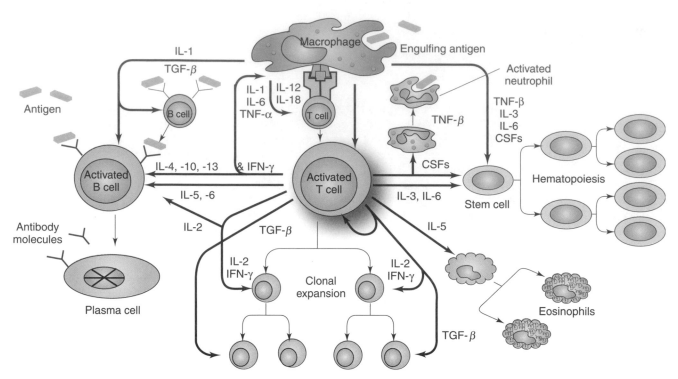

**FIGURE 9-2 A mediator regulatory network.** This figure shows some of the cytokines that make up a network of interactive signals that orchestrate inflammatory (innate) and adaptive immune responses and maintain a balance of stem cells.

names and functions and a possible mediator network (Figure 9-2). The *innate immunity cytokines* typically include: interleukin-1 (IL-1), tumor necrosis factor-α (TNF-α), IL-6, IL-12, interferon-α and -β (IFN-α/β), and IL-10. IL-1, TNF-α, IL-6, and IL-12 are also called *proinflammatory cytokines*. These macrophage- and dendritic cell-derived cytokines cause local inflammation in response to bacterial products such as lipopolysaccharide (LPS) and viral products such as double-strand RNA. Macrophages and dendritic cell can also be induced to produce these cytokines by activated T cells. As discussed in Chapter 3, NK cells also produce cytokines during innate immune responses. Many of the innate immune cells express germline-encoded receptors, such as Toll-like receptors (TLRs), which recognize a range of exogenous microbial antigens. The ligation of TLRs leads to the activation of nuclear factor κB and cytokine production, which directs the nature and magnitude of adaptive immune responses. That is, the resulting complicated cytokine cascades produced after innate immune system activation steer naïve CD4$^+$ T$_H$0 cell differentiation into effector T$_H$ cell subtypes: T$_H$1, T$_H$2, T$_H$17 and T-regulatory cells (see Chapter 10).

The other group of cytokines, the *adaptive immunity cytokines* typically include: IL-2, IL-4, IL-5, IL-13, IFN-γ, and transforming growth factor-β (TGF-β). Primarily T cells in response to specific antigen APC signals produce these cytokines, which can act during the activation phase to drive T cell proliferation and differentiation or during the effector phase by recruiting, activating, and regulating effector cells such as, monocytes, neutrophils, and esosinophils. These cytokines also mediate humoral immunity by triggering isotype switching of antibodies. The signature cytokine produced by T$_H$1 cells is IFN-γ; the signature cytokines produced by T$_H$2 cells are IL-4; and the signature cytokine produced by T$_H$17 cells is IL-17. These signature cytokines mediate cross-regulation between the three subsets (see Chapter 10), that is, they modulate the differentiation and function of one another. Cytokines such as IL-10 and TGF-β have principally anti-inflammatory or immunosuppressive effects (used by T-regulatory cells to control immune responses), while other cytokines such as IL-6 have both pro- and anti-inflammatory effects. Taken together, there is much overlap because of their associated activities.

# NONSPECIFIC CYTOKINES EXHIBIT SPECIFICITY BY BINDING EXACT RECEPTORS ON RESPONSIVE TARGET CELLS

How do cytokines target specific cells? The answer is: to mediate activities, cytokines must bind to specific target cell receptors. These transmembrane receptors consist of extracellular portions that are responsible for cytokine binding and cytoplasmic portions that are responsible for initiating intracellular signaling pathways. The expression of cytokine receptors themselves is often regulated, for example, some resting immune cells do not express cytokine receptors or only low- or intermediate-affinity receptors; this expression scenario is followed by IL-2 receptors and will be discussed shortly. The modulation of cytokine receptor expression ensures that only activated target cells will respond.

## Cytokine Receptors Are Divided into Five Families and Three Subfamilies

There are five cytokine receptor families based on their extracellular cytokine-binding domain structure (Figure 9-3). They are (1) the immunoglobulin (Ig) superfamily receptors, (2) the class I cytokine receptor family (also called the *hematopoietin receptor family*), (3) the class II cytokine receptor family (also called the *interferon receptor family*), (4) the tumor necrosis factor (TNF) receptor family, and (5) the chemokine receptor family. Class I cytokine receptors can be divided into subfamilies because they share a signal-transducing subunit. The presence of a common signaling receptor subunit suggests that two different cytokines binding to distinct receptors with a common subunit can produce a similar outcome.

The Ig superfamily receptors are so called because they contain extracellular Ig domains; therefore, they are classified in the Ig superfamily. This group contains the IL-1 receptor, which binds IL-1 one of the major cytokines of innate (inflammation) immune responses; it is a proinflammatory cytokine. There are two forms of IL-1, IL-1$\alpha$ and IL-1$\beta$, which share only 30% sequence homology yet mediate identical functions by binding to the same receptors. Two different IL-1 receptors have been characterized; both are members of Ig superfamily. The type I receptor is expressed on many different cells and the

major receptor for IL-1-mediate responses, whereas the type II receptor is expressed only on B cells. The type II receptor does not mediate IL-1 activities; therefore, it is considered a decoy that competitively inhibits IL-1 binding to the type I signaling receptor. The Ig superfamily receptors also bind macrophage colony-stimulating factor (M-CSF) and c-kit (stem cell factor).

The type I cytokine, also called *hematopoietin*, receptor family contains receptors for most of the cytokines mediating immune and hematopoietic activity. They bind cytokines that have a four $\alpha$-helical bundle structure and signal by mechanisms that include the Janus activated kinase (JAK)-signal transducer and activator of transcription (STAT) pathway. The extracellular membrane-distal domains of these receptors contain two conserved copies of cysteines (CC and CC); the membrane proximal domains contain a conserved sequence of tryptophan-serine-X-tryptophan-serine (WSXWS, where X is a nonconserved amino acid). This family is also called the *hematopoietin receptor family* because it contains most of the cytokines that function in the hematopoietic system.

Several members of the type I cytokine receptor family are grouped into subfamilies because they have an identical signal-transducing subunit. The three subfamilies are called the *IL-2 receptor subfamily* (share a common $\gamma$ subunit), the *GM-CSF receptor subfamily* (share a common $\beta$ subunit), and the *IL-6 receptor subfamily* (share a common gp130 subunit) (Figure 9-4). The sharing of signal-transducing chains clarifies the redundancy and antagonism associated with some cytokines.

The type II cytokine, also called *interferon*, receptors are similar to type I cytokine receptors because their extracellular domains also have conserved cysteines but lack the WSXWS motif (see Figure 9-4). The receptors are composed of two chains, one cytokine-binding chain and one signal-transducing chain.

The TNF receptor family also has extracellular domains that contain conserved cysteines (see Figure 9-3). When ligands bind to TNF receptors, they may stimulate gene expression or induce apoptosis depending on the adapter proteins binding to their cytoplasmic domains. For example, if the adapter protein TNF receptor-associated death domain (TRADD) binds followed by TNF receptor-associated factor (TRAF) and receptor interacting protein (RIP), it leads to new gene expression. If the adapter

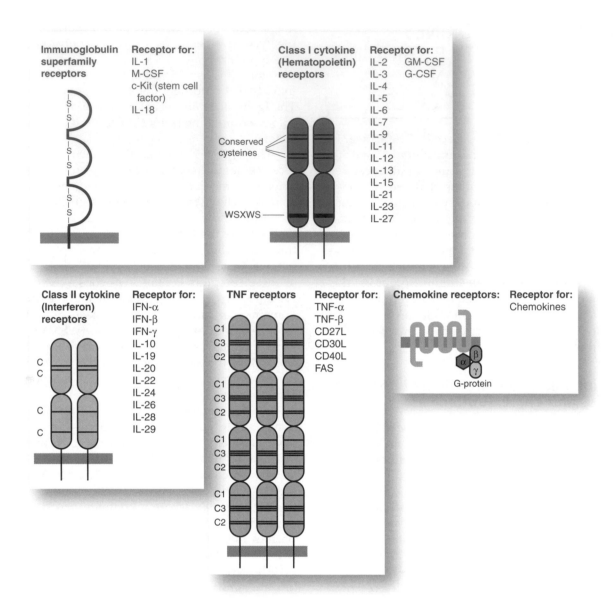

**FIGURE 9-3 Cytokine receptor families**. There are five families of receptors characterized by their structural features, which are illustrated, and the cytokines that bind to these receptors. C represents conserved cysteine (thin black lines); WSXWS motifs are presented by thick black lines.

protein Fas-associated death domain (FADD) binds to TRADD, it leads to apoptosis.

The chemokine receptors, also called *seven-transmembrane α-helical receptors* and *G-coupled receptors* because they appear to "snake" back and forth through the cell membrane, and their signal pathways are mediated through GTP-binding (G) proteins, respectively. These structurally distinct receptors mediate rapid responses when ligated by a group of cytokines called *chemokines* (discussed later).

## Cytokine Engagement of Their Counterpart Receptors Initiates Signal Transduction Pathways that Ultimately Instruct the Biologic Activity of Target Cells

The best characterized family and subfamily of receptors is the type I IL-2 cytokine receptor subfamily, in particular, the IL-2 receptor (IL-2R) due to IL-2's T cell growth factor activity for antigen-stimulated T cells and their clonal expansion following antigen

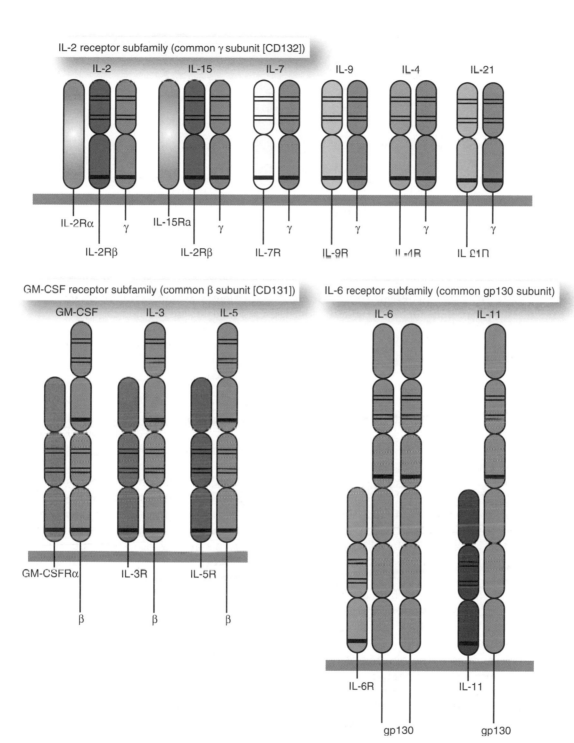

**FIGURE 9-4 Cytokine receptor subfamilies.** The class I receptor family can be divided into three subfamilies because they share an identical signaling subunit (all colored in lavender) but express a unique cytokine-specific binding subunit. The subfamily members are called *IL-2* (share common γ subunit), *GM-CSF* (share common gp130 subunit), and *IL-6* (share common β subunit).

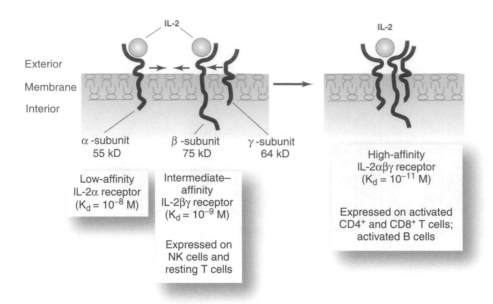

**FIGURE 9-5 IL-2 receptors come in three forms.** There is a low (α subunit), an intermediate (βγ subunits), and a high (αβγ) affinity form. The β and γ chains are required for ligand internalization and signal transduction. The γ chain is called the *common γ subunit* because it mediates signal transduction and is shared by all members of the IL-2 receptor subfamily (see Figure 9-3).

recognition. This subfamily includes receptors for IL-2, IL-4, IL-7, IL-9, IL-15, and IL-21; they share the common γ signal transducing subunit. IL-2 and IL-15 receptors are heterotrimers (β and γ subunits mediate signal transduction), whereas all of the other receptors are dimers (common γ subunit mediates signal transduction). The IL-2R consists of three noncovalently linked polypeptide chains, a cytokine-specific α-chain (p55, IL-2Rα) that alone binds IL-2 with low affinity ($K_d \approx 10^{-8}$ M), a β chain (p75, IL-2Rβ) that alone binds IL-2 with low affinity, and a γ-chain (p64, IL-2Rγ) that alone does not bind IL-2 to any measurable extent (Figure 9-5). The β chain in combination with the γ chain binds IL-2 with intermediate affinity ($K_d \approx 10^{-9}$ M). The combined αβγ molecule leads to the high-affinity ($K_d \approx 10^{-11}$ M) IL-2 binding site. Although it collaborates in the binding of IL-2, the α chain does not contribute to signal transduction, consistent with its short cytoplasmic domain. T cells and NK cells express intermediate IL-2Rs. IL-2Rα is not found on resting T cells, but it is efficiently induced by T-cell activation; therefore, it is sometimes called *T-cell activation (TAC) antigen* or *CD25*. Its high expression on CD4+ T cells may indicate the presence of T regulatory cells (see Chapter 10). IL-2Rβ is expressed constitutively by CD8+ $T_C$ cells but not by CD4+ $T_H$ cells. Like IL-2Rα, IL-2Rβ is further induced by T-cell activation. Activated human

T cells have about 5000 high-affinity binding and roughly 50,000 low-affinity sites per cell. Lymphoid cells express IL-2Rγ constitutively. The modulation in IL-2R expression guarantees that only activated CD4+ and CD8+ T cells with high levels of high-affinity IL-2Rs will response to physiologic levels of IL-2. In contrast, NK cells constitutively express β and γ chains, allowing them to be activated by bind IL-2 with intermediate affinity. The importance of the common γ signal transducing subunit is indicated by the severity of congenial X-linked severe combined immunodeficiency (see Chapter 16); it results from a defect in the IL-2Rγ gene, which maps to the X chromosome. NK cell and T cell activity are absent due to the deficit of all cytokine activity mediated by the IL-2 receptor subfamily.

To initiate cytokine-mediated biologic effects, cytokines must bind their counterpart receptors, which transduces intracellular signals leading to the assembly of active transcription factors and gene transcription (Figure 9-6). The illustrated signal transduction pertains to most, if not all, class I and class II cytokine receptors. Cytokine-receptor ligation induces dimerization of receptors juxtaposing their cytoplasmic domains, JAK-mediated phosphorylation of the receptors, recruitment and binding of inactive signal transducers and activators of transcription (STATs), phosphorylation of bound

STATs, dimerization of STATs, translocation of STATs from the cytoplasm to the nucleus, and binding to DNA promoters of genes induced by the cytokines.

The JAKs and STATs are essential intracellular mediators of IFN-α, -β, and -γ, IL-2, IL-4, IL-5, IL-6, IL-10, and IL-12 action; knockout mice that lack JAKs and STATs often have noticeable immunological defects. Nonetheless, control of the cytokine-signaling magnitude and duration is also necessary to prevent pathology. The culmination of biologic activity induced by cytokine-mediated signaling does not terminate the signaling. The dimerized STATs in the nucleus not only stimulate the transcription of cytokine-responsive genes, but those that encode suppressors of cytokine signaling (SOCS) proteins. The SOCS family is composed of eight intracellular proteins (SOCS1 through SOCS7 and the cytokine-induced SRC-homology 2 [SH2] protein CIS), which includes several key physiological regulators of cytokine responses. In fact, CIS, SOCS1, and SOCS3 seem to act in a classical negative-feedback loop to extinguish cytokine signal transduction. SOCS proteins are not expressed in unstimulated cells, but are encoded by cytokine-inducible genes that are rapidly transcribed in cytokine-exposed cells. SOCS proteins inhibit components of the cytokine-signaling cascade by direct binding, by preventing access to the signaling complex, or by targeting signal transducers for proteasomal destruction (see Figure 9-6 inset). The SOCS proteins are cytokine signal regulators essential to normal immune activity. The disruption of SOCS expression or activity is associated with several immune and inflammatory diseases, suggesting that manipulation of SOCS function may provide therapeutic options in the treatment of immunological disorders.

# MULTIPLE CYTOKINES INFLUENCE INNATE IMMUNITY

Several cytokines and chemokines are significant to the development of innate immunity and the often concomitant development of inflammatory responses. IL-1, TNF-α, IL-12, and type I IFNs facilitate innate immunity and associated inflammation, whereas IL-10 controls innate immunity and cell-mediated immunity by inhibiting activated macrophages and dendritic cells.

## IL-1, a Pleiotropic Proinflammatory Molecule, Is a Major Mediator of Inflammatory Responses to Infection

Interleukin-1 (IL-1), part of the IL-1 family with at least 10 members, is produced by activated macrophages and neutrophils and others. IL-1 has an important role in inflammation and host defense. It was originally described as an "endogenous pyrogen" because it has fever-inducing properties. The earliest cytokine description of IL-1 was by Gery and coworkers, who detected activity in the culture supernatant of human monocytes that promoted thymocyte proliferation. The activity was called *lymphocyte-activating factor (LAF)*. Every nucleated cell (except T cells) can produce IL-1, and it also seems that IL-1 affects every cell, immune or nonimmune.

The plethora of cell sources (Table 9-4), the diverse repertoire of activities, and the pleiotropic nature (Figure 9-7) of IL-1 made its characterization difficult. The varied IL-1-mediated activities on different cell types are summarized in Figure 9-7. The major function of IL-1 is to mediate and regulate innate immune responses and inflammatory reactions.

IL-1 is a polypeptide with varied ascribed molecular weights, although the predominant form is 17 kD. Two distinct genes encode two distinct forms of IL-1: *IL-1α* and *IL-1β*. They have about 30% sequence homology, yet both molecules exhibit similar biologic effects and bind to the same cell-surface receptors. IL-1 molecules are processed at the cell membrane or extracellularly to give the mature molecule. IL-1α seems to be primarily membrane-associated. Most of the IL-1 activity in circulation comes from IL-1β. Both human IL-1α and IL-1β genes are located on chromosome 2.

Production of IL-1, under physiologic conditions, occurs only in response to some stimulants (Table 9-5), even though certain cell lines are constitutive producers of IL-1. No intracellular or extracellular IL-1 production is seen in unstimulated human monocytes. Following lipopolysaccharide (LPS) stimulation, intracellular activity is detected in 30 min, and extracellular IL-1 activity is detected in 60 min. High levels of extracellular IL-1 are detected in 3 hr.

Two types of IL-1 receptors exist: an 80-kD type I (CD121a) and a 60-70-kD type II (CDw121b) (Figure 9-8). Both are members of the Ig gene superfamily. Usually the number of receptors is low (several hundred); type I IL-1 receptors are found on almost all cells, while type II IL-1 receptors are found on B cells, perhaps induced on other cells. The type I

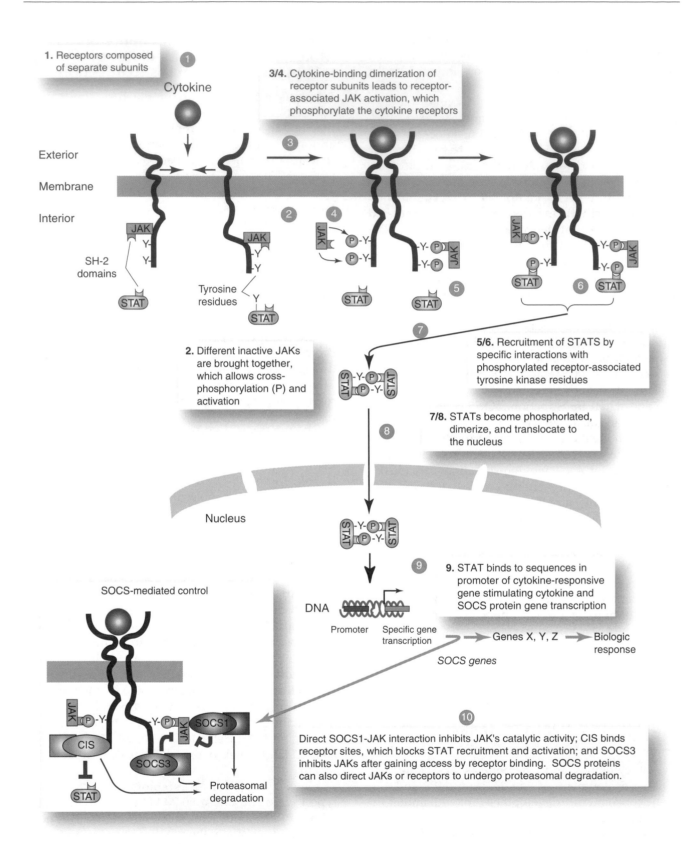

**1.** Receptors composed of separate subunits

Cytokine

Exterior

Membrane

Interior

SH-2 domains

JAK

STAT

Y-
Y-

JAK

Tyrosine residues

Y
Y

Y

STAT

**3/4.** Cytokine-binding dimerization of receptor subunits leads to receptor-associated JAK activation, which phosphorylate the cytokine receptors

JAK

P -Y-
P -Y-

Y- P
Y- P

JAK

STAT

STAT

JAK

P -Y-

Y- P

P -Y-

Y- P

JAK

STAT

STAT

**2.** Different inactive JAKs are brought together, which allows cross-phosphorylation (P) and activation

STAT -Y- P STAT
STAT P -Y- STAT

**5/6.** Recruitment of STATS by specific interactions with phosphorylated receptor-associated tyrosine kinase residues

**7/8.** STATs become phosphorlated, dimerize, and translocate to the nucleus

Nucleus

STAT -Y- P STAT
STAT P -Y- STAT

**9.** STAT binds to sequences in promoter of cytokine-responsive gene stimulating cytokine and SOCS protein gene transcription

SOCS-mediated control

DNA

Promoter   Specific gene transcription

SOCS genes

Genes X, Y, Z → Biologic response

JAK

P -Y-

CIS

STAT

Y- P

JAK

SOCS1

SOCS3

Proteasomal degradation

Direct SOCS1-JAK interaction inhibits JAK's catalytic activity; CIS binds receptor sites, which blocks STAT recruitment and activation; and SOCS3 inhibits JAKs after gaining access by receptor binding. SOCS proteins can also direct JAKs or receptors to undergo proteasomal degradation.

**FIGURE 9-6 Signal transduction through class I and II cytokine receptors—JAK/STAT pathway.** In this schematic, the receptor is a two-subunit receptor; however, others like IL-2, IL-15, and IL-6 are three-subunit receptors. Abbreviations: CIS, cytokine-induced SRC-homology 2 (SH2) protein; JAK, Janus tyrosine kinases; SOCS, suppressors of cytokine signaling protein; STAT, signal transducer and activator of transcription.

**TABLE 9-4** Some Cell Sources of IL-1 Activities

| Cell source | Inducing agents |
| --- | --- |
| IMMUNE-RELATED CELLS | |
| B-cell lines | None |
| B lymphoblasts | Lipopolysaccharide (LPS), anti-IgM |
| Dendritic cells | LPS |
| Langerhans cells | LPS |
| Monocytes, macrophages, and their cell lines | LPS, phorbol myristate acetate (PMA), muramyl dipeptide (MDP), immune complexes, tissue injury, CSF, IFN-γ, activated T cells, and UV irradiation |
| Neutrophils | Aluminum hydroxide |
| | |
| NONIMMUNE CELLS | |
| Astrocytes | LPS |
| Endothelial cells | LPS |
| Epithelial cells | LPS, PMA, and UV irradiation |
| Fibroblasts | MDP |
| Glioma cells | Cell cycle dependent |
| Mesangial cells | Cell cycle dependent |
| Microglial cells | LPS, injury, and *Staphylococcus aureus* |

IL-1 receptors are recognized by both IL-1α and IL-1β, binding by either molecule leads to the same biologic activities. When either IL-1α or IL-1β bind type II IL-1 receptors, no signaling is initiated because type II receptors lack intracellular signaling domains. This lack of response makes it a *decoy receptor*; it inhibits IL-1 activities by competing for type I receptor binding. As we saw in Chapter 3, the intracellular portion of the type I IL-1 receptor is homologous to a domain found in Toll-like receptors (TLRs); therefore, the cytoplasmic tail of TLRs is called the *Toll/IL-1R (TIR) domain*. TLRs play significant role in innate immunity to infections.

The many effects of IL-1 on diverse cell types overshadow its effects on T and B cells. At low locally produced levels, IL-1 enhances CD4$^+$ T-cell proliferation, promotes B-cell growth and differentiation, autocrinely stimulates IL-1 production, induces interleukin-6 (IL-6) synthesis, and enhances leukocyte/endothelial cell adhesion by increased expression of ligands for integrins. At high levels, IL-1 enters the circulation and causes fever, stimulates the release of acute-phase proteins from liver cells, and induces cachexia. In fact, IL-1, IL-6, and TNF-α are considered *endogenous pyrogens*, inducing fever, which helps eliminate infections. In general, IL-1 is now considered to be a mediator of inflammatory responses during innate immune reactions.

Although IL-1 enhances immune defense functions, it also triggers inflammation and tissue damage. To counter IL-1 activity, the same cells that make IL-1 produce an 18 kD cytokine called *IL-1 receptor antagonist (IL-1ra)* that blocks IL-1 activity by binding to IL-1α and IL-1β type I receptors. Thus, it functions as a competitive inhibitor of IL-1. IL-1ra has no agonist activity and does not bind to IL-1 itself. This latter characteristic makes it different from most cytokine inhibitors; most inhibitors bind to the cytokine itself. Many of the soluble cytokine inhibitors are enzymatic cleavage fragments of the extracellular domains of the cytokine's receptors for IL-2, IL-4, IL-6, IL-7, IFN-γ, and TNF.

## Tumor Necrosis Factor Is the Major Mediator of Acute Inflammatory Responses to Infection

**Tumor necrosis factor (TNF)** is also called *tumor necrosis factor-α* to distinguish it from *lymphotoxin* now called *TNF-β*. These two molecules are structurally similar and biologically indistinguishable and bind to the same receptors. The human TNF-α and TNF-β genes lie within the MHC. TNF-β, a 24-kD homotrimer cytokine, is released only by activated T$_H$1 cells and is 30% homologous to TNF-α. TNF-β also differs from TNF-α by containing N-linked oligosaccharides and by being a truly secretory protein. TNF-β is considered a paracrine-type factor. It is cytostatic and cytotoxic for some tumor cell lines and causes necrosis of certain tumors *in vivo*. TNF-β also influences the function of B cells, T cells, connective-tissue cells, and hematopoietic cells. TNF-α (17 kD) is produced mainly by activated macrophages and, to a lesser extent, by

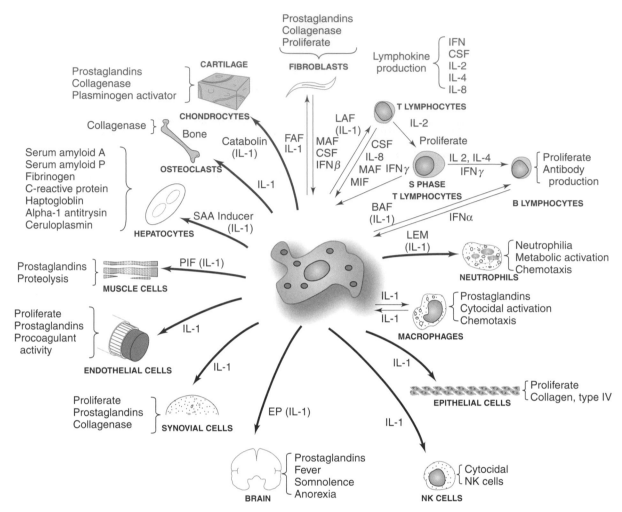

**FIGURE 9-7 IL-1 effects on target cells and tissues**. The figure shows the interactions among macrophages, other immune cells, and fibroblasts mediated by IL-1. Around the periphery are shown the responses of target cells to IL-1 and the induction and effects of other cytokines. BCGF, B-cell growth factor; CSF, colony-stimulating factor; EP, endogenous pyrogen; FAF, fibroblast activating factor; IFN, interferon; LDCF, lymphocyte-derived chemotactic factor; MAF, macrophage activating factor; MIF, macrophage inhibiting factor; PIF, proteolysis-inducing factor; SAA, serum amyloid A.

---

### TABLE 9-5 IL-1 Stimulants

**1. IMMUNOLOGIC**
   a. Activated T cells: a cell contact, class II MHC-restricted cytokine
   b. Immune complexes
   c. C5a
   d. Interferon-γ

**2. MICROBIAL**
   a. Gram-positive bacteria: cell walls, MDP, exotoxins
   b. Gram-negative bacteria: endotoxin (lipopolysaccharide [LPS])
   c. Yeast: cell walls (zymosan)
   d. Virus: hemagglutinins, double-stranded RNA

**3. OTHER**
   a. PMA
   b. Silica crystals
   c. Urate crystals

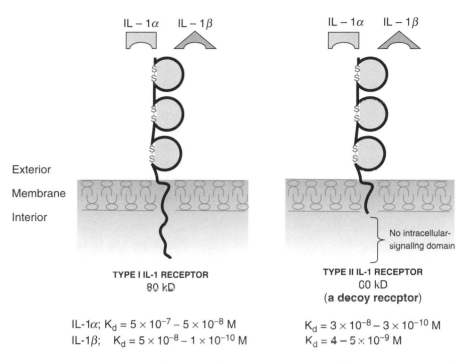

$$\text{IL-1}\alpha;\ K_d = 5 \times 10^{-7} - 5 \times 10^{-8}\ M$$
$$\text{IL-1}\beta;\quad K_d = 5 \times 10^{-8} - 1 \times 10^{-10}\ M$$

$$K_d = 3 \times 10^{-8} - 3 \times 10^{-10}\ M$$
$$K_d = 4 - 5 \times 10^{-9}\ M$$

**FIGURE 9-8 IL-1 receptors.** The two different IL-1 receptors (R), type I IL-1Rs and type II IL-1Rs, are distributed in some overlapping cell types and can bind both IL-1α and IL-1β with similar affinities. Both types of receptors are members of the Ig superfamily. Type II IL-1R binds IL-1 but does not transduce signaling pathways; it is a decoy receptor.

antigen-activated $T_H1$ cells, activated NK cells, and activated mast cells (Figure 9-9). Its chief function is to recruit neutrophils and monocytes to infection sites and activate them once they arrive. TNF-α also stimulates macrophages and vascular endothelial cells to produce chemokines, which augments adhesion by enhancing the leukocyte integrin affinity for their ligands and recruits more leukocytes to inflamed tissues. Furthermore, TNF-α induces macrophage production of IL-1. The most potent stimulus for macrophages production of TNF-α is lipopolysaccharide (LPS) derived from Gram-negative bacteria during infections. Because of activities similar to IL-1, TNF-α is also considered a proinflammatory cytokine. T-cell-derived IFN-γ induces LPS-activated macrophages to make more TNF-α. In fact, IFN-γ enhances many of the effects of TNF-α. TNF-α was originally defined as a substance that could kill tumor cells during the host's response to Gram-negative bacteria.

TNF-α is synthesized as a 25-kD, nonglycosylated transmembrane protein, whose orientation is reversed—its amino terminus is intracellular, while its carboxyl terminus is extracellular. A 17-kD membrane fragment is cleaved by macrophages and assembled into a 51-kD homotrimer secreted form. This circulating molecule's activity is concentration-dependent. At low concentrations ($10^{-9}$ M) it acts as an autocrine and paracrine regulator of immune cells and endothelial cells, while at high concentrations it acts as an endocrine hormone. For example, at low concentrations, TNF-α induces increased expression of adhesion molecules on endothelial cells, increased neutrophil adhesion, enhances neutrophil-mediated microbial killing, and stimulates macrophages to produce IL-1, IL-6, chemokines, and TNF-α itself. At high serum concentrations ($10^{-7}$ M), it induces fever, acute phase protein synthesis in liver cells, and cachexia. Severe bacterial infections by certain Gram-negative bacteria can lead to septic shock (vascular collapse and widespread intravascular coagulation), which results from bacterial endotoxin (LPS) binding TLRs of dendritic cells and macrophages and causing them to overproduce TNF-α and IL-1. TNF-α is also expressed as a homotrimer membrane form (see Figure 9-3). TNF ligands are expressed on many different immune system cells, such as, B cells, T cells, NK cells, macrophages, and dendritic cells. There are two TNF receptors, a 55-kD receptor

(CD120a) called a *type I TNF receptor (TNFRI)* and a 75-kD receptor (CD102b) called *a type II TNF receptor (TNFRII).* TNFRIs are present on all cells examined, whereas TNFRII are expressed mainly on immune cells and endothelial cells, which all have 2000 to 3000 receptors per cell. Evidence suggests that TNF-α binding to TNFRIs mediates apoptosis through the recruitment of adapter proteins that initiate caspases and triggers apoptosis, whereas binding to TNFRIIs mediates proliferation by recruitment of TNF receptor-associated factors (TRAFs) to the cytoplasmic domains of the receptors, which eventually leads to activation of transcription factors. Knockout mice deficient in either receptor obstructed most of the TNF-α-transduced signals.

## IL-6 Influences Innate and Adaptive Immunity

Another B-cell-stimulating interleukin of 19 to 26 kD is **interleukin-6 (IL-6)**. IL-6 is a multifunctional interleukin produced by mainly macrophages, endothelial cells, and activated T cells in response to IL-1 and TNF-α. IL-6 is important in host defense mechanisms and is considered an inflammatory cytokine because, like IL-1 and TNF-α, it mediates innate immunity

through inflammatory reactions. As an endogenous pyrogen, it induces fever. IL-6 also induces acute phase proteins in liver cells (see Chapter 3) and growth promotion of myeloid hematopoietic cells to neutrophils. IL-6 exerts growth-inducing, growth-inhibiting, and differentiation-inducing effects, depending on the target cells. For example, in adaptive immunity, it is the main growth factor for B cells late in their differentiation. It is also a growth factor for myeloma, plasmacytoma, and hybridoma cells. In fact, myeloma cells secrete it as an autocrine growth factor. These cells express 50 to 2000 receptors per cell. The IL-6 receptors consist of two chains, a 70-kD α chain (CD126) and a 130-kD β subunit (CD130). The α subunit is a binding chain, while the β subunit is a signal-transducing chain shared with IL-11 and other noninterleukin molecules (see Figure 9-4).

## IL-12, a Proinflammatory Cytokine that Links Innate and Adaptive Immunity

**Interleukin-12 (IL-12)**, a heterodimeric 70-kD monocyte/macrophage and dendritic cell-derived cytokine, is formed by two covalently linked chains of 35 kD (p35) and 40 kD (p40). The p35 subunit is produced

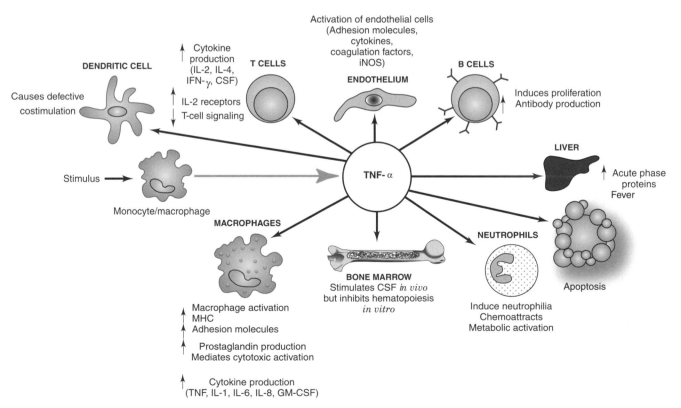

**FIGURE 9-9  The effects of TNF-α on lymphoid tissues.**

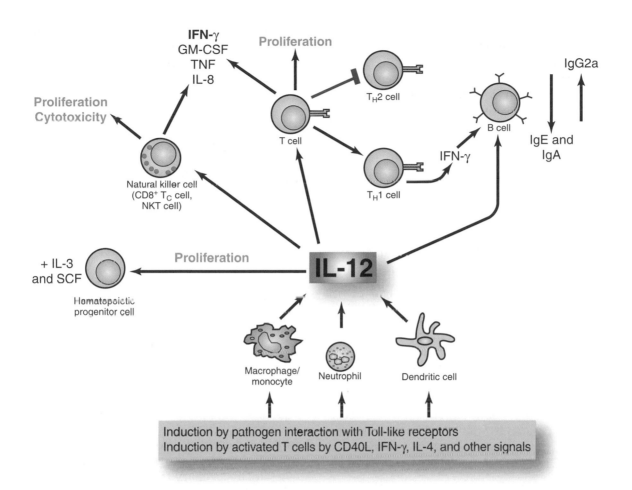

**FIGURE 9-10 Biologic activities of IL-12.** The predominant producers of IL-12 are macrophages and dendritic cells followed by neutrophils. These cells in response to pathogens through TLRs and other receptors or T cell CD40L engagement of APCs CD40 produce IL-12. IL-12 acts on hematopoietic stem cells, NK and NKT cells, T cells, and B cells. IL-12's major effect is its induction of IFN-γ production by NK cells, T$_H$1 cells, and T$_C$ cells. Abbreviations: stem cell factor, SCF; natural killer T (NKT) cell; granulocyte-macrophage colony-stimulating factor, GM-CSF. (Adapted from G. Trinchieri. 2003. *Nat. Rev. Immunol.* 3:133.)

by many immune cells and has a structure typical of other cytokines. The p40 subunit is produced by primarily APCs. The p40 subunit is homologous with the IL-6 receptor. IL-12 is the prototype member of a small family of heterodimeric cytokines, which also include IL-23 and IL-27 (structurally similar but functionally different; see Table 9-3). Figure 9-10 summarizes some of the biologic activities of IL-12. Macrophages and dendritic cells in response to microbial stimulation, such as, bacterial LPS, infection by intracellular bacteria, and fungal and virus infections, double-stranded RNA, bacterial DNA, and CpG-containing oligonucleotides, are the main producers of IL-12. IL-12, also called *NK cell stimulatory factor*, induces IFN-γ production from T$_H$1 and NK cells and augments the cytotoxic activity of both resting and cultured

NK cells. In addition to being a potent stimulator of NK cell activity, IL-12 drives the differentiation of naïve CD4$^+$ T cells into the T$_H$1 subset and CD8$^+$ T cells into functionally mature T$_C$ cells. In either case, you get increased production of IFN-γ. IL-12 has been referred to as "the jump-starter of cell-mediated immunity" and thereby linking innate immunity and adaptive immunity. That is, early in innate immunity in response to infection by intracellular microbes, macrophages and dendritic cells produce IL-12 that stimulates NK cells to produce IFN-γ and acts as a switch, with IFN-γ, nudging uncommitted CD4$^+$ T$_H$ cells to a cellular, or T$_H$1, response. T$_H$1 cells, in turn, produce IFN-γ, which activates macrophages and dendritic cells to produce IL-12. IL-12 production by dendritic cells is less dependent on the presence of IFN-γ or other enhancing cytokines than is production by macrophages. The presentation of antigen by macrophages or dendritic cells to specific T$_H$ cells leads to T-cell activation; this interaction induces T cell CD40L expression, which engages APC CD40 and causes APCs to produce IL-12. Taken together, IL-12-induced IFN-γ production mediates many of IL-12's proinflammatory activities, whereas the ability of IL-12 to polarize naïve T cells to produce a T$_H$1 cell response represents its function as an immunoregulatory cytokine that links innate immunity and adaptive immunity.

IL-12 receptor is a heterodimer composed of two chains: IL-12Rβ1 and IL-12Rβ2. Both chains are required for high-affinity binding of IL-12; the IL-12Rβ2 subunit is the signal transducer. Ligand engagement of the IL-12 receptor activates the Janus kinase (JAK)–STAT (signal transducer and activator of transcription) pathway of signal transduction (as described earlier). The IL-12 receptors are primarily expressed on activated T cells and NK cells. They are undetectable on resting T cells; however, NK cells constitutively express low levels of IL-12 receptors, which allow them to rapidly respond to IL-12. Activation of T cells through peptide-MHC molecule–TCR engagement upregulates the production of both IL-12 receptor chains, though IL-12Rβ2 expression is limited to T$_H$1 cells, which correlates with its IL-12 responsiveness.

Another cytokine functional similar to IL-12 is called *IL-18*. It is structurally related to IL-1β (member of the IL-1 superfamily) but functionally unrelated to IL-1. Also similar to IL-1β, IL-18 is synthesized as an inactive precursor (pro-IL-18) lacking a signal peptide, which is cleaved by IL-1-converting enzyme (ICE; caspase-1) to generate a biologically active, mature 18-kD moiety. Like IL-12, macrophages and dendritic cells in response to bacterial products such as LPS produce IL-18. In association with IL-12, IL-18 induces IFN-γ production by NK cells and T cells. Furthermore, IL-18 enhances T cell and NK cell maturation, cytotoxicity, and cytokine production—like IL-12, IL-18 is an inducer of cell-mediated immunity. IL-18-deficient and IL-12- and IL-18-deficient knockout mice confirm these activities; they lack IFN-γ production and T$_H$1-mediated responses to intracellular microbes.

Two new members that are structurally related to IL-12 were recently introduced; they are IL-23 and IL-27. IL-23 stimulates a previously differentiated IL-17–producing T-cell subset (T$_H$17 cells) (discussed in Chapter 10), which is highly proinflammatory and causally involved in many autoimmune diseases, whereas IL-27, a cytokine with pro- and anti-inflammatory properties, suppresses the development of T$_H$17 cells.

## Type I Interferons Are Antiviral Molecules That Mediate and Regulate Innate Immunity

We will briefly discuss type I interferons (their early antiviral activity in innate immune responses was discussed in Chapter 3). The term **interferon (IFN)** was initially used more than 50 years ago to describe an "activity" that was secreted by virus-infected cells that could protect neighboring cells from infection. All IFNs are named because of this ability to stimulate synthesis of antiviral gene products that "interfere" with viral replication and spread. Interferons are widely expressed, first defense cytokines against viral infections.

The IFN family is composed of two classes of related cytokines (see Table 3-3): type I IFNs and type II IFN. There are many type I IFNs, which include two distinct groups, IFN-α (which can be further subdivided into many different structurally related subtypes) and IFN-β. Mononuclear phagocytes are the primary source of IFN-α, whereas many cells, such as, fibroblasts, produce IFN-β. Irrespective of cellular source, double-stranded RNA produced during virus replication in infected cells stimulates IFN-α and IFN-β synthesis. In addition to their antiviral activity, type I IFNs induce increased expression of class I MHC molecules on newly infected cells thereby enhancing CD8$^+$ T$_C$ cell-mediated killing; they also enhance the expression on most uninfected cells thus enhancing their resistance to NK cell-mediated killing. Type I IFNs also promote the development of human T$_H$1 cells by inducing IL-12 receptor expression on them. Lastly, they activate NK cells, which augments early innate immunity to viral infections.

Even though IFN-α and IFN-β are structurally different, they bind a common heterodimeric cell-surface receptor, which is known as the type I IFN receptor. It is composed of two distinct subunits IFNAR1 and IFNAR2, which are associated with JAKs tyrosine kinase 2 (TYK2) and JAK1, respectively. IFN-α or IFN-β receptor binding leads to cellular activation through JAK-STAT pathways (discussed earlier).

## IL-10, an Inhibitor of Activated Macrophages and Dendritic Cells, Controls Innate Immunity

The cytokines mentioned thus far have "turned on" innate immunity and associated inflammatory responses. In closing this section we briefly discuss a cytokine that "turns down" activated macrophages and dendritic cells and thereby controls innate immunity and cell-mediated adaptive immunity. **Interleukin-10 (IL-10)** was originally described as cytokine produced by $T_H2$ cells; however, surprisingly and quickly thereafter it was realized that macrophages were major producers and to a lesser extent dendritic cells. It is an 18-kD protein that was initially called *cytokine synthesis inhibitory factor* because it inhibits cytokine synthesis by the $T_H1$ cell subset (see Chapter 10) and by activated macrophages and dendritic cells. The surprise is that the same cells that produce IL-10, activated macrophages, are the major target of its inhibitory activities.

IL-10 is the prototype cytokine for a family of cytokines with sequence homology and similar helical structure to IL-10. Like IL-10, the IL-10–related molecules (IL-19, IL-20, IL-22, IL-24, and IL-26) regulate inflammatory responses. These IL-10-related cytokines include: IL-19, a 21-kD protein produced primarily by unactivated or LPS-activated monocytes, pretreatment of monocytes with IL-4 or IL-13 but not IFN-γ increased LPS-induced monocyte IL-19 production, IL-19–treated monocytes induced IL-6 and TNF-α production and pretreatment with IL-10 blocked this production, binds to IL-20 receptor complexes, and activates STAT proteins; IL-20 a broadly expressed cytokine with proinflammatory properties for keratinocytes; IL-22 is produced by activated $T_H1$ cells and induces acute phase proteins by liver cells and reactive oxygen species in resting B cells suggesting an involvement in inflammatory responses; IL-24 is a monocyte- perhaps T cell-derived cytokine with two distinct functional characteristics, at low physiologic concentrations it acts as a cytokine at high concentrations it induces apoptosis, treatment of periphery blood mononuclear cells with IL-24 induced the production of IL-1β, TNF-α, IL-6, IL-12, IFN-γ, and GM-CSF, which is blocked by IL-10 treatment; and IL-26 a T cell-derived cytokine that is induced during viral infections but its overall function is undetermined. All of these cytokines bind to type II cytokine receptors, which initiates signals that modulate inflammatory responses, inhibit or stimulate cell proliferation, generate or hinder apoptosis, and affect many immune mechanisms.

The IL-10 receptor (IL-10R) consists of two subunits that are members of the type II (interferon) receptor family. The IL-10-specific subunit binds IL-10 with high affinity and is expressed by most hematopoietic cells. Like IFN-α and -β Rs, IL-10Rs use the other subunit for signaling and the IL-10/IL-10R engagement induces JAK1 and TYR2 tyrosine kinases–STAT pathways.

Figure 9-11 summarizes some of the biologic activities of IL-10. IL-10 is an inhibitor of $T_H1$-cytokine production, through its action on macrophages and dendritic cells, which leads to inhibition of proinflammatory cytokines and IL-12 production (IL-12 critical to $T_H1$ cell development) and in inhibition of expression of MHC class II and costimulatory molecules. IL-10 also inhibits the ability of macrophages to kill intracellular organisms and the maturation of dendritic cells from monocyte precursors. IL-10 regulates $T_H2$ responses and allergic responses. CD4⁺CD25⁺ regulatory T cells are defined by their ability to produce high levels of IL-10 and TGF-β. In sum, IL-10 is a potent anti-inflammatory cytokine, which through its suppressive effects on macrophages and dendritic cells inhibits various innate immunity and associated inflammatory activities. IL-10's crucial regulatory role is confirmed by the uncontrolled, lethal, systemic inflammatory response to various pathogens in IL-10 knockout mice.

---

### MINI SUMMARY

IL-1 is a 17-kD protein produced mainly by monocytes and macrophages during innate immune responses. Distinct genes encode the two IL-1 molecules, IL-1α and IL-1β. IL-1 has immunologic and nonimmunologic properties. IL-1 production is primarily associated with inflammation reactions to microbes. The decoy receptors and IL-1 receptor antagonist can control IL-1 activity.

Like IL-1, TNF-α is primarily produced by LPS-activated macrophages and mediates acute inflammation responses to microbes. $T_H1$ cells produce TNF-β.

IL-6 induces acute phase proteins during innate immune responses and influences B cell growth and antibody production.

IL-12 stimulates IFN-γ production by NK cells and T cells, which in turn activates APCs and polarizes naïve T cells to $T_H1$ cell responses.

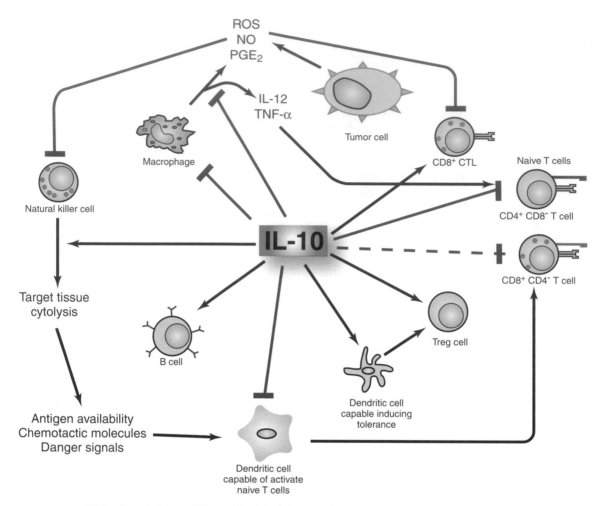

**FIGURE 9-11 Biologic activities of IL-10.** The black lines indicate stimulatory activity, whereas the solid red lines indicate inhibitory activity. The dashed red line indicates uncertainty. (Adapted from S. Mocellin et al. 2004. *Cytokine & Growth Factors Rev.* 15:61.)

IL-10 is an inhibitor of cytokine synthesis, particularly IL-12, by activated macrophages and dendritic cells, which restrains innate immunity and cell-mediated immunity.

# CHEMOKINES ARE SMALL CYTOKINES THAT SELECTIVELY CONTROL ADHESION, CHEMOTAXIS, AND ACTIVATION OF LEUKOCYTES

**Chemokines**, are a large group of low molecular weight chemotactic proteins containing 90 to 130 amino acid residues with conserved sequences, are major controllers of neutrophil, monocyte, dendritic cell, and lymphocyte traffic during development, inflammation, or immune surveillance. Chemokines are produced either by cells in inflamed tissue or sites of antigen exposure that induces adaptive immunity, which recruit leukocytes to inflammation sites and then to secondary lymphoid organs or by various normal tissues, which recruit primarily lymphocytes to healthy tissues. For example, chemokines can direct newly developed immune cells from the bone marrow to the thymus, spleen, or lymph nodes and once the cells arrive, chemokines direct their migration through the respective organs. Chemokines are classified into four subfamilies on the basis of the number and position of N-terminal conserved cysteine residues: the CC chemokine family (conserved cysteines are contiguous), the CXC chemokine family (conserved cysteines are separated by some other nonconserved amino acid [X]), and the remaining two minor families, which include the C family (lack two of the four conserved cysteines), and the CX3C family (three amino acids between the conserved cysteines). For example, using this system, CCL2 refers to chemokine ligand of the CC subfamily, number 2. A similar approach is used to label chemokine receptors, the subfamily chemokine followed by R and then an identifying number—the receptor for CCL2 is called CCR2. Chemokines are also classified according to functional activities, such as inflammatory chemokines, which are expressed by circulating leukocytes and other cells only on activation, whereas homeostatic chemokines are constitutively expressed. Table 9-6 summarizes some characteristics of the roughly 40-plus human chemokines. All but two chemokines are secreted from the cell after translation; CX3CL1 and CXCL16 are tethered to the cell surface. CXCL1 and CXCL16 are found as membrane-bound and soluble forms.

As mentioned earlier, chemokines mediate their activity by binding to serpentine, seven-transmembrane, heterotrimeric ($\alpha\beta\gamma$) G protein-coupled receptors that are grouped according to the chemokine subfamily they bind (see Table 9-6). There are at least six CXC receptors (CXCRs) for CXC chemokines, 10 CCRs for CC chemokines, one XCR for C chemokines, and one CX3CR for CX3C chemokines. Even though many chemokine receptors can recognize more than one chemokine within a family, the interaction between receptors and chemokines is strong and specific. The patterns of chemokine receptor expression on leukocytes and the production of diverse chemokines by target tissues, whether inflamed or healthy, dictate which leukocytes will respond to which chemokines, thereby accurately directing their recruitment and regulation. Activated T cells express the greatest variety of chemokine receptors—from naïve T cells expressing CXCR4 and CCR7 to activated T cells expressing CXCR5 and CCR2—CCR6, and CCR8, perhaps more. In fact, the chemokine receptor expression on T cells varies from effector T cells to effector-memory T cells to central memory T cells. The chemokine receptor profiles expressed by $T_H1$ and $T_H2$ cells differs; $T_H1$ cells frequently express CCR5, CXCR3, and CXCR6, whereas $T_H2$ cells frequently express CCR3, CCR4, and CCR8. The ligation of a receptor by its appropriate chemokine activates G protein subunits by catalyzing the replacement of guanosine diphoshate (GDP) by GTP, which stimulates phospholipase C$\beta$ isoforms, phosphoinositide

3-kinases, and c-Src family tyrosine kinases. The activation of these cellular enzymes induces the locomotion (actin polymerization) and adhesion (increasing the affinity of integrins for their ligands) by many different leukocytes to inflamed and healthy tissues, and the activation of killing mechanism in phagocytes.

## MINI SUMMARY

Chemokines are important mediators and regulators of innate immunity and inflammatory responses; they regulate cellular traffic. They act as chemoattractants and activators of leukocytes as the cells move to, arrive at, and extravasate into the site of inflammation. Chemokines are divided into four subfamilies based on the number and position of N-terminal conserved cysteine residues. Chemokines are targeted to specific cells through four subfamilies of receptors that traverse the membrane seven times, which are members of the G protein-coupled receptors that are grouped according to the chemokine subfamily they bind. Chemokine-receptor profiles mediate the differential regulation of leukocyte activities.

# MULTIPLE CYTOKINES INFLUENCE ADAPTIVE IMMUNITY

The contribution of cytokines in adaptive immunity can be divided between their activities during the activation and effector phases of adaptive immunity. During the activation phase, lymphocyte-antigen engagement, cytokines mediate lymphocyte proliferation and differentiation. During the effector phase, antigen elimination, cytokines induce the differentiation of CD4$^+$ $T_H$ cells into two subsets, which in turn produce different cytokines and activate effector T cells to kill antigens.

## IL-2 Is an Autocrine T-Cell Growth Factor

**Interleukin-2 (IL-2)**, produced by CD4$^+$ $T_H1$ cells and in lower amounts by CD8$^+$ T cells, is a 15.5-kD glycoprotein originally called *T-cell growth factor (TCGF)*. IL-2 supports the exponential growth of antigen-stimulated human T cells. IL-2 acts primarily on the T cell that produced it; it is an *autocrine*

**TABLE 9-6 Chemokines: Their Names, Receptors, and Functions**

| Classification | Systematic name | Common name | Chemokine receptors | Predominant receptor expressor | Predominant function |
|---|---|---|---|---|---|
| CXC family | | | | | |
| | CXCL1 | GROα* | CXCR2 | Neutrophils | Neutrophil recruitment, innate immunity, acute inflammation, angiogenic |
| | CXCL2 | GROβ | CXCR2 | Neutrophils | Neutrophil recruitment, innate immunity, acute inflammation, angiogenic |
| | CXCL3 | GROγ | CXCR2 | Neutrophils | Neutrophil recruitment, innate immunity, acute inflammation, angiogenic |
| | CXCL4 | PF4 | CXCR3B | Platelet | Platelet aggregation |
| | CXCL5 | ENA-78 | CXCR2 | Neutrophils | Neutrophil recruitment, innate immunity, acute inflammation, angiogenic |
| | CXCL6 | GCP-2 | CXCR1, CXCR2 | Neutrophils | Neutrophil recruitment, innate immunity, acute inflammation, angiogenic |
| | CXCL7 | NAP-2 | CXCR1, CXCR2 | Neutrophils | Neutrophil recruitment, innate immunity, acute inflammation, angiogenic |
| | CXCL8 | IL-8 | CXCR1, CXCR2 | Neutrophils | Neutrophil recruitment, innate immunity, acute inflammation, angiogenic |
| | CXCL9 | Mig | CXCR3 (CD183), CXCL3B | Activated T cells | $T_H1$ effector recruitment, adaptive immunity, $T_H1$-mediated inflammation |
| | CXCL10 | IP-10 | CXCR3, CXCR3B | Activated T cells | $T_H1$ effector recruitment, adaptive immunity |
| | CXCL11 | I-TAC | CXCR3, CXCR3B | Activated T cells | $T_H1$ effector recruitment, adaptive immunity |
| | CXCL12 | SDF-1 | CXCR4 (CD184), CXCR7 | B & T cells, monocytes, neutrophils, and some tissue cells | Leukocyte recruitment, B cell lymphopoiesis, bone marrow myelopoiesis, central nervous system and vascular development, CXCR4 is HIV coreceptor |
| | CXCL13 | BCA-1 | CXCR5 | B cells | B cell trafficking, lymphoid development |
| | CXCL14 | BRAK | Unknown | Unknown | Unknown |
| | CXCL16 | — | CXCR6 | Activated T cells | T cell and dendritic cell recruitment to spleen |
| CC family | | | | | |
| | CCL1 | I-309 | CCR8 | Monocytes, $T_H2$ cells, thymus | T cell and monocyte recruitment, innate and adaptive immunity, inflammation |
| | CCL2 | MCP-1 | CCR2 | Monocytes, $T_H2$ cells | T cell and monocyte recruitment, innate and adaptive immunity, inflammation |
| | CCL3 | MIP-1α | CCR1, CCR5 | Monocytes, macrophages, activated $T_H1$ cells | Mixed leukocyte recruitment, innate immunity |
| | CCL4 | MIP-1β | CCR5 | Monocytes, T cells, dendritic cells | T cell, monocyte, dendritic cell, NK cell recruitment; innate and adaptive immunity; CCR5 is HIV coreceptor |
| | CCL5 | RANTES | CCR1, CCR3, CCR5 | Monocytes, T cells, dendritic cells | Mixed leukocyte recruitment; innate and adaptive immunity; $T_H1$ and $T_H2$ response |
| | CCL7 | MCP-3 | CCR1, CCR2, CCR3 | Monocytes, T cells, dendritic cells | Mixed leukocyte recruitment; $T_H2$ response |

*(continued overleaf)*

**TABLE 9-6** *(Continued)*

| Classification | Systematic name | Common name | Chemokine receptors | Predominant receptor expressor | Predominant function |
|---|---|---|---|---|---|
| | CCL8 | MCP-2 | CCR2, CCR3, CCR5 | Monocytes, T cells, dendritic cells | Mixed leukocyte recruitment; $T_H2$ response |
| | CCL11 | Eotaxin | CCR3, CCR5 | Basophils, eosinophils, $T_H2$ cells | Basophils, eosinophils, $T_H2$ cells recruitment |
| | CCL13 | MCP-4 | CCR1, CCR2, CCR3 | Monocytes, T cells | Mixed leukocyte recruitment; $T_H2$ response |
| | CCL14 | HCC-1 | CCR1, CCR5 | Monocytes, macrophages, dendritic cells, T cells | Unknown |
| | CCL15 | HCC-2 | CCR1, CCR3 | Monocytes, macrophages, dendritic cells, T cells | Mixed leukocyte recruitment |
| | CCL16 | HCC-4 | CCR1, CCR2, CCR3, CCR5 | Monocytes, macrophages, dendritic cells, T cells | Mixed leukocyte recruitment |
| | CCL17 | TARC | CCR4 | Basophils, T cells | Basophil and $T_H2$ cell recruitment |
| | CCL18 | DC-CK1, PARC | Unknown | Unknown | Dendritic cell attraction of naive T cells(?) |
| | CCL19 | ELC/MIP-3β | CCR7 | T cells, dendritic cells | T cell and dendritic cell homing to lymph node parafollicular regions |
| | CCL20 | MIP-3α | CCR6 | T cells, dendritic cells | T cell and dendritic cell homing to Peyer's patches |
| | CCL21 | SLC | CCR7 | T cells, dendritic cells | T cell and dendritic cell homing to lymph node parafollicular regions |
| | CCL22 | MDC | CCR4 | Basophils, T cells | Basophil and T cell recruitment |
| | CCL23 | MPIF-1 | CCR1 | Monocytes, macrophages, dendritic cells, T cells | Unknown |
| | CCL24 | Eotaxin-2 | CCR3 | Basophils, eosinophils, T cells | Basophil, eosinophil, and $T_H2$ cell recruitment |
| | CCL25 | TECK | CCR9 | T cells | Astrocyte migration; T cell homing to gut |
| | CCL26 | Eotaxin-3 | CCR3 | Basophils, eosinophils, T cells | Basophil, eosinophil, and $T_H2$ cell recruitment |
| | CCL27 | CTACK | CCR10 | T cells | Homing of T cells to skin and gut |
| | CCL28 | MEC | CCR10 | T cells | Homing of T cells to skin and gut |
| C family | | | | | |
| | XCL1 | Lymphotactin | XCR1 | T cells, NK cells | T cell and NK cell recruitment |
| | XCL2 | SCM-1β | XCR1 | T cells | Unknown |
| CX3C family | | | | | |
| | CX3CL1 | Fractalkine | CX3CR1 | T cells, NK cells, macrophages | T cell, NK cell, and macrophage recruitment; $T_C$ cell and NK cell activation |

*Some abbreviations: BCA-1, B-cell-attracting chemokine 1; CTACK, cutaneous T-cell-attracting chemokine; ELC, Epstein-Barr-virus-induced gene 1 ligand chemokine; ENA78, epithelial-cell-derived neutrophil-activating peptide 78; GCP-2, granulocyte chemotactic protein 2; GRO, growth-regulated oncogene; IL-8, interleukin 8; IP-10, interferon inducible protein 10; I-TAC, interferon-inducible T-cell α chemoattractant; MCP, monocyte chemoattractant protein; MDC, macrophage-derived chemokine; MEC, mucosae-associated epithelial chemokine; MIG, monokine induced by interferon Y; MIP, macrophage inflammatory protein; NAP-2, neutrophil-activating peptide 2; RANTES, regulated on activation, normal T-cell expressed and secreted; SDF-1, stromal-cell-derived factor 1; SLC, secondary lymphoid-tissue chemokine; TARC, thymus and activation-regulated chemokine; TECK, thymus-expressed chemokine.

*growth factor*.[2] Originally, IL-2 was considered to be strictly a growth factor for activated T cells. However, IL-2 is also a differentiation molecule that promotes $T_C$-cell activity and B-cell activity (growth and J-chain synthesis). IL-2 also induces secretion of IFN-γ and IL-4 by T cells (discussed shortly). IL-2 synergizes with IL-12 to increase cytotoxicity by NK cells and lymphokine-activated killer (LAK) cells. Table 9-7 and Figure 9-12 summarizes some of the immunologic activities of IL-2.

Human IL-2 is a polypeptide consisting of 133 amino acid. The human IL-2 polypeptide has one intramolecular disulfide bridge between residues at positions 58 and 105. The mature glycoprotein has a molecular weight ranging from 14 to 17 kD. The gene encoding human IL-2 is located on chromosome 4.

Proliferation of activated T cells requires binding of IL-2 to its high-affinity specific cell-surface receptors; IL-2 receptors (IL-2R) are part of the type I cytokine receptors (IL-2R signaling was detailed earlier; see Figure 9-5). The IL-2R is composed of three chains, α, β, and γ. Cytokine binding is mediated by the α and β chains, whereas cytokine signaling is mediated by β and γ chains. IL-2Rβγ is expressed constitutively; IL-2Rα is not and requires certain inductive signals for expression. The inductive signals are (1) interaction of antigen with its specific TCR-CD3 complex, (2) antigen-receptor interaction associated with MHC molecules and IL-1, and (3) expression of the gene encoding IL-2. Antigen-induced proliferation is an *autocrine mechanism*. The proliferation rate of activated T cells becomes concentration-dependent when maximal IL-2R expression occurs. The presence of antigen is required for continuous IL-2R expression. Once antigen is removed, IL-2R levels decline and cell proliferation drops. IL-2 also can regulate the expression of its receptors. In fact, IL-2-receptor interaction causes the density of high-affinity IL-2Rs to diminish. Thus, the interplay between the positive effect of specific antigen-receptor triggering and the negative influence of IL-2R triggering balances

the high-affinity IL-2Rs that are determining the progression through the cell cycle, the proliferation rate, clonal growth, and the magnitude of the T-cell response. Failure to produce either IL-2R or its ligand, IL-2, leads to the absence of a T-cell-mediated immune response. The specificity of an immune response means the interaction of an appropriately presented antigen with its receptor, but the magnitude and duration of the immune response are determined by the interaction of IL-2 with high-affinity IL-2Rs. In addition to promoting the proliferation of antigen-specific T cells, IL-2 also promotes these activities in other immune cells. Like resting T cells, NK cells only express IL-2Rβγ; thus, only high levels of IL-2 can stimulate them. IL-2 is a growth factor for B cells and stimulates their antibody synthesis (see Table 9-7).

IL-2 not only promotes antigen-induced proliferation, but also stops it. IL-2 does this through a mechanism called *activation-induced cell death (AICD)*, which eliminates self-reactive T cells and through its maintenance of peripheral $CD4^+CD25^+$ regulatory T cells. Both activities control the growth of T cells that if left unchecked could lead to the pathogenesis caused by autoimmune diseases. In fact, IL-2-, IL-2Rα-, or IL-2Rβ-deficient mice develop autoimmune diseases such as hemolytic anemia and inflammatory bowel disease.

## IL-4 Is the Signature Cytokine of $T_H2$ Cells

The substances known as *B cell-stimulating factor 1 (BSF-1)*, *T-cell growth factor II (TCGF-II)*, and *mast cell growth factor II (MCGF-II)* are all encoded by a single gene found on chromosome 5. This one molecule is now called **interleukin-4 (IL-4)**. This 18-kD $CD4^+$ $T_H2$ cell- (and activated mast cells and basophils) derived factor causes activation, proliferation, and differentiation of B cells, and it increases the expression of class II MHC molecules on B cells. IL-4 also is an autocrine growth factor for $CD4^+$ $T_H2$ cells (see Chapter 10) and mast cells. It stimulates the differentiation of $CD4^+$ naïve T cells to $T_H2$ cells. IL-4 inhibits IFN-γ-induced macrophage activation and thereby restrains cell-mediated immunity, and affects erythrocyte, granulocyte, and megakaryocyte precursors; it is required for class switching to IgE production, and it regulates IgG4 isotype selection. IL-4 signals through the IL-4 receptor (IL-4R). As a type I cytokine receptor family member, IL-4Rs (140 kD) (CD124) are composed of a cytokine-binding α chain and the signaling common γ chain; the IL-4R signals through the JAK/STAT pathway. IL-4Rs are found on B and T cells, macrophages, mast

---

[2]The term *autocrine* is based on the term *endocrine* from endocrinology (the study of hormones). Hormones are made by organs distant from their targets. In an autocrine situation, the cell itself makes hormones or growth factors for which it possesses its own receptors. Thus, it is self-stimulating. The prefix "para" of *paracrine* means beside. Therefore, a paracrine system is one in which one cell has the right receptors and can respond to the stimulating factors produced by its neighboring cells. IL-2 is also a paracrine molecule because it acts on nearby $CD4^+$ and $CD8^+$ T cells, but it does not act as an endocrine growth factor.

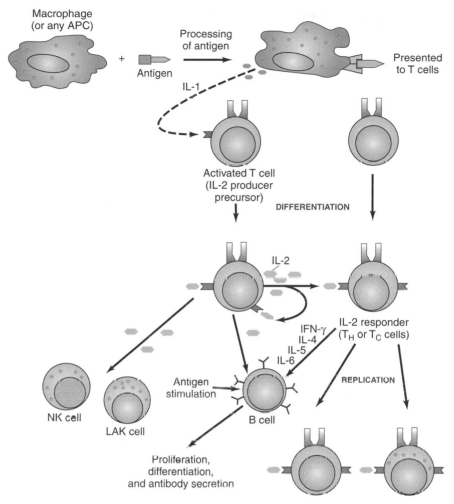

**FIGURE 9-12 Role of IL-2 in the immune response.** Resting T cells do not produce IL-2. T cells activated by antigen presented by self-MHC molecules and IL-1 rapidly synthesize and secrete IL-2. These T cells plus another, possibly overlapping, subset of T cells express high-affinity receptors for IL-2. In the presence of IL-2, these T cells proliferate, and produce other interleukins, leading to growth of the $T_H$ and $T_C$ cell populations as well as B cells.

### TABLE 9-7 Immunologic Activities of IL-2

1. Enhances proliferation of CD4$^+$ $T_H$ cells:
   a. Interaction with B cells leading to enhanced antibody production
   b. Interaction with class II MHC molecule on macrophages leading to cytokine secretion
2. Enhances proliferation of CD8$^+$ $T_C$ cells:
   a. Activation of T cells cytotoxic for tumor cells
   b. Secretion of interferon-$\gamma$ leading to macrophage activation and enhanced cytokine production
3. Enhances proliferation and cytotoxicity of NK cells and LAK cells
4. Enhances proliferation and stimulates B cell antibody production
5. Enhances apoptosis of antigen-induced T cells and maintains regulatory T cells

cells, myeloid cells, granulocytes, megakaryocytes, erythroid progenitors, NK cells, fibroblasts, and endothelial cells. When binding to endothelial cells, IL-4 stimulates the expression of adhesion molecules, leading to increased immune cell binding. About 300 IL-4 Rs are found on B and T cells, and the number increases during cell maturation. The number of IL-4 Rs expressed per cell ranges from 100 to 1000.

## IL-5 Is an Eosinophil Activation and Differentiation Factor That Links T-Cell Activation with Eosinophilic Reactions

The activities ascribed to *human T-cell-replacing factor (TRF), B-cell growth factor II (BCGF-II),* and *eosinophil differentiation factor (EDF)* are mediated by a CD4$^+$ T$_H$2 cell-derived 45-kD molecule called **interleukin-5 (IL-5)**. The IL-5 gene is found on human chromosome 5. Like IL-4, IL-5 is a B-cell activation, growth, and differentiation factor as well as an eosinophil differentiation factor. IL-5 also regulates IgA isotype selection. IL-5 seems to be a pivotal molecule in the stimulation of growth and differentiation of eosinophils and in the activation of mature eosinophils to kill helminths. B cells, basophils, and eosinophils display 500 to 1000 low-affinity receptors and 7500 to 10,000 high-affinity receptors. The IL-5 type I receptors consist of a 55-kD α chain (CD125) and a 150-kD signal-transducing β subunit shared with IL-3 and GM-CSF; the IL-5R signals through the JAK/STAT pathway.

## Interferon-γ Is a Potent Immunoregulatory Molecule with Additional Antiviral and Antiproliferative Effects

Interferons (IFNs) are a family of glycoproteins that are classically defined by their ability to protect cells against viral infections (see Table 3-3). IFN-α and IFN-γ are produced exclusively by immune cells. The third form of IFN, IFN-β, is produced by many somatic cells on challenge with virus. In addition to their antiviral effects, IFNs can suppress antibody formation, antigenic and mitogenic responses of B and T cells *in vitro*, and replication of normal and neoplastic cells. While almost all biologic effects of IFN can be produced by any of the three forms, **IFN-γ**, produced by NK cells, T$_H$1 cells, and T$_C$ cells, has greater immunosuppressive activity than do the other forms. IFN-γ is a cross-regulator between T$_H$1 and T$_H$2 cells. It downregulates T$_H$2 cell activity (see Chapter 10). IFN-γ also possesses many stimulatory activities (Table 9-8). In fact, it is the host's major activator of macrophages.

Depending on the type of antigenic stimulus, T$_H$1 CD4$^+$ T cells (it is their signature cytokine) and CD8$^+$ T$_C$ cells are the main producers of IFN-γ. T$_H$1 cells are the primary producers of IFN-γ when exposed to soluble antigens, but T$_H$ and T$_C$ cells produce IFN-γ when exposed to foreign cell-surface antigens. On appropriate stimulation, NK cells become potent IFN-γ producers. T cells independently regulate the IFN genes. To produce IFN-γ, T cells need an IL-1 and an IL-2 signal. If resting peripheral blood lymphocytes are exposed to phorbol esters, T cells are the primary producers of IFN-γ, although resting NK cells respond immediately. NK cells are the primary producers of IFN-γ when exposed to IL-2. A possible sequence of action during an immune response is

**TABLE 9-8 Biological Activities of the Interferons**

**1.** Activities of IFN-γ
   a. Potent activation of macrophages for tumor cell killing and antimicrobial activity (IFN-γ is the main *macrophage-activating factor* derived from T cells.)
   b. Induction of monocyte lineage differentiation
   c. Increased class I and II MHC molecule expression
   d. Induction of Fc receptors
   e. Inhibition of intracellular bacteria and protozoa growth
   f. Promotion and inhibition (downregulator of T$_H$2 cells) of lymphocyte proliferation
   g. Promotion of B- and T-cell differentiation
   h. Stimulation of antibody production by B cells, particularly IgG2a
   i. Stimulation of IL-1 and IL-2 synthesis
   j. Activation of neutrophils
   k. Activation of NK cells
   l. Activation of vascular endothelial cells
**2.** Activities shared by the IFNs
   a. Activation of T$_C$ cells
   b. Activation of NK cells
   c. Induction of antiviral state
   d. Induction of cell growth
   e. Increased class I MHC molecule expression
   f. Induction of protein kinase
   g. Induction of 2′,5′-oligoadenylate synthetase
   h. Stimulation of B-lymphocyte differentiation

that antigen-specific T cells recruit NK cells by IL-2 to produce IFN-γ.[3] IFN-γ also is important in the differentiation of antigen-specific $T_C$ cells.

Human IFN-γ is encoded by one gene located on chromosome 12. The 143 amino acid sequence of the IFN-γ gene is different from that of the other two forms of IFN. The two forms of the IFN-γ molecule are caused by the posttranslational modification, the 50-kD form of IFN-γ is glycosylated, whereas the homodimer consists of 21- to 24-kD subunits. The extent of glycosylation is variable, but neither species needs to be glycosylated to be biologically active.

---

[3]NK cells comprise 10 to 19% of circulating lymphocytes; thus, they outnumber antigen-specific T cells.

Like other cytokines, IFN-γ mediates its activity by binding to specific membrane receptors. Receptors for the three forms of IFN are different. The receptors (CD118) for IFN-α and IFN-β are shared, while the IFN-γ receptor (CD119) is specific for IFN-γ. Binding assays suggest about 2400 high-affinity ($K_d = 10^{-10}$ to $10^{-11}$ M) binding 90 to 100 kD IFN-γ receptors per human fibroblast and about 12,000 receptors per murine macrophage. All human cells tested to date bear IFN-γ receptors, and the number of receptor sites per cell ranges from 200 to 10,000.

Taken together, IFN-γ activates macrophages and neutrophils thereby facilitating their killing of intracellular microbes; it stimulates NK cell-mediated cytotoxicity; it increases the expression of APC class I and class II MHC molecules and costimulators

**TABLE 9-9** Immunoregulatory Properties of the TGF-βs

| Properties | Inhibits (↓) or Stimulates (↑) | |
|---|---|---|
| | *In vitro* | *In vivo* |
| Allograft rejection | — | ↓ |
| Angiogenesis & tissue repair | — | ↑ |
| Cytokine production | | |
| IFN-γ | ↓ | |
| IL-1 | ↑* | |
| IL-1β | ↓ | |
| IL-1, IL-2, & IL-3 | * | |
| IL-6 | ↓ & ↑ | |
| Platelet-derived growth factor | ↑ | |
| TGF-β | ↑ | |
| TNF α | ↓ & ↑ | ↓ & ↑ |
| c-*myc* expression | ↓ | |
| Cytotoxic macrophage generation | ↓ | ↓ |
| Epithelial cell growth | ↓ | |
| FcRIII expression | ↑ | |
| Fibroblast chemotaxis | — | ↑ |
| Hematopoiesis | ↓ & ↑ | ↓ |
| HLA-DR expression | ↓ | |
| $H_2O_2/O_2$ production | ↓ | |
| IgA production | ↑ | |
| IgG, IgM production | ↓ | |
| IL-2 receptor p55 expression | ↓ | |
| Macrophage chemotaxis | ↑ | |
| Monocyte TGF-β receptors | ↓ | |
| mRNA expression for IL-1α, IL-1β, TGF-α, TNF-α | ↑ | |
| NK cell activity | ↓ | ↓ |
| $PGE_2$ synthesis | ↑ | |
| $T_C$ cell generation | ↓ | ↓ |
| T-cell/B-cell proliferation | ↓ | ↓ |
| Thymocyte proliferation | ↓ | |

*TGF-β antagonizes IL-1, IL-2, and IL-3 activity.

making them better APCs; through IL-12 induction, IFN-γ indirectly drives the differentiation of CD4$^+$ naïve T cells to T$_H$1 cells and counteracts the proliferation T$_H$2 cells; and IFN-γ also affects B cells by causing them to switch to IgG2a and blocks switching to IgG1 and IgE.

## Transforming Growth Factor-β, an Inhibitor and a Stimulator Molecule, Is Important to the Initiation, Progression, and Resolution of an Immune Response

Most cytokines described so far are only upregulatory; thus, in closing our discussion of interleukins that influence adaptive immunity, it seems appropriate to mention briefly another cytokine that could limit an immune response. One such molecule is **transforming growth factor-β (TGF-β)**. TGF-β was initially identified and characterized based on its ability to promote the transformation of nonneoplastic cells (hence its name). However, TGF-β has many other biologic activities (Table 9-9). It is actually a family of molecules, made primarily by activated CD4$^+$ T cells, particulary T$_H$17 cells, but like IL-1, it seems to be made by all cells. Regulatory T cells are also major producers of TGF-β (see Chapter 10 and Figure 10-16). TGF-β is usually secreted in an inactive form that is activated by acids and proteases. Macrophages and possibly T cells can immediately activate TGF-β after it is secreted. Platelets, important in wound repair, are a major storage site for TGF-β. There are three TGF-β family members, TGF-β1, TGFβ2, and TGF-β3, and TGF-β1 is the prototypic molecule and produced by immune cells. The genes for human TGF-β are found on chromosome 19. From 10,000 to 40,000 high-affinity ($K_d$ of $1-6 \times 10^{-12}$ M) TGF-β receptors are found on all cells, normal or malignant. TGF-β signals through heteromeric signaling complexes composed of TGF-β type I and type II receptors. First TGF-β binds the extracellular domain of type II TGF-β receptor homodimers with high affinity. Second, the ligand-bound type II TGF-β receptor complex then binds and transactivates a type I TGF-β receptor, which leads to the phosphorylation of a glycine serine-rich region kinase that phosphorylates transcription factors called *mothers against decapentaplegic homologue (SMAD)* proteins. Some SMADs can transduce the signal to the nucleus.

TGF-β is a homodimer polypeptide (roughly 25 kD) that has potent, widespread activity as a growth inhibitor and as a stimulator of fibrosis and tissue repair. TGF-β secreted at an inflammatory or immune site resulting from a wound may be beneficial in limiting immune cell function (inhibits B, T, and NK cell activities) while promoting extracellular matrix formation and the growth of new blood vessels, a process called *angiogenesis*. However, TGF-β is produced by some cancers and therefore may contribute to tumor-mediated immunosuppression. TGF-β inhibits T$_H$ cell proliferation and inhibits T$_C$-cell development. It also inhibits macrophage activation. Signals (such as from a growing tumor) that cause T cells and macrophages to produce TGF-β may convert neighboring CD4$^+$ T cells to regulatory T cells (see Chapters 10 and 15). TGF-β usually is thought of as a molecule that shuts down all immune responses. However, it also has a positive effect in mucosal immunity by switching B cells to produce the IgA isotype.

## IL-13 Is More Than Another T$_H$2 Cell-Derived Cytokine

**Interleukin-13 (IL-13)**, a 15-kD highly pleiotropic cytokine structurally similar to IL-4 that is produced by activated human T$_H$2 cells, inhibits activation of macrophages through antagonizing IFN-γ–mediated activities. This property is shared by IL-4 and IL-10. IL-13 synergizes with IL-2 in regulating IFN-γ synthesis in NK cells. IL-13 also increases B-cell proliferation, class II MHC molecule expression, and promotes IgE synthesis. IL-13 also has activities that are unique to it, such as, mediating resistance to most gastrointestinal nematodes and intracellular organisms including *Leishmania major*, *Leishmania mexicana*, and *Listeria monocytogenes*, and allergic asthma (infiltration of eosinophils, mucus secretion, and airway hyperresponsiveness). An IL-13 receptor is expressed primarily on macrophages and shares a component with the IL-4 receptor because both cytokines can signal through the IL-13 receptor.

> ## MINI SUMMARY
>
> Interleukin-2 (IL-2), formerly called T-cell growth factor (TCGF), is a 15.5-kD glycoprotein. Its activity includes the generation of T$_C$ cells and antibody production by B cells. T cells that have reacted with foreign antigen and IL-1 are stimulated to produce IL-2. These activated T cells express IL-2 receptors. IL-2 is regulated in an autocrine manner. IL-2 receptors consist of three noncovalently linked chains. The combined αβγ molecule leads to the highest-affinity IL-2 binding site.
>
> IL-4 is an autocrine growth factor for T$_H$2 cells, drives the differentiation of CD4$^+$ naïve T cells to T$_H$2 cells, and induces IgE production. IL-5 activates eosinophils. IFN-γ activates

macrophages and dendritic cells, increases the expression of class I and class II MHC and costimulatory molecules, and increases antigen presentation. TGF-β inhibits the proliferation of T cells the activation of macrophages.

$T_H1$ cell-derived IFN-γ activates macrophages for tumor cell killing, suppresses antibody formation, decreases antigenic responses of B and T cells, and inhibits replication of normal or neoplastic cells. $T_H$ and $T_C$ cells produce IFN-γ, and on appropriate stimulation NK cells also will produce IFN-γ. Because of its inhibitory activity, IFN-γ has been used as an immunotherapeutic agent in cancer treatment, but with disappointing results.

TGF-β is another immunoinhibitory cytokine, but it also promotes matrix formation (wound repair) and angiogenesis.

IL-13 is key to regulation of gastrointestinal parasite expulsion, tissue eosinophilia, and airway hyperresponsiveness.

# CYTOKINES STIMULATE THE GROWTH AND DIFFERENTIATION OF HEMATOPOIETIC STEM CELLS

The first step in the development of blood cells from stem cells is the formation of progenitor cells committed irreversibly to one or more of the six main hematopoietic differentiation lineages.[4] The proliferation and differentiation of these committed hematopoietic cells is under the control of specific growth glycoproteins commonly called **colony-stimulating factors** (**CSFs**). The name comes from the fact that CSFs can be monitored by the formation of colonies of maturing progeny cells in semisolid culture systems. CSFs have multiple and overlapping functions (Table 9-10). They cause activation, proliferation, and differentiation of many different cell types. CSFs also affect the functional activities of the mature immune cells.

Hematopoiesis begins with the binding of the pluripotent stem cell tyrosine-kinase receptor *c-kit*

with the cytokine *c-kit ligand* (also called *stem cell factor*) (see Chapters 2 and 10). Bone marrow stromal cells constitutively produce stem cell factor as either a transmembrane protein or secreted protein. Receptor-ligand binding induces stem cell and progenitor survival and proliferation; stem cell factor also drives the differentiation of mast cells.

Several CSFs have been identified and isolated:[5] **granulocyte-macrophage colony-stimulating factor** (**GM-CSF**), **granulocyte colony-stimulating factor** (**G-CSF**), **macrophage colony-stimulating factor** (**M-CSF**), and IL-3.

GM-CSF stimulates the formation of mixtures of granulocyte-macrophage and granulocyte, macrophage, and eosinophil colonies from pluripotent, hematopoietic stem cells. Activated T cells and macrophages, vascular endothelial cells, and fibroblasts produce GM-CSF. All cells in the eosinophil, neutrophil, and monocyte series bind GM-CSF by some 100 receptors per cell. This number increases as the cells mature. The GM-CSF receptor consists of two chains, a 70 to 85 kD α chain (CD116) and a common 150-kD β chain (CD131) shared with IL-3 and IL-5. T-cell-derived GM-CSF, like IFN-γ, activates macrophages. The CSFs also can induce each other; for example, macrophages can be induced by GM-CSF to produce M-CSF and by M-CSF and IL-3 to produce G-CSF. GM-CSF is a locally acting molecule not found in circulation.

G-CSF is produced by activated macrophages and by endothelial cells and fibroblasts. G-CSF preferentially stimulates the formation of granulocytic and granulocyte-macrophage colonies from pluripotent, hematopoietic stem cells. Unlike GM-CSF, G-CSF is found in circulation. All cells of the neutrophilic granulocytic series bind G-CSF. In contrast, cells of the erythroid, lymphoid, eosinophilic, and megakaryocytic lineages do not bind G-CSF.

Fibroblasts, endothelial cells, and macrophages produce M-CSF, which is found in circulation. M-CSF is the only CSF that is constitutively produced. It stimulates the formation of macrophage colonies from pluripotent, hematopoietic stem cells. From 3000 to 15,000 receptors for M-CSF are found on normal monocytes and macrophages, while no receptors are found on erythroid, lymphoid, eosinophilic, or

---

[4]These lineages are designated according to their end-cell names: erythrocytic, thrombocytic, granulocytic, monocytic, B-lymphocytic, T-lymphocytic, and dendritic cells that can be either lymphocytic or monocytic. A flow chart of hematopoiesis is presented in Figure 2-3 of Chapter 2.

[5]The distinction between CSFs and interleukins is an artificial one because all CSFs can be produced by immune cells and can affect immune cells, and many interleukins can be produced by nonimmune cells and can act on nonimmune cells. Considerable overlap exists in the spectrum of CSF and interleukin activities.

megakaryocytic cells. Low numbers are expressed on neutrophils. The number of receptors increases as cells mature. The M-CSF receptor is an intracytoplasmic tyrosine kinase that was first identified as the proto-oncogene (c-*fms*) of its viral counterpart, v-*fms*. The receptors for the other three CSFs also are transmembrane glycoproteins, but they lack a tyrosine kinase domain.

Activated $T_H1$, $T_H2$ cells, and macrophages produce **interleukin-3** (**IL-3**), also called *multilineage colony-stimulating factor*. IL-3 was originally called *burst-promoting activity, pluripotential hematopoietic cells-stimulating activity, multicolony stimulating factor, mast cell growth factor*, and *histamine-producing cell stimulating factor*. Glycosylation accounts for most of the heterogeneity in the charge of IL-3. Molecular weight determinations suggest a mean molecular weight ranging from 20 to 26 kD.

IL-3 has many different bioactivities. It stimulates the growth of mast cells (and mast-cell lines) and promotes the development of hematopoietic progenitor cells into neutrophils, macrophages, megakaryocytes, and mast cells. IL-3 also acts on macrophages and well-differentiated mast cells. Maintenance of local levels of IL-3 is required for an *in vivo* increase in mast cell numbers. IL-3 may be a link between the immune system and the hematopoietic system. The hematopoietic system provides some of the auxiliary and accessory cells needed for an efficient immune and repair response. IL-3 plays an important role in chronic allergic diseases and perhaps in hematopoietic disorders. It interacts with myeloid precursors, basophils, mast cells, macrophages, and megakaryocytes through IL-3-specific receptors. The IL-3 receptors consist of two chains, a 70-kD α chain (CD123) and a common 150-kD β chain shared with IL-5 and GM-CSF). When activated T cells release IL-3 *in vivo*, its effects are usually restricted to the site of immunization or sites to which activated T cells migrate. IL-3 is found only in the serum with severe immunologic stimuli, such as graft-versus-host disease or parasitic infestations. The half-life of IL-3 in the blood is about 40 min.

**Interleukin-5** (**IL-5**) was discussed earlier; it is produced by activated $T_H2$ cells and is involved in eosinophil development. **Interleukin-6** (**IL-6**) was also discussed earlier; it is produced by activated T cells, monocytes endothelial cells, and fibroblasts and is involved in progenitor-cell stimulation.

Another hematopoietic cytokine is the bone marrow and lymphoid stromal cell-derived, 25-kD molecule called **interleukin-7** (**IL-7**). IL-7 is required for the early development and expansion of precursor B and T cells. IL-7 also appears to promote protection from apoptosis and T cell receptor gene rearrangement among thymic pre-T cells. Genetic deficiencies in the IL-7 pathway lead to severe lymphopenia; however, humans that lack the IL-7 pathway produce B cells. The IL-7 receptor consists of two chains, IL-7Rα binding chain (also know as CD127) and the signaling common γ-chain (also known as CD132); the intracellular domains are associated with JAK1 and JAK3, respectively. IL-7R is expressed on bone marrow lymphoid precursors, pro-B-cells, and mature T cells. Natural killer T cells and γδ T cells require IL-7Rα for their development, whereas NK cells do not. Mature naïve peripheral T cells also require IL-7 for their survival and for the induction of a memory phenotype, particularly in $CD4^+$ T cells.

**Interleukin-9** (**IL-9**) is a 30 to 40 kD $T_H$-cell-derived T-cell growth factor that supports the growth of some T-cell lines and mast cell progenitors. IL-9 activity is mediated by binding to a heavily glycosylated protein receptor of 64 kD. **Interleukin-11** (**IL-11**) is a 20-kD bone marrow stromal cell-derived cytokine that is a growth factor for megakaryocytes.

## MINI SUMMARY

Colony-stimulating factors (CSFs) are glycoproteins produced by stromal cells, macrophages, lymphocytes, endothelial cells, and fibroblasts that induce the proliferation and differentiation of particular cell populations. Three CSFs

### TABLE 9-10 Characteristics of CSFs

1. CSFs are synthesized by bone marrow stromal cells, endothelial cells, fibroblasts, macrophages, and lymphocytes.
2. CSF production is boosted by endotoxin, antigen, and phorbol esters.
3. CSFs are required continuously to stimulate cellular division.
4. CSFs commit cells irreversibly.
5. CSFs stimulate functional activity of mature, nondividing end cells.
6. CSFs have no amino acid sequence homology among five murine CSFs.
7. CSFs have extensive functional overlaps.

have been isolated: (1) granulocyte-macrophage colony-stimulating factor (GM-CSF), (2) granulocyte colony-stimulating factor (G-CSF), and (3) macrophage colony-stimulating factor (M-CSF). All stimulate hematopoietic colony formation of bone marrow cells and some control the functional activities of the mature cells finally produced.

IL-3 is a T-cell-derived, heavily glycosylated protein considered to be one of the colony-stimulating factors. The most generally recognized activities of IL-3 are its ability to stimulate stem cell, myeloid progenitor cell, and mast cell growth. It does not act on T cells. IL-3 also plays an important role in chronic allergic diseases and hematopoietic disorders. Other hematopoietic factors include IL-5, IL-6, IL-7, IL-9, and IL-11.

# SUMMARY

Once immune cells are activated by antigen, they need more signals to reach functional maturity. These signals are generally called *cytokines*—the chemical messengers of the immune system. Cytokines are produced by immune and nonimmune cells and act on various cell types. Cytokines are divided into five families that mediate their activities in an *autocrine, paracrine*, or *endocrine* manner by binding to high-affinity receptors. Cytokine receptors are grouped into five families and three subfamilies that transduce signals through specialized pathways, such as the JAK/STAT pathway.

Cytokines play a major role in mediating and regulating innate and adaptive immunity. Innate immunity-associated cytokines are primarily produced by activated macrophages. They include IL-1, TNF-$\alpha$, IL-6, IL-12, IFN-$\alpha$/$\beta$, and IL-10 but are not limited to controlling only innate immune responses. *IL-1* and *TNF-$\alpha$* are the primary mediators of acute inflammatory responses to microbes. During innate immune responses, *IL-6* induces the production of acute phase proteins; it also is important in adaptive immunity, where it induces proliferation and antibody secretion by B cell lineage. *IL-12* induces NK cells to produce IFN-$\gamma$, which in turn activates macrophages; it is also the "jump-starter of cell-mediated immunity" by promoting $T_H1$ cell development. *Type I IFNs (IFN-$\alpha$ and -$\beta$)* mediate antiviral activity. *IL-10* inhibits macrophages and dendritic cells' ability to produce IL-12 and express class II MHC and costimulatory molecules. IL-10 is part of a large family that controls innate immunity and associated inflammatory response.

During inflammatory responses, a superfamily of small cytokine, *chemokines*, acts as chemoattractants recruiting leukocytes to the site of inflammation, once there chemokines activate them to promote their adhesion and extravasation. Chemokines are divided into four subgroups (CC, CXC, XC, and CX3C) accord to the position of conserved cysteine residues. The cellular chemokine-receptor profile dictates leukocyte activity. Chemokine receptors are grouped in four groups according to the cytokines they bind, either CC receptors (CCRs), CXCRs, XCRs, or CX3CRs.

The primary cytokine players during adaptive immune responses include IL-2, IL-4, IL-5, IL-13, IFN-$\gamma$, and TGF-$\beta$ but are not limited to these nor do these cytokines limit their activities to adaptive immune responses. In contrast to innate immune responses, antigen-activated T cells primarily produce cytokines associated with adaptive immunity. *IL-2* is a T cell growth factor derived from activated $T_H1$ cells, which promotes cytotoxic activity in T cells, antibody production by B cells, and causes T cells to secrete many other cytokines. IL-2 typically regulates in an autocrine manner. T-cell IL-2 receptors are composed of three noncovalently linked $\alpha$, $\beta$, and $\gamma$ chains. The combination of the three chains leads to a high-affinity IL-2 receptor. *IL-4* promotes the development of naïve T cells to $T_H2$ cells and induces the isotype switch to IgE production. *IL-5* activates eosinophils and acts as a hematopoietic cytokine by inducing the generation of eosinophils. Antigen-activated $T_H1$ and $T_C$ cells produce *IFN-$\gamma$*. Activated NK cells can also produce IFN-$\gamma$. The biologic activities of IFN-$\gamma$ are many and varied, including antiviral and antitumor activity, immunosuppression, growth inhibition, and the differentiation of antigen-specific $T_C$ cells. The most important characteristic of IFN-$\gamma$ is its ability to activate macrophages. *Transforming growth factor-$\beta$ (TGF-$\beta$)* inhibits T cell proliferation and other immune cells but can activate some leukocytes; it also induces isotype switching to IgA production. $T_H2$ cell-derived *IL-13* is a B cell growth and differentiation factor that inhibits macrophage cytokine production and $T_H1$ cell activity. It induces allergic reactions and asthma.

The proliferation and differentiation of hematopoietic cells is under the control of specific growth glycoproteins commonly called *colony-stimulating factors (CSFs)*. These factors can induce proliferation in many cell types but are limited to specific cell types when causing differentiation. CSFs have been identified and isolated: *granulocyte-macrophage colony-stimulating factor (GM-CSF), granulocyte colony-stimulating factor (G-CSF), macrophage colony-stimulating factor (M-CSF),* and *IL-3.* Other hematopoietic factors include *c-Kit ligand, IL-5, IL-6, IL-7, IL-9,* and *IL-11.*

# SELF-EVALUATION

## RECALLING KEY TERMS

Autocrine
Chemokines
Colony-stimulating factors (CSFs)
   Granulocyte CSF (G-CSF)
   Granulocyte-macrophage CSF (GM-CSF)
   Macrophage CSF (M-CSF)
Cytokines
Endocrine
Hematopoietic cytokines
   CSFs
   IL-3
   IL-5
   IL-6
   IL-7
   IL-9
   IL-11
Interleukins (IL)
   IL-1, -2, -3, -4, -5, -6, -7, -9, -10, -11, -12, -13
Lymphokines
Monokines
Paracrine
Transforming growth factor-β (TGF-β)
Tumor necrosis factor-α (TNF-α)
Type I interferons (IFNs)
   IFN-α
   IFN-β
Type II interferon
   IFN-γ

## MULTIPLE-CHOICE QUESTIONS

*(An answer key is not provided, but the page[s] location of the answer is.)*

1. Which of the following is produced by macrophages and dendritic cells, and is essential for activities subsequent to antigen-presentation to $T_H$ cells? (a) IFN-γ, (b) IL-1, (c) IL-2, (d) TNF-α, (e) prostaglandins, (f) none of these. *(See pages 298–300 and 302–304.)*

2. Which of the following is produced by $T_H$ cells and helps $T_C$ cells to proliferate? (a) IL-1, (b) IL-2, (c) IL-3, (d) TNF-β, (e) lysozyme, (f) none of these. *(See pages 309–311.)*

3. TNF-α is a (a) factor produced by B cells, (b) factor produced by tumor cells that kills T cells, (c) factor produced by macrophages that activates B cells, (d) factor produced by macrophages that kills tumor cells, (e) factor produced by cytotoxic T cells at the time of killing target cells, (f) none of these. *(See pages 301 and 302.)*

4. IFN-γ is a (a) B cell product that activates T cells, (b) T-cell product that activates B cells, (c) T-cell product that activates macrophages, (d) macrophage product that activates T cells, (e) none of these. *(See pages 311–313.)*

5. Which lymphokine activates LAK cells? (a) IL-1, (b) IL-2, (c) IL-3, (d) IL-4, (e) TNF-α, (f) none of these. *(See page 309.)*

6. Which of the following is a CSF? (a) IL-1, (b) IL-2, (c) IL-3, (d) IL-4, (e) IL-5, (f) none of these. *(See page 316.)*

7. Which of the following statements is/are false concerning IL-2? It (a) promotes the proliferation and differentiation of $T_C$ cells, (b) promotes the proliferation and differentiation of $T_H$ cells, (c) is released by macrophages, (d) can be a B-cell growth factor, (e) none of these. *(See pages 309–311.)*

8. IL-1 (a) is produced by T cells, (b) acts only on cells sharing identical MHC molecules with the producing cell, (c) has a limited range of cells it can affect, (d) is released by nonspecific stimulation of the producing cell, (e) none of these. *(See pages 298–301.)*

9. IL-2 receptors are expressed on (a) resting T cells, (b) activated T cells, (c) activated macrophages, (d) resting B cells, (e) none of these. *(See pages 296 and 311.)*

10. IL-12 is produced mainly by T cells and is an important activator of NK cells. (a) true, (b) false. *(See page 302.)*

11. Generally, TGF-β acts as an inhibitory cytokine but it also can promote wound repair and angiogenesis. (a) true, (b) false. *(See page 313.)*

## SHORT-ANSWER ESSAY QUESTIONS

1. Distinguish the terms: *cytokines, lymphokines, monokines, interleukins,* and *chemokines.*

2. Briefly discuss the significance of the three forms of the IL-2 receptor.

3. What is the sequence of the generic cytokine signaling transduction pathway?

**4.** The difficulty in characterizing IL-1 is caused by the fact that it seems to be made by every cell and seems to be able to affect every cell. Explain. What is IL-1's primary function in immune cell interactions?

**5.** Distinguish between IL-1α and IL-1β.

**6.** Describe TNF-α's contributions to innate immunity and associated inflammatory responses.

**7.** What do we mean when we say IL-12 is the "jump-starter of cell-mediated immunity?"

**8.** How do type type I interferons differ from type II interferons?

**9.** How does IL-10 control innate immunity?

**10.** Because some cancer cells can make TGF-β, explain how these cancer cells could be immunosuppressive.

**11.** Breifly describe the two main chemokine families.

**12.** Briefly discuss some important immune functions of IL-2.

**13.** IL-2 is an autocrine T-cell growth factor. Explain.

**14.** Why do you think IFN-γ was considered to be a "magic bullet"?

**15.** Briefly describe hematopoietic cytokines.

## FURTHER READINGS

Allen, S.J., S.E. Crown, and T.M. Handel. 2007. Chemokine: Receptor structure, interactions, and antagonism. *Annu. Rev. Immunol.* 25:787–820.

Bono, M.R., R. Elgueta, D. Sauma, K. Pino, F. Osorio, P. Michea, A. Fierro, and M. Rosenblatt. 2007. The essential role of chemokines in the selective regulation of lymphocyte homing. *Cytokine & Growth Factor Rev.* 18:33–43.

Dinarello, C.A. 2003. Interleukin-1 family and receptors. In *Fundamental Immunology*, 5th ed. W.E. Paul, ed. Philadelphia: Lippincott Williams & Wilkins. p. 775–800.

Leonard, W.J. 2003. Type I cytokines and interferons and their receptors. In *Fundamental Immunology*, 5th ed. W.E. Paul, ed. Philadelphia: Lippincott Williams & Wilkins. p. 701–748.

Leonard, W.J., and R. Solski. 2005. Interlukin-21: A modulator of lymphoid proliferation, apoptosis and differentiation. *Nat. Rev. Immunol.* 5:688–698.

Li, M.O., Y.Y. Wan, S. Sanjabi, A-K.L. Robertson, and R.A. Favell. 2006. Transforming growth factor-β regulation of immune responses. *Annu. Rev. Immunol.* 24:99–146.

Ma, A., R. Kola, and P. Burkett. 2006. Diverse functions of IL-2, IL-15, and IL-7 in lymphoid homeostatsis. *Annu. Rev. Immunol.* 24:657–679.

Mantovani, A., R. Bonecchi, and M. Locati. 2006. Tuning inflammation and immunity by chemokine sequestration: Decoys and more. *Nat. Rev. Immunol.* 6:907–918.

Malek, T.R. 2008. The biology of interleukin-2. *Annu. Rev. Immunol.* 26:553–579.

Moldawer, L.L. 2003. The tumor necrosis factor superfamily and its receptors. In *Fundamental Immunology*, 5th ed. W.E. Paul, ed. Philadelphia: Lippincott Williams & Wilkins. p. 749–774.

Murphy, P.M. 2003. Chemokines. In *Fundamental Immunology*, 5th ed. W.E. Paul, ed. Philadelphia: Lippincott Williams & Wilkins. p. 801–840.

Paunovic, V., H.P. Carroll, K. Vandenbroeck, and M. Gadina. 2008. Crossed signals: The role of interleukin (IL)-12, -17, -23 and -27 in autoimmunity. *Rheumatology* 47:771–776.

Pesta, S., C.D. Krause, D. Sarkar, M.R. Walter, Y. Shi, and P.B. Fisher. 2004. Interleukin-10 and related cytokines and receptors. *Annu. Rev. Immunol.* 22:929–979.

Rot, A., and U.H. von Andrian. 2004. Chemokines in innate and adaptive host defense: Basic chemokinese grammar for immune cells. *Annu. Rev. Immunol.* 22:891–928.

Spolski, R., and W.J. Leonard. 2008. Interleukin-21: Basic biology and implications for cancer and autoimmunity. *Annu. Rev. Immunol.* 26:57–79.

Waldmann, T.A. 2006. The biology of interleukin-2 and interleukin-15: Implications for cancer vaccine and vaccine design. *Nat. Rev. Immunol.* 6; 595–601.

Worbs, T., and R. Forster. 2007. A key role for CCR7 in establishing central and peripheral tolerance. *Trends Immunol.* 28:274–280.

# CHAPTER TEN

Help

TCR

Class II
molecule

Antigen

Antigen
processing

# CELLULAR INTERACTIONS: DEVELOPMENT OF EFFECTOR FUNCTIONS AND THEIR REGULATION

Peptide

Antigen Presentation

## CHAPTER OUTLINE

1. The immune response develops sequentially.

2. B lymphocyte development occurs in the absence and presence of antigen, the latter usually requires T lymphocytes.

   a. B cells are generated from hematopoietic stem cells and develop in the bone marrow.

   b. Immunoglobulin-gene rearrangements mark B-cell development stages.

   c. B-cell receptors engage antigen but signal transduction is through Ig$\alpha$–Ig$\beta$ molecules.

3. The development of a humoral immune response requires cellular cooperation.

   a. Early experimental observations showed the importance of lymphocytes in the immune response.

   b. Complex cooperative interactions among immune cell populations lead to antibody production.

      1) T- and B-cell cooperation is needed to produce antibody.

      2) Helper T-cell subsets regulate antibody production through differences in cytokine production patterns.

         a) In cross-regulation, the collection of cytokines positively regulates the $T_H$ subset that produces them and negatively regulates other subsets.

         b) The cytokine environment controls CD4$^+$ $T_H$ subset differentiation.

         c) Distinct CD4$^+$ T cells negatively regulate immune responses.

         d) The immune response can be regulated by antigen.

         e) Antibodies, the end products of humoral immune responses, also regulate through feedback inhibition.

      3) Antibody production occasionally occurs in the absence of help (T-independent antigens).

4. The development of CD8$^+$ T cell-mediated cytotoxic immune response also requires cellular cooperation; cytotoxic T and natural killer cells mediate killing.

   a. CD4$^+$ helper T-cell and CD8$^+$ cytotoxic T-cell cooperation is needed to develop cellular immunity but the mechanism(s) are debated.

   b. Effector cytotoxic T cells kill target cells in two ways.

   c. Natural killer cells recognize and are activated differently by target cells than cytotoxic T cells but kill target cells similarly.

---

**OBJECTIVES**

The reader should be able to:

1. Realize that the immune response develops sequentially.
2. Describe B-cell development in the absence of antigen and as it correlates with immunoglobulin-gene rearrangements.
3. Sequence the signal transduction activity following the antigen–cross-linking of B-cell receptors.
4. Comprehend how immune responses develop through cellular interactions.
5. Draw a simple model for T- and B-cell interaction; describe antigen processing and antigen presentation by B cells.
6. Outline the sequence of CD4$^+$ effector helper T (T$_H$)-cell involvement in antibody production.
7. Describe the interplay between CD4$^+$ effector T$_H$ cell subsets in the development of immune responses; distinguish the conditions needed during the initial response of naïve T$_H$ precursors to determine whether a T$_H$1 or T$_H$2 response will result; what are the contributions of T$_H$17 cells and regulatory T cells to adaptive immunity.
8. Describe how antigen removal contributes to immune regulation.
9. Understand the concept that antigen-specific antibodies can regulate the antibody response to the appropriate antigen through negative feedback.
10. Understand how T$_H$ cells and cytotoxic T cells cooperate in the development of cellular immunity; realize the importance of dendritic cells in the development of T cell-mediated cytotoxicity.
11. Illustrate how natural killer cells recognize and distinguish altered-self cells from normal host cells.

---

As discussed in previous chapters, the introduction of antigen into an immunologically naïve host starts several events that lead to an immune response (see Chapter 4). Traditionally, these mechanisms are classified as either **humoral** or **cell-mediated immunity**. *Whereas humoral immunity mediates protection strictly through antibodies, cell-mediated immunity mediates protection through sensitized T cells* (see Chapter 2). Irrespective of the type immune response, immune cells need to collaborate to have a successful humoral or cell-mediated response.

The main function of the immune response is protection of the host against disease. When foreign antigens such as bacteria, fungi, viruses, parasites, or allogeneic tissue are introduced into an individual, the individual responds (1) by producing antibodies against the antigens and (2) by mobilizing cells that can react against and destroy them. The first part of this chapter describes the development of B cells, the cellular interactions required to develop humoral immunity from antigen-independent to -dependent B-cell development and the modifications of the immune response that are downregulatory, while the second part of the chapter describes the cellular interactions required to achieve cell-mediated immunity

(cytotoxicity), and its mediation by cytotoxic T (T$_C$) cells and natural killer (NK) cells.

# THE IMMUNE RESPONSE DEVELOPS SEQUENTIALLY

*Despite its complexity, the immune response can be divided into three sequential phases* (Figure 10-1). The initial phase involves innate immunity (see Chapter 3) and includes the events between the entry of antigen and antigen contact with specific receptors on lymphocyte membranes. The mononuclear phagocyte system is essential to this facet of the immune response. Macrophages are especially critical for engulfing, degrading, and removing antigen. Any perturbations in phagocytic functions significantly disrupt the initial phase. Other components including neutrophils, dendritic cells, and NK cells, and soluble factors such as defensins, lysozyme, complement, acute phase proteins, and interferon are important in this phase.

The central phase of the immune response involves cell cooperation among lymphocyte populations. The central phase includes the

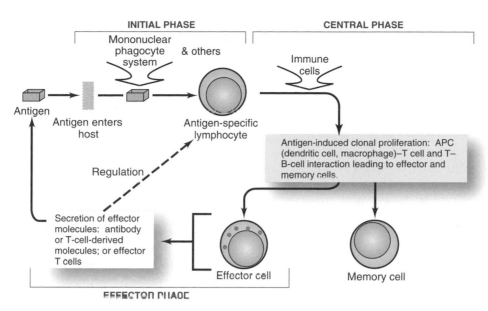

**FIGURE 10-1 The sequential development of immunity.** The immune response can be arbitrarily divided into three phases called the *initial, central,* and *effector phases.*

interactions between antigens, B and T lymphocytes, dendritic cells, cytokines, and antibody. When antigen-stimulated lymphocytes proliferate and differentiate, both antibody-secreting cells and specifically sensitized T cells are produced. Functionally, however, these cells are either memory cells (primed) or effector cells (activated). Memory cells become activated only during reexposure to antigen, but effector cells express their activity irrespective of the presence of antigen. Effector cells have short half-lives (days) in comparison to the long-lived (months to years) memory populations.

The last phase, called the *effector phase,* involves the differentiated B and T cells generated during the central phase. Antibody-secreting plasma cells release antibody irrespective of the presence of antigen. Effector CD4$^+$ helper T (T$_H$) cells mediated immune activities through the release of cytokines and B-cell help. Differentiated effector T cells, such as CD8$^+$ T$_C$ cells, are especially important during viral infections. Except as a target for destruction, antigen has no importance in the effector phase.

**MINI SUMMARY**

The introduction of antigen into a host starts sequential reactions that lead to the production of antibodies (humoral immunity) to the mobilization of sensitized T cells (cellular immunity), and to store memory cells.

# B LYMPHOCYTE DEVELOPMENT OCCURS IN THE ABSENCE AND PRESENCE OF ANTIGEN, THE LATTER USUALLY REQUIRES T LYMPHOCYTES

As discussed in Chapter 2, the primary immune organs (bone marrow and thymus), in particular, the bone marrow, are where all leukocytes start their maturation (hematopoiesis). They start as pluripotent, self-renewing stem cells that are driven by growth factors and their counterpart receptors to divide and differentiate into the full complement of functional blood cells. During the different stages of hematopoiesis, going from stem cells to progenitor cells to mature cells, the cells become more restrictive in their cellular potential. This restriction is evidenced by stem cells that differentiate into lymphocytes; they acquire receptors with single antigen specificity, coreceptors, cytokine receptors, and costimulatory adhesion molecules. T lymphocytes complete their development in the thymus, whereas B lymphocytes almost complete their entire development in the bone marrow. This stage of B and T cell development does not require antigen; hence, it is called *antigen-independent development.* Once antigen-independent development is completed, T cells migrate to peripheral immune organs, such as, the lymph nodes, spleen, and gut-associated lymphoid tissues. B cells exit the bone marrow as functionally immature cells with high levels of membrane IgM but little IgD and migrate to the spleen, where they develop into mature B cells with low levels of membrane IgM and high levels of membrane IgD. Like naïve mature T cells, mature B cells can move to other peripheral immune organs. In the peripheral immune organs, B and T cells can interact with antigen and antigen-presenting cells (APCs) and develop into plasma cells or effector T cells, respectively. This stage of development is called *antigen-dependent development* and requires cellular cooperation (discussed later).

## B Cells Are Generated from Hematopoietic Stem Cells and Develop in the Bone Marrow

During embryogenesis, B-cell development occurs first in the yolk sac, then liver, and finally in the bone marrow, after birth it occurs in the bone marrow and continues throughout life. As all lymphocytes, B cells develop in complex bone-marrow microenvironments called *niches* from hematopoietic stem cells (HSCs) through common lymphocyte and numerous lineage-restricted precursors. These niches are created by bone-marrow stromal cells to support hematopoiesis and B-cell development. The earliest stages in the developmental pathway from HSCs to early B cell precursors suggests that there are several precursor-cell subsets with progressively more limited potential, which need further documentation; the current consensus is that human **B cell-lineage–restricted cells** mature from HSCs through multipotent progenitors (MPPs), then through common lymphoid progenitors (CLPs) to the earliest distinctive B-lineage cell, the **early B cells** (also called *pre-progenitor B cell [pre-pro B cell]*), followed by **progenitor B cells (pro-B cells)**, **precursor B cells (pre-B cells)**, **immature B cells**, **mature B cells**, and **plasma cells** (Figure 10-2).

The earliest steps in human B-cell development require $CD34^+CD45R^+CD19^-$ early B cells to interact with stromal cells in the bone-marrow niches. Some stromal cells express CXC-chemokine ligand 12 (CXCL12; stromal-cell-derived factor 1), vascular cell-adhesion molecule 1 (VCAM-1), and secrete IL-7, whereas others express CXCL12 and VCAM-1 but do not secrete IL-7; early B cells, expressing CXC-chemokine receptor 4 (CXCR4), very late antigen 4 (VLA-4), and IL-7 receptor, move toward stromal cells expressing their counterpart ligand CXCL12. The pro-B cells now express CD19 and move to IL-7–expressing stromal cells; the pro-B cells use the

cell adhesion molecule VLA-4 to contact its counterpart stromal cell ligand VCAM-1. This contact drives the interaction of the pro-B cell receptor c-Kit to interact with the stromal cell-surface molecule called *stem cell factor* (*SCF*; also called *c-Kit ligand*). c-Kit ligation induces its tyrosine kinase activity, causing the pro-B cells to divide and differentiate into pre-B cells. The stromal cells secrete IL-7, which binds to pro-B cell IL-7 receptors augmenting pro-B cell maturation into pre-B cells, downregulation of adhesion molecules, the disengagement of pre-B cells from the stromal cells, and lost of IL-7 receptor expression. (In contrast to the requirement for IL-7 in B-cell development in mice, humans do not need IL-7 for B-cell development.) The proliferation and differentiation of pre-B cells leads to the development of immature B cells, their signature is the expression of membrane IgM. The IgM-expressing immature B cells have completed their bone-marrow phase of B-cell development. The functionally immature B cells exit the bone marrow expressing high levels of membrane IgM and low levels of membrane IgD. Once they reach the spleen, to survive the rigors of further development, immature B cells require cytokines and positive signals through their antigen receptors. If they survive, they express high levels of membrane IgD along with low levels of membrane IgM—they are now long-lived, mature, recirculating naïve B cells (for further details read below).

## Immunoglobulin-Gene Rearrangements Mark B-Cell Development Stages

B-cell development, as assessed by membrane-immunoglobulin (Ig) expression, can be divided into antigen-independent and -dependent phases (the latter phase is detailed later in the chapter). As described in the preceding section, the surrounding microenvironmental influences of the bone marrow drives early antigen-independent development of B cells.

Although it is uncertain whether the bone marrow has exclusive B-cell domains, identifiable migration occurs from the edge of the marrow, where precursors develop, toward the center, where maturer B cells congregate. Reminiscent of thymic T-cell development, roughly 90% of the developing B-cell population is culled; which B cells survive culling depends not only on the cells' ability to rearrange their Ig genes productively but also on selection, which is subject to the specificity and affinity of the displayed Ig.

B-cell development moves through several stages marked by the rearrangement of Ig genes (see Chapter 6). Bone-marrow stromal cells influence all of these

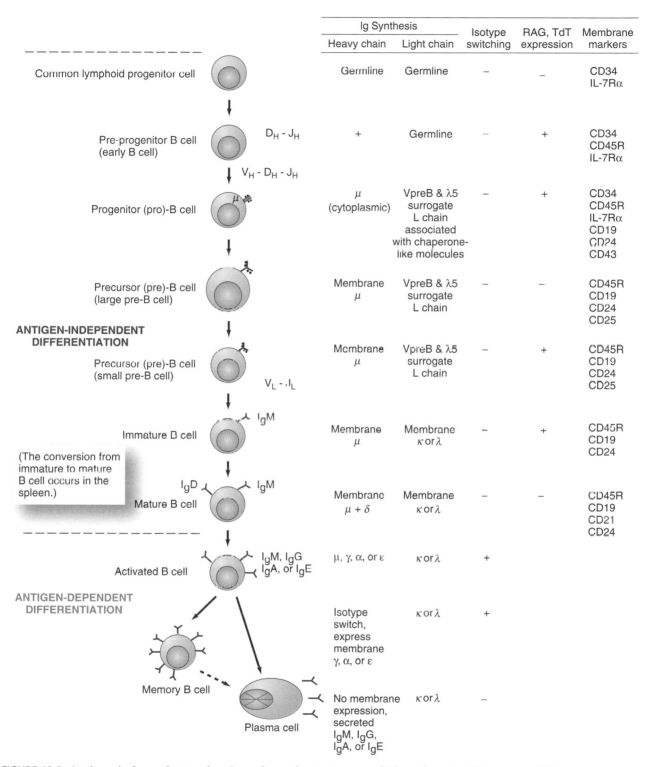

| | | Ig Synthesis | | Isotype switching | RAG, TdT expression | Membrane markers |
|---|---|---|---|---|---|---|
| | | Heavy chain | Light chain | | | |
| Common lymphoid progenitor cell | | Germline | Germline | – | – | CD34 IL-7Rα |
| Pre-progenitor B cell (early B cell) | $D_H$ - $J_H$ | + | Germline | – | + | CD34 CD45R IL-7Rα |
| Progenitor (pro)-B cell | $V_H$ - $D_H$ - $J_H$ | $\mu$ (cytoplasmic) | VpreB & λ5 surrogate L chain associated with chaperone-like molecules | – | + | CD34 CD45R IL-7Rα CD19 CD24 CD43 |
| Precursor (pre)-B cell (large pre-B cell) | | Membrane $\mu$ | VpreB & λ5 surrogate L chain | – | – | CD45R CD19 CD24 CD25 |
| **ANTIGEN-INDEPENDENT DIFFERENTIATION** Precursor (pre)-B cell (small pre-B cell) | $V_L$ - $J_L$ | Membrane $\mu$ | VpreB & λ5 surrogate L chain | – | + | CD45R CD19 CD24 CD25 |
| Immature B cell | IgM | Membrane $\mu$ | Membrane $\kappa$ or $\lambda$ | – | + | CD45R CD19 CD24 |
| (The conversion from immature to mature B cell occurs in the spleen.) IgD IgM Mature B cell | | Membrane $\mu + \delta$ | Membrane $\kappa$ or $\lambda$ | – | – | CD45R CD19 CD21 CD24 |
| Activated B cell | IgM, IgG IgA, or IgE | $\mu$, $\gamma$, $\alpha$, or $\varepsilon$ | $\kappa$ or $\lambda$ | + | | |
| **ANTIGEN-DEPENDENT DIFFERENTIATION** | | Isotype switch, express membrane $\gamma$, $\alpha$, or $\varepsilon$ | $\kappa$ or $\lambda$ | + | | |
| Memory B cell Plasma cell | | No membrane expression, secreted IgM, IgG, IgA, or IgE | $\kappa$ or $\lambda$ | – | | |

**FIGURE 10-2  Antigen-independent and antigen-dependent ontogeny of B lymphocytes**. This process follows a sequence of immunoglobulin (Ig) gene rearrangements that lead to RNA processing of the resulting DNA transcripts. See text for further information.

stages. Figure 10-2 illustrates the membrane-Ig that changes during the above-described B-cell differentiation. B lymphocytes differentiate from stem cells to early B cells, where cytokines induce the synthesis of terminal deoxyribonucleotidyl transferase (TdT) and recombinase enzymes RAG-1 and RAG-2. These B cells undergo some heavy-chain V-region gene rearrangements ($DJ_H$) and convert to pro-B cells. Pro-B cells can experience complete heavy-chain V-region gene rearrangements ($V_H DJ_H$) and contain cytoplasmic $\mu$ chains (but do not express stable membrane Ig). Pro-B cells are the first cells to exhibit complete heavy chain rearrangement, initially $D_H$-to-$J_H$, then $V_H$-to-$DJ_H$. (Somatic recombination is discussed in Chapter 6.) Rearrangements can be productive (that is, leads to synthesis of a functional Ig heavy or light

chain) or nonproductive due to deletions, frame shifts, or mutations that lead to stop codons. If heavy-chain gene rearrangement is nonproductive on the first chromosome, it moves to the second chromosome. Failure to successfully rearrange gene segments in the second chromosome leads to apoptosis of the developing B cell. For light-chain gene rearrangements, the B cells have four overall opportunities to productively rearrange them (paternal and maternal $\kappa$ and $\lambda$ loci) (see Figure 6-11 in Chapter 6).

Like T-cell development, when T cells express $\beta$ chains associated with pre-T$\alpha$ chains to form the pre-TCR (discussed in Chapter 8), pro-B cells become pre-B cells when they express membrane $\mu$ heavy chains associated with **surrogate light chains** in the **pre-B cell receptor** (Figure 10-3). These surrogate

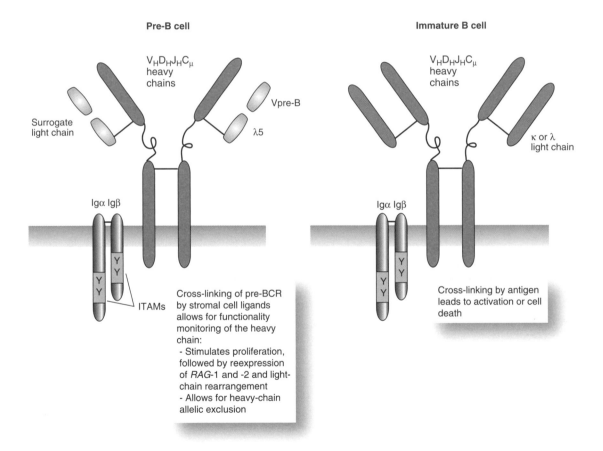

**FIGURE 10-3 The pre-B cell receptor.** The pre-B cell expresses a complex that consists of membrane-bound $\mu$ heavy chains associated with surrogate light chains and the Ig$\alpha$-Ig$\beta$ heterodimer. The surrogate light chains are composted of nonrearranged gene products, a variable (V)-like sequence, called *VpreB* and constant (C)-like sequence, called $\lambda 5$, which are noncovalently associated to form a light-chain-like structure. Pre-B cell receptor cross-linking initiates proliferation (generates pre-B cells with all the same receptor that can undergo rearrangement), cessation of surrogate light-chain synthesis, initiation of light-chain gene rearrangement, and halts further heavy-chain gene rearrangement. Disruption of surrogate light-chain genes blocks differentiation of pre-B cells to immature B cells. Immature B cells express IgM molecules with either $\kappa$ or $\lambda$ light chains; naïve mature B cells express IgM and IgD molecules.

light chains, encoded by non-rearranging genes not found in the antigen-receptor loci, consist of two proteins with a V-region-like sequence called **Vpre-B** and a C-region-like sequence called $\lambda 5$, which non-covalently associate with each other to form a light chain-like structure. The expression of surrogate light chains is induced by the transcription factors E2A and early B-cell factor (EBF); its chain expression indicates that heavy-chain gene recombination was successful. The inability to express surrogate light chains halts further B-cell maturation. The surrogate light chains are identical on all pre-B cells. The disulfide-linked signal transducing molecules Ig$\alpha$ (CD79a) and Ig$\beta$ (CD79b) chains also associate with the pre-B CR to form the pre-B CR complex. Stromal cell ligand–pre-B CR binding leads to phosphorylation of the cytoplasmic tails of the Ig$\alpha$–Ig$\beta$ molecules, which initiates a signaling cascade (detailed below) causing cessation of heavy-chain gene recombination and induction of several cycles of division into a clone of descendents with the same $\mu$ chain, which serves to increase the number of B cells that have productive recombinations of the Ig heavy-chain V-region gene. Because dividing cells are larger than nondividing cells, they are called *large pre-B cells*. Once proliferation stops, the small pre-B cells shut down surrogate light chain synthesis and first attempt to undergo $\kappa$ light-chain gene rearrangement (V$_L$-J$_L$) on one chromosome; if successful, it is expressed with the $\mu$ chain. If $\kappa$-chain gene rearrangement is not successful on either chromosome, $\lambda$-chain gene rearrangement is attempted. This is rare because nonproductive light-chain gene rearrangement can be reversed by additional gene rearrangements. In fact, if the $\kappa$ light-chain locus V-J rearrangement fails to produce a functional light chain, the rearrangements can be repeated with the unused V and J gene segments up to five times (humans have five J$\kappa$ gene segments) on each chromosome before moving on to the other chromosome and attempting $\lambda$ light-chain gene rearrangement. If neither $\kappa$- nor $\lambda$-chain gene rearrangements are productive, the cell undergoes apoptosis in the bone marrow. The successful cells are called *immature B cells* and express both $\mu$ heavy chains and light chains as membrane IgM molecules. Immature B cells can recognize and respond to foreign antigen but they are functionally incomplete, that is, if they react with multivalent ligands (antigen) it induces apoptosis or anergy rather than proliferation and differentiation, which occur when mature BCR are cross-linked.

As for T-cell receptor gene rearrangements, B-cell receptor gene rearrangements are random; thus, the process generates receptors that can bind to any antigen, self or nonself—B cells with self-reactive receptors must be culled.[1] As T cells, B cells experience *positive* (binding to the antigen receptor leads to cell survival) and *negative* (binding to the antigen receptor usually leads to cell death) *selection* in primary lymphoid organs—leading to foreign antigen-specific, self-tolerant B cells. Developing pre-B cells are positively selected when their pre-BCR binds its appropriate ligand. The underlying mechanisms for positive selection are less well characterized than negative selection but like the T-cell avidity model, it is probably associated with tonic BCR signaling and additional responsiveness to the follicle-derived antiapoptotic cytokine B-cell–activating factor (BAFF) belonging to the tumor necrosis factor (TNF) family. In fact, mutants lacking BAFF receptors are mostly immature B cells. The immature B-cell stage marks the expression of a complete B-cell receptor (membrane Ig associated with Ig$\alpha$ and Ig$\beta$), which makes self reactive B cells subject to negative selection through *clonal deletion, anergy*, and *receptor editing*. This is the first testing for self-antigen tolerance and the tolerance produced at this stage is called *central tolerance* (see Chapter 13). Immature B-cell binding to multivalent bone-marrow stromal cell self-molecules induces B-cell apoptosis and clonal deletion. Binding to small self-soluble molecules (non-cell-surface molecules) inactivates, rather than kills, the B cells. These cells are permanently anergic (unresponsive), but do not immediately die. Anergic B cells can move to the periphery and express IgD but only modest amounts of IgM; they cannot react to antigen and have a short life span. Even though many autoreactive B cells are clonally deleted, this is not the only outcome for autoreceptor-positive B cells. Some undergo further somatic recombination by reactivating the their V(D)J recombinase, which leads to new receptor V$_L$ combinations that are not self-reactive. This process is called *receptor editing* and rescues some autoreactive B cells by arresting their further development while they edit the receptor light-chain V-region genes, that is, they undergo secondary rearrangements using unrearranged V and J segments The editing may change their self-specificity to nonself-specificity, thereby rescuing them from deletion or anergy. If the BCR remains autoreactive, the cell continues to attempt rearrangements until non-self-reactive receptors are expressed or V and J gene segments are expended. The remaining autoreactive B cells die by apoptosis.

---

[1] Murine bone marrow generates roughly $2 \times 10^7$ immature B cells daily of which only roughly 10% exit to the periphery. Of the emigrants, only about a third advances to the mature B cell pool.

These selection processes ensure an emerging peripheral repertoire that is reasonably free of self-reactive B cells. Use of transgenic mice, show that mature, naïve self-reactive B cells can undergo anergy or be clonal deleted in the periphery. Not unexpected, because some self antigens are not expressed in, or do not have access to the bone marrow (see Chapter 13).

The immature B cell stage ends the bone marrow phase of B-cell development; they exit the bone marrow and proceed through the circulation to the spleen. (The overall spleen organization is depicted in Figure 2.16.) The immature B cells emigrating from the bone marrow are designated *transitional B cells* and are partitioned into two (perhaps three) subpopulations called *transitional 1 (T1)* and *T2 B cells* based on their surface phenotype, functional characteristics, and splenic localization. T1 B cells are IgM$^{high}$IgD$^-$ CD21$^-$CD23$^-$, whereas T2 B cells are IgM$^{high}$IgD$^+$ CD21$^+$CD23$^+$ and localize in the red pulp outer periarteriolar lymphoid sheath and splenic B cell follicles, respectively. (T3 B cells resemble T2 B cells but express lower levels of membrane IgM.) T1 B cells do not proliferation on B-cell receptor cross-linking by antigen, whereas T2 B cells do proliferate and differentiate into plasma cells but only in association with T-cell help (discussed later in the chapter). T1 and T2 B cells are subjected to another round of negative selection before they become mature B cells. Mature B cells can be divided into two main groups: *long-lived follicular B cells* and a smaller group (10% of mature splenic B cells) of *marginal-zone B cells*. Marginal-zone B cells are found only in the spleen, do no recirculate, and their function is unknown. The long-lived follicular B cells continue circulating to splenic follicles, to lymph nodes, and to the bone marrow until they either die or encounter antigen. Once stimulated by antigen (antigen-dependent B-cell development) and usually with T-cell help, they undergo further maturation. A portion of the cells becomes memory cells. The majority of antigen-activated B cells progress into plasma cells that secrete the class of Ig last represented on their surfaces. The antibodies secreted by a progeny plasma cell and the antigen receptors on its parent B cell are an accurate reflection of one another. The only difference is that one is a membrane-bound receptor and the other is a circulating form of the receptor.

## B-Cell Receptors Engage Antigen but Signal Transduction Is Through Igα–Igβ Molecules

Cross-linking of membrane Igs provides antigen recognition and starts a cascade of events that leads to cellular activation and differentiation (Figure 10-4).

Although each heavy chain of membrane IgM and membrane IgD possesses cytoplasmic domains incapable of signal transduction (the domains of Ig classes are too short to associate with tyrosine kinases and G proteins to transmit antigen-binding signals), two Ig-associated accessory molecules together with Ig form the *B-cell antigen receptor complex*, which transduce the activation signals that follow antigen receptor ligation. The complex is composed of an antigen-binding, membrane Ig noncovalently associated with a second substructure involved in signal transduction. This transducer/transporter substructure consists of a heterodimer composed of disulfide-linked Igα (CD79a) and Igβ (CD79b) chains, associated with heavy chains of the membrane Ig. The 32-kD Igα and the 37-kD Igβ subunits are transmembrane proteins with single extracellular Ig-like domains and therefore are members of the Ig superfamily. Igα–Igβ molecules have 18-amino acid residue, cytoplasmic immunoreceptor tyrosine-based activation motifs (ITAMs), which become phosphorylated by receptor-associated tyrosine kinases on antigen–B-cell receptor ligation. (ITAMs are not limited to B-cell receptors; they are also associated with T-cell receptors, NK cell receptors, and Fc receptors.) Briefly, after antigen cross-linking of two adjacent B-cell receptors, membrane Ig and Igα–Igβ translocate to the glycolipid and cholesterol-rich membrane regions called *lipid rafts* wherein Src family kinases are constitutively present and become activated; they phosphorylate two tyrosine residues in each of the Igα–Igβ heterodimers' cytoplasmic tails, which creates docking sites for cytoplasmic spleen tyrosine kinase *Syk*. Activated Syk phosphorylates the adaptor protein B-cell-linker protein (BLNK), which provides docking sites for Bruton's tyrosine kinase (Btk) and phospholipase Cγ2 (PLCγ2). These events induce activation of PLCγ2, which converts the membrane phospholipid phosphatidylinositol-4,5 biphosphate (PIP$_2$) into diacylglycerol (DAG) and inositol (1,4,5)-triphosphate (IP$_3$) and causes Ca$^{2+}$ release. DAG along with Ca$^{2+}$ activates protein kinase C, which induces additional pathways, one of which includes NF-κB production. B-cell receptor cross-linking also instigates signals that trigger small G protein pathways. Irrespective of B-cell receptor activation signal-transduction pathways that are induced, they lead to B-cell activation.

Like T cells, B cells have *coreceptors* that enhance antigen signaling; they include CD19, CD21, and CD81 (Figure 10-5). As mentioned above for Ig and Igα–Igβ migration into lipid rafts after antigen-binding, coengagement of B-cell

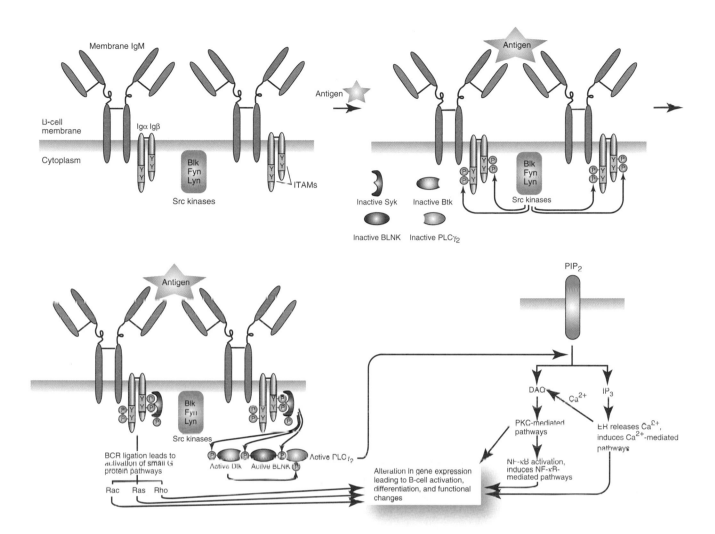

**FIGURE 10-4 Antigen-induced B-cell signaling.** Receptor cross-ligation of adjacent immunoglobulins (Igs) initiates a phosphorylation cascade of the protein kinases Blk, Fyn, and Lyn, which phosphorylate Igα-Igβ tyrosine residues in the ITAMs and recruits the kinase Syk to the cluster of molecules. Activated Syk recruits and activates adapter protein B-cell–linker protein (BLNK), which forms a complex of active kinase Btk and phospholipase Cγ (PLCγ). The activation of PLCγ leads to hydrolysis of the membrane phospholipid phosphatidylinositol-4,5 biphosphate (PIP$_2$) into diacylglycerol (DAG) and inositol (1,4,5)-triphosphate (IP$_3$) and causes Ca$^{2+}$ release from the endoplasmic reticulum (ER), which leads to the activation of protein kinase C (PKC). The activation of PKC induces additional signal transduction pathways, such as ones that produce NF-κB. Cross-linking of the BCR also induces signals that activate the small G protein pathways Rac, Ras, and Rho, the activation of these intracellular signaling pathways causes transcription factors to enter the nucleus promoting the transcription of Ig and cytokine genes.

receptor and complement receptor CD21 (also called *CR2*) with C3d bound to antigen promotes CD19-CD21-CD81 translocation into lipid rafts, which induces phosphorylation of CD19 leading to augmented and potentiated signal transduction. In fact, it increases B-cell sensitivity to antigen by 1000–10,000-fold. After stimulation, Lyn rapidly initiates a negative regulatory feedback loop by phosphorylating immunoreceptor tyrosine-based

inhibitory motifs (ITIMs) in the cytoplasmic domains of the inhibitory B-cell receptor CD22. ITIMs bind phosphatases that dephosphorylate signal molecules (CD22 inhibits CD19 phosphorylation by the tyrosine phosphatase SHP-1), which inactivate the signal molecules thereby facilitating downregulation of the B-cell response. Similar mechanisms occur in T-cell inactivation through cytotoxic T-lymphocyte antigen 4 (CTLA-4)–associated ITIMs.

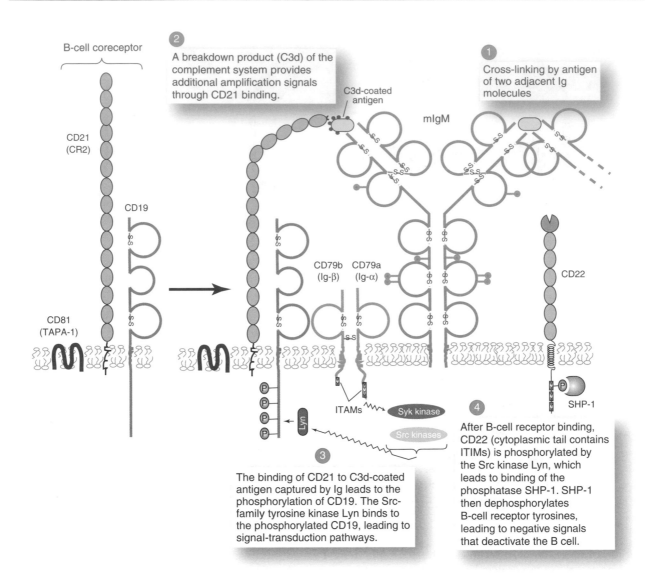

**B-cell coreceptor**

CD21 (CR2)

CD19

CD81 (TAPA-1)

② A breakdown product (C3d) of the complement system provides additional amplification signals through CD21 binding.

C3d-coated antigen

mIgM

① Cross-linking by antigen of two adjacent Ig molecules

CD79b (Ig-β)  CD79a (Ig-α)

CD22

ITAMs  Syk kinase

Lyn  Src kinases

③ The binding of CD21 to C3d-coated antigen captured by Ig leads to the phosphorylation of CD19. The Src-family tyrosine kinase Lyn binds to the phosphorylated CD19, leading to signal-transduction pathways.

④ After B-cell receptor binding, CD22 (cytoplasmic tail contains ITIMs) is phosphorylated by the Src kinase Lyn, which leads to binding of the phosphatase SHP-1. SHP-1 then dephosphorylates B-cell receptor tyrosines, leading to negative signals that deactivate the B cell.

SHP-1

**FIGURE 10-5 B-cell coreceptor complex can amplify B-cell responses**. The B-cell co-receptor complex, analogous to CD4 and CD8 function on T cells, consists of the transmembrane molecules CD19, CD21 (complement receptor 2 [CR2]), and CD81 (TAPA-1) enhances the binding of antigen thereby decreasing the amount of antigen needed to trigger the B cell. CD19 phosphorylation and association with the BCR adds signals for B cell activation. For example, antimicrobial responses required 100- to a 1000-fold less antigen to stimulate an antibody response by activating B cells through the BCR plus coreceptor than by the BCR alone. The immunoreceptor tyrosine phosphate inhibitory motif (ITIM)-containing CD22, which includes a SHP-1 docking site, delivers deactivating to the B cell.

**MINI SUMMARY**

Antigen-independent differentiation of B cells from HSCs, through four stages, to mature cells occurs in the blood marrow with final touches accomplished in the spleen, whereas antigen-dependent differentiation occurs in the periphery. Antigen-induced activation of B cells leads to antibody-secreting plasma cells or memory cells.

During antigen-independent differentiation of B cells, they undergo sequential Ig-gene rearrangements that convert pro-B cells to immature B cells, which express antigen-specific membrane IgM. Finally maturation occurs in the spleen with the development of mature naïve B cells expressing membrane IgM and IgD, yet remaining specific for a single antigen. The molecular mechanisms that generate Ig receptor diversity also constitute checkpoints in the development of B cells.

Random Ig-gene rearrangements can lead to self-reactive B cells; these cells are culled by positive and negative selection in the bone marrow. Negative selection causes deletion of self-reactive cells by apoptosis or receptor editing, which leads to cells that convert their self-reactive receptors to nonself-reactive membrane Ig. Peripheral self-reactive B cells are rendered anergic.

Even though B-cell activation is started by the engagement of antigen–cross-linked B-cell receptors, the Ig receptors cannot directly convey signal transduction; two Ig-associated molecules, Igα and Igβ, which together with Ig form the B-cell antigen receptor complex, transduce the activation signals that follow antigen ligation. These signals initiate activation of membrane-associated protein tyrosine kinases, assembly of protein tyrosine kinase signaling complexes, and activation of signal transduction pathways, leading to expression of specific genes.

Primary B-cell activation can be amplified by B-cell coreceptor participation during antigen cross linkage of membrane Ig. Membrane molecules, such as CD22, can downregulate B-cell activation.

# THE DEVELOPMENT OF A HUMORAL IMMUNE RESPONSE REQUIRES CELLULAR COOPERATION

A host's ability to distinguish self from nonself is the essence of humoral and cell-mediated immunity. The ability to react against any foreign substances and not against self-antigens is due to specificity. How the immune system accomplishes this task is the subject, in part, of the remainder of this chapter. As described in the first section of this chapter and later in the text (see Chapter 17), that exposure to antigen sequentially leads to immunity that is both humoral and cell-mediated. Humoral immunity is associated with antibody secretion by plasma cells that are derived from developing stem cells in the bone marrow (described earlier), whereas cell-mediated immunity is associated with sensitized T cells that are derived from bone marrow stem cells and develop in the thymus (see Chapter 8). *Humoral immunity requires*

*complex interactions among at least three cell types: B cells, T cells, and dendritic cells; the historical foundations for these interactions are presented first, followed by discussion of T$_H$ cell differentiation and resulting regulatory network. The last section of the chapter deals with the more clouded aspect of adaptive immunity, cell-mediated immunity, which requires interactions between effector T cells, target cells, and perhaps APCs, and ends describing the cytotoxic effector mechanisms of T cells and NK cells.*

## Early Experimental Observations Showed the Importance of Lymphocytes in the Immune Response

The pioneering work of Gowans in the 1960s showed the importance of lymphocytes in the immune response. In 1962, he reported that depletion of the recirculating pool of lymphocytes led to the loss of immune responsiveness and that reconstitution by the same cells restored immunologic competence. These results instigated a series of approaches to identify the lymphocytes responsible for immunity. Two general experimental approaches were taken: (1) those that manipulated the intact animal, and (2) those that characterized how antigens induce immune responses. The first experimental observations, using thymectomized mice, revealed the importance of the thymus in immunity. The second group of experimental observations, using haptens and carriers, suggested a compartmentalization of cells and antigen. These experiments collectively suggested that different kinds of lymphocytes collaborate during a successful immune response and that the participating lymphocytes recognize different parts of the same antigen molecule.

Some enlightening conclusions were drawn from deletion experiments. If hosts were thymectomized or bursectomized during early stages of development and later exposed to antigen, two interesting results occurred: (1) bursectomy eliminated humoral immunity, with no effect on cell-mediated immunity, and (2) thymectomy eliminated both humoral and cell-mediated immunity. These results suggested that, in its simplest form, an immune system includes B cells (from the *b*ursa in birds) for humoral immunity and T cells (from the *t*hymus) for cell-mediated immunity. This uncomplicated scheme of immunity was not enough, however, to explain the data. The use of immunologic restoration experiments helped to answer the question of why the removal of either B or T cells affected humoral immune responses.

In 1965, Playfair and Papermaster developed an adoptive transfer method for cells that established the basis for immunologic restoration. They showed that lethally irradiated mice could be reconstituted with the right number of syngeneic bone marrow cells; otherwise, the mice would have died of hematopoietic insufficiency. When the thymectomy and reconstitution approaches were coupled, further experimentation showed the need for the thymus in the full expression of humoral responses. Lethally irradiated, thymectomized hosts could not be restored to immunologic competence by receiving bone marrow cells because the host lacked an environment for prothymocyte maturation. These irradiation experiments helped to identify the T- and B-cell collaborative mechanisms needed for humoral responses.

By the mid-1960s, several immunologists had concluded that thymus-derived and bone marrow-derived cells must cooperate for successful antibody synthesis. They had also concluded that the bone marrow and the thymus orchestrate distinct immune activities. However, the way in which these separate organ systems accomplished their tasks was unclear. By the early 1970s, immunologists had explained how two populations of lymphocytes, controlled by distinct organs, interact to produce a successful antibody response. In a series of benchmark experiments, they showed that immune cells cooperate and determined that bone marrow-derived cells were the source of antibody-producing cells and T cells assist B cells during humoral immunity; hence, they are called *helper (T$_H$) cells*.

Even though evidence at this time strongly supported that immune cells cooperate, immunologists did not know whether the cooperating cells recognized different determinants on the same antigen. Several experiments evaluated whether interacting T and B cells recognized the same or different antigenic determinants during an antibody response. A hint that T and B cells recognized different regions of the same antigen came from an observation by Ovary and Benacerraf in 1963: *to get a secondary response to a hapten, the host must be immunized with the same hapten-carrier conjugate. This phenomenon is called the* **carrier effect** (Figure 10-6). The carrier effect offered strong evidence that immune cells recognize different determinants (here hapten and carrier molecules) on the same antigen during an antibody response. This was confirmed in 1969 using immunologic restoration of irradiated mice. Using similar restoration experiments, but pretreating the cells with T cell-specific antibodies before cell-transfer, showed that the remaining cells were T cells, which recognize carrier determinants.

**MINI SUMMARY**

Thymectomy, immunologic restoration, and carrier specificity testing helped to define the function of lymphocytes. Results suggested a correlation between specific immune organs (and their cells) and immune functions. From the mid-1960s to the early 1970s, a series of experiments by different immunologists led to the conclusion that T and B cells collaborate during antibody production. T cells help antibody-producing B cells. T and B cells recognize different epitopes of the same antigen during antibody responses.

## Complex Cooperative Interactions Among Immune Cell Populations Lead to Antibody Production

As we saw in Chapter 8, peripheral naïve CD4$^+$ and CD8$^+$ T cells are derived from the thymus in roughly a two-to-one ratio of CD4$^+$ T cells to CD8$^+$ T cells. The CD4$^+$ T cells are key to antibody production; however, as newly thymus-exiting T cells that have not encountered antigen and therefore are unactivated and unable to provide help, they start their recirculation process in search of antigen. Naïve T cells persistently travel between the blood, lymph systems (peripheral lymph nodes and gut-associated lymphoid tissue), and spleen but are mostly barred from extralymphoid tissues; the trek takes 12 to 24 hours. This naïve T-cell tropism for secondary lymphoid organs is driven by the expression of homing receptors such as L-selectin and CCR7 to interact with their counterparts on secondary lymphoid tissue high endothelial venules (see Chapter 2). Part of the time, they reside in secondary lymphoid tissues such as the lymph nodes, where they wait to encounter antigen from either peripheral tissue that is collected by dendritic cells, which then migrate through the afferent lymphatics into the draining lymph nodes, or lymph node-resident dendritic cells that process antigen trapped in the lymph node, and present the antigen to the appropriate naïve T cells. If the naïve T cells do not encounter the appropriate APC-associated MHC molecule-antigen complexes, they exit via the efferent lymphatics, progress into the thoracic duct, and rejoin the blood to repeat the process. This recirculation increases the chances that the low numbers (1 in 10$^4$ to 1 in a million cells) of antigen-specific naïve T cells will encounter the

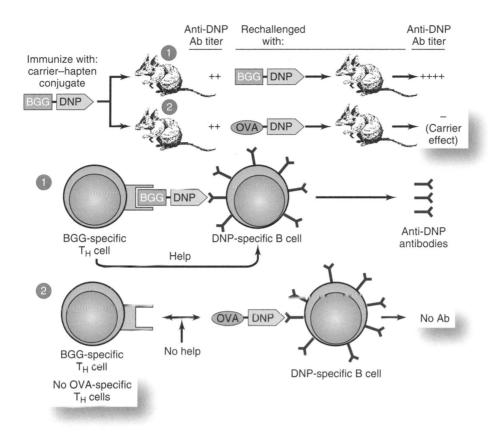

**FIGURE 10-6 The carrier effect.** A secondary antibody response to the hapten dinitrophenyl (DNP) is obtained only when immune cells are primed to the carrier (bovine gamma globulin, BGG) and hapten. (1) Priming with BGG-DNP conjugate and rechallenging with the same conjugate gives a secondary anti-DNP response. Because BGG-DNP-primed mice have BGG-specific T cells and DNP-specific B cells, they can form a bridge between each other. This association allows T cells to help B cells produce anti-DNP antibodies. (2) If BGG-DNP-primed mice are rechallenged with DNP on a different carrier, ovalbumin (OVA), there is no secondary anti-DNP antibody response. This occurs because existing BGG-specific T cells cannot interact with OVA to provide help to the DNP-specific B cells. OVA induces a new set of helper T cells that provides primary help to DNP-specific B cells. As a result, only a low antibody response occurs.

correct antigen. If the naïve T cells do recognize the appropriate APC-associated MHC molecule-antigen complexes (signal 1) followed by costimulatory signals (signal 2), they will be activated, which leads to blast cell formation, repeated rounds of cell division, and clones of progeny cells that differentiate into effector and memory cells.

### T- and B-Cell Cooperation Is Needed to Produce Antibody

The immune system is tightly regulated. Its main regulators are the CD4+ effector T cells called **helper T ($T_H$) cells**, which permit small signals to be rapidly amplified. Help is provided by antigen-induced proliferation of precursor effectors and by the outcome of helper activity by helper cells mostly through their secreted cytokines, which either act on the cells that produce them in an autocrine fashion or other cells in a paracrine fashion.

Certain antigens can trigger antibody synthesis only in the presence of T cells; others do not need T cells. These antigens are called **thymus (T)-dependent** and **thymus (T)-independent antigens**, respectively. Most protein antigens fall into the T-dependent category and are discussed here. T-independent antigens are mentioned later.

The mechanism by which T-dependent antigens trigger antibody synthesis remained unclear until the mid-1980s. Until then, T-cell help was thought to be conveyed by some form of an antigen bridge, a *cognate interaction* in which two functionally different cells recognize different antigenic determinants on the

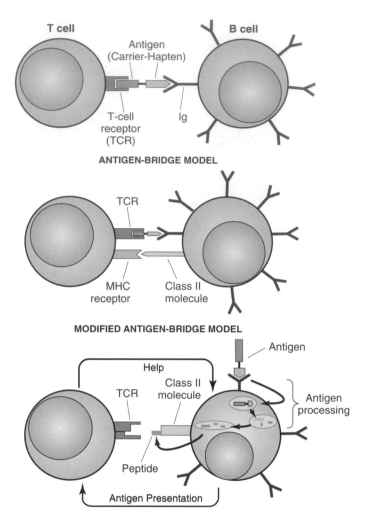

**ANTIGEN-BRIDGE MODEL**

**MODIFIED ANTIGEN-BRIDGE MODEL**

**T–CELL RECEPTOR–PROCESSED ANTIGEN–CLASS II MOLECULE BRIDGE MODEL**

**FIGURE 10-7  Models for T cell help**. In the *antigen-bridge model* the T cell binds to a carrier determinant on the antigen, while the B cell binds to a distinct haptenic determinant. The *modified antigen-bridge model* incorporates MHC restriction. The T cell expresses another receptor (MHC receptor) with which to bind B-cell class II MHC molecules. In the current model, the T cells have one receptor, which recognizes a complex of processed antigen and class II MHC molecules on the B-cell surface. Antigen processing starts by attachment of native antigen to the antibody receptor.

same molecule. This cellular interaction hypothesis was used to explain the recognition of carrier by T cells and the recognition of hapten by B cells on a carrier-hapten conjugate. This interaction or bridge would enable transmission of regulatory effects from the T cell to the B cell. Because antigen-specific T-B cell interactions are MHC-restricted, the antigen-bridge model incorporated MHC restriction. However, this modified model raised a significant question: How could processed antigen in association with a class II MHC molecule (a bimolecular complex on a

macrophage's surface) resemble processed antigen associated with both surface antibody and a class II MHC molecule (a trimolecular complex on a B cell's surface)? The answer is that the processed antigen is *not* bound to the antibody but is associated only with the B cell's class II MHC molecules.

Resolution of this paradox led to the formulation of a new model of how T cells offer help (Figure 10-7). The new model requires that B cells, using their membrane Igs, bind specific antigen by recognizing topographic conformational epitopes and internalize the antigen for processing. However, the processed antigen (peptide) must be presented to $T_H$ cells using class II MHC molecules. The implication is that the B-cell–recognized epitope and the T-cell–recognized epitope need not be the same; in fact, they are generally distinct. The Ig's reactivity to an epitope is defined by the random recombination of Ig-gene segments and the epitope can be almost anywhere on the antigen. The T-cell's reactivity to an epitope is limited by antigen processing machinery, which is why B cells and the other two professional APCs dendritic cells and macrophages can display the same peptide-MHC complexes. However, *even though B cells can process and present antigens like dendritic cells and macrophages, they can bind only an epitope that specifically locks into their membrane-bound Ig receptors.*

The separation of B-cell and T-cell epitopes is best exemplified by the earlier discussed *carrier effect.* To get a good immune response to a hapten, it is usually conjugated to a *carrier* (such as BSA or OVA) that contains many potential T-cell epitopes (a hapten alone cannot be a T-cell epitope) (see Figure 10-6). The B cell internalizes the complex using a hapten-specific surface antibody molecule, and presents carrier-derived epitopes on class II MHC molecules to the appropriate carrier-primed T cells. The T cells were primed by dendritic cells (or macrophages) that internalize the carrier-hapten complex nonspecifically. The B cells then receive T-cell help to differentiate into hapten-specific plasma cells, undergoing isotype switching and antibody secretion (Figure 10-8).

Another sign of the interaction of membrane-bound Ig with a specific antigen is **capping** (Figure 10-9). *Capping is the redistribution of antibody-antigen complexes to one area of the B-cell plasma membrane.* B-cell processing of endocytosed antigen and the presentation to a $CD4^+$ $T_H$ cell of an antigen fragment bound to class II MHC molecules occurs within 1 to 6 hr of binding of protein antigen to the B cell. The B cell appears to undergo several cycles of capping over the next 6 to 24 hr, after which the receptors are internalized. Receptor regeneration promotes cell division and differentiation.

$CD4^+$ $T_H$ cells are required during antibody production. How do $CD4^+$ $T_H$ cell–B cell interactions occur? The sequence is detailed in the following paragraphs.

1. *Antigen internalization and processing by APCs:* $T_H$ cells do not react to soluble nominal antigen; the protein antigen must be processed and presented in an immunogenic form (antigenic peptide associated with class II MHC molecules) by the professional APCs, dendritic cells, macrophages, and B cells (see Chapter 7). The experiments of Mosier helped to show clearly that APCs are required for both humoral and cell-mediated immune responses. Only T and B cells are capable of specific immune responses against an antigen, but responses occur only if T lymphocytes interact with APCs, such as dendritic cells or macrophages. APC presentation of nominal antigen plus class II MHC molecules is tightly MHC-restricted. This restriction was proved by Rosenthal and Shevach in 1973 when they observed that T-cell activation happened only when histocompatible APCs and T cells were cocultured.

*Migratory dendritic cells* reside in peripheral tissues as immature "sentinel" cells specialized in the sampling of their surrounding environment—sites of potential pathogen entry—using endocytic mechanisms. They constitutively express low levels of class II MHC molecules and T-cell costimulatory molecules (B7 family members) but are outfitted with pattern recognition receptors (PRRs) and secondary inflammatory compound receptors such as Toll-like receptors (TLRs), nucleotide-binding oligomerization domain (NOD) receptors, C-type lectin receptors, and cytokine and chemokine receptors (see Chapter 3). Ligand (antigen) binding of these receptors signals the dendritic cells to migrate through afferent lymphatics to the local draining lymph nodes. As they arrive, the dendritic cells mature. Maturation is accompanied by downregulation of endocytosis and phagocytosis, increased expression of class II MHC molecules and T-cell costimulatory molecules, presentation of peripherally captured antigen, and the inability to present newly encountered antigens. These mature migratory dendritic cells are divided into two groups, constitute roughly 50% of all lymph node dendritic cells, and are called *interstitial dendritic cells* if they migrate from the dermis or *Langerhans cells* if they migrate from the skin epidermis. The other 50% of lymph node dendritic cells are *lymphoid-organ-resident dendritic cells.* They develop in the lymphoid organs themselves and remain in an immature state unless they encounter antigen or inflammatory signals, which induces their maturation. Resident dendritic cells represent all the dendritic cells in the spleen. Resident dendritic cells can also be subdivided into subsets based on surface phenotype and function.

Dendritic cells lie upstream in the $T_H$ cell development pathway and provide an initial reaction to infection; they orchestrate immune

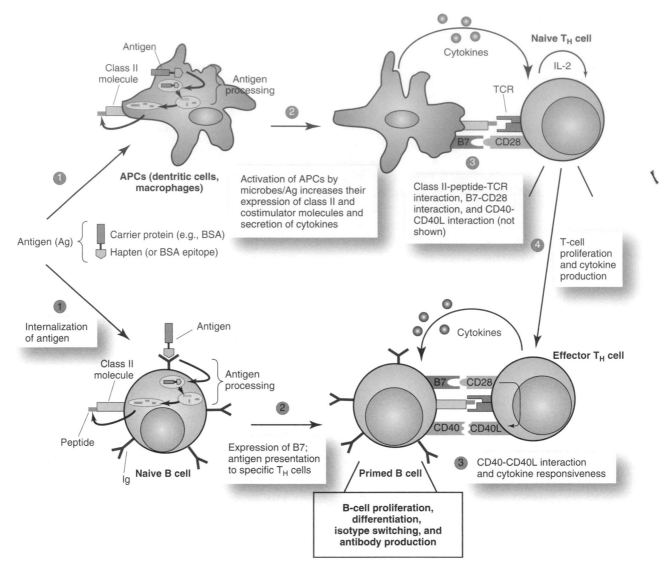

**FIGURE 10-8 Help for B-cell activation: Requires two cells recognizing two different epitopes on the same antigen**. Early experiments, demonstrating the carrier effect (see Figure 10-6), suggested immune cells recognized different types of epitopes. Contemporary data indicate that the B cell uses membrane Ig receptors that recognize topographic conformational epitopes but the processed antigen must be displayed linear antigenic peptides associated with class II MHC molecules to a T cell. This interaction allows for B-cell activation, leading to proliferation, differentiation, and antibody production.

responses. This role primarily relies on the ligation of dendritic cell-priming receptors, such as, PRRs and receptors that bind tissue factors associated with infection. The ligation initiates and modulates dendritic cell maturation leading to the development of functionally different effector dendritic cell subsets (such as human mature dendritic cell-1 and -2 [mDC1 and mDC2]; the mouse equivalents are CD8$\alpha^+$ DC and CD8$\alpha^-$ DC, respectively) that selectively promote T$_H$ subset responses through the transmission of cytokine signals—dendritic cells control pathogen-driven T-cell polarization. Dendritic cell-derived polarizing molecules include IL-12, IL-18, IL-27, type I interferons (IFN-$\alpha$ and IFN-$\beta$), and cell-surface-expressed ICAM-1 for T$_H$1, CC-chemokine ligand 2 (CCL2) and Notch ligand for T$_H$2, IL-6, transforming growth factor-$\beta$ (TGF-$\beta$), and IL-23 for T$_H$17, or IL-10 and TGF-$\beta$ for regulatory T (T$_{reg}$) cells. (These T$_H$ subsets are discussed shortly.) For example, the polarizing signals IL-12 and CCL2 derived from mDC1 and mDC2, respectively, promote the development of T$_H$1 and T$_H$2 cells and mDC-derived IL-23 expands previously differentiated T$_H$17 cells. Dendritic cells and macrophages favor T$_H$1 cell growth, whereas B

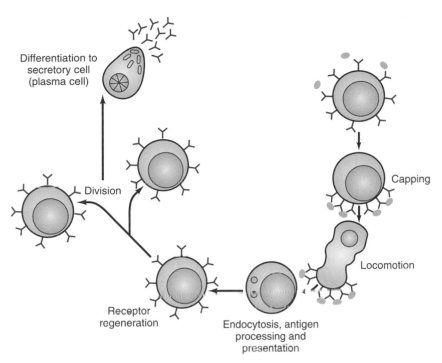

**FIGURE 10-9 Antigen-induced B-cell differentiation**. The first sign of B-cell-antigen interaction is *capping* and the directed movement of the B cells. The cells then undergo several cycles of capping and regeneration of antibody receptors. This cycling causes proliferation of the cells. To continue proliferation and differentiation, these B cells require interaction with $T_H$ cell-derived cytokines.

cells favor $T_H2$ cell growth. Dendritic cell-derived IL-12 favors the generation of $T_H1$ cells through the induction of IFN-γ production, whereas TGF-β alone induces various subsets of $T_{reg}$ cells or in combination with IL-6 induces $T_H17$ cell development. In addition, dendritic cell- and macrophage-derived IL-12 and TNF-α elicit NK cell IFN-γ production. Taken together, the overarching feature that defines dendritic cells is their ability as immature cells to capture and process antigen initiating their migration to lymph nodes and conversion to mature cells, which then can present antigen—a prerequisite for T-cell activation.

2. *Antigen presentation by APCs to naïve specific CD4$^+$ $T_H$ cells:* The three types of professional APCs (dendritic cells, macrophages, and B cells) play different roles in CD4$^+$ $T_H$ cell responses. Dendritic cells are the most effective APCs for initiating T-cell responses because they constitutively express both class II MHC molecules and costimulatory molecules; the expression of both molecules increases with maturation. Macrophages and B cells do not constitutively express costimulatory molecules; on activation they increase expression

of class II MHC molecules and express costimulatory molecules—they now can interact with effector $T_H$ cells, which leads to macrophage activation in cell-mediated immunity and B-cell activation and antibody production in humoral immunity.

The professional APCs, dendritic cells, have the intrinsic ability to capture, process, and present protein-antigen complexed with class II MHC molecules and deliver costimulatory signals principally by B7-1 (CD80) and B7-2 (CD86) and CD40. Naïve $T_H$ cells are activated when they "corecognize" foreign peptides associated with class II MHC molecules plus use costimulatory molecules CD28, CD40L, and others to interact with their respective APC counterparts (see Chapter 8), which leads to their clonal expansion and differentiation into effector $T_H$ cells.

In number 1 above, we describe that the ligation of dendritic cell receptors initiates their migration and concomitant maturation leading to the development of functionally different effector dendritic subsets. These subsets parlay this information into unique T-cell–polarizing molecules (sometimes called *signal 3*) that selectively promote antigen-specific $T_H$ cell responses—$T_H1$-,

$T_H2$-, $T_H17$-, or $T_{reg}$-cell responses. The variable expression of T-cell–polarizing molecules, mostly cytokines, by dendritic cells orchestrates the various forms of immune responses. The next few paragraphs discuss some examples.

In the absence of infectious antigens, dendritic cells still take up self-antigens and ferry them to secondary lymphoid organs; however, regulatory activities prohibit the development of adaptive immune responses to these antigens—they generate tolerance to these antigens. How? These dendritic cells synthesize and release TGF-β and little or no IL-6; this combination does not induce naïve T-cell differentiation but does inhibit the proliferation and differentiation of $T_H17$, $T_H1$, and $T_H2$ cells. Naïve T-cell interaction with self-antigenic peptide–MHC molecule complexes and TGF-β induces the expression of transcription factor FOXP3, which converts these cells to *induced $T_{reg}$ cells* that can block autoreactive T cells.

During the earliest phases of an infection, the activation and differentiation pathway of naïve $CD4^+$ T-cell development is significantly influenced by dendritic cell-derived cytokines. Dendritic cells that just snapped up antigen produce high levels IL-6 and IL-23 along with high levels of TGF-β before other cytokines such as IL-12 take over. IL-6 and TGF-β drive naïve $CD4^+$ T cells to express the transcription factor retinoic-acid-receptor-related orphan receptor γt (RORγt) and differentiate into the newly characterized cells called *$T_H17$ cells* (detailed shortly); the $T_H17$ cells leave the lymph node and migrate to sites of infection. Interaction with pathogenic antigens induces them to synthesis IL-17 family member cytokines such as IL-17 (also called *IL-17A*) and IL-17E (also called *IL-25*). IL-17 receptors are expressed on epithelial cells, fibroblasts, and keratinocytes, ligation of the IL-17 receptors induces these cells to synthesize and release various cytokines, such as IL-6, chemokines such as CXCL8 and CXCL2, and hematopoietic factors such as granulocyte colony-stimulating factor (G-CSF) and granulocyte-macrophage colony-stimulating factor (GM-CSF). The chemokines attract neutrophils and the CSFs inform the bone marrow to manufacture more neutrophils and macrophages. In addition to making IL-17, $T_H17$ cells produce IL-22, which collaborates with IL-17 to induce epidermal keratinocytes to synthesize and release the antimicrobial peptides called *β-defensins* (see Chapter 3).

The cytokines produced by dendritic cells in later stages of infection contain little or no IL-6 ad TGF-β. The cytokines that are present influence naïve $CD4^+$ T cells to differentiate into $T_H1$ or $T_H2$ cells. For example, intracellular pathogens such as bacteria and viruses induce dendritic cells to express IL-12 and NK cells to express IFN-γ. These cytokines induce the expression of transcription factors that drive the differentiation of $CD4^+$ T cells to become $T_H1$ cells, and IFN-γ inhibits the development of $T_H2$ cells. The chemokines CCL3, CCL4, and CCL5, released by cells in infection sites, bind to the dendritic cell chemokine receptors CCR5 and CCR1 (see Chapter 9). These ligations plus the bacterial ligands that interact with dendritic cell TLRs (see Chapter 3) cause dendritic cells to produce IL-12. Because $T_H1$ cells also express receptors for these chemokines, they are recruited to infection sites. $T_H1$ cells, induced by IL-12, produce IL-2, TNF-β, and their signature cytokine IFN-γ, which in turn induces dendritic cells to make IL-12. These collaborative interactions lead to a $T_H1$ cell-dominated response.

The dendritic cell role in naïve T-cell differentiation to $T_H2$ cells or the development of $T_H2$ cell responses in general is not as well characterized as $T_H1$ cell responses to pathogens. Naïve $CD4^+$ T cells activated in the presence of IL-4 differentiate into $T_H2$ cells; however, the source of IL-4 in this reaction is unclear. Pathogens such as helminths and other extracellular parasites consistently induce $T_H2$ cell responses and IL-4 signaling is required in driving this $T_H2$ cell development. Possible sources for the IL-4 include NKT cells (see Chapters 2 and 15) and mast cells (see Chapter 12). Dendritic cells produce CCL2 and express Notch-1 ligand (Jagged-1) that bind to their corresponding CCR2 and CCR4 and Notch-1 receptors (see Chapter 3) on naïve $T_H$ cells, inducing their production of IL-4, which in turn favors $T_H2$ cell development and down-regulates $T_H1$ and $T_H17$ cell development. Unclear in humans, but in mice the presence of IL-25 causes naïve $T_H$ cells produce IL-4.

3. *Differentiation and clonal growth of effector $CD4^+$ $T_H$ cells:* Interaction of naïve $T_H$ cells with dendritic cell-presented antigenic peptide plus dendritic cell-derived cytokines drives T cells through rapid rounds of proliferation, causing differentiation, and acquisition of the ability to secrete effector cytokines needed to confront pathogens (Figure 10-10). Collectively, this cascade of events is called *T-cell activation* (see Chapter 8), leads to the development of effector and memory T cells,

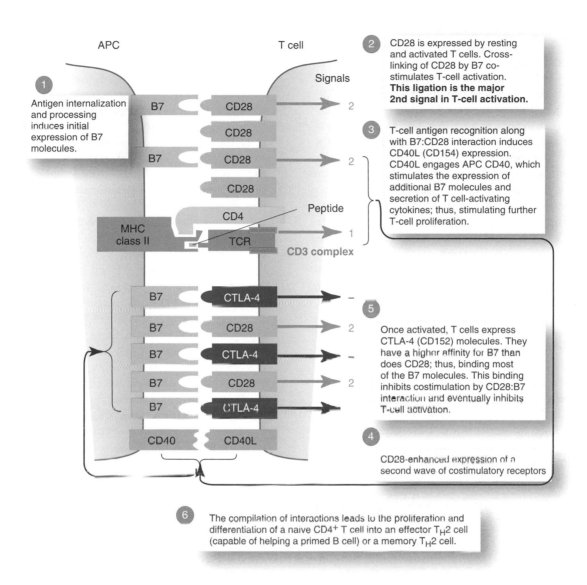

**1** Antigen internalization and processing induces initial expression of B7 molecules.

**2** CD28 is expressed by resting and activated T cells. Cross-linking of CD28 by B7 co-stimulates T-cell activation. **This ligation is the major 2nd signal in T-cell activation.**

**3** T-cell antigen recognition along with B7:CD28 interaction induces CD40L (CD154) expression. CD40L engages APC CD40, which stimulates the expression of additional B7 molecules and secretion of T cell-activating cytokines; thus, stimulating further T-cell proliferation.

**5** Once activated, T cells express CTLA-4 (CD152) molecules. They have a higher affinity for B7 than does CD28; thus, binding most of the B7 molecules. This binding inhibits costimulation by CD28:B7 interaction and eventually inhibits T-cell activation.

**4** CD28-enhanced expression of a second wave of costimulatory receptors

**6** The compilation of interactions leads to the proliferation and differentiation of a naive CD4+ T cell into an effector $T_H2$ cell (capable of helping a primed B cell) or a memory $T_H2$ cell.

**FIGURE 10-10** Two signals needed for naïve T-cell activation: TCR-peptide-MHC molecule complex (signal 1) plus costimulatory molecule ligation (signal 2) leading to T-cell proliferation and differentiation.

and initiates *a primary response*. However, note that clonal growth is maintained by cytokines produced by APCs and lymphocytes. These cytokines are discussed in Chapter 9. The daughter cells of this clonal growth differentiate into fixed effector cells, which change their homing-receptor profile, allowing some to migrate toward the B-cell follicle to provide help to B cells (follicular B helper T cells) and others to leave the lymph node and enter various extralymphoid tissues, where they coordinate inflammatory and immune responses in the periphery. As mentioned in Chapter 2 and detailed later in this chapter, CD4+ effector $T_H$ cells were divided into two dominant functional effector

subsets based on their cytokine-expression profiles and immunoregulatory function: $T_H1$ cells, which produce IL-2, TNF-β, and large quantities of IFN-γ and regulate cellular immunity, whereas $T_H2$ cells produce IL-4, IL-5, IL-10, and IL-13 and mediate humoral immunity and allergic responses. Recent studies show a greater diversification of the CD4+ T-cell effector repertoire than represented by the $T_H1/T_H2$ paradigm. Effector CD4+ $T_H$ cells, which produce IL-17, have been characterized; they represent a new, completely separate naïve CD4+ T cell-derived lineage called *$T_H17$ cells*, which provide protection against extracellular bacteria and some fungi and can induce severe autoimmunity.

Effector cells are derived from both naïve and memory cells after activation; memory cells are discussed next.

One of the cardinal features of adaptive immunity is the development of antigen-specific immune memory—the rapid and heightened protection to reexposure of the same antigen, *a secondary response*. Long-lived, quiescent memory T cells are derived from naïve T cells after their encounter with APC-presented antigen and from antigen-activated effector T cells. Homing capacity and effector function categorize CD4$^+$ memory T cells into two populations: recirculating *central memory T ($T_{cm}$) cells* and *tissue-homing effector memory T ($T_{em}$) cells*. The expression of the chemokine receptor CCR7 controls homing to secondary lymphoid organs; $T_{cm}$ cells express CCR7, home to lymph nodes, lack immediate effector function, but they proliferate and become effector cells on secondary stimulation; whereas, $T_{em}$ cells do not express CCR7, home to peripheral tissues, rapidly expression effector function by producing IFN-$\gamma$ after antigenic challenge, but have limited proliferative capacity. Taken together, $T_{cm}$ cells mediate secondary responses, provide long-term immunity, and are found in lymphoid tissues, whereas $T_{em}$ cells afford immediate immunity and reside in nonlymphoid tissues. Both populations may persist for years and the $T_{cm}$ cells give rise to $T_{em}$ cells on secondary challenge. At the systemic level, the frequency of antigen-specific memory B and T cells is much higher than that of naïve cells and memory cells have the capacity for selective migration to sites of infection, leading to rapid contact with pathogens. At the per-cell level, memory T-cell activation has fewer requirements than activation of naïve T cells; the latter cells required dendritic cells, whereas any of the APCs can activate memory T cells. The increased expression of adhesion molecules by memory T cells may facilitate their binding to APCs. Memory T cells also have accelerated synthesis of cytokines.

4. *Delivery of effector CD4$^+$ $T_H$ cell augmentation to antigen-primed B cells:* Direct contact between the effector CD4$^+$ $T_H$2 cell and the B cell by an antigen-bridging class II MHC molecule complex is the initial conveyance signal for B-cell activation; that is, mature, antigen-naïve B cells need two distinct types of signals to drive their proliferation and differentiation: interaction with antigen (signal 1) and interaction with effector CD4$^+$ $T_H$ cells and their cytokines (signal 2). The production of specific antibody directed against T-dependent antigen starts with the binding of antigen to clones of B cells displaying complementary membrane-Ig receptors (see Chapter 6 and earlier in this chapter). This binding is by naïve B cells, involves the cross-linking of membrane-Ig by antigen, but does not cause the B cells to move into the early stages of the cell cycle or to gain responsiveness to cytokines that drive their growth and differentiation. However, the binding and processing of antigen, which takes roughly 30 to 60 minutes, increases the expression of class II MHC molecules and induces the expression of B7-1 (CD80) and B7-2 (CD86)—it primes the B cell for interaction with effector $T_H$ cells. The interaction with effector CD4$^+$ $T_H$2 cells provides B cells with the cellular and humoral requirements for growth and differentiation.

The delivery of T-cell help is divided into a *recognition phase* and an *effector phase*. The recognition phase is a class II-restricted, antigen-specific interaction, while the effector phase is a class II-unrestricted, antigen-nonspecific interaction. During the *recognition phase*, the appropriate effector CD4$^+$ $T_H$ cells recognize the complexes of processed antigen-class II MHC molecule displayed on the surface of B cells. Figure 10-11 shows the pairs of cell-surface coreceptors involved in interactions between B cells and $T_H$2 cells. The $T_H$2 cell–B cell conjugate is further stabilized by the binding of CD54 to CD11a/CD18 and by the binding of CD4 to monomorphic domains of the class II MHC molecules. These interactions lead to the clustering of T-cell surface molecules (TCR, CD4, CD11a/CD18, CD28—major components of the *immunological synapse* [see Chapter 8]) and subsequent induction of $T_H$2 cell effector functions. The TCR–class II MHC interaction also sends an activation signal to the T cell and to the B cell (Figure 10-12). It induces the T cell's expression of CD40 ligand (CD40L [CD154]) that interacts with constitutively expressed CD40 on the B cell, which promotes B-cell expression of B7-1/B7-2 (CD80/CD86) that interact with constitutively expressed T-cell CD28 and induced CTLA-4 molecules. Another pair of T-B cell interacting receptors important for B-cell activation by $T_H$ cells is inducible T-cell costimulator (ICOS), which is rapidly induce on TCR engagement, enhanced by CD28 stimulation, and binds to constitutively expressed B-cell ICOS ligand. However, B-cell induction into the cell cycle occurs only after a constitutively expressed B-cell surface molecule known as *CD40* interacts with a transiently expressed T-cell surface glycoprotein called *CD40L* on activated T cells. Thus, CD40 engagement by CD40L is considered the

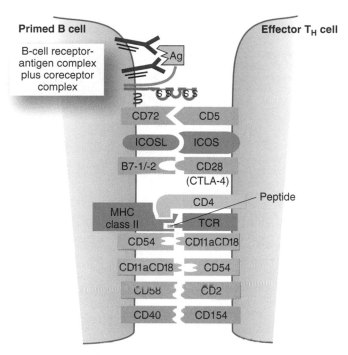

**Primed B cell**

B-cell receptor-
antigen complex
plus coreceptor
complex

Ag

**Effector T_H cell**

| CD72 | CD5 |
| ICOSL | ICOS |
| B7-1/-2 | CD28 (CTLA-4) |
| | CD4 |
| MHC class II | TCR — Peptide |
| CD54 | CD11aCD18 |
| CD11aCD18 | CD54 |
| CD58 | CD2 |
| CD40 | CD154 |

**FIGURE 10-11 The pairs of cell-surface molecules interacting between primed B cells and effector helper T cells during B cell activation.** See text for description. Ag, antigen; TCR, T-cell receptor.

second signal. This engagement induces Ig isotype switching and affinity maturation, promotes the formation of germinal centers and memory B cells, encourages increased costimulatory molecule expression, contributes to B-cell proliferation, and inhibits B-cell apoptosis. B cells stimulated by CD40 ligation by CD40L can proliferate but they fail to differentiate unless they received cytokine signaling; B cells are progressing through competence levels (Figure 10-13).

The entry of B cells into the cell cycle initiates the second phase, known as the *effector phase*. As this phase proceeds, the dominant interaction becomes the recognition of nonpolymorphic domains of B-cell class II MHC molecules by T-cell CD4 molecules. During this stage, the T cell's Golgi apparatus and microtubular-organizing components migrate toward the junction with the B cell, which aids in the directional release of cytokines toward the interacting B cell. The increase in occupancy of CD4 molecules, not soluble factor signaling, triggers B cells to progress from the $G_0$ stage of the cell cycle to $G_1$, and increases B-cell mRNA synthesis and B-cell responsiveness to $T_H2$ cell-derived cytokines. Now the cytokine-dependent part of the effector phase of help begins. IL-4 helps to promote the

transition from $G_1$ to S, while other cytokines, such as IL-5 and IL-6, participate as differentiation factors and facilitate transition through the $G_2$ stage of the cell cycle (Figure 10-14).

Taken together, these findings show that B-cell contact with antigens and cooperative interactions with effector CD4+ $T_H$ cells, which initially interacted as naïve T cells with dendritic cells, start antigen-dependent differentiation. The result is the activation and proliferation of B cells and their differentiation into plasma cells.

5. *Clonal growth and differentiation of antigen-primed B cells:* B-cell activation involves the differentiation of a B cell into a plasma cell. The cell switches from using antibody as a receptor to synthesizing a soluble form of the antibody. This process can be described in three steps (see Figure 10-14). Interaction of primed B cells with antigen-activated T cells starts some B-cell clonal growth, but effector $T_H2$ cells also give significant help by releasing cytokines. Many of these cytokines act sequentially to guide B cells through activation, proliferation, differentiation, and isotype switching (see Figure 10-14). For example, IL-4 provides help only to B cells that have differentiated to a certain stage in response to antigenic stimulation. IL-4 starts these B cells into the cell cycle and stimulates B-cell

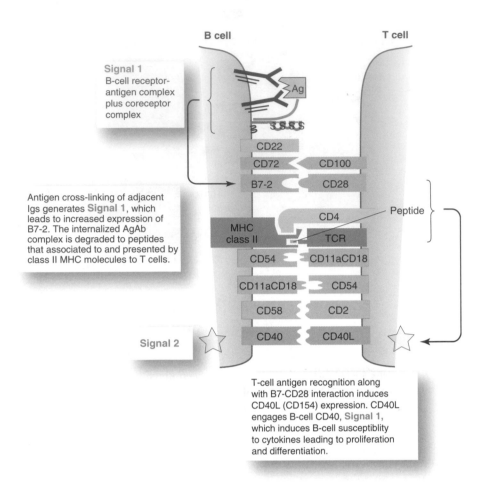

**FIGURE 10-12 Interaction molecules between B and T Cells: Mainly CD40-CD40L (CD154) engagement provides second signal**.

proliferation. IL-4 also promotes isotype switching from IgM to IgE and IgG$_1$ and reduces IgG$_{2a}$ production. B cells become better APCs in response to IL-4 by increasing their expression of class II MHC molecules. IFN-$\gamma$ antagonizes the effects of IL-4 because it inhibits IL-4-induced B-cell proliferation, blocks isotype switching, and enhances IgG$_{2a}$ production. IL-5 promotes DNA synthesis in B cells but does not induce production of antibody-secreting cells unless IL-2 and IL-4 are present. IL-4 and IL-5 are the most potent inducers of mouse antibody production. In humans, IL-2 and IL-6 have the same effect. Both IL-5 and TGF-$\beta$ positively regulate IgA production. T-cell–derived and macrophage-derived IL-6 affects only activated B cells in the G$_2$ phase of the cell cycle. Along with IL-4, IL-6 may contribute to somatic hypermutation, which leads to affinity maturation and the development of B-cell memory provided by quiescent memory B cells and long-lived plasma cells.

Collectively, the cascade of cytokine signals received by the B cell promotes clonal proliferation and differentiation, and leads to the development of immunologic memory and the secretion of antibodies. The development of mature plasma cells takes several days, but once they are mature, they can secrete thousands of antibody molecules per second for 4–5 days.

### Helper T-Cell Subsets Regulate Antibody Production Through Differences in Cytokine Production Patterns

As described above, migrant dendritic cells endocytose antigen (such as a pathogen), enter lymph nodes with evidence that they have encountered antigen in infected tissues, present it in class II molecules to rare, recirculating, naïve, antigen-specific CD4$^+$ T$_H$ cells that must then divide and differentiate to a critical mass suitable to defend against the pathogenic opponent. Furthermore, dendritic cells instruct the T$_H$ cells in the nature and location of the threat by

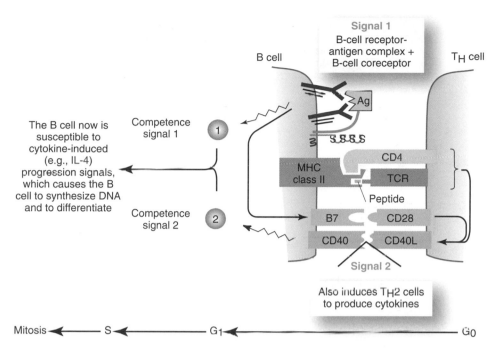

The B cell now is susceptible to cytokine-induced (e.g., IL-4) progression signals, which causes the B cell to synthesize DNA and to differentiate

Competence signal 1 ①

Competence signal 2 ②

Signal 1
B-cell receptor-antigen complex + B-cell coreceptor

B cell

$T_H$ cell

Ag

MHC class II

CD4

TCR

Peptide

B7 — CD28

CD40 — CD40L

Signal 2

Also induces $T_H2$ cells to produce cytokines

Mitosis ← S ← $G_1$ ← $G_0$

**FIGURE 10-13** Two competence signals are required to drive B cells from $G_0$ to mitosis.

their ability to recognize differences among various classes of microbes by their pattern-recognition receptors and then translate this information into unique signals to the specific T cells. The key signals that direct the maturing $T_H$ cell's various patterns of gene expression are cytokines. The cytokine actions that stimulate $T_H$ cell maturation range from the induction and repression of lineage-specific transcription factors to that of growth factors for specific lineages. Cytokines are also how mature $T_H$ cells mediate their influence on other cells during the immune response. That is, unlike other lymphocytes, $CD4^+$ $T_H$ cells orchestrate inflammation and adaptive (humoral and cellular) immune responses by rallying other cell types to do their bidding. To react to diverse types of microbes, diverse effector mechanisms are activated, the latter is accomplished by using more than one type of $CD4^+$ effector $T_H$ cell; they include functionally distinct $CD4^+$ $T_H$ cell subsets: **$T_H1$, $T_H2$, $T_H17$**, and **regulatory T ($T_{reg}$) cells**. They coordinate immunity by producing unique sets of cytokines that determine through an autocrine or paracrine mechanism, which immune cells are mobilized to perform distinct effector functions. IFN-γ, IL-4, and IL-17 are the signature cytokines of $T_H1$, $T_H2$, and $T_H17$ cells, respectively. The cytokine produced by a certain subset often is a differentiation inducer of that subset as well as a downregulator of the other subsets.

*In cross-regulation, the collection of cytokines positively regulates the $T_H$ subset that produces them and negatively regulates other subsets.* As suggested earlier, $CD4^+$ effector T cells have long been characterized into two subsets: $T_H1$ and $T_H2$. It no longer is a two $T_H$ subset paradigm. A new effector T-cell subset that produces IL-17 (and IL-22 and other cytokines), thus called *$T_H17$ cells*, has been identified. They are the subject of intense current study (discussed shortly). So the twin middlemen of the immune system, $T_H1$ and $T_H2$ cells, are really triplets, $T_H1$, $T_H2$, and $T_H17$ cells. $T_H1$ cells and $T_H2$ cells direct cellular and humoral immune (and allergy) responses, respectively, through the secretion of distinct cytokines (Table 10-1). The $T_H1$ and $T_H2$ cells were also called *inflammatory* and *helper $CD4^+$ T cells*, respectively. As the $T_H1$-associated name implies, $T_H1$ cells were considered pathogenic, while $T_H2$ cells are thought to be protective of tissue inflammation and the development of autoimmune diseases. This concept is being reconsidered with the discovery of distinct IL-17–producing $CD4^+$ T cells called *$T_H17$ cells*. $T_H1$, $T_H2$, $T_H17$, and $T_{reg}$ cells develop from naïve precursor cells, $T_Hp$, that secrete only IL-2. The function and growth characteristics of $T_H1$ and $T_H2$ cells are markedly different (Figure 10-15). Activated $T_H1$ cells produce IL-2, IFN-γ, and TNF-β, use IL-2 as an autocrine growth factor, IFN-γ mediates cytotoxicity (promotes the differentiation

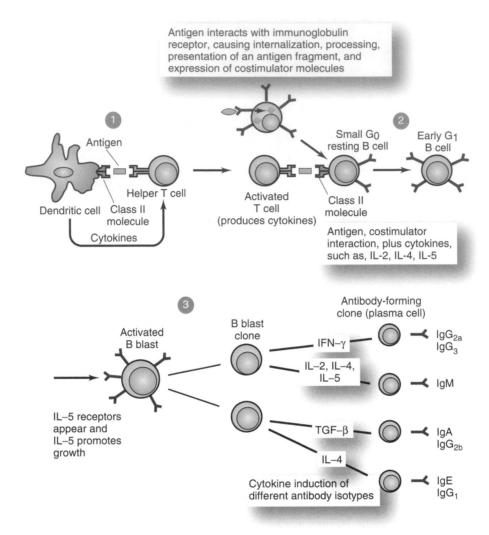

**FIGURE 10-14 The stages of B-cell activation.** The first step (1) involves uptake of antigen by macrophages, reappearance of processed antigen with class II MHC surface protein, and presentation of this antigen–class II MHC complex to CD4$^+$ T$_H$ cells, leading to the production of mediators by macrophages and T$_H$ cells. In the second step (2), the excitation of B cells from their resting state (from the G$_0$ to the G$_1$ phase of the cell cycle) is accomplished by the binding of antigen to a surface antibody and its final presentation in association with class II MHC molecules, and to the interaction of macrophage-derived IL-1 with T$_H$ cells, which then interact with the B cell. In the third step (3), the B cell replicates and matures to a plasma cell capable of antibody secretion.

of CD8$^+$ precursor to fully mature T$_C$ cells) and delayed-type hypersensitivity responses, and activate macrophages, which are highly effective in clearing intracellular pathogens. Even though T$_H$1 cells do not initiate antibody formation, they can induce isotype switching to certain isotypes, such as IgG$_{2a}$, which are important in opsonization-promoting activities, such as, antibodies that bind to phagocyte Fc receptors or interact with the complement system. In contrast, activated T$_H$2 cells produce IL-4, IL-5,

IL-10, and IL-13, use IL-4 for autocrine growth, and fail to induce delayed-type hypersensitivity responses but induce the production of large amounts of IgM, IgE, and noncomplement-activating IgG isotypes, stimulate eosinophilic attack on helminth (roundworm) infections, and support allergic reactions. T$_H$2 cells primarily provide help to B cells. Despite these differences in growth characteristics and cytokine profiles, both CD4$^+$ T$_H$ cell subtypes recognize foreign antigen in association with class

**TABLE 10-1** Cytokine, Growth, and Functional Characteristics of CD4$^+$ T Cell Subsets

| | $T_H1$ | $T_H2$ | $T_H17$ |
|---|---|---|---|
| **Cytokine released** | | | |
| IL-2 | + | – | – |
| IL-3 | + | + | – |
| IL-4 | – | + | – |
| IL-5 | – | + | – |
| IL-10 | – | + | – |
| IL-13 | – | + | – |
| IL-17 | – | – | + |
| IL-17F | – | – | + |
| IL-21 | – | – | + |
| IL-22 | – | – | + |
| IL-26 (in humans) | – | – | + |
| IFN-$\gamma$ | + | – | – |
| Lymphotoxin (TNF-$\beta$) | + | – | – |
| Granulocyte-macrophage colony-stimulating factor (GM-CSF) | ++ | + | + |
| Priming cytokines | IL-12 | IL-4/IL-25 (IL-17E) | In mice: TGF-$\beta$ & IL-6; in humans: IL—1$\beta$ & IL-23, not TGF-$\beta$ |
| **Autocrine growth** | | | |
| IL-2 | + | – | – |
| IL-4 | – | + | – |
| IL-10 | – | + | – |
| IL-21 | – | – | + |
| IFN-$\gamma$ | + | – | – |
| **Cytokine/chemokine receptors** | | | |
| IL-2 | I | – | – |
| IL-4 | – | + | – |
| IL-12 | + | – | – |
| IL-18 | + | – | – |
| CCR2 (binds CCL2, CCL7, CCL8, CCL13) | + | – | + |
| CXCR3 (binds CXCL9—11) | + | – | ? |
| CCR4 (binds CCL17, CCL20, CCL22) | – | + | + |
| CCR5 (binds CCL3—5, CCL8) | + | – | – |
| CCR6 (binds CCL20) | + | + | + (also produces CCL20) |
| Ligands for E- and P-selectins | + | – | + (express E-selectins) |
| STAT regulators | STAT1 & STAT4 | STAT6 | STAT3 |
| Lineage-specific transcriptional regulators | T-bet | GATA3 | ROR$\alpha$ & ROR$\gamma$t |
| **Functions** | | | |
| Help B-cell proliferation | No | Yes | No |
| Help for total antibody production | Yes but<$T_H2$ | Yes | No |
| Help for specific antibody production | | | No |
| IgG$_{2a}$ | Yes (mouse) | No | No |
| IgE | No | Yes | No |
| Eosinophil and mast cell production | No | Yes | |
| T$_C$ cell activation | Yes | No | |
| Mediate delayed-type hypersensitivity | Yes | No | ? (Depends on intracellular organism) |
| Macrophage activation | Yes | No | ? |
| Recruit neutrophils and macrophages to infected tissues | Yes | No | Yes |
| Matrix modification | No | No | Yes |
| Proinflammatory/autoimmune diseases | Yes | No | Yes |
| IFN-$\gamma$ inhibits the expansion of: | No | Yes | Yes |
| IL-4 and IL-10 inhibits the expansion of: | Yes | No | Yes |

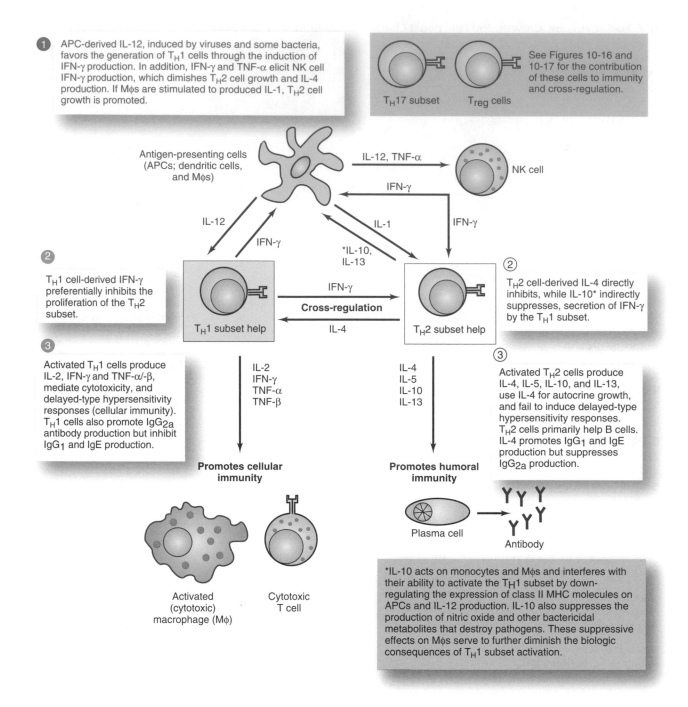

**1** APC-derived IL-12, induced by viruses and some bacteria, favors the generation of T$_H$1 cells through the induction of IFN-γ production. In addition, IFN-γ and TNF-α elicit NK cell IFN-γ production, which dimishes T$_H$2 cell growth and IL-4 production. If Mφs are stimulated to produced IL-1, T$_H$2 cell growth is promoted.

See Figures 10-16 and 10-17 for the contribution of these cells to immunity and cross-regulation.

T$_H$17 subset    T$_{reg}$ cells

Antigen-presenting cells (APCs; dendritic cells, and Mφs)

IL-12, TNF-α    NK cell

IFN-γ

IL-12    IFN-γ    IL-1    IFN-γ

*IL-10, IL-13

**2** T$_H$1 cell-derived IFN-γ preferentially inhibits the proliferation of the T$_H$2 subset.

IFN-γ

**Cross-regulation**

IL-4

T$_H$1 subset help    T$_H$2 subset help

**2** T$_H$2 cell-derived IL-4 directly inhibits, while IL-10* indirectly suppresses, secretion of IFN-γ by the T$_H$1 subset.

**3** Activated T$_H$1 cells produce IL-2, IFN-γ and TNF-α/-β, mediate cytotoxicity, and delayed-type hypersensitivity responses (cellular immunity). T$_H$1 cells also promote IgG$_{2a}$ antibody production but inhibit IgG$_1$ and IgE production.

IL-2
IFN-γ
TNF-α
TNF-β

IL-4
IL-5
IL-10
IL-13

**3** Activated T$_H$2 cells produce IL-4, IL-5, IL-10, and IL-13, use IL-4 for autocrine growth, and fail to induce delayed-type hypersensitivity responses. T$_H$2 cells primarily help B cells. IL-4 promotes IgG$_1$ and IgE production but suppresses IgG$_{2a}$ production.

**Promotes cellular immunity**

**Promotes humoral immunity**

Activated (cytotoxic) macrophage (Mφ)    Cytotoxic T cell

Plasma cell    Antibody

*IL-10 acts on monocytes and Mφs and interferes with their ability to activate the T$_H$1 subset by down-regulating the expression of class II MHC molecules on APCs and IL-12 production. IL-10 also suppresses the production of nitric oxide and other bactericidal metabolites that destroy pathogens. These suppressive effects on Mφs serve to further diminish the biologic consequences of T$_H$1 subset activation.

**FIGURE 10-15  T Helper cell-mediated cross-regulation of antibody production (and cell-mediated immunity).** See text for more details.

II MHC molecules. Furthermore, both T$_H$1 and T$_H$2 cells have the same antigen specificity and MHC-restriction elements (both types conjugate with a single antigen-specific immune cell).

Factors such as the density of the antigen-MHC ligand, the cytokines elicited by antigen, the type of APC, and the MHC haplotype influence the differentiation of naïve CD4$^+$ T cells into specific effector T$_H$ subsets. The mechanism whereby one subset is activated over the other is continuing to be resolved, but low-affinity interactions between T cells and APCs presenting low densities of peptide-MHC ligands induce naïve CD4$^+$ T cells to differentiate into T$_H$2 cells, while high-affinity interactions between

T cells and APCs presenting high densities induce them to differentiate into $T_H1$ cells. $T_H2$ cells seem less susceptible to being turned off by inappropriate stimulation than are $T_H1$ cells; therefore, if the amount of antigen is low or too high, $T_H2$ cells have the advantage. Because antigen-specific B cells efficiently acquire antigen by their specific Ig receptors and dendritic cells constitutively express class II MHC molecules and costimulatory molecules, these cells have an advantage in presenting antigen at low concentrations.

The new member of the effector $T_H$ team is the $T_H17$ cell, which is characterized by IL-17 production. IL-17's existence has been known for more than 10 years. Even so, its production by a distinct CD4$^+$ $T_H$ subset has only recently been recognized and is under active research. $T_H17$ cells exist in mice and humans but their phenotypic, functional, and developmental characteristics seem to differ. This subset is highly proinflammatory and induces severe autoimmunity. In the mouse, IL-6 plus TGF-β induce the differentiation of $T_H17$ cells from naïve precursor CD4$^+$ T cells and IL-23 is an essential survival factor that expands previously differentiated $T_H17$ cells; IL-23 is not required during their differentiation. The origin of human $T_H17$ cells differs from mice; some combination of IL-1β, IL-6, IL-21, IL-23, and TGF-β are responsible for their development. Murine $T_H17$ cells and transcription factor FOXP3$^+$ CD4$^+$ $T_{reg}$ cells share a common origin because both require TGF-β to develop. Nonetheless, the combined involvement of TGF-β and IL-6 in the induction of $T_H17$ cells suggests a dichotomy between them and transcription factor FOXP3-positive CD4$^+$ $T_{reg}$ cells. TGF-β alone induces FOXP3 and generates induced $T_{reg}$ cells, whereas IL-6 inhibits TGF-β-induced FOXP3 expression, but jointly TGF-β and IL-6 induces $T_H17$ cell development. In addition to their implicated activities in autoimmune and inflammatory conditions, $T_H17$ cells bring some unique contributions to the immune armamentarium; they appear to mediate tissue inflammation by supporting neutrophil recruitment and survival, matrix degradation, and induction of proinflammatory cytokines in structural cells. They also protect the host from bacteria and fungi. IL-17, a member of a cytokine family that shares little homology with other cytokines, which is comprised of IL-17A–F (IL-17A is called *IL-17* and is the hallmark cytokine of the $T_H17$ subset), acts as a potent proinflammatory cytokine by eliciting secretion of chemokines and matrix proteins to yield neutrophil recruitment. IL-17 and IL-22 (an IL-10 family member) are implicated in barrier formation by inducing proliferation, differentiation, and junctional integrity of junctional epithelia. $T_H17$

cells also express high levels of IL-21, which sustains them in an autocrine manner and establishes their transcriptional program (see below). $T_H17$ cells also express high levels of IL-21 (an IL-2 family member), which sustains them in an autocrine manner and establishes their transcriptional program (see below). IL-27, an IL-12 family member, curbs $T_H17$ responses by limiting $T_H17$ effector cell development.

***The cytokine environment controls CD4$^+$ $T_H$ subset differentiation.*** The cytokine environment in which naïve CD4$^+$ T cells are activated and proliferate plays the most prominent role in regulating their commitment along the $T_H1$, $T_H2$, $T_H17$, or $T_{reg}$ effector pathways (Figure 10-16). The signature cytokines IFN-γ and IL-4 profoundly influence $T_H1$ and $T_H2$ cell development (see also Figure 10-15). $T_H1$-derived IFN-γ supports the generation of $T_H1$ cells, upregulates macrophage and dendritic cell IL-12 production, facilitates the activation of IL-12 receptors on activated T cells through the expression of the IL-12β1 chain, and suppresses the development and effector functions of $T_H2$ and $T_H17$ cells, whereas $T_H1$-derived TNF-β enhances $T_H17$ cell activities. $T_H2$-derived IL-4 supports the generation of $T_H2$ cells, and IL-4, IL-10, and IL-13 suppress the development of $T_H1$ cells and oppose the effects of IFN-γ on macrophages and dendritic cells. TGF-β plus IL-6–containing milieu drive $T_H17$ cell differentiation, which is augmented by IL-23. TGF-β alone induces $T_{reg}$ cell development.

As discussed, antigen-primed, costimulator-induced CD4$^+$ $T_H$ cell differentiation leads to low levels of cytokine and cytokine receptor expression, and these cells can be polarized toward various subsets depending on the surrounding cytokine milieu. This polarization has a molecular basis, that is, cytokine engagement of the appropriate receptors and subsequent activation of transcription factors drives one subset to promote its own growth and development while inhibiting the development of its opposing counterpart. That is, each $T_H$ cell ($T_H1$, $T_H2$, and $T_H17$ cell) differentiation program is driven by specific transcription factors called *master regulators or master transcription factors*; they include **T-box expressed in T cells (T-bet)**, **GATA-binding protein 3 (GATA-3)**, and **retinoic-acid-receptor-related orphan receptor-γt (RORγt)** and **RORα**, respectively (see Figure 10.16). IL-12 receptor engagement with its corresponding priming cytokine leads to the activation of signal transducer and activator of transcription 4 (STAT4) that through STAT1 induces IFN-γ production, which rapidly induces expression of the $T_H1$-cell-specific transcription factor (T-bet), which, in turn, potentiates expression the *IFNg* gene

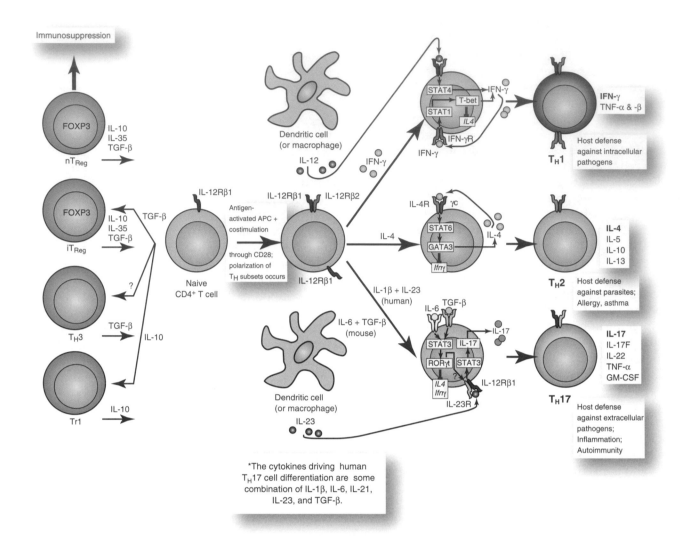

**FIGURE 10-16 CD4$^+$ T$_H$cell development** Naïve CD4$^+$ T$_H$ cells (sometimes called *T helper precursor [T$_H$p] cells*) can be induced to differentiate toward at least four mutually exclusive types of effector T$_H$ cells, T$_H$1, T$_H$2, T$_H$17, and regulatory (T$_{reg}$) phenotypes based on mode of stimulation, antigen concentration, costimulation, and most importantly, the "bathing" cytokine environment. IL-12 signaling through signal transduction and activator of transcription 4 (STAT4) skews toward T$_H$1, IL-4 (signaling through STAT6) toward T$_H$2, depending on species IL-6 plus transforming growth factor-β (TGF-β) toward T$_H$17 (in humans, the combination of cytokines that drive T$_H$17 cell development is uncertain), and TGF-β alone toward T$_{reg}$ lineage (nT$_{reg}$, naturally occurring T$_{reg}$ cell; iT$_{reg}$, induced T$_{reg}$ cell; Tr1, T regulatory cell). Once differentiated, each lineage is characterized by its own archetypal cytokine profile with interferon-γ (IFN-γ) being the cytokine of T$_H$1, IL-4 of T$_H$2, IL-17 of T$_H$17, and TGF-β of T$_{reg}$ cells and signature transcription factors, T-box expressed in T cells (T-bet) for T$_H$1, GATA-binding protein 3 (GATA-3) for T$_H$2, retinoic-acid-receptor-related orphan receptor-γt (RORγt) for T$_H$17, and forkhead box (FOXP3) for T$_{regs}$ cells. IL-17 has a proinflammatory role and is implicated in many inflammatory and autoimmune conditions, while T$_{reg}$ cells have an antiinflammatory role and maintain tolerance.

and upregulates the inducible IL-12 receptor chain IL-12Rβ 2. T-bet promotes T$_H$1 lineage commitment and suppresses their development to T$_H$2 cells. The upregulation of IL-12R expression enables IL-12 signaling through STAT4, which further potentiates IFN-γ production and induces expression of IL-18Rα. The latter expression confers responsiveness to IL-18

by mature T$_H$1 cells, which leads to effector cells that can produce IFN-γ through a TCR-dependent or -independent (IL-12 plus IL-18) pathways. The coordinate signaling through the TCR and IL-4 receptor engagement with its corresponding cytokine leads to the activation of STAT6 that induces expression of the T$_H$2-cell-specific transcription factor (GATA-3), which, in turn, enables expression of *Il4*, *Il5*, and *Il13* genes, while repressing the expression of T-bet. GATA-3 promotes $T_H2$ lineage commitment and suppresses their development to $T_H1$ cells. T-bet and GATA-3 are the "master switches" that control $T_H1$- and $T_H2$-cell development, respectively. In addition, the respective signaling pathways can downregulate expression of GATA-3 and IFN-$\gamma$, thereby enhancing one response by inhibiting the other response. The involvement of $T_H17$ transcription factors in cross-regulation is under current study. The antigen-induced differentiation of $T_H17$ cells does not require $T_H1$ or $T_H2$ transcription factors and $T_H17$ cells do not express T-bet or GATA-3. In fact, T-bet may actively antagonize $T_H17$ cell differentiation. $T_H17$ cell differentiation is initiated by STAT3 through IL-6 and TFG$\beta$ priming plus IL-21–induced signaling. Activated STAT3 induces the expression of the lineage-specific transcription factors ROR$\gamma$t and ROR$\alpha$. These transcription factors establish the $T_H17$ cell-associated transcriptional programs—production of IL-17, IL-17F, and IL-21 (and IL-26 in humans). ROR$\gamma$t expression blocks $T_H1$ and $T_H2$ cell differentiation; however, the $T_H1$ and $T_H2$ differentiation signaling pathways remain functional in $T_H17$ cells, suggesting that the $T_H17$ lineage may be transient and unstable.

Figure 10-17 illustrates an oversimplified view of how antagonistic cytokines may choreograph host immunity. The following example catalogs the role of certain cytokines as downregulators of particular T-cell responses. IFN-$\gamma$ from $T_H1$ cells suppresses $T_H2$-cell responses and therefore antibody formation. IL-4 from $T_H2$ cells suppresses $T_H1$-cell responses directly, whereas $T_H2$-derived IL-10 suppresses $T_H1$ cell responses by downregulating APC class II MHC molecule expression and blocking APC IL-12 synthesis, which alters $T_H1$ cell IFN-$\gamma$ production and therefore cell-mediated immunity, including both the cytotoxic and inflammatory forms. Furthermore, IL-10 suppresses macrophage production of nitric oxide, other bactericidal metabolites, and inflammation mediators, such as, IL-1, IL-6, CXCL8 (IL-8), TNF-$\alpha$, G-CSF, and GM-CSF. $T_H1$ and $T_H2$ cells become a "tag-team," that is, both IFN-$\gamma$ and IL-4 inhibit $T_H17$ cells. IFN-$\gamma$'s inhibitory role may vary during the course of information. TGF-$\beta$ seems to suppress everything, paradoxically it plus IL-6 initiates the differentiation of $T_H17$ cells, sustained by autocrine IL-21 production, which enhances expression of the IL-23 receptor, promoting IL-23–mediated expansion of $T_H17$ cells. In contrast, TGF-$\beta$ alone stimulates $T_{reg}$ cell differentiation—the latter cells inhibit immune responses. (Whether human $T_H17$-cell development is similar to the mouse still needs to be established; for example, in humans, IL-1$\beta$ induces and IL-6 enhances $T_H17$-cell development whereas TGF-$\beta$ and IL-12 inhibit. Human $T_H17$ cell differentiation is driven by some combination of IL-1$\beta$, IL-6, IL-21, IL-23, and TGF-$\beta$.

The flipside is that all of these T cells also can be helpers in the right context: IFN-$\gamma$ for increased class II MHC molecule and costimulatory molecule expression on dendritic cells and macrophages, for increased expression of IL-12 receptors on $T_H1$ cells, for macrophage, dendritic cell, NK cell, $T_C$ cell activation in cell-mediated immunity, for increased IL-12 production, and for IgG$_{2a}$ production, IL-4 for B-cell activation and increased class II MHC molecule expression on B cells, IL-4 and IL-10 for IgE and IgG$_1$ production, and TGF-$\beta$ for IgA production. Therefore, the magnitude and duration of an immune response is largely determined by the cross-regulation between antagonistic CD4$^+$ effector T cell-derived signals. The bottom line is that *cross-regulation*, or reciprocal regulation, occurs between CD4$^+$ effector T cell subsets. *The magnitude and duration of an immune response is largely determined*

---

**FIGURE 10-17 Cross-regulation network between CD4$^+$ effector and regulatory T cells.** T cell-polarizing capacity correlates with the patterns of cytokines produced, or cell-cell contact, by various types of dendritic cells when activated by microbial stimuli and T cell help—the dendritic cell–precursor T ($T_H$P) cell interaction drives $T_H$P cells to develop into different subsets. The early production of IL-12 promotes the development of $T_H1$ cells (leads to cellular immunity), whereas the early production of IL-4 favors the development of $T_H2$ cells (leads to humoral immunity and allergy). In contrast, IL-12 inhibits $T_H2$ cell development and IL-4 inhibits $T_H1$ cell development while either IL-12 or IL-4 inhibit $T_H17$ cell differentiation. The high production of IL-6 (or IL-1$\beta$ or autocrine IL-21) and TGF-$\beta$ drives the development of IL-17–producing $T_H17$ cells and IL-1$\beta$ has an enhancing effect on development (leads to autoimmune and inflammatory diseases and protection against various pathogens). TGF-$\beta$ and IL-6 lead to the expression of IL-21, which boosts expression of the IL-23 receptor, which in turn promotes the expansion of antigen-primed $T_H17$ cells by IL-23, whereas another IL-12 family member, macrophage-derived IL-27, negatively regulates $T_H17$ cell development. High TGF-$\beta$ production alone induces the transcription factor FOXP3, which promotes the development of T regulatory ($T_{reg}$) cells, an outcome that is inhibited by IL-6. In many instances, the production of $T_{reg}$ cell-derived TGF-$\beta$ (and IL-10) leads to immunosuppression. Green arrows indicate promoting activity, whereas red lines indicate inhibitory activity. (Also see Figure 10-16 and text for additional detail.)

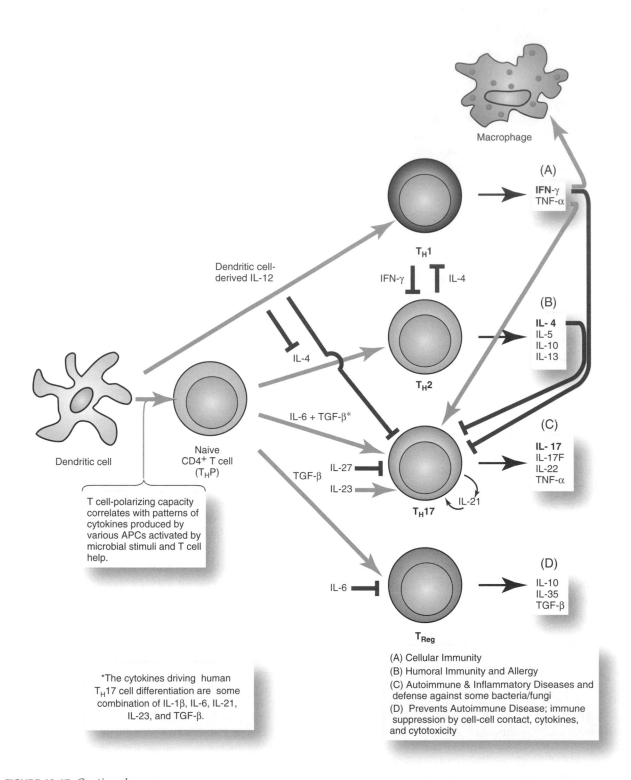

Macrophage

(A)

**T_H1**

Dendritic cell-
derived IL-12

IFN-γ ⊥ T IL-4

**IFN-**γ
TNF-α

(B)

**IL- 4**
IL-5
IL-10
IL-13

IL-4

**T_H2**

IL-6 + TGF-β*

Naive
CD4⁺ T cell
(T_HP)

Dendritic cell

TGF-β

IL-27 ⊥

IL-23

IL-21

(C)

**IL- 17**
IL-17F
IL-22
TNF-α

**T_H17**

T cell-polarizing capacity
correlates with patterns of
cytokines produced by
various APCs activated by
microbial stimuli and T cell
help.

IL-6 ⊥

(D)

**T_Reg**

IL-10
IL-35
TGF-β

(A) Cellular Immunity
(B) Humoral Immunity and Allergy
(C) Autoimmune & Inflammatory Diseases and
defense against some bacteria/fungi
(D) Prevents Autoimmune Disease; immune
suppression by cell-cell contact, cytokines,
and cytotoxicity

*The cytokines driving human
T_H17 cell differentiation are some
combination of IL-1β, IL-6, IL-21,
IL-23, and TGF-β.

**FIGURE 10-17** *Continued*

*by the cross-regulation between antagonistic cytokine signals. The balance between these signals is a key determinant of the in vivo effectiveness of a particular responder to antigen.*

### Distinct CD4$^+$ T cells negatively regulate immune responses.

During the early 1970s, investigators suggested that downregulation of the immune response was mediated by a group of lymphocytes distinct from $T_H$ and $T_C$ cells called *suppressor T* ($T_S$ *cells*), their phenotype was thought to be CD8$^+$. At the time, there were no reliable ways to study the phenotype or function of these cells; therefore, they fell out of favor. The advent of molecular immunology led to a re-emergence of the $T_S$ cell concept in the 1990s. This raised the question, is T-cell regulation a special job or everyone's responsibility? The "old" concept of T suppressors has not returned, at least not under that name. It has re-emerged, under the guise of **regulatory T ($T_{reg}$) cell**, perhaps modulated by $T_H17$ cells. $T_{reg}$ cells are characterized as CD4$^+$, not CD8$^+$, cells and constitutively express high levels of CD25 (the IL-2 receptor α-chain), CTLA-4, glucocorticoid-induced TNF receptor (GITR), and OX40; these molecules characterize activated T cells. However, the high level expression of transcription factor forkhead box p3 (FOXP3) distinguishes this $T_{reg}$ lineage. There are several subsets of $T_{reg}$ cells, including *naturally occurring $T_{reg}$ cells* generated in the thymus from CD4$^+$ thymic precursor cells expressing receptors with intermediate to high affinity for self-antigens (their phenotype is CD4$^+$CD25$^+$FOXP3$^+$), and *induced $T_{reg}$ cells* with the same phenotype, *IL-10-secreting Tr1 cells*, and *TGF-β-secreting $T_H3$ cells* all generated in the periphery (see Figures 10–16 and 10–17; also see Chapter 13). The forkhead-family transcription factor FOXP3 is essential for the development and function of $T_{reg}$ cells. In fact, the expression of FOXP3 is the main difference between effector and $T_{reg}$ cells; evidence suggests that $T_{reg}$ cells and effector T cells respond differently to T-cell receptor stimulation and that these differences in responses are mediated by FOXP3. In the periphery, the most important $T_{reg}$ cells are considered natural and induced $T_{reg}$ cells because they maintain tolerance by inhibiting autoimmunity, and control excessive effector T cell responses against foreign antigens (chronic inflammatory diseases, such as asthma and inflammatory bowel disease), when they become dangerous to the host. However, they also limit beneficial responses by preventing immunity to certain pathogens and limiting antitumor immunity. $T_{reg}$ cell activation is antigen-specific; however, they

can inhibit both CD4$^+$ and CD8$^+$ effector T cells and APCs in an antigen-nonspecific manner. $T_{reg}$ cells suppress effector T cells in a contact-dependent manner ($T_{reg}$ cell CTLA-4 and lymphocyte-activating gene 3 protein [CD223] interactions with APC B7 and class II MHC molecules, respectively), through the production of IL-10, IL-35, and TGF-β, and through perforin/granzyme-mediated cytotoxicity. Tr1 and $T_H3$ cells (discussed in Chapter 13) also produced IL-10 and TGF-β, respectively. (The focus in this text is naturally occurring or induced CD4$^+$ CD25$^+$ FOXP3$^+$ $T_{reg}$ cells and they are referred to as $T_{reg}$ cells throughout.) The production of TGF-β alone promotes the development of $T_{reg}$ cells, while in combination with IL-6 contributes to the development of $T_H17$ cells but inhibits $T_{reg}$ cells. Taken together, $T_{reg}$ cells restrain immunogenic (or autoreactive) responses by assorted pathways depending on the context, depending on cytokine milieu (IL-12 *vs.* IL-6 and/or TGF-β), the activation status of APCs (immature *vs.* mature dendritic cells), and the strength of antigen stimulation (see next section).

### The immune response can be regulated by antigen.

Antigens are the primary initiators of immune responses because antigens or antigens/MHCs are the first signals to trigger lymphocyte activation. The chemical nature of the antigen, the dose of antigen, the frequency of antigen exposure, the route of antigen exposure, and the genetic makeup of the host dictate whether an immune response develops, the type of response, and its magnitude (see Table 4-1 in Chapter 4).

Most protein antigens are recognized by both B cells and T cells, and induce both humoral and cell-mediated immunity. In contrast, polysaccharide and lipid antigens are unable to associate with MHC molecules for display to antigen-specific αβ$^+$ T cells, leading to a failure to stimulate cell-mediated immunity. The T-independent antibody responses to polysaccharide and lipid antigens elicit primarily low-affinity IgM antibodies, whereas the T-dependent antibody responses to protein antigens lead to antibody class switching, affinity maturation, and memory B cells.

Optimal antigen doses lead to optimal immune responses, whereas too large doses of polysaccharide and lipid antigen or protein induce B-cell and T-cell tolerance, respectively. Antigen administered intradermally or intramuscularly is usually immunogenic. Orally and intravenously administered antigen can induce tolerance. Another important influence on antigen elimination is the host's genetic constitution.

That is, no matter how immunogenic an antigen is, it will not induce an immune response if the host does not have the MHC haplotype for the antigen's particular epitopes.

In sum, the interaction between antigen and the immune system and the resulting regulation is seen at the cellular level. Antigen-MHC molecules trigger T-cell activation, leading to the expression of cytokine receptors and cytokines needed for T-cell proliferation. The resulting T-cell help causes B cells to make specific and appropriate antibody, which leads to antigen elimination. Antigen disappearance removes any initial signals to trigger B-cell activation. Likewise, antigen-MHC molecule disappearance removes any initial signals to trigger T-cell activation. *The immune system returns to a resting state by eliminating the inducer of an immune response—the antigen.*

### Antibodies, the end products of humoral immune responses, also regulate through feedback inhibition.

Antibodies, in addition to their effector functions such as cytotoxicity (by complement) and opsonization, are important in controlling immune responses through *antibody-mediated end-product feedback*. IgG antibodies are downregulators of the normal antibody response, and the removal of antigen-specific antibodies leads to their increased production. Rather than removing the appropriate antibodies, introducing antigen-specific antibodies into a recipient either shortly before immunization or during an antibody response reduces subsequent antibody formation. Antibody, therefore, can inhibit antibody formation during a conventional humoral response through a feedback mechanism called **antibody feedback**. This phenomenon is not limited to humoral responses, it also affects cell-mediated immune responses. Negative feedback mediated by antibody occurs during (1) antigen removal and (2) Fc receptor ligation. Antibody-mediated negative feedback occurs during antigen removal and Fc receptor ligation.

1. *Antigen removal:* The complexing of IgM and certain subclasses of IgG with antigen during an immune response leads to activation of the complement system. Antibodies and complement fragments opsonize or coat target antigens to make them more palatable to Fc receptor- and complement receptor-displaying phagocytes. Red blood cells also have receptors for complement that appear to pick up complement-coated antigen-antibody complexes and deliver them to the phagocytes in the liver. Antigen removal by enhanced phagocytosis, a major effector function

of antibodies, leads to the absence of the triggering substance for the immune response. Furthermore, antibodies block antigen access to the antibody receptors on the appropriate B cells. This blockage limits B-cell activation by neutralizing the triggering ability of antigens.

2. *Fc receptor ligation:* IgG antibody against an antigen suppresses the antibody response to that antigen. This suppression depends on the ability of antibody to bind antigen and on functions associated with the antibody's having an intact Fc portion. Antibody-mediated end-product feedback depends on the cross-linking of Fc receptors by antigen-antibody complexes (a process that stops B-cell activation). FcγRII (CD32) seems to be the major player in Fc-mediated suppression. The antigen-binding portion of IgG molecules allows for the antigen-specific nature of suppression. The immunosuppression is antigen-specific but not epitope-specific. For example, IgG antibodies binding to one epitope on a red blood cell can suppress the antibody response to all epitopes on the cell. All subclasses of IgG can mediate suppression. IgG-mediated immunosuppression affects the primary IgM and IgG responses and can occur in the absence of T cells. B cells are activated when they interact with antigen by their membrane Ig; however, the concomitant binding of the Fc portions of the antigen-specific secreted IgG antibodies to the B cells' Fcγ receptors inactivates the B cells (Figure 10-18). The Fcγ receptor cytoplasmic domains have associated phosphatases, which are brought into close proximity of B-cell receptor cytoplasmic signaling complexes during cross-linking of antigen-antibody complexes. The phosphatases can then dephosphorylate the signaling molecules that must stay phosphorylated to sustain B-cell activation. As the amount of Fcγ receptor-bound IgG increases, the B-cell activity is increasingly suppressed. Thus, the biological relevance of Fcγ receptors on B cells may be their role in antibody feedback.

### Antibody Production Occasionally Occurs in the Absence of Help (T-Independent Antigens)

Many antigens stimulate antibody production in T-cell-deficient animals such as athymic and neonatally thymectomized mice. These antigens are called *thymus-*, or *T-independent antigens*. T-independent antigens are large polymer molecules composed of repeating subunits of either proteins (such as bacterial

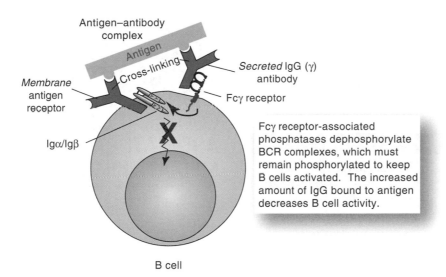

Antigen–antibody complex

Antigen

Cross-linking

*Secreted* IgG (γ) antibody

*Membrane* antigen receptor

Fcγ receptor

Igα/Igβ

Fcγ receptor-associated phosphatases dephosphorylate BCR complexes, which must remain phosphorylated to keep B cells activated. The increased amount of IgG bound to antigen decreases B cell activity.

B cell

**FIGURE 10-18 Antibody feedback inhibition.** The simultaneous cross-linking of B cell antigen receptors (BCRs) and Fc receptors causes B-cell inhibition. This cross-linking occurs when membrane antibodies and secreted antibodies bind to the stimulatory antigen. The antigen-attached, soluble antibodies are available for interaction with Fc receptors on the B cells.

**TABLE 10-2 Properties of T-independent Antigens**

1. They are molecules with high molecular weights and repeating antigenic determinants.
2. They are generally carbohydrates associated with bacterial cell walls.
3. They are slowly metabolized.
4. They induce tolerance in large doses or in a soluble form.
5. Some T-independent antigens are mitogenic (induce proliferation of cells of a particular class) or polyclonal B-cell activators.
6. Some T-independent antigens activate the alternative complement pathway.
7. They usually generate antibody responses of IgM and particular subclasses of IgG.
8. They induce little or no antibody class switching.
9. They are ineffective in inducing memory B cells.

flagellin) or polysaccharides (dextran). Some properties of T-independent antigens are listed in Table 10-2. T-independent antigens can be subdivided into two groups, *type 1 antigens* and *type 2 antigens*, according to their degree of independence from T cells and their physiochemical properties. Type 1 antigens, such as the bacterial cell-wall molecule lipopolysaccharide (LPS), can activate B cells in a polyclonal fashion (that is, all B cells are activated irrespective of their antigen specificity; type 1 antigens are B-cell mitogens). B cells can interact with LPS using TLR4 and the B-cell receptor (membrane Ig). Type 1 antigens can activate immature and mature B cells, whereas type 2 antigens inactivate immature B cells and activate mature ones. All B cells express TLR4, whereas a low percentage of B cells express LPS-specific B-cell receptors. LPS-specific B cells are stimulated to proliferate, differentiate, and secrete LPS-specific antibody by independent activation pathways initiated by Ig receptors and TLR4. In contrast, non-LPS–specific B cells are stimulated to proliferate and differentiate into antibody-producing cells by interacting with LPS through TLR4. The combination of these activation pathways leads to a varied production of antibodies. Type 1 antigens can be considered totally T cell-independent because T$_H$-cell-derived cytokines are not required during type 1 antigen-induced B-cell activation. Because T-cell-derived cytokines are absent, B cells produce only high levels of IgM antibodies and class switching does not occur. In contrast, type 2 antigen-induced B-cell activation and antibody production require some T-cell help mediated through cytokines. Type 2 antigens are highly repetitious molecules, such as dextran, capsular polysaccharides and polymeric proteins (flagellin), which do not induce polyclonal B-cell activation (that is, type 2 antigens are not B-cell mitogens) and cytokines are required for efficient B-cell activation. The antibody response to type 2 antigens is mainly IgM; however, class switching can occur. Both type 1 and type 2 antigens are biologically important because they constitute many of the surface antigens on bacteria. Even though humoral immunity is a primary defense against bacterial infections, the response to their T-independent antigens is weaker, lacks memory, and is mediated predominantly by IgM antibodies, which is in contrast to humoral immunity developed against T-dependent antigens. The latter scenario is driven by $T_H$ cell influences.

## MINI SUMMARY

The generation of memory B cells and antibody-secreting plasma cells against T-dependent antigens requires dendritic cell and effector $CD4^+$ $T_H$ cell involvement—need to activate $CD4^+$ naïve $T_H$ cells to effector T cells, which in turn can activate antigen-primed B cells. T- and B-cell activation, proliferation, and differentiation involve surface antibody recognition of antigen, accessory molecule interactions, MHC-restricted antigen presentation and recognition, and a cascade of antigen-nonbinding, antigen-nonspecific amplification signals mediated by cytokines. Naïve T cells required two signals to become activated to help B cells; naïve B cells also require two signals to become antibody-secreting plasma cells. Two subsets of $T_H$ cells, $T_H1$ and $T_H2$, antagonistically regulate humoral and cellular immunity—the balancing between antagonistic cytokines regulates the type, magnitude, and duration of an immune response. A newly discovered third $T_H$ subset called $T_H17$ is also involved. The cytokine environment, through the induction of transcription factors, drives the polarization of $T_H$ cells to the appropriate subset to counteract a pathogen threat. $CD4^+CD25^+$ $FOXP3^+$ $T_{reg}$ cells inhibit autoimmunity and protect against tissue injury.

Exposure to antigen supplies the first signal in immune cell activation. The removal of antigen downregulates the immune system.

During humoral immune responses, immune complexes are formed that can indirectly regulate in at least two ways. Immune complex formation enhances phagocytosis, leading to antigen removal. Immune complexes cause Fc receptor interaction with antigen-bound antibody, leading to B-cell inactivation. Both results lead to inhibition of further antibody production.

In contrast to T-dependent antigens, T-independent antigens require little or no $T_H$-cell involvement. T-independent antigens activate B cells in a polyclonal fashion and do not induce memory B cells.

# THE DEVELOPMENT OF $CD8^+$ T CELL-MEDIATED CYTOTOXIC IMMUNE RESPONSE ALSO REQUIRES CELLULAR COOPERATION; CYTOTOXIC T AND NATURAL KILLER CELLS MEDIATE KILLING

Antibody production provides humoral immunity. As just described, B cells, T cells, and dendritic cells all affect antibody production. B cells recognize free extracellular antigen through surface anibody receptors but need effector $T_H$ cells for final activation, and naïve $T_H$ cells need assistance from dendritic cells. Antibodies cannot detect intracellular antigen; the role of cell-mediated immunity is to detect and remove cells infected by intracellular pathogens. In this section, interactions between helper and effector cells will be demonstrated—the helper and effector cells during cellular immune responses are T cells (effector $CD4^+$ $T_H$ cells and $CD8^+$ precursor and effector $T_C$ cells). Dendritic cells are also involved; they are "licensed" by $T_H$ cells, which allows for the induction of $T_H$-cell-dependent $T_C$ cell responses. Irrespective of cellular collaboration mechanism(s), activated $T_C$ cells kill targets cells in two ways. Cytotoxic-mediated backup comes in the form of natural killer (NK) cells. NK cell-mediated killing is similar to $T_C$ cell-mediated killing; the recognition and activation is not.

## $CD4^+$ Helper T-Cell and $CD8^+$ Cytotoxic T-Cell Cooperation Is Needed to Develop Cellular Immunity but the Mechanism(s) Are Debated

As the title of this section suggests, the importance of $CD4^+$ $T_H$ cells in $T_C$ cell responses is questioned. This doubt arises from studies using mice in which the *CD4 gene* was disrupted.[2] The following discussion is not meant to overemphasize the importance of $CD4^+$ $T_H$ cells in $T_C$-cell responses, but rather to show the plasticity in the immune system.

The traditional examples of $T_C$-cell-mediated immunity are allograft rejection and tumor rejection,

---

[2]"Knocked out" in laboratory vernacular. Mice possessing the knock out mutation in the *CD4 gene* are depleted of mature $CD4^+$ T cells but still show cytotoxic responses to some viruses. However, these mice confirm the need for $CD4^+$ $T_H$ cells in antibody responses.

even though the physiologic function of $T_C$ cells is the eradication of altered-self cells (such as virus-infected cells). **$T_C$ cells**, usually identifiable by the CD8 marker, are killer cells that respond to antigenic peptide bound to self-class I MHC molecules on target cells. Class I MHC molecules are expressed on all nucleated cells in the body; therefore, $T_C$ cells can recognize and kill any cell infected by intracellular pathogens because they exhibit pathogen-derived peptides associated with class I MHC molecules. To ensure that only infected cells are killed, the processing of proteins, such as virus-derived proteins, synthesized within the cell is restricted to the class I MHC (or cytosolic) pathway, excluding exogenous proteins captured from the extracellular environment. Consequently, virus-infected cells can display viral peptides on their class I MHC molecules, which are recognized for $T_C$ cell-mediated destruction; however, neighboring cells that merely internalize viral debris cannot process such antigens to form antigenic peptide–class I MHC complexes, thereby negating $T_C$ cell-targeting. This restriction in processing endogenous versus exogenous antigen is not as exact for dendritic cells. They have the ability to process exogenous antigens into the class I MHC pathway; this ability is called *cross-presentation* (discussed shortly).

$T_C$ cell-mediated immunity occurs in two stages. In the first stage, naïve or precursor $T_C$ cells are activated in a complex interaction with $T_H$ cells and licensed dendritic cells, and differentiate into effector $T_C$ cells. In the second stage, the effector $T_C$ cells identify specific target cells by their expression of antigenic peptide–class I MHC complexes, and the recognition leads to target cell destruction.

In the 1970s, investigators discovered that CD4$^+$ and CD8$^+$ cell types interacted cooperatively (Figure 10-19) by treating lymph node cells with anti-CD antibodies plus complement before exposing the cells to antigen. Treatment with anti-CD4 antibodies removed all CD4$^+$ cells, whereas treatment with anti-CD8 antibodies removed all CD8$^+$ cells. When only CD4$^+$ cells remained, they were incapable of generating a cytotoxic response. When CD8$^+$ cells remained, they were capable of generating a cytotoxic response, but at only 30% of the control value. If the two cell populations were mixed, they generated control-level cytotoxic responses. Anti-CD8 treatment was the only one that abolished cytotoxic activity because CD8$^+$ cells are the effector cells that require CD4$^+$ cells as helper cells. Once CD8$^+$ cells interacted with antigen, they converted from naïve precursors to mature effector $T_C$ cells. *These experiments show that the main cell (effector cell)*

*mediating cellular immunity is the CD8$^+$$T_C$ cell, but the CD4$^+$ $T_H$1 cell is needed for complete reactivity.*

What these experiments do not show are the chronological events needed for the development of a functional $T_C$ cell—the goal of cellular immunity. Why is this point important? The answer lies in the fact that proliferation leads to clonal growth and differentiation of immune cells—to have a functional cell-mediated reaction, or immunity in general, requires proliferation of immune cells. To identify the events required for cellular immunity, the mixed lymphocyte reaction (MLR) assay is used (see Chapter 14 for the mechanics on the MLR). Because $T_C$ cells result from cellular events that happen in the MLR, this assay serves as the *in vitro* precursor reaction for development of cell-mediated lympholysis (CML). One cannot have total CML without the MLR or a similar type of reaction. Cell-depletion experiments using anti-CD4 and anti-CD8 antibodies showed that the proliferating cells in the MLR were CD4$^+$ (Figure 10-20), and they were needed for a CD8$^+$ T cell cytotoxic responses to develop (Group 2 results). Group 3 had high MLR activity but no cytotoxicity; anti-CD8 antibodies removed the CD8$^+$ $T_C$ cells. Other experiments, using antibody blocking and transfection studies, showed that CD4$^+$ T cells recognized class II MHC molecules, whereas CD8$^+$ T cells recognized class I MHC molecules.

The nature of effector CD4$^+$ T cell-provided help in the development of $T_C$ cells is not completely resolved. Nonetheless, a breakthrough in understanding CD4$^+$–CD8$^+$ T-cell cooperation came with the realization of the central role of dendritic cells in stimulating cytotoxicity responses (Figure 10-21). The dendritic cell contribution is not unexpected because naïve T cells do not traffic throughout the body but recirculate through different secondary lymphoid organs waiting to encounter dendritic cell-associated antigen. In contrast, dendritic cells are ubiquitous, capture antigen, transport it to draining lymph nodes, and present it to naïve T cells. What if the antigen is not associated with APCs, such as virus-infected or tumor cell targets? These non-APCs do not express costimulatory molecules, therefore to kill these targets naïve CD8$^+$ T cells need to recognize antigenic peptide–class I MHC molecule complexes (signal 1) plus encounter costimulatory molecules on APCs (signal 2). To resolve this quandary, the immune system can take extracellular antigens, contrary to the belief that class I MHC molecules presented peptides exclusively derived from intracellular antigens, and present them with class I MHC molecules; the process is called **cross-presentation** (see Figure 10-21). The principal cells endowed with

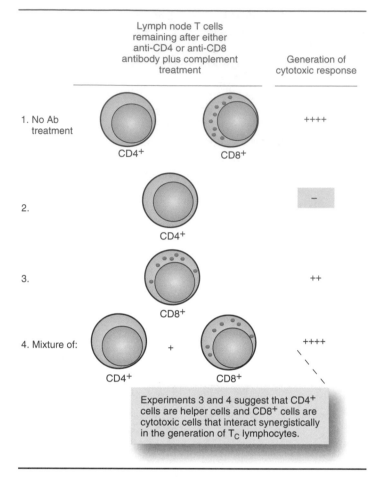

**Lymph node T cells remaining after either anti-CD4 or anti-CD8 antibody plus complement treatment**

**Generation of cytotoxic response**

1. No Ab treatment

CD4+    CD8+    ++++

2.    CD4+    −

3.    CD8+    ++

4. Mixture of:    CD4+   +   CD8+    ++++

Experiments 3 and 4 suggest that CD4+ cells are helper cells and CD8+ cells are cytotoxic cells that interact synergistically in the generation of T_C lymphocytes.

**FIGURE 10-19 T-cell cooperation in generating cytotoxic T cells.** Lymph node T cells are treated with antibody plus complement, and the remaining cells are mixed with allogeneic target cells. After 4 to 5 days of coculture, another aliquot of allogeneic cells is added and cytotoxicity is assessed. Only test groups 1 and 4 are able to cooperate, providing the necessary cellular interactions for development of $T_C$ cells.

this ability are dendritic cells. They can acquire cellular antigen by phagocytosis of necrotic or apoptotic cells or virally infected cells that carry class I MHC- and class II MHC-restricted antigens. The dendritic cell-internalized antigen is presented to CD4+ $T_H1$ cells, which provide permission to intentionally kill infected cells through a process called *licensing*, that is, dendritic cells become licensed through CD40–CD40L interactions and in turn promote effector and memory CD8+ T-cell development. Help may be exerted directly by CD40–CD40L interactions between CD4+ and CD8+ T cells while associated with the same dendritic cell; evidence suggests that the major contribution is by effector CD4+ T cell-licensed dendritic cells. Nonetheless, exposure to certain infectious agents might circumvent the

need for CD4+ T cell-recognition of dendritic cell-associated antigen by stimulating dendritic cells directly through their TLRs (see Chapter 3).

How the trio of dendritic cells, $T_H$ cells, and $T_C$ cells collaborates to control cellular reactions is complex and not completely known. Naïve $T_C$ cells are immature cells, called *precursor-$T_C$ cells*, when they exit the thymus. These cells are CD8+, have functional CD3-associated $\alpha\beta$ TCRs, and recognize specific antigen, but they cannot lyse target cells (lack both cytoplasmic granules and their contents). Also, they do not express IL-2 or IL-2 receptors and are unable to proliferate. After activation, it takes 5 to 10 days for pre-$T_C$ cells to differentiate into functionally mature $T_C$ cells capable of mediating cytotoxicity. This conversion from a pre-$T_C$ cell to a

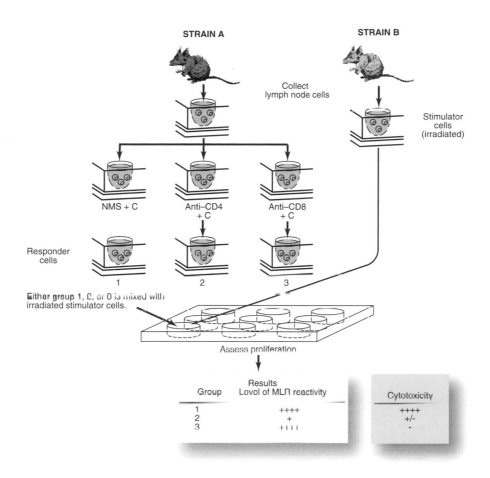

**FIGURE 10-20 The precursor cells of the mixed lymphocyte reaction are CD4$^+$, which provide help for T$_C$ cell development**. Lymph node cells are treated with antibody plus complement, and the remaining responder cells are mixed with allogeneic stimulator cells. After a 4-day incubation period, the proliferation (MLR reactivity) is assessed by measuring the amount of radiolabel incorporated.

functionally cytotoxic T$_C$ cell occurs in the peripheral lymphoid tissues. Although no special microenvironment is required for pre-T$_C$-cell differentiation, there are sequential signals required to transform naïve pre-T$_C$ cells into functional effector T$_C$ cells. The first signal is interaction of TCR with a protein antigen fragment bound to class I molecules on a target cell. The second signal is the licensing of dendritic cells by CD4$^+$ T cells. The third signal consists of T$_H$ cell-derived cytokines (such as, IL-2 and IFN-$\gamma$) and expression of high-affinity IL-2 receptors binding autocrinely produced IL-2, leading to the proliferation and differentiation of pre-T$_C$ cells into effector T$_C$ cells. This differentiation process causes T$_C$ cells to develop membrane-bound cytoplasmic granules filled with *perforins* and *granzymes* (discussed shortly) and to develop the ability to transcribe and secrete cytokines such as IFN-$\gamma$ and TNF-$\beta$ and, to a lesser extent, IL-2. See Figure 10-21 for models of T-cell

interaction proposed in the development of effector antigen-specific CD8$^+$ T$_C$ cells.

## Effector Cytotoxic T Cells Kill Target Cells in Two Ways

As their name implies, mature CD8$^+$ T$_C$ cells are cytotoxic to target cells. This cytotoxicity is antigen-specific, requires cell contact, and does not injure the T$_C$ cells themselves during the killing of the target cells. T$_C$-cell-mediated killing is a complex, multistep process (Figure 10-22) that involves (1) antigen recognition and conjugate formation between the T$_C$ cell and target cell; (2) activation of the T$_C$ cell; (3) delivery of the lethal hit by cytotoxic proteins or Fas ligand-Fas interaction; (4) T$_C$-cell detachment from the target cell; (5) target cell death by apoptosis; and (6) reinitiation of the killing cycle.

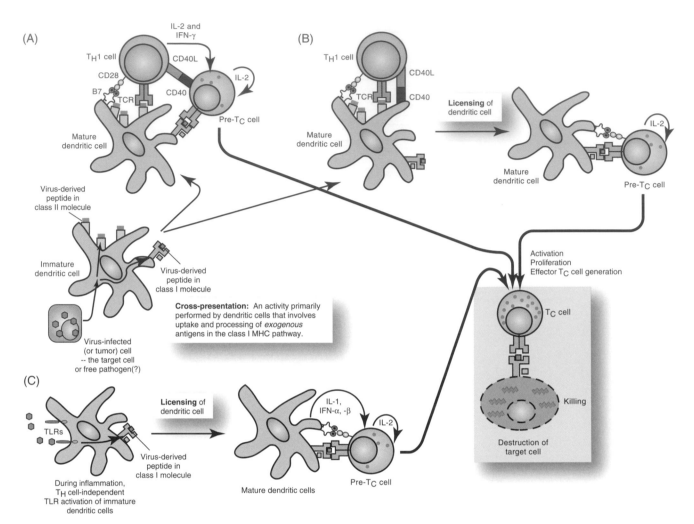

**FIGURE 10-21 Costimulation in the induction of CD8$^+$ T-cell effector function: Cytotoxicity of virally infected cell.** Dendritic cells acquire cellular antigen by phagocytosis of infected cells thereby express T$_H$ cell-specific peptide–class II MHC molecule complexes and T$_C$ cell-specific peptide–class I MHC molecule complexes through a process of cross-presentation. The dendritic cells are not virally infected. (**A**) Tripartite interaction: To prime naïve pre-T$_C$ cells, dendritic cells require a CD4$^+$ effector T$_H$ cell-dependent signal through CD40/CD40L interaction. The process is called *licensing*; without licensing, naïve pre-T$_C$ cells cannot be primed by dendritic cells. (**B**) Licensing the dendritic cell: The phagocytosed antigen is cross-presented to T$_H$1 cells, which activates (*licenses*) the dendritic cell through CD40/CD40L interactions and gives it the ability to trigger the pre-T$_C$ cell to express IL-2 receptors, produce IL-2, and develop into an effector T$_C$ cell. (**C**) T$_H$ cell-independent T$_C$ cell activation (no T$_H$1 cell-derived licensing signal): Dendritic cells could be licensed directly by interacting with bacteria or viruses through Toll-like receptors (TLRs). Most evidence suggests that the most prominent way is through the licensing of dendritic cells by T$_H$1 cells. Irrespective of method, dendritic cells must be licensed before they can prime naïve T$_C$ cells.

The two mechanisms of T$_C$-cell-mediated killing are that effector CD8$^+$ T$_C$ cell-target cell interactions trigger a programmed process of cell death (apoptosis) of the target cell by either (1) directionally secreted cytotoxic molecules, called *perforin* and *granzymes*, into the intercellular space, forming lytic pores in the target cell plasma membrane and endosome membranes or (2) the interaction of T$_C$ cell Fas ligand with target cell Fas receptor or TNF with target cell

TNF receptor (both mechanisms involve receptors of the TNF receptor family coupled to extrinsic factors).

*The first, and principal, mechanism of T$_C$-cell-mediated death,* **granule exocytosis-mediated apoptosis,** *involves the delivery of the lethal hit by T$_C$ cell-derived cytoplasmic storage granules that contain cytotoxic proteins to the intercellular space at the site of contact between the T$_C$ cell and the target cell, which leads to apoptosis of the target cell (Figure 10-23).*

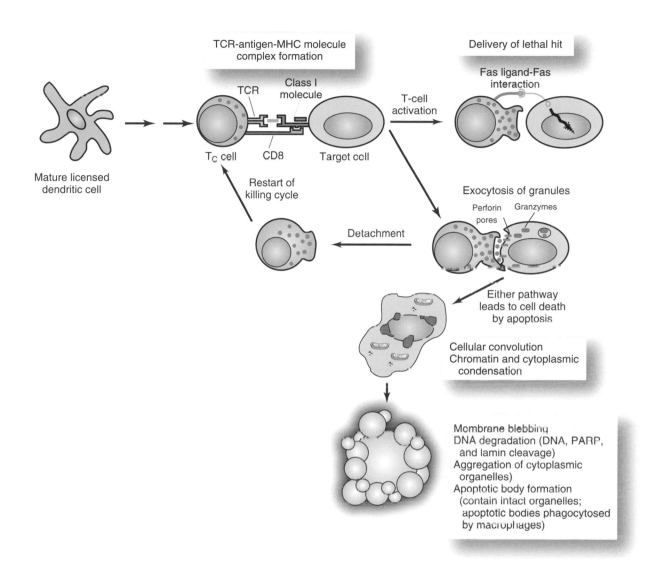

**FIGURE 10-22** The sequence for cytotoxic T-cell-mediated lysis.

**FIGURE 10-23 Two pathways of T$_C$ cell-mediated apoptosis of target cells.** (**A**) The granule exocytosis mechanism occurs when an effector T$_C$ cell interacts with a target cell (virus-infected or transformed cell) and there is a directed release of granule contents, granzyme B and perforin, into the cleft between the two cells. Granzyme B enters the target cell through two paths. Perforin either polymerizes in the target cell membrane forming a pore through which granzyme B enters the cell or granzyme B binds to target cell mannose-6-phosphate receptors and enters through receptor-mediated endocytosis. Perforin enters the target cell cytosol and perforates endosome membranes, releasing the granzyme B molecules. Cytoplasmic granzyme B cleaves procaspase-8, which activates the caspase cascade leading to apoptosis. (**B**) Effector T$_C$ cell-expressed Fas ligand engagement with target cell Fas receptor leads to recruitment of procaspase-8 by interaction with the adapter protein Fas-associated death domain (FADD) protein with Fas death domains. The interaction leads to procaspase-8 conversion to active caspases-8. Caspase-8 activation by either Fas-FasL interaction or granzyme B leads to cleavage of BID, the insertion of BID and BAX into mitochrondrial membrane and release of cytochrome *c*, which combines with apoptotic protease-activating factor 1 (APAF-1) to form the apoptosome complex. At the apoptosome, inactive procaspase-9 is activated. Active caspase-9 converts procaspase-3 into its active state. Caspase-3 initiates a series of reactions that lead to apoptosis.

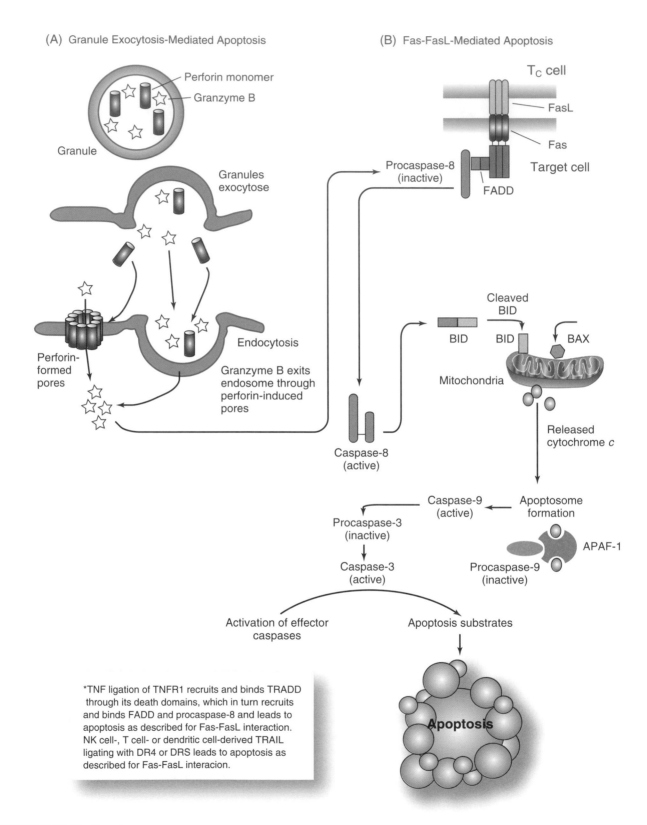

(A) Granule Exocytosis-Mediated Apoptosis

(B) Fas-FasL-Mediated Apoptosis

*TNF ligation of TNFR1 recruits and binds TRADD through its death domains, which in turn recruits and binds FADD and procaspase-8 and leads to apoptosis as described for Fas-FasL interaction. NK cell-, T cell- or dendritic cell-derived TRAIL ligating with DR4 or DRS leads to apoptosis as described for Fas-FasL interacion.

**FIGURE 10-23** *Continued*

Cytotoxicity begins when the $T_C$ cell's TCR-CD3 complex recognizes class I MHC molecule-associated antigenic peptide on a target cell; this interaction induces the binding of $T_C$ cell LFA-1 to target cell ICAM-1, leading to conjugate formation. The $T_C$ cell–target cell conjugate formation causes the $T_C$ cell's granules to concentrate at the junction with the target cell. The granules release their contents by *exocytosis* (a membrane fusion event between the granule membrane and plasma membrane causing an opening between the granule interior and the extracellular space) into the pocket formed between the cells. The granules kill targets without specificity, and the lesions that appear on the target cell's surface closely resemble those formed by the membrane attack complex of complement. Purified granules produce the same circular lesions as whole $T_C$ cells or NK cells. The granule constituents are **perforin** and serine esterases called **granzymes**. Both perforin and granzymes are needed for efficient $T_C$ cell killing of target cells. Perforin, a membrane-perturbing protein, is activated by surrounding $Ca^{2+}$. The $Ca^{2+}$ allows polymerization of perforin on the target cell's surface. Once perforin is on the membrane, it depolarizes the membrane and perforates it. These pores facilitate granzymes entry into the target cell. Another mode of perforin-mediated death shows that granzyme B moves out of the $T_C$ cell, binds to the mannose 6-phosphate receptor found on many target cell surfaces, and then the complex is endocytosed. Perforin forms pores in the target membrane, enters, permeabilizes the endosome, which releases endosome-sequestered granzymes into the target cell's cytosol, leading to cleavage and activation of an apoptotic protein, and activation of a cascade of *caspases*.[3] Caspases promote apoptotic cell death.

The second mechanism of target cell killing, **Fas–Fas ligand-mediated apoptosis**, involves receptors of the TNF receptor family coupling with extrinsic signals, as well as the delivery of the lethal hit by conjugate formation between the $T_C$ cells and target cells (see Figure 10-23). It is mediated by the interaction of **Fas ligand** (**FasL** [CD178]), a member of the TNF family expressed on membranes of activated $T_C$ cells, and the protein receptor **Fas** (CD95) a member of the TNF receptor family of death receptors expressed on many target cell types. This interaction triggers target cell enzymes to degrade target cell nuclear DNA. *The fragmentation of nuclear DNA leads to concomitant fragmentation of the target cell's nucleus, a process called* **programmed cell death**. The morphologic changes (decreased cell volume, membrane blebbing, condensation of chromatin, and degradation of the DNA into fragments) associated with programmed cell death are collectively called **apoptosis**. Phosphatidylserine, normally found on the cytosolic surface of plasma membranes, is redistributed during apoptosis to the extracellular surface. Phagocytic cells, such as macrophages, recognize this aberrant placement; they internalize the cells, thereby removing the dying cells without inducing inflammation. Apoptotic target-cell removal is followed by recycling of the $T_C$ cell to start another cytotoxic interaction. In sum, $T_C$ cell-mediated death mechanisms are initiated differently but the end is the same, death of the target cell by apoptosis.

## Natural Killer Cells Recognize and Are Activated Differently by Target Cells Than Cytotoxic T Cells But Kill Target Cells Similarly

**Natural killer** (**NK**) **cells** are lymphocyte-like cells that develop from bone-marrow precursors (their precise lineage needs further study), which function as important mediators of the innate immune responses against viruses, other intracellular parasites, and tumors (see Chapter 3). They constitute roughly 15% of circulating lymphocytes and are also found in the liver and peritoneum. NK cells were discovered because of their ability to spontaneously kill tumor-cell targets—that is, mediate immediate, nonspecific cytotoxicity without prior sensitization, hence, named *natural killer cells*. NK cells also promptly mediate noncytolytic activities through the secretion of cytokines, such as IFN-γ and TNF, and chemokines. These cytokines and chemokines have regulatory properties and influence innate and adaptive immune responses; therefore, NK cells are a crucial link between innate and adaptive immunity. NK cells are significant early producers of IFN-γ, which can augment innate immunity through activation of macrophages and shift the $T_H$ cell populations by inhibiting $T_H2$ cell growth while boosting $T_H1$ cell development. NK cells also produce TNF, which can influence $T_H17$ cell activity. NK cells interact with dendritic cells, that is, dendritic cells prime NK cells, which, in turn, secrete cytokines (IFN-γ and TNF) that can induce dendritic cell maturation, thereby promoting adaptive immune responses. The function

---

[3] The term is derived from cysteine, *asp*artatem and prote*ase* because it is a family of intracellular cysteine proteases that cleaves after aspartate residues. These proteases are important in the chain of reactions that lead to apoptosis.

of NK cells in the elimination of virus- and intracellular bacteria-infected cells is an important component of the early immune response. During a viral infection, the rapid increase in IFN-$\alpha$ and -$\beta$, and IL-12, rouses NK cell activity, which peaks within 3 days. This quick development compensates for the slower growth (roughly 7 days to a week) associated with virus-specific $T_C$ cells. NK cells are poised as immediate effector cells; killing can be triggered within minutes, without requiring transcription, translation, or cell proliferation. Nonetheless, they share common killing mechanisms—the exocytosis of granules containing perforin and granzymes, FasL–Fas interaction, or TNF-related apoptosis-induced ligand (TRAIL) binding to TRAIL receptor leading to apoptosis of the target cell.

NK cells express numerous membrane molecules, some of the ones that highlight NK cells are CD16 (also known as Fc$\gamma$RIII) a receptor for the Fc portion of IgG, CD56, CD25, the high affinity IL-2 receptor, and many activating and inhibitory receptors. The latter molecules are at the heart of how NK cells recognize and distinguish altered-self cells from normal host cells. Because NK cells do not express antigen receptors encoded by genes that undergo recombination-activating gene–dependent recombination, they accomplish recognition by binding to potential target cells with killer cell Ig-like receptors (KIRs), which recognize MHC class I molecules and block the cytotoxic function of NK cells and activating NK-cell receptors (such as, CD94/NKG2D [natural-killer group 2, member D]), which recognize glycoproteins with carbohydrate moieties and stimulate cytotoxic function. NK-cell activation depends on the set of activating and inhibitory ligands that the target cell presents, the number of activating and inhibitory receptors on the NK cell, and, ultimately, the balance of signaling through the activating versus inhibitory receptors. NK cell-activating receptors bind ligands on virus-infected, transformed, or otherwise stressed cells, and when unopposed by signals from inhibitory receptors, they signal NK cells to kill the target cells (Figure 10-24). The altered cells might also express more activating ligands such that inhibition delivered by inhibitory receptors is overwhelmed.

Later, during humoral response to a virus infection when antiviral antibodies are present, NK cells can also mediate killing by antibody-dependent cell-mediated cytotoxicity (ADCC) (see Chapter 15). NK cells, alone with macrophages, neutrophils, and eosinophils can mediate ADCC because they express CD16, the Fc$\gamma$RIII for the Fc region of IgG molecules. Target cells coated with IgG bound to an epitope are susceptible to binding by NK cells through their expressed Fc receptors, leading to increased metabolic activity and granule exocytosis-mediated killing.

## MINI SUMMARY

Cooperation between $T_H$ and $T_C$ cells, through a CD4$^+$ T cell-licensed dendritic cell, is required for the development of cellular immunity. Although CD8$^+$ $T_C$ cells are the primary cell type responsible for cellular immunity, CD4$^+$ $T_H$-cell-derived cytokines and costimulatory molecule interaction either between CD4$^+$ and CD8$^+$ T cells or more likely between CD8$^+$ T cells and licensed dendritic cells, using the process of cross-presentation, is required for complete reactivity. Whereas CD4$^+$ $T_H$ cells recognize exogenous processed antigen in association with class II MHC molecules on the surfaces of class II$^+$ APCs, CD8$^+$ $T_C$ cells respond to antigens of cellular origin (such as viral antigens) in association with class I MHC molecules on the surfaces of target cells. Effector $T_C$ cells kill target cells through apoptosis by delivery of cytotoxic proteins (perforin and granzymes), $T_C$ cell Fas ligand (FasL) or TRAIL interaction with target cell Fas or TRAIL receptor, respectively.

NK cells are poised to participate in early immune responses that can directly eliminate virally infected, transformed, or stressed cells through target-cell–mediated killing (as $T_C$ cells through the delivery of cytotoxic proteins, FasL or TRAIL), and/or recruit neutrophils and macrophages, activate dendritic cells, and prime T cells and B cells through the release of soluble amplifying factors. The balance of activating and inhibitory signals received by NK cells determines the outcome of interactions with target cells.

# SUMMARY

All specific immune responses start with the introduction of antigen into a host, its recognition, and dendritic cell or macrophage processing. Usually both pathways of immunity, humoral and cell-mediated, are activated. The first includes antibody production by daughter B cells called plasma cells. The second, cell-mediated immunity, involves activated T cells capable of killing virally infected and aberrant target cells and even needed transplanted tissues and organs. The development of either type of immunity

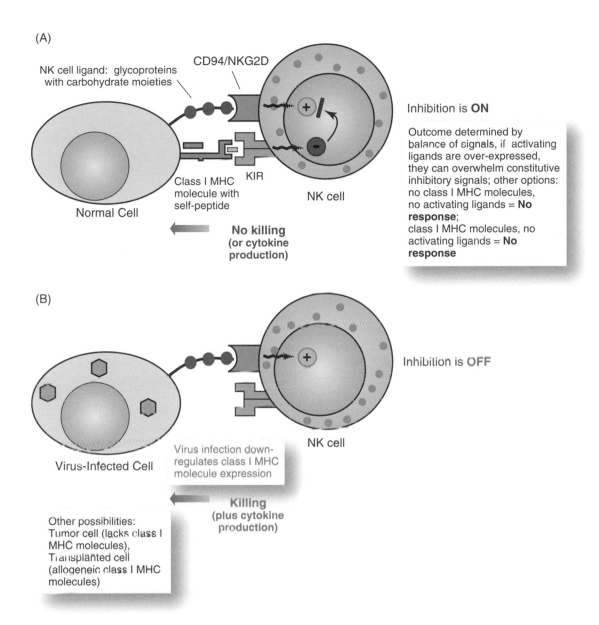

(A)

NK cell ligand: glycoproteins with carbohydrate moieties

CD94/NKG2D

Class I MHC molecule with self-peptide

KIR

Normal Cell

NK cell

**No killing (or cytokine production)**

Inhibition is **ON**

Outcome determined by balance of signals, if activating ligands are over-expressed, they can overwhelm constitutive inhibitory signals; other options: no class I MHC molecules, no activating ligands = **No response**; class I MHC molecules, no activating ligands = **No response**

(B)

Virus-Infected Cell

Virus infection down-regulates class I MHC molecule expression

NK cell

Inhibition is **OFF**

**Killing (plus cytokine production)**

Other possibilities: Tumor cell (lacks class I MHC molecules), Transplanted cell (allogeneic class I MHC molecules)

**FIGURE 10-24 NK cell recognition of target cells.** According to the classical model of NK cell activation, whether a NK cell-mediates killing is determined by the balance of signals received from activating and inhibitory receptors. (**A**) When a NK cell interacts with a normal, autologous target cell it receives activating signals through receptors such as CD94/NKG2D, however, because the target cell expresses the appropriate self-MHC molecules, the NK cell does not lyse the target cell. The inhibitory signal from the bound MHC-binding receptor (KIR) at the NK cell surface is on. (**B**) During viral infections or transformation of cells, the target cells have reduced expression, or an absence, of class I MHC molecules; thus, there is little or no engagement of the KIRs. The NK cell's inhibitory signals are off, leading to lyse of the target cell. In the latter scenario, the NK cell perceives that the target cell is missing self, which reduces the strength of inhibitory signals and thereby facilitates NK cell activation. See text for more details. Abbreviations: killer cell immunoglobulin-like receptors (KIRs); activating NK-cell receptors (CD94/NKG2D); major histocompatibility complex (MHC).

follows a set sequence of events. These events are highly *specific* and lead to antigen removal and, later, immunologic memory for the antigen.

B lymphocytes differentiate from stem cells to *early B cells, progenitor B cells (pro-B cells)*, and *precursor B cells (pre-B cells)* that contain cytoplasmic IgM but do not express stable cell-surface Ig. Early B and pro-B cells are marked by Ig-gene rearrangements. Pre-B cells do not express Fc receptors or C3b receptors. The next stage is represented by immature B cells that express membrane IgM. The appearance of surface Ig signals the beginning of B-cell differentiation, which goes through a series of stages leading to *immature B cells* (express only IgM). At this time, the B cells move to the spleen where they become *mature B cells*, expressing both IgM and IgD. These Ig receptors engage specific antigen but signal transduction occurs through adjacent Igα–Igβ heterodimers.

B-cell activation is initiated by signal transduction events that are prompted by the engagement of the B cell receptor, which leads to the expression of specific genes that translate into functional changes. The signal transduction pathways include signaling through Ig- companioned molecules (Igα–Igβ heterodimers), which are activated by membrane-associated tyrosine kinases (Src kinases), assembled into signaling complexes with protein kinase activity (Btk, BLNK, and PLCγ2), and recruitment of other signal transduction pathways (Rac, Ras, and Rho).

Primary B-cell activation can be amplified by B-cell coreceptor (CD19, CD21, and CD81) participation during antigen cross-linkage of membrane Ig with low concentrations of antigen. Membrane molecules, such as, CD22, can downregulate B-cell activation through protein tyrosine phosphatases docked to CD22 ITIMs that dephosphorylate B-cell receptor complexes.

Immune responses are dominated by interactions and cooperation among three cell types: dendritic cells (and macrophages), T lymphocytes, and B lymphocytes—which may use positive or negative controls. Early experiments showed that successful antibody synthesis required cooperation between T and B cells. The continuing experiments showed that the antibody-producing cell is the B cell and that T cells and B cells recognize different antigenic determinants on the same antigen molecule (the *carrier effect*).

B cells can endocytose and degrade antigen the same way that dendritic cells and macrophages do—the first signal. B-cell antibody receptors act as an antigen capturing-concentrating device but are not directly involved in antigen presentation. B cells present processed antigen to CD4$^+$ effector T$_H$ cells using class II MHC molecules; this plus costimulatory signals activate the T$_H$ cells—the helped, help the helpers. The costimulatory molecules that mediate collaborative signals include T$_H$ cell CD28 and CD40L and B cell B7 and CD40. The T$_H$ cells start to express CD40L, which leads to interaction with B cell CD40—the second signal; the collaborating cells are concomitantly undergoing B7–CD28 interactions, which provides costimulation to T$_H$ cells. They then secrete cytokines that drive B cells to proliferate, differentiate, produce antibody, and form memory cells.

T cells are divided into two subsets: helper T (T$_H$) and cytotoxic T (T$_C$) cells. The "controller" cells are the CD4$^+$ *helper T cells*. T$_H$ cells not only affect B cells but also activate dendritic cells and macrophages and enable T$_C$ cells to respond to antigen. T$_H$ cells that augment B-cell responses to T-dependent antigens can be subdivided into subsets, *T$_H$1, T$_H$2, T$_H$17*, and *T$_{reg}$cells*, based on their functional responses and cytokine production profiles. T$_H$1 cells mediate cell-mediated immunity, while T$_H$2 cells mediate humoral immunity. The new members of the team, T$_H$17 cells, mediate inflammation and autoimmune responses.

CD4$^+$ T$_H$ cell–dendritic cell interactions and CD4$^+$ effector T$_H$ cell–B cell interactions are *MHC-restricted*. T$_H$-cell proliferation is maintained by dendritic cell- and lymphocyte-derived cytokines. The T$_H$ cell–dendritic cell interaction can be regarded as mutually stimulatory. Once activated by interaction with dendritic cell-presented antigen, T$_H$2 cells can go on to collaborate with primed B cells. The different T$_H$ subsets exhibit characteristic cytokine-secretion profiles, which allow them to promote their development and inhibit the development of opposing subsets; this activity is called *cross-regulation*. Surrounding cytokine environment drives the differentiation of T$_H$ subsets. The molecular basis for subset commitment and cross-regulation involves the transcription factors *T-bet, GATA-3, RORγt*, and *FOXP3*. T-bet expression drives naïve T cells to differentiate into T$_H$1 cells and blocks their development along the T$_H$2 pathway. In contrast, GATA3 expression drives naïve T cells into T$_H$2 cells and suppresses their development along the T$_H$1 pathway. RORγt and FOXP3 expression drive the development of T$_H$17 and T$_{reg}$ cells, respectively.

Removal of antigen, a substance that turns on an immune response, downregulates or returns the immune system to a resting state.

Antibodies have a role in controlling immune responses through antigen removal and *antibody feedback*. Soluble IgG molecules mediate this control through enhanced phagocytosis and Fc receptor ligation, respectively.

Antigens can be classified by their ability to trigger antibody synthesis in the presence or absence of T cells (called *T-dependent antigens* and *T-independent antigens*, respectively). Complete B cell differentiation requires interaction with free antigen, B-cell-$T_H$ cell interactions, and $T_H$ cell-derived cytokines.

Cooperation is also required for the development of cellular immunity. The effector cell in cell-mediated immunity is the CD8$^+$ *cytotoxic T ($T_C$) lymphocyte*. These cells kill foreign or virally infected target cells but must recognize the foreign antigen in association with class I MHC molecules. $T_H$-cell help is required in the generation of $T_C$ cells through the *cross-presentation* by, and licensing of, dendritic cells by $T_H$ cells. $T_C$ cells can destroy virally infected cells, allograft cells, and tumor cells directly by **apoptosis** through *granule exocytosis-mediated killing* or *Fas–Fas ligand-mediated killing*. **NK cells** also kill target cells by apoptosis through granule exocytosis but recognize targets differently than $T_C$ cells. Unlike $T_C$ cells, NK cells do not express antigen-specific receptors; they recognize target cells using two different types of receptors: one is called an inhibitory receptor that binds class I MHC molecules and conveys an inhibition signal that counteracts the other receptor called an activating receptor (activates NK cells to kill). Simultaneous ligation of inhibitory and activating receptors blocks killing of target cells. In contrast, binding of activating receptors alone or expression of overwhelming numbers of activating receptors induces NK cells to kill target cells. The expression of class I MHC molecules on normal host cells protects them from NK cell-mediated death.

# SELF-EVALUATION

## RECALLING KEY TERMS

Affinity maturation
Antibody feedback
Apoptosis
B cell-lineage–restricted cells
  Early B cells
  Progenitor B cells (pro-B cells)
  Precursor B cells (pre-B cells)
  Immature B cells
  Mature B cells
  Plasma cells
Capping
Carrier effect

Cell-mediated immunity
Cross-presentation
Cross-regulation
Cytotoxic T ($T_C$) cells
Fas
Fas ligand
Fas–Fas ligand-mediated killing
Granule exocytosis-mediated killing
Helper T ($T_H$) cells
  $T_H$ 1 cells
  $T_H$ 2 cells
  $T_H$ 17 cells
  $T_{reg}$ cells
Humoral immunity
Natural killer (NK) cells
Perforin
Pre-B cell receptor
  Surrogate light chains
    Vpre-B
    $\lambda$ 5
Primary antibody response
Programmed cell death
Thymus (T)-dependent antigens
Thymus (T)-independent antigens
Transcription factors
  FOXP3
  GATA-3
  ROR$\gamma$t
  T-bet

## MULTIPLE-CHOICE QUESTIONS

*(An answer key is not provided, but the page[s] location of the answer is.)*

1. The earliest event in B cell differentiation is (a) the expression of membrane IgD, (b) the expression of membrane IgM, (c) the expression of cytoplasmic $\mu$ chain, (d) $\mu$-chain V-region gene rearrangements, (e) the synthesis of light chains, (f) none of these. *(See page 325.)*

2. The immunologic restoration of lethally irradiated mice can be fully accomplished with syngeneic bone marrow. (a) true, (b) false. *(See page 331.)*

3. Neonatal thymectomized animals have (a) no antibody response, (b) no cell-mediated immune response, (c) a limited antibody response and no cell-mediated immune response, (d) a normal immune response, (e) none of these. *(See page 331.)*

4. In the hapten-carrier complex model, antigen recognition and processing involves (a) T cells binding to the hapten, while B cells respond to the carrier determinant, (b) T and B cells binding to the hapten, (c) T cells binding to the carrier

portion, while B cells respond to the hapten determinant, (d) T and B cells binding to the carrier determinant, (e) none of these. *(See pages 332 and 335.)*

5. In the induction of an immune response, (a) dendritic cell presentation of antigen is necessary to induce $T_H$ cells, (b) T and B cell interactions are initially through MHC molecules, (c) release of cytokines by $T_H$ cells, (d) all of these, (e) none of these. *(See pages 333–341.)*

6. In the immune response, (a) effector $CD4^+$ T cells provide help to B cells after dendritic cell presentation of the antigen, (b) T cells recognize free antigen and respond by providing help to B cells, (c) class I molecules allow immune cells to collaborate with one another, (d) B cells present antigen using their immunoglobulin molecules, (e) none of these. *(See pages 333 and 339.)*

7. B cells serve as APCs to $T_H$ cells. (a) true, (b) false. *(See pages 336 and 337.)*

8. Cytokines can downregulate the cell-mediated immune response by (a) $T_H1$ cell release of IL-4 and IL-10, (b) $T_H2$ cell release of IL-4 and IL-10, (c) $T_H2$ cell release of IFN-$\gamma$, (d) $T_H1$ cell release of IFN-$\gamma$, (e) none of these. *(See pages 345–347.)*

9. The simultaneous binding of membrane antibody and Fc receptors (a) induces B-cell activation, (b) augments B-cell activation, (c) is cytotoxic to the B cell, (d) inhibits B-cell activation, (e) none of these. *(See page 352.)*

10. Which of the following is not true about T-cell-independent antigens? (a) they are usually polysaccharides or LPS with identical units repeated in sequence, (b) they induce only IgM production, (c) they act as polyclonal B-cell mitogens, (d) the antibody response to them is affected by the presence of T cells, (e) none of these. *(See page 353.)*

11. The main proliferating cell in the MLR is the $T_C$ cell. (a) true, (b) false. *(See pages 355 and 356.)*

12. The main effector cell in the MLR is the $T_H$ cell. (a) true, (b) false. *(See pages 355 and 356.)*

13. It takes roughly _____ after antigen contact for pre-$T_C$ cells to differentiate into functional $T_C$ cells. (a) 1 minute, (b) 30 minutes, (c) 24 hours, (d) 2–3 days, (e) 5–10 days. *(See page 357.)*

14. $T_C$ cells mediate death of target cells by stimulating them to express Fas on their membranes. (a) true, (b) false. *(See page 358.)*

15. Natural killer (NK) cells mediate target cell death by: (a) Fas–Fas ligand interaction, (b) being stimulated through carbohydrate-binding receptors, (c) recognizing increased levels of class I MHC molecules, (d) recognizing class II MHC-associated viral peptide, (e) none of the above. *(See pages 361–362.)*

## SHORT-ANSWER ESSAY QUESTIONS

1. Briefly discuss the sequential development of an immune response.

2. List in correct chronological sequence the events leading to the synthesis of $\lambda$ light chains and their incorporation into an antibody molecule (do not forget to include heavy and other light chains).

3. Draw the B-cell signaling pathways induced by membrane-immunoglobulin binding by antigen.

4. Early experiments showing the importance of lymphocytes to immunity followed two approaches. What were they, and how did they differ? What were some of the initial observations that arose from these two approaches?

5. Describe the carrier effect. How did the study of the carrier effect resolve whether T and B cells needed to react specifically with the same epitope on an antigen molecule, and whether T cells and B cells are specific for distinct antigenic determinants on a complex antigen?

6. Show how the fact that B cells can internalize and process antigen resolves the following question: How could $T_H$ cells with one receptor for both an antigen fragment and a class II molecule on the surface of a antigen-presenting cell provide antigen-specific help to a B cell bearing antigen in its antibody receptor?

7. Discuss the molecules that are key to providing the second signal in B-cell activation.

8. Helper T cells can be divided into subsets based on their cytokine secretion profile. Explain.

9. How do dendritic cells contribute to antibody production?

10. Briefly describe cross-regulation between $T_H$ subsets and cytokine production.

11. Describe the transcription factors that are key $T_H$ subset development.

12. As an immune response progresses, it needs to limit itself and decrease in intensity. How does antibody feedback accomplish this?

13. How were the mixed lymphocyte reaction and the cytotoxicity reaction used to explain how T cells helped other T cells, and which cell provided help and which cell mediated cytotoxicity?

**14.** Explain the connection between cross-presentation and licensed dendritic cells.

**15.** Even though T$_C$ and NK cells recognize target cells differently, they mediate death similarly. Explain.

## FURTHER READINGS

Ansel, K.M., I. Djuretic, B. Tanasa, and A. Rao. 2006. Regulation of TH2 differentiation and *Il4* locus accessibility. *Annu. Rev. Immunol.* 24:607–656.

Barry, M., and R.C. Bleackley. 2002. Cytotoxic T lymphocytes: All roads lead to death. *Nat. Rev. Immunol.* 2:401–409.

Basta, S., and A. Alatery. 2007. The cross-priming pathway: A portrait of an intricate immune system. *Scand. J. Immunol.* 65:311–319.

Behrens, G., M. Li, C.M Smith, G.T. Belz, J. Mintern, F.R. Carbone, and W.R. Heath. 2004. Helper T cells, dendritic cells and CTL Immunity. *Immunol. Cell Biol.* 82:84–90.

Bevan, M.J. 2004. Helping the CD8$^+$ T-cell response. *Nat. Rev. Immunol.* 4:1–8.

Busslinger, M. 2004. Transcriptional control of early B cell development. *Annu. Rev. Immunol.* 22:55–79.

Castellino, F., and R.N. Germain. 2006. Cooperation between CD4$^+$ and CD8$^+$ T cells *Annu. Rev. Immunol.* 24:519–540.

Claman, H.N., E.A. Chaperon, and R.F. Triplett. 1966. Thymus-marrow cell combinations. Synergism in antibody production. *Proc. Soc Exp. Biol. Med.* 122:1167–1171.

Dal Porto, J.M., S.B. Gauld, K.T. Merrell, D. Mills, A.E. Pugh-Bernard, and J. Cambier. 2004. B cell antigen receptor signaling 101. *Mol. Immunol.* 41:599–613.

Dong, C. 2006. Diversification of T-helper-cell lineages: Finding the family root of IL-17-producing cells. *Nat. Rev. Immunol.* 6:329–333.

Forster, R., A.C. Davalos-Misslitz, and A. Rot. 2008. CCR7 and its ligands: Balancing immunity and tolerance. *Nat. Rev. Immunol.* 8:362–371.

Hagman, J., and K. Lukin, 2006. Transcription factors drive B cell development. *Curr. Opin. Immunol.* 18:127–134.

Hardy, R.R. 2003. B-lymphocyte development and biology. In *Fundamental Immunology*, 5th ed. W.E. Paul, ed. Philadelphia: Lippincott Williams & Wilkins. p. 159–194.

Henkart, P.A., and M.V. Sitkovsky. 2003. Cytotoxic T lymphocytes. In *Fundamental Immunology*, 5th ed. W.E. Paul, ed. Philadelphia: Lippincott Williams & Wilkins. p. 1127–1150.

Lanzavecchia, A. 1985. Antigen-specific interaction between T and B cells. *Nature* 314:537–539.

Lanier, L.L. 2005. NK cell recognition. *Annu. Rev. Immunol.* 23:225–274.

McHeyzer-Williams, M. 2003. B-cell signaling and activation. In *Fundamental Immunology*, 5th ed. W.E. Paul, ed. Philadelphia: Lippincott Williams & Wilkins. p. 195–226.

Mitchell, G.F., and J.F.P. Miller. 1968. Cell to cell interaction in the immune response. II. The source of hemolysin-forming cells in irradiated mice given bone marrow and thymus or thoracic duct lymphocytes. *J. Exp. Med.* 128:821–837.

Mitchison, N.A. 1971. The carrier effect in the secondary response to hapten-protein conjugates. II. Cellular cooperation. *Eur. J. Immunol.* 1:18–27.

Mosier, D.E. 1967. A requirement for two cell types for antibody formation *in vitro. Science* 158:1573–1575.

Mosmann, T.R., and R.L. Coffman. 1989. TH1 and TH2 cells: Different patterns of lymphokine secretion lead to different functional properties. *Ann. Immunol.* 7:145–173.

Nitschke, L., and T. Tsubata. 2004. Molecular interactions regulate BCR signal inhibition by CD22 and CD72. *Trends Immunol.* 25:543–550.

Reiner, S.L. 2007. Development in motion: Helper T cells at work. *Cell* 129:33–36.

Rock, K.L., and T Shen. 2005. Cross-presentation: Underlying mechanisms and role in immune surveillance. *Immunol. Rev.* 207:166–183.

Romagnani, S. 2006. Regulation of the T cell response. *Clin. Exp. Allergy* 36:1357–1366.

Rothenberg, E.V., and T. Taghon. 2005. Molecular genetics of T cell development. *Annu. Rev. Immunol.* 23:601–649.

Rothenberg, E.V. 2007. Cell lineage regulators in B and T cell development. *Nat. Immunol.* 8:441–444.

Shevach, E.M. 2003. Regulatory/suppressor T cells. In *Fundamental Immunology*, 5th ed. W.E. Paul, ed. Philadelphia: Lippincott Williams & Wilkins. p. 935–964.

Smith, C.M., N.S. Wilson, J. Waithman, J.A. Valladangos, F.R. Carbone, W.R. Heath, and G.T. Belz. 2004. Cognate CD4$^+$ T cell licensing of dendritic cells in CD8$^+$ T cell immunity. *Nat. Immunol.* 5:1143–1148.

Stinchcombe, J.C., and G.M. Griffiths. 2007. Secretory mechanisms in cell-mediated cytotoxicity. *Annu. Rev. Cell Dev. Biol.* 23:495–517.

Vignali, D.A.A., L.W. Collison, and C.J. Workman. 2008. How regulatory T cells work. *Nat. Rev. Immunol.* 8:523–532.

Voskoboinik, I., M.J. Smyth, and J.A. Trapani. 2006. Perforin-mediated target-cell death and immune homeostasis. *Nat. Rev. Immunol.* 6:940–952.

Weaver, C.T., R.D. Hatton, P.R. Mangan, and L.E. Harrington. 2007. IL-17 family of cytokines and the expanding diversity of effector T cell lineages. *Annu. Rev. Immunol.* 25:821–852.

Weiss, A., and L.E. Samelson. 2003. T-lymphocyte activation. In *Fundamental Immunology*, 5th ed. W.E. Paul, ed. Philadelphia: Lippincott Williams & Wilkins. p. 321–364.

Williams, M.A., and M.J. Bevan. 2007. Effector and memory CTL differentiation. *Annu. Rev. Immunol.* 25:171–192.

Ziegler, S.F. 2006. FOXP3: Of mice and men. *Annu. Rev. Immunol.* 24:209–226.

Zuniga-Pflucker, J.C. 2004. T-cell development made simply. *Nat. Rev. Immunol.* 4:67–72.

# CHAPTER ELEVEN

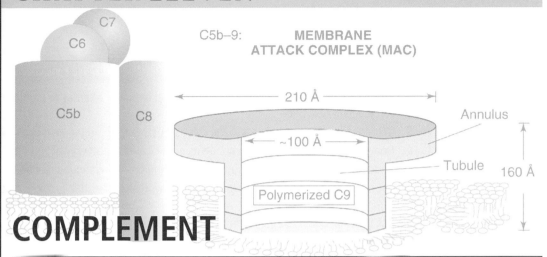

C5b–9:     **MEMBRANE ATTACK COMPLEX (MAC)**

# COMPLEMENT

*Immunology: Understanding the Immune System,  Second Edition*, by Klaus D. Elgert
Copyright © 2009 John Wiley & Sons, Inc.

## OBJECTIVES

The reader should be able to:

1. Define complement.
2. Understand the nomenclature of complement components.
3. Describe some of the unique characteristics and properties of complement.
4. Appreciate the differences between the classical pathway, alternative pathway, and lectin pathway of complement activation.
5. Name the three distinct phases in the classical pathway of complement activation; discuss each phase.
6. Name the biologically active components in the classical pathway of complement activation.
7. Understand why the amplification phase is so important in immune reactions.
8. List the components of the alternative pathway; realize that this pathway and the classical pathway come together at C3.
9. List the components of the lectin pathway; realize that this pathway and the classical pathway come together at C4 and C2.
10. Recognize how complement activation is controlled; name the regulatory proteins.
11. Specify the major sources of complement; comment on the genetic control of complement proteins.

The interactions between antibodies and antigens can lead to precipitation and agglutination, but these reactions have no *in vivo* protective function. One of the three phenomena discussed in this chapter also is an antigen-antibody interaction, but it *activates a complex, potent series of blood enzymes known as the* **complement system**. *This system "complements" the activity of the antibodies in destroying pathogens, either by easing phagocytosis or by puncturing the microbial cell wall.* Activation of the complement system is not limited to induction by only antigen-antibody complexes; the interaction of complement components directly with microbial surfaces or the interaction of mannan-binding lectins (MBLs) with pathogen-associated molecular patterns (PAMPs) (see Chapter 3) activates the complement system. Different molecules can activate the complement system, but many of the components and all of the effectors' functions are identical. The complement system represents a chief part of innate immunity but it also participates in enhancing adaptive immunity. Many attributes of the complement system give the host a powerful auxiliary defense mechanism.

*Complement* is a collective term designating a series of plasma proteins whose activation is responsible for certain aspects of the host defense and for many features of the inflammatory response. Because complement is such a potent inflammatory agent, it is tightly regulated. Complement is not antigen-specific, is activated instantly in the presence of pathogens,

but it also can be activated by antibody; therefore, it is considered part of innate and humoral immunity. The complement system is a bridge between the cellular and humoral immune systems because it entails the production of molecules that influence cellular immune mechanisms, such as enhanced phagocytosis. Complement molecules, constitutively produced by heptocytes and macrophages, circulate in the blood in an inactive form, but activation of the first complement component sets in motion a ripple effect. As each component is activated, it acts in turn on the next component in a precise sequence known as the *complement cascade*. As cleavage fragments are formed, they interact with one another and assemble complex enzymes that link the stages of the reaction sequence. Many of the smaller fragments formed have important immunologic properties that require tight control and that augment the immune response. Follicular dendritic cells express high levels of complement receptor 1 (CR1 [CD35]) and CR2 (CD21), which provide an effective mechanism for retention of C3b-coated immune complexes in germinal centers of B cell follicles. On B cells, CR2, as part of the B cell receptor complex, forms a signaling complex with CD19 and CD81 (see Chapter 10); CR2 binds the complement fragment C3d. The coengagement of C3d-coated antigen with the CD21-CD19-CD81 coreceptor and the B cell receptor increases the sensitivity of the B cell to antigen by as much as a

1000-fold; thereby, lowering the threshold of B cell activation.

Complement molecules have four important activities in the immune response: (1) *cell lysis*—the later complement component complexes disrupt the lipid bilayer of biological membranes, (2) *stimulation of an inflammatory response*—the cleavage products of several complement components regulate the activities of cells and tissues through chemotactic and anaphylatoxic fragments, (3) *opsonization*—several complement component fragments coat target cells (opsonization) to make them more palatable to phagocytic cells, which carry receptors for some complement fragments, and (4) *removal of antigen-antibody (immune) complexes*—complement fragments reduce tissue-damaging immune complexes to small, soluble aggregates while in the circulation and facilitate clearance of circulating immune complexes by the spleen and liver.

Thus, **complement** *is a group of nonimmunoglobulin plasma proteins that are sequentially activated by antigen-antibody complexes, microbial cell-surface molecules, or soluble pattern-recognition receptors such as MBL that bind PAMPs and cause irreversible damage to membranes of cellular targets. Complement proteins also carry out several important functions related to the host's defense mechanisms.*

# SCIENTISTS HAD TO SOLVE A CONUNDRUM: THE FACT THAT SOME *IN VIVO* AND SOME *IN VITRO* INTERACTIONS ARE OPPOSITE

Evidence of the complement system arose from studies in the late 1800s. When mixed with the right bacteria or blood cells *in vitro*, serum from immunized hosts contained antibodies that could agglutinate but not kill the immunizing agents. The anomaly was that the host was protected *in vivo*, yet *in vitro* the antibody did not mediate cell death. However, fresh serum addition to a mixture of specific antibody and antigen often led to death of the bacteria or foreign cells.

Pfeiffer first described the complement system during the 1890s. He found that peritoneal fluid or serum from animals immunized with *Vibrio cholera* lysed the bacteria, but lysis was not observed using body fluids from nonimmune animals. At the same time, Bordet showed that bactericidal activity was lost (without a loss in antibody-binding activity) when

serum was heated to 56°C. Bordet received the 1919 Nobel Prize for his work on complement.

Continuing research on this lytic phenomenon showed that the substance responsible for lysis was actually a complex group of materials. In 1907, data showed that serum dialyzed against water produced two fractions. Neither fraction alone could mediate lysis, but when the fractions were recombined, lytic ability was restored. To characterize the reactions leading to cell death, new experimental model systems were developed. Bordet designed the most successful model system, which included the *in vitro* use of an antigen (sheep red blood cells, SRBC), an antibody (anti-SRBC produced in rabbits), and a source of complement (fresh guinea pig serum). Sensitization (coating with specific antibody) of SRBC, followed by addition of fresh guinea pig serum, led to SRBC lysis.

Years later, workers fractionated fresh serum into several groups of distinct proteins that are specific intermediates of the complement components. These intermediates were reacted with sensitized SRBC and later tested to determine whether the newly isolated complement component would lead to lysis. Mixing and matching each of the newly defined complement molecules from each group showed that proteins from each group were needed for lysis. By 1926, the first four complement components had been described. It was not until 1958 that research groups identified five more complement components. They also showed that some of the complement proteins could be split into subcomponents. In fact, nine distinct complement components working in a precise sequential cascade are required for lysis by the classical pathway. The classical complement pathway is sometimes considered to be made up of 11 components. The three subcomponents of C1 are thought of as individual molecules. The complement system is complicated because it involves nearly 30 plasma and membrane proteins.

Complement components are designated by the letter C. Individual proteins are designated *1* and a numeral corresponding to the sequence in which the protein components are activated. The sequence of activation is C1 to C9, except for C4, which is activated after C1 and before C2 (C1, C4, C2...C9). The reason for this anomaly is that the numbers were assigned before the activation sequence was completely known. C1 consists of three distinct subcomponents designated by C followed by numbers and letters (C1*q*, C1*r*, and C1*s*). Fragments resulting from enzymatic cleavage of components are designated by the name of the component followed by a lowercase letter (for example, C3*a* and C3*b*). The first letters of the alphabet are used for fragments to distinguish them from the subcomponents of C1. Enzymatic components are designated with a horizontal bar over the number of the component (for example, C$\overline{1}$). Complement components formed by joining two or more components that have enzymatic activity also have a bar over the numbers and letters (for example, C$\overline{4b2a}$). Fragments that have lost biologic activity are inactive and have the lowercase letter "i" preceding the abbreviation (for example, iC3b).

# THERE ARE THREE PATHWAYS FOR COMPLEMENT ACTIVATION: ONE BY ANTIGEN-ANTIBODY COMPLEXES, TWO BY MICROBIAL CONSTITUENTS

Activation of the complement cascade occurs through three mechanisms. *The phylogenetically newer pathway, the* **classical pathway**, *is activated by the interaction of certain antibody classes with antigen.* The classical pathway differs from the alternative and lectin pathways in that antigen-antibody interaction (antigen-bound IgM and IgG) activates the early-acting complement components. *The phylogenetically older mechanism is called the* **alternative pathway**. *It is activated by several surface substances, particularly those with repeating units such as those found in the cell walls of bacteria (lipopolysaccharide [LPS] and teichoic acid) and fungi (zymosan) but also nonmicrobial substances like human IgG, IgA, and IgE in complexes and cobra venom factor. The phylogenetically oldest pathway is the* **lectin pathway**, *which is triggered by binding of MBL to microbial repetitive polysaccharide structures, such as, PAMPs.* Through the alternative and lectin pathways of complement activation, complement also participates in innate immunity. Although the origins of the three pathways are different, they converge at the cleavage of C3. The two resulting enzymatic activities can cleave C5, allowing the continuation of the complement cascade. Figure 11-1 presents a simplified flowchart for the three complement pathways.

## Complement Has Some Unique Characteristics and Properties

Complement has several characteristics that are summarized in Table 11-1. Table 11-2 lists some properties of the complement components of the classical, alternative, and lectin pathways and their regulatory molecules. Complement proteins are synthesized

at a constant rate by all normal vertebrate animals. Individuals maintain the complement proteins characteristic of their species. In contrast to antibody levels that increase following natural exposure or immunization by antigen, complement levels do not increase during an immune response. During an immune response, complement is activated by either soluble or insoluble antigen molecules that are bound by antibodies. Complement activation is not limited to antigen-antibody interactions, it can be activated by microbial cell-surfaces (such as LPS from Gram-negative organisms, teichoic acid from Gram-positive organisms, and zymosan from fungal and yeast cells) and sugar moieties on microbial cell-surfaces (such as mannose and N-acetyl glucosamine). However, antigen susceptibility to complement-mediated lysis varies. Erythrocytes, Gram-negative bacteria, enveloped viruses, and lymphocytes are very susceptible to lysis by complement, while Gram-positive bacteria, yeast, molds, and many nucleated mammalian cells are weakly susceptible or nonsusceptible. Nonetheless, complement protects because it leads to increased phagocytosis of these foreign cells. Complement proteins from one species may be activated by antigen-antibody complexes in which the antibodies are of another species. Activation of complement by antibodies from another species has no biologic relevance in the intact host but is important in diagnostic tests. Table 11-3 lists some biologic effects of complement components and activation products.

## MINI SUMMARY

Complement consists of more than 30 distinct serum proteins; some bind antigen-antibody complexes, pathogen cell-surfaces, and microbial cell-surface pathogen-associated molecular patterns (PAMPS), while others control complement activation. When complement interacts with these complexes, it is activated in a sequential, cascade reaction. Complement activation is the result of the assemblage of individual components, each of which activates the next component. When all nine complement (C) components are activated in sequence (C1, C4, C2, C3 to C9), the cascade is complete. This activation can lead to the neutralization of virus, the promotion of phagocytosis, and the lysis of bacteria and other antigenic cells. Three pathways, the classical, the alternative, and the lectin, activate complement components.

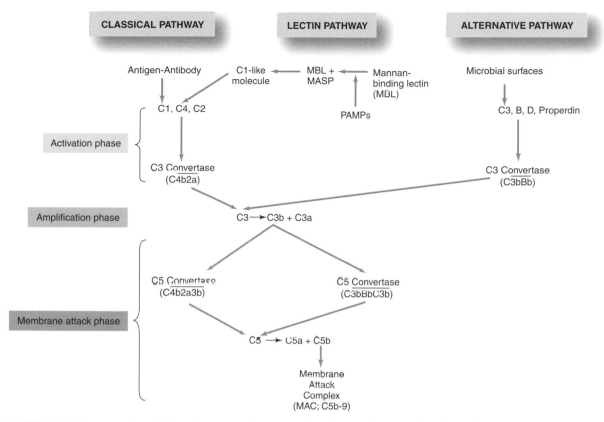

**FIGURE 11-1 An overview of the three complement activation pathways.** The classical pathway is activated by antigen-antibody complexes when C1 binds the antibody in the complex. Activation by this pathway requires the development of humoral immunity against the target antigen. The alternative pathway of activation of the complement system occurs by microbial cell wall materials. No specific antibody is involved and this is a totally nonspecific mechanism of complement activation. It bypasses the first three complement components (C1, C4, and C2) of the classic pathway but meets at C3, like the classic pathway; the remainder of the lectin pathway is the same as the classical pathway. This pathway is part of the innate immune system. The lectin pathway of complement activation, like the alternative pathway, occurs in the absence of antibodies. It is initiated by the binding of plasma protein mannose-binding lectin (MBL) to mannose-containing components of microbial cell walls. The binding of MBL, which is structurally similar to C1q and like C1q, activates the C1r-C1s enzyme complex; it leads to the development C3 convertase activity. The remaining steps are similar to the classical and alternative pathway of complement activation, which leads to formation of the membrane attack complex (MAC). Abbreviations: MASP, MBL-associated serine proteases; PAMPs, pathogen-associated molecular patterns.

## There Are Three Distinct Stages in the Classical Complement Pathway; It Is Initiated by Antigen-Antibody Binding

*The classical pathway cascade can be divided into three stages: (1) initiation, (2) amplification, and (3) membrane attack.* In the **initiation** (or **activation**) **phase**, the complement system recognizes *antigen-antibody complexes*. Because complement is nonspecific, it will react with antigen-antibody complexes displaying IgG or IgM antibodies. Recognition is followed by the generation of proteases from enzymatically inactive complement precursors. These enzymes cleave and activate later complement proteins. This stage generates little protection, but it helps generate later protective

substances. In the next phase, the **amplification phase**, the few protease molecules generated during the initiation phase cause the activation of thousands of C3 molecules. Protection is generated by increased phagocytosis of target substances. The last phase, the **membrane attack phase**, builds a multimolecular complex constructed from the later complement components. These complexes lyse susceptible cells.

### The Activation Phase Involves Components C1, C4, and C2

*C1.* The first event in the activation of the classical complement pathway is the noncovalent binding of **C1** to sites on the Fc region of IgG- and IgM-antigen

**TABLE 11-1 The Complement System**

1. Complement of the classical pathway is not one substance but nine proteins or *components* (C1 through C9). In fact, the complement system (classical and alternative pathways) encompasses 25 plasma glycoproteins, plus 7 more plasma control proteins and 4 more cell membrane control proteins.
2. Complement proteins are not immunoglobulins.
   a. Complement components do not share antigenic determinants with immunoglobulins.
   b. They are α- and β-globulins.
3. Complement proteins must be *activated*. They ordinarily exist in a biologically inactive form.
   a. Activation is *sequential*. Proteins of the complement system become activated in a fixed sequence. One becomes activated and activates the next protein in the sequence. Therefore, complement activation is a *cascade* mechanism.
   b. Activation of complement (or complement fixation) is followed by inactivation.
4. Three pathways can activate complement.
   a. *Classical pathway*: Complement proteins are activated by antigen-antibody complexes when C1q binds in the complex. IgM- or IgG1-, IgG2-, or IgG3-antigen complexes can initiate the classical pathway. Activation of this pathway requires the development of humoral immunity against the target antigen.
   b. *Alternative pathway*: Activation of the complement system is by microbial cell wall materials. No specific antibody is involved, although aggregated IgA can activate complement through the alternative pathway. This pathway is a completely nonspecific mechanism of complement activation; therefore, it can mediate innate immunity.
   c. *Lectin pathway*: Activation of this pathway requires the synthesis of the soluble pattern-recognition receptor mannose-binding lectin (MBL) in the liver in response to macrophage cytokines. MBL and MBL-associated serine proteases (MASPs) function like C1 to cleave and activate C4 and C2 to form a C3 convertase activity. Like the alternative pathway, the lectin pathway does not use antibody (mediates innate immunity); however, like the classical pathway, lectin pathway uses C4 and C2 to form C3 convertase.

complexed antibodies. C1 is in serum as a macromolecular (750 kD) assembly of three noncovalently bound glycoproteins, **C1q, C1r,** and **C1s.** They are in a molar ratio of 1:2:2 ($C1qr_2s_2$). C1 subunits are held together in the presence of ionic calcium. The C1q subcomponent binds to an antigen-antibody complex by the $C_H2$ domains of two adjacent IgG antibodies bound to antigen or by the $C_H3$ domain of a single, nonadjacent IgM antibody molecule bound to antigen. C1q binding with the different IgG subclasses varies in efficiency. In humans, the four IgG subclasses' order of ability to bind complement (C1q) is

$IgG_3 > IgG_1 > IgG_2 > IgG_4$. C1q consists of 18 chains in three chain types (A, B, and C chains) with six copies of each per molecule (6A, 6B, and 6C). Figure 11-2 schematically depicts C1q.

C1r and C1s are made up of similar polypeptide chains and form a $C1r_2s_2$ complex, which exists in two arrangements. In its free unattached form, $C1r_2s_2$ assumes a rod-like S-shaped molecule. Its other arrangement occurs when $C1r_2s_2$ attaches to C1q, where it wraps around the arms of C1q and promotes interaction with C1q or each other. C1r and C1s are proenzymes that become active serine proteases after the C1q terminal globular heads bind bivalently to antigen-complexed antibody (Figure 11-3). Monovalent binding of C1q to free IgG triggers dissociation before activation of C1r and C1s. If C1q binds two or more adjacent IgG molecules, the binding constants increase and the C1q-2IgG complex remains associated long enough to activate the C1r and C1s proenzymes. Thus, C1 activation by IgG occurs only when IgG is part of an antigen-antibody complex.

C1 activation by IgM-antigen complexes is different. Single IgM molecules bound to antigen can fix complement, but C1q binding sites on IgM are unavailable when IgM is free in solution. Binding of C1q to free IgM shows a low binding constant. The binding half-life, which is only a few seconds, is not long enough to activate C1r and C1s. By a still incompletely understood mechanism, conformational changes occur after antigen-binding that expose binding sites for C1q globular heads, allowing bivalent attachment between two monomers of IgM. This attachment allows activation of C1r and C1s.

The mechanism of C1 activation is not completely known (Figure 11-4). Cleavage of the single-chain C1r protein generates a large amino-terminal peptide disulfide linked to a smaller carboxyl-terminal fragment. The smaller fragment bears the enzymatic site for C1r cleavage. The substrate for $\overline{C1r}$ is C1s. $\overline{C1r}$ cleaves C1s to activate this subcomponent by conversion of the single-chain protein to a disulfide-linked heterodimer. Binding and activation of C1 (C1 or $\overline{C1qrs}$ complex) leads to a protease enzyme with trypsin-like activity (cleaves lysine, arginine, or tyrosine) called *C1 esterase*. The natural substrate for C1 or $\overline{C1s}$ is the next two complement components of the sequence, C4 and C2 (in that order).

*C4.* The second component in the complement cascade is **C4.** It is a three-chain glycoprotein. The three chains are called α, β, and γ. $\overline{C1s}$ cleaves a 77-amino-acid-long piece from the amino-terminal end of the α chain (Figure 11-5). Cleavage of C4 (and

**TABLE 11-2** **Properties of Complement Components**

| Component | Plasma concentration (μg/ml) | Activation product | Molecular weight (kD) | Chain structure |
|---|---|---|---|---|
| | | CLASSICAL PATHWAY *Initiation Phase* | | |
| C1q | 150 | | 460 | 6 × 3 chains |
| C1r | 50 | C1r | 85 | 1 chain |
| C1s | 50 | C1s | 85 | 1 chain |
| C4 | 300 | | 205 | α, β, γ |
| | | C4a | 8 | |
| | | C4b | 200 | |
| C2 | 20 | | 102 | 1 chain |
| | | C2a | 70 | |
| | | C2b | 30 | |
| | | *Amplification Phase* (common to the classical and alternative pathways) | | |
| C3 | 1200 | | 185 | α, β |
| | | C3a | 9 | |
| | | C3b | 185 | α', β |
| | | IC3b | 176 | |
| | | C3d, g | 41 | |
| | | C3c | 145 | |
| | | C3d | 33 | |
| | | C3g | 8 | |
| | | *Membrane Attack Phase* (common to the classical and alternative pathways) | | |
| C5 | 80 | | 190 | α, β |
| | | C5a | 11 | |
| | | C5b | 180 | |
| C6 | 45 | | 110 | 1 chain |
| C7 | 90 | | 100 | 1 chain |
| C8 | 55 | | 150 | α, β, γ |
| C9 | 60 | | 70 | 1 chain |
| | | ALTERNATIVE PATHWAY | | |
| Factor B | 200 | | 93 | 1 chain |
| | | Ba | 30 | |
| | | Bb | 63 | |
| Factor D | 2 | D | 24 | 1 chain |
| Properdin | 25 | | 110–200 | 3 chains |
| | | LECTIN PATHWAY | | |
| MBL | 0.05–3 | ? | 200–600 | 2-6 subunits (1 subunit = 3 chains, each 32 kD) |
| MASP-1 | 2–12 | ? | 100 | |
| MASP-3 | ? | | 42 | |
| MASP-2 | ? | | 76 | |
| sMAP/Map19 | ? | | 19 | |

*(continued overleaf)*

**TABLE 11-2** *(Continued)*

| Component | Plasma concentration (μg/ml) | Activation product | Molecular weight (kD) | Chain structure |
|---|---|---|---|---|
| | | REGULATORY MOLECULES | | |
| *In Plasma* | | | | |
| Anaphylatoxin inactivator | 35 | | 310 | |
| C1-INH | 240 | | 105 | 1 chain α |
| C4b-BP | 250 | | 550 | 7 identical α chains, 1 β chain |
| Factor H | 300–450 | | 150 | 1 chain |
| Factor I | 35 | | 88 | α, β |
| S protein | 500 | | 84 | 1 chain |
| SP-40,40 | 50 | | 70 | 2 chains |
| | | *On Cell Membrane* | | |
| CR1 (CD35) | | | 190–280 | 1 chain |
| DAF (CD55) | | | 70 | 1 chain |
| MCP (CD46) | | | 45–70 | 1 chain |
| MIRL (CD59) | | | 18–20 | 1 chain |

Abbreviations: C1-INH, C1 inhibitor; CR1, complement receptor 1; DAF, decay-accelerating factor; MCP, membrane cofactor protein; MIRL, membrane inhibitor of reactive lysis.

**TABLE 11-3** Biologic Properties of Complement Components and Activation Products

| Complement component | Activity |
|---|---|
| C4a | Some anaphylatoxin activity (induction of histamine release from mast cells and basophils leading to vasodilation and smooth muscle contraction) |
| C4b | Opsonization (enhanced phagocytosis) |
| C3a | Anaphylatoxin activity (degranulation of mast cells, basophils, and eosinophils) Aggregation of platelets |
| C3b | Opsonization (enhanced phagocytosis) Inhibits immune complex formation Promotes clearance of immune complexes Viral neutralization |
| C3c | Release of neutrophils from bone marrow |
| C5a | Anaphylatoxin activity Chemotaxis of neutrophils Immune adherence to vascular endothelium through specific macrophage receptors |
| Bb | Migration inhibition Induction of monocyte and macrophage spreading (nonspecific) |
| C5b-9 (membrane-attack complex [MAC]) | Membrane damage (lysis of target cell) Viral neutralization |

C2) occurs in the plasma near the $\overline{\text{C1s}}$ catalytic site. *The small molecule, termed* **C4a**, *has anaphylatoxin activity.* **Anaphylatoxins** *are hormone-like peptides, which bind to complement receptors on mast cells and basophils signaling their degranulation (releasing histamine) that induce smooth muscle contraction, trigger vasoactive amine release, and enhance vascular permeability.* The remainder of C4 (called **C4b**) binds to antigen by covalent linkage of amino or carboxyl groups to reactive groups in C4 molecules that are generated by splitting of a thioester bond in the α chain. The clusters of C4b that bind to the cell membrane near the antibody-$\overline{\text{C1qrs}}$ complex continue the complement cascade. Some C4b molecules can react with specific host cell receptors that recognize C4b. In fact, the "simple" binding of C4b to certain substances may directly change their biologic activity. For example, certain viruses are neutralized because C4b molecules bind to them and prevent their attachment to host cells.

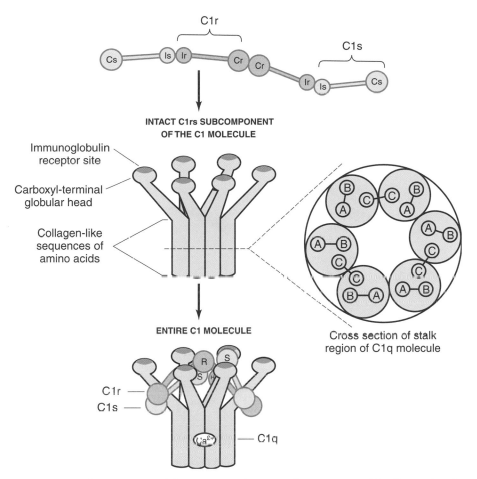

**FIGURE 11-2  The structure of the C1q complement subcomponent.** The C1q molecule consists of 18 polypeptide chains arranged in three subunits of six chains each. Each subunit is held together at the stem, forming a Y-shaped-like structure ending in a globular head. The globular heads contain the receptors for immunoglobulin attachment. Because there are six globular regions, each C1q molecule, by assuming a figure-eight form, can bind six $C_H2$ domains or up to six different IgG molecules. This multiple C1q-antibody binding determines the firmness of binding. The arms are collagen-like triple helical units. Rich in glycine, hydroxyproline, and hydroxylysine, C1q resembles collagen. Collagen-like regions bind the two other C1 subcomponents, consisting of two C1r and two C1s components.

*C2.* The third component in the complement cascade is **C2**. It is a single-chain peptide (Figure 11-6). C2 is cleaved by $\overline{C1s}$ into two fragments, **C2a** and **C2b**. In the presence of $Mg^{2+}$ ions, the bound C4b interacts with the carboxyl-terminal C2a fragment to continue the cascade. *The enzyme activity of $\overline{C4b2a}$ complex is called **C3 convertase** because C3 convertase can cleave and interact with C3. C3 convertase continues the complement cascade.* In the $\overline{C4b2a}$ complex, C4 functions only to anchor the complex to the cell membrane; it has no enzymatic function. In contrast, C2 acts as an enzyme in the hydrolytic activation of C3. After $\overline{C4b2a}$ is formed, the earlier-reacting complement components are no longer needed to continue the complement cascade. The enzymatic site of $\overline{C4b2a}$ resides on the C2a part of the complex. The C4b molecule of the $\overline{C4b2a}$ complex binds to the C3 molecule to make it more accessible to C2a cleavage. C3 convertase ($\overline{C4b2a}$), an unstable enzyme, undergoes rapid decay; it has a half-life of 5 min at 37°C. The short half-life is caused by the physical loss and decay of C2a from C4b into a fluid phase as an enzymatically inactive fragment (C2d). However, the C4b remaining on the cell can bind another C2 molecule that, on splitting by C1, will again form the bimolecular $\overline{C4b2a}$ complex (C3 convertase). These early steps (antigen-antibody

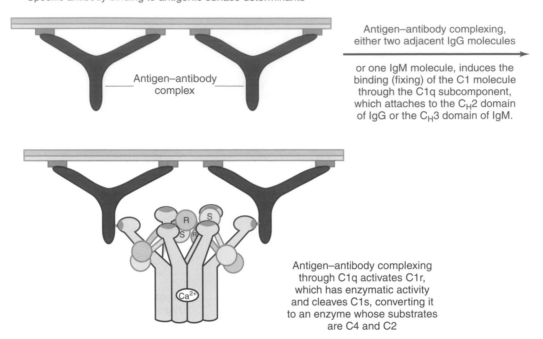

Specific antibody binding to antigenic surface determinants

Antigen–antibody complex

Antigen–antibody complexing, either two adjacent IgG molecules

or one IgM molecule, induces the binding (fixing) of the C1 molecule through the C1q subcomponent, which attaches to the $C_H2$ domain of IgG or the $C_H3$ domain of IgM.

Antigen–antibody complexing through C1q activates C1r, which has enzymatic activity and cleaves C1s, converting it to an enzyme whose substrates are C4 and C2

**FIGURE 11-3 Initiation of the complement cascade—C1 activation**. The complement cascade starts with a pair of adjacent IgG molecules that bind to a protein antigen (here a cell-surface antigen). The antigen-antibody complex causes the exposure of a complement receptor in the $C_H2$ domain of IgG, allowing C1q to bind to two adjacent IgGs or to the $C_H3$ domain of a single IgM. This causes the folding of the rod-like $C1r_2s_2$ around the arms of C1q, causing the C1r (R) and C1s (S) catalytic domains to contact one another. Binding activates the complement cascade.

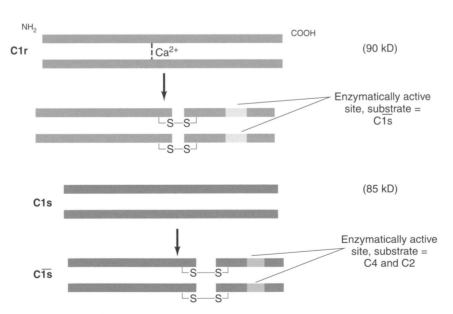

NH$_2$          COOH

**C1r**          Ca$^{2+}$          (90 kD)

Enzymatically active site, substrate = C1s

(85 kD)

**C1s**

**C1̄s**

Enzymatically active site, substrate = C4 and C2

**FIGURE 11-4 C1 activation—Cleavage of C1r and C1s**. Binding of two IgG molecules to antigen causes a conformational change that is transmitted to C1r. C1r changes to reveal an enzymatic site which cleaves a peptide bond in C1s. C1s is converted into an enzymatic molecule (C1̄s).

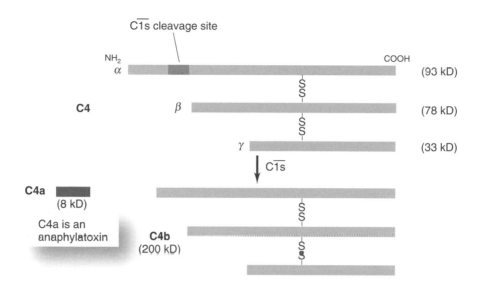

**FIGURE 11-5 C4 activation—Cleavage of C4.** C4 is cleaved by activated $\overline{C1s}$, leading to two molecules, C4a (anaphylatoxin) and C4b. The C4b molecule binds to the antigen surface near the C1 molecule and acts as an anchor for the complex $\overline{C4b2a}$.

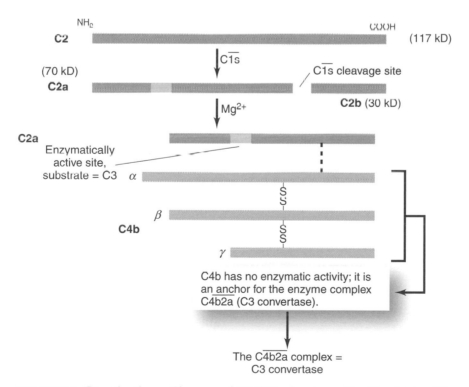

**FIGURE 11-6 C2 activation—Cleavage of C2.** C2 is also cleaved by C1, which splits it into C2a and C2b. C2a binds to C4b to generate the enzymatic complex C4b2a. This molecule can cleave C3 and is therefore called *C3 convertase*.

**CLEAVAGE OF C4**

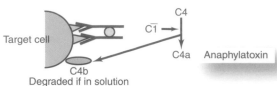

Target cell

C4b
Degraded if in solution

C4a    Anaphylatoxin

**CLEAVAGE OF C2**

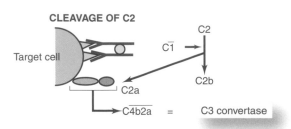

Target cell

C2b

C2a

$\overline{C4b2a}$  =  C3 convertase

**FIGURE 11-7 Summary of the activation phase.** Formation of antibody complexes with cellular antigens activates $\overline{C1}$, which cleaves C4 into C4a and C4b. C4b binds to antigen after C1 cleaves C2 into C2a and C2b, and C2a binds to C4b to form the enzymatic complex $\overline{C4b2a}$ (C3 convertase).

complexing with activation of C1, C4, and C2 of the classical complement pathway) finish the initiation phase of the reaction (Figure 11-7).

---

## MINI SUMMARY

The classical pathway of complement activation starts with the binding of C1q to the antibody of an antigen-antibody complex. C1 is a $Ca^{2+}$-dependent union of three subcomponents: (1) C1q, which activates (2) C1r, and then (3) C1s, a serine protease that goes on to attack C4 and then C2. C4 is split by $\overline{C1s}$ into C4a (small) and C4b (large) fragments. C2 is the third component of the pathway and is also split by C1s into C2b (small) and C2a (large) fragments. C4b and C2a then join and attach to the antigen-antibody complex, forming C3 convertase ($\overline{C4b2a}$). C4a is an anaphylatoxin.

---

### The Amplification Phase Involves Only C3

The amplification phase of the complement cascade is so called because one antigen-antibody complex can generate several C3 convertases. The C3 component is the natural substrate for C3 convertase. Each C3 convertase can cleave hundreds to thousands of C3 molecules into C3a and C3b. The latter molecule

---

is deposited on the microbe surface and recognized by complement receptors on phagocytic cells. *Enhanced phagocytosis is the most important action of complement.*

**C3.** The third component of complement, **C3**, is the fourth in the reaction sequence and is the most important of the complement system. C3 is:

1. the most abundant complement component in plasma (1 to 2 mg/ml);
2. the converging point for the classical, alternative, and lectin complement pathways;
3. capable of forming a covalent linkage with the target of complement activation;
4. associated with impaired host resistance to bacterial infection when the host has a genetic deficiency of C3; and
5. cleaved into fragments that can bind to different receptors residing on cells participating in inflammatory and immunologic reactions (Table 11-4).

Human C3 is a globular glycoprotein that consists of an α chain and a β chain. C3 convertase cleaves a 77-amino-acid-long fragment from the amino-terminal end of the α chain.[1] *smaller fragment,* **C3a,** *is an anaphylatoxin.* The larger fragment, **C3b,** remains covalently linked by disulfide bonds to the β chain. The cleavage of C3 to C3a and C3b, like C4, exposes an internal thioester in the α polypeptide of the C3b molecule (Figure 11-8). Cleaved C3 can interact covalently with cell surfaces. Most of the C3b molecules fail to attach to the cell membrane and are degraded in solution, but several hundred bind to the cell surface near the $\overline{C4b2a}$ attachment site. C3b molecules are arranged radially around the site. The binding of C3b-coated antigen to surfaces such as blood vessel walls is called **immune adherence.** It makes the particulate antigen easy prey for circulating phagocytic cells. The coating of particulate antigens by C3b also allows for binding of C3b receptor (CR1)-bearing cells (see Table 11-4). If the interacting cells are neutrophils, monocytes, or macrophages, phagocytosis will be enhanced. This enhancement is called **opsonization.** CR2, CR3, and CR4 bind to the inactive forms of C3b that remain attached to the microbe surface, thereby stimulating phagocytosis.

---

[1]Even though C3 activation does not stop here, it is not discussed further. Briefly, however, C3f is removed from C3b to form iC3b. Then iC3b is changed to C3dg and C3c. C3dg can be cleaved into C3d and C3g. iC3b also can be lysed by kallikrein, a vasodilator, to give C3dk.

**TABLE 11-4 Receptors for Complement Fragments**

| Receptor | Ligands | Cellular distribution |
|---|---|---|
| Complement receptor Type 1 (CR1, C3b receptor, CD35) | C3b and C4b | Erythrocytes, eosinophils, neutrophils, monocytes, macrophages, B cells, some T cells, follicular dendritic cells |
| Complement receptor Type 2 (CR2, C3d receptor, CD21) | C3dg, C3d, iC3b, Epstein-Barr virus | B cells, follicular dendritic cells, nasopharyngeal epithelial cells |
| Complement receptor Type 3 (CR3, iC3b receptor, Mac-1, CD11bCD18) | iC3b | Neutrophils, NK cells, monocytes, macrophages, follicular dendritic cells |
| Complement receptor Type 4 (CR4, p150,95, CD11cCD18) | iC3b | Neutrophils, monocytes, macrophages, platelets |
| C3a/C4a receptor | C3a, C4a | Basophils, granulocytes, mast cells |
| C5a receptor | C5a | Basophils, granulocytes, mast cells, monocytes, macrophages, platelets, and endothelial cells |

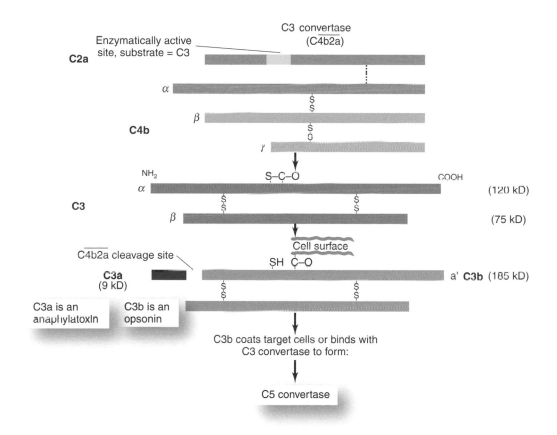

**FIGURE 11-8 The amplification phase—C3 activation.** The amplification phase starts with cleavage of C3 by C3 convertase. C3a and C3b are released. C3a has anaphylatoxin activity. The C3b molecule is the biologically active form of C3, and it starts the remainder of the pathway. C3b can act as an opsonin, thereby enhancing immune adherence and leading to increased phagocytosis of the antigen by phagocytic cells. C3b also leads to the solubilization of trapped immune complexes and to the clearance of circulating immune complexes. C3b can also bind with C3 convertase (C4b2a) to form C5 convertase.

C3b molecules also contribute to the removal of immune complexes (1) by binding to immunoglobulin and thereby interfering with immune complex formation (keeps complexes in small soluble aggregates) and (2) by promoting the clearance of C3b-coated, soluble immune complexes bound to C3b receptor-bearing erythrocytes. These complexes are cleared from circulation by phagocytic cells as they pass through the liver and spleen.

The complement component needed to continue the complement cascade is C5. Activation of C5 happens when another region of the C3b molecule allows the C3b molecules to attach to the $\overline{\text{C4b2a}}$ complex (C3 convertase) and form a trimolecular complex, $\overline{\text{C4b2a3b}}$. This complex is called **C5 convertase**, cleaving C5 into C5a and C5b (Figure 11-9).

---

## MINI SUMMARY

C3 is the central component of all complement reactions and is the only component in the amplification phase. During the amplification phase (1) C3 convertase cleaves hundreds to thousands of C3 molecules; (2) C3a molecules (anaphylatoxins) induce the release of mediators from mast cells; (3) C3b molecules coat target cells to promote immune adherence, opsonization, and solubilization and clearance of immune complexes; and (4) C3b molecules bind to C3 convertase ($\overline{\text{C4b2a}}$) to form a new enzyme called C5 convertase ($\overline{\text{C4b2a3b}}$).

---

### The Membrane Attack Phase Involves Components C5b, C6, C7, C8, and C9

*Activation of C5 leads to the sequential interaction of the remaining complement molecules and their assembly into an endpoint macromolecular structure called the* **membrane attack complex** (**MAC**). This fusion of the terminal complement components starts at hydrophobic sites through which the MAC inserts itself into the lipid bilayer of bacteria or eukaryotic cells. The insertion of the MAC leads to the formation of transmembrane channels. These channels permit the exchange of small molecules and ions as well as water, which enter the cell, causing it to swell and burst.

***C5, C6, C7, C8, and C9.*** Formation of the MAC starts with the activation of **C5**, a molecule consisting of two disulfide-linked chains, $\alpha$ and $\beta$. C5 is activated when a small polypeptide splits off from the amino-terminus of the $\alpha$ chain (Figure 11-10). Two biologically active fragments are formed, **C5a** and **C5b**. The smaller C5a molecule exhibits anaphylatoxin and chemotactic activity, increases neutrophil adhesiveness through increased CR1 and CR3 expression, stimulates neutrophil oxidative metabolism, induces IL-1 production by macrophages and induces mast cells to release mediators with similar activities. In fact, of the three anaphylatoxins C4a, C3a, and C5a, C5a is the most biologically active. The C5b fragment is unstable and short-lived (2.3 min at 37°C). During the cleavage reaction, C5b acquires both a site for attachment to the target cell membrane and sites for

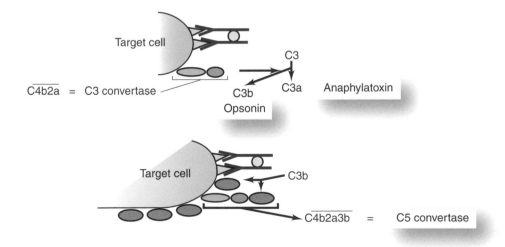

**FIGURE 11-9 Summary of the amplification phase.** C3 convertase ($\overline{\text{C4b2a}}$) cleaves C3 into C3a and C3b. The cleaving of C3 is the most abundant reaction (amplification phase) of the classical complement pathway. C3a is an anaphylatoxin. An internal thioester bond is exposed on the C3b molecule, causing it to bind near C3 convertase. The new complex $\overline{\text{C4b2a3b}}$ is an enzyme called *C5 convertase.*

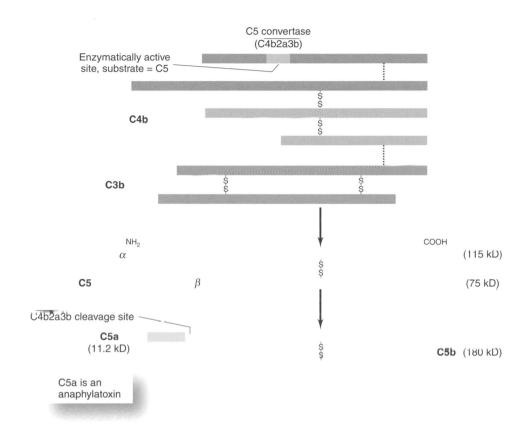

**FIGURE 11-10 C5 activation—Cleavage of C5.** The C5 molecule is cleaved by C5 convertase into C5a and C5b. C5a is an anaphylatoxin. C5b binds to the antigen and provides the attachment site for intact C6 and C7.

the binding of C6 and C7. C5b can bind to C6 and C7 either in solution or when membrane-bound. If the fluid-phase C5b67 complex is deposited on "innocent bystander" cells, they may be lysed without the earlier complement components. The phenomenon is known as *reactive lysis*. The primary attack mechanism, however, depends on the deposit of C5b on the membrane near the C5 convertase (C4b2a3b) attachment site. When C5b binds C6, it forms the stable C5b6 complex.

The **C6** and **C7** molecules are similar: each consists of one polypeptide chain. The stable, hydrophilic, bimolecular C5b6 complex is loosely bound to C5 convertase until it binds C7 and exposes hydrophobic binding regions for phospholipid. The C5b67 complex is then endowed with a membrane-binding site. This complex constitutes the receptor for C8.

The **C8** component is a peculiar molecule because of its structure and its resistance to irreversible denaturation. It consists of three nonidentical polypeptide chains. The $\alpha$ and $\beta$ chains are covalently linked, but the $\gamma$ chain is noncovalently associated with the other two. When C5b67 binds with C8, it processes C8 so

that the C8$\alpha$ chain can enter the membrane of the target cell. The C5b678 complex has limited lytic activity. It can lyse erythrocytes but is unable to lyse nucleated cells, which endocytose a "puncture wound" and repair the damage unless there are multiple wounds. With C5b678 formation, the C8 part of the molecule binds C9 and nonenzymatically catalyzes C9 polymerization. **C9** consists of one polypeptide chain. The polymerization of C9 leads to the strong attachment of tubular poly C9 to the polymerizing unit C5b678. The C5b-9 organization is the *membrane attack complex (MAC)* that creates the large complement channels. The size and composition of the MAC are heterogeneous because multiple copies of C9 can be incorporated in C5b - 9. In fact, the MAC is arranged according to the formula $C5b_1, C6_1, C7_1, C8_1, C9_n$, where $n$ can vary from 10 to 16. The C5b - 8 complex concentrates C9 on its surface and thereby eases its polymerization. It is called *poly-C9*, when the MAC contains between 12 and 15 C9 molecules associated with one C5b - 8 complex. The MAC now forms pores in the target cell membrane. How the C5b - 8 complex catalyzes the self-association of C9 is unknown, but there is

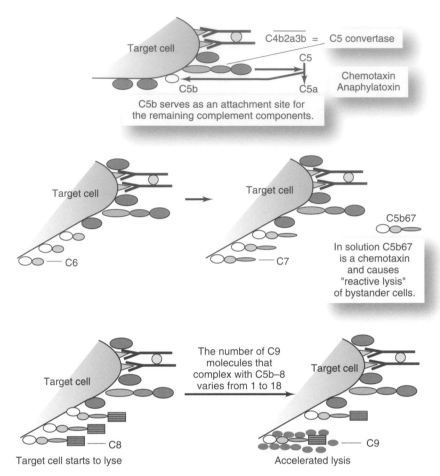

**FIGURE 11-11 Summary of the membrane attack phase.** Following the cleaving of C5 by C5 convertase into C5a and C5b, the C5b molecule attaches to antigen, providing an anchor for intact C6 and C7 to bind to. The C5b67 complex interacts with C8, forming the next complex, C5b678. This complex mediates some of the lytic effect on the cellular antigen membrane. C5b678 also causes the polymerization of C9 to form holes in the membrane. The C9 complex is called the *membrane attack complex* (see Figure 11-12).

no doubt that the electron microscopic image of the cylinder-like, complement-induced membrane lesion is elicited by poly C9. Figure 11-11 summarizes the membrane attack phase.

The doughnut model of MAC-mediated cell lysis is so-called because the MACs appear as doughnuts or ringed pores when viewed in electron micrographs. These channels or pores traverse the target cell membrane and permit osmotic leakage from the cell. The lesion results when the MAC contains a hydrophilic protein transmembrane channel. Figure 11-12 schematically depicts how the MAC acts through the doughnut model.

After C8 binding, circular lesions (about 110 Å in diameter) start to appear on the target cell membrane. The MAC ($\overline{C5b-9}$) disrupts the phospholipid arrangement in the cell membrane through a detergent-like attack. Hydrophobic sites on $\overline{C5b-9}$ interact with nonpolar (hydrophobic) parts of the membrane phospholipids. The integrity of the membrane surrounding the MAC is disrupted because phospholipids associate with the complex rather than with other phospholipids in the outer layer of the membrane. Funnel-shaped transmembrane hydrophilic or polar channels are formed. These channels allow small molecules and ions to leak out of the cell and allow water to go in, so that cells are killed and lysed by osmotic shock. The circular lesions are multimolecular MACs surrounded by rearranged phospholipids. These lesions are similar to the larger diameter (160 Å) perforin pores caused by $T_C$ cells and NK cells. Gram-negative bacteria and enveloped viruses are susceptible to complement-mediated lysis.

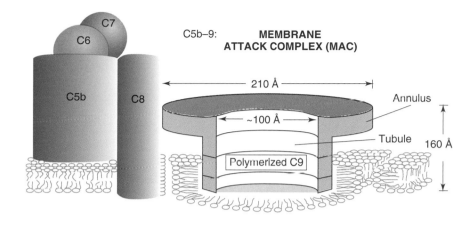

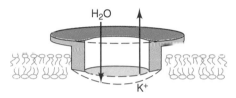

The central channel of the MAC allows small molecules to diffuse freely; thus, the cell cannot maintain osmotic stability. The influx of water and loss of electrolytes kills the cell.

**FIGURE 11-12 Complement-mediated membrane damage caused by the membrane attack complex.** Poly C9 of the membrane attack complex is an 160-Å tubule, with 120 Å extending above the surface of the membrane. The inner diameter of the cylinder is 110 Å. The cylinder ends at its external, hydrophilic end in a 30-Å thick annulus (a thick rim) that has an outer diameter of 210 Å. The 50- to 140-Å-wide, elongated C5b - 8 subunit is attached to the poly C9 and extends about 180 Å above C9's annulus. The length of the membrane attack complex is about 340 Å, with 300 Å above the membrane surface. The funnel-shaped lesion caused by the membrane attack complex (C5b-9) disrupts the lipid bilayer enough to allow the free exchange of water and electrolytes. The entrance of water and $Na^+$ into the cell eventually leads to lysis.

## MINI SUMMARY

The membrane attack mechanism involves C5 through C9. C5 is a protein that is split by C5 convertase (C4b2a3b) into C5a (small) and C5b (large) fragments. C5a is an anaphylatoxin and a chemoattractant that also can activate neutrophil oxidative metabolism. C5b starts the assembly of one molecule each of C6, C7, and C8 and up to 16 molecules of C9 into the MAC. This complex creates a channel through the cell membrane allows small molecules and ions to leak out of the cell and water to flow in. Cells are killed and lysed by osmotic shock.

## There Are Also Distinct Stages in the Alternative Complement Pathway; It Is Initiated by Microbial Surfaces in the Absence of Antibodies

In 1954, Louis Pillemer described a *mechanism of activation for the complement system in the absence of antigen-antibody reactions. This alternative mechanism or pathway of complement activation was designated the* **alternative pathway** *and generates both soluble and membrane-bound C3 convertases to cleave C3.* Because antibody is not needed, this mechanism of complement activation is nonspecific and considered a form of innate immunity.

Pillemer mixed zymosan, a yeast cell wall polysaccharide, with fresh serum, a complement source. This zymosan-treated serum was no longer able to lyse a susceptible cell reacted with specific antibody. Similar results were seen with several other microbial polysaccharides. Closer examination of the alternative pathway revealed that the C3 through C9 components were activated by zymosan but C1, C4, and C2 were not. Pillemer called this alternative mechanism the *properdin system*.

In the 1960s, each component of the classical complement pathway was purified, and *functional assays* for each component were developed. These functional assays led to the rediscovery of the properdin or alternative pathway. Using functional assays, scientists showed that some humans and animals lack C1, C4, or C2. Therefore, these individuals should be susceptible to bacterial infections because the sequence of complement reactions is stopped before much protection is generated. However, these individuals appeared normal. Thus, either (1) complement is not important in protection or (2) another mechanism exists to activate C3 through C9. In 1967, different groups described an alternative mechanism for complement activation, the details of which later revealed that this alternative pathway is the properdin system described by Pillemer.

Activation of the alternative pathway can be started by Gram-negative bacterial endotoxins or bacterial products such as dextrans and levans, complex microbial and plant polysaccharides such as zymosan and inulin, rabbit erythrocytes, human erythrocyte stroma, aggregated human IgA, and aggregated $F(ab')_2$ fragments of guinea pig $IgG_1$. Human IgG and IgM do not activate the alternative pathway. Even though some human antibodies can activate the alternative pathway, they are not required for this activation, as they are for activation of the classical pathway. The importance of the alternative complement pathway is that it amplifies the effects of the classical complement pathway through bound C3b.

Four normal serum proteins are important in the initiation of the alternate pathway. They are C3 itself, *Factor B, Factor D,* and *properdin*.

The alternative pathway to complement activation starts with C3 (Figure 11-13). Soluble C3 possesses an inherently unstable, highly reactive thioester group, which is prone to spontaneous activation. This activation leads to soluble C3b, called *C3b($H_2O$)*. Because of this C3 "tickover" phenomenon, C3b($H_2O$) is produced continuously in trace amounts. These trace amounts are enough to form *alternative pathway C3 convertase*, which in turn

cleaves C3 to supply more C3b. A trace endogenous pool of C3b occurs even in patients deficient in C1, C2, and C4. Host cells, which express high levels of sialic acid, inactivate C3b if it binds, whereas bacteria with lower levels of external sialic acid bind C3b without inactivating it. One of the two altered forms of C3 triggers the alternative pathway: membrane or antibody-bound C3b generated by the classical pathway or C3b($H_2O$) generated by C3 tickover. Once C3b is available, it binds Factor B. Binding of Factor B to C3b requires $Mg^{2+}$. The binding of Factor B to C3b exposes a site that is the substrate for Factor D. Factor D is a protease that cleaves Factor B when B is bound to C3b. Cleavage leads to two fragments, Ba and Bb. Ba floats away and has no known function. In contrast, Bb is a protease and remains bound to C3b. Bb alone has no enzymatic activity, but the resulting bimolecular complex, C3bBb, acts as the C3 convertase of the alternative pathway. C3b in the alternative pathway C3 convertase (C3bBb) is similar to C4b of the classical pathway C3 convertase. Both native and activated properdin are important for normal C3bBb function. Properdin decreases the rate of C3bBb dissociation and thereby stabilizes enzymatic activity. C3bBb amplifies the alternative pathway. The resulting C3b molecules have several functions. Some may bind to other zymosan molecules, and serve as anchors for Factor B to amplify the pathway. Others may bind to C3bBb, forming the alternative pathway C5 convertase (C3bBb3b), which cleaves C5. On C5 activation, the alternative pathway converges with the classical pathway, and the two pathways use the common lytic sequence of C5b to C9, the formation of the MAC C5b - 9. The beginnings of the pathways may be different, but the results are the same.

**Factor B** (formerly called *C3 proactivator*) is a single-chain polypeptide whose importance in the alternative pathway is similar to that of C2 in the classical pathway. Factor B and C2 are similar in size, structure, cleavage fragments, natural substrate (C3), and mechanism of action. They may represent gene duplications. Factor B is cleaved by Factor D into two fragments, Ba and Bb. Ba has no known biologic function. When Factor B binds to C3b, it becomes susceptible to Factor D.

**Factor D** (formerly called *C3 proactivator convertase*) is the smallest complement component and may be similar to C1s. It is found naturally as an enzyme in serum; however, Factor D has no activity on Factor B until Factor B binds to C3b.

**Properdin** (L. *perdere*, to destroy) is a γ-globulin consisting of identical subunits held together noncovalently. Properdin can take two forms, native or

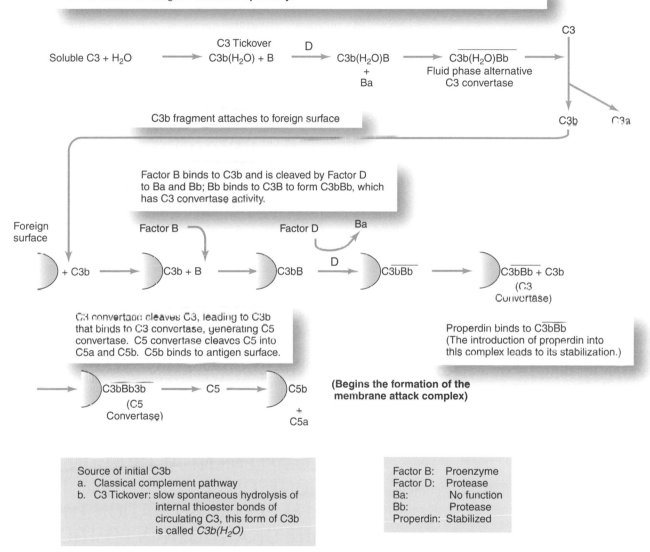

FIGURE 11-13 **The alternative pathway.** C3b is generated either by the classical complement pathway or C3 tickover. Following the interaction, for example, of zymosan (antigen) with C3b, C3b and factor B combine to form C3bBb and Ba by the action of factor D. $\overline{\text{C3bBb}}$ is an enzyme called *C3 convertase*. C3 convertase converts more C3 to C3b, which complexes with C3bBb (C3 convertase) to become C5 convertase ($\overline{\text{C3bBb3b}}$), which begins the formation of the membrane attack complex.

activated, which differ from each other only by a small conformational change. Native properdin can bind to C3bBb but not to C3b alone. Its function is to retard dissociation of Bb from C3b and thus promote activation of the alternative pathway. Activated properdin can bind to C3b in the absence of Factor B and thereby promote the assembly of C3bBb.

**MINI SUMMARY**

The main features distinguishing the alternative pathway from the classical pathway are the lack of dependence on calcium ions, the lack of requirement for C1, C4, or C2, and the lack of need for specific antigen-antibody interactions. The alternative pathway may be started directly by LPS and other bacterial products, leading to a rapid defense against certain pathogens. The complement component common to the three pathways, C3, reacts with Factor B in combination with Factor D to generate C3b$\overline{\text{Bb}}$ (a C3 convertase). C3 convertase converts more C3 to C3b, complexing with C3b$\overline{\text{Bb}}$ to become C5 convertase (C3bBb3b). This enzyme activates C5, which in turn activates C6 through C9. These last components make up the MAC, which can lyse a target cell.

### The Activation Stage of the Lectin Pathway Is Unique; It Is Initiated by Mannan-Binding Lectin Attaching to Microbial Polysaccharides in the Absence of Antibodies

The human collectin, mannan-binding lectin (MBL), an acute phase protein, is a pattern recognition molecule of the humoral innate immune system (see Chapter 3). Lectins are proteins made by the liver in response to macrophage proinflammatory cytokines induced by macrophage-pathogen binding, which recognize and bind to specific carbohydrates. MBL recognizes and binds to a range of sugars (such as, mannose, *N*-acetyl-D-glucosamine, fucose, and glucose), which permits it to interact with a wide selection of bacteria, viruses, fungi, and protozoa adorned with such sugars. When MBL binds with cell or microbial surface sugars, it is able to activate complement in an antibody- and C1-independent manner. In fact, MBL is structurally similar to, and functions like, C1q. When MBL binds cellular or microbial carbohydrates, a family of MBL-associated serine proteases (MASPs) called *MASP-1*, *MASP-2*, *MASP-3*, and a truncated version

of MASP-2 called *MAp19* interact with MBL. Most evidence suggests that MASP-2 is the most important in complement activation. The minimum functional unit MBL:MASP-2 to activate the lectin pathway is a MASP-2 dimer bound to two MBL trimeric units. Ligand engagement by MBL induces a conformational change in MASP-2 that activates the terminal serine protease domain (enzyme activity identical to C1 esterase), which then sequentially cleaves C4 and C2. The generated C4b fragments bind covalently to the microbial surface and then interact with MASP-2–cleaved C2 fragments C2a. The C$\overline{\text{4b2a}}$ complex, expresses C3 convertase activity, which is indistinguishable from classical and alternative pathway C3 convertases. The MBL pathway provides protect in the first hours to days of a primary immune response to pathogens, long before the adaptive immune response is operative.

**MINI SUMMARY**

The lectin pathway is initiated by the recognition and binding of PAMPs (such as, N-acteyl glcosamine and mannose) by soluble pattern-recognition receptors, lectin proteins called mannan-binding lectin (MBL). MBL is structurally similar to C1q and binds N-acteyl glucosamine and mannose, which are common sugars among microbes. When MBLs bind mannose, they become associated with MBL-associated serine proteases (MASPs), which bind C1r and C1s of the classical pathway, activating C4 and C and forming C3 convertase. The remainder of the lectin pathway is identical to the classical pathway.

## COMPLEMENT ACTIVATION IS CONTROLLED BY LIMITING THE EFFECTS OF ACTIVATION TO THE SITE OF ANTIGEN DEPOSITION

Complement activation may lead to potent biologic effects systemically, but activation is limited to the microenvironment surrounding a foreign invader. The host possesses regulatory proteins that restrain the extent of complement activation and prevent systemic activation.

Complement components can be inactivated by one of three mechanisms: (1) spontaneous decay, (2) stoichiometric inhibition, or (3) enzymatic degradation. C4, C3, and C5 rapidly decay unless the binding site is stabilized through attachment to a membrane. Stoichiometric inhibition involves inhibition by interaction of two molar equivalent molecules without enzymatic cleavage but with consumption by the reaction. Molecules such as C1 inhibitor, Factor H, and C4-binding protein are stoichiometric inhibitors. The final mechanism for complement inactivation is enzymatic degradation of the complement component by the inhibitor (such as Factor I).

Homeostatic maintenance of complement activation is mediated by the regulatory proteins *anaphylatoxin inactivator, C1 inhibitor (C1-INH), Factor H (H), Factor I (I), C4b-binding protein (C4b-BP), S-protein*, and *SP-40,40* in plasma and, on cells, the *complement receptor 1 (CR1 [CD35]), the decay-accelerating factor (DAF), membrane cofactor protein (MCP [CD46])*, and *membrane inhibitor of reactive lysis (MIRL [CD59]; also called homologous restriction factor (HRF)*. C4b-BP, CR1, Factor H, MCP, and MIRL contain repeating amino acid motifs of 60 residues, called *short consensus repeats*, which are encoded in a single region in Chromosome 1 called the *regulators of complement activation* (RCA) gene cluster. RCA proteins prevent C3 convertase assembly in the classical and lectin pathways. Figure 11-14 summarizes the control mechanisms regulating the classical and alternative pathways.

**Anaphylatoxin inactivator**, the plasma enzyme carboxypepidase N, inactivates the anaphylatoxins C4a and C3a and decreases the activity of C5a by cleaving the carboxy-terminal arginine residue from each peptide.

The **C1 inhibitor (C1-INH)** is a single-chain α-globulin with an unusually high carbohydrate content (35 to 40%). C1-INH combines with the active site on activated C1r and destroys its protease activity. This prevents C1s from cleaving C4 and C2 in the classical pathway. The importance of C1-INH is seen in its autosomal dominant deficiency called *hereditary angioneurotic edema* (see Chapter 16). These individuals have uncontrolled local activation of C2 that undergoes conversion to kinin, leading to excessive edema in the skin of the face and the laryngeal and intestinal mucosa.

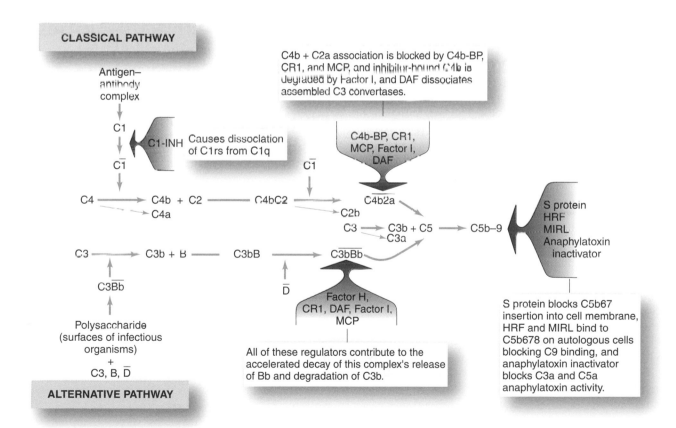

**FIGURE 11-14 Regulators of the classical and alternative pathways.** Abbreviations: C1-INH, C1 inhibitor; C4b-BP, C4b-binding protein; CR1, complement receptor 1; DAF, decay-accelerating factor; HRF, homologous restriction factor; MCP, membrane cofactor protein; MIRL, membrane inhibitor of reactive lysis.

**Factor H** is a single-chain plasma polypeptide that binds fluid-phase and membrane-bound C3b. Factor H binds to C3b and increases the susceptibility of C3b to cleavage by Factor I. It also dissociates Bb from C3bBb complexes, which mediate decay acceleration of the alternative pathway C3 convertase. Factor H exhibits no enzymatic activity.

**Factor I** is a two-chain β-globulin. The two chains are held together by disulfide bonds. Factor I acts enzymatically on C3b by making two cuts in the α-chain and converting C3b to iC3b. The active site is found on the smaller chain. The activity of Factor I is probably controlled by the need for configurational changes in its substrates (C3b or C4b) and is mediated by the cofactors H and C4-binding protein. This change happens before exposure of the site for cleavage. The mechanism is similar to that of Factor D enzymatic cleavage of Factor B.

**C4b-binding protein (C4b-BP)** is a multiple-subunit plasma glycoprotein that consists of several identical disulfide-bridged subunits. C4b-BP binds C4b in the fluid and membrane-bound phases. C4b-BP is a cofactor for Factor I-mediated cleavage of the C4b α-chain. It also mediates decay acceleration of the classical pathway C3 convertase. C4b-BP control of C4b and C4b-containing convertases is similar to Factor H control of C3b and C3b-containing convertases.

A single-chain glycoprotein called **S-protein** (also called *vitronectin*) is the primary MAC inhibitor. S-protein competes for the C5b67 binding site and prevents C9 polymerization. S-protein-mediated inhibition of binding causes the formation of the soluble SC5b67 complex. By binding to the complex, the S-protein prevents its attachment to the cell surface. This complex allows the binding of C8 and three molecules of C9 to form hydrophilic SC5b-9, but it will not allow C9 polymerization.

**SP-40,40** (also called *clusterin*) like S-protein, it is a fluid-phase protein, which inhibits MAC formation just as S-protein does by binding to C5b6, C5b67, C5b678, and C5b6789.

**Complement receptor 1 (CR1 [CD35])** is an intrinsic membrane glycoprotein that can bind to C3b and C4b in the fluid and membrane-bound phases. CR1 has three functions: (1) it exhibits cofactor activity for Factor I-mediated cleavage of C3b and C4b; (2) it mediates C3b and C4b rosette formation; and (3) it mediates decay acceleration of C3 convertases (see Chapter 19 for complement receptor deficiencies).

**Decay-accelerating factor (DAF [CD55])** is a single-chain intrinsic membrane glycoprotein. Because it has binding specificity for C4b2a and C3bBb, it is able to accelerate the decay of the classical and alternative pathway C3 convertases. DAF has no cofactor activity. DAF binds to C3b/C4b only when these molecules are on the membrane of the same cell as DAF. DAF's function may be to prevent assemblage of the convertases or to disassociate already-formed enzyme complexes.

**Membrane cofactor protein (MCP [CD46];** a glycoprotein of 45 to 70 kD), is present on platelets and peripheral blood leukocytes but not on erythrocytes. MCP may control C3b or C3b-containing enzymes by modulating their activation on cell surfaces. Surface expression of CR1 and MCP appears to be a reciprocal relationship, suggesting that MCP may have some of the same functional activities as CR1.

**Membrane inhibitor of reactive lysis (MIRL [CD59];** also called *homologous restriction factor* [HRF]) inhibits lysis by MACs that are deposited on self-tissue. MIRL is a glycolipid-anchored protein that binds both C8 and C9 and blocks membrane attack complex formation after C7 binding.

# MACROPHAGES AND HEPATOCYTES ARE THE MAJOR SOURCES OF COMPLEMENT; COMPLEMENT DEFICIENCES ARE ASSOCIATED WITH AN INCREASED TENDENCY TO PYOGENIC INFECTIONS

The main sources for the complement proteins are the hepatocytes (liver cells), epithelial cells of the gut, blood monocytes, and tissue macrophages. More than 90% of plasma C3, C6, C8, and C9 is synthesized in the liver. Even though most of the complement synthesized is by hepatocytes, local production by tissue macrophages may be important at sites of inflammation. For example, C3 serum levels increase by 50% during acute phase response. IL-1, IL-6, and TNF-α stimulate synthesis of C3 in hepatocytes, monocytes, and several other cell types. In contrast, IFN-γ inhibits monocyte C3 synthesis, while it enhances C3 synthesis by astrocytes and human glomerular epithelial cells. Table 11-5 lists the producers of complement proteins.

Complement deficiencies (see Chapter 16), although uncommon, have been described for all complement proteins except C9 and regulatory complement proteins, including C1-INH, Factor I, Factor H, DAF, and MIRL. Inherited deficiencies

**TABLE 11-5** Source of Complement Components

| Complement components | Source |
| --- | --- |
| C1q | Macrophages |
| C1r | Macrophages |
| C1s | Blood monocytes, tissue macrophages, and epithelial cells |
| C2 | Macrophages |
| C3 | Hepatocytes (not immune cells) |
| C4 | Macrophages |
| C5 | Macrophages |
| C6 | Hepatocytes |
| C7 | Hepatocytes |
| C8 | Cells in spleen |
| C9 | Hepatocytes |
| Factor B | Macrophages, lymphocytes, and hepatocytes |
| Factor D | ? |

of complement components are associated with an increased prevalence of pyogenic infection by *Staphylococcus*, *Streptococcus*, and *Neisseria* organisms, due to decreased opsonization and phagocytosis, and immune complex diseases typified by systemic lupus erythematosus and glomerulonephritis, which are due to complement-mediated inflammation in response to persistent antigen-antibody complexes. Deficiencies in C1 through C2 lead to similar symptoms. Deficiencies in the early components of the alternative pathway seem to be associated with *Neisseria* infections. The inability to produce MBL leads to pyogenic infections and increased respiratory tract infections. The most serious clinical manifestations are associated with C3 deficiencies. In the absence of complement regulators, complement components decrease at accelerated rates. As described earlier, congenital C1-INH deficiencies gives rise to the condition called *hereditary angioedema*. Factor H, DAF, and MIRL deficiencies cause complement-mediated lysis of erythrocytes leading to hemoglobin in the urine.

# THE GENES FOR SOME COMPLEMENT PROTEINS ARE IN THE MAJOR HISTOCOMPATIBILITY COMPLEX

Loci for several of the complement components and regulatory proteins have been identified. The gene for human C3 is found on Chromosome 19. C8 is encoded at two unlinked loci on Chromosome 1, one

gene encoding the α- and γ-chains and one gene encoding the β-chain, whereas a single locus encodes the individual chains of the multichain C3, C4, or C5 molecules. Thus, the genetic information is transcribed into a single mRNA and translated into one polypeptide chain. Cutting of chains to form the final products occurs only after translation. An intriguing aspect of complement genetics is the association of some loci encoding complement proteins in the MHC. Human genes encoding the complement components C2, C4, and Factor B lie near the HLA-B locus on chromosome 6, whereas C3, C5, C6, C7, C8, and are not linked to the HLA complex. The genes for C6, C7, C8, and C9 are on Chromosome 1. RCA proteins are also encoded by cluster of genes found on Chromosome 1. A similar association of genes encoding complement proteins and the MHC has been demonstrated in the mouse. The murine S locus of the H-2 complex includes the genes for C4, Factor B, and C2.

## MINI SUMMARY

Because complement activation has potent biologic effects, accurate control mechanisms must be in operation. Spontaneous decay starts at the same time that new components are generated. Control is also mediated by regulatory proteins found in the plasma or on cells.

Liver cells are the primary producers of complement proteins, but monocytes and macrophages also synthesize many complement proteins. This latter activity may be important at the local site of antigen-antibody interaction.

Many complement molecule genes are localized in the MHC.

# SUMMARY

The **complement system** is a complicated group of about 30 serum proteins that act in cooperation with *complexed* antigen and antibody in a predetermined sequence. Classically, when specific antibody of the proper class (IgG or IgM) and subclass (IgG1, IgG2, or IgG3) binds with antigen, the complex that forms binds (or fixes) the first component of complement, called *C1*. The antigen-antibody-C1 complex *activates* more components with unique enzymatic activities, in the order *C1, C4, C2, C3, C5, C6, C7, C8, C9*. Four main effects occur that help defend the host against infection: (1) release of vasoactive peptides active in *inflammation*, (2) deposition of C3b, a promoter (an **opsonin**) for *phagocytosis*, (3) removal of antigen-antibody complexes, and (4) membrane damage leading to *lysis*.

Activation of the complement cascade can occur through three distinct routes: (1) the *classical pathway* starts by the combination of specific IgG or IgM antibodies with their right antigens, (2) the *alternative pathway* starts directly by polysaccharides on the surfaces of infectious organisms and by aggregates of IgA, and (3) the *lectin pathway* is initiated by MBL binding to pathogen surface.

Lysis of red blood cells exemplifies the classical pathway of complement activation. The classical pathway has three phases: (1) the *initiation phase* (includes components C1, C4, and C2), (2) the *amplification phase* (involves C3), and (3) the *membrane attack phase* (involves components C5b, C6, C7, C8, and C9). Activation starts when antibody binds to a specific antigen. This binding exposes a C1 binding site in the Fc portion of the antibodies. The C1 molecule is a $Ca^{2+}$-dependent union of three polypeptides: (1) C1q, a protein with six immunoglobulin-binding sites linked by collagen-like fibrils, which in turn activates through rearrangement of the structure of (2) C1r and (3) C1s, a serine esterase which goes on to alter C4 and then C2. The combination of antigen-antibody-C1 leads to C1s, which is the first enzymatic complement component; it is designated C$\overline{1s}$. C$\overline{1s}$ converts native C4 and then C2 into activated states. C4 is split into C4a and C4b. C4a is anaphylatoxin. The C4b molecule attaches to the surface of the target cell near the antigen-antibody-C1 complex. C4b acts as an anchor for C2a. *C2* is split by C$\overline{1s}$ into C2a and C2b fragments. C2a binds to C4b, forming C$\overline{4b2a}$ (or *C3 convertase*). C3 convertase splits *C3* into C3a and C3b fragments, plus several other fragments. Some of C3b is deposited on the membrane of the target cell, where it serves as a site for the attachment of phagocytic cells and acts as an *opsonin*. Other C3b becomes associated with C$\overline{4b2a}$ (C3 convertase) to form C$\overline{4b2a3b}$ (or *C5 convertase*). C3b also is involved in solubilization and clearance of circulating immune complexes. C3a is an *anaphylatoxin*. C5 convertase activates C5, C6, and C7. C5 is split into C5a and C5b subcomponents. C5a is an anaphylatoxin and a chemoattractant. C5b starts the assembly of C6, C7, C8, and C9 by acting as an anchor for C6. One molecule each of C6, C7, and C8 unite with C5b and with 10–16 C9 molecules to form the *membrane attack complex (MAC)*. This complex forms channels through the plasma membrane, causing damage to the membrane. The lipid bilayer is disrupted enough to allow the free exchange of water and electrolytes. The influx of water and $Na^+$ eventually leads to lysis.

Lysis by the MAC is due to mechanisms described by the doughnut model.

The other routes of complement activation are called the *alternative* and *lectin pathways*. The main features distinguishing alternative pathway from the classical pathway are dependence on $Mg^{2+}$ and bypass of C1, C4, and C2. Specific antigen-antibody interaction is not required for the alternative pathway. Activation of the alternate pathway involves different molecules able to activate C3 into its subcomponents. The remaining pathway (C5 through C9) is the same as the classical pathway. Substances that can activate the alternative pathway include certain complex polysaccharides such as endotoxins (LPS) and aggregates of some kinds of antibodies such as IgA. The biologic relevance of the alternate pathway is its ability to provide an amplification loop for the classical pathway. The alternative pathway is in a continuous cycle that is held in check by control molecules whose effects are counteracted by different initiators.

The first three components of the alternative pathway are *Factor B, Factor D*, and *properdin*. Factor B complexes with C3b, whether produced by the alternate or classical pathway. Factor B is structurally and functionally similar to C2. Factor B is cleaved by Factor D into two fragments, called *Ba* and *Bb*. Ba has no known biologic function. Bb binds to C3b and thereby becomes susceptible to Factor D.

Factor D may be similar to C$\overline{1s}$. Factor D has no activity on Factor B until Factor B binds to C3b. The latter combination produces the C3 convertase of the alternative pathway.

Properdin is a γ-globulin consisting of identical subunits held together noncovalently. Properdin can take two forms, native or activated, which differ from each other only by a small conformational change. Native properdin cannot bind to C3b alone but can retard dissociation of Bb from C3b. Properdin merely stabilizes the C3bBb complex so that it can act on further C3. Activated properdin can bind to C3b in the absence of Factor B and thereby promote the assembly of C$\overline{3bBb}$. This interaction is a positive feedback loop with amplifying potential, held in check by the C3b inactivator.

The phylogenetically oldest pathway is the *lectin pathway*. As the alternative pathway, the lectin pathway is part of the innate immune system and does not involve antibodies. It is activated by the binding of the plasma pattern-recognition molecule, *mannose-binding lectin* (MBL; it structurally resembles C1q) to mannose residues in microbial proteins and polysaccharides but not in mammalian molecules. The binding of cellular or microbial polysaccharides to plasma lectins MBL, causes MBL-associated serine proteases, MASP-1 and MASP-2, to attach to MBL; MASP-1 and MASP-2 are structurally and functionally similar to C1r and C1s. The tripartite association forms an active complex that cleaves and activates C4 and C2, which triggers the lectin pathway of complement activation. Apart from being activated without antibody (like the alternative pathway), the remainder of the lectin pathway is the same as the classical pathway.

Because complement activation has potent biologic effects, it is tightly controlled. Complement activation is limited to the microenvironment surrounding a foreign invader. The host has regulatory proteins that control the extent of complement activation and prevent systemic activation. Complement components can be inactivated by one of three mechanisms: (1) spontaneous decay, (2) stoichiometric inhibition, and (3) enzymatic degradation.

Homeostatic maintenance of complement activation is mediated by the regulatory proteins: in plasma, *anaphylatoxin inactivator, C1 inhibitor (C1-INH), Factor H (H), Factor I (I), C4b-binding protein (C4b-BP), S-protein* and *SP-40,40*; and, on cells, the *complement receptor (CR1), decay-accelerating factor (DAF), membrane cofactor protein (MCP)* and *membrane inhibitor of reactive lysis (MIRL [CD59])*.

The main sources of the complement proteins are the hepatocytes (liver cells), epithelial cells of the gut, blood monocytes, and tissue macrophages. More than 90% of plasma C3, C6, C8, and C9 is synthesized in the liver. Monocytes and macrophages also synthesize many complement proteins. Even though most of the complement is synthesized by liver hepatocytes, local production by tissue macrophages may be important at sites of inflammation. Complement deficiencies are associated with an increased tendency to pyogenic infections.

Some complement components are encoded in the MHC. Human genes encoding the complement components C2, C4, and Factor B lie near the HLA-B locus, whereas C3, C5, C6, C7, and C8 are not linked to the HLA complex. The murine S locus of the H-2 complex includes the genes for C4, Factor B, and C2.

# SELF-EVALUATION

## RECALLING KEY TERMS

Alternative pathway
Anaphylatoxin inactivator
Anaphylatoxins

C1
  C1q
  C1r
  C1s
C1 inhibitor (C1-INH)
C2
  C2a
  C2b
C3
  C3a
  C3b
C3 convertase
Complement receptor 1 (CR1)
C4
  C4a
  C4b
C4b-binding protein (C4b-BP)
C5
  C5a
  C5b
C5 convertase
C6
C7
C8
C9
CD59
Classical pathway
  Amplification phase
  Initiation (or activation) phase
  Membrane attack phase
Complement
Complement system
Decay-accelerating factor (DAF)
Factor B
Factor D
Factor H
Factor I
Immune adherence
Lectin pathway
Mannose-binding lectin (MBL)
Membrane attack complex (MAC)
Membrane cofactor protein (MCP)
Membrane inhibitor of reactive lysis (MIRL)
Opsonization
Properdin
S-protein
SP-40,40

## MULTIPLE-CHOICE QUESTIONS

*(An answer key is not provided, but the page[s] location of the answer is.)*

1. Which of the following cells synthesize substantial amounts of complement components? (a) mast cells, (b) macrophages, (c) hepatocytes, (d) *b* and *c* are correct, (e) none of these. *(See page 388.)*

2. Chemotaxins generated during the complement cascade are (a) C3a and C5a, (b) C3a and C2a, (c) C3a and C3b, (d) C5a, (e) none of these. *(See page 374).*

3. In the membrane attack phase of the classical complement pathway, the role of C5b is to (a) attach to the target cell and bind the remaining complement components, (b) cause lysis of the cell membrane, (c) attract immune cells, (d) *a* and *c* are correct, (e) none of these. *(See pages 380 and 381.)*

4. Concerning the classical complement pathway, which of the following is true? (a) C1r is the recognition site of the C1 complex and binds to the antibody, (b) activation of C1 is dependent on magnesium ions, (c) activated C1 (C1 esterase) cleaves C2 and C3, (d) activated C3 (C3 convertase) cleaves C4 and C5, (e) none of these. *(See pages 371 and 372.)*

5. Which of the following is true concerning complement? (a) activation of one C1 molecule can lead to cell lysis, (b) the alternative pathway is not dependent on antibody for activation, (c) it can be activated by IgG or IgM antibodies complexed with antigen, (d) it is heat stable, (e) *a*, *b*, and *c* are correct, (f) none of these. *(See pages 369, 370 and 384.)*

6. Properdin (a) initiates the complement cascade of the alternative pathway, (b) stabilizes the alternative pathway C3 and C5 convertases, (c) cleaves factor D, (d) cleaves factor B, (e) *b* and *d* are correct, (f) none of these. *(See pages 384 and 385.)*

7. The complement protein that recognizes the IgM or IgG antibodies in antigen-antibody complexes is (a) C1q, (b) C1r, (c) C1s, (d) C4, (e) none of these. *(See page 372.)*

8. The complement component or fragment that binds the C3 convertases of both the classical and alternative pathways and alters their specificity so that they become C5 convertases, is (a) C4b, (b) C3b, (c) C3a, (d) C5b, (e) C2a, (f) none of these. *(See pages 378 and 384.)*

9. Complement proteins (a) increase in concentration during an immune response, (b) are ordinarily gamma globulins, (c) ordinarily exist in an active form, (d) share antigenic determinants with antibodies, (e) none of these. *(See page 370.)*

10. The molecules in the complement system that have anaphylatoxin activity are (a) C4a, (b) C5b, (c) C2a, (d) *a* and *b* are correct, (e) *a* and *c* are correct, (f) none of these. *(See pages 374 and 380.)*

11. Which of the following is not true concerning C3b? (a) it is part of the amplification phase, (b) it is an anaphylatoxin, (c) it is an opsonin, (d) it binds with C3 convertase, (e) none of these. *(See page 379.)*

12. The natural substrates of C1s include (a) C2, (b) C4, (c) C3, (d) B, (e) *a* and *b* are correct, (f) none of these. *(See page 372.)*

13. The membrane attack phase begins when C5 is cleaved by C4b2a3b into two pieces, C5a and C5b. C5a functions as a(n) (a) anaphylatoxin, (b) chemotaxin, (c) convertase, (d) *a* and *b* are correct, (e) *a* and *c* are correct, (f) none of these. *(See page 380.)*

14. The complement fragment responsible for immune adherence is (a) C4b, (b) C5b, (c) C3b, (d) Bb, (e) D, (f) none of these. *(See page 378.)*

15. Which of the following is a component of the alternative complement pathway? (a) C1, (b) C2, (c) Factor B, (d) Properdin, (e) *c* and *d* are correct, (f) none of these. *(See pages 384 and 385.)*

16. The lectin pathway involves the binding MBL with microbial mannose moieties, MASP-2 association with bound MBL, which leads to a MBL:MASP complex that cleaves C4 and C2 forming a C5 convertase activity. (a) true, (b) false. *(See page 386.)*

17. C1 inhibitor, by blocking C1r activity, inhibits the classical pathway. (a) true, (b) false. *(See page 387.)*

18. Complement protein or regulator deficiencies can lead to (a) frequent infections, (b) immune complex disease, (c) blood in the urine, (d) all of the above, (e) none of the above. *(See pages 388 and 389.)*

## SHORT-ANSWER ESSAY QUESTIONS

1. Complement is involved in antigen-antibody interactions, yet there is no resulting precipitation or agglutination. What does happen?

2. Complement has four important functions. What are they?

3. If complement activation can lead to lysis of antibody-tagged cellular antigens, what is the purpose of complement activation by antibody-tagged noncellular antigens?

4. Briefly distinguish between the classical pathway, the alternative pathway, and the lectin

pathway of complement activation. How do the pathways differ in substances that initiate them?

5. Briefly discuss the three stages in the classical pathway of complement activation. What stage is most important and why?

6. What is the difference between complement activation by antigen-IgM complexes and antigen-IgG complexes?

7. What is the biologic importance of C4a?

8. What complement components make up C3 convertase, and what does it do?

9. Macrophages display receptors for C3b. What is the biologic significance of this fact?

10. What is the last complement component to be split into two biologically active fragments, and what are their functions?

11. If the complement cascade is stopped before the membrane attack phase, has complement fulfilled its function in an immune response? If yes, why? If no, speculate on the reason for having the membrane attack phase.

12. What components of the complement system are shared between the classical pathway, the alternative pathway, and the lectin pathway?

13. Why is it important to tightly control complement activation?

## FURTHER READINGS

Arlaud, G.J., P.N. Barlow, C. Gaboriaud, P. Gros, and S.V. Narayana. 2007. Deciphering complement mechanisms: The contributions of structural biology. *Mol. Immunol.* 44:3809–3822.

Carroll, M.C. 2004. The complement system in regulation of adaptive immunity. *Nat. Immunol.* 10:981–986.

Davis, A.E., S. Cai, and D. Lui. 2007. C1 inhibitor: Biologic activities that are independent of protease inhibition. *Immunobiology* 212:313–323.

Degn, S.E., S. Thiel, and J.C. Jensenius. 2007. New perspectives on mannan-binding lectin-mediated complement activation. *Immunobiology* 212:301–311.

Dommett, R.M., N. Klein, and M.W. Turner. 2006. Mannose-binding lectin in innate immunity: Past, present and future. *Tissue Antigens* 68:193–209.

Guo, R-F., and P.W. Ward. 2005. Role of C5a in inflammatory responses. *Annu. Rev. Immunol.* 23:821–852.

Holmskov, U., S. Thiel, and J.C. Jensenius. 2003. Collectins and ficolins: Humoral lectins of innate immune defense. *Ann. Rev. Immunol.* 21:547–578.

Muller-Eberhard, H.J. 1988. Molecular organization and function of the complement system. *Annu. Rev. Biochem.* 57:321–347.

Pillemer, L., L. Blum, I.H. Lepow, O.A. Ross, E.W. Todd, and A.C. Wardlaw. 1954. The properdin system and immunity. I. Demonstration and isolation of a new serum protein, properdin, and its importance in immune phenomena. *Science* 120:279–285.

Prodinger, W.M., R. Wurzner, H. Stoiber, and M.P. Dierich. 2003. Complement. In *Fundamental Immunology*, 5th ed. W.E. Paul, ed. Philadelphia: Lippincott Williams & Wilkins. p. 1077–1104.

Roozendaal, R., and M.C. Carroll. 2007. Complement receptors CD21 and CD35 in humoral immunity. *Immunol. Rev.* 219:157–166.

Takahashi, K., W.K. Eddie, I.C. Michelow, and R.A.B. Ezekowitz. 2006. The mannose-binding lectin: A prototypic pattern recognition molecule. *Cur. Opin. Immunol.* 18:16–23.

The September 1991 issue of *Immunology Today* is entitled *The Biology of Complement* and is devoted entirely to complement. *Immunol. Today.* 12:291–342.

Walport, M.J. 2001. Complement (two parts) *N. Engl. J. Med.* 344:1058–1066, 1140–1144.

# CHAPTER TWELVE

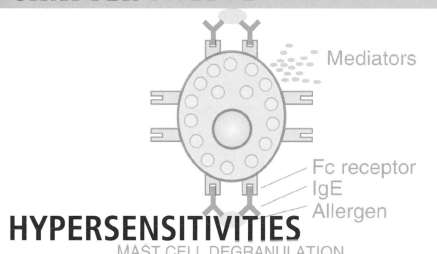

Mediators

Fc receptor
IgE
Allergen

# HYPERSENSITIVITIES

MAST CELL DEGRANULATION

    d. There are systemic and localized consequences of type I hypersensitivity.

       1) Systemic anaphylaxis is a life-threatening hypersensitivity reaction.

       2) Atopic allergies are usually the wheezing, sneezing, runny nose, watery eyes, and itching kinds of hypersensitivity reactions.

    e. Sensitivity testing is done to determine if an individual has immunity or hypersensitivity.

    f. Treatments for type I hypersensitivities consider only the symptoms, not the causes.

       1) Antigen avoidance is the best but not always possible treatment.

       2) Desensitization, hyperimmunization that leads to hypoimmunity, is the oldest form of treatment.

       3) Medication is the other mode of treatment.

**3.** Type IV: Cell-mediated (delayed-type) hypersensitivity is mediated by T cells and activated macrophages, not antibodies.

    a. Mechanisms for DTH induction and development involve sensitization rather than immunization.

    b. There are different kinds of DTH reactions.

       1) Contact sensitivity (dermatitis) is a DTH caused by an antigen touching the skin.

       2) The tuberculin reaction is a classical example of a DTH reaction.

       3) Tuberculosis is the classic example of a DTH disease.

## OBJECTIVES

The reader should be able to:

**1.** List the Coombs and Gell classification for hypersensitivity reactions; give examples of each type.

**2.** Appreciate the fact that in type I hypersensitivity reactions, the immune system itself provokes tissue damage by responding to a false alarm.

**3.** Define allergy, anaphylaxis, atopy, desensitization, hypersensitivity, immediate versus delayed-type hypersensitivity, sensitization, and shocking dose.

**4.** Appreciate the difference between primary and secondary exposure to antigen in immunity and in hypersensitivity.

**5.** Discuss the structural and functional characteristics of IgE; comment on the cytotropic nature of IgE.

**6.** Describe the role of mast cells in immediate hypersensitivity reactions; explain degranulation; distinguish between release of preformed and newly formed mediators from mast cells; list examples of each type of mediator.

**7.** Appreciate the difference between the cyclooxygenase and lipoxygenase pathways of mediator production.

**8.** Give an account of skin testing; describe the triple response.

**9.** Recognize that the combination of avoidance, desensitization, and medication is used to reduce allergic reactions temporarily; explain desensitization.

**10.** Understand the differences between systemic anaphylaxis and atopic allergies.

**11.** Discuss the hallmarks of DTH.

**12.** Explain the mechanisms for DTH induction and development.

**13.** Distinguish between the different types of DTH reactions; describe tuberculosis.

# PREAMBLE: THE COOMBS AND GELL CLASSIFICATION DIVIDES IMMUNE FUNCTIONS INTO FOUR CATEGORIES OF HYPERSENSITIVITY

The immune system is *not* infallible. It can malfunction; that is, a pathogenic consequence of having an adaptive immune response elicited by noninfectious, harmless antigens such as animal dander, drugs, food, house dust, and pollen can cause a disease—a hypersensitivity. According to Coombs and Gell, there are four classes of immune malfunction or hypersensitivity, in addition to autoimmune reactions (Figure 12-1):

1. Type I: immediate (anaphylactic) hypersensitivity
2. Type II: antibody-dependent cytotoxic hypersensitivity
3. Type III: immune complex-mediated hypersensitivity
4. Type IV: cell-mediated (delayed-type) hypersensitivity

The first three types of hypersensitivity are mediated by antibodies (type I mediated by IgE; types II and III mediated by IgG and IgM), and the last is mediated by activated T helper 1 ($T_H1$) cells and their derived cytokines or cytotoxic T ($T_C$) cells themselves. All four types of hypersensitivity are briefly discussed in the next few pages, but only types I and IV are discussed in detail. Examples of type II and type III hypersensitivities are given where appropriate in the remaining chapters.

## Type I: Immediate (Anaphylactic) Hypersensitivity Involves Cell-Bound IgE Antibodies

**Type I hypersensitivity**—*exemplified by allergic asthma, allergic rhinitis (hay fever), atopic dermatitis (eczema), acute urticaria (hives), and food allergies—is manifested within minutes after a second exposure to certain types of offending innocuous antigens called allergens.* Exposure to these innocuous allergens induces the production of IgE antibodies, which sensitizes the individual to the allergens. Individuals exhibiting these immediate allergic responses are called *atopic* and their hyperresponsive (hypersensitivity) state is called *atopy*. These atopic reactions occur after basophil or mast cell *Fc receptor-bound IgE antibodies* are cross-linked with the second-exposure allergen leading to basophil and mast cell *degranulation*

(Figure 12-2). Mediator substances subsequently are released from the mast cells or basophils granules or actively synthesized, and these mediators, *histamine* and *leukotrienes*, cause blood vessel dilation and leakage, smooth muscle contraction, sensory nerve stimulation (itching, sneezing, and coughing), mucus secretion, and impaired breathing (asphyxia). Once the hypersensitivity subsides, the mediators that were released during the acute reaction can cause a localized inflammation called a *late phase response*. Type I hypersensitivities are synonymous with *allergies*.

Given the sometimes dire consequences of IgE production against common, harmless environmental antigens—what is IgE's normal physiological role on exposure to dangerous infectious antigens—it provides protective immunity against parasitic worms (helminths), which are widespread in less developed countries. In fact, individuals from these countries exhibit little or no allergies; however, roughly 40% of individuals in industrialized countries that are not threatened by parasitic worms exhibit allergies. The prevalence of allergies over the last two decades has doubled in industrialized countries. The reason why is not totally clear.

## Type II: Antibody-Dependent Cytotoxic Hypersensitivity Involves Antibody Responses Against Antigens on Cells

**Type II hypersensitivity** *is also an immediate reaction that generally involves harmful antibody-mediated responses to surface antigens of red blood cells or platelets, which causes complement-mediated lysis or antibody-dependent cell-mediated cytotoxicity (ADCC).* Usually, however, only one type of blood element is involved in a single episode. Tissue injury also can result from recruitment and activation of neutrophils and macrophages. A type II response is exemplified by an incompatible blood transfusion (see Chapter 5). The recipient of the incompatible blood rapidly destroys the red cells in that blood because of existing IgM (called *isohemagglutinins*) in the host plasma. IgM antibodies bind to the cells and activate the complement sequence, which leads to enhanced phagocytosis or eventual lysis of the target cells. A similar mechanism results from Rh blood incompatibility due to anti-Rh IgG antibodies. Type II reactions can result from the attachment of a drug to a cell surface or from immune complexes absorbing to cell surfaces. Autoimmune diseases such as immune hemolytic anemia and thrombocytopenia can result from drug treatment with penicillin, cephalosporin, and streptomycin

(A)

### Type I -- Immediate (anaphylactic) hypersensitivity

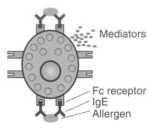

MAST CELL DEGRANULATION

On primary exposure to allergen excess amounts of IgE are produced that bind to mast cells by their Fc receptors. Secondary exposure of allergen leads to crosslinked IgE molecules, causing degranulation and vasoactive mediator release.

(B)

### Type II -- Antibody-dependent cytotoxic hypersensitivity

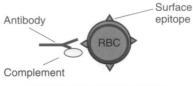

COMPLEMENT–MEDIATED LYSIS

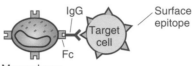

MACROPHAGE– OR NK CELL–MEDIATED CYTOTOXICITY

Antibodies bind to epitopes on cells, inducing activation of complement, phagocytic cells, or cytotoxic cells, leading to cell lysis.

(C)

### Type III -- Immune complex-mediated hypersensitivity

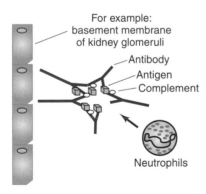

Interactions between antibodies and antigens can lead to immune complexes that are deposited in the tissue. Complement is often fixed, inducing inflammatory reactions because of neutrophil attraction to the site of deposition, causing tissue damage.

(D)

### Type IV -- Cell-mediated (delayed-type) hypersensitivity

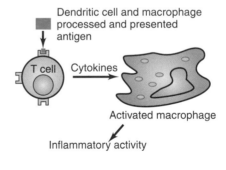

Following secondary exposure to the same antigen, this tissue damage is mediated by antigen-sensitized $T_H1$ cells through release of cytokines and chemokines. The chemokines and cytokines attract and activate macrophages that release mediators, leading to inflammatory reactions.

**FIGURE 12-1** *Continued*

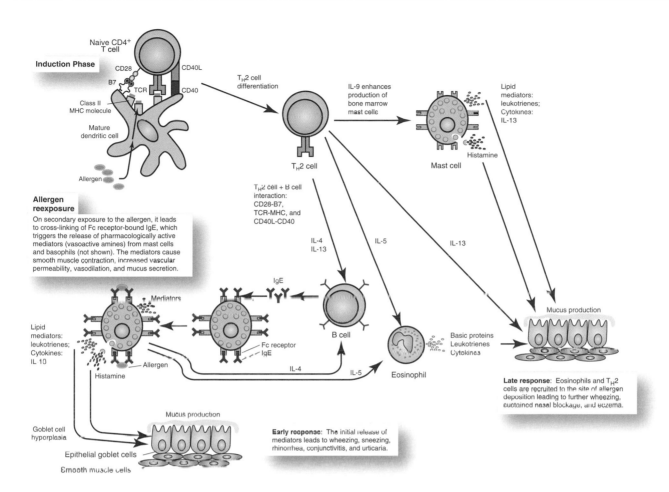

**FIGURE 12-2** Induction of an allergic response.

(see Chapter 13). These antibiotics absorb nonspecifically to erythrocyte membrane proteins, forming hapten-carrier complexes. IgG antibodies reacting against the hapten induce complement-mediated lysis of the red blood cells, causing anemia. Drug withdrawal leads to cessation of hemolytic anemia. Penicillin can induce all four types of hypersensitivities. Other examples of type II hypersensitivity that mediate autoimmune diseases are when antagonistic autoantibodies are produced to membrane proteins such as, the acetylcholine receptors in the motor end plates of skeletal muscles causing muscular weakness associated with myasthenia gravis or conversely, the autoantibodies produced against thyroid-stimulating hormone receptors act as agonists, which leads to the hyperthyroidism associated with Graves' disease (see Chapter 13). Hyperacute graft rejection is considered a type II hypersensitivity. Type II

**FIGURE 12-1** **Immune malfunctions leading to tissue damage**. The four panels represent classification of hypersensitivity reactions (after Coombs and Gell). *Panel A: type I—immediate (anaphylactic) hypersensitivity*. On primary exposure to antigen (allergen), excess amounts of IgE are produced, which bind to mast cells by their Fc receptors. Secondary exposure of allergen leads to cross-linked IgE molecules, causing degranulation and vasoactive mediator release. *Panel B: type II—antibody-dependent cytotoxic hypersensitivity*. Antibodies bind to antigenic determinants on cells, inducing activation of complement, phagocytic cells, or cytotoxic cells, leading to cell lysis. *Panel C: type III—immune complex-mediated hypersensitivity*. Interactions between antibodies and antigens can lead to immune complexes that are deposited in the tissue. Complement is often fixed, inducing inflammatory reactions because of neutrophil attraction to the site of deposition, causing tissue damage. *Panel D: type IV—cell-mediated (delayed-type) hypersensitivity*. Following secondary exposure to the same antigen, this tissue damage is mediated by antigen-sensitized $T_H1$ cells through release of cytokines. The cytokines attract and activate macrophages that release mediators, leading to inflammatory reactions.

hypersensitivity also can be mediated by ADCC reactions.

Treatments of type II hypersensitivities include prevention of blood and tissue mismatches, discontinuing the offending drug, and immunosuppressants. Autoimmune diseases initiated by type II hypersensitivities are more difficult to treat because the offending antigen cannot be removed.

## Type III: Immune Complex-Mediated Hypersensitivity Involves Formation of IgG Antibody-Antigen Aggregates

**Type III hypersensitivity** *is typified by the hives of serum sickness and other manifestations due to soluble immune complexes that may deposit themselves anywhere in the body, where the classical complement system activation leads to tissue damage.* Type III hypersensitivities can be systemic or localized; however, the mechanism of injury is the same irrespective of systemic or localized immune complex deposition. Typically the formation of antigen-antibody complexing (also called *immune complexes*) facilitates phagocytic cell clearance of antigen, through the binding of such complexes to IgG Fc receptors (CD16) expressed on the phagocytic cells. In addition, most of the complexes that are too small to bind Fc receptors are removed from the circulation by binding to CR1-expressing erythrocytes that are trapped in the liver and removed by phagocytic Kupffer cells. Serum sickness is a systemic type III hypersensitivity, which occurs when large amounts of IgG antibodies and antigen combine. This interaction sometimes leads to large aggregates of IgG-antigen complexes that are deposited on blood vessel walls, joints, skin, or in the kidney glomeruli. These complexes then activate the complement system and subsequently induce fever and an intensive inflammatory reaction in the area. Rashes may include palpable purpura and/or urticaria. The syndrome starts to subside when the offending antigen or its pathogenic metabolite is completely removed from the body. *Serum sickness,* a term originally used to describe reactions to heterologous antiserum (such as therapeutic serum from horses immunized against snake venom), may be a misnomer in many cases because therapy with many drugs, such as penicillins, sulfonamides, and streptomycin, can cause serum-sickness–like syndromes.

The type III response is similar to the type I response because some of the same effects (such as blood vessel dilation, itching, sneezing, coughing, and impaired breathing) are caused by the release of histamine. The difference is how histamine is released. Central to injury associated with type III responses is the fixation of complement, which leads to the formation of anaphylatoxins (vasoactive mediators released in plasma during complement activation) C3a and C5a. Anaphylatoxins cause mast cells to release histamine and chemokines. In addition to increased vascular permeability, complement activation via chemokines also attracts neutrophils (and other immune cells such as basophils, eosinophils, and macrophages) to the sites of immune complex deposition and stimulates the neutrophils to engulf the immune complexes. The internalization of the immune complexes by neutrophils damages the neutrophils, and they, in turn, release lysosomal enzymes and large amounts of oxidizing agents that damage the surrounding tissues. Localized macrophages produce tumor necrosis factor-α (TNF-α) and interleukin-1. Type III hypersensitivity is implicated in certain autoimmune diseases such as systemic lupus erythematosus (see Chapter 13), resulting from autoantibodies reacting against endogenous antigen such as DNA, leading to tissue damage. The rheumatoid factor detected in patients with the autoimmune disease rheumatoid arthritis is an IgM anti-IgG antibody that contributes to arthritic joint inflammation. Another example of a type III hypersensitivity, a localized immune complex disease, is the *Arthus reaction*. This is a local skin reaction characterized by redness and swelling occurring a few hours after intradermal inoculation of antigen into a host who has already produced IgG antibodies to the same antigen. The antibodies diffuse out of the capillaries and bind to antigen. The antigen–IgG complexes do not remain soluble but bind to FcγRIII on neutrophils, which in turn release lytic enzymes into the surrounding environment as they internalize immune complexes. The immune complexes also activate complement, releasing C5a that increases capillary permeability. C5a also binds to and sensitizes mast cells to respond to immune complexes. Binding immune complexes activates mast cell FcγRIIIs, which in turn induces mast cell degranulation. A local inflammation occurs with the observed redness, and blood vessel occlusion swelling. A clinical example of localized type III hypersensitivity disease is the occupational disease called *Farmer's Lung,* in which large amounts of IgG are produced to the thermophilic actinomycetes spores that grow on rotting hay that are encountered repeatedly—it resembles an Arthus reaction of the skin but in the lung.

Treatments of type III hypersensitivities include plasmapheresis to reduce immune complex levels, supportive therapy as the patient clears the immune complexes, and use of immunosuppressants.

## Type IV: Cell-Mediated (Delayed-Type) Hypersensitivity Involves T Cells and Activated Macrophages, Not Antibodies

**Type IV hypersensitivity** *differs from the preceding three types of hypersensitivity in two important ways: (1) the hypersensitivity is mediated by antigen-specific effector $T_H1$ cells and their activated macrophages rather than by antibody, and (2) as the name implies, the hypersensitivity starts after a latent period of several hours and peaks at 48 to 72 hr.* The reaction of specific $T_H1$ cells to the appropriate antigen starts a series of cellular interactions culminating in activation of $T_H1$ cells and release of chemokines, which attract macrophages and cytokines such as interferon γ ($IFN-\gamma$) that activates macrophages. The activated macrophages produce $TNF-\alpha$, which upregulates adhesion molecules on local blood vessels facilitating further cell recruitment, binding, and extravasation into surrounding tissues. Delayed-type hypersensitivity, discussed in the second half of this chapter, is an important part of the process of immunity to many intracellular infectious agents, such as those that cause tuberculosis. This response also is involved in graft rejection, tumor immunity, and is seen in allergic reactions to poison ivy and metals. As described for type I hypersensitivity, the initial response in type IV hypersensitivity is called *sensitization* and may not lead to symptoms.

# TYPE I: IMMEDIATE (ANAPHYLACTIC) HYPERSENSITIVITY IS MEDIATED BY IgE ANTIBODIES

*Allergy* ("altered reaction"), or *hypersensitivity*, and related disorders constitute a large group of antigen-induced diseases characterized by abnormally intense immune responses to a harmless antigen. In an allergic reaction, the immune system itself provokes tissue damage by responding to an antigen "threat" that would usually go unnoticed. Immunity gone wrong: invasion by a normally innocuous substance such as ragweed pollen can lead to symptoms that range from merely annoying to life-threatening.

The most widely recognized tissue damage disorders are the type I hypersensitivities mediated by IgE antibodies. Hay fever (*allergic rhinitis*), a primary example of such a disorder, is a respiratory disease that occurs on reexposure to proteins in inhaled pollen grains. The proteins diffuse across the respiratory epithelium where they bind submucosal mast cell-expressed IgE, activating the mast cells. The mast cells degranulate and release mediators that cause the disease. *Hay fever* is a misnomer because hay is not the causative agent and an increase in body temperature is not one of its symptoms. The symptoms of hay fever show the most familiar type I hypersensitivity reactions of respiratory allergic reactions: the wheezing, sneezing, runny nose, and watery eyes caused by inhaled substances from growing trees, grasses and weeds, molds, house dust mites, house dusts, and animal dander. Another example of a respiratory disease sometimes associated with allergy (about a 40% correlation) is asthma. However, allergies are not limited to the respiratory tract; many allergies strike the skin or can occur through ingestion of certain foods. An itchy rash appearing in the crook of the arms or legs, or even over the entire body, is eczema, an atopic dermatitis. Yet, all in all, the most dire type I hypersensitivity reaction is anaphylactic shock.

## The Definitions of Hypersensitivity Reactions Are the Opposite of Those Used to Define Immune Reactions

Individuals with type I hypersensitivities do not develop immunity when exposed to certain antigens. **Hypersensitivity** is an increased state of reactivity that involves a detrimental immune response (the word **allergy** is derived from the Greek word *allos* which means "other" or "altered response"). Instead of immunization after the first exposure to an offending antigen (or **allergen**), **sensitization** occurs. The sensitization is usually noticed on the second exposure to the allergen because the second exposure functions as a **shocking dose** rather than as a booster dose. The individual exhibits **anaphylaxis** (meaning "without protection") rather than an anamnestic (nonforgetting) response.

**Immediate (Type I) hypersensitivity** reactions occur quickly (within seconds to minutes) after a second exposure to the allergen. Usually only after the second exposure to the allergen is the hypersensitivity manifested. If only one exposure occurs, individuals usually do not realize they have a sensitivity. From 2 to 4 hr after some immediate hypersensitivity reactions, a second **late phase reaction** occurs, peaks at 6–9 hours, and may persist for a day or two. During this phase, mast cells release mediators including chemokines to attract leukocytes (particularly eosinophils and T helper [$T_H2$] cells), cytokines such as interleukin-4 (IL-4) and IL-13 to activate eosinophils, and leukotrienes to promote increase blood flow, smooth muscle contraction, and mucus secretion. Under the influence of chemokines and cytokines, this inflammation reaction consists of an accumulation of basophils, eosinophils, macrophages, neutrophils, and $T_H2$ cells. This accumulation of cells may be part of the protective function of IgE-mediated responses in the removal of parasites. For example, IgE-coated helminths are killed by eosinophils. The most severe form of type I hypersensitivity is **systemic** or **generalized anaphylaxis**, which can lead to **anaphylactic shock**. Most individuals only make increase amounts of IgE in responses to parasitic infections. The genetic tendency to develop immediate hypersensitivities, production of increased amounts of IgE, against common environmental antigens is called **atopy** (unusual, strange disease); hence, the disease states such as asthma and hay fever are called **atopic allergies**.

The opposite of hypersensitivity is **hyposensitivity**. Hyposensitization occurs when repeated small doses of an allergen are administered to reduce a hypersensitivity. This clinical approach helps to **desensitize** individuals to an allergen. This is different from *anergy*, a general loss of immune responsiveness due to deficient T-cell function.

## Experimental Observations of the Early 1900s Showed That Immune Responses to Innocuous Substances Can Be Harmful

Early investigators, in their search for ways to induce immunity, found that immunity is not always protective. In 1902, Richet[1] and Portier were studying the antitoxic immunity of dogs to a poison obtained from sea anemones. They found that dogs previously exposed to the poison collapsed and died within a few minutes after reinoculation with doses of the poison that were nontoxic to unexposed dogs. The paradoxical result was not immunity or a prophylactic state, but a reversed state, which they called *anaphylaxis*. Prausnitz showed the importance of antibodies in immediate hypersensitivities 20 years later. He injected himself with serum from an individual named Kustner, who was sensitized to fish. Prausnitz then took a fish extract and inoculated it into the same site that had received the serum. He observed redness within minutes. The reaction is called the *Prausnitz-Kustner (P-K) reaction* or, descriptively, *passive cutaneous anaphylaxis*. Not until 1967,

when Johansson described an IgE myeloma, did Ishizaka and coworkers isolate IgE; their work led to our understanding of the immunochemical basis of type I (immediate) hypersensitivities, which are related to the antibody known as *IgE*. Later, the importance of mast cells and basophils was shown, followed by the description of the allergens that provoke a type I hypersensitivity. This information permitted a more complete description of the mechanism for IgE-mediated immediate hypersensitivities.

## The First and Second Exposures to an Allergen Can Be Called a Sensitization and a Shocking Exposure Rather Than a Primary and a Secondary Antibody Response

The tendency to develop type I hypersensitivities is familial, but the exact method of inheritance is unknown. If both parents have atopy, there is a 75% chance that their child may have atopic reactions. The probability drops to 50% if only one parent has atopy. However, 38% of patients with atopic allergies have no parental history of atopy. The IgE levels in serum are under genetic control; the trait for low levels of IgE is dominant.

The genetic tendency to atopic allergies is associated with several susceptibility loci. For example, one locus on chromosome 5 is associated with disease, which is linked to a region that encodes the IL-4 family of cytokines such as IL-4, IL-5, IL-9, IL-13, and granulocyte-monocyte colony-stimulating factor (GM-CSF), all of which encourage IgE production. IL-4 gene polymorphism correlates with high serum IgE levels and enhanced IL-4 gene expression. Also, some atopic patients express a gain-of-function mutation in the α subunit of the IL-4 receptor, which leads to increased signaling following ligation of the receptor.

Another group of susceptibility genes found in this region of chromosome 5, is the *T* cell, *i*mmunoglobulin domain and *m*ucin domain (*TIM*) gene family, which encodes T cell surface proteins that regulate adaptive immune responses. TIM proteins are not limited to activated CD4+ T cells; dendritic cells also express them (TIM-3 and -4). Three of the family members (TIM-1, TIM-3, and TIM-4) are conserved between mice and humans. High levels of TIM-1 are expressed on activated $T_H2$ cells and promote $T_H2$ cell responses; TIM-1 plays a major role as a human susceptibility gene for allergy, asthma, and autoimmunity. TIM-2 in mice is a negative regulator of $T_H2$ cell responses. Fully differentiated $T_H1$ cells and dendritic cells express TIM-3; it has

---

[1]Charles Richet received the 1913 Nobel Prize in Medicine for his studies on anaphylaxis.

opposing roles in innate (synergizes with Toll-like receptors to induce inflammation) and adaptive (negative regulator of $T_H1$ cell responses by ligation with T cell-expressed galectin-9) immunity. Unlike the other TIM proteins, TIM-4 is only expressed by dendritic cells. It promotes $T_H2$ cell proliferation and survival by providing a costimulatory signal.

Alterations in the transcription factors STAT6 and GATA-3, master switches in the development of $T_H2$ cells and the region that encodes the p40 chain of IL-12, are associated with increased allergic responses. Clearly, there is an association with aberrant expression of genes needed for $T_H2$ cell development and $T_H2$ cell polarization in atopic diseases. Alterations in the opposing $T_H1$ pathways are also associated with atopic disorders; impaired IL-12 production is correlated with all atopic disorders. This is important because IL-12 directly primes $CD4^+$ T cells for $T_H1$ differentiation; its lack promotes $T_H2$ cell polarization. There is a susceptibility locus for asthma and atopic dermatitis on chromosome 11 that is linked to a region that encodes the high-affinity IgE receptor β chain. An association also exists between the expression of different HLA gene-encoded molecules and the ability to develop atopic responses to the five purified fractions of ragweed pollen (fractions E and K are consider major allergens, whereas fractions Ra3, Ra4, and Ra5 are considered minor allergens). These atopic responses to allergens, listed in Table 12-1, are caused by HLA-linked genes on chromosome 6. The hyper-responsiveness of atopic patients seems to correlate mainly with the expression of two HLA molecules, B8 and Dw3. Also, the DR2, DR3, and DR5 HLA alleles are associated strongly with IgE responses.

Environmental factors also contribute to the development of atopic allergies. One such factor is associated with the lack of early childhood exposure to microbial pathogens, presented as the *hygiene hypothesis* in 1989. The hypothesis (it is a hypothesis, not fact) goes something like this: inappropriate or defective development of immunologic regulatory controls in early childhood results from inadequate exposure to environmental microbes. Other contributing factors include allergen sensitization

(such as, house dust mites and cockroaches), lack of older siblings, widespread use of antibiotics, urban environment, excessive hygiene, and prevention of disease. The implication is that in early childhood the $T_H2$ cell responses predominate by default over $T_H1$ cell responses. Environments that predispose children to infections, reprogram them to a dominant $T_H1$ response by the cytokine response to these early infections. There is supportive and non-supportive evidence for this hypothesis. The dendritic cells of infants do synthesize and release less IL-12; consequently, $T_H1$ cells release less IFN-γ than in older children which would favor a $T_H2$ response. Children from developing countries who are treated with antihelminthic drugs have increased prevalence of atopy, while their untreated counterparts have significant parasitic infections but low prevalence of atopy. This is difficult to reconcile when helminth infections induce $T_H2$ cell responses.

$CD4^+CD25^+$ natural regulatory T ($T_{reg}$) cells (see Chapter 10) also contribute to the control atopic allergies. For example, $T_{reg}$ cells from atopic individuals are unable to inhibit $T_H2$ cell cytokine production, while their non-atopic counterparts can. In a mouse model, transcription factor FOXP3-deficient mice are unable to develop $T_{reg}$ cells; they exhibit symptoms associated with allergies. These symptoms could be partially reversed in mice that had a simultaneous deficiency in STAT6.

Irrespective of the measures that coerce the development of atopic allergies, antigen-antibody binding has two results: (1) the eventual destruction of the foreign substance and (2) the harmful results associated with allergies. For allergy-prone individuals who produce abnormal levels of IgE but normal levels of all other classes of antibodies, these two results occur through the same mechanisms as for normal immune responses. *However, the first exposure to a foreign environment substance that is an allergen (for that individual) is a* **sensitizing dose**. The resulting immune response follows the normal immune processing mechanisms (such as performed by skin dendritic cells called *Langerhans cells*) except that more IgE is made and it binds to mast cells (in tissues) and basophils (in the circulation), and it binds to these cells almost immediately after secretion.[2] If there is only one exposure to the allergen, the clinical signs of the type I hypersensitivity do not always arise. *However, if after an immunologic waiting period of about 10 days or more there is reexposure to the allergen*

**TABLE 12-1 Association of HLA Molecule Expression and Allergen Reactivity**

| HLA antigen | Allergen |
| --- | --- |
| A2, A28 | Ra3 |
| Dw2, B7 | Ra5 |
| A1, B8, Dw3 | Rye I |
| B8, Dw3 | Rye II |
| B7 | Timothy A3 |

---

[2]Because mast cells are located in the lungs, skin, tongue, and linings of the nose and intestinal tract, they can immediately act during hypersensitivity reactions.

*(the shocking dose), the hypersensitivity is triggered within seconds to minutes.* Hypersensitivity represents immune responses that show both specificity and memory, yet are protective against a harmless invader. The substances and mechanisms responsible for this rapid, yet seemingly unuseful, response are described in the remainder of the chapter.

### It is Unclear What Makes Antigens Allergens for Atopic Individuals

The terms *antigen* and *immunogen* are used to describe a substance that elicits an immune response. However, the term *allergen* is sometimes more appropriate than *antigen*. *An allergen is a common, harmless environmental substance (an antigen) that elicits an allergic response rather than an immune response.* Is there a difference between an antigen and an allergen? Frequently, no difference exists. Why ragweed pollen induces strong $T_H2$-mediated allergic responses, whereas other pollens like nettle pollen do not, is unknown. An allergen generally originates in plants, animals, or fungi; in contrast, bacteria (viruses can initiate some asthmas) do not induce allergies. Allergens are always proteins or are bound to protein as haptens because only proteins induce T-cell responses. IL-4-producing $CD4^+$ $T_H2$ cells are required for IgE production. These molecules, except haptenic allergens, are small and have molecular weights between 15 and 40 kD and are very soluble proteins associated with dried particles such as animal dander, mite feces, and pollen grains. The major allergens in the US are Der p1[3] and Der p 2 from fecal pellets of the house dust mite *Dermatophagoides pternyssimus*, Fel d 1 from the cat, several tree allergens, and many grasses and pollens. Allergies from latex and peanut proteins are significant problems. There is no clear-cut biological characteristic that can be ascribed to allergens. Nonetheless, allergens induce potent $T_H2$ cell responses; the following paragraph gives some suggestions why.

Exposure to allergens is either artificial (by injection) or natural. Routes of natural exposure include inhalation, ingestion, and contact with the skin or eyes. Type I hypersensitivity usually requires more than mere contact, but it does not require many exposures to the allergen or large amounts of it. In fact, microgram quantities are adequate. Low doses of antigen favor $T_H2$ cells (see Chapter 11 and the next section). The upper respiratory tract APCs bind allergen and transport it to local lymph nodes. These APCs are poorly phagocytic, do not produce IL-12, but are strongly costimulatory; therefore, they are unable to drive $T_H1$ responses, so by default they favor $T_H2$ responses. In atopic dermatitis, a type I hypersensitivity and in contact dermatitis, a delayed-type hypersensitivity, the hypersensitivity results after the allergen comes into contact with the skin.

### As in a Normal Immune Response, T and B Cells Are Involved in Type I Hypersensitivity Responses

The activation of precursors of IgE-secreting B cells is $T_H2$–cell–dependent; they drive IgE responses through the release of particular cytokines: IL-4, IL-5, and IL-13. *In fact, $T_H2$ cell-derived IL-4 and IL-13 have overlapping activities that stimulate $T_H2$ responses and thereby increase B-cell IgE production; IL-4 causes isotype switching to IgE; and IL-5 promotes eosinophil recruitment and activation.* Atopic individuals may have more allergen-specific IL-4-producing $T_H2$ cells, and these cells may make more IL-4 than their normal counterparts. In fact, the magnitude and duration of IgE responses are determined by crossregulation between antagonistic IL-4 and $T_H1$–cell-derived IFN-γ signals. The balance between these cytokines is an important determinant in a host's expression of the IgE-responder phenotype (see Chapter 10). (Another source of IL-4, IL-5, and IL-13 is the mast cell, which contributes to more IgE synthesis on allergen exposure.) $CD4^+$ $T_H1$ cell-derived cytokines downregulate the IgE response because they control B-cell differentiation, that is, low levels of IgE are maintained through the tight control of IgE class switching. The control is exerted through inhibition by cytokines (IFN-γ and IL-12), B-cell surface receptors (CD45 and CTLA-4 ligation), and transcription factors (BCL-6 and ID2), which converge on the regulation of $T_H2$–type cytokine–induced ε-chain constant-region germline DNA transcription.

### IgE Antibodies Act as Antigen Receptors Through Mast Cell and Basophil Fc Receptors

Of the five classes of antibody, IgE is found in the lowest concentration in plasma. The normal adult level of IgE is about 10 to 250 ng per milliliter of blood, while severely allergic individuals have about 700 to 1000 ng/ml. These levels of IgE in atopic individuals are still roughly 1000-fold less than that of plasma IgG. Table 12-2 lists some of the structural and biologic characteristics of the IgE antibody molecule.

---

[3]Many allergens are enzymes. Der p 1 is a cysteine protease, which cleaves occludin (a protein in intercellular tight junctions) thereby facilitating Der p 1 access to subepithelial regions. Dendritic cells in these regions take up Der p1 and present it to $T_H2$ cells, which drive Der p1-specific IgE production. IgE fixes to mast cells and waits for further Der p 1 interactions

**TABLE 12-2 Structural and Biological Characteristics of Human IgE**

| Structural | Biological |
|---|---|
| Two light chains (κ or λ) | Serum concentration: 10–250 ng/ml |
| Two heavy chains (ε) | Half-life in serum: 2–4 days, several weeks when bound to mast cells |
| Molecular formula: $\kappa_2\varepsilon_2$ or $\lambda_2\varepsilon_2$ | Species-specific binding to mast cells: homocytotropic |
| Molecular weight: 190,000 | Positive P-K test with 0.2 nanograms antibody |
| Carbohydrate content: 10–20% | |
| One more heavy-chain constant domain (total of 5 domains) | |

The function of IgE is controversial, but IgE-mediated responses may be important during parasitic worm (Helminth) infections (as mentioned at the beginning of the chapter). The mediators released during IgE-related responses are vasoactive amines that both increase vascular permeability and cause smooth muscle contraction. Thus, IgE may help to expel the parasitic worms from the body. However, the deleterious effects of type I hypersensitivity induced by nonparasitic, environmental allergens overshadow the benefits of IgE-associated parasite control.

IgE is different from the other antibody classes because it acts as an antigen receptor on the surface of mast cells and basophils. The additional IgE constant-region domain (Cε2) may stabilize IgE's binding to receptors on the surface of mast cells and basophils. This additional domain gives the IgE molecule a mw of 190,000. IgE also differs from other antibody isotypes by its limited selection of variable segments that contribute to the variable region. IgE associates with either high-affinity ($K_d = 1-2 \times 10^{-9}$ M) Fc receptors (called **FcεRI**) constitutively expressed on mast cells, basophils, and activated eosinphils or low-affinity ($K_d = 1-2 \times 10^{-6}$ M) Fc receptors (called *FcεRII* or *CD23*) on eosinophils, B cells, activated T cells, platelets, follicular dendritic cells, and monocytes. FcεRI is abundantly expressed (200,000 molecules per cell) on mast cells and basophils. Human FcεRI has a wider distribution than mast cells and basophils; it is also found on monocytes, myeloid and plasmacytoid dendritic cells, Langerhans cells, and eosinophils but at lower levels. The FcεRI are glycoproteins consisting of a four-polypeptide chain complex (Figure 12-3): an α and β chain and two identical disulfide-linked γ chains. Platelets and monocytes that express high-affinity Fc receptors lack the β chain. The FcεRI interacts with both $C_H3$ domains of a single IgE molecule through the two Ig-like domains of the α chain; the FcεRI contact sites for IgE are the α2 domain and the linker region between α1 and α2. The β and γ chains have associated immunoreceptor tyrosine-based motifs (ITAMs); the γ chains are responsible for intracellular signal transduction and are homologous to the B-cell receptor Igα/Igβ and T-cell receptor complex ζ chains. Cross-linking of FcR-bound IgE by allergen induces ITAM tyrosine phosphorylation, activates mast cells leading to their degranulation.

Figure 12-3 also shows the low-affinity Fc receptor FcεRII (CD23), which is structurally unrelated to FcεRI but also binds to the $C_H3$ domains of IgE. As mentioned above, FcεRII is expressed by several immune cell types, including B cells and may contol IgE levels. FcεRII is expressed by several immune cell types, including B cells. CD23-bound IgE facilitates allergen uptake by B cells and enhances presentation to T cells, leading to augmented IgE production.

**MINI SUMMARY**

Type I, or immediate, hypersensitivity involves individuals genetically predisposed to make large amounts of IgE. When initially exposed to an allergen, these individuals produce large amounts of IgE antibodies that bind to the surface of mast cells or basophils by Fc receptors. Clinical manifestations of immediate hypersensitivity appear after reexposure to the same allergen. The allergen binds and cross-links two adjacent mast cell FcεRI-bound IgE molecules, leading to mast cell degranulation and the release of mediator molecules that cause the symptoms of immediate hypersensitivity.

### Mast Cells and Basophils Degranulate After Allergen Cross-Links IgE Antibodies on Their Surfaces

*The IgE molecule sensitizes* **mast cells** *and* **basophils.** The main effector cells are mast cells and

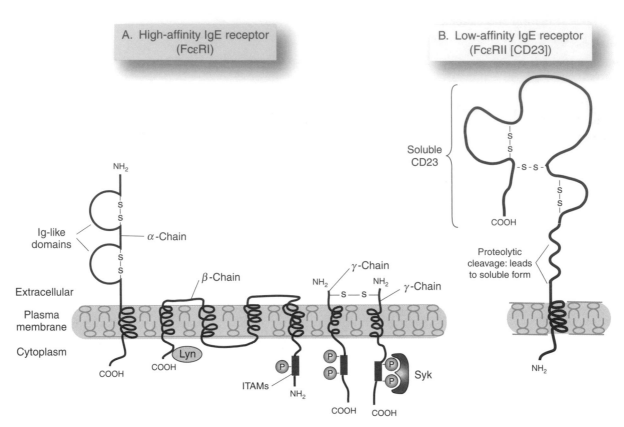

**FIGURE 12-3 The polypeptide chain structure of the mast cell high-affinity and low-affinity IgE Fc receptors.** The two immunoglobulin-like domains of the α chain bind IgE. The β and γ chains are mostly transmembrane and cytoplasmic and thus are thought to mediate signal transduction when IgE binds to its receptor.

basophils, mast cells were first described by Paul Ehrlich in 1877. He noticed that mast cells are filled with about 1000 large granules that stain with basic dyes because they contain acidic proteoglycans. The granules contain the chemical mediators of type I hypersensitivity reactions. Mast-cell precursors develop in the bone marrow during hematopoiesis but mature locally. The c-kit ligand, IL-3 IL-4, and IL-9 are important in driving mast cell development. Mast cells have two subpopulations that vary in the mediators they produce, named according to their tissue distribution, *mucosal mast cells* (respiratory and gastrointestinal tracts) and *connective tissue mast cells* (ubiquitous, mainly associated with blood vessels). In atopic individuals, these cells are coated heavily with allergen-specific IgE. The type of allergen-induced IgE response depends on which type of mast cell is activated. Allergens that are administered intravenously or subcutaneously activate connective tissue mast cells, which release histamine and other mediators systemically (causing anaphylaxis) or locally (causing a wheal-and-flare), respectively. Allergens that are inhaled or ingested activate mucosal mast cells, which release histamine and other mediators in the upper respiratory tract (causing allergic rhinitis) or the intestinal tract (causing vomiting), respectively. If the ingested allergen is released into the bloodstream, it causes urticaria (hives). The severity of allergic responses corresponds to the exposure levels of allergen: low levels transduce strong signals that lead to strong allergic responses; in contrast, high levels of allergen transduce the production of immunoregulatory cytokines such as IL-10 and TGF-β and milder allergic responses. Table 12-3 summarizes the characteristics of mast cells and basophils.

When allergen encounters IgE sitting on a mast cell or the basophil surface, it bridges several IgE molecules and cross-links the corresponding Fc receptor sites. Receptor cross-linking activates mast cells and basophils, but monomeric IgE alone does not trigger mediator release. Once activated, mast cells and basophils expel the preformed contents of their granules by a process called **degranulation**. Activated mast cells also release newly synthesized lipid mediators, cytokines, chemokines, and enzymes. The

**TABLE 12-3 Comparison of Mast Cells and Basophils**

| Parameter | Mast cell subpopulation | | Basophil |
| --- | --- | --- | --- |
| | Mucosal mast cell (MMC) | Connective tissue mast cell (CTMC) | |
| Origin | Bone marrow | Bone marrow | Bone marrow |
| Distribution | Gut and lungs | Ubiquitous | Blood (0.5–1.0% of circulating human leukocytes) |
| T cell-dependent | Yes | No | No |
| Life span | <40 days | Months to years | 8–12 days |
| Mitosis in mature cell | Yes | Yes | Yes |
| Size | <CTMC | 10–30 μm | 10–14 μm |
| Locomotion | No | No | Yes |
| Histamine content | <CTMC | 20–30 pg/cell | 1–2 pg/cell (rat) |
| Cytoplasmic IgE | Yes | No | — |
| IgE receptors | Yes | Yes | Yes |
| IgG4 receptors | ? | Yes | Yes |
| Number of FcεRI | $2 \times 10^5$ | $2 \times 10^4$ | <CTMC |
| Degranulation | Yes | Yes | Yes |
| Granule proteoglycan | Chondroitin sulfate | Heparin | Chondroitin sulfate |
| Theophylline inhibits histamine release | No | Yes | — |
| Major arachidonate metabolite | $LTC_4$ | $PGD_2$ | $LTC_4$ |

IgE molecule acts as an allergen recognition unit, and the Fc receptor is the degranulation-triggering unit (Figure 12-4). After cross-linking, the complexes undergo capping (localization of allergen-antibody complexes to one pole of the cell) and are either internalized or shed into the medium.

The release of mediators from mast cells starts within 15 to 20 sec after the cross-linkage of cell-bound IgE by the application of allergen. The series of biochemical events is summarized in Figure 12-5. The intracellular signaling events that initiate mast cell activation and degranulation revolve around the activation of Lyn, which phosphorylates the ITAM-associated tyrosines of the FcεRI β and γ chains. This instigates a series of phosphorylation reactions including phospholipase Cγ1 (PLCγ1), which induces the production of the secondary messenger molecules inositol triphosphate ($IP_3$) and diacylglycerol (DAG). $IP_3$ boosts intracellular $Ca^{2+}$ levels and the DAG-$Ca^{2+}$ duet activates protein kinase C (PKC), which contributes to the events that surround degranulation. Another part of this reaction involves the metabolism of membrane phospholipids leading to the activation of phospholipase $A_2$, which, in turn, interacts with membrane substrates and generates phospholipid by-products. These by-products participate in the fusion of the granule and the cell membrane. The activated lipase is important in the production of the newly formed mediators, such

as prostaglandin and leukotrienes. Simultaneously, membrane enzymes convert phosphatidylserine (PS) to phosphatidylethanolamine (PE), which is methylated to form phosphatidylcholine (PC). The accumulation of PC on the exterior of the cell's plasma membrane causes the formation of $Ca^{2+}$ channels. Within in 2 min of FcεRI cross-linkage, the combination of extracellular $Ca^{2+}$ influx and the liberation of intracellular stores of $Ca^{2+}$ promotes PKC activation of mitogen-activated protein kinase (MAPK)—leads to cytokine synthesis, the activation of phospholipase $A_2$—leads to the conversion of PC to lysophosphatidylcholine (Lyso-PC) and arachidonic acid, the latter is the source for potent mediators, and the assembly of microtubules and contraction of microfilaments—leads to degranulation. The importance of $Ca^{2+}$-increases to mast cell degranulation is underscored by using disodium cromoglycate, a blocker of $Ca^{2+}$ influx, as a treatment for allergies.

Concomitant with the transmethylation of phospholipids, the bridging of two FcεRIs, through allergen binding to two adjacent IgE antibodies, stimulates adenylate cyclase, which, in the presence of $Ca^{2+}$, leads to the conversion of cytosolic ATP to cAMP. Cyclic AMP levels peak within 15 sec and parallel phospholipid methylation occurs. Feedback suppression of further influx of $Ca^{2+}$ and of histamine release results from the increased level of cAMP. The entry

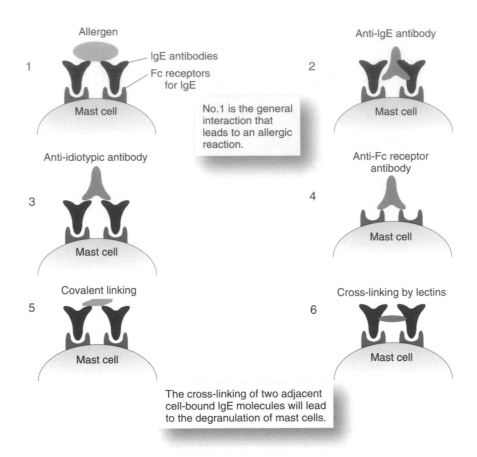

**FIGURE 12-4 Triggering mediator release from mast cells—mechanisms for cross-linking cell-bound IgE molecules**. When two adjacent IgE molecules bound to mast cell Fc receptors are cross-linked, the mast cells are triggered to degranulate and release vasoactive mediators. Six possible mechanisms of cross-linking Fc receptors are illustrated: (1) multivalent antigen bridging two adjacent IgE molecules, (2) anti-IgE antibodies reacting with Fc portions of IgE molecules, (3) anti-idiotypic antibodies against IgE idiotope, (4) anti-Fc receptor antibodies, (5) chemical covalent linking of adjacent IgE molecules, and (6) lectins reacting with carbohydrates on IgE molecules.

of $Ca^{2+}$ causes the granule to swell by increasing its membrane permeability and activates enzymes that release energy as ATP molecules. This energy promotes assembly of microtubules and contraction of microfilaments, leading to movement of the swollen granules to the mast cell surface. The fusogens then induce the fusion of the granules to form secretory granules, which in turn merge with the mast cell plasma membrane. This fusion leads the granules to disgorge their preformed mediators, such as histamine, heparin, and eosinophil chemotactic factor of anaphylaxis (ECF-A) and others.

In addition to mast cells and basophils, several other cells are implicated in allergic reactions. Human platelets contain serotonin. Rabbit platelets contain serotonin plus heparin and histamine. Platelets also

produce arachidonic acid metabolites. The main cyclooxygenase product of human platelets is thromboxane $A_2$, a potent vasoconstrictor and platelet agonist (inducer of platelet aggregation). Macrophages and neutrophils are not target cells in allergic reactions but are major producers of prostaglandins and leukotrienes. Another blood cell involved in allergic reactions without being a direct target cell is the eosinophil. In nonatopic persons, eosinophils represent about 1 to 3% of circulating leukocytes, while in atopic patients their percentage may rise to 10 to 20%. Eosinophils are mostly found in connective tissues associated with the intestinal, respiratory, and urogential epithelium. Eosinophils are attracted to the allergic inflammatory site by chemotactic factors released by mast cells and basophils. Eosinophils

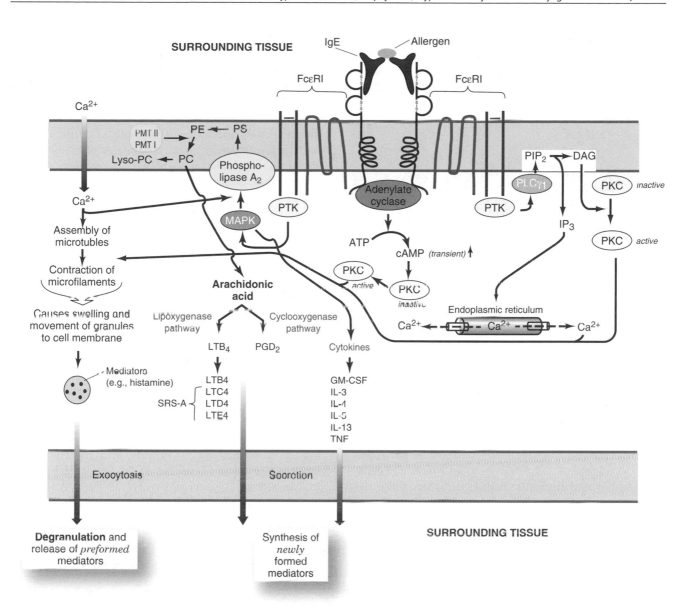

**FIGURE 12-5 Triggering of mast cell degranulation—release of preformed and newly synthesized mediators.** The process of mast-cell degranulation starts when two adjacent IgE molecules, associated on the cell's surface by Fc receptors (FcεRI), are cross-linked by an allergen (antigen) molecule. This cross-linking induces three membrane-associated events. One leads to the activation of protein tyrosine kinase (PTK), which phosphorylates phospholipase Cγ1 (PLCγ1). PLCγ1 converts phosphatidylinositol-4,5 biphosphate (PIP$_2$) into diacylglycerol (DAG) and inositol triphosphate (IP$_3$). DAG activates protein kinase C (PKC); it along with Ca$^{2+}$ drives microtubule assembly and fusion of granules with the cell's membrane. The intracellular Ca$^{2+}$ stores are mobilized by IP$_3$. Cross-linking also induces membrane-associated serine proesterase to form serine esterase. Serine esterase converts phosphatidylserine (PS) into phosphatidylethanolamine (PE). PE is methylated in two steps by PMT I & II to form phosphatidylcholine (PC). As PC accumulates on the exterior surface of the plasma membrane, it changes the cell membrane so that there is an increased influx of Ca$^{2+}$ into the cell. The influx of Ca$^{2+}$ and PTK-activated mitogen-activated protein kinase (MAPK) activates phospholipase A$_2$, which promotes the breakdown of PC to lysophosphatidylcholine (Lyso-PC) and arachidonic acid. Arachidonic acid is converted by two pathways into potent mediators, the leukotrienes (LT) and prostaglandins (PG) (see Figure 12.5). The activation of MAPK leads to cytokine gene expression and secretion of cytokines. Cross-linking also activates membrane adenylate cyclase, leading to the transient increase in cAMP (see text for further detail). The increased Ca$^{2+}$ influx also promotes degranulation by regulating the enzymes that control microfilaments. This influx leads to the movement of the granules to the mast cell membrane and fusion of the granules to form secretory granules that disgorge their contents. Newly formed mediators: the leukotrienes, slow reactive substance-anaphylaxis (SRS-A), prostaglandins, and cytokines. Preformed mediators: histamine and heparin. PMT I & II, phospholipid methyltransferase I & II.

limit allergic reactions by releasing arylsulfatase B and histaminase, which cleave leukotrienes and histamine, respectively, thus decreasing the local mediator concentration. Eosinophils also can remove the allergic antigen-antibody complexes by phagocytosis. Thus, eosinophils are important in modulating allergic reactions.

---

## MINI SUMMARY

The main effector cells of type I hypersensitivity reactions are mast cells and basophils. They display FcεRIs for IgE molecules and possess granules that contain histamine, heparin, and chemotactic factors. The second exposure (shocking dose) to the homologous allergen cross-links cell-surface FcεRI-bound IgE molecules and initiates degranulation, which releases preformed mediators, and the synthesis of new mediators and cytokines.

---

### Preformed and Newly Synthesized Mediators Are the Effector Molecules of Type I Hypersensitivity Reactions

During type I hypersensitivity reactions, activation of tissue mast cells or peripheral basophils leads to the release of preformed and newly synthesized, pharmacologically active, effector molecules (Table 12-4 and Table 12-5). The preformed mediators include *histamine, heparin* (the predominate proteoglycan in human mast cells), a group of peptide chemotactic factors (*ECF-A* and neutrophil chemotactic factor of anaphylaxis or *NCF-A*), the proteoglycans chondroitin sulfates, and several acid-hydrolases and proteolytic enzymes. The newly formed effector molecules include arachidonic acid metabolites such as *prostaglandins, thromboxanes, and slow-reacting substance of anaphylaxis (SRS-A, a mixture of three leukotrienes), bradykinins, platelet-activating factor, and various cytokines and chemokines. Serotonin*, found in human platelets, is another molecule with physiologic effects similar to those of histamine. These mediators act on local tissues and cells, such as, eosinophils, monocytes, neutrophils, platelets, and $T_H2$ cells.

The mast cell granule is water-insoluble and remains intact for a time after discharge. Histamine, a short-lived vasoactive amine, is a positively charged molecule electrostatically complexed with negatively charged heparin-proteoglycan on the granule surface. After dissolution of the granule, positively charged sodium from the surrounding environment exchanges with the histamine in the histamine-heparin complex. Histamine mediates its activity through specific receptors on smooth muscle, endothelial cells, and nerves. There are four different histamine receptors: $H_1$, $H_2$, $H_3$, and $H_4$. Histamine ligation of $H_1$ and $H_2$ receptors mediates the majority of the allergic effects with $H_1$ receptors-histamine association predominating. The free histamine acts

---

**TABLE 12-4 Preformed Mediators of Type I Hypersensitivity**

| Mediator | Characteristics | Biologic effects |
|---|---|---|
| Histamine | 111 mw | Contraction of smooth muscle and increase in vascular permeability |
| Serotonin | 176 mw | Increase in vascular permeability |
| ECF-A | ≈380 mw | Chemotactic for eosinophils |
| Heparin | Proteoglycan of ≈750,000 mw | Anticoagulant |
| Chymase | Protein of 29,000 mw | Chymotrypsin |
| Arylsufatase | Protein of 116,000 mw | Inactivation of SRS-A |

---

**TABLE 12-5 Newly Formed Mediators of Type I Hypersensitivity**

| Mediator | Characteristics | Biological effects |
|---|---|---|
| Prostaglandins | Arachidonic acid metabolites, such as $PGD_2$, $PGE_2$, $PGI_2$, $TxA_2$ with mw of ≈400 | Bronchial muscle contraction and relaxation, vasodilation, and platelet aggregation |
| Leukotrienes $B_4$; $C_4$, $D_4$, $E_4$ (SRS-A) | Arachidonic acid metabolites with mw of ≈400 | Contraction of smooth muscle and increase in vascular permeability |
| Platelet-activating factor (PAF) | Lipid-like with mw of 523 and 551 | Aggregation of platelets and release of vasoamines |
| Cytokines and chemokines | IL-3, IL-4, IL-5, IL-13, GM-CSF, and TNF-α; CXCL8 and CCL2 | Activate endothelial cells, recruit inflammatory cells, and drive the growth and differentiation of eosinophils |

immediately on the blood vessel endothelial cells and smooth muscles in the immediate vicinity of the mast cell. Histamine causes smooth muscle contractions of bronchioles and small blood vessels, increases capillary permeability, increases mucus secretions from nasal and bronchial globlet cells, and increases the release of stomach acid. The earliest manifestations of allergen exposure in atopic individuals are caused by histamine-mediated bronchial and tracheal contractions but within minutes contractions are mediated by leukotrienes and prostaglandins.

The molecules synthesized during mast cell activation are classified as lipids. Most lipid mediators result from the metabolism of arachidonic acid through both the *cyclooxygenase* and *lipoxygenase pathways* (Figure 12-6). Activation of mast cells changes the specific geometric orientation of the phospholipids in the membranes and activates phospholipase $A_2$, phospholipase C, and diglyceride lipase, which generate arachidonic acid for oxidative metabolism.

Arachidonic acid is the precursor of leukotrienes, which constitute the SRS-A mediators. By another pathway, arachidonic acid can be metabolized into prostaglandins and thromboxane (see Figure 12-6).

The biologic activities of these mediators are relevant to some end-organ effects. The $PGD_2$ and $PGF_{2\alpha}$ molecules have bronchospastic effects in humans. In addition, $PGD_2$ is an enhancer of random granulocyte migration. The administration of $PGI_2$ (prostacyclin) by the intravenous or inhalation routes causes vasodilatory and platelet antiaggregation effects in humans. $PGE_2$ can inhibit macrophage spreading

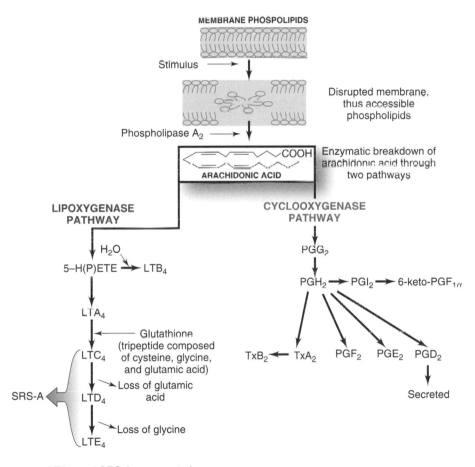

**FIGURE 12-6 The cyclooxygenase and lipoxygenase pathways of mediator production.** The mediators of immediate hypersensitivities result from the breakdown of cell membrane phospholipid molecules into arachidonic acid. Arachidonic acid is, in turn, metabolized by the cyclooxygenase and lipoxygenase pathways to form the prostaglandins (PG) and leukotrienes (LT), respectively. $LTC_4$, $LTD_4$, and $LTE_4$ constitute the slow-reacting substance of anaphylaxis (SRS-A). 5-H(P)ETE, 5-hydroperoxyeicosatetraenoic acid; $TxA_2$, thromboxane $A_2$; $TxB_2$, thromboxane $B_2$.

and surface adherence. In humans, $PGE_2$ has bronchodilatory effects. The HETEs are chemotactic for human granulocytes. The leukotrienes are vasodilators, bronoconstrictors, and inducers of mucus production. In fact, leukotrienes are 10–1000 times more potent than histamine in mediating these activities. Thromboxane $A_2$ is a platelet aggregator and potent vasoconstrictor.

In addition to prostaglandins and leukotrienes, mast cell-synthesized *platelet-activating factor (PAF)* serves as a potent mediator possessing a spectrum of inflammatory and physiologic activity. PAF stimulates platelets to produce prostaglandins and thromboxanes, and causes aggregation and secretion of granules from these cells. It also causes neutrophils to aggregate and, in the presence of cytochalasen B, starts the release of enzymes from granules of neutrophils. PAF is 100 to 1000 times more potent than histamine in causing cutaneous erythema and increasing vascular permeability. In animal tests using monkeys, the intravenous infusion of microgram quantities of PAF induces all the clinical sequelae associated with IgE-induced systemic anaphylaxis in humans. Some of these changes include (1) intravascular platelet aggregation, pulmonary localization, and secretion of granular constituents such as thromboxane $B_2$; (2) neutropenia and basopenia; (3) prolonged systemic hypotension; and (4) in the most severe cases, complete apnea (cessation of breathing) with subsequent death. PAF may act independently of platelets because in the rabbit the depletion of platelets does not change its physiologic effects. These findings suggest that PAF is one of the most potent mediators yet described for immediate hypersensitivity reactions.

Mast cells also synthesize nonlipid mediators such as, the cytokines IL-3, IL-4, IL-5, IL-6, IL-13, GM-CSF, and TNF-$\alpha$ and chemokines such as CXC-chemokine ligand 8 (CXCL8), CXCL10, CC-chemokine ligand 2 (CCL2), CCL2, CCL4, and CCL5 (see Chapter 9). (Mast cells also contain preformed stores of IL−1$\alpha$, IL-6, CXCL8, and TNF-$\alpha$.) These cytokines and chemokines, along with earlier mentioned mediators, in particular ECF-A and NCF-A, contribute to a second wave of type I hypersensitivity activity, the **late phase reaction**, its clinical manifestations appear a few hours after allergen exposure, peak by 6–9 hours, and have resolved themselves by 24–48 hours. It occurs in roughly 50% of the patients who exhibit an immediate phase response. The classical signs of inflammation, edema, erythema, warmth, and pain characterize the clinical manifestations of the late phase reactions in tissues. In contrast, lung reactions are characterized by airway narrowing and mucus hypersecretion. The tissue edema results from the recruitment and infiltration of inflammatory cells such as basophils, eosinophils, macrophages, neutrophils, and $T_H2$ cells to the sites of allergen exposure. The migration of $T_H2$ cells to these sites, reactivates them, and causes their clonal expansion. Localized IgE-facilitated dendritic cells increase $T_H2$ cell activation. Local IgE production occurs in allergic rhinitis and asthma but not in atopic dermatitis. Eosinophils constitute up to 50% of the infiltrating cells in the lungs of asthmatic individuals, whereas only 1–2% of the cellular infiltrate of individuals with atopic dermatitis is represented by eosinophils. Locally released IL-3, IL-5, and GM-CSF drive the growth and differentiation of eosinophils. Since eosinophils express Fc$\epsilon$RII and Fc receptors for IgG, the binding of either will activate them, causing degranulation, and the release of leukotrienes, PAF, major basic protein (MBP), which kills schistosomes by affecting their mobility and damaging their surface, and eosinophil cationic protein (ECP), which is a potent neurotoxin and anti-heminthic toxin. MCP and ECP may play a role in anti-parasitic infections but during allergic reactions they mediate the late phase reaction. MCP causes degranulation of mast cells. Eosinophils also release a diverse array of cytokines, which enhance their own activation and perpetuate the associated inflammatory response. NCF-A– and CXCL8–recruited neutrophils activated by localized antigen-antibody complexes, degranulate, and release lytic enzymes, PAF, and leukotrienes that exacerbate the late phase reaction. The production of IFN-$\gamma$ and TNF-$\alpha$ and expression of Fas ligand (CD95) by localized $T_H1$ cells contributes to their induction and apoptosis of skin keratinocytes, bronchial epithelial cells, and pulmonary smooth-muscle cells. The activation of localized mast cells and basophils also add to the late phase allergic reaction.

## MINI SUMMARY

During degranulation, the breakdown of arachidonic acid through both the cyclooxygenase and lipoxygenase pathways leads to the formation of prostaglandins (and thromboxanes) and leukotrienes, respectively. Histamine, serotonin, prostaglandins, and leukotrienes are smooth muscle contractors and vasodilators. Another potent mediator is platelet-activating factor (PAF); it causes aggregation of platelets, and release of platelet granules and stimulates platelets to produce prostaglandins. Mast cells also synthesize another group of potent molecules that mediate the late phase reaction, which includes cytokines and chemokines to attract leukocytes and activate eosinophils, and leukotrienes to perpetuate increased blood flow, smooth muscle constriction, and mucus secretion.

## There Are Systemic and Localized Consequences of Type I Hypersensitivity

Fifty million Americans suffer from allergies. These disease states are clinically important to the physician and patient, but to the experimental scientist they are merely curiosities or artificially induced animal situations. From an economic standpoint, allergic disorders affect everyone indirectly through lost schooldays and workdays and required medical treatment.

### Systemic Anaphylaxis Is a Life-Threatening Hypersensitivity Reaction

Systemic anaphylaxis may occur after insect stings and after using certain medications, especially those given by intravenous injection. Similar but milder reactions may occur from certain foods. Though the exact incidence is unknown, roughly 2000 preventable deaths occur each year.

In each patient, a sensitizing exposure has taken place, probably without notice, with an offending allergen introduced directly into the bloodstream or absorbed from the gut or skin. This priming experience elicits the development of cytotropic IgE antibodies that fix to target tissue (mast) cells and circulating basophils. On the second or shocking exposure with the appropriate allergen, the combination of the allergen with mast cell-bound IgE antibodies causes release of vasoactive mediators, which activate a sequence of events that lead to a systemic increase in vascular permeability causing a significant drop in blood pessure, to asphyxia or the shock syndrome of anaphylaxis—**anaphylactic shock**. In severe cases without medical intervention, the patient may die within 30 min. The shock organs involved in systemic anaphylaxis in different species are listed in Table 12-7. It is usually treated by an immediate injection of epinephrine, which relaxes smooth muscle and counteracts the cardiovascular effects of anaphylactic shock. Shock organs are the target sites in the body where a type I hypersensitivity reaction occurs.

Various antigens can trigger an anaphylactic shock in atopic individuals; they include bee, wasp, and hornet venom and ant bites; drugs, such as

**TABLE 12-6  Approaches to Intervention in Type I Hypersensitivity Reactions**

1. Avoid allergen contact
2. Prevent allergen from reaching mast cells or basophils
3. Reduce IgE antibody production
4. Prevent IgE binding to mast cells or basophils
5. Interfere with intracellular events needed for degranulation
   a. Raise cAMP levels
   b. Prevent lowering of cAMP levels
   c. Prevent raising of cGMP levels
6. Prevent synthesis of mediators (histamine, prostaglandins, leukotrienes)
7. Antagonize specific mediators (histamine, prostaglandins, leukotrienes)
8. Enhance degradation of mediators once synthesized
9. Prevent or reverse biologic effects of mediator action

penicillin and antitoxins; and foods, such as eggs, shellfish, and peanuts. Allergic reactions to drugs can take many forms and can result from immediate or delayed-type hypersensitivity reactions (only IgE-mediated reactions will be discussed). Nonetheless, the pattern of reaction to a drug is usually fairly consistent.

Approximately 1 to 3% of patients treated with penicillin have a type I hypersensitivity reaction; penicillin is the most common cause of drug allergy. Many individuals show drug allergy to alternative antibiotics and are placed at risk by what are otherwise easily treatable infections. It is estimated that allergic reactions occur in 0.1 to 1% of drug treatment regimens, and 5% of the adult population may be allergic to one or more drugs.

The drug or a chemical breakdown product of the drug often causes the allergic reaction after it has combined with some protein of the body. The drug or its derivative is known as an *autocoupling hapten*, which spontaneously binds to self-proteins and is considered a complete antigen on drug–protein combination. The complete antigen or allergen stimulates the production of specific IgE antibodies, and the later interaction leads to allergic tissue damage or drug reactions, such as systemic anaphylaxis.

For most drugs, the immunologic mechanism is poorly understood. However, a drug can convert into many complex products during its breakdown in the body. For example, penicillin G can be degraded to four different haptens. These haptens combine with self-proteins and induce $T_H2$ cells specific for penicillin-modified self-peptides. These cells activate penicillin-binding B cells to produce penicillin-specific IgE antibodies.

**TABLE 12-7** Systemic Anaphylaxis in Different Species

| Species | Principal pharmacologic mediator | Shock organ(s) | Manifestations |
|---|---|---|---|
| Dog | Histamine | Hepatic veins | Hepatic engorgement, vomiting, diarrhea |
| Guinea pig | Histamine, SRS-A | Lungs | Bronchiolar constriction, breathing difficulties (dyspnea), hyperinflation of lungs |
| Human | Histamine, SRS-A | Lungs | Respiratory distress, low blood pressure, circulatory collapse |
| Mouse | Serotonin<br><br>Histamine | Intestine, lungs | Intestinal hyperemia, respiratory distress, hyperinflation of lungs |
| Rabbit | Histamine<br><br>Serotonin<br><br>SRS-A<br><br>PAF | Heart, pulmonary vessels | Heart failure, liver and lung congestion |
| Rat | Serotonin<br><br>Histamine | Intestine | Circulatory collapse and intestinal bleeding |

### Atopic Allergies Are Usually the Wheezing, Sneezing, Runny Nose, Watery Eyes, and Itching Kinds of Hypersensitivity Reactions

Atopic allergies occur in genetically predisposed individuals. The genetic defect of these individuals does not allow them to control the physiologic IgE response; thus, they exhibit a pathologic response. The person with atopy is sensitized, but the sensitization is the result of a *natural exposure to common, harmless environmental antigens* such as by inhalation, ingestion, or contact with the skin. Atopy cannot be induced in normal individuals.

Some classic examples of atopy are (1) allergic rhinitis (commonly called *hay fever*), (2) asthma, (3) atopic dermatitis, (4) atopic urticaria (hives), and (5) food allergies. *Hay fever* is commonly seasonal, occurring when certain fungal spores, pollens, and grasses are abundant. The nonseasonal forms are caused by inhalation of common airborne allergens, such as pet danders, house dust, dust mites, and molds that interact with sensitized mast cells in the conjunctivae and nasal epithelium. The released mediators cause localized vasodilation and increased capillary permeability, leading to sneezing, coughing, and watery exudate from the eyes and nose. Hay fever affects nearly 10% of the American population. Antihistamines reduce its symptoms.

*Asthma* is a term used for several conditions in which the common factor is a constriction of the bronchioles of the lung. The lungs demonstrate increased susceptibility to histamine and SRS-A. The tissue surrounding the capillaries of the lung contains many mast cells, which, when stimulated by allergen-antibody interactions, release their pharmacologically active mediators, causing contraction of the smooth muscles surrounding the smaller airways, which leads to bronchoconstriction manifested by episodes of wheezy breathlessness. Other clinical signs include development of mucus and buildup of proteins and fluids leading to airway edema, sloughing of the epithelium, and occlusion of bronchial lumens. Asthmatic attacks may be triggered by exposure to dust, plant pollens, animal dander, insect products (cockroach calyx is a major asthma-inducing allergen in children), or viral antigens in which case asthma usually coexists with allergic rhinitis. Exercise and cold temperatures independent of allergens may also induce asthma; this type of asthma is called *intrinsic asthma*.

An asthma that first appears in adults is sometimes called *infective* or *adult-onset asthma*; it strikes adults over the age of 40. This type of asthma usually appears after an apparent respiratory infection. Childhood asthma is usually preceded by atopic dermatitis, but frequently this disease disappears by puberty. Patients with juvenile asthma usually exhibit positive skin tests, while those with infective asthma may not. Because asthma is a family of diseases with a common symptom, the results of skin tests with allergens differ. In severely sensitive patients, skin testing may provoke an asthmatic attack. Even though asthma is defined as a localized anaphylaxis, asthmatic attacks can be fatal.

Irrespective of the type of asthma, immuno-histopathology suggests that inflammation is a major component of asthma. As allergic rhinitis, asthma initially involves the results instigated by degranulation of mast cells but occurs in the lower respiratory tract. A few hours later, cytokines and chemokines from lung epithelial cells induce expression of endothelial cell adhesion molecules and recruit large numbers of particularly eosinophils but also neutrophils and $T_H2$ cells into the bronchial tissue. As the eosinophils enter the airway matrix, their survival is prolonged by IL-5 and GM-CSF. The accumulation and activation of eosinophils and their release of oxygen radicals, nitric oxide, and cytokines injure airway tissues. Eosinophils can produce GM-CSF to prolong and potentiate their survival and contribute to a variable degree of airflow obstruction, bronchial hyperresponsiveness, and airway inflammation. $T_H2$ cell-derived IL-9 and IL-13 cause airway epithelial cells to differentiate into goblet cells, leading to increased secretion of mucus.

*Atopic dermatitis* (also called *allergic eczema*) is a condition affecting the epidermis of young children; it usually persists until puberty. Atopic dermatitis is characterized by itching and a red rash, consisting of tiny papules, that affects especially the skin in the folds of the elbows and knees, but much of the body may be affected. Atopic dermatitis does not follow a constant course, and sudden flare-ups preceded by intense irritation may occur, often at times of emotional tension. The association between mental state and atopic dermatitis or asthma has long been evident, but its basis is unknown. Atopic dermatitis tends to run in the family, but no simple method of inheritance has been found. Affected patients have abnormally high levels of IgE. The inciting allergen is unknown, the skin lesions are erythematosus, and contain $T_H2$ cells and eosinophils. The lesions may contain pus, if bacterial superinfections have occurred. Both atopic dermatitis and asthma respond well to treatment with corticosteroids.

In contrast to atopic dermatitis, which is the appearance of swellings in the epidermis, *atopic urticaria* (*hives*) is a skin condition characterized by intensely itching, elevated and circumscribed eruptions (wheals) caused by swellings of the dermis. The wheals can vary in size from small and pimple-like to much larger welts. The hives can last for hours to years but usually subside within 2 days, and most single exposure-induced urticaria resolves within 1 to 2 weeks. Hives arise from vasodilation and increased capillary permeability of the venules of the dermis caused by release of vasoactive amines from the surrounding tissue mast cells. Drugs, allergy to foods, and allergy to food additives can cause atopic urticaria. Other common causes include physical stimuli such as cold and heat.

Food allergies, which affect 1–4% of Americans, are caused by ingestion of certain foods, such as peanuts, eggs, shellfish, and milk by individuals with allergies to them. Rougly 25% of all food allergies is instigated by peanuts. IgE cross-linking on sensitized mast cells situated in the upper and lower gastrointestinal tract induces degranulation, mediator release and localized smooth muscle contraction and vasodilation, often causing vomiting and diarrhea. Mast cell degranulation can cause increased mucous membrane permeability, which allows the food allergen to leak into the bloodstream. As mentioned in the preceding paragraph, the food allergen can be deposited by mast cells in the skin leading to atopic urticaria (commonly called hives)—swollen and red eruptions called the *wheal-and-flare response*.

## Sensitivity Testing Is Done to Determine if an Individual Has Immunity or Hypersensitivity

If the symptomatic history of a patient suggests sensitivity to some allergen, skin testing is used to confirm specific sensitivities. The skin reacts to allergen in most patients with type I hypersensitivities, even though their symptoms occur in other organs. Skin testing is a convenient, reliable, and safe way to diagnose allergic disease. Care must be taken, however, to correlate the skin test findings with the patient's clinical history.

*Skin testing is an established way of determining if an individual suffers from an atopic condition. There are three different approaches to sensitivity testing, but all look for a* **local triple response (erythema, edema,** *and* **wheal-and-flare)**, which appears in less than 30 minutes. A wheal-and-flare is an elevated, circumscribed eruption (welt) caused by swelling of the dermis due to dilation of local blood vessels that then become leaky (a wheal: redness and local swelling). Further dilation of blood vessels on the edge of the swelling leads to a red rim (the flare). Skin testing is accomplished by scratch, patch, or intradermal skin testing. In the scratch test, several scrapes are made on the skin and a small amount of the suspected offending allergen is applied to the area. A triple response shows that the individual has an atopic sensitivity to the allergen. In the patch test, a piece of paper or cloth is impregnated with the test allergen and taped to the skin (normally on the back). The patch is removed after

24 hr and the area is observed for the triple response. The patch test is a convenient method for skin testing of children because no pain is involved. The third kind of skin testing involves injecting the test allergen intradermally and looking for the triple response. Present skin tests often fail to show which substances are responsible for the atopic disease because of the complex nature of the allergen being used. A patient sensitive to elm pollen, for example, may often cross-react with many other types of pollen, and only by prolonged observation is the offending allergen identified. Also, the true allergen may be a breakdown product rather than the complete molecule. Furthermore, reintroducing of the allergen by skin testing may aggravate the sensitivity. Skin testing may also sensitize the patient to new allergens. *In vitro* assays have been developed to avoid *in vivo* problems and to attain the sensitivity needed to measure nanogram amounts of IgE accurately. Radioimmunoassays give precise quantitative measurements of the total or specific IgE present in the serum without the problems related to skin testing. Figure 12-7

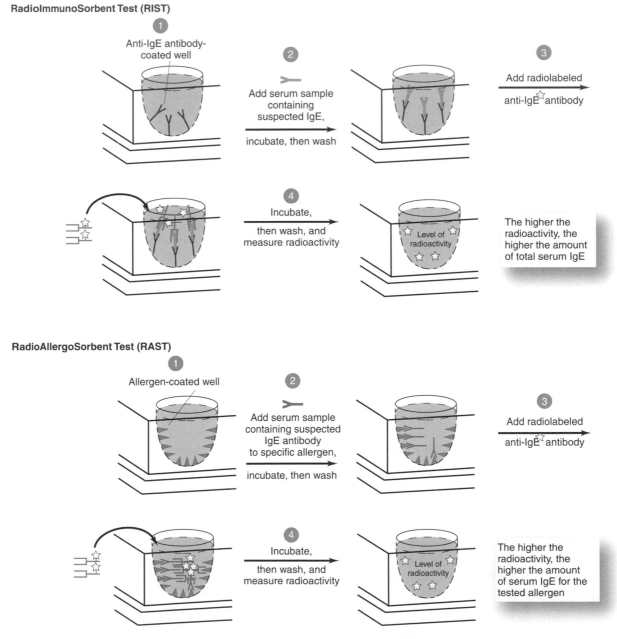

**FIGURE 12-7** *In vitro* **assessment of type I hypersensitivities**. The RadioImmunoSorbent Test (RIST) measures total serum IgE amounts, whereas the RadioAllergoSorbent Test (RAST) measures allergen-specific IgE amounts.

shows the **radioimmunosorbent test (RIST)**, which measures total serum levels of IgE antibody and the **radioallergosorbent test (RAST)**, which measures the amount of serum IgE specific for a particular allergen.

## Treatments for Type I Hypersensitivities Consider Only the Symptoms, Not the Causes

Allergy treatments (Table 12-6) attempt to suppress IgE production or IgE-mediated hypersensitivity reactions. Many drugs accomplish this suppression or intervention, but they all introduce undesirable side effects (especially after prolonged use) and treat the symptoms of the allergies rather than the causes. Therefore, immunologic approaches such as *avoidance* and *desensitization* often are used to treat immediate hypersensitivities.

### Antigen Avoidance Is the Best but Not Always Possible Treatment

Once the offending allergen has been identified, suggestions for its avoidance are made. Avoidance is entirely effective. Many people have found it desirable or necessary to change their occupation or their place of residence, or even to give up their pets, to escape exposure to offending allergens. The elimination of inhalant allergens, such as pollens is impossible.

### Desensitization, Hyperimmunization That Leads to Hypoimmunity, Is the Oldest Form of Treatment

The current approach to intervention in atopic disorders stresses identification of allergens and treatment with drugs. When drugs fall short, the patient may be a candidate for desensitization with allergy shots. *Desensitization*, or more correctly *hyposensitization*, is one of the oldest forms of immunotherapeutic treatment of any immunologic disorder. It reduces the severity of, or in some cases eliminates, allergic rhinitis in atopic patients. Atopic individuals receive, over an extended time, repeated subcutaneous injections of increasing doses of the offending allergen, usually as an extract. This repeated exposure to the allergen induces the production of circulating IgG antibodies. These antibodies intercept the allergen before it reacts with the membrane-bound IgE, hence the name *blocking antibodies*. The IgG-allergen complex is removed by cells of the mononuclear phagocyte system and leads to a *temporary unresponsiveness* to the allergen. Another possibility for the shift to IgG

production is a switch from $T_H2$ to $T_H1$ cells and the production IFN-$\gamma$, which blocks B-cell differentiation and turns off IgE production in response to allergen. Whether either of these mechanisms or others mediate the reduction in hypersensitivities following allergen-specific immunotherapy remains incompletely defined. Nonetheless, successful allergen-specific immunotherapy is associated with several characteristics, including increases in allergen-specific IgG1, IgG4 and, to a lesser extent, IgA, reduced $T_H2$—cell proliferative responses to allergens, and modified cytokine-secretion profiles, leading to an increased ratio of $T_H1$-cell to $T_H2$-cell responses and in the induction of functional $T_{reg}$ cells secreting IL-10 and TGF-$\beta$, which direct the antibody response away from IgE production.

Other approaches to immunotherapy of allergic rhinitis and asthma include the use of humanized anti-IgE monoclonal antibody. These antibodies are engineered to bind to the IgE heavy-chain domain that contacts the Fc$\epsilon$RI thereby binding free IgE. This interaction leads to decreased IgE production and expression of Fc$\epsilon$RI on mast cells and basophils. Other immunologic interventions include the administration of: hypoallergenic allergens and allergen derivatives that do not combine with preexisting IgE in allergen-specific immunotherapy; IL-12 to shift $T_H2$ to $T_H1$-type responses; anti-cytokine antibodies to deplete for example IL-4 and IL-5 and; cytokine receptor antagonists.

### Medication Is the Other Mode of Treatment

Some treatments of atopic conditions interfere with intracellular biochemical events needed for degranulation. Because an increase in the cellular cAMP level inhibits degranulation of mast cells, drugs that can pharmacologically modulate cAMP levels, such as theophylline, which modifies the mediator release reaction and directly relaxes bronchi and pulmonary blood vessel smooth muscles. It is used to prevent severe attacks of bronchial asthma. Other treatments of atopic disorders prevent synthesis or release of mediators. Sodium cromoglycate (*Nasalcrom*) inhibits or decreases mast cell degranulation by stabilizing lysosomal membranes and preventing $Ca^{2+}$ influx. Many corticosteroids, such as budesonide, flunisolide, fluticasone propionate, hydrocortisone, methylprednisone, prednisolone, and prednisone are potent anti-inflammatory drugs with immunosuppressive activity that when administered in high doses also effectively treat allergic reactions. Some therapies antagonize specific mediators. Both antihistamines (when smooth muscle are affected) and diethycarbamazines, such as

Zafirlukast, Zileuton, and Singulair (which block the effect of leukotrienes) are effective in the treatment of asthma. Drugs that inhibit the biological effects of histamine are called either $H_1$ or $H_2$ receptor antagonists. The $H_1$ receptor antagonists are represented by antihistamines, such as cetirizine (Zyrtec), fexofenadine (Allegra), and loratidine (Claritin); the $H_2$ receptor antagonists include cimetidine, metiamide, and burimamide.

The last approach to treating atopic conditions reverses or prevents the biologic effects of mediator action. Smooth muscle contraction and vasodilation can be countered with blocking agents called β-agonists, such as atropine (an anti-cholinergic drug) and phentolamine (an anti-α-adrenergic drug), or by stimulation with epinephrine. Cholinergic stimulation causes smooth muscle contraction and increased vasopermeability; α-adrenergic stimulation also causes smooth muscle contraction, but vasoconstriction. Preloaded epinephrine syringes, called epinephrine auto-injectors or EpiPens, are available for self-administration.

---

### MINI SUMMARY

The most severe form of type I hypersensitivity is a life-threatening, systemic anaphylactic reaction. The classic examples of type I hypersensitivity reactions, which are more of an annoyance and discomfort, are the atopic allergies, such as allergic rhinitis (hay fever), asthma, atopic eczema, atopic urticaria (hives), and food allergies.

Skin tests determine if a suspected allergen causes an allergic reaction. Skin testing is done by applying the allergen by a scratch, a patch, or an intradermal injection. At the site of application or injection, a small, circular welt will appear within 24 hr if the patient is allergic to the test substance. The welt exhibits a triple response consisting of erythema, edema, and wheal-and-flare.

The combination of avoidance, desensitization, and medication is used to reduce allergic reactions temporarily. Desensitization is done by hyposensitization, leading to the production of IgG-blocking antibodies, shifting from $T_H2$-type to $T_H1$-type responses, and induction of regulatory T cells. Drugs such as antihistamines, inhibitors of mast cell degranulation (sodium cromoglycate), and blockers of leukotrienes reduce the symptoms of type I hypersensitivity. β-agonists are antagonists of histamine; they relax smooth muscle and decrease vascular permeability.

---

## TYPE IV: CELL-MEDIATED (DELAYED-TYPE) HYPERSENSITIVITY IS MEDIATED BY T CELLS AND ACTIVATED MACROPHAGES, NOT ANTIBODIES

The preceding sections of the chapter dealt with detrimental antibody-mediated immune responses that appear shortly after a secondary antigen exposure. The remainder of this chapter deals with T-cell-mediated harmful responses that occur on secondary antigen challenge but take 1 to 3 days to appear. *These cell-mediated reactions (in which the ultimate effector cells are* activated macrophages*) are called* type IV hypersensitivity *or* **delayed-type hypersensitivity (DTH)**. *They start in a sensitized individual after a latent period of at least 8 hr and reach a peak 24 to 72 hr after a secondary exposure to the sensitizing antigen.* The hypersensitivity is characterized by an inflammatory reaction at the site of antigen deposition. The inflammatory reaction is characterized by erythema *(redness)* and induration *(hardening)* caused by vascular dilation and increased permeability of the postcapillary venules. DTH is dependent on the activity of $T_H1$ cells rather than on antibody. When specific $T_H1$ cells react with foreign protein antigen present in or bound to one's own cells or tissues, a series of interactions activate $T_H1$ cells to secrete cytokines (TNF-β and IFN-γ) that stimulate the expression of adhesion molecules on endothelial cells, increase vascular permeability at the site, and recruit and activate macrophages. (Additional cytokines and chemokines participate in DTH reactions; they are discussed shortly.) The accumulation of macrophages and lymphocytes at a site of antigen deposition sometimes leads to the formation of *granulomas*, a collection of lymphocytes and macrophages lying between strands of fibrous connective tissue. The combination of these characteristics distinguishes DTH from immediate hypersensitivity. Table 12-8 summarizes the hallmarks of DTH. DTH is part of the process of graft rejection, tumor immunity, and, most important, immunity to many intracellular infectious microorganisms, especially those causing chronic diseases such as tuberculosis. During his studies of tuberculosis, around 1900, Koch was the first to describe increased skin reactivity of tuberculous animals and humans to tuberculin. The reaction to tuberculin, the *Mycobacterium tuberculosis* product,

## TABLE 12-8 Hallmarks of DTH

1. DTH is induced by polypeptides or glycopeptides but not polysaccharides.
2. The optimal route for induction of DTH is by intradermal injection of antigen.
3. DTH develops slowly (8–24 hr) after a secondary exposure (shocking dose) and peaks between 24 and 72 hr.
4. In contrast to type I hypersensitivity, there is no tissue specificity in DTH reactions.
5. DTH does not depend on antibodies but rather on adoptive transfer by T cells.
6. A DTH reaction requires $T_H1$ cells and their products, which are collectively called *cytokines*.
7. The antigen deposition sites of DTH reactions are characterized by mononuclear cell infiltrates which give cutaneous manifestation of erythema and induration.
8. DTH reactions can be treated with steroids.
9. There is no desensitization for DTH; once positive for DTH reactions, always positive.
10. Disease manifestations include contact sensitivity, tuberculin reaction, granuloma formation, graft rejection, graft-versus-host reaction, and tumor rejection.

is the classic example of DTH, and the increased reactivity is termed the *Koch phenomenon*.

Humoral immunity is involved only indirectly during DTH. Although a 1000- to 10,000-fold increase in phagocytosis occurs in the presence of antibodies, some pathogens multiply within phagocytes, where antibodies cannot neutralize them. $T_H1$ cells promote macrophage accumulation and activation at the infective foci and later interact with opsonized pathogens to mediate quick destruction of the invading agent. Phagocyte activation inhibits intracellular parasite growth, and $T_H1$ cells play the central role in this activation process.

Landsteiner and Chase in 1942 showed that lymphocytes are involved in DTH. They demonstrated that unprimed, naïve animals acquire DTH after the adoptive transfer of lymphocytes from animals exposed either to a contact-sensitizing agent or to tuberculin. DTH can be transferred by washed cell suspensions from which macrophages and B cells have been removed. DTH cannot be transferred by serum. The lymphocytes that mediate DTH are CD4+ T lymphocytes (see Chapters 2 and 10), they are denoted as $T_H1$ cells (also called *inflammatory T cells*) and are restricted by MHC class II molecules.

## Mechanisms for DTH Induction and Development Involve Sensitization Rather than Immunization

The induction (or sensitization) of DTH can involve many natural and synthetic proteins and autocoupling haptens. Polysaccharides do not cause DTH. The method of induction is important in the stimulation of DTH; a natural disease accompanied by DTH is usually characterized by a chronic condition that includes the formation of granulomas. In the experimental situation, DTH occurs because the antigen injected (usually intradermally) is in a complete adjuvant (see Chapter 4). The injection of the same antigen in a saline solution can induce an immune response but might not induce DTH. Why? The antigen within the adjuvant emulsion is only slowly cleared; this delay allows for buildup of phagocytes. The dose of antigen needed to induce DTH reactions is less (1 to 3 µg of antigen in complete adjuvant) than that required for non-DTH reactions.

Once DTH is induced, the precise mechanism for the development of a DTH response is multifaceted (Figure 12-8). The interaction of macrophage-processed and -presented antigen with specific receptors on CD4+ $T_H1$ cells leads to the formation of sensitized $T_H1$ cells. A portion of these cells become memory cells, and on a second intradermal exposure of antigen, a more vigorous response follows. As the antigen diffuses through the skin into the small blood vessels, it can be presented to circulating sensitized $T_H1$ cells by epidermis-resident Langerhans cells, by dermis-resident macrophages, and by endothelial cells lining the postcapillary venules, causing the restimulated $T_H1$ cells, and probably IL-17–producing T helper ($T_H17$) cells (see Chapter 10), to release cytokines and chemokines. The most prominent cytokines and chemokines are:

1. IL-2, causing autocrine and paracrine proliferation of antigen-primed $T_H1$ cells;
2. IL-3 and GM-CSF induce localized hematopoiesis of monocytes and neutrophils.
3. IL-12 (plus IL-18) activates $T_H1$ cells and triggers their IFN-γ production while suppressing $T_H2$ cell development.
4. IL-17, derived from the recently characterized $T_H17$ cells, acts as a potent mediator of tissue inflammation by supporting neutrophil recruitment and survival, matrix degradation, and

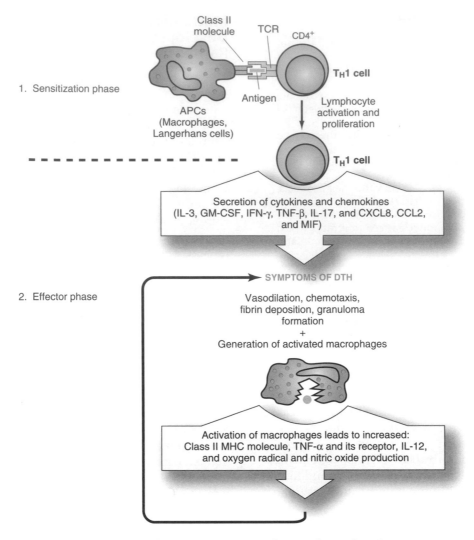

1. Sensitization phase

Class II molecule  TCR  CD4+

T$_H$1 cell

APCs
(Macrophages,
Langerhans cells)

Antigen

Lymphocyte
activation and
proliferation

T$_H$1 cell

Secretion of cytokines and chemokines
(IL-3, GM-CSF, IFN-γ, TNF-β, IL-17, and CXCL8, CCL2,
and MIF)

2. Effector phase

SYMPTOMS OF DTH

Vasodilation, chemotaxis,
fibrin deposition, granuloma
formation
+
Generation of activated macrophages

Activation of macrophages leads to increased:
Class II MHC molecule, TNF-α and its receptor, IL-12,
and oxygen radical and nitric oxide production

**FIGURE 12-8 The immunologic events in DTH**. See text for explanation.

induction of proinflammatory cytokines (such as IL-1, IL-6, TNF-α, and GM-CSF) and the chemokine CXCL8 and the IFN-inducible chemokines CXCL9, CXCL10, and CXCL11 by epidermal keratinocytes (see Chapter 9 and Table 9.6).

5. TNF-α and -β (lymphotoxin), augmenting endothelial cell binding and activation of, leukocytes; and

6. IFN-γ[4], causing increased expression of class II MHC molecules on endothelial cells or macrophages and activation of macrophages.

Chemokines (see Chapter 9), such as CXCL8 (IL-8) and CCL2 (monocyte chemoattrantant protein 1 [MCP-1]), attract neutrophils and monocytes to the blood vessels near the foci of antigen deposition. The recruitment of leukocytes is augmented by venular endothelial cells and their products, which regulate leukocyte movement out of blood vessels. TNF-β (reinforced by macrophage-derived TNF-α and IL-1), acting with IFN-γ through endothelial cells, sequentially regulates this movement in four ways:

1. TNF-β induces endothelial cells to increase their production of vasodilator molecules such as prostacyclin, which increases blood flow and delivery of leukocytes to the site of antigen deposition.

---

[4]The use of knock-out mice deficient in IFN-γ strongly supports the necessity of IFN-γ in DTH responses. The IFN-γ knock-out mice, infected with *M. bovis*, died within 60 days of infection. Their normal counterparts survived.

2. Once leukocytes arrive, TNF-β has made the endothelial cells "sticky," and the leukocytes adhere to the blood vessel walls. This increased stickiness results from increased expression of endothelial leukocyte adhesion molecule-1 (*ELAM-1*, also called *CD62E*), which selectively binds neutrophils. Later, after ELAM-1 wanes, endothelial cells instead express intercellular adhesion molecule-1 (*ICAM-1*, also called *CD54*) and vascular adhesion molecule-1 (*VCAM-1*, also called *CD106*). The leukocyte ligands for ICAM-1 and VCAM-1 are lymphocyte function-associated antigen-1 (*LFA-1*, also called *CD11aCD18*) and very late activation antigen-4 (*VLA-4*, also called *CD29*), respectively.

3. Under the influence of TNF-β, endothelial cells secrete chemokines, such as CXCL8 and CCL2, which increase the mobility of neutrophils and monocytes.

4. TNF-β, acting with IFN-γ, reshapes endothelial cells, leading to leaky vessels and to ease of leukocyte movement out of blood vessels.

To summarize, neutrophils, followed later by lymphocytes and monocytes, force themselves through the blood vessel walls by a process called *diapedesis* and enter the antigen-containing tissue. The morphologic transformation of monocytes to macrophages leads to the characteristic accumulation of mononuclear cells seen in the typical DTH skin reaction. A cytokine called *migration-inhibition factor (MIF)* keeps the macrophages at the DTH reaction site. During diapedesis, monocytes come in contact with IFN-γ and differentiate into activated macrophages, which eliminate antigen. If antigenic stimulation persists, however, the macrophages become chronically activated and release additional cytokines, growth factors, and lysosomal enzymes that attack and destroy the surrounding tissue. The reason the skin reaction is delayed may be the time required for the reaction to amplify to a noticeable level. This scenario explains the three main features of the DTH skin reaction: (1) *hardening*, the result of the large accumulation of mononuclear cells to a circumscribed area; (2) *reddening*, the result of local blood vessel damage and blood leakage into the surrounding tissues; and (3) *necrosis* (death of tissue), the result of enzyme degradation of the surrounding tissues.

## MINI SUMMARY

Type IV, or delayed-type, hypersensitivity (DTH) is the only hypersensitivity directly mediated by T cells through activated macrophages. DTH is characterized by late (24 to 72 hr) clinical signs after reexposure to the sensitizing antigen. The inflammatory reaction seen at the site of antigen deposition, usually the skin, is characterized by redness, hardness, and mononuclear cell infiltration. The accumulation of macrophages at the site of infection can lead to the formation of granulomas.

## There Are Different Kinds of DTH Reactions

There are three general types of DTH, distinguished by the place where antigen is applied (surface, intradermally) and by the extent of the latent period after a challenge exposure. The three types of DTH discussed here are (1) contact sensitivity (dermatitis), (2) the tuberculin skin reaction, and (3) systemic granuloma formation (tuberculosis).

### Contact Sensitivity (Dermatitis) Is a DTH Caused by an Antigen Touching the Skin

During **contact sensitivity**, the major target cells are in the skin. The most common causes of contact sensitivity are poison ivy (pentadecacatechol), poison oak, metals (nickel chromate), chemicals in rubber, and medications. Contact sensitivity is commonly induced by experimental cutaneous exposure to chemicals (haptens) such as 2,4-dinitrochlorobenzene (DNCB), and 2,4-dinitrofluorobenzene (DNFB). These compounds spontaneously and covalently couple with free amino groups of skin proteins (particularly the ε-amino groups of lysine) to form neoantigens. The modified self-proteins, or neoantigens, are taken up and processed by skin dendritic cells (Langerhans cells) into peptides that associate with class II MHC molecules, which can be presented to, and recognized by, specific T$_H$1 cells in the draining lymph nodes. If animals are challenged later or if individuals are reexposed accidentally to the offending chemical, sensitized T$_H$1 cells release CCL2, MIF, IL-17, and IFN-γ, which stimulates the epidermal keratinocytes to release proinflammatory cytokines and the chemokines CXCL8, CXCL9, CXCL10, and CXCL11. These cytokines and chemokines recruit monocytes, then limit their movement, induce their maturation to macrophages, and finally activate macrophages that release lytic enzymes and cytotoxins such as TNF-α leading to an inflammatory reaction that can be recognized by the rough, scaly appearance of the exposed skin. The skin reaction reaches its peak intensity at 24 to 48 hr. Similar mechanisms occur when pentadecacatechol from the poison ivy plant contacts skin.

Histologically, the dermis (deep layer of the skin) becomes infiltrated with mononuclear cells. These cells start to appear at 6 to 8 hr after contact and peak by 12 to 15 hr. Contact dermatitis gives a different reaction in the epidermis (superficial layer of the skin) than does tuberculin. The epidermis is hyperplastic; it is invaded by mononuclear cells, and intraepidermal vesicles form. These vesicles can coalesce to form large blisters filled with serous fluid, granulocytes, and mononuclear cells. The primary APCs in contact sensitivity are dendritic cells (called *Langerhans cells*) that express class II MHC molecules. These cells migrate to, and carry antigen to, the lymph nodes for presentation to naïve $T_H1$ cells.

Cytotoxic T cells can also be involved in contact sensitivity. For example, the rash that occurs by contact with poison ivy is due to the T cell response to the lipid-soluble compound pentadecacatechol, which can cross the cell membrane and modify cytosolic proteins. These modified cytosolic proteins are processed, translocated to the endoplasmic reticulum, and delivered to the cell surface by class I MHC molecules, where they are recognized by $CD8^+$ cytotoxic T cells and the cells displaying the self-peptide–MHC class I molecule complexes are killed.

### The Tuberculin Reaction Is a Classical Example of a DTH Reaction

The **tuberculin skin reaction**, the classic example of a DTH reaction, was originally described by Koch and is also known as the *Koch phenomenon*. Koch observed that in tuberculous patients subcutaneous exposure to tuberculin, a lipoprotein of *M. tuberculosis*, caused a generalized illness accompanied by an inflammatory reaction at the site of inoculation.

Tuberculin was first made by taking culture filtrates of *M. tuberculosis* and concentrating them by boiling and removing cellular debris. This preparation is now called "old tuberculin." The current preparation of active proteins from *M. tuberculosis* cultures is made by concentrating autoclaved cultures by precipitation with ammonium sulfate. This product is called *purified protein derivative (PPD)*.

The intradermal inoculation of PPD (PPD skin test discussed shortly) into a sensitized individual (exposed to *M. tuberculosis* bacteria or immunization with BCG vaccine) or animal leads to a T cell-mediated inflammatory reaction was called the *tuberculin reaction*. No observable changes are seen for the first 8 hr. Then a red, hard swelling gradually appears, which reaches a maximal intensity and size (as large as 7 cm in diameter) in 24 to 72 hr. The response then subsides over the next few days. The reaction is due to $T_H1$ cells that infiltrate the antigen injection site and recognize APC-presented peptide-MHC complexes, which cause them to release IFN-$\gamma$ and TNF-$\beta$.

Histologically, the tuberculin skin reaction is characterized by massive accumulation of inflammatory cells. Early in the reaction (about 12 hr), neutrophils are present around blood vessels, but at peak reactivity the lesions are composed exclusively of mononuclear cells: 10 to 20% are lymphocytes, and 80 to 90% are macrophages. Depending on the sensitivity of individuals, the injection of PPD can cause a granulomatous reaction with necrosis, ulceration, and scarring at the site of inoculation. The systemic formation of granulomas is associated with tuberculosis and is described later in the chapter. Table 12-9 summarizes some of the characteristics of two types of DTH reactions.

### Tuberculosis Is the Classic Example of a DTH Disease

Several chronic diseases exhibiting DTH are caused by intracellular infectious agents such as bacteria (such as *M. tuberculosis, M. leprae, Brucella abortus,* and *Listeria monocytogenes*), fungi (such as *Candida albicans, Cryptococcus neoformans, Histoplasma capsulatum,* and *Pneumocystis carinii*), viruses (such as Herpes simplex virus, Measles virus, and Variola virus), and protozoa (such as *Leishmania* sp.). Even though many diseases are represented in this group, such as **tuberculosis**, leprosy, listeriosis, blastomycosis, leishmaniasis, and schistosomiasis,

**TABLE 12-9 Characteristics of DTH Skin Reactions**

| | Contact sensitivity reaction | Tuberculin reaction |
|---|---|---|
| Antigen | Epidermal: pentadecacatechol from poison ivy plant | Dermal: tuberculin from mycobacteria |
| Reaction time | 48 hr | 24–72 hr |
| Clinical manifestations | Eczema | Redness and hardness |
| Histological picture | Mononuclear cells and edema | Mononuclear cells, lymphocytes, and macrophages |

only tuberculosis will be discussed. Like type I hypersensitivity, DTH is not always synonymous with protective immunity.

An infection by *M. tuberculosis* starts when the bacteria are inhaled and reach the lungs. One or more of these bacteria lodge within an air sac and are rapidly internalized by alveolar macrophages. In contrast to what is expected, the mycobacteria are not destroyed but grow slowly in the macrophages. An inflammatory response occurs, and the air sacs fill with fluid and neutrophils from leaky capillaries. A small nodule called an *exudative lesion* forms. Fluid containing bacteria is drained away by lymphatic vessels. These bacteria are localized in the draining lymph nodes, but are not destroyed by the standard immune mechanisms and eventually reach the bloodstream. Once in circulation, the bacteria can localize in different parts of the body. Usually, for still unknown reasons, these transplanted mycobacteria are destroyed and do not lead to secondary foci. As the mycobacteria slowly grow at the primary focus of infection in the lungs, the macrophages break down some of the organisms into peptides that appear on the surface of macrophages. The macrophages "present" the nominal antigen to specific $T_H1$ cells. The interaction between the macrophage-presented antigen and specific T cells stimulates the macrophages to secrete IL-12 and IL-18. Because tuberculosis is a chronic infection, the supply of macrophages at the focus of infection becomes abundant. The IL-12 induces proliferation of neighboring $T_H1$ cells, which in turn secrete IFN-$\gamma$ and CCL2. CCL2 acts as a chemotaxin that attracts monocytes to the site of infection and IFN-$\gamma$ as a macrophage-activating factor that converts resting monocytes into activated macrophages while suppressing $T_H2$ cell development. Because activated macrophages have increased amounts of lysosomes and hydrolytic enzymes, they keep the mycobacteria from growing and multiplying but do not kill them. Other cytokines either directly or indirectly hold macrophages at the site of inflammation. Once macrophages arrive at the site of infection, they cannot leave the site—another reason for macrophage accumulation.

The result of this accumulation of macrophages is the formation of nodules called **granulomas**. The granulomas that occur in tuberculosis are called **tubercles**. A histologic cross section of a tubercle shows mycobacteria at the center (within macrophages), concentric layers of macrophages around the bacteria, and an outer mantle of $T_H1$ cells. Many of the macrophages, under the influence of cytokines, become elongated and weakly phagocytic.

They are then called *epithelioid cells* and make up most of the tubercle. Some macrophages also may fuse with each other and become giant cells with multiple nuclei. The mycobacteria remain dormant within the tubercle if the patient's resistance is high. DTH stops the infection from developing further, and it remains in a subclinical state. However, if the patient's resistance is low, the DTH may not arrest the growth of the mycobacteria, and the disease progresses to *primary clinical tuberculosis*.

During primary clinical tuberculosis, more tubercles appear and grow larger. Within the tubercle, some macrophages may die because of toxic lipids from the mycobacteria or lack of oxygen circulation. The dead macrophages fuse, forming an amorphous mass called *caseation necrosis*. The tubercles continue to increase in size and start to fuse, causing an area of dead tissue in the lungs. When enough tubercles have coalesced, the damaged tissue can be detected by a chest X-ray. At this point, the disease may continue further or undergo a healing process. The healing process involves calcium deposition in the tubercles, converting them to hard, friable bodies, which may become encapsulated and completely walled off from the surrounding tissue. This process is called *calcification*. If calcification does not occur, however, the disease continues to spread.

As the caseation necrosis continues, the patient starts to show the clinical signs of tuberculosis, such as loss of appetite, fatigue, loss of weight, night sweats, and a persistent, worsening cough. As a result of necrosis, a bronchus may erode, discharging thousands of mycobacteria into the bronchi. At this point, the mycobacteria appear in the patient's coughed up sputum. Blood vessels then erode, further aggravating the situation, and the sputum may be streaked with blood. The blood vessel erosion allows discharge of many of the mycobacteria directly into the blood vessels. In contrast to the first invasion of the blood at the onset of the infection, the patient's resistance is now low. Thus, wherever the blood-borne bacteria localize, new tubercles arise. Thousands of tubercles appear throughout the body, and the disease is now considered generalized. Generalized tuberculosis leads to damage of vital organs, which can cause death.

The most prevalent type of tuberculosis in the United State is *reactivation tuberculosis*. In this type of tuberculosis, dormant bacilli from an old subclinical primary infection are no longer held in check and start to multiply rapidly, causing clinical tuberculosis. Reactivation tuberculosis occurs most often in elderly persons with lowered resistance caused by malnutrition and other environmental stresses.

The first sign that a person may have been or is infected by *M. tuberculosis* is the conversion from a PPD-negative to a PPD-positive skin test, which is evidence of the development of DTH to the mycobacterial antigens. Approximately 3 weeks after the infection has started, tuberculin reactivity occurs and is detected by the tuberculin skin test. When PPD, a protein extract from *M. tuberculosis*, is injected intradermally, an infected individual responds by development of a circumscribed, hard red zone in 48 to 72 hr. The histology of a tuberculin skin reaction was described earlier in the chapter.

Three methods exist for cutaneous tuberculosis testing: (1) In the von Pirquet test, PPD is rubbed into scarified skin; variations of this test include the Tine or multiple puncture technique; (2) in the Mantoux test, the test antigen is injected intradermally; and (3) in the Vollmer patch test (used for children), a square of gauze is impregnated with PPD and held to the skin with a piece of tape. Forty-eight hours later, the appearance and size of the inflammation site are noted. In the Mantoux test, the skin reaction must be at least 6 mm in diameter to be considered a positive test.

A positive skin test for PPD means only that the individual has been infected. In 10% of the cases, the infection may become clinical, while in the remaining cases it remains subclinical. Even if it is a subclinical infection, it does not have to be a recent infection because the mycobacteria of a dormant tubercle are alive. The person remains skin test positive as long as the bacteria are present. Only certain types of treatment can eliminate them, and only then does the skin reaction turn negative. Thus, patients whose skin reactivity becomes positive are treated for several months with antibacterial drugs to ensure that their infections will not progress to clinical tuberculosis.

The patient with clinical tuberculosis is treated for a year or more because of the chronic nature of tuberculosis and the walling off of the mycobacteria by tubercle formation. The best drugs are isoniazid, streptomycin, *p*-aminosalicylic acid, and rifampin.

The development of immunity to tuberculosis is controversial. In most countries except the United States, people are immunized with an attenuated vaccine. Killed mycobacteria are not effective. To stimulate cellular immunity (DTH), a live vaccine called *Bacillus Calmette-Guérin (BCG)* is used. BCG is an attenuated strain of *M. bovis* antigenically identical to *M. tuberculosis*. BCG was initially highly virulent, but after 231 serial subcultures over a period of 11 years, it lost its virulence.

BCG bacilli persist in tissue for long periods and can induce DTH against virulent strains of *M. tuberculosis* or *M. bovis*. The BCG vaccine's efficacy is questionable. In addition, vaccinated individuals give a false-positive skin test; therefore, minimizing the use of skin testing to determine *M. tuberculosis* exposure. Nonetheless, many countries do vaccinate with BCG.

---

**MINI SUMMARY**

A disease (such as tuberculosis) that exhibits DTH is usually a chronic condition and involves the formation of granulomas. The inability of macrophages to degrade or kill intracellular microorganisms or parasites leads to the localized chronic inflammation. The inflammatory response is characterized by accumulation and proliferation of leukocytes and granuloma formation. On secondary exposure to the sensitizing antigen, a more vigorous response follows. As the antigen diffuses through the skin into the small blood vessels, circulating sensitized $T_H1$ cells interact with the antigen and release IFN-$\gamma$. The skin reaction shows three main features: hardening, reddening, and necrosis.

---

# SUMMARY

Immune malfunctions, according to Coombs and Gell, are divided into four classes: (1) *type I: immediate (anaphylactic) hypersensitivity*, (2) *type II: antibody-dependent cytotoxic hypersensitivity*, (3) *type III: immune complex-mediated hypersensitivity*, and (4) *type IV: cell-mediated (delayed-type) hypersensitivity*.

*Hypersensitivity* is a state existing in a previously *sensitized* individual, which leads to tissue damage on later exposure to the *allergen*. The allergic individual has an immune system that reacts to material that is harmless to the nonallergic individual.

The tendency to develop type I hypersensitivities is familial, but the exact mode of inheritance is unknown. There is a relationship between HLA MHC molecule expression and the appearance of type I hypersensitivities. The first encounter with an allergen is the *sensitization*. Exposure to an allergen can be artificial or natural. The exposure of an allergic individual to an allergen prompts the formation of mainly *IgE antibodies*. The clinical signs of type I hypersensitivity do not arise until after the second exposure to the allergen (the *shocking dose*). Clinical signs are manifested within minutes.

*Mast cells* and *basophils* mediate type I hypersensitivity reactions. These cells are filled with granules, which contain preformed mediators, such as *histamine, heparin*, and *chemotactic factors*. The mast cells and basophils make newly formed effector molecules, including *prostaglandins, thromboxanes, leukotrienes (slow-reacting substance of anaphylaxis [SRS-A])*, and *cytokines*. Cell-fixed IgE antibodies act as allergen-specific cell receptors. Type I hypersensitivity reactions start when allergens bind to two adjacent IgE molecules and form an IgE-allergen-IgE bridge. This cross-linking promotes *degranulation*, a process during which mast cell granules fuse with the plasma membrane and extrude their contents to the surrounding tissue. All soluble mediators (such as histamine, serotonin, prostaglandins, and leukotrienes) have overlapping effects that generally consist of smooth muscle contraction and increased vascular permeability. Other mediators, such as heparin and platelet-activating factor (PAF), reduce blood clotting and aggregate platelets and cause the release of vasoamines, respectively.

Some allergic patients require professional medical help. A positive diagnostic skin test is represented by a *triple response (erythema, edema*, and *wheal-and-flare)*.

The best way to treat type I hypersensitivities is to avoid the causative agent. The next best solution is *desensitization* and medication to relieve the symptoms. Prescription (antihistamines, cromolyn sodium) and nonprescription (antihistamines) drugs reduce immediate hypersensitivity symptoms.

Type I hypersensitivity disease states can range from the minor *atopic allergy* symptoms of hay fever to a systemic, life-threatening hypersensitivity reaction called *anaphylaxis*. Atopic allergies are usually associated with pollens, grasses, house dust, house dust mites, animal danders, certain foods, and drugs. These substances can cause systemic anaphylaxis in patients with severe hypersensitivities. Some classic examples of atopy are (1) allergic rhinitis (hay fever), (2) asthma, (3) atopic dermatitis, (4) atopic urticaria (hives), and (5) food allergies.

*Type IV*, or *delayed-type, hypersensitivity (DTH)* is cell-mediated and is caused by the reaction of sensitized CD4$^+$ T$_H$1 cells to the shocking antigen. DTH manifestations appear after 12 hr and peak by 48 to 72 hr. The classic example of DTH is the tuberculin-type skin reaction, exemplified by *redness* and *hardness*, and, if there is continued antigen stimulation, leads to granuloma formation. After sensitized T cells are reexposed to the antigen, they proliferate and divide, forming a clone of cells, which release cytokines. Koch gave the first account of DTH around 1900, when he

described the increased skin reactivity of tuberculous animals and humans to the *M. tuberculosis* product *tuberculin*. This heightened reactivity is called the *Koch phenomenon*.

The distinctive characteristics of DTH include the following: (1) DTH is mediated by T cells; (2) effector molecules are cytokines; (3) adoptive transfer is accomplished with lymphocytes; (4) DTH is induced only by protein antigens; (5) inflammatory manifestations are seen between 24 to 72 hr; (6) cutaneous reactions are exemplified by redness, hardness, and mononuclear cell infiltration; (7) complement is not involved; and (8) DTH is suppressed by corticosteroids.

DTH can be grouped into three general types: (1) contact sensitivity, (2) tuberculin skin reaction, and (3) tuberculosis. *Contact sensitivity* (dermatitis) is an eczematous skin reaction occurring in a sensitized individual within 48 hr of antigen contact. The antigen couples with normal skin tissue, creating a new antigen recognized as foreign by T cells. The reaction can occur from contact with poison ivy (an example of a contact sensitivity). The *tuberculin skin reaction* follows a subcutaneous injection of purified protein derivative (PPD) into tuberculous patients.

*Tuberculosis* is a good example of a disease associated with DTH. The disease occurs when *M tuberculosis* is internalized by alveolar macrophages. The mycobacteria slowly grow in the macrophages and induce an inflammatory reaction. The accumulation of macrophages at the site of infection leads to the formation of a *granuloma* (or *tubercle*). As tuberculosis progresses, more tubercles are formed and grow larger. A chest X-ray can detect the surrounding damaged tissue. Skin testing can also be used to determine the presence of infection. Chemotherapy is used to treat tuberculosis. Most countries, other than the United States immunizes against tuberculosis using an attenuated vaccine. The live vaccine is called *Bacillus Calmette-Guérin (BCG)*.

# SELF-EVALUATION

## RECALLING KEY TERMS

**Allergen**
**Allergy**
**Anaphylactic shock**
**Anaphylaxis**
**Anergy**
**Atopic allergies**
**Atopy**

Basophils
Contact sensitivity
Degranulation
Delayed-type hypersensitivity (DTH)
Desensitize
FcεRI
Granulomas
Homocytotropic antibodies
Hypersensitivity
    Type I hypersensitivity
    Type II hypersensitivity
    Type III hypersensitivity
    Type IV hypersensitivity
Hyposensitivity
Immediate hypersensitivity
Late phase reaction
Mast cells
Sensitization
Sensitizing dose
Shocking dose
Systemic (or generalized) anaphylaxis
Triple response
    Edema
    Erythema
    Wheal-and-flare
Tubercles
Tuberculin skin reaction
Tuberculosis

## MULTIPLE-CHOICE QUESTIONS

*(An answer key is not provided, but the page[s] location of the answer is.)*

1. Common causes of anaphylaxis in humans include the following agents except (a) penicillin, (b) local steroid injections, (c) stinging insects, (d) allergen extract injections, (e) none of these. *(See page 413.)*

2. What substance(s) other than histamine are important in type I hypersensitivity? (a) serotonin, (b) prostaglandins, (c) leukotrienes, (d) all of the above, (e) none of these. *(See pages 410 and 411.)*

3. An example of an atopic allergic disease is asthma. (a) true, (b) false. *(See pages 413 and 414.)*

4. Interaction of antigen and IgE on the surface of mast cells, with subsequent release of histamine occurs in (a) asthma, (b) serum sickness, (c) DTH, (d) contact sensitivity, (e) tuberculosis, (f) none of these. *(See pages 406, 407, and 408.)*

5. Anaphylaxis refers to (a) the severe reaction following intravenous reinjection of the antigen in a sensitized animal, (b) the severe reaction following primary injection of protein solutions, (c) the state of immunity developed by repeated injections of any foreign substance, (d) the severe reaction resulting from sensitivity to common allergens, (e) none of these. *(See pages 413 and 414.)*

6. Antihistamines are usually effective in preventing type III hypersensitivity. (a) true, (b) false. *(See pages 417 and 418.)*

7. Which of the following conditions is not mediated by antibodies? (a) anaphylaxis, (b) contact sensitivity, (c) serum sickness, (d) hay fever, (e) none of these. *(See pages 421 and 422.)*

8. IgE differs from (a) all other immunoglobulins in that IgE binds to mast cells, (b) IgM in that IgE will pass the placental barrier, (c) IgG in that IgE has only κ light chains, (d) IgA in that IgE has no carbohydrate, (e) IgD in that IgE is much more plentiful in serum, (f) none of these. *(See pages 405 and 406.)*

9. The triple response will show a site with redness, edema, and a wheal-and-flare. (a) true, (b) false. *(See page 404.)*

10. In the Gel and Coombs classification of hypersensitivities, which corresponds to the immune complex group? (a) type I, (b) type II, (c) type III, (d) type IV, (e) none of these. *(See page 399.)*

11. Which of the combinations contributes exclusively to type I hypersensitivity? (a) histamine, serotonin, steroids, SRS-A, (b) mast cells, histamine, IFN-γ, IgE, (c) mast cells, histamine, skin contact, (d) histamine, tuberculin, heparin, (e) none of these. *(See pages 404–411.)*

12. Adrenergic drugs (a) relax smooth muscle, (b) are true antihistamines, (c) contract smooth muscle, (d) are exemplified by heparin, (e) help alleviate the symptoms of anergy, (f) none of these. *(See page 418.)*

13. The reaction to poison ivy is classified as a delayed-type hypersensitivity. (a) true, (b) false. *(See page 421.)*

14. Degranulation (a) leads to the release of heparin and histamine, (b) is the lymphocytic destruction of cells to which the lymphocytes have non-antibody-related reactivity, (c) refers to mast cell lysis by antibodies to mast cells, (d) is an *in vitro* correlate of immediate hypersensitivity, (e) none of these. *(See pages 406–411.)*

15. In the Gel and Coombs classification of hypersensitivities, which corresponds to the delayed group? (a) type I, (b) type II, (c) type III, (d) type IV, (e) none of these. *(See page 397.)*

16. A positive tuberculin skin test suggests that the patient has some immunity to *M. tuberculosis*. (a) true, (b) false. *(See page 422.)*

**17.** A positive DTH skin reaction involves a complex interaction of (a) antigen, complement, and histamine, (b) antigen, antigen-sensitive lymphocytes, and macrophages, (c) homocytotropic antibody, complement, and serotonin, (d) antigen-antibody complexes, complement, and histamine, (e) none of these. *(See page 422.)*

**18.** Contact sensitivity is a skin reaction that can be transferred passively with IgE antibody. (a) true, (b) false. *(See page 422.)*

**19.** The tuberculin/PPD reaction (in skin) is the (a) triple skin reactions seen in tuberculous patients, (b) historical prototype of delayed skin reactions, (c) historical prototype of immediate skin reactions, (d) skin reaction easiest to eliminate by desensitization, (e) none of these. *(See page 422.)*

**20.** Histamine is clearly linked to DTH. (a) true, (b) false. *(See page 410.)*

## SHORT-ANSWER ESSAY QUESTIONS

**1.** By derivation, what does allergy mean and what does hypersensitivity mean? Are they synonymous?

**2.** The main difference between immediate and delayed types of hypersensitivity is the time of appearance of reactions. True or false? If false, name the main differences.

**3.** What is the type II reaction described by Coombs and Gell? Does this reaction require complement?

**4.** Describe some characteristics of a type III reaction. What are some examples of autoimmune diseases that are caused by this type of hypersensitivity?

**5.** Is there a hereditary tendency to type I hypersensitivity reactions? Explain.

**6.** Distinguish between an antigen and an allergen.

**7.** What immune and nonimmune cells are involved in type I hypersensitivity?

**8.** What class of antibody is responsible for type I hypersensitivity? Describe some structural and biologic characteristics of this antibody. What do we mean by homocytotropic antibodies?

**9.** Briefly describe the result of IgE interaction with mast cells. What are the chemical mediators of type I hypersensitivity reactions?

**10.** Some effector molecules of type I hypersensitivity reactions are preformed mediators; others are newly synthesized mediators. Distinguish between the two. Briefly describe the two pathways for the production of newly synthesized mediators.

**11.** How can you determine whether a person is allergic to a foreign protein? What is the triple response? Name two *in vitro* tests.

**12.** What is the mechanism for desensitization for type I hypersensitivities? Is this desensitization lifelong? If not, speculate on the reasons. What are some other modes of treatment for type I hypersensitivity?

**13.** Describe the differences between systemic anaphylaxis and atopy.

**14.** Are the mechanisms of cell-mediated immunity and DTH the same? Name the effector cells in DTH. What are some of hallmarks of DTH reactions?

**15.** Describe contact sensitivity. How does contact sensitivity differ from the tuberculin skin reaction?

**16.** What is the mechanism of the tuberculin skin test? If the test is positive, what causes the induration (hardening) of the test site? What substances are used in this test? Name three different types of tuberculin skin tests.

## FURTHER READINGS

Calandra, T., and T. Roger. 2003. Macrophage migration inhibitory factor: A regulator of innate immunity. *Nat. Rev. Immunol.* 3:791–800.

Cohn, L., J.A. Elias, and G.L. Chupp. 2004. Asthma: Mechanisms of disease persistence and progression. *Annu. Rev Immunol.* 22:789–815.

Devereux, G. 2006. The increase in the prevalence of asthma and allergy: Food for thought. *Nat. Rev. Immunol.* 6:869–874.

Galli, S.J., J. Kalesnikoff, M.A. Grimbaldeston, A.M. Piliponsky, C.M.M. Williams, and M. Tsai. 2005. Mast cells as "tunable" effector and immunoregulatory cells: Recent advances. *Annu. Rev. Immunol.* 23:749–786.

Gould, H.J., B.J. Sutton, A.J. Beavil, R.L. Beavil, N. McCloskey, H.A. Coker, D. Fear, and L. Smurthwaite. 2003. The biology of IgE and the basis of allergic disease. *Annu. Rev. Immunol.* 21:579–628.

Hawrylowicz, C.M., and A. O'Garra. 2005. Potential role of interleukin-10–secreting regulatory T cells in allergy and asthma. *Nat. Rev. Immunol.* 5:271–283.

Jacobsen, E.A., A.G. Taranova, N.A. Lee, and J.J. Lee. 2007. Eosinophils: Singularly destructive effector cells or purveyors of immunoregulation? *J. Allergy Clin. Immunol.* 119:1313–1320.

Kraft, S., and J-P. Kinet. 2007. New developments in FcεRI regulation, function and inhibition. *Nat. Rev. Immunol.* 7:365–378.

Larche, M., C.A. Akdis, and R. Valenta. 2006. Immunological mechanisms of allergen-specific immunotherapy. *Nat. Rev. Immunol.* 6:761–771.

Ravetch, J.V. 2003. Fc receptors. *Fundamental Immunology*, 5th Ed. Philadelphia: Lippincott Williams & Wilkins.

Schmidt-Weber, C.B., M. Akdis, and C.A. Akdis. 2007. $T_H17$ cells in the big picture of immunology. *J. Allergy Clin. Immunol.* 120:247–254.

Szabo, S.J., B.M. Sullivan, S.L. Peng, and L.H. Glimcher 2003. Molecular mechanisms regulating $T_H1$ immune responses. *Annu. Rev. Immunol.* 21:713–758.

Ulrich, B., and J. Rivera. 2004. The ins and outs of IgE-dependent mast-cell exocytosis. *Trends Immunol.* 25:266–273.

van Beelen, A.J., M.B.M. Teunissen, M.L. Kapsenberg, and E.C. de Jong. 2007. Interleukin-17 in inflammatory skin disorders. *Curr. Opin. Allergy Clin. Immunol.* 7: 374–381.

Vukmanovic-Stejic, M., J.R. Reed, K.E. Lacy, M.H.A. Rustin, and A.N. Akbar. 2006. Mantoux Test as a model for a secondary immune response in humans. *Immunol. Lett.* 107:93–101.

Wills-Karp, M., and G.K.K. Hershey. 2003. Immunological mechanisms of allergic disorders. *Fundamental Immunology*, 5th Ed. Philadelphia: Lippincott Williams & Wilkins.

# CHAPTER THIRTEEN

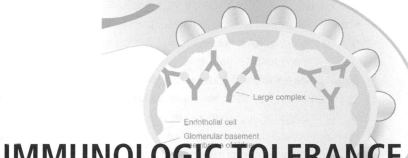

# IMMUNOLOGIC TOLERANCE AND AUTOIMMUNITY

## CHAPTER OUTLINE

1. The study and understanding of tolerance began around 1900.
2. The major characteristic of tolerance is a secondary "nothing" response.
   a. The dose of antigen affects tolerance induction.
   b. The physicochemical nature of the antigen affects tolerance induction.
   c. The immunogenicity of an antigen affects tolerance induction.
   d. The route of antigen administration affects tolerance induction.
3. The principal mechanisms that induce self-tolerance are clonal deletion, clonal anergy, or regulated inhibition of self-reactive T and B cells.
   a. Central tolerance induction occurs at the level of developing lymphocytes in primary lymphoid organs.
   b. Peripheral tolerance induction occurs at the level of mature self-reactive lymphocytes in secondary lymphoid tissues.
4. Autoimmunity, in which the body turns against itself, leads to autoimmune diseases and even self-destruction.
   a. Even though there are multiple etiologies for autoimmune diseases, $CD4^+$ T cells are central to the activation of autoimmune responses.
5. Autoimmune diseases are either organ-specific or systemic and are a consequence of either a predominance of T lymphocyte or B lymphocyte dysfunction.
   a. Autoimmune diseases are caused by self-reacting T cells.
      1) Hashimoto's thyroiditis results when T cells react against unmasked self-antigens.
      2) Insulin-dependent diabetes mellitus results from an autoimmune attack of the pancreas' insulin-producing cells.
      3) Multiple sclerosis results either from an immune response to exposed sequestered antigen myelin basic protein (MBP) or from molecular mimicry to MBP following a virus infection.
   b. Autoimmune diseases are caused by self-reacting antibodies.
      1) Myasthenia gravis results when blocking antibodies bind self-acetylcholine receptors.

2) Graves' disease results when antibodies stimulate inappropriate thyroid activity rather than destroying thyroid tissue.

3) Systemic lupus erythematosus involves antibodies that react primarily against self-nuclear components.

4) Rheumatoid arthritis involves antibodies that react against self-constituents in joints.

   a) The etiology of RA is not understood, but the pathology is known.

   b) The therapy for RA is palliative.

5) Autoimmune hemolytic diseases result when normal cells are affected as innocent bystanders.

   c) Autoimmune hemolytic anemia results when antibodies react against self red blood cells.

   d) Thrombocytopenic purpura results when antibodies react against self-platelets.

6) Poststreptococcal diseases result when antibodies against bacteria cross-react with self-antigens.

   e) Acute rheumatic fever results when antibodies against streptococcal antigens cross-react with heart muscle tissue.

   f) Glomerulonephritis results when antibodies react against self-antigens and the resulting antigen-antibody complexes localize in the glomeruli of the kidney.

6. Treatments of autoimmune diseases are moving from counteracting the effects of autoimmunity with nonspecific treatments to specifically preventing the causes.

## OBJECTIVES

*The reader should be able to:*

1. Define and conceptualize immunologic tolerance.
2. Describe an experiment that shows tolerance induction.
3. Categorize the conditions that influence tolerance induction.
4. Outline the mechanisms that induce tolerance.
5. Define autoimmunity.
6. Discuss the concept of *horror autotoxicus*; list and explain how contemporary results invalidate this concept.
7. Realize that the origin of autoimmune diseases may lie in the immune process, the self-antigens, or both; describe two major events that may lead to autoimmune disease; list the other factors that may lead to autoimmune disease.
8. Distinguish between organ-specific and systemic autoimmune diseases; give two examples of cell-mediated and antibody-mediated autoimmune diseases and discuss each.
9. Discuss some of the approaches used in the treatment of autoimmune diseases.

The interaction of antigen with specific immunologically competent lymphocytes may elicit either induction of an immune response or a state of antigen-specific unresponsiveness. The lack of *specific* responsiveness is called **immunologic tolerance** or **self-tolerance**. *Specific immunologic tolerance is defined as the acquired inability of a host to express specific humoral or cell-mediated immunity to a self-antigen to which it would otherwise respond.* Self-tolerance induction is an "immune response" that shows specificity and memory for an antigen, but nothing happens. It represents negative immunologic memory. The lack of responsiveness is not caused by a host's genetic control of immunity or by the nonimmunogenicity of an antigen. Under normal conditions, the host would be competent to respond to the specific antigen. Immunologic tolerance is the principal mechanism of discrimination between self and nonself. The mechanism of tolerance is divided into **central tolerance** and **peripheral tolerance**. Central tolerance is associated with the events in the early life of *immature* lymphocytes in the primary lymphoid organs, the bone marrow for B lymphocytes and the thymus for T lymphocytes, where B and T cell clones are deleted if they express receptors that bind self antigen with greater than low affinity. The central tolerance mechanism in its attempts to eliminate all self-reactive lymphocytes is not always successful; it is successful only for the self-antigens expressed in the primary lymphoid organs. These surviving newly emigrated self-reactive lymphocytes move into the secondary (peripheral) lymphoid tissues. However, a backup layer of tolerance mechanisms exists to counteract the escapees of central tolerance—it is peripheral tolerance. Its principal mechanism (others discussed later) renders *mature* self-reactive lymphocytes that encounter peripheral self-antigens for the first time anergic (that is, functionally unresponsive to self-antigen). Even under the strict control of central and peripheral tolerance, potentially harmful self-reactive lymphocytes are present in the periphery of normal individuals that are occasionally activated, leading to inappropriate humoral or cell-mediated immune responses against self-antigens—literally, *an attack on self. This activity is called* **autoimmunity**—it results from failures in self-tolerance mechanisms that can lead to **autoimmune diseases** characterized by tissue damage. Autoimmune diseases occur in hosts because the ability to recognize nonself is tightly linked to recognition of self. This kind of recognition has to stay under strict control. If lymphocytes are activated by **autoantigens**, they quickly turn against the body's healthy cells and tissues. This chapter first describes the mechanisms that limit an adaptive immune response against self-antigens, presents the different concepts and mechanisms involved in the development of autoimmune diseases, then discusses different disease states, and ends with approaches to treating autoimmune disease states.

# THE STUDY AND UNDERSTANDING OF TOLERANCE BEGAN AROUND 1900

The idea of immunologic tolerance began in the discussions on *horror autotoxicus*. Paul Ehrlich, the 1908 Nobel laureate, wrote that "the organism possesses certain contrivances by means of which the immune reaction...is prevented from acting against the organism's own elements...These contrivances are naturally of the highest importance for the individual." These "contrivances" are represented by immunologic tolerance. The recognition of self-antigens—that is, horror autotoxicus, the inbuilt tendency to avoid attack of self-antigens—by the immune system (autoimmunity) is incompatible with life. Proof of immunologic tolerance was offered in 1939 when Traub reported that mice infected *in utero* with the nonpathogenic lymphocytic choriomeningitis virus can carry it throughout life and never show an immune response to the virus. In contrast, mice infected first in adult life have a normal antiviral antibody response leading to virus elimination. This phenomenon was not correlated with immunologic tolerance at that time.

The word *tolerance* was introduced to the immunologic community in 1945 by Owen, who described a naturally induced state of unresponsiveness in cattle. He reported that Freemartin cattle are fraternal (dizygotic) twins, which share a common placenta. These types of twins allow cross-transfusion of blood cells during pregnancy, and individual animals contain erythrocytes of two different genotypes. As adults, these animals are unable to respond immunologically to skin grafts from their fraternal twin. These results established that tolerance is an acquired characteristic.

In 1949, Burnet and Fenner used Traub's and Owen's data to offer a formal theory for the study of immunologic tolerance. They suggested that exposure to self-antigens during embryonic life (before immunologic maturity) prevented a host from responding to its own tissues. They further predicted that *in utero* exposure to foreign antigen would cause the adult host's immune system to regard the antigen as self. Although Burnet was unsuccessful in providing experimental data to support this theory, in 1953 Billingham, Brent, and Medawar demonstrated acquired immunologic tolerance. Billingham and coworkers showed that the *in utero* exposure of mice to viable allogeneic spleen cells led to the adults' toleration of skin grafts from the same strain of mice that provided the allogeneic spleen cells. If syngeneic spleen cells, immune to the allogeneic cells, are transferred into the tolerant animal, the state of unresponsiveness is terminated. Figure 13-1 illustrates an experiment similar to Billingham's, which shows how neonatal tolerance is induced experimentally. This study spurred intensive research on the subject. Taken together, these experiments involved analysis of tolerance at the cellular level and established that unresponsiveness was a property of antigen-specific lymphocytes.

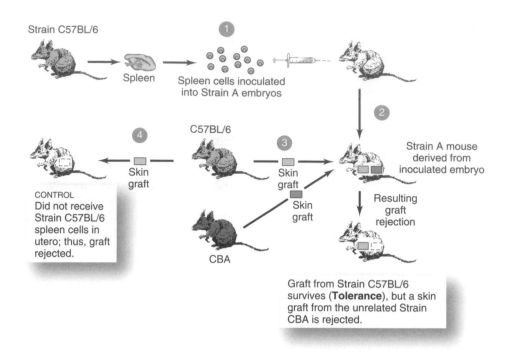

**FIGURE 13-1 Assessment of tolerance induction using skin grafts.** Spleen cells from an adult C57BL/6 mouse are injected into Strain A embryos. As adults, these mice receive a skin graft from strains C57BL/6 and CBA. The Strain A mice reject the CBA graft, but the C57BL/6 graft survives. Strain A mice are tolerant to C57BL/6 antigens. The adult Strain A mouse is chimeric, that is, T cells and APCs are derived from both the host (recipient) and the donor spleen; therefore, mature Strain A T cells would become tolerant to donor cell MHC molecules because the developing T cells in these mice would be negatively selected on APCs from the donor animal. Strain A control mice, which have not been tolerized to C57BL/6 antigens, reject them.

Burnet's clonal selection theory lent support to the idea of tolerance. If each lymphocyte was predisposed to react with its specific antigen, the deletion of self-reactive clones would account for self-tolerance. This culling of self-reactive lymphocytes was postulated to occur during early embryonic life. At that time, the host would take inventory of its antigens. If specific lymphocytes could react against autologous antigens, they were deleted. Burnet's hypothesis and Medawar and coworkers' results, however, could not completely explain tolerance. Their model maintained that a host has one chance to secure nonresponsiveness to antigens early in its development. Thus, the model could not explain why adult hosts can be made tolerant to foreign antigens. Burnet's hypothesis can be modified to explain adult tolerance induction if the maturity status of the lymphocytes (rather than the developmental stage of the animal) is presumed to be the cardinal feature responsible for tolerance induction. We now know that tolerance induction is a 24/7 process that can occur in immature and mature lymphocytes.

Fast-forwarding to the 1990s, the use of transgenic mice eloquently showed that central and peripheral tolerance occurs by deletion or inactivation of self-reactive lymphocytes. Briefly, transgenic mice expressing hen egg-white lysozyme (HEL) were mated with transgenic mice expressing immunoglobulin receptors against HEL; the $F_1$ progeny express HEL and possess B cells with anti-HEL specific receptors. During development in the bone marrow, $F_1$ progeny B cells encounter HEL and are negatively selected (central tolerance), which leads to most HEL-reactive B cells being deleted but some B cells undergo *receptor editing* (rearranging a replacement anti-HEL light chain, leading to a less self-reactive receptor; receptor editing is discussed later). Non-HEL–reactive B cells leave the bone marrow. Using the same system, peripheral tolerance was demonstrated by introducing syngeneic anti-HEL B cells into mice that express soluble HEL as self-antigen; the anti-HEL B cells encounter HEL in the periphery and become anergic (they are unresponsive to self-antigen; are not activated, do not proliferate, and do not migrate to lymph nodes or splenic follicles) due to lack of help from $T_H$ cells. The latter results confirm the need for two levels of tolerance; central tolerance is not an absolute mechanism for culling all possible self-reactive lymphocytes. The survivors appear in the periphery, where they encounter peripheral tolerance. These survivors are not unexpected because purging of autoreactive immune cells in central lymphoid organs is mainly effective against autoantigens found in these organs.

---

### MINI SUMMARY

If a host is exposed to antigen at two different times and no response occurs against the specific antigen, the antigen has induced immunologic tolerance. Acquired immunologic tolerance was demonstrated in 1939 by Traub, in 1945 by Owen, and in 1953 by Medawar and coworkers. Medawar exposed embryos to allogeneic spleen cells; as adults, these animals did not reject skin grafts of the same allogeneic type administered *in utero*. Most of the current work on immunologic tolerance deals with its induction in adult transgenic or knockout animals.

---

# THE MAJOR CHARACTERISTIC OF TOLERANCE IS A SECONDARY "NOTHING" RESPONSE

*Self-tolerance* is the essence of the immune system's operation; the immune system must distinguish between self and nonself. The seemingly twisted approach to study the mechanisms of *self*-tolerance is to study *acquired tolerance* to *foreign* antigens. Therefore, most studies dealing with tolerance involve experimental model systems using foreign antigen to induce in the immune system a state of nonreactivity. Experimental model results may or may not represent the physiologic situation of a host's maintaining nonreactivity against autologous tissues (avoiding autoimmune reactions). Nonetheless, the advent of monoclonal antibodies and molecular biology approaches provided convincing evidence showing that: maturing T and B cells are clonally deleted in the thymus and bone marrow, respectively; clonal deletion and clonal anergy of self-antigen recognizing T and B lymphocytes could be credibly demonstrated using transgenic mice; tolerance induction could occur by editing self-reactive

receptor genes where only the offending receptor development is aborted; and a dedicated lineage of thymus-derived CD4$^+$CD25$^+$Foxp3$^+$ regulatory T ($T_{reg}$) cells (discussed below; also see Chapter 10) suppress peripheral autoreactive lymphocytes.

Manipulation of certain parameters can force a host to consider a foreign substance as a **tolerogen** rather than an immunogen. *A tolerogen is a substance that induces nonresponsiveness rather than immunity.* The common thread during the manipulation of these parameters is that any reduction in the immune response favors the induction of tolerance.

## The Dose of Antigen Affects Tolerance Induction

Doses of antigen higher than needed for immunization are tolerogenic. The higher the antigen dose, the more profound the tolerance and the longer its duration is. This relationship changes as the B cell matures. In fact, the tolerogenic dose of antigen needed to tolerize mature B cells is 100- to 1000-fold higher than that needed for mature T cells. Changes in binding avidity and in the number of antibody receptors from low to high in maturing B cells may be responsible for the increased requirement for antigen.

Tolerance is easily induced by exposure to antigen early in fetal life (the first trimester in humans) because the antigen is recognized as self. In adults, the induction of tolerance is difficult. Two main factors influence tolerance induction in adults: the amount of antigen given and its form. Soluble antigens are not always tolerogenic. The amount of soluble antigen given determined whether tolerance or immunity is induced. Two types of tolerance are recognized in adults—*low* and *high dose* (Figure 13-2). When mice are given repeated doses of bovine serum albumin (BSA), ranging from $10^{-12}$ g/ml to 10 g/ml, two zones of tolerance are observed—low zone tolerance,

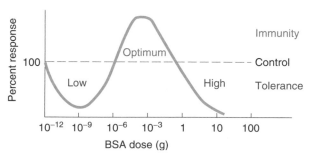

**FIGURE 13-2 Low and high dose tolerance.** Exposure to extreme doses of antigen causes tolerance. Only an optimal dose range between the extremes leads to an immune response.

peaking at $10^{-9}$ g per animal, a median of $10^{-6}$ to $10^{-3}$ g per animal leading to immunity, and a high dose tolerance range of about 10 g per animal. The T cell is the target for tolerance at low antigen levels, and T and B cells are made unresponsive at high antigen doses. The mechanisms of low and high dose tolerance induction, however, are poorly understood. Antigens are more tolerogenic when in a soluble rather than an aggregated or particulate form, which is readily taken up by antigen-presenting cells (APCs). Antigens, therefore, are *tolerogenic* if they react directly with lymphocytes but *immunogenic* if they are first processed by APCs before presentation to lymphocytes. The basic line of thinking is that only professional APCs can induce tissue-specific responses because they express costimulatory molecules. As described in Chapter 10, T-cell activation requires more than just antigen triggering. T cells also require costimulation. T cells that recognize antigen without costimulation become anergic or undergo apoptosis—tolerance is induced. Because tissue cells do not express costimulatory molecules such as B7 or others, T cells are self-tolerant to self-tissues.

The *in situ* situation reflects *in vitro* high-dose tolerance, that is, high and constant concentrations of self-antigens, which can provide strong signals to lymphocytes. These persistent signals tolerize lymphocytes. In contrast, foreign pathogenic antigens appear suddenly and initially their concentrations increase rapidly, a combination that activates lymphocytes.

## The Physicochemical Nature of the Antigen Affects Tolerance Induction

The form in which antigen is administered influences tolerance induction in adult animals. Antigen is more tolerogenic when in a soluble, monomeric form rather than in an aggregated or particulate form, which is highly immunogenic.

The inability to break down antigen greatly eases tolerance induction. For example, polypeptides composed primarily of D-amino acids, or polysaccharides consisting of many repeated units, are highly tolerogenic. If the dose of either of these substances is increased 10- to 100-fold above that needed for immunization, the increase in dose leads to profound, long-lasting tolerance. The early experiments of Dresser, using aggregate-free human gamma globulin (HGG), eloquently showed that the physicochemical nature of antigen is pivotal in determining whether a foreign substance is considered immunogenic or tolerogenic by the host. Nossal and collaborators also used aggregate-free HGG to show that

low doses tolerize immature B cells but that higher doses are needed to make mature splenic B cells tolerant. They went on to show that $T_{reg}$ cells (then called *suppressor T cells*) are not involved in nonresponsiveness to HGG and that the unresponsiveness cannot be adoptively transferred. These results support the idea of clonal deletion of immature lymphocytes when they run into self-antigen.

The molecular weight of an antigen also influences its tolerogenic ability. If the molecular weight of an antigen is decreased without changing its specificity, its ability to induce tolerance is increased. For example, the protein of bacterial flagella called *flagellin* can be divided into three molecular weight fractions: (1) the 10 kD polymerized flagellin, (2) the 40 kD monomeric flagellin, and (3) the 18 kD fragment A from monomeric flagellin. These three molecules have identical antigenic determinants. Moving from highest to lowest molecular weight flagellin, a reversal from good immunogen to poor tolerogen to good tolerogen to poor immunogen is observed. Similar results occur with polysaccharides of less than 10 kD. The lower limit of molecular weight for a tolerogen seems to be between 1.5 and 5 kD.

Besides an antigen's degradability, physical form, and molecular weight, the density of its determinants is a determining factor in tolerance induction. Using T-dependent antigens, a direct relationship between antigenic determinant density and tolerogenicity is seen. If determinant density increases, the ease of tolerance induction is enhanced. The threshold determinant density required for a molecule to be an immunogen is lower than for a tolerogen.

## The Immunogenicity of an Antigen Affects Tolerance Induction

The more immunogenic a substance, the more difficult it is to use as a tolerogen. Soluble proteins such as albumins are better tolerogens than are foreign erythrocytes because soluble proteins are difficult to trap in lymphoid organs. In contrast, erythrocytes are rapidly internalized by phagocytic cells of the lymph nodes and spleen. To study whether the inherent immunogenicity of a substance dictates its ability to serve as a tolerogen, nonimmunogenic or weakly immunogenic substances (carriers) can be conjugated to haptens and injected into animals. The conjugation of hapten to carrier usually leads to hapten-specific tolerance. Carriers that have been tried are (1) syngeneic antibodies and lymphoid cells, (2) foreign substances to which the host is genetically unable to respond, and (3) substances nonimmunogenic to particular species. Tolerance appears due to clonal

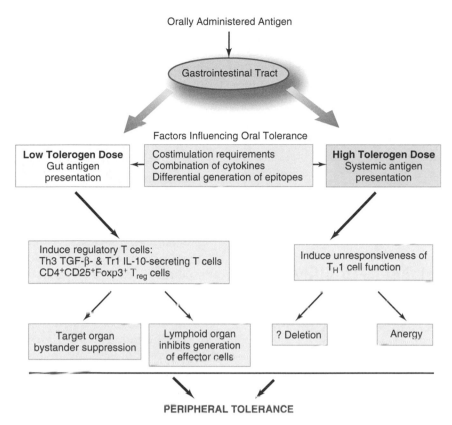

**FIGURE 13-3 Immunologic mechanisms of oral tolerance.** See text for explanation.

deletion in all cases except when hapten-labeled, syngeneic lymphoid cells are used. The latter case of tolerance induction appears due to activation of $T_{reg}$ cells.

## The Route of Antigen Administration Affects Tolerance Induction

Two principal routes of antigen administration favor tolerance induction: the oral and intravenous routes. Orally administered antigen inhibits the later immune response when the animal is challenged systemically with the same antigen. Oral tolerogens induce tolerance through the generation of active suppression or clonal anergy (Figure 13-3). Low doses of orally given antigen favor active suppression, whereas higher doses favor clonal anergy. Low-tolerogen doses stimulate gut-associated lymphocytes of the MALT. At least three types of regulatory lymphocytes are associated with oral tolerance, $T_H3$ *cells*, following triggering by the oral tolerogen, secrete high amounts of the suppressive cytokine TGF-β. $T_H3$ cells also produce variable amounts of IL-10 and IL-4, which is responsible for their growth. *Tr1 cells* secrete IL-10, which enhances Th3 cell TGF-β production. The localized TGF-β production drives the expression of Foxp3 and the development of CD4+CD25+ $T_{reg}$

cells. The tolerogen-induced regulatory cells are triggered in an antigen-specific manner but suppress in an antigen-nonspecific manner. These cells mediate *bystander suppression* when they meet the fed antigen at the target organ by suppressing autoimmune disease through release of downregulatory TGF-β. In addition to regulatory cell-derived TGF-β, the small intestine tissue is known to constitutively express large amounts of TGF-β—the combination of TGF-β and the vitamin A metabolite retinoic acid promotes *de novo* generation of CD4+CD25+Foxp3+ $T_{reg}$ cells. Induction of these CD4+ T cells is influenced by costimulation needs, surrounding cytokines, and retinoic acid all provided by specialized mucosal dendritic cells. High oral tolerogen doses lead to systemic antigen presentation because the antigen passes through the gut and enters the systemic circulation as either intact protein or fragmented protein antigen. These antigens induce $T_H1$ unresponsiveness, mainly through clonal anergy. Orally administered antigens may have clinical importance. For example, fed autoantigens control some experimentally induced autoimmune diseases, such as experimental autoimmune encephalomyelitis, whereas orally administered alloantigens suppress alloreactivity and prolong graft survival.

If hapten-labeled, syngeneic macrophages are injected intradermally, contact sensitivity is induced, while their inoculation intravenously leads to tolerance. The reasons for these reactions are unclear, but tolerance with intravenous antigens is due mainly to a combination of clonal deletion and clonal anergy.

> **MINI SUMMARY**
>
> Tolerance induction in adult hosts involves the dose of antigen, the form of antigen, the immunogenicity of antigen, and the route of antigen administration.

# THE PRINCIPAL MECHANISMS THAT INDUCE SELF-TOLERANCE ARE CLONAL DELETION, CLONAL ANERGY, OR REGULATED INHIBITION OF SELF-REACTIVE T AND B CELLS

Tolerance is a complex process involving changes in the function of the T- and B-cell compartments of the immune system. These changes generally involve physically, functionally, or suppressively purging lymphocytes that react to self-antigens (Figure 13-4). The mechanisms of tolerance induction are not mutually exclusive. *The mechanisms of tolerance induction either (1) physically eliminate (clonal deletion), (2) functionally inactivate (clonal anergy), or (3) regulatively inhibit the clones of autoreactive T and B cells that otherwise would react against self-antigen.* Clonal deletion mechanisms are generally associated with *central tolerance*, which occurs in the thymus and bone marrow, whereas clonal anergy and suppression by $T_{reg}$ cells are associated with tolerance induction in secondary lymphoid tissues (the site of *peripheral tolerance*). Peripheral tolerance accounts for the failure of central tolerance mechanisms to cull self-antigen reactive lymphocytes, which are specific for peripheral tissue-restricted self-antigens that may not be expressed in or have access to the thymus or bone marrow (there are exceptions, as mentioned below).

## Central Tolerance Induction Occurs at the Level of Developing Lymphocytes in Primary Lymphoid Organs

Central tolerance mechanisms accompany V(D)J recombination events in maturing T and B lymphocytes. Central tolerance is achieved partly through **clonal deletion** as part of the process of negative selection (see Chapters 8 and 10) and **receptor editing** in T lymphocytes and B lymphocytes during their maturation in the thymus and bone marrow, respectively. Positively selected cortical thymocytes continually move to the medulla, where their TCR self-reactivity continues to be tested; they are triggered to undergo apoptosis on engagement of TCRs that bind strongly with self-peptides presented in association with the appropriate self-MHC molecules. In fact, negative selection of self-reactive thymocytes occurs mainly in the thymic medullary compartment. It is now know that medullary thymic epithelial cells (mTECs) promiscuously express a large number of genes, which encode peripheral tissue-restricted self-antigens (pTAs) that are normally present only in specialized peripheral organs. During negative selection, the copy of peripheral self in mTECs encodes pTAs, which are presented to differentiating thymocytes, either directly by mTECs, or indirectly by thymic dendritic cell internalizing and displaying mTEC released antigens, leading to tolerance induction by apoptotic clonal deletion of the self-reactive T cells. What allows this promiscuous expression of pTAs in mTECs? To date, only the *autoimmune regulator (AIRE)* gene does (an autoimmune disease due to mutated *AIRE* is discussed shortly). It encodes the AIRE protein, which promotes the ectopic transcriptional activity of many chromosomal locations, thereby enhancing the expression by mTECs of genes that would normally only be expressed in peripheral specific tissues. These mechanisms foretell the absence of autoimmune attack of peripheral organs. Whether AIRE is expressed in the periphery is under intense research.

A limited number of self-reactive T cells prompt receptor editing, which leads to stoppage of receptor production with continued *recombination-activating gene 1 (RAG-1)* and *RAG-2* expression, and replacement of the self-reactive TCR α-chain with a less reactive one. Although deletion is the predominant process of T-cell central tolerance, the selection of $T_{reg}$ cells is also important (discussed in the next section).

As T cells in the thymus, most B cells in the bone marrow are polyreactive and capable of binding self-antigen, but only a small percentage enter the mature peripheral B cell pool. If immature B cells express self-reactive receptors in the bone marrow that bind with a cross-linking strength that exceeds a certain threshold, the immature B cells internalize the self-reactive receptors and halt their maturation program. The consequence of this stoppage is that

## CENTRAL TOLERANCE

**CLONAL DELETION**

Normal antigen-reactive cells are kept (positive selection). In the absence of positive selection, the cells die. Next, the immature self-reactive T and B cells can be clonally deleted (negative selection) during maturation in the central immune organs, thymus, and bone marrow, respectively. Self-reactive B cell receptors can be edited to ones that are not self-reactive. Mature self-reactive T and B cells can be intrinsically or extrinsically inactivated (anergy or regulated, respectively; see below).

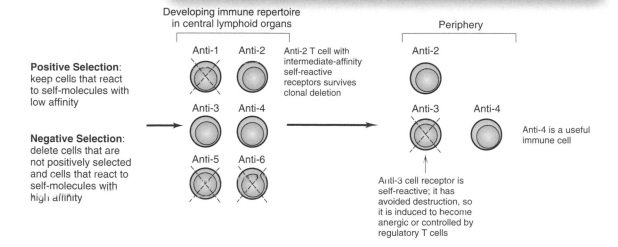

**Positive Selection:**
keep cells that react to self-molecules with low affinity

**Negative Selection:**
delete cells that are not positively selected and cells that react to self-molecules with high affinity

## PERIPHERAL TOLERANCE

**CLONAL ANERGY**

Activation of mature T and B cells requires at least two signals, the first antigen-binding, the second costimulatory signals from antigen-presenting cells. Therefore, a mechanism for induction of clonal anergy would be the absence of costimulatory signals required for cellular activation when stimulated by self-antigens.

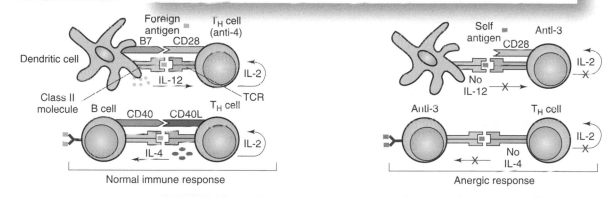

**REGULATED INHIBITION**

Intermediate-affinity self-reactive T cells, driven by FOXP3 upregulation, differentiate into specialized regulatory T cells: $CD4^+CD25^+Foxp3^+T_{reg}$ cells.

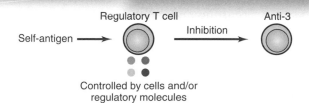

**FIGURE 13-4 Mechanisms for the development of self-tolerance.** Self-tolerance is divided into central tolerance and peripheral tolerance. The primary mechanism of central tolerance is clonal deletion. Mature self-reactive T and B cells in the periphery can be physically eliminated (apoptotic cell death; not shown), functionally inactivated (shown), or regulatively inhibited (shown). See text for details.

the homing receptors CD62 ligand are not expressed (required by B cells to enter lymph nodes), B-cell activating factor (BAFF) receptors are limited (BAFF is a cytokine needed to sustain B cell survival), and *RAG-1* and *-2* continue to be expressed (allowing new immunoglobulin light chain genes to be edited by rearrangement). If a self-reactive B cell fails to edit its receptor to a less reactive one, it dies in the bone marrow or shortly after arriving in the spleen. Receptor editing plays a more predominant role in B-cell tolerance development than in T cells.

## Peripheral Tolerance Induction Occurs at the Level of Mature Self-Reactive Lymphocytes in Secondary Lymphoid Tissues

B and T lymphocytes that evade negative selection during central tolerance and enter the periphery face another level of tolerance induction—*peripheral tolerance*. Peripheral tolerance mechanisms include clonal anergy (that is, functional unresponsiveness), deletion by activation-induced cell death (AICD), and suppression by $T_{reg}$ cells.

During a normal immune response, activation of mature T and B cells requires two signals, antigen binding followed by costimulatory molecule interactions (see Chapter 10). B cell responses to T-dependent antigen require help from $CD4^+$ $T_H2$ cells; B-cell receptor cross-linking by antigen provides the first signal, B-cell CD40 ligation by T-cell CD40L provides the culmination of the second signal (see Figure 13-5). Like B cells, T-cell activation requires two signals; the first signal is TCR engagement of peptide fragments of antigen bound to MHC molecules, the second signal is APC B7-1 (CD80) or B7-2 (CD86) joining with T cell CD28. The second signal induces IL-2 secretion (see Figure 13-5), which leads to T-cell proliferation and cytokine and cytokine receptor production.

The predominant peripheral tolerance mechanism is **clonal anergy**. It occurs when B cells encounter soluble antigen that cross-links their antigen receptors, and T cells encounter processed antigen through their TCR, in the absence of costimulatory signals. For example, cells derived from the kidneys, liver, pancreas, and other organs do not commonly express costimulatory molecules; therefore, they induce anergy rather than activation of self-reactive T cells. Autoreactive B cells encountering antigen in the absence of T-cell help become anergic. The autoreactive T cells remaining after anergy and deletion may be subjected to induction of inhibitory receptors triggering anergy or death and active suppression by $T_{reg}$ cells.

As we saw, antigen-primed T cells required CD28–B7 molecule interactions for full activation. The normal downregulation by the T-cell inhibitory receptor cytotoxic T lymphocyte antigen 4 (CTLA-4) binding the costimulatory molecules B7 shuts off T-cell responses and induces anergy. *CTLA-4* knockout mice (gene encoding CTLA-4 is deleted) demonstrate the significance of CTLA-4 in maintaining peripheral tolerance; these mice develop a fatal systemic autoimmune disease characterized by massive proliferation of lymphocytes leading to severe enlargement of lymph organs and lymphocytic infiltration of multiple organs.

Cell death by apoptosis plays an important role in removing mature self-reactive B and T lymphocytes. The Fas–Fas ligand (FasL; also called CD95 and CD178, respectively) pathway provides the deletion mechanism. Fas and FasL are transmembrane proteins that belong to the tumor necrosis factor (TNF) receptor family and TNF family of membrane proteins, respectively. In fact, Fas is the prototype death receptor of the TNF receptor family. Fas is expressed on many cell types including T cells, whereas FasL is expressed mainly on activated T cells. The ligation of Fas with FasL initiates AICD leading to apoptosis of the self-reactive cell (see Figure 10-23)—the deletion of mature T and B cells that recognize self-antigens. The biological importance of Fas–FasL interactions in the development of autoimmune diseases was established in naturally occurring mutations of either Fas or FasL in mice. The genetic lesions lead to massive T-cell proliferation in the lymph nodes and spleen; the mouse strain with the lesion in the gene encoding Fas is called *lpr* (for lymphoproliferative) and its counterpart with a lesion in the gene encoding FasL is called *gld* (for general lymphoproliferative disease). These mice are unable to induce the AICD pathway, leading to autoimmune disease early in life. A human disease, which mimics the disease associated with *lpr/lpr* and *gld/gld* mice, called *autoimmune lymphoproliferative syndrome (ALPS)* is caused by mutations in Fas. Anergized autoreactive B cells can also under apoptosis by Fas–FasL interactions.

Characterization of other human, naturally occurring mutations that block tolerance and lead to autoimmune diseases such as *autoimmune polyendocrinopathy-candidiasis-ectodermal dystrophy (APECED)* and *immune dysregulation, polyendocrinopathy, enteropathy, X-linked syndrome (IPEX)* have enhanced our understanding of tolerance—lethal autoimmune lymphoproliferative diseases. Currently, APECED is the only known autoimmune disease inherited in a Mendelian fashion, which is characterized by multiple autoimmune endocrinopathies, chronic mucocutaneous candidiasis, and ectodermal dystrophies. APECED is also known as *autoimmune polyendocrine syndrome 1 (APS1)*. The APECED gene encodes a protein called *autoimmune regulator (AIRE)*, which is restricted to a subset of medullary thymic epithelial cells (described earlier) and dendritic cells. These cells promiscuously express a wide array of peripheral-tissue antigens derived from nearly all organs in the body. The transcription factor AIRE regulates the transcription of genes encoding peripheral-tissue antigens; thus, AIRE controls the development of central tolerance and consequently autoimmunity. In fact, mutations in AIRE cripple thymic negative selection of organ-specific T cells. *Aire* knockout mice confirmed this; these *aire*-deficient mice have normal immune systems but develop multi-organ infiltrates and autoantibodies—the thymus's ability to display the body's repertoire of self-antigens is extinguished when the AIRE gene is defective.

Another rare, fatal, systemic autoimmune disease known by the acronym IPEX mirrors a disease of a natural mutation that occurs in *scurfy* mice, an early autoimmunity (including type 1 diabetes and thyroiditis) directed against a variety of tissues caused by the lack of $T_{reg}$ cells. The genetic mapping of the mutation in IPEX patients and in *scurfy* mice showed that both conditions resulted from mutations in the *Foxp3* gene. Foxp3 is the transcription factor required for the development of CD4$^+$CD25$^+$T$_{reg}$ cells, whether it fulfills the role of a master controller of $T_{reg}$ cell-differentiation, at least at the level of $T_{reg}$ cell transcriptional programs, is under intense investigation. Nonetheless, alterations in Foxp3 affect the development and/or function of CD4$^+$CD25$^+$ Foxp3$^+$ $T_{reg}$ cells and subsequently autoimmune disease development. Scurfy mice can be cured by the exogenous provision of $T_{reg}$ cells; an effective treatment for IPEX requires a bone marrow transplant from an HLA-identical sibling.

$T_{reg}$ cells also maintain peripheral tolerance; these T cells are CD4$^+$CD25$^+$Foxp3$^+$ and can transfer tolerance. They are a unique subset of CD4$^+$ T cells (representing roughly 10% of peripheral CD4$^+$ cells) that express high levels of the IL-2 receptor α-chain (CD25; see Chapter 10). $T_{reg}$ cell development and function depend on the expression of the transcription factor forkhead fox 3 (Foxp3)—a regulator that programs CD4$^+$CD25$^+$Foxp3$^+$ $T_{reg}$ cell development in the thymus as in the periphery. CD4$^+$CD25$^+$ $T_{reg}$ cells can be derived from two sources, specifically those that develop in the thymus and those that are generated in the periphery (at least in gut-associated lymphoid tissue and perhaps

other places). The thymus-derived $T_{reg}$ cells are called *natural $T_{reg}$ cells*, in contrast to peripheral naïve T cells that acquire Foxp3 expression and $T_{reg}$ cell function, and are called *adaptive* or *induced $T_{reg}$ cells*. During thymic development, $T_{reg}$ cells arise from intermediate-avidity, self-reactive T cells. The binding of self-peptide–MHC complexes induces Foxp3 expression, which drives $T_{reg}$ cell development. CD4$^+$CD25$^+$ $T_{reg}$ cells, like their CD4$^+$CD25$^-$ T cell counterparts, have a diverse TCR repertoire, and are not restricted to self-antigens. CD4$^+$CD25$^+$ $T_{reg}$ cells can directly (and perhaps) indirectly suppress the activation and proliferation of T cells, B cells, dendritic cells, NK cells, and NKT cells. $T_{reg}$ cells mediate control through three potential pathways: cell contact–dependent inhibition of the activation and proliferation of APCs and effector T cells, and B cells; the killing of either APCs or T cells or both; and suppression by cytokines such as IL-10 and TGF-β that may lead to bystander suppression. The ability of $T_{reg}$ cells to control autoimmune diseases is illustrated in nonobese diabetic (NOD) mice, which spontaneously develop type 1 diabetes. Transfer of $T_{reg}$ cells blocks islet destruction in NOD mice. How $T_{reg}$ cells mediate regulation is uncertain but it is regulated, in part, by the production IL-10 and TGF-β; however, this is not a prerequisite for their suppressive activity. $T_{reg}$ cells constitutively express the inhibitory receptor CTLA-4 and the chemokine receptors CCR4 and CCR8; the latter receptors facilitate their migration to inflamed tissues and draining lymph nodes. *De novo* induced Foxp3$^+$ $T_{reg}$ cells from naïve CD4$^+$ precursors in the periphery, that is, cells resembling thymus-derived $T_{reg}$ cells, can be generated at least in gut-associated lymphoid tissues and perhaps other places. These cells acquire suppressive activity after *in vitro* TCR stimulation in the presence of TGF-β and IL-2, and *in vivo* exposure to subimmunogenic doses of antigen and the endogenous expression of foreign antigen in a lymphopenic environment.

Two additional types of inducible CD4$^+$ $T_{reg}$ cells have received attention: *type 1 regulatory T (Tr1) cells* and $T_H3$ *cells*. Neither cell type constitutively expresses CD25 nor Foxp3 and is distinguished by their cytokine profile. Tr1 cells produce high levels of IL-10, which represents the true hallmark of Tr1 cells (thus, also called *IL-10-secreting Tr1 cells*); their cytokine profile varies with TGF-β, IFN-γ, and/or IL-5 production, which are all secreted at lower levels than IL-10; IL-4 production is undetectable. Unlike their natural $T_{reg}$-cell counterpart development, Tr1 cells are dependent on surrounding cytokines and chronic activation in the presence of IL-10, but like natural $T_{reg}$ cells, Tr1 cells are similar in their ability to mediate suppression or proliferate in response to antigenic stimulation. $T_H3$ cells, distinct from $T_H1$, $T_H2$, or $T_H17$ CD4$^+$ cells, are induced primarily after oral or intravenous antigen application; the resulting tolerance is mediated by TGF-β. $T_H3$ cells also produce IL-10 and perhaps IL-4, both are thought to contribute to their differentiation. Numerous other immunoregulatory cell types have been described.

---

### MINI SUMMARY

The mechanisms of tolerance are varied and complex. Many mechanisms combine to supplement one another. Mechanisms for tolerance may include physical (clonal deletion) or functional (clonal anergy) purging of autoreactive T and B cells, as well as regulated inhibition of autoreactive T and B cells by $T_{reg}$ cells.

---

# AUTOIMMUNITY, IN WHICH THE BODY TURNS AGAINST ITSELF, LEADS TO AUTOIMMUNE DISEASES AND EVEN SELF-DESTRUCTION

At the heart of the immune system is its ability to discriminate between self and nonself substances. As mentioned above, *immunologic tolerance is the acquisition of unresponsiveness to self-antigens, mainly through clonal deletion, clonal anergy, and active suppression mechanisms; as such, the proper working of these mechanisms is essential to the preservation of the biologic integrity of the host.* The expression of self-antigens is preprogrammed in the germline, while unresponsiveness or self-tolerance to self-antigens is not preprogrammed but is acquired somatically by mechanisms that delete, functionally inactivate, or control autoreactive lymphocytes. If these mechanisms that maintain self-tolerance break down, autoimmune diseases result—a specific activation of autoreactive lymphocytes by autoantigens. Due to the spontaneous nature of this activity, it is difficult to prove and identify the eliciting autoantigen.

As mentioned earlier, the concept of *horror autotoxicus* implies that immune responses against self do not occur normally and, if they do occur, the outcome is harmful to the host. If the immune system can recognize almost any antigen, why not the antigens

that belong to self? The counterintuitive answer is that immune cells *must* recognize self before they can react to nonself. This recognition implies that it is normal for the immune system to react with self. In one case the result is immunity; in the other it is autoimmunity. What tips the balance in favor of autoimmunity is uncertain. Autoimmune diseases can be characterized by abnormal or excessive anti-self immune responses that cause harmful effects to the host. Despite the huge repertoire of self-antigens that could act as a source for relentless lymphocyte stimulation, more than half of the lymphocyte antigen receptors that are generated by random V(D)J recombination react to self-antigens, and the production of roughly $10^{11}$ new lymphocytes daily, activation by self-antigens is infrequent and sporadic, as confirmed by the low incidence of autoimmune diseases (1 to 2% of the U.S. population).

## Even Though There Are Multiple Etiologies for Autoimmune Diseases, CD4$^+$ T Cells Are Central to the Activation of Autoimmune Responses

Individuals with autoimmune diseases have antibodies or T cells that attack their own bodily proteins. *The origin of this autoimmune disorder may lie in the immune process, the self-antigens, or both. Thus, the disease may be caused by (1) an abnormal immune response to normal self-antigens, (2) a normal immune response to abnormal self-antigens, or (3) an abnormal immune response to abnormal self-antigens.* The progress of an autoimmune disease state appears to be three-tiered. The first tier is *hereditary susceptibility* (an inactive "time bomb" in the host's genetic machinery). The second tier is a *triggering* vehicle—the environment, such as a virus, that starts this "bomb." The third tier is *immune system malfunction* brought about, in part, by a foul-up in the body's physical defenses. In sum, it usually is not a single agent that initiates autoimmune diseases, as we saw exceptions exist.

Evidence strongly suggests a multifactorial etiology for many autoimmune diseases, including genetics and environmental influences. However, most diseases probably result from two major events: (1) change in self-antigens, leading to the formation of neoantigens, and (2) exposure to cross-reactive antigens.

The use of experimental animal models of autoimmune diseases suggests that CD4$^+$ $T_H$ cells are the primary mediators of disease. Autoimmune disease can be transferred into naïve recipients using autoreactive T-cell clones and can be reversed in sick hosts by deleting $T_H$ cells with anti-CD4 antibodies plus complement or adding back $T_{reg}$ cells. Because CD4$^+$ $T_H$ cells recognize antigen only when presented by class II MHC molecules, the activation of autoimmune responses by autoreactive $T_H$ cells requires that class II molecules and TCRs bind self-antigens. Direct evidence using animal models and the indirect association between human autoimmune diseases and the higher frequency of certain HLA alleles and susceptibility genes suggest that the MHC haplotype correlates with susceptibility to autoimmunity (see Table 13-2 and associated text). The TCR-autoimmunity connection is observed in *experimental autoimmune encephalomyelitis (EAE)*. EAE is a CD4$^+$ IL-23/$T_H$17—cell—mediated autoimmune disease of the central nervous system inducible in rodents by immunization with autologous or foreign myelin basic protein (MBP) or its peptides. These T cells produce unwanted IFN-$\gamma$ in response to MBP. Because of the similarities in symptoms and pathology, a demyelination of the nerves, EAE is a model for the human disease *multiple sclerosis (MS)*, which is one of the most frequent causes of neurological impairment in young adults (discussed later). Mouse collagen-induced arthritis (CIA) is a model for human rheumatoid arthritis; the method of CIA induction and immune mechanism mirror EAE, only the target tissue differ, that is, joints of the hands, wrists, and knees as oppose to central nervous system tissues. Figure 13-5 lists, and the following paragraphs briefly discuss, nine ways to bypass self-tolerance, mainly through alterations in $T_H$ cells. Other mouse models for human autoimmune diseases are mentioned during discussion of the diseases.

1. CD4$^+$ T cells are needed for most humoral immune responses, but autoreactive T cells controlling the generation of autoantibodies are made harmless through tolerance induction. Thus, T- and B-cell collaboration in the development of autoantibodies is restricted if not impossible. If T cells, however, are exposed to neoantigens, this self-tolerance fails or is broken, and this breakdown leads to autoantibody production, the first important method of causing an autoimmune disease. Chemicals or viruses may combine with normal self-constituents and change them. This change, although slight, when recognized by the immune system, may start an immune response directed against the changed tissue or cellular constituents. This mechanism may occur during autoimmune hemolytic anemia in patients treated with $\alpha$-methyldopa.[1]

The $\alpha$-methyldopa changes the surface antigens of red blood cells, thereby eliciting an autoimmune response, whether or not the drug is present.

2. Autoimmunity may be induced by exposure to exogenous antigens bearing a close structural resemblance to normal tissue components (**molecular mimicry**). These antigens may stimulate the immune system and cause damage because the immune response also cross-reacts with the normal tissue that has been mimicked. Rheumatic fever may occur after a group A *Streptococcus* infection (and others) caused by the development of autoantibodies cross-reactive with streptococcal cell wall antigens and heart muscle antigens. Another compelling example of molecular mimicry that may lead to MS is the mimicry between MBP and viral peptides from measle virus P3 and numerous others.

3. For induction of tolerance to self-constituents, contact between self-antigens and the immune system must occur early in ontogeny. Certain tissue antigens are sequestered or masked during ontogeny so that tolerance to them is never established. If these self-antigens are exposed to the immune system during adult life, through tissue damage because of infections or injuries, an immune response may be started. This immune response is characterized by the production of autoantibodies to these released, formerly sequestered self-antigens. However, there are probably few, if any, truly sequestered self-antigens. In fact, the injection of unmodified extracts of "sequestered" antigens does not easily induce antibody formation. Two possible exceptions to this situation are the immune responses to sperm after vasectomy or to eye lens protein after eye injury. In most of these cases the autoimmunity is transient, but chronic autoimmune disease can occur. One theory is that tolerance is best maintained when self-antigens are accessible to the circulation and to lymphocytes. If this theory is true, and admittedly it is a simplistic view, (a) autoimmunity to circulating serum proteins is never found, (b) development of autoantibodies to intracellular (hidden) components is easy, and (c) autoreactivity to many self-constituents is possible only if strong immunization measures are taken, such as changing autologous proteins so that they appear foreign or immunizing with a mixture of autologous tissue and complete Freund's adjuvant. Nonetheless, autoantigens play a mandatory role in autoimmune disease, as suggested by the suppression of animal autoreactive responses following autoantigen withdrawal.

---

[1]$\alpha$-Methyldopa is an antihypertensive drug used in the treatment of Parkinson's disease.

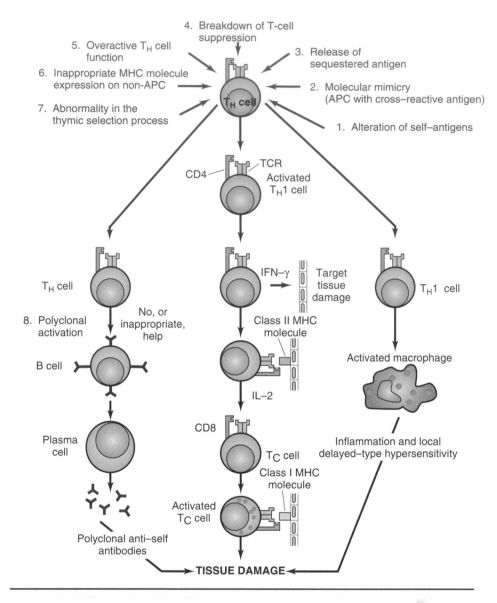

1. Alteration of self-antigens by chemicals or viruses
2. Cross-reactive antibody production
3. Exposure to sequestered self-antigens
4. Decrease in regulatory T-cell number or function
5. Overactive or absence of $T_H$ cell function (polyclonal B-cell activation)
6. Inappropriate class II MHC molecule expression on non-APCs
7. Thymic defects
8. Polyclonal activation
9. Genetic factors (not shown but discussed in text)
10. Hormonal factors (not shown but discussed in text)

**FIGURE 13-5 Possible Contributing Factors in Autoimmune Diseases.** This list provides ways to activate normal $T_H$ cells and bypass control mechanisms (self-tolerance), thereby losing the restraint that leads to tissue damage by elements of the immune system. See text for details.

4. The immune system is a dynamic system kept in balance by $T_{reg}$ cells. These cells dampen the response to foreign and autologous antigens. Thus, if autoantigen-specific $T_{reg}$ cells are lost, the result can be the development of harmful autoantibodies or autoreactive T cells. For example, we saw earlier that $T_H17$ cells mediate EAE in mice, in part, by IL-17 and IL-23 production. Reports also show that feeding MBP to these mice induces $CD8^+$ T cells that produce TGF-$\beta$ and IL-4, which protect against the disease. The flip-side to $CD8^+$ dysregulation is the possibility that autoimmune disease is associated with immune dysregulation due to a $T_H$ subset imbalance as suggested by alternations in the IL-23/$T_H17$ cell axis (see Chapter 10). In fact there has been a paradigm shift in our understanding of autoimmune inflammation pathogenesis—many autoimmune diseases are now thought to be driven by a non-$T_H1$ cell pathway. TGF-$\beta$ and IL-6, together with IL-23, collectively polarize and expand and sustain a distinct $CD4^+$ $T_H17$ inflammation effector cell subset that produces IL-17 and other inflammatory cytokines and chemokines. The combination of TGF-$\beta$ and IL-6, in the absence of IFN-$\gamma$ and IL-4, drives the differentiation of naïve T cells to $T_H17$ cells and upregulates their expression of IL-23 receptors. IL-23 is an expansion and survival factor to already differentiated $T_H17$ cells. The development of $T_H17$ and $T_{reg}$ cells require the presence of TGF-$\beta$ but the presence of IL-6 skews the response toward a $T_H17$ phenotype (see Figures 10-16 and 10-17). The inappropriate or continuous activation of this $T_H17$ subset can lead to autoimmune diseases. Indeed, this pathogenic $T_H17$ subset is now considered to represent the population responsible for mediating autoimmune pathogenesis once attributed to $T_H1$ cells.

5. Tolerance to self-antigens seems to be maintained at the $T_H$-cell level. Autoreactive B cells exist, yet are unable to be activated by self-antigens because of the lack of help from tolerant $T_H$ cells. Thus, autoimmune disorders could result from (a) the direct stimulation of autoreactive B cells by polyclonal activators, (b) the bypassing of tolerant T cells by nonspecific helper factors, or (c) the activation of the tolerant T cells by changed antigens or cross-reactive antigens. In fact, there are many known nonspecific B cell polyclonal activators (Table 13-1), such as Gram-negative bacteria, cytomegalovirus, and Epstein-Barr virus, which induce the proliferation of multiple B-cell clones that produce IgM in the absence of $T_H$

**TABLE 13-1 Some Polyclonal Activators of B Cells**

Lymphokines

Lipopolysaccharide

Some viruses (such as cytomegalovirus and Epstein-Barr virus)

Parasites

Purified protein derivative (PPD) of *Mycobacterium tuberculosis*

Fc fragment of IgG

cells. If autoreactive B cells encounter these polyclonal activators or are ligated via their receptors for pathogen-associated molecular patterns (PAMPs) (see Chapter 3), autoantibody production can occur. If we speculate that B cells not tolerant to self-antigens exist, but are inhibited either by $T_{reg}$ cells or by not being helped by $T_H$ cells, then any substance supplying the second (nonspecific) signal for B-cell stimulation, either directly or by substituting for $T_H$ cells, may trigger such B cells to produce autoantibodies. For example, the administration of lipopolysaccharide into mice induces the production of autoantibodies against DNA, immunoglobulins, thymocytes, and red blood cells. The diverse antibodies produced during polyclonal lymphocyte activation lead to systemic lesions. Hypergammaglobulinemia and autoantibody production may result and lead to a generalized autoimmune disease such as systemic lupus erythematosus (SLE).

6. Some autoimmune diseases may be the result of aberrant expression of class II MHC molecules on cells where they are normally absent. For example, the $\beta$ cells of patients diagnosed with insulin-dependent diabetes mellitus (type 1 diabetes) display high levels of both class I and class II MHC molecules. Normally, healthy $\beta$ cells express low levels of class I molecules and no class II molecules. This change in expression, and the resulting diabetes, are observed in mice transgenic for the IFN-$\gamma$ gene coupled to the insulin promoter. These mice express the IFN-$\gamma$ gene only in $\beta$ cells. If these mice are treated with anti-IFN-$\gamma$ antibodies, diabetes is prevented. These results suggest that the hyperexpression of class II MHC molecules, in part, leads to type 1 diabetes. High levels of serum IFN-$\gamma$ are also present in patients with active SLE. In another autoimmune disease, Graves' disease, thyroid acinar cells express high levels of class II MHC molecules. This aberrant expression of class II MHC molecules on non-APCs could allow the presentation of peptides derived from $\beta$ cells and

acinar cells to CD4$^+$ T$_H$ cells. This presentation would lead to the activation of B cells, T$_C$ cells or T$_H$1/T$_H$17 cells to self-antigens. Other factors also must be contributing to this activation because TCR recognition of peptide-MHC complexes (the first signal in T-cell activation) is insufficient to lead to T-cell proliferation or effector function. For full T-cell activation, a second signal is required from costimulatory receptor-counter-receptor interactions by APC B7 and T cell CD28 (see Chapter 10). Because self-tissues do not express costimulatory molecules, self-tissues normally induce tolerance. Therefore, autoimmunity may be the result of T-cell activation by APCs expressing a tissue-specific peptide together with costimulatory molecules. These autoantigen-activated T cells home to the tissues where they mediate their autoreactivity.

7. The thymus is needed for the maturation and differentiation of immature T cells. Any dysfunction also indirectly affects humoral immunity because T cells are required for full expression of immunity. Studies of mouse SLE and of autoimmune strains of mice suggest the importance of the thymus in the expression of autoimmune diseases. For example, all SLE-prone mice develop early thymic atrophy, particularly involving the thymic cortex, where 70 to 90% of the cells die in animals 2 to 6 months of age. The autoimmune strain MRL/1 expresses an SLE-like disease only in the presence of a thymus, irrespective of its genotype, and thymectomized animals do not exhibit the disease. The chicken model for Hashimoto's thyroiditis shows that neonatal thymectomy accelerates the disease, although neonatal bursectomy prevents the disease. Whether thymic dysfunction is the result or the cause of autoimmune diseases is unclear. In some cases, thymic ablation in myasthenia gravis patients is helpful.

8. Autoimmune diseases are genetically and environmentally determined. Autoimmune reactions, like other immune responses, are influenced by the genes of the MHC. Many patients with autoimmune disease have particular histocompatibility types. For example, many persons with autoimmune diseases are associated with the MHC alleles that encode the class II molecules DR2, DR3, DR4, and DR5 (Table 13-2); fewer autoimmune diseases are associated with class I MHC molecules. An association exists between the amino acid sequences of the class II MHC molecule binding cleft and the development of autoimmune disease. In patients with type 1 diabetes, a single amino acid change at residue 57 in the HLA-DQβ chain

**TABLE 13-2 MHC Genes Associated with Autoimmune Diseases**

| Disease | HLA alleles |
|---|---|
| **Organ-specific diseases** | |
| Addison's disease | DR3 |
| Autoimmune hemolytic anemia | * |
| Graves' disease | B8/DR3 |
| Pemphigus vulgaris | DR4, DR6 |
| Hashimoto's thyroiditis | DR5 |
| Idiopathic thrombocytopenic purpura | * |
| Insulin-dependent diabetes mellitus | DR3 and DR4 |
| Myasthenia gravis | DR3 |
| **Systemic diseases** | |
| Ankylosing spondylitis | B27 |
| Goodpasture's syndrome | DR2 |
| Rheumatoid arthritis | DR4 |
| Sjögren's syndrome | DR3 |
| SLE | DR3 (Japanese: DR2) |

*Alleles unknown

correlates with resistance or susceptibility to diabetes. An aspartic acid at position 57 correlates with resistance, while an alanine, serine, or valine at position 57 correlates with susceptibility. The differences in amino acids at this position probably affect self-peptide binding to this class II MHC molecule. Some autoimmune diseases are associated with certain genes encoding the variable (V) and constant (C) regions of immunoglobulins or for the expression of certain autoimmune diseases such as rheumatoid arthritis, Hashimoto's thyroiditis, myasthenia gravis, and SLE. For example, in experimental rheumatoid arthritis, the expression of certain autoantibodies depends in part on a gene linked to the constant locus for production of an immunoglobulin heavy chain. Thus, high levels of these autoantibodies are found in sera of animals with a particular homozygous haplotype, while these autoantibodies are depressed in heterozygous animals. Other susceptibility genes that predispose to autoimmune diseases are associated with genetic variations that lead to (1) lymphocyte signaling aberrations: deficient expression of CTLA-4 (blocks inhibitory signal leading to prolonged T-cell activation), TCR ζ chain (leads to over-excitable T cells) or IL-2 (T cells escape AICD and T$_{reg}$ cells are unable to inhibit autoreactivity); alteration in *protein tyrosine phosphatase-22 (PTPN22) gene* (encodes a dysfunctional inhibitor of spontaneous T-cell activation), *programmed cell death 1 (PD-1) gene* (encodes protein unable to block inhibitor signal leading to overactive T cells), and the *AIRE, Fas,* and *FasL genes* (discussed earlier); over-expression of Cox-2 (increases T cell survival by preventing AICD), CD40 ligand by T cells (upregulates T–B cell interactions leading to autoantibody production), and B-cell activation factor (BAFF; survival factor for maturing B cells that at high levels rescues autoreactive B cells); and dysfunctional inhibitory Fc receptor FcγRIIb on B cells (contributes to B cell overactivity); and (2) abnormal function of soluble mediators: deficiency in C1q, C4, C2, mannan binding lectin, C-reactive protein, and serum amyloid P protein (dysfunctional immune-complex and apoptotic cell debris clearance); and deficiency in DNase I (ineffective clearance of apoptotic material).

9. The sex hormones and X-chromosome or Y-chromosome-linked genes are implicated in the expression of some autoimmune diseases. Most of the studies have dealt with SLE. The results suggest that postpubescent women are about 10 times more susceptible to the disease than men. We do not know why the difference in sex leads to this increased susceptibility. However, women and castrated men have levels of immunoglobulin and of specific immune responses higher than those of sexually normal men. Whether this difference is caused by the suppressive effects of testosterone or by the enhancing effects of estrogen is uncertain.

## MINI SUMMARY

Autoimmunity is an immune response against self-constituents, sometimes causing autoimmune diseases. The idea of autoimmunity had its origins with the concept of *horror autotoxicus* proposed by Ehrlich in 1901. Animal models of autoimmune disease require the demonstration of autoantibodies or sensitized, autoreactive T cells.

Autoimmune disease may involve either an immune response to self-antigens changed by infection or drugs or self-antigens after exposure to cross-reactive antigens. Other possible origins of autoimmune diseases include sequestered antigens, a decrease in $T_{reg}$ cell number or function, enhanced $T_H$ cell function, inappropriate expression of MHC molecules on nonantigen-presenting cells, polyclonal B-cell activation, thymic defects, genetic factors, and hormonal factors. Autoimmune diseases have a multifactorial basis.

# AUTOIMMUNE DISEASES ARE EITHER ORGAN-SPECIFIC OR SYSTEMIC AND ARE A CONSEQUENCE OF EITHER A PREDOMINANCE OF T LYMPHOCYTE OR B LYMPHOCYTE DYSFUNCTION

Without knowing the causative mechanisms that instigate autoimmune diseases, it is difficult to classify them. Nonetheless, to reduce some of the complexity involved in analyzing autoimmune diseases using their clinical aspects, they can be classified as either organ-specific or systemic. Table 13-3 lists some examples of each class; in general, the autoantigens themselves seem to be organ-specific and systemic. Note that almost any organ can be affected, and a systemic form may develop after an initial organ has been affected. Autoimmune diseases also may be arbitrarily divided into diseases resulting from which lymphocytes play a predominant role in mediating organ injury.

## Autoimmune Diseases Are Caused by Self-Reacting T Cells

### Hashimoto's Thyroiditis Results When T Cells React Against Unmasked Self-Antigens

Hashimoto's disease (or Hashimoto's thyroiditis) is a form of thyroid disease with a 1 to 2% incidence in the United States. Patients with Hashimoto's disease, usually women between the age of 30 and 60, have general malaise lasting for several years and a moderately enlarged thyroid, which slowly progresses to *hypothyroidism*. On histologic examination, the thyroid is characteristically infiltrated with lymphocytes and the ectopic formation of lymphoid follicles with germinal centers. The severe lymphocytic infiltration causes the destruction of the thyroid follicles and subsequent hypothyroidism. The autoantibodies against the thyroid autoantigens *thyroid peroxidase* and *thyroglobulin* are clinically the most important tool for diagnosis of the disease. Both thyroid molecules affect iodine uptake, autoantibody binding obstructs uptake leading to decreased thyroid hormone production.

Hashimoto first described a lymphomatous goiter in 1912, but not until 1956 did Roitt and coworkers show it to be an autoimmune disease. At the same time, autoimmune thyroiditis was induced in an animal model by immunization with autologous

**TABLE 13-3 Examples of Autoimmune Diseases**

| Disease | Organ or tissue | Antigen |
|---|---|---|
| **Organ-specific diseases** | | |
| Addison's disease | Adrenals | Adrenal cell |
| Autoimmune hemolytic anemia | Red blood cells | Rh blood group antigens, I antigens |
| Graves' disease | Thyroid | Thyroid stimulating receptor |
| Bullous pemphigoid | Skin | Basement membrane zone of skin |
| Pemphigus vulgaris | Skin | Epidermal cadherin |
| Hashimoto's thyroiditis | Thyroid | Thyroglobulin, thyroid peroxidase |
| Idiopathic thrombocytopenic purpura | Platelets | Platelet integrin GpIIb:IIIa |
| Insulin-dependent diabetes mellitus | Pancreas | Pancreatic β cell antigen (glutamic acid decarboxylase) |
| Myasthenia gravis | Muscle | Acetylcholine receptor |
| **Systemic diseases** | | |
| Goodpasture's syndrome | Kidneys, lung | Basement membrane collagen type IV |
| Rheumatoid arthritis | Joints | Unknown synovial joint antigen, IgG |
| Sjögren's syndrome | Salivary and lacrimal glands | Salivary duct antigens, SS-A, SS-B nucleoproteins |
| Systemic lupus erythematosus | Kidney, brain, skin, and other organ systems | Nuclear antigens, DNA, RNA, histones, ribosomes |

thyroid extract and complete Freund's adjuvant. The immunization of animals with thyroglobulin produces chronic inflammation of the thyroid closely resembling thyroiditis in humans. Both humoral and cellular responses against thyroglobulin appear necessary for maximum injury; however, T cells primarily mediate the disease with antibodies contributing to the progression of the disease. Animal models revealed that immunologic processes are important in thyroiditis and that these processes are under genetic control (linked to the class II region in the H-2 and HLA complexes). The pathogenic importance of CD4$^+$ T$_H$1 cells is strongly suggested, in that thyroglobulin-specific T cells taken from susceptible mice and introduced into normal mice start experimental autoimmune thyroiditis. These autoreactive T cells recognize and proliferate on exposure to self-thyroglobulin—a type IV (delayed) hypersensitivity reaction occurs characterized by a mononuclear infiltration by B cells, T cells and macrophages. The resulting effector cells and autoantibodies cause hypothyroiditis with symptoms of intolerance to cold, dry skin, fatigue, weight gain, and in a worst-case scenario the development of a goiter. Hashimoto's disease is treated with orally taken, daily hormone replacement therapy with synthetic thyroid hormones, such as levothyroxine (Synthroid).

### Insulin-Dependent Diabetes Mellitus Results from an Autoimmune Attack of the Pancreas' Insulin-Producing Cells

**Insulin-dependent diabetes mellitus** (also called **type 1 diabetes**) is a major health problem in most developed countries; it affects roughly 1% of the population. Diabetes mellitus is a pathologic state defined by high levels of blood glucose (hyperglycemia), ketoacidosis, and increased urine production. Late stages of the disease can lead to atherosclerotic vascular lesions. Type 1 diabetes results from the destruction of insulin-producing β cells of the islets of Langerhans in the pancreas. Disease development is caused by a multifactorial process in which metabolic, genetic, and environmental factors may trigger an autoimmune reaction against β cells in genetically predisposed people. The major autoantigens are insulin, glutamic acid decarboxylase, and islet-specific glucose-6-phosphatase catalytic subunit-related protein. The usual diabetes treatment is replacement therapy through daily insulin injections. Transplantation of islet cells offers a possible cure for type 1 diabetes.

Type 1 diabetes is a T cell-mediated disease characterized by lymphocytic infiltration of the islets of Langerhans, detection of autoantibodies against islet cells at the onset of disease, and the expression of class II MHC molecules by islet cells suggest that an immune response is involved. The presence of insulitis, the specific lesion of the disease, observed in newly diagnosed patients, results from infiltration of the islets of Langerhans mainly with CD8$^+$ T cells and, to a much lesser extent, CD4$^+$ T cells. Concomitant with T$_C$ cell-mediated killing of β-cells, significant levels of IL-1, TNF-α, and IFN-γ are found—reminiscent of a delayed-type hypersensitivity response. Even though autoantibodies against islet cells are characteristic of type 1 diabetes, they are not considered a cause of islet cell destruction. These antibodies can be used as a predictive tool because they precede the onset of disease. Antibodies against the β-cell autoantigen *glutamic acid decarboxylase* occur in roughly 80% of newly diagnosed patients. The association of genetic factors in diabetes susceptibility includes the insulin gene on chromosome 11, HLA class II region genes, and at last count 11 non-HLA linked diabetes susceptibility genes. In fact, the expression of class II MHC molecules on islet cells is well established; approximately 50% of diabetic patients are HLA-DR3/DR4 heterozygotes versus only 5% of the healthy population expressing these molecules. Furthermore, individuals that express HLA-DQ1*0602 rarely develop type 1 diabetes. Preventing or halting a turncoat immune system is paramount to curing the disease, despite evidence the presence of genes outside the MHC that confer susceptibility to type 1 diabetes.

As mentioned earlier, NOD mice are a model for human type 1 diabetes; they exhibit the characteristic lymphocytic infiltration of the islets of Langerhans in the pancreas, the transfer of CD4$^+$ T cells (probably T$_H$1 cells) from diabetic to nondiabetic mice confers the disease, and a strong link to the expression of class II MHC molecules and development of diabetes. One notable difference is a greater incidence of diabetes in female mice when compared to human disease.

### Multiple Sclerosis Results Either from an Immune Response to Exposed Sequestered Antigen Myelin Basic Protein (MBP) or from Molecular Mimicry to MBP Following a Virus Infection

**Multiple sclerosis** (MS) is an inflammatory demyelinating disease of the central nervous system, characterized by the formation of focal demyelinated plaques in the white matter of the brain and spinal cord. The disease course usually begins as relapsing–remitting followed after some years by a progressive form; in some patients, the disease is progressive from the onset. Activated CD4$^+$ T$_H$1 cells, their derived IFN-γ, and activated macrophages or microgia dominate the inflammation. Sclerotic plaque macrophages express proinflammatory

cytokines, chemokines, and release proteases—a delayed-type hypersensitivity response to the basic protein of myelin, the protective sheath of nerves, causes demyelination—subsequent variable degree of acute axonal injury and axonal loss. Antibodies to nerve tissue can be found, but they do not correlate with disease induction. Among MS's symptoms are motor weakness, incoordination, and jerking movements of the arms and legs. MS patients are treated with corticosteroids, IFN-β, myelin protein decoys (such as Copaxone), and immunosuppressive drugs.

An animal model provides indirect evidence that MS is an autoimmune disease. Rodents immunized with nerve tissue protein, such as MBP or proteolipid protein in complete Freund's adjuvant, develop a neurologic disease within 2 to 3 weeks called *experimental autoimmune encephalomyelitis (EAE)*. The similarity of EAE and MS is obvious; EAE shows a cellular infiltrate of the myelin sheaths of the central nervous system leading to demyelination and paralysis. When MBP-specific CD4$^+$ T cells, initially thought to be T$_H$1 cells, are transferred to normal recipients, most develop EAE and die; an exception, IL-23–deficient mice, suggests that T$_H$17, not T$_H$1, cells are the culprits. These mice lack IL-17–producing T$_H$17 cells and are resistant to induction of EAE. Also, anti-IL-17 vaccine or IL-27, a negative regulator of T$_H$17 cell differentiation, administered to mice protected them against EAE induction, whereas IL-27–deficient mice were hyperresponsive to myelin-induced EAE. The IL-23/T$_H$17 cell pathway is essential for EAE development; evidence for this pathway in MS patients is emerging. MS patient-derived dendritic cells produce more IL-23, and roughly 40% of MS patients have higher numbers of IL-17 mRNA-positive peripheral blood mononuclear cells, than their normal counterparts. The trend is similar for MS patients in remission versus those in clinical exacerbation.

Using T$_{reg}$ cells in the preceding mouse model suggests that they dictate whether EAE can be induced; for example, if T$_{reg}$ cells are given before disease induction, lesions do not present. If the T$_{reg}$ cells are myelin-specific, lesion suppression is more evident. Treatment of EAE-resistant mice with anti-CD25 antibodies renders them more susceptible to EAE induction.

## Autoimmune Diseases Are Caused by Self-Reacting Antibodies

### Myasthenia Gravis Results When Blocking Antibodies Bind Self-Acetylcholine Receptors

First described in 1672, **myasthenia gravis** is an autoimmune disease characterized by muscular weakness and excessive fatigue, which is improved by anticholinesterase drug and corticosteroid treatment. Thymic abnormality is common in myasthenia gravis patients, thymoma occurs in roughly 15% of them, and thymectomy is often beneficial in those patients without thymoma. The disease is more common in women and usually appears early in adult life but can present at any age. An animal model, using rabbits immunized with acetylcholine receptors, showed that the symptoms of the experimental disease and its human counterpart were mediated by antiacetylcholine receptor autoantibodies. Acetylcholine receptors are at the tips of skeletal muscle fibers; receptor binding of acetylcholine helps trigger muscle contraction. In myasthenia gravis, autoantibodies attach to acetylcholine receptors blocking acetylcholine binding and also induce complement-mediated lysis of cells; subsequently the number of receptors is reduced, leading to transmission failures at many of the motor units in a muscle (Figure 13-6).

The mechanism initiating or regulating the autoimmune response during myasthenia gravis is unknown. Myasthenia gravis-mediated pathologic changes are attributed to binding of autoantibodies to postsynaptic membranes, which fix complement, causing alteration of the folded structure of the membrane or loss of acetylcholine receptors. Receptor loss leads to the symptoms of the disease, and the loss in receptors seems to be caused by complement-mediated lysis and antigenic modulation of the receptor. The latter effect may be caused by a cross-linking of receptors by the autoantibodies, which increases their normal rates of both endocytosis and breakdown by lysosomal enzymes.

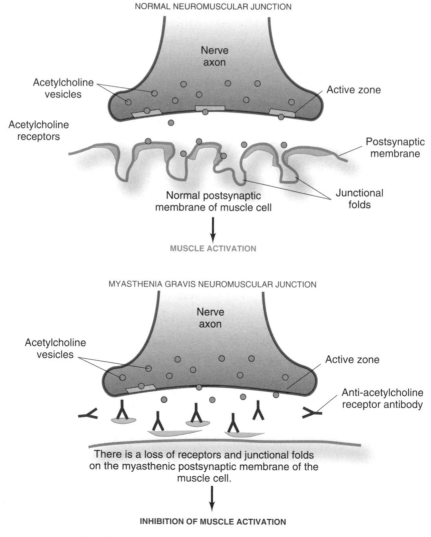

**FIGURE 13-6 The decrease in neuromuscular junctions during myasthenia gravis.**

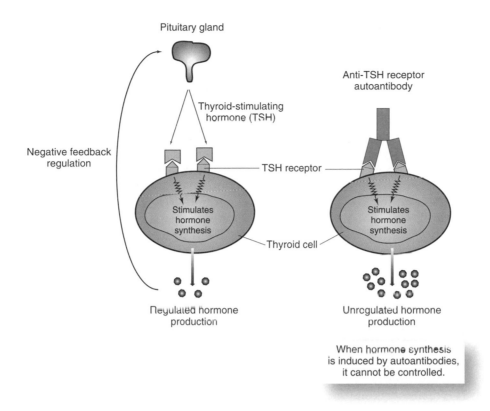

**FIGURE 13-7** Graves' disease: Autoantibodies to thyroid-stimulating hormone receptor.

### Graves' Disease Results When Antibodies Stimulate Inappropriate Thyroid Activity Rather Than Destroying Thyroid Tissue

**Graves' disease** is a common disorder of the thyroid gland, occurring in roughly 0.5% of the population, mainly women in their 30s and 40s. As with Hashimoto's thyroiditis, Graves' disease is characterized by lymphocytic infiltration of the thyroid parenchyma but the infiltration is mild and induces production of autoantibodies that bind to thyroid-stimulating hormone (TSH) receptor (Figure 13-7). It is unique among autoimmune disorders because it is caused by autoantibodies that stimulate thyroid cellular activity by displacing TSH binding. It demonstrates that not all autoreactivities destroy tissue. The autoantibodies act as agonists and stimulate the overproduction of two thyroid hormones, thyroxine and triiodothyronine, by mimicking the pituitary hormone TSH. Graves' disease is the direct consequence of autoantibody production against TSH receptors on thyroid epithelial cells. Normally, TSH binds to TSH receptors, activates adenylate cyclase, and stimulates the production of thyroid hormones by epithelial cells. The autoantibodies do the same thing as TSH but are unregulated, leading to extended overproduction of

thyroid hormones; therefore, Graves' disease is called *hyperthyroidism*. The associated symptoms include intolerance to heat, warm moist skin, weight loss, irritability, and goiter development. Short-term treatment for Graves' disease involves drugs that inhibit thyroid function, whereas long-term treatment involves thyroid ablation by surgery or [131]I uptake, followed by thyroid hormone replacement therapy. As an antibody-mediated autoimmune disease, it can be passed from mother to fetus during pregnancy, and is called *transient neonatal hyperthyroidism*. The latter disease is the best evidence that Graves' disease is an antibody-mediated autoimmune disease. Other evidence supports the autoimmunity connection: the expression of HLA class II genes *DRB1*, *DQB1*, and *DQA1* has significant risk factor association with Graves' disease, as do the susceptibility genes *CD40*, *CTLA-4*, and *protein tyrosine phosphatase-22 (PTPN22)*.

### Systemic Lupus Erythematosus Involves Antibodies That React Primarily Against Self-Nuclear Components

**Systemic lupus erythematosus (SLE)** is a multisystem, autoimmune, connective-tissue (arthritis) disorder with a broad range of clinical features. It is primarily a chronic disease of young women (women to men ratio of roughly 10:1) with a peak onset between their late teens and early 40s. SLE is potentially fatal when either the kidneys or the central nervous system are affected, but it usually leads to chronic debilitating ill health. SLE is an inflammatory connective tissue disease of unknown cause. During the disease, the immune system produces autoantibodies capable of binding nuclear antigens such as double-stranded or single-stranded DNA, RNA, nuclear proteins (such as nucleosomes and ribosomes), histones, and protein-nucleic acid complexes; the increased levels of anti-DNA antibodies, elevated circulating immune complexes, and complement consumption correlates with disease activity. These immune complexes mainly composed of IgG and IgM circulate in the blood and are eventually deposited in the kidneys, which fix complement and mediate an inflammation known as *glomerulonephritis*. The pattern is that of a type III hypersensitivity response. Whether anti-DNA autoantibodies are the cause or the result of the disease is still unknown—that is, the pathogenesis of SLE remains unclear.

Even though SLE pathogenesis is blurred, the impaired clearance of early apoptotic cells suggests how the immune system might recognize predominately intracellular antigens. Cell death is the likely source for these immunologically sequestered autoantigens. Autoantigens are released from necrotic and apoptotic cells; however, in normal settings they are quickly removed by macrophages, neutrophils, and dendritic cells. If apoptotic cells are not cleared in a timely manner (frequently observed in SLE patients), they lose their membrane integrity, become secondarily necrotic, and release large amounts of nuclear and cytoplasmic material that becomes assessable to tissue dendritic cells. The dendritic cells produce proinflammatory cytokines and present the autoantigens with costimulatory molecules to autoreactive T cells, which in turn provide help to autoreactive B cells—autoimmunity gets started. Irrespective of the intracellular antigens that induced the autoimmune response, as SLE progresses more cells are killed and more antigens, normally not present outside the cell, are released. These released self-antigens now provide *de novo* activation of autoreactive T cells, this cellular "spilling" leads to **determinant spreading**—the generation of autoreactive T cells and antibodies to other local molecules.

The discovery that the New Zealand Black (NZB) strain of mice and the $F_1$ progeny of NZB mice crossed with NZ White (NZW) mice spontaneously develop a disease that duplicates human SLE has provided a model to study the clinical aspects of the disease and the genetic control and mechanisms of gene action in autoimmunity. These mice consistently lose tolerance to self-antigens and have a mortality rate of 50% by 16 to 25 months of age due to autoimmune disease complications. The NZB mice also exhibit hemolytic anemia. In the $F_1$ progeny, antigen-autoantibody complexes accumulate in the kidneys and lead to glomerulonephritis. Results from crossing NZB and NZW mice showed that the NZW mouse contributes two genes and the NZB mouse contributes one gene to the susceptibility to disease. One of the three genes is in the H-2 complex, and one is linked to the H-2. Their influence on the disease is unknown. Even though the animal model has provided valuable information on SLE, it has not shown whether autoantibodies are the cause of the disease or result from damaged tissue. Also, the model has not identified the antigenic stimulus of the disease, although the cause seems to be multifactorial. SLE is no different in humans; hormonal (such as estrogen) and environmental (such as sunlight) factors, interact with a multitude of gene products (such as HLA-DR molecules, Fcγ receptors, complement components, C-reactive protein, CTLA-4, and PD-1) leading to an increased risk for the development of SLE.

### Rheumatoid Arthritis Involves Antibodies That React Against Self-Constituents in Joints

**Rheumatoid arthritis (RA)** is a common, chronic disease afflicting about 3 million people in the United States. RA produces a crippling inflammation of the joints, especially of the hands, wrists, and knees but also can have systemic manifestations. Large growths of tissue form in the affected joints and eat into the cartilage and bone. These growths decrease the person's ability to move the affected joints. RA affects three females to every male, usually strikes when the victims are 35 to 45 years of age, and progressively worsens over 10 to 30 years. In addition to the joints, the eyes, lungs, heart, spleen, skin, muscles, and peripheral nerves may be affected. Usually, autoantibodies known as *rheumatoid factors* are present. They are antibodies (or antiantibodies) against the Fc portion of normal self-IgG molecules. However, not all RA patients have rheumatoid factor, and not all people with rheumatoid factor have RA.

The arthritic joint fluid contains rheumatoid factors (either IgM or IgG) and normal IgG, which together form antigen-antibody complexes—it is a type III hypersensitivity. Inflammation results, and the synovium or lining membrane becomes heavily infiltrated by dendritic cells, macrophages, T and B lymphocytes, NK cells, and clumps of plasma cells. Thus, two of the symptoms are usually synovitis and vasculitis. The causes of the formation of rheumatoid factor are unknown. Signs of immune reactions proceeding in the affected synovium are seen when the immune cells of the cultured synovium produce gamma globulin, and complement levels in the synovial fluid are depleted.

***The Etiology of RA Is Not Understood, but the Pathology Is Known.*** Although the etiology of RA is unknown, the pathology (progression) of the disease is reasonably well understood. RA starts with an inflammatory reaction within the joint. Speculation about the nature of the antigenic stimulus has ranged from bacteria to *Mycoplasma* to viruses. The cause may be any, all, or none of these. The severity of the inflammatory response may depend on the genetic background of the host because people with the MHC gene product HLA-DR4, in particular HLA-DRB1 alleles, are statistically more likely to develop RA than are those without this gene. The resulting antigen-antibody complexes are deposited in the joint tissue, and macrophages and neutrophils are drawn to the joint space by chemotactic factors. In attempts to clear the joint of undesirable immune complexes, the phagocytic cells do more damage than help. The proteolytic enzymes released by macrophages and neutrophils during phagocytosis start to degrade the surrounding tissue. The activated macrophages also release IL-1 and TNF-α, which activates T lymphocytes, which in turn produce interferons and other mediators that favor further macrophage activation and chemotaxis. Thus the self-perpetuating "immunologic juggernaut" is born. The downregulation that would normally dampen any antigen-clearance process fails to function adequately in RA. The repeated inflammatory bouts cause fibrin deposition and replacement of cartilage with fibrous tissue, eventually leading to ankylosis (fusing of the joints).

***The Therapy for RA Is Palliative.*** Current therapy is palliative. Most drugs treat symptoms of RA but do not stop or reverse the inexorable progression of chronic, systemic bone erosion and joint destruction. Medication consists of several lines of treatment, with each successive treatment posing successively greater risks to the patient.

Nonsteroidal anti-inflammatory drugs are the first line of treatment. These drugs (aspirin, indomethacin, and naproxen) control the inflammation and pain associated with RA but do not slow disease progression. Because RA is usually not

a life-threatening disease in itself, physicians are reluctant to prescribe harsher medication if these drugs alone will allow the patient to maintain a bearable quality of life.

If the nonsteroidal anti-inflammatory drug treatment fails or causes side effects (usually gastrointestinal complications), disease-modifying anti-rheumatic drugs are prescribed. These compounds appear to slow the progression of RA. They fall into three classes: (1) antimalarials, like chloroquine and Plaquenil; (2) gold compounds, like auranofin and gold sodium thiomalate; and (3) D-penicillamine, a copper chelator. These compounds have no better than a 50% chance of causing measurable improvement. They also have potentially serious side effects ranging from retinopathy (chloroquine) to leukopenia (D-penicillamine) to severe skin rashes (gold).

The most intractable cases of RA are treated with immunosuppressive drugs like cyclophosphamide. This treatment nonspecifically short-circuits all immunologic activity, which leaves the body open to infections.

Advances in genetics, immunology, and molecular biology have provided a greater understanding of the immunoregulatory mechanisms (especially TNF α release) involved in RA. Cyclosporin-A, used to dampen the immune system's graft rejection mechanism, is now being used to dampen the immunologic activity associated with RA. Other compounds such as IL-1 receptor antagonists and TNF-α inhibitors have reached the marketplace. The TNF-α blockers include Enbrel, Remicade, and Humira; they are also used in the treatment of psoriasis, Crohn's disease, and ankylosing spondylitis. The class of anti-cholesterol drugs called *statins*, recently also shown to reduce C-reactive protein serum levels, shows promise in the treatment of RA (and MS), as does the anti-CD20 monoclonal antibody Rituxan (currently approved for treatment of B cell lymphomas).

### Autoimmune Hemolytic Diseases Result When Normal Cells Are Affected as Innocent Bystanders

Red blood cell disorders resulting from autoimmune processes are generally called **autoimmune hemolytic diseases**—they are a type II hypersensitivity. Two groups of autoimmune hemolytic diseases will be briefly discussed: anemias involving either red blood cells or platelets. The former are grouped into warm antibody, cold antibody, or drug-induced autoimmune hemolytic anemias. The other autoimmune hemolytic disease involves the destruction of platelets and is called *autoimmune* *(idiopathic) thrombocytopenic purpura.* In some cases, the autoantibodies are directed against the platelet GpIIb:IIIa fibrinogen receptor.

Although drugs such as aspirin or penicillin have beneficial effects, their effect on some individuals may be fatal, similar to an immediate hypersensitivity response. Drug-antidrug antibody reactions may clinically lead to anemia or purpura (hemorrhage) when red cells or platelets, respectively, are involved. Some individuals may be severely and even fatally affected. Some clinically important and commonly used drugs—penicillin in hemolytic anemia and quinine in purpura—may be involved in this reaction; most cases resolve in a few weeks after the drug is withdrawn.

*Autoimmune Hemolytic Anemia Results When Antibodies React Against Self Red Blood Cells.* **Warm antibody autoimmune hemolytic anemia** is the most common form of autoimmune anemia. Patients with this disorder have antibodies on their red blood cells; these antibodies are detected by using anti-immunoglobulins at an incubation temperature of 37°C. This anti-immunoglobulin test is called the *direct Coombs test.* Major symptoms of the disease are anemia, fever, jaundice, splenomegaly associated with hemolysis, and congestive heart failure. Autoimmune hemolytic anemia may be idiopathic or secondary to lymphoreticular malignancy or other autoimmune diseases.

**Cold antibody autoimmune hemolytic anemia** is associated with high titers of autoagglutinating IgM antibodies that react optimally at temperatures below 37°C. This disease can be idiopathic or secondary to infections or lymphomas. The immune specificity of the IgM autoagglutinins is usually to the I or II red blood cell antigen. The onset of disease correlates with exposure of patients to cold temperatures. Thus, treatment involves keeping the patient warm and waiting for spontaneous resolution.

Many forms of **drug-induced autoimmune hemolytic anemias** exist. Different drugs induce autoimmunity by different mechanisms, which can be divided into four groups: (1) immune complex formation, exemplified by quinidine; (2) drug adsorption to red cell membranes, exemplified by penicillin and cephalosporin; (3) modification of the red cell membrane, exemplified by cephalosporins; and (4) idiopathic (unknown etiology) mechanisms, exemplified by α-methyldopa.

The drug-antidrug immune complexes sensitize red blood cells. This interaction is called the *immune* or *innocent bystander phenomenon.* A second situation arises when the drug acts as a hapten (appearance of a new antigenic determinant) and the red cell as a carrier, leading to antibody production against the hapten or drug. Cephalosporins modify the red cell membrane so that it absorbs proteins nonspecifically and leads to a positive Coombs test. Lastly, autoimmune hemolytic anemias, appearing in some patients treated with α-methyldopa, are called *idiopathic* because the mechanisms of induction are unknown.

*Thrombocytopenic Purpura Results When Antibodies React Against Self-Platelets.* The autoimmune form of thrombocytopenia, **thrombocytopenic purpura**, is caused by increased platelet destruction primarily following coating of platelets with antibody. Platelet destruction is mediated by IgG autoantibodies, which sensitize circulating platelets. Splenic macrophages rapidly remove the antibody-coated platelets, but the antigenic stimulus initiating the disease is unknown. A drug-induced form of thrombocytopenic purpura appears to have mechanisms of causation similar to that for drug-induced autoimmune hemolytic anemia. Similar drugs cause the two diseases.

### Poststreptococcal Diseases Result When Antibodies Against Bacteria Cross-react with Self-Antigens

*Acute Rheumatic Fever Results When Antibodies Against Streptococcal Antigens Cross-react with Heart Muscle Tissue.* **Acute rheumatic fever**, a collagen vascular disease affecting many different organs, follows a group A streptococcal pharyngitis (throat infection). A hereditary predisposition to rheumatic fever may exist; 2 to 3% of a normal population are susceptible. The disease, which occurs most commonly in children between the ages of 5 and 15 years, arises because antibodies to streptococcal cellular and extracellular antigens are formed. These antibodies cross-react with different host tissues. T-cell reactivity also may be important. The clinical signs of the disease include inflammation of the joints, heart, brain, and skin. The cardiac involvement is the most serious sign of acute rheumatic fever. Some other organisms that cause infections associated with autoimmune disease include *Chamydia trachomatis* (Reiter's syndrome), *Borrelia burgdorferi* (chronic arthritis in Lyme disease), and *Shigella flexneri* or *Champylobacter jejuni* (arthritis).

*Glomerulonephritis Results When Antibodies React Against Self-Antigens and the Resulting Antigen-Antibody Complexes Localize in the Glomeruli of the Kidney.* Immune complex diseases provide a basis for the understanding of autoimmune diseases such as **glomerulonephritis**, RA, and SLE. When immune complexes are trapped in vessel walls, they cause inflammation. The interlocking of antibody with antigen sets in motion the complement cascade. Various fragments that are flung off during the cascade stimulate and attract neutrophils. Still another fragment coats the antigen-antibody complexes to make them more palatable to phagocytes. The accumulation of these cells leads to engulfment of some of the complexes, but also to the death of neutrophils and the release of hydrolytic enzymes. These enzymes can degrade the surrounding tissues.

Glomerulonephritis results from the overload of circulating antigen-antibody complexes being deposited in the glomeruli of the kidney (Figure 13-8). Some antigens that have been implicated in human glomerulonephritis include drugs, foreign serum, streptococcal antigens, and hepatitis and measles viruses. Thus, glomerulonephritis is caused by self-injury arising from the immune response to foreign antigen.

---

**MINI SUMMARY**

Autoimmune diseases can be classified as either organ-specific or systemic. They can be further classified as diseases initiated by T cells or by antibodies. Hashimoto's thyroiditis, insulin-dependent diabetes mellitus, and multiple sclerosis are cell-mediated autoimmune diseases. Myasthenia gravis, Graves' disease, systemic lupus erythematosus (SLE), rheumatoid arthritis, autoimmune hemolytic diseases, and poststreptococcal diseases are antibody-mediated autoimmune diseases.

---

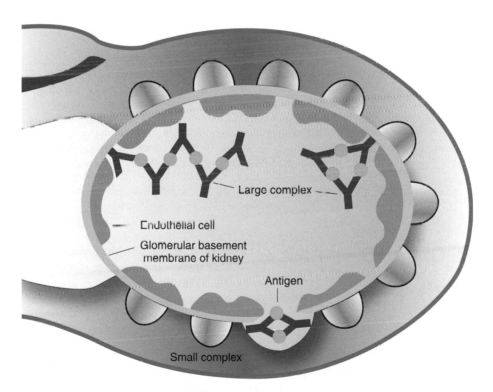

KIDNEY GLOMERULUS

**FIGURE 13-8 Glomerulonephritis.** Immune complex diseases are caused by clusters of interlocking antigens and antibodies. Under normal conditions, immune complexes are rapidly removed from the bloodstream by macrophages in the spleen and liver. In some instances, these complexes continue to circulate and eventually become trapped in the tissues of the kidneys (or joints, lung, skin, or blood vessels), where they set off reactions leading to inflammation and tissue damage. The tissue damage is caused by the release of hydrolytic enzymes from the phagocytic cells involved in removing these complexes.

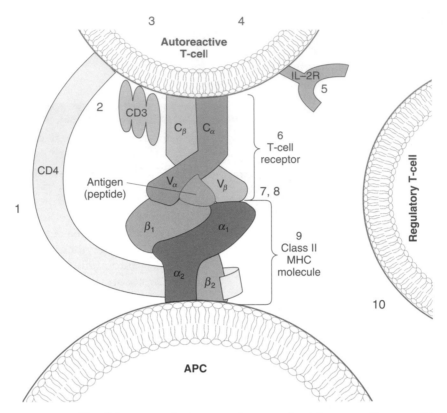

**FIGURE 13-9 Possible targets for immunotherapy of autoimmune diseases.** (1) Removal of CD4$^+$ T cells with anti-CD4 antibodies, (2) removal of CD3$^+$ T cells with anti-CD3 antibodies, (3) inhibition of gene transcription, (4) uncoupling of signal transduction, (5) removal of activated T cells with anti-IL-2 receptor (R) antibodies or IL-2 toxins, (6) removal of T cells with TCRs for self-constituents, (7) competition for autoantigen presentation, (8) tolerance induction, (9) blockage of MHC binding of self-antigens, and (10) activation of regulatory T cells through TCR idiotypes and antigen. Not shown, but anti-cytokine and -cytokine R agents (such as, anti-TNF-α and anti-TNF-αR) are in the marketplace and show promise in the treatment of RA. See text for more information.

# TREATMENTS OF AUTOIMMUNE DISEASES ARE MOVING FROM COUNTERACTING THE EFFECTS OF AUTOIMMUNITY WITH NONSPECIFIC TREATMENTS TO SPECIFICALLY PREVENTING THE CAUSES

Therapeutic treatment of autoimmune diseases remains mostly palliative. Nonetheless, several therapeutic options targeting the trimolecular complex of antigen, TCR, and MHC molecule, the associated accessory/adhesion molecules, and the associated cytokines and their receptors may provide cures for autoimmune diseases (Figure 13-9). The following paragraphs present some possible immunotherapeutic strategies, including: (1) nonspecific immunointervention, (2) induction of autoantigen-driven tolerance, (3) anti-TCR immunotherapy, and (4) MHC blockade.

1. Nonspecific treatments are the most widely used for therapy of autoimmune diseases, but they cannot distinguish between normal and abnormal immune responses and thus lead to serious side effects. Examples of nonspecific immunointervention treatments include (a) immunosuppressive drugs (such as corticosteroids, cyclophosphamide, and azathioprine); (b) anti-CD3 antibodies to eliminate all T cells; (c) anti-cytokine receptor antibodies, cytokine-toxin conjugates or cytokine blockers to eliminate activated T cells;

(d) cyclosporin A and FK506 (tacrolimus) to inhibit T-cell activation; (e) specific anti-signal transduction drugs to inhibit signal transduction by kinases, phosphatases, and G proteins; and (f) anti-accessory/stimulatory molecule (B7, CD2, CD4, CD8, CD11a/CD18, CD20, CD28) antibodies to inhibit lymphocyte activation.

2. Induction of autoantigen-specific tolerance is probably the most effective treatment approach because it causes few side effects and is specific for the autoreactive T cells. This approach involves oral administration of autoantigens (mice fed MBP do not develop EAE) or intravenous injection of autoantigens coupled to syngeneic lymphoid cells.

3. Anti-TCR therapy using T-cell vaccination, anti-TCR antibodies, and TCR peptides could overcome autoaggressive T-cell activity. The attenuated (by irradiation or chemical fixation), autoaggressive T cells elicit clonotype-specific $T_{reg}$ cells to confer resistance to the disease. Another approach uses anti-idiotypic monoclonal antibodies directed against TCR structures used by autoaggressive T cells (this protocol can reverse EAE). A third approach is immunization with synthetic peptide sequences of TCR complementarity-determining regions from autoimmune disease-mediating T-cell clones.

4. Because certain MHC alleles are associated with autoimmune disease, blocking the autoantigen-presenting activity of disease-associated MHC molecules could interfere with disease. For example, anti-class II MHC molecule antibody would prevent activation of class II MHC-restricted autoreactive T cells by preventing these cells from interacting with autoantigen-presenting cells (this protocol can reverse EAE). An alternative approach is to block the MHC-binding site with peptide competitors.

---

## MINI SUMMARY

New approaches in the prevention and therapy of autoimmune diseases are becoming available. Nonselective treatments are currently the mainstay of autoimmune disease treatment, but they cause serious side effects. Immunotherapeutic approaches such as the application of anti-cytokine or -cytokine receptors, the induction of autoantigen-driven tolerance, the physical or functional deletion of autoaggressive T cells, the blockade of MHC molecules, and the induction of regulatory T cells are being developed.

# SUMMARY

The immune system needs to be prevented from reacting to self-tissues. A mechanism must be in place to prevent a host from destroying self-antigens; otherwise, we would not survive (*horror autotoxicus*). The host must distinguish among foreign antigens, whereby exposure leads to specific immunity, and self-antigens, whereby exposure leads to specific lack of immunity. The inducing molecules are called *immunogens* and **tolerogens**, respectively. The first phenomenon is called *immunity*, the second is called **immunologic tolerance**.

Tolerance can be induced in fetal, newborn, and adult animals. Difficulty in tolerance induction increases with age. The exchange of blood cells between fraternal embryos *in utero* was the first recognized example of naturally acquired immunologic tolerance. As adults, these animals can tolerate each other's tissues. Tolerance can also be acquired in adult life by oral administration or injection of antigen under the appropriate conditions. Numerous animal models of autoimmune diseases are available.

T and B cells are susceptible to tolerance induction at two levels: **central tolerance** of immature lymphocytes in primary lymphoid organs (T cells in the thymus, B cells in the bone marrow) and **peripheral tolerance** of mature lymphocytes in the peripheral lymphoid organs, the spleen and lymph nodes. Immunologic tolerance induction may hinge on different, overlapping mechanisms, the principal ones are: (1) **clonal deletion** (and B and T cell **receptor editing**), (2) **clonal anergy**, and (3) suppression of autoreactive T and B cells, by **regulatory T ($T_{reg}$) cells**. The most generally accepted of mechanisms involve opposite extremes: either actual removal of autoreactive cells (clonal deletion) or functional removal of autoreactive cells (clonal anergy). In the latter situation, the cells remain but are unable to respond. Another mechanism is the regulated inhibition of autoreactive cells by $T_{reg}$ cells. Experiments using transgenic and knockout mice confirm these mechanisms.

*Autoimmunity* is the mirror image of tolerance; self-tolerance is the lack of reactivity to self, while autoimmunity is reactivity to self or the loss of tolerance to self. Reactivity to foreign antigen associated with self-MHC molecules in the presence of costimulation normally leads to immunity, whereas self-reactivity in the presence of costimulation if not controlled leads to abnormal or excessive antiself responses that cause harm to the host—**autoimmune diseases**.

Autoimmune diseases have a multifactorial etiology. The causes of autoimmunity may be an abnormal immune response to normal self-antigens, a normal immune response to abnormal self-antigens, or an abnormal immune response to abnormal self-antigens. Two major mechanisms lead to autoimmunity: (1) change of self-antigens leading to the formation of neoantigens and (2) exposure to antigens that induce cross-reactive antibodies. Many other conditions can lead to autoimmunity, such as exposure to sequestered antigens, decrease in $T_{reg}$-cell number or function, overactive helper T-cell function, aberrant expression of MHC molecules on non-APCs, polyclonal B-cell activation, thymic defects, genetic factors, and hormonal factors.

Autoimmune diseases can be divided into *organ-specific* and *systemic*. These two groups can be further divided into diseases that result from humoral or cell-mediated immune dysfunction. Examples of cell-mediated autoimmune diseases are *Hashimoto's thyroiditis, insulin-dependent diabetes mellitus*, and *multiple sclerosis*. Antibody-mediated autoimmune diseases include *myasthenia gravis, Graves' disease, systemic lupus erythematosus (SLE), rheumatoid arthritis (RA), autoimmune hemolytic anemia, thrombocytopenic purpura, acute rheumatic fever*, and *glomerulonephritis*.

The most widely used treatments for autoimmune diseases are still nonspecific and palliative, but anti-cytokine or -cytokine receptor agents are a significant step forward. Some new immunotherapeutic strategies that target the trimolecular complex of antigen, TCR, and MHC molecule and associated structures or cytokines or their receptors may change the conventional approaches.

# SELF-EVALUATION

## RECALLING KEY TERMS

**Acute rheumatic fever**
**Autoantigens**
**Autoimmune diseases**
**Autoimmune hemolytic diseases**
    **Cold antibody autoimmune hemolytic anemia**
    **Drug-induced autoimmune hemolytic anemia**
    **Warm antibody autoimmune hemolytic anemia**
**Autoimmunity**
**Clonal anergy**
**Clonal deletion**
**Determinant spreading**
**Glomerulonephritis**
**Graves' disease**

**Hashimoto's disease (Hashimoto's thyroiditis)**
*Horror autotoxicus*
**Immunologic tolerance**
**Insulin-dependent diabetes mellitus (type 1 diabetes)**
**Myasthenia gravis**
**Multiple sclerosis**
**Organ-specific autoimmune diseases**
**Regulatory T ($T_{reg}$) cells**
**Rheumatoid arthritis (RA)**
**Systemic autoimmune diseases**
**Systemic lupus erythematosus (SLE)**
**Thrombocytopenic purpura**
**Tolerogen**

## MULTIPLE-CHOICE QUESTIONS

*(An answer key is not provided, but the page[s] location of the answer is.)*

1. Tolerance induction is specific and has memory. (a) true, (b) false. *(See page 430.)*

2. Tolerance induction of T cells is quicker than that of B cells. (a) true, (b) false. *(See page 433.)*

3. In tolerance induced with small concentrations of antigen, or low-dose tolerance, (a) T cells are predominantly affected, (b) only B cells are unresponsive, (c) the duration of the tolerant state is short, (d) both B and T cells are unresponsive, (e) none of these. *(See page 433.)*

4. Which of the following mechanisms participate in the induction of immunologic tolerance? (a) clonal deletion, (b) $T_{reg}$ cells, (c) anergy, (d) all of the above, (e) none of these. *(See pages 436 and 437.)*

5. An experiment was conducted with three genetically different strains of mice, designated A, B, and C. Tissue from Strain A was injected into an embryo of Strain B. When the Strain B embryo became an adult, it received skin grafts from Strain A and Strain C mice. Skin graft rejection was observed. Which of the following is the correct result? (a) the recipient Strain B mouse rejected the skin graft from Strain A but accepted the skin graft from Strain C, (b) the recipient Strain B mouse rejected the skin graft from Strain C but accepted the skin graft from Strain A, (c) the recipient Strain B mouse rejected skin grafts from Strain A and Strain C, (d) the recipient Strain B mouse accepted skin grafts from Strain A and Strain C, (e) none of these. *(See pages 431 and 432.)*

6. Normally, the immune system does not respond to self-antigens since it develops tolerance to self-antigens, one reason is because these

antigens are present during embryonic life. (a) true, (b) false. *(See page 432.)*

7. To induce tolerance, immunization with which of the following is preferred? (a) aggregated antigen intradermally, (b) aggregated antigen intramuscularly, (c) aggregated antigen intravenously, (d) deaggregated antigen intramuscularly, (e) deaggregated antigen intravenously, (f) none of these. *(See pages 433 and 434.)*

8. Tolerance induction includes changes that involve purging the repertoire of those cells that react with self-antigens. The mechanisms can include (a) clonal deletion, (b) clonal anergy, (c) regulated inhibition, (d) all of these, (e) none of these. *(See page 436.)*

9. Which of the following is not a common immunologic symptom shared by most autoimmune diseases? (a) autoantibodies, (b) hypergammaglobulinemia, (c) IgE antibodies, (d) T cells reactive with autoantigens, (e) none of these. *(See pages 441–444.)*

10. Which of the following is not an explanation for the origin of autoimmune diseases? (a) deficiencies of IL-23, (b) hidden antigen release, (c) neoantigens, (d) autocoupling haptens, (e) mutation of an immunocompetent cell, (f) none of these. *(See pages 441 and 442.)*

11. _____ secretion can polarize naïve T cells toward a regulatory phenotype, _____ whereas secretion can polarize naïve T cells toward an autoaggressive phenotype. (a) IL-12 and IL-18; IFN-γ and IL-2, (b) IL-6 and TGF-β; IFN-γ, (c) IL-6; TGF-β, (d) TGF-β; IL-6 and TGF-β, (e) none of these. *(See page 442.)*

12. Which of the following is generally classified as a T cell-associated autoimmune disease? (a) SLE, (b) poststreptococcal glomerulonephritis, (c) rheumatic fever, (d) thrombocytopenic purpura, (e) multiple sclerosis, (f) none of these. *(See pages 446 and 447.)*

13. Hashimoto-type thyroiditis (a) cannot be induced in animals, (b) is due to antibody against thyroglobulin, (c) is seen in newborn infants of mothers who have the disease, (d) was the first described autoimmune diseases, (e) none of these. *(See pages 445 and 446.)*

14. The cold antibodies involved in autoimmune hemolytic disease are (a) primarily IgG, (b) primarily IgM, (c) non-complement-fixing antibodies, (d) incomplete antibodies, (e) none of these. *(See page 451.)*

15. An immune complex disease (a) is difficult to understand from an immunological basis, (b) is caused by a T cell reaction, (c) frequently exhibits symptoms of glomerulonephritis, (d) is exemplified by postvaccinal or postinfectious encephalomyelitis, (e) is exemplified by thrombocytopenic purpura, (f) none of these. *(See page 449.)*

16. Rheumatic fever is best classified as an autoimmune disease originating from which of the following mechanisms? (a) neoantigen, (b) shared antigen, (c) sequestered antigen, (d) mutation in the immune response, (e) none of these. *(See page 452.)*

17. Lupus erythematosus is (a) actually caused by antibodies against cell ribosomes, (b) free from an immune complex disease component, (c) associated with antibodies against nucleic acid, (d) a disease of red and white blood cells, (e) none of these. *(See page 449.)*

18. Myasthenia gravis is a neuromuscular disease caused by (a) production of autoantibodies against acetylcholine receptors, (b) generation of T cells against acetylcholine receptors, (c) production of autoantibodies against acetylcholine, (d) excessive production of acetylcholine, (e) none of these. *(See pages 447 and 448.)*

19. One of the following autoimmune diseases is caused by T cells: (a) SLE, (b) RA, (c) experimental allergic encephalomyelitis, (d) myasthenia gravis, (e) none of these. *(See pages 441 and 447.)*

20. Immunotherapy based on specific modulation of the TCR could use T-cell vaccination, anti-TCR monoclonal antibodies, and TCR peptide competitors. (a) true, (b) false. *(See page 454.)*

## SHORT-ANSWER ESSAY QUESTIONS

1. How does immunodeficiency differ from immunologic tolerance?

2. Design an experiment showing that *in utero* exposure to foreign antigens leads to tolerance in the adult animal.

3. The clonal selection theory lends support to the idea of immunologic tolerance. Explain.

4. Briefly discuss some of the conditions that affect the initiation of immunologic tolerance. What is common among all these conditions? What are some of the basic differences between an antigen and a tolerogen?

5. Compare and contrast low- and high-dose tolerance. Speculate on how this type of tolerance occurs.

6. Tolerance to self-antigens seems to be permanent, while experimentally induced tolerance is not. Explain.

7. The idea of clonal deletion suggests that self-reactive cells are eliminated (no cells to react to self-antigens; therefore, we tolerate self-antigens), yet autoimmune diseases occur (react to self-antigens). Explain.

8. The idea of *horror autotoxicus* was proposed in 1901 to suggest that reactions against self could not occur. Current evidence suggests otherwise. Explain.

9. Other than the characteristic of foreignness, self-antigens and exogenous antigens are not inherently different. Explain.

10. The origin of an autoimmune disorder may lie in the immune process, the self-antigens, or both. Explain. What are the two major events that could lead to an autoimmune disease? List some other possibilities.

11. In Hashimoto's disease, high levels of antibodies against thyroglobulin are found. Yet, these antibodies do not seem to cause the disease. Explain.

12. The description of SLE includes three mechanistic elements; what are they?

13. Compare and contrast the three lines of treatment for RA.

14. Briefly discuss some autoimmune diseases that can follow bacterial infections.

15. Why would the induction of tolerance to an autoantigen, which is causing disease, be one of the most effective treatment approaches for autoimmunity?

## FURTHER READINGS

Anderton, S.M., and D.C. Wright. 2002. Selection and fine-tuning of the autoimmune T-cell repertoire. *Nat. Rev. Immunol.* 2:487–498.

Bell, E., and L. Bird. 2005. Autoimmunity. *Nature* 435:582–627. (A series of six review articles)

Cambier, J.C., S.B. Gauld, K.T. Merrell, and B.J. Vilen. 2007. B-cell anergy: From transgenic models to naturally occurring anergic B cells? *Nat. Rev. Immunol.* 7:633–643.

Chernajovsky, Y., D.J. Gould, and O.L. Podhajcer. 2004. Gene therapy for autoimmune diseases: *Quo vadis? Nat. Rev. Immunol.* 4:800–811.

Cohen, P.L. 2003. Systemic autoimmunity. In *Fundamental Immunology*, 5th ed. W.E. Paul, ed. Philadelphia: Lippincott Williams & Wilkins. p. 1371–1400.

Cheng, M.H., A.K. Shum, and M.S. Anderson. 2007. What's new in the Aire? *Trends Immunol.* 28:321–327.

Feldman, M., and L. Steinman. 2005. Design of effective immunotherapy for human autoimmunity. *Nature* 435:612–619.

Gregersen, P.K., and T.W. Behrens. 2006. Genetics of autoimmune diseases—disorders of immune homeostasis. *Nat. Rev. Genetics* 7:917–928.

Gonzalez-Rey, E., A. Chorny, and M. Delgado. 2007. Regulation of immune tolerance by anti-inflammatory neuropeptides. *Nat. Rev. Immunol.* 7:52–63.

Goodnow, C.C., et al. 2005. Cellular and genetic mechanisms of self tolerance and autoimmunity. *Nature* 435:590–597.

von Herrath, M.G., and D. Homann. 2003. Organ-specific autoimmunity. In *Fundamental Immunology*, 5th ed. W.E. Paul, ed. Philadelphia: Lippincott Williams & Wilkins. p. 1401–1438.

Hogquist, K.A., T.A. Baldwin, and S.C. Jameson. 2005. Central tolerance: Learning self-control in the thymus. *Nat. Rev. Immunol.* 5:772–782.

Kyewski, B., and L. Klein. 2006. A central role for central tolerance. *Annu. Rev. Immunol.* 24:571–606.

Lassmann, H., W. Bruck, and C.F. Lucchinetti. 2007. The immunopathology of multiple sclerosis: An overview. *Brain Pathol.* 17:210–218.

Marshak-Rothstein, A. 2006. Toll-like receptors in systemic autoimmune disease. *Nat. Rev. Immunol.* 6:823–835.

Mathis, D., and C. Benoist. 2007. A decade of AIRE. *Nat. Rev. Immunol.* 7:645–650.

Mayer, L., and L. Shao. 2004. Therapeutic potential of oral tolerance. *Nat. Rev. Immunol.* 4:407–419.

McInnes, I.B., and G. Schett. 2007. Cytokines in the pathogenesis of rheumatoid arthritis. *Nat. Rev. Immunol.* 7:429–442.

Pan, P-Y., J. Ozao, Z. Zhou, and S-H. Chen. 2008. Advancements in immune tolerance. *Adv. Drug Deliv. Rev.* 60:91–105.

Paust, S., and H. Cantor. 2005. Regulatory T cells and autoimmunity. *Immunolog. Rev.* 204:195–207.

Rioux, J.D., and A.K. Abbas. 2005. Paths to understanding the genetic basis of autoimmune disease. *Nature* 435:584–589.

Schwartz, R.H., and D.L. Mueller. 2003. Immunological tolerance. In *Fundamental Immunology*, 5th ed. W.E. Paul, ed. Philadelphia: Lippincott Williams & Wilkins. p. 901–934.

Vincent, A. 2002. Unraveling the pathogenesis of myasthenia gravis. *Nat. Rev. Immunol.* 2:797–804.

# CHAPTER FOURTEEN

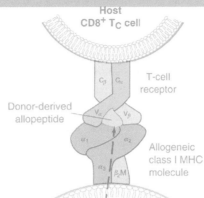

# TRANSPLANTATION IMMUNOLOGY

b) Antimetabolites are impostor molecules that cause faulty cell metabolism.

c) Folic acid analogs include methotrexate and aminopterin.

d) Purine analogs include azathioprine and 6-mercaptopurine.

e) Pyrimidine analogs include cytosine arabinoside, 5-fluorouracil, 5-bromodeoxyuridine, and leflunomide.

3) Microbial peptides have immunosuppressive activity.

4) Some antibiotics can suppress the immune response.

b. Downregulating the immune system with specific polyclonal or monoclonal antibodies.

1) Polyclonal antilymphocyte serum: killing T lymphocytes with the immune system's own antibodies.

2) Monoclonal antibodies are made to react to specific epitopes and minimize their own immunogenicity.

5. Privileged transplants survive because they are inaccessible to the immune system; the fetus is an almost perfect allograft.

6. Many human organs and tissues can be transplanted, including blood, kidneys, hearts, livers, lungs, pancreata, corneas, skin, and bone marrow.

## OBJECTIVES

The reader should be able to:

1. Realize that the cell-mediated immune response to transplants is no different from the immune response to any other foreign antigen.

2. Name the different types of grafts.

3. List the five transplantation laws; note the contribution of sex to these laws.

4. Distinguish between first-set rejection and second-set rejection; distinguish between acute and chronic graft rejection; differentiate between a host-versus-graft reaction and a graft-versus-host reaction.

5. Recognize that MHC genes encode the antigens responsible for graft rejection; compare the contribution of class I and class II antigens to graft rejection; comment on which T cells are responsible for graft rejection.

6. Gain perspective on the phenomenon of alloreactivity.

7. Describe serologic tissue typing; describe tissue typing using the mixed lymphocyte reaction (MLR); understand why you would want to use the MLR in tissue typing.

8. Distinguish between specific and nonspecific immunosuppression.

9. Identify chemical and biologic immunosuppressants.

10. Differentiate between the ways in which the four different types of immunosuppressants cause immunosuppression; give examples of each type of immunosuppressant.

11. Distinguish between privileged sites and privileged tissues; discuss how a developing fetus defies the basic tenets of transplantation immunology.

12. Appreciate the many different tissues and organs that can be transplanted.

One of the main functions of the immune system is to recognize and attack foreign invaders of the body (including foreign tissues). The attack is adverse if the foreign tissue is a transplanted kidney but advantageous if the foreign tissue is self-cells that are cancerous. Whether a transplant is accepted or rejected depends on the stubbornness of the immune system. The immune system is not versatile enough to discriminate in favor of intruders that are beneficial. For a transplant to "take," the recipient's body must suppress its natural tendency to get rid of a foreign invader. Immunologists have tackled this problem in two ways. First, tissue typing ensures that the tissue of the donor and recipient are as similar as possible.

**TABLE 14-1** Transplantation Terminology

| Term | Type of tissue | Definition |
|---|---|---|
| **Autograft** | Autogenic, autologous | Grafts taken from and placed on the same individual—for example, transfer of healthy skin to a burned area of a burn patient or blood vessels to replaced blocked coronary arteries |
| **Syngraft** Isograft | Syngeneic Isologous | Grafts transplanted between identical individuals— for example, between syngeneic mice within the same inbred strain or between identical (monozygotic) twins in humans |
| **Allograft** Homograft | Allogeneic | Grafts transplanted between genetically different individuals of the same species—for example, between two different strains of mice or between two humans |
| **Xenograft** Heterograft | Xenogeneic Heterologous | Grafts transplanted between individuals of two different species—for example, between a mouse and rat or human and baboon (pig tissue has been transplanted into humans) |

Second, the immune system is bombarded with powerful immunosuppressive drugs. This assault is very costly to the well-being of the patient. The first successful kidney transplant in 1954 and the transplants that followed were a rarity. The combination of now "routine" surgical procedures with immunologic understanding makes transplants common, and now organ availability has become rare.

**Transplantation** or **grafting** *is the transfer of cells, tissues, or organs from one part of the body to another or from one individual to another. The transferred material is called the* **transplant** *or* **graft. Transplantation immunity** *is the consequence of an immune response to cell-surface antigens or transplantation antigens, precisely called major histocompatibility complex (MHC) antigens* (**histocompatibility** *refers to tissue compatibility). The individual providing the graft is the* donor, *and the individual receiving the graft is the* recipient *or* host. This chapter describes how the molecules encoded by the MHC, displayed on body cells that when transferred as cells, tissues or organs are instrumental in causing graft rejection—*transplantation immunology.* Next, the chapter shows how immunologic testing is performed, along with immunosuppression, to increase the success of transplants. The chapter closes with a discussion of the importance of placement and type of graft to its survival, followed by some examples of transplantation.

# GENETICISTS, IMMUNOLOGISTS, AND SURGEONS CONTRIBUTED THE TERMINOLOGY USED TO DESCRIBE TRANSPLANTATION IMMUNOLOGY

Geneticists, immunologists, and surgeons have formulated transplantation terminology. The trend is

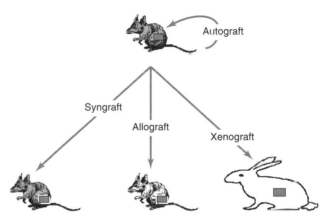

**FIGURE 14-1** The four types of grafts are represented by the direction of the arrows.

toward the use of the geneticist's nomenclature, as defined in Table 14-1 and illustrated in Figure 14-1. Not included in either Table 14.1 or Figure 14.1 is *blood transfusion*, which is the earliest and most common form of tissue transplantation. Matching for MHC molecules is not necessary because erythrocytes or platelets express little or no class I MHC molecules and do not express class II MHC molecules. The absence of MHC molecules eliminates the recipient's T cells from targeting the donated erythrocytes or platelets; however, the blood must be matched for ABO and Rh blood group antigens (see Chapter 5).

Additional terms, not included in the preceding table and figure, define the physical placement and growth properties of grafts. If the graft is transplanted from one place on the donor to the same place on the recipient, it is called *orthotopic*. If the graft is transplanted from one place on the donor to a different site on the recipient, it is called *heterotopic*. If growth does not occur, the graft is called *homostatic* (tissues such as bone or cornea). If tissue growth occurs after transplantation, the graft is called *homovital*.

# GRAFT REJECTION IS IMMUNOLOGIC; IT IS IMMUNITY AGAINST GOOD NONSELF

The transplant rejection process is treated as a normal immune response to **alloantigens**—the histocompatibility antigens on nucleated cells that vary between genetically different members from the same species. The response may be either cell- or antibody-mediated, but cell-mediated predominates. An individual's immune system will not respond against self-antigens or self-transplants, but will react against nonself antigens or nonself transplants. The goal for the transplantation immunologists is to inhibit or at least reduce the latter reaction.

The fate of a graft is determined by the genetic relationship between the donor and the recipient. Each species has a group of histocompatibility genes that encode transplantation or histocompatibility antigens. These antigens are cell surface structures on nucleated cells that are highly polymorphic within a species (see Chapter 7) and are immunogenic enough to elicit a rejection reaction. Histocompatibility genes are almost always *codominantly expressed*. That is, if a $F_1$ progeny inherits the paternal histocompatibility gene *a* and the maternal histocompatibility gene *b*, the products from both genes will be expressed on the cell surface. The $F_1$ progeny expresses the two alleles at each histocompatibility locus. Antigens encoded by histocompatibility genes determine the compatibility or incompatibility of transplants. In humans there are many histocompatibility loci. The most important MHC locus of humans is called the **human leukocyte antigen (HLA) complex** (see Chapter 7; detailed later). Any difference between a donor and recipient at the MHC leads to an immune response directed at the non-self MHC molecules expressed on the graft. Even in a "perfect" match where there is no detectable difference between a related donor and recipient at the MHC, genetic differences at other loci can instigate rejection. This response is due to *minor histocompatibility antigens*, which are self-peptides derived from polymorphic cellular protein bound to graft class I MHC molecules that vary in amino-acid sequence between individuals; this dissimilarity gives rise to minor histocompatibility antigen differences between donor and recipient. If the peptide is different, the recipient's T cells recognize it as foreign leading to eventual rejection of the graft. In fact, these self-peptides are required for the structural integrity of class I molecules and for their successful delivery to the cell surface (see Chapter 7). Examples of minor histocompatibility antigens are proteins encoded on the male-specific Y chromosome. Because females do not produce these proteins, Y antigen peptides are foreign alloantigens that elicit immune responses.

## There Are Transplantation Laws or Commandments for Graft Survival, Which Were Initially Described by Skin Transplantation

Whenever a graft possesses histocompatibility antigens new to the recipient, they are recognized and attacked and the graft is rejected. This genetic "rule" can be divided into five laws of transplantation based on results of experimental transplantation between inbred strains of mice, which are summarized in Figure 14-2. These results show that polymorphic MHC gene products are codominantly expressed on a graft and are the molecules used by immune system's T cells to distinguish between a foreign and a self-graft. The results of experiment 3 in Figure 14-2 show codominant expression, where an $(A \times B)F_1$ animal expresses both Strain A and Strain B alleles; therefore, this animal is tolerant to both Strain A and B grafts, but both Strain A and Strain B animals recognize $(A \times B)F_1$ grafts as foreign.

In certain circumstances, exceptions to the laws of transplantation exist. These exceptions include (1) exposure to transplanted tissue during neonatal life or after some immunopharmacologic manipulation leading to tolerance to the donor tissue; (2) the transfer of immunocompetent cells into an immuno*in*competent recipient, leading to a graft-versus-host reaction (discussed shortly); and (3) the transplant of tissue between genetically identical individuals of different sexes. Because X and Y chromosomes determine histocompatibility antigens, grafts from females to males (within an inbred strain) are accepted, though grafts from males to females may be rejected. Transplants from the maternal parent to a male or female $F_1$ recipient are accepted, but transplants from the paternal parent to a male or female $F_1$ recipient may be rejected.

## The First Set and Second Set Rejections Are Primary and Secondary Immune Responses

Graft rejection is immunologically mediated; the response exhibits two features of immunity—specificity and memory. Mechanisms of allograft rejection for an organ or tissue transplant are separated into the first set rejection and the second set rejection (Figure 14-3); these mechanisms were first explained by skin

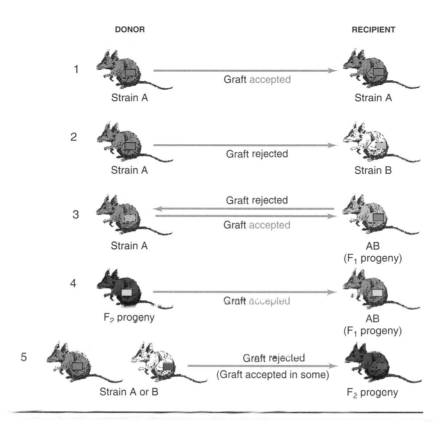

DONOR                                      RECIPIENT

1    Strain A    ——— Graft accepted ———▶    Strain A

2    Strain A    ——— Graft rejected ———▶    Strain B

3    Strain A    ◀——— Graft rejected ———    AB
                 ——— Graft accepted ———▶    (F₁ progeny)

4    F₂ progeny  ——— Graft accepted ———▶    AB
                                            (F₁ progeny)

5    Strain A or B   ——— Graft rejected ———▶   F₂ progeny
                     (Graft accepted in some)

1. Transplants within inbred strains (syngraft) are accepted.
2. Transplants between inbred strains (allografts) are rejected.
3. Transplants from either inbred parental strain to an F₁ progeny are accepted, but transplants in the reverse direction are rejected.
4. Transplants from F₂ or later generation animals to F₁ animals are accepted.
5. Transplants from either parental strains are accepted in some F₂ animals, but fail in most.

**FIGURE 14-2 Immunologic nature of the transplantation rejection response.** *Panel I—immunity.* This panel depicts the immune reactivity to a skin graft (foreign antigen) by strain A mouse. The skin is rejected at the time when a primary immune response is fully developed. *Panel II—memory.* This panel shows that when the strain A mouse is exposed to a strain B mouse skin graft for a second time, it shows accelerated rejection. The increased reactivity is known as a *memory response* or *secondary immune response.* The immune response also is specific because it treats the skin graft from a strain C mouse as a new foreign antigen.

transplantation between inbred strains of mice. The **first set rejection** occurs about 10 days (skin grafts are rejected faster than kidney or heart) after a first graft from an allogeneic donor. In this rejection, sensitized T cells are found in the lymph nodes that drain the site of the graft; they appear 6 to 10 days after the graft has been placed into the recipient. Foreign antigens expressed on the grafted cells stimulate the T cells that mediate graft rejection. Immune cells infiltrate the graft in large numbers, leading to vascular changes resulting in thrombosis and eventual death of the graft. This time sequence of events is the

same as for the typical immune response or primary immune response to conventional foreign antigens. T-cell involvement of graft rejection is confirmed with the transplant of skin to an athymic mouse, it leads to graft survival. Reconstitution of the athymic mouse with normal T cells restores graft rejection.

The **second set rejection** is more accelerated than its first set counterpart if a patient receives a second graft such as a skin graft derived from the same donor or genetically identical donors. The accelerated nature of the response is similar to the secondary or anamnestic response after exposure to the same antigen—*an*

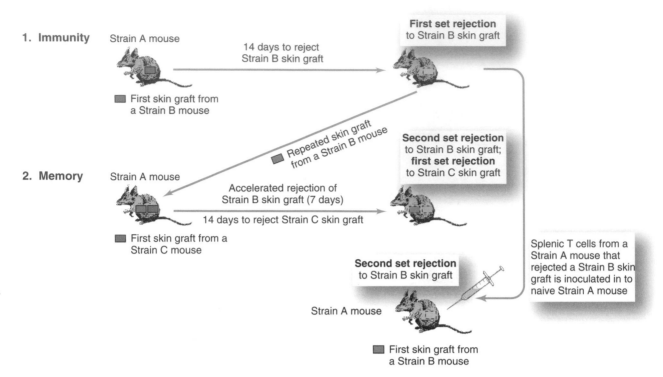

1. **Immunity**    Strain A mouse

14 days to reject
Strain B skin graft

**First set rejection**
to Strain B skin graft

■ First skin graft from
a Strain B mouse

Repeated skin graft
from a Strain B mouse

**Second set rejection**
to Strain B skin graft;
**first set rejection**
to Strain C skin graft

2. **Memory**    Strain A mouse

Accelerated rejection of
Strain B skin graft (7 days)

14 days to reject Strain C skin graft

■ First skin graft from a
Strain C mouse

Splenic T cells from a
Strain A mouse that
rejected a Strain B skin
graft is inoculated in to
naive Strain A mouse

**Second set rejection**
to Strain B skin graft

Strain A mouse

■ First skin graft from
a Strain B mouse

**FIGURE 14-3 Transplantation Laws**. Mouse A and mouse B are members of two inbred strains. The $F_1$ and $F_2$ are individuals of the first and second filial generations, respectively. The five laws of transplantation are presented schematically in sequence from 1 to 5.

*example of immunologic specificity and memory*. These patients often have high circulating titers of cytotoxic anti-graft IgG antibodies (but T cells also are involved because experimentally the response can be adoptively transferred). These antibodies appear after the rejection of the first graft and have little or no importance in first set rejection. They are capable, however, of immediate cytotoxic effects and immune complex formation in the presence of complement after the second transplant. Immune complexes can cause occlusion of blood vessels and inhibition of the entrance and removal of nutrients. Because of the rapid nature of the second set rejection process, the graft never becomes vascularized. Taken together, the first- and second-set rejections are mainly mediated by CD8$^+$ T cells and CD4$^+$ T cells.

## Preformed Recipient Antibodies Mediate the Quickest Graft Rejection, a Hyperacute Rejection

**Hyperacute graft rejection** occurs within a few minutes to hours after transplantation. The reaction is due to the recipient having preformed antibodies against the donor's tissue endothelium; cell-mediated immunity is not involved, in fact, it is a type III hypersensitivity reaction. (That is not to say, if hyperacute rejection is prevented the graft would not be subject to cell-mediated rejection.) The antibodies activate complement; the complement products rigorously recruit neutrophils and induce the clotting cascade, which results in an inflammatory reaction that leads to thrombotic occlusion of the graft vasculature. The graft is rejected so quickly that it never becomes vascularized. The preformed antibodies are against foreign MHC alloantigens or vascular endothelial cell alloantigens and arise from prior exposure to alloantigens through earlier transplantation, repeated blood transfusions, multiple pregnancies, or wrong ABO blood typing and cross-matching (determining whether the recipient has antibodies against donor leukocytes). If the second graft expresses alloantigens similar to an earlier graft, the recipient's existing antibodies can react immediately with the second graft, inducing a hyperacute rejection reaction. Patients that have received multiple blood transfusions can develop numerous anti-HLA antibodies; this increases their risk of reacting with potential grafted tissues or organs. One of the most common ways of developing circulating anti-HLA class I and class II antibodies is through a previous pregnancy.

During the trauma of childbirth, the mother can be exposed to fetal cells that express paternal HLA molecules, leading to anti-HLA antibodies. With successive pregnancies, the levels anti-HLA antibodies increase. In fact, multiparous women are the primary source for HLA typing sera. Because ABO blood antigens (see Chapter 5) are also expressed on vascular endothelial cells, a mistake in ABO blood typing and cross-matching can lead to hyperacute rejection of grafted organs, such as, kidneys. For example, if a recipient with type O blood (they have naturally occurring anti-A and anti-B antibodies) received a kidney from a donor with type A blood, the recipient's anti-A antibodies would immediately react with the A antigens expressed throughout the kidney graft's blood vessels. Pretransplantation testing for these preformed antibodies has eliminated the problem of hyperacute rejection responses. This is important because there is no dependable method to reverse hyperacute rejection.

Because the need for transplants significantly outpaces organ donations (Table 14-2), one proposed solution is the use of animal organs—*xenotransplantation*. Irrespective of the zoonotic or ethical issues, experimentation using pig organs is underway. In fact, pig heart valves have been used in humans for years. However, there are some serious problems associated with using pig organs. For example, were a human to receive a pig kidney graft, the graft would rapidly fail due to a hyperacute rejection reaction. The reason is that pigs, most other mammal cells, and microorganisms express a disaccharide antigen (galactosyl-1,3-α-galactose) that is not expressed on human cells; therefore, the presence of this antigen on many microorganisms means everyone has been exposed and has formed antibodies against the antigen. These preexisting antibodies bind to the pig cells, fix complement, and rapidly lysis the cells. Furthermore, because pig cells lack human regulators of complement activity, such as decay accelerating factor (DAF), CD59, and human membrane cofactor, complement-mediate lysis intensifies (see Chapter 11). To circumvent this problem, pigs are genetically engineered. In some pigs, the gene for the enzyme that synthesizes α1,3-galactosyltransferase is knocked out; thus, they do not express galactosyl-1,3-α-galactose. Others are made transgenic and express human DAF, which dampens the complement response. Additional antigenic differences between human and pig cells that intensify NK cell and macrophage activities need to be overcome. Nonetheless, recent advances have moved xenotransplantation closer to clinical application.

**TABLE 14-2** **August 2008 Waiting List Candidates Statistics\***

| Candidates | Number |
|---|---|
| All candidates\*\* | 99,298 |
| Heart | 2,633 |
| Heart/Lung | 98 |
| Intestine | 231 |
| Kidney | 76,561 |
| Kidney/Pancreas | 2,281 |
| Liver | 16,160 |
| Lung | 2,109 |
| Pancreas | 1,582 |

\*Obtained from United Network for Organ Sharing (UNOS) website.
\*\* All candidates will be less than the sum due to candidates waiting for multiple organs.

## Effector T Cells Mediate the Acute Graft Rejection

Most organ transplants are completed between individuals that have some HLA class I and/or class II antigen differences; therefore, the recipient's T cell population includes alloreactive T cells against the differing HLA antigens. **Acute graft rejection** is mediated by effector $CD8^+$ and $CD4^+$ T cells, which respond to class I and class II HLA antigens, respectively, and occurs in a recipient that has not been previously sensitized to the graft. Unlike a hyperacute rejection, the acute rejection process starts roughly 10 days after transplantation and can be lessened or averted by immunosuppressive intervention before transplantation and maintenance with them after transplantation. The histologic picture of a graft undergoing acute rejection is reminiscent of a type IV delayed-type hypersensitivity reaction; there is intense infiltration of lymphocytes and macrophages. If acute rejection is not reversed, in the case of a kidney transplant, it leads to loss of kidney function 10–14 days after transplant.

## The Chronic Graft Rejection Is a Smoldering Immune Response

The second set rejection or acute graft rejection is almost an expected phenomenon. However, **chronic graft rejection** is now receiving more attention because of the expanded importance of organ grafts and the judicious use of immunosuppressive drugs. Long-range follow-up of kidney recipients has allowed the description of chronic graft rejection. Rejection occurs months to years after the seemingly successful transplant. Short-term 1-year survival for kidney grafts has increased significantly since the 1970s; however, chronic rejection is unchanged, it is responsible for more than 50% of all kidney graft rejections within 10 years after transplantation. Rejection usually results from thickening of graft blood vessels and a narrowing of their lumina—*arteriosclerosis*. Although acute rejection episodes do not occur, the kidney gradually loses its function, and biopsy reveals the evidence of a long-smoldering rejection process. The biopsy specimen shows the loss of normal kidney morphology, perivascular infiltration of immune cells, replacement of the kidney parenchyma with fibrotic tissues, thickening of the small arteries and their luminal narrowing, and widespread infiltration by lymphocytes and plasma cells. The cumulative result is blood supply becomes inadequate, leading to ischemia, loss of kidney function, and death of the graft. Chronic graft rejection is generally caused by alloreactivity (discussed shortly), ischemic-reperfusion injury during transplantation, chronic toxicity of immunosuppressive drugs, and infection by cytomegalovirus.

## In the Graft-Versus-Host Reaction, the Graft Rejects the Host

The more common type of graft rejection process, and the main concern in transplantation immunology, is the *host-versus-graft reaction*, or the immune response of the recipient's immune cells to the graft's antigens. However, the reverse situation, in which the graft rejects the host's tissues, called the **graft-versus-host reaction** (**GvHR**), occurs when immunocompetent cells (the *graft*—such as in bone marrow transplantation) are transferred into an immuno*in*competent recipient (the *host*). This kind of graft leads to an unopposed attack by the graft on the host's tissues; it leads to **graft-versus-host disease** (**GvHD**). GvHR occurs under the following conditions: (1) histoincompatibility between the donor (graft) and recipient (host), (2) adoptive transfer of immunocompetent cells (particularly T cells), and (3) immunodeficiency of the recipient (neonatal individual, congenital or acquired immunodeficiency, or clinical immunosuppression). The GvHR frequently occurs after bone marrow transplantation for stem cell replacement in thalassemia major, aplastic anemia, acute leukemia, lymphoma, and combined immunodeficiencies. In fact, the GvHR is the major limitation on the use of bone marrow transplantation. The resulting GvHD can be acute or chronic. Acute GvHD is a progressive, systemic disease characterized by epithelial cell necrosis mainly in the gastrointestinal tract, the liver, and the skin. In contrast, chronic GvHD, which is a pleiotropic

syndrome characterized by fibrosis and atrophy of the same organs, but with no sign of epithelial cell necrosis; it has similarities to autoimmune diseases, such as, scleroderma.

Allogeneic bone marrow is obtained by needle aspirations from a healthy donor (usually an HLA-identical sibling), the graft, bone marrow, contains pluripotent stem cells, which are intravenously inoculated into the recipient. These stem cells can reconstitute the recipient's immune system and erythrocytes and platelets. The recipient has usually undergone a preparative treatment called *conditioning regiment*, which can consist of chemotherapy, irradiation, and specific immunosuppressive therapy that must lead to disease eradication (in the case of cancer, such as, leukemia) and overcome host rejection (suppression of T cell-mediated anti-graft responses) of donor graft. Because the recipient is now immunoincompetent, the primary problem is the donor's mature alloreactive CD4$^+$ and CD8$^+$ T cells in the grafted bone marrow that can respond to the recipient's HLA antigens. These effector T cells migrate into the recipient's circulation and enter and attack tissues (GvHR) damaged by the conditioning regiment, the skin, intestines, and liver. To prevent GvHR, the bone marrow graft is depleted of mature T cells. Within a few weeks after a successful bone marrow transplant, the recipient starts to produce new circulating blood cells; a sign that pluripotent stems have colonized the bone marrow—a successful *engraftment* has occurred. As the recipient's hematopoietic system is restored, granulocytes and NK cells recover first, followed by B and T cells. The chimeric patient now has the donor's hematopoietic cell genotype with the remaining cells of the recipient's genotype. The new immune system now becomes tolerant of donor and recipient HLA molecules.

Experimental GvHR can be induced in adult F$_1$ mice by injecting parental strain T cells, which respond to allogeneic MHC antigens and induce symptoms of systemic GvHD. The GvHR is similar to a delayed-type hypersensitivity reaction mediated by T cells reacting against cellular surface antigens of recipient tissues. If T cells are removed by antibody treatment, no GvHR occurs. The first stages of a GvHR involve the proliferation of donor T cells, which generally localize in the spleen. This localization leads to an increase in spleen size called *splenomegaly*. As the GvHR progresses to its peak response, the skin and intestinal walls become heavily infiltrated by immune cells, leading to skin rash and diarrhea. During this phase of the reaction, most of the proliferating cells are of host origin, consisting of T and B cells, monocytes, and macrophages.

The recipient's cells probably proliferate in response to nonspecific mitogenic and differentiation factors released by the stimulated T cells. Even though T cells seem to initiate a GvHR, the effector cells that cause epithelial cell necrosis are uncertain. Histologically, NK cells are found attached to dying epithelial cells, suggesting that NK cells, recruited and primed by $CD4^+$ T-cell-derived interleukin (IL)-2 and interferon-$\gamma$ (IFN-$\gamma$), are the effector cells of acute GvHD.

## MINI SUMMARY

Grafting of tissue within an individual (autograft), between identical twins, or between inbred animals within the same strain (syngraft) succeeds if the recipient is tolerant. However, grafting between genetically nonidentical host and donor, either between those within the same species (allograft) or between species (xenograft), leads to graft rejection. The rejection is the result of a cell-mediated immune response caused by T cells reacting with foreign cell-surface class I and class II MHC antigens. There is no difference between graft rejection and the usual immune response to conventional foreign antigen. Several different rejection reactions can take place after a transplant: first set rejection (the immune system handles the graft as it would any first exposure to any foreign antigen); second set rejection (the immune system handles the graft as it would any secondary exposure to the same antigen); hyperacute graft rejection (preformed antibodies against the graft); acute graft rejection (rapid recipient T-cell–mediated response against unshared MHC antigens); chronic graft rejection (a weak, long-term immune response to foreign tissue); and a graft-versus-host reaction (the graft contains lymphocytes that can reject the host).

# TRANSPLANTATION, OR HISTOCOMPATIBILITY, ANTIGENS ARE FOREIGN ANTIGENS ON THE DONOR'S LIFE-SAVING "INVADER" TISSUE THAT LEAD TO ITS DESTRUCTION

What makes grafted tissue appear immunologically foreign? In the early 1930s, Peter Gorer showed that molecules on the surface of foreign tissue that are immunogenic cause tissue rejection. All persons have these unique self-markers on all of their nucleated cells. It is almost impossible for any unrelated two individuals to have identical self-markers; therefore, transplants between two unrelated individuals always fail. Immunologists discovered that these self-markers are encoded by a special set of genes. These genes, which lie close together in a region on chromosome 6, are called the *major histocompatibility complex* (*MHC*). The first two words in the name, *major* and *histocompatibility* (the prefix *histo-* means "tissue"), suggest the importance of this region in graft rejection; the third word, *complex*, suggests that the region consists of many genes closely linked to each other and mediating different functions (see Chapter 7). (Minor histocompatibility antigens were mentioned earlier.) At least six pairs of MHC genes encode the different HLA-encoded self-markers (half inherited from a person's father and half from the mother). Each member of the pair is expressed. This results because the MHC is so polymorphic; therefore, most individuals are heterozygous at each locus. Both alleles are expressed and both their products are found on all nucleated cells. Because each one of these genes may come in 100s or more varieties (polymorphism),[1] many possible MHC combinations exist. The chance that two unrelated individuals will share the same combination is less than 1 in 100,000. Although the chances of two unrelated persons having identical self-markers are slim to nonexistent, the odds of a complete match between siblings are roughly 1 in 4.

## The Class I MHC Molecules Are Known as the Traditional Transplantation Antigens

The murine H-2 complex K, D, and L regions or the human HLA complex B, C, and A regions encode the **class I molecules** (in this context, they are called **class I antigens**), also called *serologically defined* (*SD*) *antigens* or, traditionally, **transplantation antigens**. Products of these MHC genes determine the cell membrane antigens that are expressed on all nucleated cells. These membrane molecules function as the MHC antigens involved in transplantation reactions. MHC antigens also stimulate cytotoxic T ($T_C$)-cell responses and antibody responses, and under physiologic conditions MHC antigens are involved in determining the specificity of $CD8^+$ T cells, most of which are $T_C$ cells.

---

[1]In the context of the MHC, polymorphism refers to the number of variants at a single gene locus; individual variants are called *alleles* (see Chapter 7).

Even though antibodies are produced against class I (and II) MHC molecules, as we have seen antibodies are not the primary mediators of graft rejection. They can mediate detrimental effects during hyperacute (and second set) rejection by occluding the graft's blood vessels or by forming immune complexes, which can activate the complement system.

## Class II MHC Molecules Are the Interaction Entities on Immune Cells That Are the Primary Instigators in Graft Rejection

The murine I (letter, not Roman numeral) region or the human D region (DP, DQ, and DR subregions) encodes the **class II molecules** (in the case of graft reactions, they are called **class II antigens**), also called *lymphocyte-defined (LD) antigens*. Class II MHC molecules stimulate the *mixed lymphocyte reaction* (discussed below), which is the proliferative response of T cells *in vitro* to allogeneic lymphocytes. This lymphocyte-induced proliferation is the reason they are called LD antigens. Class II MHC molecules are important in the activation of CD4+ T cells, most of which are helper T ($T_H$) cells, probably through the presentation of class II MHC antigens by donor passenger leukocytes (discussed shortly). Table 14-3 summarizes the tissue distribution of mouse and human MHC antigens.

## T Lymphocytes Are Responsible for Allograft Rejection

The immune system's involvement in graft rejection was confirmed by studies in the early 1950s, which showed that adaptive transfer of lymphocytes, but not serum, conferred allograft immunity. Later studies using athymic (nude) mice, which lack functional T cells, demonstrated that they fail to reject allogeneic and even xenogeneic grafts. Inability to reject foreign grafts can be reversed by administering T cells. Therefore, T-cell involvement in allograft rejection is proven using congenitally athymic mice. B cells make antibodies against alloantigens that are indirectly involved in graft rejection through complement activation. However, neonatally bursectomized chickens, which lack B cells, are capable of rejecting foreign grafts. This direct evidence suggests no role for B cells in graft rejection. Using anti-CD4 and anti-CD8 monoclonal antibodies to depleted one or both types of T cells, showed that anti-CD8 antibody treatment had no affect on should read on graft survival, anti-CD4 antibody treatment extended graft survival, and treatment with both antibodies extended graft survival even further. This proved that the CD4+ and CD8+ T cells collaborate in graft rejection.

Most evidence to date, from *in vitro* tests as well as histologic studies, suggests that $T_H$ cells are the primary cells involved in allograft rejection. The site of rejection is infiltrated by many small lymphocytes, which precedes the destruction of the graft by several days. Studies comparing the classes of MHC antigens show that the differences between recipient and donor class II MHC antigens are more important than the differences between their respective class I MHC antigens. Because CD4+ T cells recognize class II MHC antigens, the CD4+, or $T_H$1, cells must be the cells primarily involved in allograft rejection. The presence of high levels of IL-2, IFN-$\gamma$, and tumor necrosis factor $\beta$ (TNF-$\beta$), but the lack of IL-4, in graft-infiltrating T cells also supports $T_H$1 subset involvement. IL-2 promotes $T_H$ cell proliferation and drives the development of pre-$T_C$ cells to effector $T_C$ cells. IFN-$\gamma$, along with the vascular endothelial cell-derived chemokines such as CCL5, recruits monocytes that mature into macrophages into the graft; once there, it activates them into more destructive anti-graft cells. TNF-$\beta$ adds to the destructive effect by directly lysing the graft cells. These cytokines plus IFN-$\alpha$ and IFN-$\beta$ and TNF-$\alpha$ contribute to the increased expression of class I MHC molecules on graft cells. IFN-$\gamma$ also increases the expression of class II MHC molecules and adhesion molecules, particularly in the graft's vascular endothelial cells. This increased MHC molecule expression promotes graft rejection. The $T_H$ cells that dispense these cytokines are thought to be equivalent to the T cells involved in delayed-type hypersensitivity (DTH) reactions because, on histologic examination, one sees many macrophages and lymphocytes at the graft site, similar to the cells seen in inflammatory reactions at DTH sites. (Because these T cells mediate DTH and are found in DTH sites, they are also called $T_{DTH}$ or $T_D$ *cells*.)

### The Molecular and Cellular Basis of Reacting to Tissues We Do Not Encounter Normally

Why do hosts have such aggressive graft rejection reactions? Clones responsive to a specific conventional antigen and self-MHC protein appear at low frequency (0.01 to 0.0001%), but many (1 to 3%) T cells are responsive to allo-MHC molecules alone. This intriguing feature of T-cell recognition is the phenomenon of **alloreactivity**—the T cell's ability to recognize peptide–allogeneic-MHC complexes that were not encountered during thymic development, which manifests itself clinically as transplant rejection. Why do so many T cells recognize foreign

**TABLE 14-3 Tissue Distribution of MHC Antigens**

| MHC regions | | |
|---|---|---|
| **Murine H-2** | **Human HLA** | |
| K, D, L | B, C, A | All nucleated cells, platelets, and mouse erythrocytes |
| I-A and I-E | DP, DQ, DR | B lymphocytes, monocytes, macrophages, dendritic cells, melanoma cells, activated human T cells (but not activated mouse T cells), and human vascular endothelial cells |

MHC molecules? Initially, alloreactivity was interpreted to mean that a host was primed to MHC antigens. However, germ-free animals also possess a high frequency of alloreactive T cells. The current hypothesis is that T cells see a foreign MHC molecule much the same as a self-MHC molecule and foreign peptide complex. That is, TCR specificity is defined by the peptide and by the MHC molecule displaying the peptide (see Chapter 10). The TCRs of MHC-restricted, antigen-specific cloned T cells also can bind allo-MHC antigens. This observation implies that heightened allogeneic responses are a matter of cross-reactivity. Alloreactive T cells arise as a secondary consequence of MHC-restricted recognition, and allo- and MHC-restricted recognition are mediated by the same basic mechanism. Recent evidence suggests that allorecognition results from the recognition of peptides derived from processed cellular proteins presented in association with self-MHC molecules. Thus, CD8+ T$_C$-cell recognition of allogeneic MHC antigens proceeds by an MHC-restricted mechanism. This scenario implies that the ligand is an MHC molecule complexed to particular peptide derived either from the local environment or from the target cell or APC itself. This suggests that *recognition of foreign MHC molecules is a cross-reactivity at the TCR level for a self-MHC molecule plus foreign peptide.* Allogeneic MHC antigens appear to the recipient's T cells as a foreign peptide-altered self-MHC molecule complex. Evidence suggests that different self-peptides can bind with one foreign MHC molecule to create determinants recognized by different cross-reactive T-cell clones.

*In vitro* models useful in testing alloreactivity are **mixed lymphocyte reactions (MLRs)**. MLRs serve as (1) *in vitro* correlate reactions to the *in vivo* detection of foreign MHC molecules, (2) precursor reactions for cytotoxicity, and (3) prototype reactions for T-T-cell interaction. MLRs occur when lymphoid cells from genetically distinct individuals or strain of the same species are mixed in tissue culture. In order to proliferate, the T cells in an MLR do not need earlier immunization to the stimulating cell-surface MHC antigens. In fact, the MLR is the only *in vitro* reaction, which results from the proliferation of antigen-specific T

cells without their prior immunization to the stimulating antigen. Most of the alloreactive T cells are not specific for the allogeneic MHC antigens but proliferate in response to cytokines, such as IL-2, produced by specifically stimulated, alloreactive T cells.

Cells that act as stimulators are made incapable of cell division (Figure 14-4), which simplifies measuring of the reactivity of the *responder cells* (recipient) against the *stimulator cells* (donor). The greater the difference, the higher the proliferation or MLR reactivity (see Chapter 10) and, thus the greater the chance of the recipient's rejecting the donor tissue or organ. The responder cells in an allogeneic MLR are CD4+ and CD8+ T cells; CD4+ T cells are stimulated by cells that express class II MHC molecules and provide costimulatory signals, while CD8+ T cells are stimulated by class I molecules and CD4+ T-cell-derived cytokines. Alloreactive CD4+ and CD8+ T cells, like their self-MHC-restricted, antigen-specific counterparts, can be stimulated only by cells that express class II and I MHC molecules, respectively. Because all class II and I MHC alleles inherited from both parents are codominantly expressed (no allelic exclusion), one stimulator cell can activate several different T$_H$ cells that have different class II MHC specificities. Likewise, one target cell can be lysed by several different T$_C$ cells that have different class I MHC specificities.

### Passenger Leukocytes, the Antigen-Presenting Cells That Contaminate Graft Tissue, Contribute to Graft Rejection

The artificial transfer of cells, tissues or organs between genetically disparate individuals elicits a specific adaptive immune response; the response is like that against a conventional antigen, such as, microorganisms. This response is orchestrated by T cells recognizing MHC molecules expressed on the transferred graft. CD4+ T$_H$ cells, which respond to APC-presented class II MHC molecule-peptide complexes, are not activated until they receive a second signal (Figure 14-5), such as APC costimulatory molecule expression and IL-12 production. Conversely, CD8+ T$_C$ cells respond to class I MHC antigens as their first signal but also are not activated

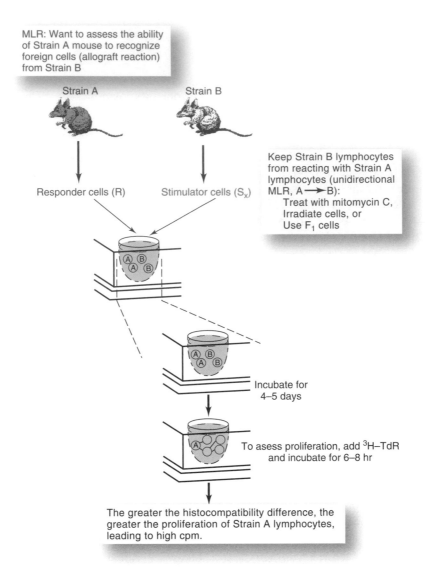

**FIGURE 14-4 Unidirectional MLR**. See text for further explanation.

until they receive a second "help" signal, CD40L and IL-2 and IFN-γ, which can be produced by the activated T$_H$ cells or directly accomplished by dendritic cells that have undergone cross-presentation and been licensed by activated T$_H$ cells (see Figure 10-21).

How do T$_H$ cells become activated and, in turn, activate T$_C$ cells when virtually every cell within a graft expresses donor class I MHC molecules, which are a target for both host CD8$^+$ T$_C$ cells and alloantibody, yet few graft cells express donor class II MHC molecules to present alloantigen directly to prime host CD4$^+$ T$_H$ cells. Host T cells are activated in draining lymph nodes by two pathways of graft HLA antigen recognition: **direct** and **indirect** (Figure

14-6). To prime host CD4$^+$ T$_H$ cells, if comparing an allograft response to an immune response to conventional antigen, recipient dendritic cells must acquire, process, and *indirectly* present donor alloantigen in the context of recipient class II MHC molecules. That is, for T$_C$ cells to eventually mediate cytotoxicity, there must be *direct* presentation of donor alloantigen to CD8$^+$ pre-T$_C$ cells typically accompanied by the *indirect* presentation of donor alloantigen to CD4$^+$ T$_H$ cells. In the context of an allograft, how these T$_H$ cells assist CD8$^+$ T$_C$ cells and B cell responses to distinct *directly* presented class I MHC molecules is the question. Evidence shows a role for donor dendritic cells, so-called **passenger leukocytes** that contaminate a graft, in *directly* initiating and priming the immune

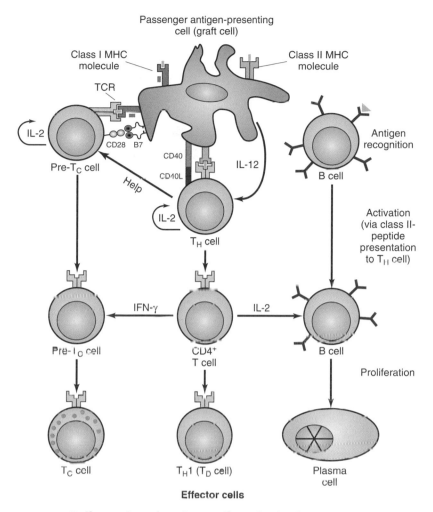

**FIGURE 14-5** Generation of a primary allograft rejection response.

response to alloantigens. These cells are trapped in tissue and blood vessels of the grafted organ. Human vascular endothelial cells also exhibit costimulatory activity through class II MHC molecule expression and thereby the cells lining the graft's blood vessels can activate T$_H$ cells.

Direct recognition of alloantigens was thought to be the only route by which alloantigens could be recognized in a graft, and this recognition is of high frequency (*alloreactivity* was discussed earlier). The vigorous and immediate nature of direct allorecognition is because there is no need for processing and presentation by self-MHC molecules. There is now also considerable evidence for indirect recognition of alloantigens. The latter mechanism is dominated by CD4$^+$ T$_H$ cells, leading to the development of multiple allogeneic peptides and thereby amplification of the rejection response, but the response is slower than direct allorecognition. The indirect response may be responsible for long-term reactivity to grafts once

passenger APCs and direct responses are exhausted. To summarize, in either case, allograft rejection results from activated alloreactive CD4$^+$ T cells that proliferate and secrete various cytokines, which serve to recruit and activate macrophages, causing graft rejection through a DTH response; to activate alloreactive CD8$^+$ T cells that directly lyse graft cells; and drive the growth and differentiation of B cells to produce alloantibodies that activate the complement system or ADCC and injure the endothelium of graft blood vessels (Figure 14-7).

## MINI SUMMARY

MHC genes encode class I and class II antigens that influence the fate of grafted tissues. The two best-characterized MHCs are the mouse H-2 and the human HLA complexes. Activation of CD4$^+$ T$_H$ cells is caused by class II MHC antigens

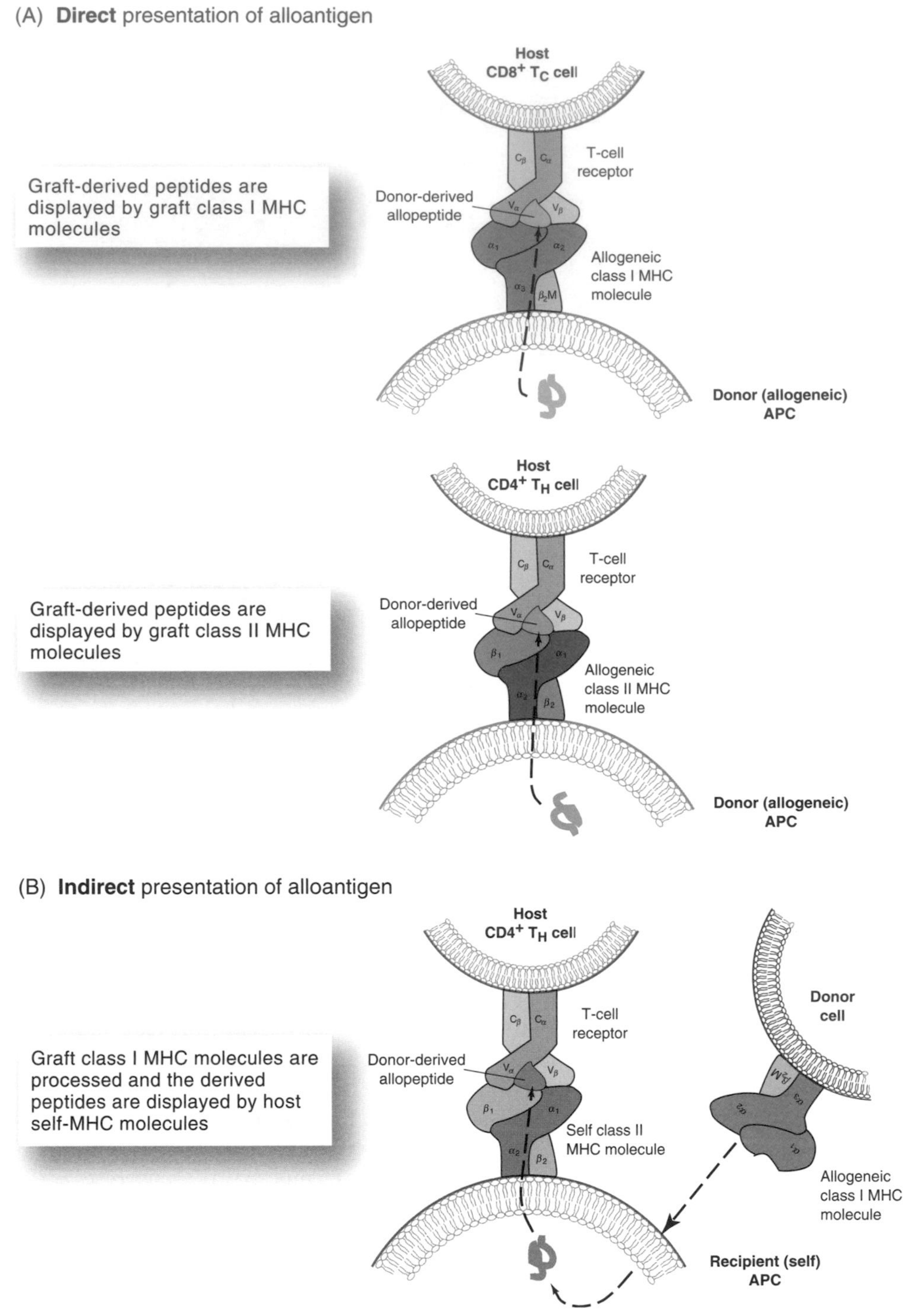

(A) **Direct** presentation of alloantigen

Graft-derived peptides are displayed by graft class I MHC molecules

Graft-derived peptides are displayed by graft class II MHC molecules

(B) **Indirect** presentation of alloantigen

Graft class I MHC molecules are processed and the derived peptides are displayed by host self-MHC molecules

**FIGURE 14-6 Two possible pathways of alloantigenic peptide recognition: (A) direct vs. (B) indirect.** See text for explanation.

expressed on APCs found within the graft. A host's cells seem to be obsessed with reactivity to foreign class I MHC antigens. This phenomenon is called alloreactivity.

## Histocompatibility Testing, the Matching of Nonself to Self, Equals Graft Survival

Despite the problems with rejection, organs and tissues obtained from live, unrelated donors and from

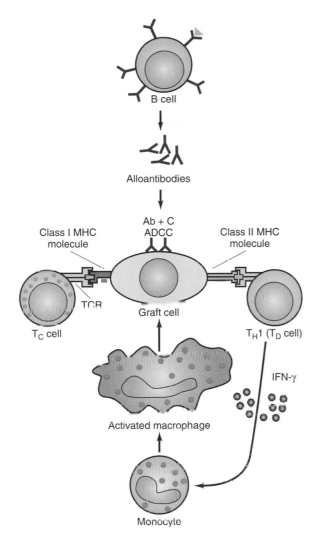

**FIGURE 14-7 Mechanisms of allograft rejection.** Ab, antibody; C, complement; ADCC, antibody-dependent cell-mediated cytotoxicity; T$_C$ cell, cytotoxic T cell; T$_H$ cell, helper T cell; IFN-$\gamma$, interferon-$\gamma$.

cadavers have been successfully transplanted. Careful matching through histocompatibility testing helps to insure success. Two approaches can be used to compare HLA antigens. The first approach analyzes the known HLA antigens (100s have been described) of the two individuals, using an *antibody-mediated cytotoxic test* also called a *microcytotoxicity test*. In practice, a panel of donor and recipient target cells (lymphocytes) is reacted with each of the anti-HLA antibodies plus complement. Figure 14-7 summarizes this approach. However, this method can test only for known HLA antigens and the same antibody may bind two similar but nonidentical HLA molecules.

The second approach involves mixing lymphocytes from both the donor and the recipient, or mixing cells from each with homozygous typing cells,

to determine compatibility (the MLR, discussed earlier). This approach (*a predictive test of graft rejection*) accounts for any HLA antigens that may be present. Figure 14-9 shows how the MLR is used in tissue typing. Lastly, the donor and recipient blood groups (ABO and Rh) are matched to determine if the recipient has preformed antibodies against the donor's cells (blood type antigens are also present on the graft organ's vascular endothelium).

# IMMUNOSUPPRESSIVE PREVENTION OF GRAFT REJECTION IS THE INHIBITION OF THE RESPONSE TO NONSELF

Transplantation, when successful, is one of the most dramatic forms of treatment in modern medicine. The recipient of an HLA-identical kidney can reasonably expect discharge from the hospital within a few weeks and a return to productive life within a few months. To avoid failure, recipients are immunosuppressed to allow them to retain grafts. Most transplant patients are saddled with a lifetime of immunosuppressive drugs, which protect their substitute organs from rejection. Because most immunosuppressive drugs are not antigen-specific, causing a generalized suppressed immune response to all antigens, the recipient has increased risk for infections and lymphoid cancers, plus nephrotoxicity and metabolic bone disease. These drugs also affect rapidly dividing nonimmune cells, such as epithelial cells lining the gut, hair follicle cells, and bone marrow hematopoietic stem cells.

To delay or prevent graft rejection, immunosuppressive therapy relies on agents that destroy immunocompetent cells or inhibit the proliferation and differentiation of lymphocyte responses to MHC antigens. Immunosuppression can be divided into antigen-nonspecific and antigen-specific forms. The three most common drugs used to disarm anti-graft immune responses are (1) corticosteroids, (2) azathioprine, and (3) cyclosporin A and/or FK506 (also called *tacrolimus*). Clinically, cyclosporin A and FK506 are the most important immunosuppressants used. They moved the chances for transplantation success from marginal to significant. It blocks IL-2-dependent proliferation and differentiation of T cells (detailed later). Studies evaluating the use of antibodies are providing new approaches to specific immunosuppression. The ideal strategy for preventing allograft rejection would be to remove the immune response to antigens on the graft while leaving intact the response

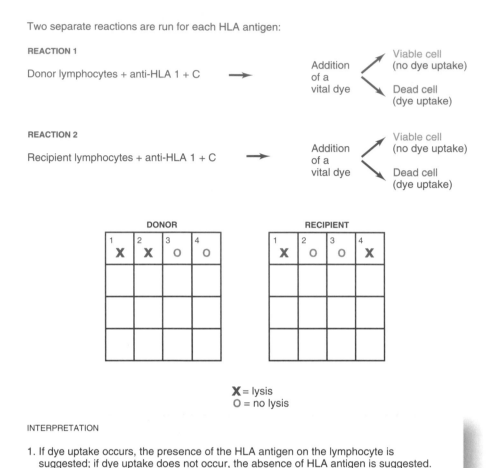

Two separate reactions are run for each HLA antigen:

REACTION 1

Donor lymphocytes + anti-HLA 1 + C ⟶ Addition of a vital dye ⟋ Viable cell (no dye uptake) ⟍ Dead cell (dye uptake)

REACTION 2

Recipient lymphocytes + anti-HLA 1 + C ⟶ Addition of a vital dye ⟋ Viable cell (no dye uptake) ⟍ Dead cell (dye uptake)

DONOR

| 1 | 2 | 3 | 4 |
|---|---|---|---|
| X | X | O | O |
| | | | |
| | | | |
| | | | |

RECIPIENT

| 1 | 2 | 3 | 4 |
|---|---|---|---|
| X | O | O | X |
| | | | |
| | | | |
| | | | |

**X** = lysis
O = no lysis

INTERPRETATION

1. If dye uptake occurs, the presence of the HLA antigen on the lymphocyte is suggested; if dye uptake does not occur, the absence of HLA antigen is suggested.
2. Compatible tissue is implied when there is either dye uptake in both reactions (presence of HLA antigen in both) or no dye uptake in either (no HLA antigen in either).

**FIGURE 14-8 Serologic tissue typing**. Wells of tissue typing plates contain typing antisera of defined specificity (such as anti-HLA 1 through 4, numbered 1 through 4 in the upper left corners of both square grids). Lymphocytes from the donor or recipient are added and incubated, complement is added, the cells are incubated further, and the viability dye trypan blue is added. Cell death (dye uptake leads to a "blue cell") confirms that the lymphocyte expresses the antigen in question.

to all other antigens. Although the current strategies potentially leave graft recipients vulnerable to opportunistic infections and some cancers, many of them lead normal, active lives.

## Downregulating the Immune System with Nonspecific Immunosuppressive Drugs

*Chemical immunosuppressants used to prolong graft survival can be placed in four main groups:* **corticosteroids, antiproliferatives, immunophilin inhibitors**, and **antibiotics**. Table 14-4 lists some popular chemical

immunosuppressive agents. All these agents are either directly or indirectly *antiproliferative* and, as such, affect the amplification both of the immune response so necessary for production of antibodies and of effector T cells needed in cell-mediated immune reactions. Furthermore, chemical immunosuppressants are effective in the treatment of cancer and autoimmune diseases (see Chapters 13 and 15). Immunosuppressive therapy cannot discriminate between immune and nonimmune cells or, more precisely, antigen-specific immune cells; therefore, the entire immune system is suppressed. Thus, the patient is not protected against explosive bacterial

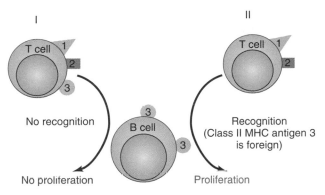

**FIGURE 14-9 Human tissue typing using the MLR.** Human homozygous typing cells (B lymphocytes), expressing known HLA-D class II antigens such as antigen 3, are mixed with test T lymphocytes. If the test cells (Group II) recognize foreign antigen, they undergo proliferation and transformation, signifying histoincompatibility.

and viral infections, an important cause of death in many immunosuppressed patients.

### Corticosteroids Are Anti-inflammatory Agents That Suppress the Immune Response

**Corticosteroids**, such as prednisone, hydrocortisone, and dexamethasone, are potent anti-inflammatory agents, which mediate their effects through binding intracellular steroid receptors found in most cells of the body. Once bound to the intracellular receptor, the complex translocates itself into the cell nucleus, interacts with specific transcription factors, and regulates gene transcription. The resulting immunosuppression is due to the decrease in multiple proinflammatory cytokine gene expressions, leading to diminished IL-1 through IL-5, IL-8, TNF-$\alpha$, and granulocyte-macrophage colony-stimulating factor (GM-CSF) production. Corticosteroids also downregulate all aspects of inflammation, from adhesion to migration to phagocytosis to killing mechanisms of phagocytes. They also diminish the expression of class II MHC molecules—corticosteroids suppress humoral and cell-mediated immunity. Unlike many of the other immunosuppressants, corticosteroids are effective whether or not the cell is in the replicative cycle.

As all other immunosuppressive drugs, corticosteroids are not without side effects and risks. The side effects include fluid retention, weight gain, diabetes, increased skin fragility, and reduced bone density. The corticosteroid efficacy is augmented and side effects reduced when corticosteroids are combined with other drugs. Currently, the corticosteroid prednisone, together with azathioprine, and

**TABLE 14-4 Chemical Immunosuppressants That Are Used to Delay or Prevent Graft Rejection**

**Steroids (corticosteroids)**
1. Prednisone
2. Hydrocortisone
3. Dexamethasone

**Antiproliferatives**
Alkylating Agents
1. Cyclophosphamide (Cytoxan)
2. Chlorambucil

Antimetabolites
1. Folic acid analogs
   a. Methotrexate (Amethopterin)
   b. Aminopterin
2. Purine analogs
   a. 6-Mercaptopurine (6-MP)
   b. Azathioprine (Imuran)
   c. Mycophenolate mofetil*
3. Pyrimidine analogs
   a. Leflunomide
   b. Cytosine arabinoside
   c. 5-Fluorouracil
   d. 5-Bromodeoxyuridine

**Immunophilin inhibitors**
1. Cyclosporin A
2. FK506 (tacrolimus)
3. Rapamycin (sirolimus)

**Antibiotics**
1. Actinomycin D
2. Mitomycin C
3. Puromycin

cyclosporin A, are the mainstays of organ transplantation immunosuppression. The latter two substances are discussed below.

### Chemical Anti-proliferative Drugs Strike at the Heart of an Immune Response, the Proliferation of Lymphocytes

These groups of drugs inhibit cell division; most of them derive their origin in the chemotherapeutic treatment of malignant diseases. Nonetheless, many are important to the delay and prevention of graft rejection. In the context of the development of a normal immune response, lymphocytes must go from few to many cells to provide immunity—they must proliferate. In contrast during transplantation, this process must be prevented to allow the survival of a lifesaving antigen, the graft. The potent drugs mentioned below target lymphocyte proliferation.

*Alkylating Agents Inhibit Cellular Division by Cross-Linking DNA Strands.* **Alkylating agents** interfere with some basic metabolic processes needed for cell division, differentiation, or protein synthesis. Alkylating agents are lymphocytolytic and antiproliferative, while the antimetabolites primarily inhibit cell division. Alkylating agents transfer alkyl groups to other substances such as nucleic acids and proteins. Their main effect is on DNA synthesis. The most vulnerable DNA site for attack by an alkylating agent is guanine. Alkylation of DNA can (1) cause guanine to behave as an analog of adenine (pairing errors); (2) break guanine from its sugar-phosphate backbone (purine gaps in the DNA); and (3) cross-link DNA strands (block DNA replication). Alkylating agents are sometimes called *radiomimetic agents* because they cause biologic actions similar to those caused by X-irradiation. Alkylating agents block proliferation and differentiation by tying DNA strands together. They are effective in the inductive phase or throughout the immune response.

Alkylating agents were the first known immunosuppressants. These agents were discovered in World War I when sulfur mustards were used in chemical warfare. A direct result was the development of *nitrogen mustard*. Nitrogen mustard is used infrequently because it is too toxic for oral administration. **Cyclophosphamide** is probably one of the most potent immunosuppressive drugs. To avoid side effects, another, less toxic alkylating agent is used: **chlorambucil**. Cyclophosphamide and chlorambucil have drastic effects on lymphoid tissues and can produce necrosis of lymphoid tissues in a few hours. Even though cyclophosphamide acts on both T and B cells, its selectivity for B cells makes it one of the most powerful inhibitors of antibody production (humoral immunity). Its action on cell-mediated immunity is less dramatic.

### Antimetabolites Are Impostor Molecules That Cause Faulty Cell Metabolism.

Antimetabolites function as antagonists of folic acid, purines, or pyrimidines. They resemble natural molecules but lead to faulty cell metabolism because they are unable to carry out their counterparts' function.

### Folic Acid Analogs Include Methotrexate and Aminopterin.

Folic acid is a widely distributed vitamin. Derivatives of folic acid are involved in one-carbon transfer reactions required for DNA synthesis, such as the conversion of deoxyuridylic acid to thymidilic acid. Examples of folic acid analogs are *methotrexate* (*amethopterin*) and *aminopterin*. Methotrexate and aminopterin compete for the substrates required by enzymes involved in the production of the folic acid derivative tetrahydrofolic acid, a carrier of one-carbon units essential to the synthesis of purines. Thus, methotrexate and aminopterin inhibit DNA synthesis. Methotrexate is better known as a cancer drug because it causes temporary remission of certain leukemias. The drug primarily suppresses cellular immunity but has some effects on humoral immune responses. The drug is more effective when given after antigen exposure. Aminopterin is structurally similar to methotrexate and has similar effects, but its therapeutic index (that is, the most effective dose of a drug) is lower.

### Purine Analogs Include Azathioprine and 6-Mercaptopurine.

Purines are nitrogenous bases found in nucleotides and nucleic acids. The two main purines are adenine and guanine. Synthetic purine analogs appear to block a stage of lymphocyte differentiation. They can act either as substitutes in base sequences or as competitive enzyme inhibitors. The results are a decreased rate of cell replication. Development of immunoblasts is affected because of the general changes in cellular DNA, RNA, and protein synthesis.

The two most common purine antimetabolites used in clinical practice are **azathioprine (Imuran)** and **6-mercaptopurine**, an analog of the purine guanine. Azathioprine and 6-mercaptopurine preferentially suppress primary antibody responses. They also are used successfully in the prevention of allograft rejection reactions.

### Pyrimidine Analogs Include Cytosine Arabinoside, 5-Fluorouracil, 5-Bromodeoxyuridine, and Leflunomide.

Pyrimidines, like purines, are nitrogenous bases. The three pyrimidines are thymine (found in DNA), cytosine (found in DNA and RNA), and uracil (found in RNA). Pyrimidine analogs (like purine analogs) (1) compete with enzymes involved in nucleotide synthesis, or (2) substitute for natural bases in nucleic acids. Pyrimidine analogs are **cytosine arabinoside, 5-fluorouracil,** and **5-bromodeoxyuridine. Leflunomide** is a pyrimidine synthesis inhibitor belonging to the disease-modifying anti-rheumatic drug (DMARD) class of drugs used in the treatment of rheumatic diseases. It inhibits dihydroorotate dehydrogenase, an enzyme involved in *de novo* pyrimidine synthesis. Recently, leflunomide was assigned orphan drug status for the prevention of solid organ rejection when co-administered with commonly used first-line agents. Interestingly, leflunomide also exhibits antiviral activity against cytomegalovirus, which is a hazard to immunosuppressed transplant patients.

### Microbial Peptides Have Immunosuppressive Activity

The most widely used immunosuppressants in anti-graft therapy are fungal metabolites. **Cyclosporin A**, used since 1983, is a cyclic polypeptide metabolite of the fungus *Tolypocladium inflatum*. Cyclosporin A differs from the other conventional immunosuppressive drugs because it is not lymphocytic and has no antimitotic activity. Another unique feature is its selectivity. Cyclosporin A's principal target is the $T_H$ cell. It specifically inhibits transcription of the IL-2 gene (other T-cell genes affected are c-*myc* and *IFN-γ*) by blocking a late stage of the signal pathway started by TCR engagement (discussed below) and thereby suppresses T-cell growth and differentiation without directly affecting antibody production or impairing marrow function. This result also prevents $T_C$-cell induction. In fact, cyclosporin A is more immunosuppressive than azathioprine, the drug most commonly used to suppress graft rejection. However, immunosuppression is reversible once cyclosporin A treatment is stopped. Cyclosporin A is not without toxicities and side effects. Toxicities are usually dose-dependent and reversible. Common side effects include nephrotoxic activity, hirsutism, tremors, hypertension, and gingival hypertrophy. Two additional microbial metabolites, **FK506** (also called *tacrolimus*) derived from soil *Streptomyces tsukubaensis* and **rapamycin** (also called *sirolimus*) derived from *Streptomyces hygroscopicus*, can prolong the survival of transplanted grafts. Although FK506 is totally different in structure from cyclosporin A, it functions in remarkably similar ways; however, its immunosuppressive potency is much greater than that of cyclosporin A and has less pronounced side effects. Specifically, cyclosporin A and FK506 block T-cell activation by first binding to molecules called *immunophilins* (peptidyl-prolyl *cis-trans* isomerases), the *cyclophilins* and *FK-binding proteins*, respectively. Either of the drug-immunophilin complexes can bind to the serine/threonine-specific phosphatase *calcineurin*, preventing its activation by calcium. Inactive calcineurin cannot dephosphorylate the cytosolic component of the transcription factor NF-AT, which is then unable to migrate to the nucleus and induce transcription of the IL-2 gene—the T cell activation, proliferation, and differentiation program is shutdown. Although rapamycin is structurally similar to FK506 and binds to the immunophilin FK-binding protein and then calcineurin, its immunosuppressive effects are distinct from those of FK506. The ultimate target protein for rapamycin is called the *mammalian target of rapamycin (mTOR)*; it inhibits T-cell proliferation by blocking the signaling pathway initiated by the IL-2 receptor ligation, rather than by the TCR. This blockade inhibits the transition of the cell cycle from $G_1$ to S phase. Rapamycin is used in combination with either FK506 or cyclosporine, thus minimizing its side effects.

### Some Antibiotics Can Suppress the Immune Response

Certain **antibiotics** (normally considered as antimicrobial agents) have immunosuppressive activity. They are **actinomycin D, mitomycin C**, and **puromycin**. These antibiotics inhibit DNA-directed synthesis of RNA (interfere with formation of mRNA), DNA replication (cross-link DNA strands), and protein synthesis (as an analog of esterified tRNA, they interfere with translation of mRNA), respectively.

## Downregulating the Immune System with Specific Polyclonal or Monoclonal Antibodies

One may also use biologic products of normal immune reactions, such as antibody, to suppress an immune response. Biologic agents of immunosuppression do not have the generalized toxic effects that chemical immunosuppressants do because they target specific lymphocytes.

### Polyclonal Antilymphocyte Serum: Killing T Lymphocytes with the Immune System's Own Antibodies

Antilymphocyte serum is an immune reagent that selectively reacts with lymphocytes. It is prepared by injecting rabbits or horses with human thymocytes or thoracic duct lymphocytes; therefore, antilymphocyte serum is also called *antithymocyte globulin* or *antilymphocyte globulin*. The combination of low toxicity and high potency endows antilymphocyte serum with a high therapeutic index. Because of its side effects (allergy-like symptoms and antigen-antibody complex localization in the kidneys), it has limited use in humans. Fractionating the serum into its IgG fraction can reduce these side effects. Also, *chimeric antibodies*, monoclonal antibodies (discussed next) engineered with mouse antigen-combining sites and human Fc, avoid the above problems. In addition, they are administered with other immunosuppressant to reduce their dosage and toxicity. Antilymphocyte serum acts primarily by two mechanisms: (1) depletion of circulating T cells and (2) inactivation of lymphocytic recognition receptors (coating of surface receptors). The administration of antilymphocyte serum is still used today to treat acute graft rejection.

### *Monoclonal Antibodies are Made to React to Specific Epitopes and Minimize their Own Immunogenicity*

The first mouse monoclonal antibody (OKT3), approved for human use, targeted T lymphocytes. It is an anti-human CD3 monoclonal that prevents T-cell activation and proliferation by binding the TCR complex, which leads to T cell depletion. Because of its potent immunosuppressive activity, it is clinically used to control the corticosteroid and/or polyclonal antibodies resistant acute rejection episodes. To reduce the immunogenicity of mouse monoclonal antibodies, mouse-human chimeric antibodies are engineered. Two such antibodies with specificity for the high-affinity IL-2 receptor α-chain (CD25), called *basiliximab* and *daclizamab*, are used clinically. Because only activated T cells express high-affinity IL-2 receptors, their use provides a selective immunosuppressive treatment that causes decreased survival of IL-2–activated T cells. Either antibody provides prophylactic treatment of acute organ rejection following bilateral kidney transplantation with few side effects.

The experimental use of monoclonal anti-CD4 antibodies induces long-lasting, antigen-specific tolerance. Other monclonal antibodies to cell-surface molecules, used to suppress antigraft reactivity, include anti-TCR Vβ domains, anti-adhesion molecules (such as, LAF-1, ICAM-1, and ICAM-2), and anti-B7-1 (CD80) and anti-B7-2 (CD86) antibodies; the latter antibodies block their ability to interact with CD28 to provide costimulatory activity to T cells. Fusion protein antibodies of CTLA-4 and the Fc portion of human immunoglobulin have been used to prolong graft survival, because when interacting with B7 molecules, CTLA-4 delivers inhibitory signals to the responding T cells. The blocking of another costimulatory molecule, CD40L (CD154) with CD40, by a chimeric mouse anti-CD40L monoclonal antibody prevents acute graft rejections. The last two approaches limit anti-graft rejection because they lead to anergic T cells.

Table 14-5 lists some ways in which immunosuppressants can act on the immune response. There are ongoing efforts to identify the dominant immunologic mechanism(s) involved in rejection of organ and tissue grafts and in autoimmune diseases. The ultimate goal is to develop pharmacologic agents that can suppress the specific immunologic mechanisms involved without bringing about more generalized suppression.

**TABLE 14-5 Possible Mechanisms for Immunosuppressant Alteration of the Immune Response**

1. Negate formation of precursor cells.
2. Inhibit immunocompetent cell production.
3. Block or destroy the immunocompetent cells.
4. Prevent or restrict effective contact.
5. Block phagocytic activity.
6. Inhibit biosynthesis of nucleic acids.
7. Block proliferation and differentiation.
8. Induce a regulatory cell response.

---

### MINI SUMMARY

There are four principal groups of chemical immunosuppressants used to prolong graft survival: (1) corticosteroids, (2) antiproliferatives, (3) immunophilin inhibitors, and (4) antibiotics. All are nonspecific suppressants that have limited effectiveness because of their dangerous side effects. The corticosteroid prednisone probably mediates its immunosuppressive activity by blocking cytokine production of susceptible lymphocytes and anti-inflammatory action. Cyclophosphamide and chlorambucil are alkylating agents, which cross-link DNA strands to prevent cellular division. Antimetabolites are represented by folic acid analogs such as methotrexate and aminopterin, purine analogs such as azathioprine and 6-mercaptopurine, and pyrimidine analogs such as cytosine arabinoside, 5-fluorouracil, 5-bromodeoxyuridine, and leflunomide. Antimetabolites mediate immunosuppression by acting as impostors of natural metabolites needed in the synthesis of DNA. Microbial peptides like cyclosporin A, FK506, and rapamycin selectively inhibit $T_H$ cell activation. Some antibiotics are immunosuppressants.

Biologic means of immunosuppression can involve antilymphocyte serum. Biologic agents such as antilymphocyte and antithymocyte serum are used as immunosuppressants because they do not have the generalized toxic effects of chemical immunosuppressants. Newer modalities of antibody treatment for graft rejection use chimeric mouse-human monoclonal antibodies to precisely target anti-graft lymphocytes and minimize their immunogenicity.

## PRIVILEGED TRANSPLANTS SURVIVE BECAUSE THEY ARE INACCESSIBLE TO THE IMMUNE SYSTEM; THE FETUS IS AN ALMOST PERFECT ALLOGRAFT

The rejection process is influenced not only by the immunogenicity of the grafted tissue but also by the location of the graft site. Sites such as the anterior eye chamber, the central nervous system, testes, placenta, and the cheek pouch of hamsters are called **privileged sites** because they allow prolonged to permanent survival of incompatible grafts. Grafts in these locations survive probably because of the lack of draining lymphatics and the scarcity of blood vessels in tissues surrounding these sites. Privilege was assumed to exist at these sites because of their anatomic location; however, more than physical barriers maintain the immune privilege, active immunosuppressive mechanisms play a role. Another reason may be that some tissues, **privileged tissues**, do not stimulate an immune response. Corneal grafts and cartilage grafts possess sialomucin, which masks their antigenic determinants.

The ultimate example of a privileged site and privileged tissue is the uterus and the fetus, respectively. A fetus carries both immunologically compatible self-antigens from its mother and foreign antigens from its father. Mothers can produce antibodies against fetal antigens, as seen in the production of anti-Rh antibodies by Rh⁻ mothers. Multiparous women have antibodies to the father's HLA. However, a fetus usually is not rejected—the mother's $T_C$ cells are kept in check.

The human embryo invades the highly vascular uterus and establishes a complex maternal parasitic relationship. Maternal acceptance results from the presence of a physical barrier (the placenta) and the placenta's ability to produce many immunosuppressive factors. Thus, the placenta presents an elaborate physical defense and modulates the mother's response to fetal tissues. As the fetal cell mass begins to penetrate the maternal decidua, the outermost trophoblasts seem to lose their class I and class II MHC antigens but expressed the HLA class Ib molecules, called *HLA-G*, and the apoptotic FasL. This loss of MHC, and the expression of HLA-G, antigens may permit penetration of the uterine wall without recognition of the cell mass as foreign. The fetal trophoblasts do not sensitize cell-mediated immune responses associated with allograft rejection. HLA-G is a ligand for the mother's NK cell inhibitory receptors (KIRs); therefore, her NK cells are preventing from killing fetal cells (see Chapter 10). HLA-G and FasL can induce apoptosis in maternal anti-fetal–reactive immune cells. There is a protective expansion of maternal CD4⁺CD25⁺ $T_{reg}$ cells during pregnancy, which can suppress an aggressive allogeneic response directed against the fetus. There is also an absence of placental dendritic cells. As placental development continues, the trophoblast differentiates into cytotrophoblasts and giant cells, which reside deep within the

decidua. Because of the large resulting area, which is continuously bathed by maternal blood, there is extensive exchange of nutrients and wastes and a region over which paternal antigens are exposed to the maternal immune system. This physical barrier, the differentiated trophoblast wall, may be the most important protective portion of the fetoplacental unit.

Control of the mother's immune response to the developing fetus's paternal antigens may be regulated by (1) nonspecific immunosuppressive molecules, (2) hormonal mediators, (3) blocking mechanisms, and (4) $T_{reg}$ cells. Nonspecific factors of immunosuppression include α-fetoprotein, hormones (cortisol, estrogen, and progesterone), pregnancy-associated glycoproteins (α₂-macroglobulin, β₁-glycoprotein, fetulin, and ovomucoid), and uromodulin. These molecules may all nonspecifically inhibit and decrease the general tone of maternal immune responses at the placental interface, where many of these substances are found in high concentrations. Because nonspecific suppressors may not be sufficient to stop presensitized effector T cells, specific blocking mechanism may be present. The absence of classical HLA antigens (class I and class II molecules) in the presence of inhibitory molecules (HLA-G and FasL) found on trophblasts, which inhibit maternal lymphocytes responding to paternal antigens. These blocking devices could obstruct the interaction of antigen with its appropriate immune cell and prevent or decrease sensitization. In fact, antigen-presenting placental dendritic cells are absent, which also could directly suppress the development of effector cell function. Lastly, the mother may suppress immune reactivity to the fetus's paternal antigens by inducing $T_{reg}$ cells. These cells would protect the fetus by suppressing $T_C$-cell activity, by decreasing antibody production, and by decreasing cytokine production.

## MINI SUMMARY

The closer the histocompatibility between recipient and donor, the easier it is to overcome the genetic rules of transplantation rejection. Differences in histocompatibility are determined by serologic (anti-class I MHC antigen antibodies plus complement, called a microcytotoxicity test) and *in vitro* (MLR) testing.

Because the recipient is receiving foreign antigens expressed by the graft, a normal functioning immune response must be suppressed. To prolong graft survival or prevent graft rejection, nonspecific and specific immunosuppressive drugs are used. The most used immunosuppressive cocktail to delay or prevent graft rejection includes corticosteroids, azathioprine, and cyclosporine A and/or FK506.

Some privileged sites and some privileged tissues allow successful transplantation or grafts (the eye chamber, the brain, and the uterus/fetus).

# MANY HUMAN ORGANS AND TISSUES CAN BE TRANSPLANTED, INCLUDING BLOOD, KIDNEYS, HEARTS, LIVERS, LUNGS, PANCREATA, CORNEAS, SKIN, AND BONE MARROW

Almost 400 years before the biologic basis of histocompatibility was established, the famous surgeon Gaspare Tagliacozzi of Bologna wrote "the singular character of the individual entirely dissuades us from attempting this work [organ transplantation] on another person." Therefore, it is not unlikely that since ancient times there have been attempts to replace worn-out or deformed parts with new ones obtained from unrelated donors. The grafts never survived. The immune system is the major obstacle to such grandiose ideas. Nonetheless, defective organs and tissues are being replaced with healthy ones. Usually, organs such as the heart, kidney, or liver or certain combinations of organs (heart/lung or kidney/pancreas) are acquired from just-deceased donors, but often a healthy living donor can contribute one kidney to someone else (see Table 14-2).

Transfusion of blood and blood products is the most familiar and most successful clinical application of transplantation in medicine to date (roughly 14 million units are used each year). Blood transfusion is an example of a transplant that is not from the dead to the living. Safe transfusion was not practical until physicians learned to identify and match the major blood cell antigens of the donor and recipient in such a way that the transfused cells were not seen as foreign and destroyed. The basic research defining the ABO blood group system supplied the basis for the development of typing technology. Such studies also constituted the basis for our understanding of the genetic compatibility needed for successful organ transplantation.

More than 40,000 transplants of the cornea are done in the United States each year. Improved microsurgery has made this a highly successful procedure for curing one form of blindness. Unlike most tissues, the cornea is not perfused with blood and lacks lymphatic drainage. However, some of these operations fail because of immunologic rejection. If the rejection response is treated early, injury to the transplanted cornea is frequently temporary. Several problems familiar to all transplantation operations pertain to corneal transplants. Choosing a donor (cadaver) that is right for the recipient, early testing to detect graft rejection, prompt treatment for any rejection reaction, and preserving of corneas at low temperature (eye bank) are measures guaranteeing an improved success rate.

Skin transplantation (perhaps the oldest form of tissue transplantation) is now used extensively in the treatment of burns. Autografts are commonly successful, and several recent advances provide promise of superior results using allografts. These include tissue typing, the donation of skin from family members to take advantage of genetic compatibility, improved control of infection, and the prudent use of drug therapy.

Thousands of patients die each year because of loss of function in a single organ. Innumerable other patients are disabled. Although prevention of the original disease would be preferable, a successful transplant can return the recipient to a near-normal condition of health and even to complete rehabilitation. General steps taken to evade rejection include the preservation of donor organs until suitable recipients are located and prepared for surgery, improved procedures for selection of donor-recipient pairs to lessen the likelihood of rejection (histocompatibility testing procedures were discussed earlier), and increasing the potential donor pool by improved exchange between distant transplant centers. These procedures apply to all forms of organ transplantation.

End-stage kidney disease kills more than 67,000 Americans each year; there were 17,092 and 924 kidney and kidney/pancreas transplants, respectively, performed in 2006. Dialysis by the artificial kidney can maintain patients with renal failure for extended periods but at considerable psychological, medical, and economic cost. Kidney transplantation has proved to be the preferable form of therapy when rehabilitation of the patient, amount of time (including medical attendants needed for patient upkeep), and costs are considered. When the donor is a sibling sharing the identical set of HLA antigens, more than 90% of the transplants survive for more than 2 years. Unfortunately, few kidney patients have an eligible sibling to act as a donor and must rely on high doses of potent drugs to restrain the immune response to protect the incompatible cadaver graft from rejection. Nonetheless, the usual five-year survival value for kidneys is 80–90%.

The proportion of incompatible kidneys surviving depends on many variables, including the age and clinical state of the patient. Success rates of over 70% for kidneys transplanted from cadaveric donors are reported in certain series.

The constant improvement in kidney transplant survival in recent years is due to many factors: (1) improved medical care for the patient before and after the transplant; (2) the use of tissue typing procedures to match donor and recipient and thus lessen rejection; (3) early detection and care of rejection occurrences; and (4) more skillful use of new drugs to avert rejection.

Heart transplants are not as successful as kidney transplants; there are roughly 2000 heart transplants per year in the United States (2,192 in 2006). Early heart transplants were not very successful; however, today, more than 7 out of 10 heart transplant recipients live for at least 5 years. Problems of impending rejection of heart transplants are compounded because end-stage heart disease patients do not have a support system comparable to hemodialysis, which will sustain a kidney transplant patient until a suitable donor can be found. The use of artificial devices is now of limited value.

Bone marrow is the source of cells giving rise to the red blood cells, lymphocytes, and other cells of the blood. Transplanting bone marrow (roughly 2,500 were done in 2004) is a procedure with widespread applicability, but it is not without risk to the patient. Allogeneic bone marrow transplantation has been used to treat aplastic anemia, congenital immunodeficiencies, and drug-resistant leukemia, most bone marrow transplants are done for leukemia.

Bone marrow cells are acquired with a needle from the pelvic bone while the volunteer donor is under anesthesia; the cells are then injected into a vein of the recipient. If the transplant is successful, the injected cells locate an environment inside the bones of the patient, multiply rapidly, and replenish the blood of the patient. An important problem with bone marrow transplantation is the development of a GvHR against the recipient's tissues. This problem can be reduced, if not eliminated, by cleansing the donor bone marrow of potentially dangerous mature T cells, leaving primarily hematopoietic stem cells.

Other organs have been transplanted, but with less overall success (even though a 70% success rate has been achieved at some medical centers), and such operations are usually empirical and last-ditch attempts. These organs include the liver

(6,650 transplants in 2006 with a 1-year survival rate of approximately 65%), lungs (1,405 transplants in 2006 with a 1-year survival rate of approximately 60%), intestines (175 transplants), and pancreas (462 transplants in 2006 with a 1-year survival rate of approximately 55%; offers a cure for type 1 diabetes). The lack of success with these organs is not due to difficulties in surgical techniques; instead, as with all transplants, the big problem is immune rejection. Patients needing these organs, however, usually face certain death without the transplant.

## MINI SUMMARY

Many examples exist of transplants in humans; the most familiar and most successful is blood transfusion. Many human organs are now successfully transplanted, particularly kidneys and hearts. Cornea, skin, and bone marrow transplants are also widely performed, but other organs have a less successful transplant record.

# SUMMARY

Many situations demand transplanting of a tissue or an organ to a recipient whose tissue or organ is nonfunctional. The most important barrier to a successful transplant is the immunologic recognition and rejection of the graft. The immune system treats a kidney as a foreign invader rather than a life-saving organ. Transplantation immunologists usually use two approaches to reduce immune reactivity: selection of recipient-donor combinations in which predictable immunogenic differences and the resulting immune response are minimal and suppression of the immunologic responsiveness of the recipient. The latter protocol involves detrimental effects.

Grafts are defined according to the genetic relationship between donor and recipient. Transplants on the same individual or between identical twins, known as *autografts* and *syngrafts*, respectively, are usually successful. All other grafts—*allografts* between nonidentical members of the same species and *xenografts* between species—are usually rejected.

Cell-surface antigens (*alloantigens*) responsible for eliciting rejection are called *transplantation antigens* or *class I MHC antigens*. These highly polymorphic antigens are found on all nucleated cells. Genes that code for these antigens are found in the MHC, the H-2, or the *HLA complexes* of mice and humans, respectively.

Graft rejection is an immune response that exhibits memory and specificity, a primary response called *first set rejection* and secondary response called *second set rejection*. Rejection of transplanted tissue or an organ can take four different forms: *hyperacute graft rejection, acute rejection, chronic graft rejection*, and *graft-versus-host reaction (GvHR)*; the latter can lead to *graft-versus-host disease (GvHD)*. The MHC determines the fate of a transplant because this complex contains the genes that encode the class I and class II antigens. Class I MHC antigens also are called *serologically defined (SD) antigens*. Even though antibodies are produced against class I MHC molecules, they are not the primary mediators of graft rejection. Class II MHC antigens also are called *lymphocyte-defined (LD) antigens* because they are detected by their ability to stimulate the mixed lymphocyte reaction (MLR). Class II MHC antigens are primarily found in antigen-presenting cells (APCs), such as, B cells, macrophages, and dendritic cells. If $T_C$ cells need help from $T_H$ cells, and if $T_H$ cells are activated by class II MHC antigens, what activates $T_H$ cells when exposed to a graft? Activation may be caused by immune cells called *passenger leukocytes*, the APCs, that is, dendritic cells that contaminate a graft.

Cytotoxic T cells do not need to recognize foreign class I MHC antigens in association with self-MHC molecules to be stimulated. Obsession of T cells with foreign MHC antigens is called *alloreactivity*. Alloreactivity seems to be a matter of cross-reactivity. The *in vitro* model for alloreactivity is the *mixed lymphocyte reaction (MLR)*. The MLR measures the histocompatibility antigen difference between recipient and donor. The greater the difference, the higher the proliferation or MLR reactivity and the greater the chance of the recipient's rejecting the donor tissue or organ.

To minimize rejection, before transplantation the HLA antigens of the donor and the recipient must be identified to determine how closely they match. First, they are blood typed and cross-matched. Second, there are two important methods of detecting histoincompatibility. Class I MHC antigens are determined by serologic methods using antigen-specific antibody plus complement. The MLR is used to mimic the cell-cell interactions determined by LD antigens (class II MHC molecules). In either approach, the closer the similarity of class I and class II MHC antigens, the better the chance of graft survival. In addition to the immunogenicity of grafted tissue, the grafting site (*privileged site*) and the type of tissue grafted (*privileged tissue*) affect the rejection process.

Allograft survival is prolonged by *nonspecific* and *specific immunosuppression*. Immunosuppression may occur by inoculation of chemical or biologic agents. Many drugs reduce immunologic responsiveness. The chemical immunosuppressants or drugs that prolong graft survival can be divided into four groups: (1) *corticosteroids*, (2) *antiproliferatives*, (3) *immunophilin inhibitors*, and (4) *antibiotics*. Biologic immunosuppression of an antigraft response can occur by treatment with antilymphocyte serum. Biologic agents such as antilymphocyte sera are potent immunosuppressive agents that have the added benefit of directly affecting only lymphocytes. Chimeric mouse-human monoclonal antibodies maintain precise immune cell targeting but reduce their immunogenicity.

Many human organs and tissues can be transplanted. Blood transfusions are the most familiar and successful, followed by kidney transplants; other transplants include hearts, corneas, skin, and bone marrow. Because most graft antigens between the recipient and donor are not identical, the recipient receives immunosuppressive therapy which can limit or, even better, prevent graft rejection. Immunosuppression is nonspecific and affects all dividing cells. This characteristic is responsible for the noxious effects of immunosuppressive drugs.

# SELF-EVALUATION

## RECALLING KEY TERMS

**Acute graft rejection**
**Allograft**
**Alloreactivity**
**Antibiotics**
    **Actinomycin D**
    **Mitomycin C**
    **Puromycin**
**Antiproliferatives**
    **Alkylating agents**
        **Chlorambucil**
        **Cyclophosphamide**
    **Antimetabolic agents**
        **Folic acid analogs**
            **Aminopterin**
            **Methotrexate (or amethopterin)**
        **Purine analogs**
            **Azathioprine (or Imuran)**
            **6-Mercaptopurine**
        **Pyrimidine analogs**
            **Cytosine arabinoside**
            **5-Bromodeoxyuridine**

5-Fluorouracil
Leflunomide
Autograft
Chronic graft rejection
Class I MHC antigens
Class II MHC antigens
Corticosteroids
First set rejection
Graft-versus-host disease (GvHD)
Graft-versus-host reaction (GvHR)
Histocompatibility
Human leukocyte antigen (HLA) complex
Hyperacute graft rejection
Immunophilin inhibitors
    Cyclosporin A
    FK506
    Rapamycin
Immunosuppression
    Nonspecific
    Specific
Mixed lymphocyte reaction (MLR)
Passenger leukocytes
Privileged sites
Privileged tissues
Second set rejection
Syngraft
Transplant or graft
Transplantation (or grafting)
Transplantation immunity
Xenograft

## MULTIPLE-CHOICE QUESTIONS

*(An answer key is not provided, but the page[s] location of the answer is.)*

1. Which of the following is not an immunologically privileged site? (a) brain, (b) glomerulus of the kidney, (c) hamster cheek pouch, (d) cornea, (e) none of these. *(See page 479.)*

2. Which of the following grafts is most likely to be rejected by a host-versus-graft rejection? (a) a heterotopic autograft, (b) a syngraft, (c) an adult lymphocyte graft into a neonatally thymectomized mouse, (d) a graft of an $F_1$ to an $F_2$ from a highly inbred strain of mice, (e) a skin graft of a boy onto his twin sister, (f) none of these. *(See pages 461 and 463.)*

3. Histocompatibility testing before human grafts (a) is related to the HLA antigens, (b) may be performed by the mixed lymphocyte culture technique, (c) may be performed using specific antisera to histocompatibility antigens, (d) all of these, (e) none of these. *(See pages 469, 471, and 473.)*

4. Purified lymphocytes from the donor and the recipient are mixed in a tissue culture medium for the (a) triple response, (b) MLR, (c) agglutination assay, (d) none of these. *(See page 469.)*

5. Which of the following is true concerning donor-recipient matching for transplantation? (a) failure of a graft from an identical twin is never due to HLA mismatch, (b) matching of HLA-D is less important than matching of HLA-A or HLA-B, (c) a potential donor is suggested if the recipient has preexisting antibodies to the donor's HLA antigens, (d) ABO erythrocyte compatibility is not essential, (e) none of these. *(See pages 462 and 463.)*

6. Tissue grafts, except those between genetically identical individuals, (a) are generally rejected in 5–7 days, (b) are rejected due to the formation of antibodies, (c) can survive for months even if not matched at all histocompatibility antigens, (d) are prolonged by bursectomy in the fowl, (e) are called syngrafts, (f) none of these. *(See pages 463, 464, and 478.)*

7. The responder cells in an MLR culture are normally irradiated or treated with mitomycin-C. (a) true, (b) false. *(See page 470.)*

8. Which of the following statements does not apply to tissue grafting? (a) if tissues from the same donor are then reapplied to the same recipient, the rejection occurs more quickly, (b) graft rejections reveal the specificity characteristic of immunologic phenomena, (c) the rejection state can be transferred from an immune subject to a normal recipient using phagocytic cells, (d) none of these. *(See pages 461–463.)*

9. A patient needs to find a kidney donor. Several donor types are listed below. Whom would you recommend? (a) father, (b) mother, (c) siblings, (d) distant relative, (e) friend, (f) none of these. *(See pages 463 and 467.)*

10. Consider two inbred strains of mice; their mother has the genotype AA and their father has the genotype BB. In this example, grafts transplanted from the mother or father to the $F_1$ generation are accepted. (a) true, (b) false. *(See page 463.)*

11. In humans, grafts from parents to children are usually rejected. (a) true, (b) false. *(See pages 463 and 467.)*

12. In human kidney transplants, which of the following has the best survival rate? (a) when the donor is HLA-DR matched and unrelated, (b) when the donor is a HLA-matched sibling, (c) when the donor is a HLA-mismatched sibling,

(d) when the donor is HLA-mismatched and unrelated, (e) none of these. *(See pages 463 and 467.)*

**13.** Antimetabolites function as antagonists of (a) folic acid and adenylic acid, (b) purines and pyrimidines only, (c) thymine and thymidilic acid, (d) folic acid, purines, and pyrimidines, (e) none of these. *(See pages 475 and 476.)*

**14.** Cyclosporin A (a) is cytotoxic for CD4$^+$ T cells, (b) induces a decrease in the number of T cells, (c) primarily affects helper T cells, (d) competes with IFN-$\gamma$ and IL-2, (e) none of these. *(See pages 476 and 477.)*

## SHORT-ANSWER ESSAY QUESTIONS

**1.** What do we mean when we say that the immune system is the greatest obstacle to most transplants?

**2.** What is the difference between an autograft and a syngraft? Give examples of both.

**3.** How do we know that the immune system is involved in allograft rejection? Are antibodies or T cells the main mediators of rejection?

**4.** Summarize the five transplantation laws for graft survival. Briefly discuss an exception: the transplant of tissue between genetically identical individuals of different sexes. In the following examples, the two strains of mice are: strain 1 = AA genotype, strain 2 = BB genotype. Will the grafts be accepted (indicate if only some would be) or rejected (indicate if only some would be) in each of the following?

| Donor | Recipient |
| --- | --- |
| Strain 1 | F$_1$ progeny |
| F$_1$ progeny | Strain 2 |
| Strain 1 | Strain 1 |
| Strain 1 | Strain 2 |
| F$_2$ progeny | F$_1$ progeny |
| F$_1$ progeny | Strain 1 |
| Strain 1 | F$_2$ progeny |
| F$_1$ progeny | F$_2$ progeny |

**5.** Compare and contrast first set rejection and second set rejection. What does second set rejection suggest about the similarity of transplantation antigens?

**6.** What conditions could lead to a GvHR?

**7.** Even though class II MHC molecules are found mainly on immune cells, they can still contribute to graft rejection. How?

**8.** Discuss the controversy about whether cytotoxic T cells are the cells responsible for graft rejection.

**9.** What may be the biologic significance of alloreactivity?

**10.** Describe serologic tissue typing.

**11.** Describe the MLR. Why is this test done in addition to serological tissue typing?

**12.** What is the difference between specific and nonspecific immunosuppression? List some complications of nonspecific immunosuppression.

**13.** Most immunosuppressive drugs are also used as anticancer drugs. Explain.

**14.** Why is antilymphocyte serum considered to be the first truly immunosuppressive agent? What are some of the problems in using it?

**15.** Distinguish between privileged sites and privileged tissues.

## FURTHER READINGS

Afzali, B., G. Lombardi, and R.I. Lechler. 2008. Pathways of major histocompatibility complex allorecognition. *Curr. Opin. Organ Transplant.* 13:438–444.

Alegre, M.L., D.R. Goldstein, and A.S. Chong. 2008. Toll-like receptor signaling in transplantation. *Curr. Opin. Organ Transplant.* 13:358–365.

Clift, R., and R. Storb. 1987. Histoincompatible bone marrow transplants in humans. *Annu. Rev. Immunol.* 5:43–64.

Dinavahi, R., and P.S. Heeger. 2008. T-cell immune monitoring in organ transplantation. *Curr. Opin. Organ Transplant.* 13:419–424.

Halloran, P.F. 2004. Immunosuppressive drugs for kidney transplantation. *New Engl. J. Med.* 351:2715–2729.

Hunt, S.A., and F. Haddad. 2008. The changing face of heart transplantation. *J. Am. Coll. Cardiol.* 52:587–598.

Lafferty, K., S.J. Prowse, C.J. Simeonovic., and H.S. Warren. 1983. Immunobiology of tissue transplantation: A return to the passenger leukocyte concept. *Annu. Rev. Immunol.* 1:143–173.

Lechler, R.I., O.A. Garden, and L.A. Turka. 2003. The complementary roles of deletion and regulation in transplantation tolerance. *Nat. Rev. Immunol.* 3:147–158.

Martin, P.J., J.A. Hannen, R. Storb, and E.D. Thomas. 1987. Human marrow transplantation: An immunological perspective. *Adv. Immunol.* 40:379–438.

Mason, D.W., and P.J. Morris. 1986. Effector mechanisms in allograft rejection. *Annu. Rev. Immunol.* 4:119–145.

Murray, J.E. 1992. Human organ transplantation: Background and consequences. *Science* 256:1411–1416.

Ricordi, C., and T.B. Strom. 2004. Clinical islet transplantation: Advances and immunological challenges. *Nat. Rev. Immunol.* 4:259–268.

Sayegh, M.H., and C.B. Carpenter. 2004. Transplantation 50 years later—progress, challenges, and promises. *New Engl. J. Med.* 351:2761–2766.

Schiopu, A., and K.J. Wood. 2008. Regulatory T cells: Hypes and limitations. *Curr. Opin. Organ Transplant.* 13:333–338.

Sherman, L.A., and S. Chattopadhyay. 1993. The molecular basis of allorecognition. *Annu. Rev. Immunol.* 11:385–402.

Shevach, E. 1985. The effects of cyclosporin A on the immune system. *Annu. Rev. Immunol.* 3:397–423.

Starzl, T.E., and R.M. Zinkernagel. 2001. Transplantation tolerance from a historical perspective. *Nat. Rev. Immunol.* 1:233–239.

Sykes, M., M. Auchincloss Jr., and D.H. Sachs. 2003. Transplantation immunology. In *Fundamental Immunology*, 5th ed. W.E. Paul, ed. Philadelphia: Lippincott Williams & Wilkins. p. 1481–1556.

Turnquist, H.R., and A.W. Thomson. 2008. Taming the lions: Manipulating dendritic cells for use as negative cellular vaccines in organ transplantation. *Curr. Opin. Organ Transplant.* 13:350–357.

Waldmann, H., and S. Cobbold. 2004. Exploiting tolerance processes in transplantation. *Science* 305:209–212.

Walsh, P.T., T.B. Strom, and L.A. Turka. 2004. Routes to transplant tolerance versus rejection: Role of cytokines. *Immunity* 20:121–131.

Yang, Y-G., and M. Sykes. 2007. Xenotransplantation: Current status and a perspective on the future. *Nat. Rev. Immunol.* 7:519–531.

# CHAPTER FIFTEEN

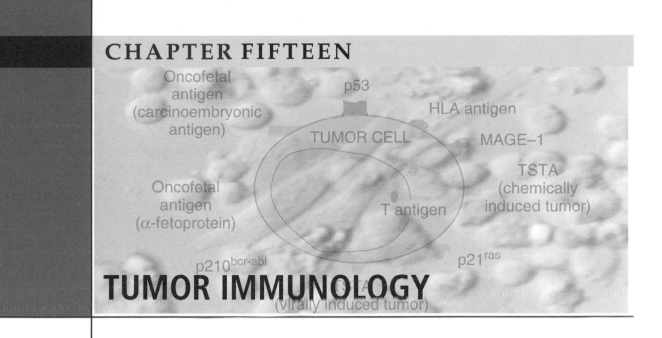

Oncofetal antigen (carcinoembryonic antigen)

p53

HLA antigen

TUMOR CELL

MAGE–1

TSTA (chemically induced tumor)

Oncofetal antigen (α-fetoprotein)

T antigen

p210^bcr-abl

p21^ras

# TUMOR IMMUNOLOGY
(virally induced tumor)

## CHAPTER OUTLINE

1. Early theories about the connections between tumor growth and tumor immunity were supported by later studies.

2. While cancers are made up of immortal cells, they usually are not deadly until they move.

3. Even though environmental factors are identifiable causes of cancer, cancers are mainly a dysfunction of genes.

   a. Human cancers can be caused by chemicals, radiation, and viruses.

   b. Cancer genes derail normal cell growth.

      1) Oncogene-associated activities established the existence of a genetic component to cancer.

      2) Even though oncogenes are cancer-causing genes and proto-oncogenes are not, they both function as cell-growth regulators.

      3) Are oncogenes villains or accomplices in tumor progression?

      4) The loss or inactivation of the oncogene's mirror image, the tumor suppressor gene, can lead to cancer.

4. Genetic dysregulation of immune cells can lead to immune system neoplasms.

5. Tumors are characterized by their associated antigens.

   a. There are three types of experimental tumors: chemically and physically induced, virally induced, and spontaneously occurring.

   b. There are two general types of antigens associated with tumor cells: tumor-specific and tumor-associated.

6. Immune surveillance refined, now called immunoediting, explains how the immune system both protects against, and promotes, cancer development.

7. Cellular immunity against tumors involves different cells and their weapons.

   a. Cytotoxic T lymphocytes are specific killers.

   b. NK cells are natural, nonspecific tumor killers.

   c. Macrophages are nonspecific killers "activated" to pursue tumor cells but are subverted to promote tumor initiation and progression.

    d. Dendritic cells are more than sentinels that sense tumor cells and alert effector cells; they can be directly tumoricidal.

    e. B lymphocytes are indirect killers through antibody production.

**8.** Tumors camouflage themselves to evade antitumor defenses.

**9.** Immunotherapy involves fighting cancer by using our built-in pharmacy of molecules and cells.

    a. Specific immunotherapy uses tumor vaccines or "magic bullets".

    b. Nonspecific immunotherapy works by boosting existing host mechanisms.

## OBJECTIVES

The reader should be able to:

**1.** Understand the relationship between cancer and immunology.

**2.** Describe an experiment that shows immunity to syngeneic tumors.

**3.** Define tumor, neoplasm, transformation, malignancy, and metastasis.

**4.** Differentiate between a benign tumor and a malignant tumor.

**5.** List the causes of cancers and briefly describe.

**6.** Understand the idea that cancer is a dysfunction of genes; differentiate between oncogenes and proto-oncogenes; differentiate between oncogenes and tumor suppressor genes.

**7.** Realize that transfection of DNA demonstrated the link between cancer and DNA.

**8.** Describe how oncogene-encoded proteins may act; explain the importance of protein kinases.

**9.** Distinguish between tumor-specific antigens (TSA) and tumor-associated antigens (TAA); discuss the major difference between virally induced and chemically induced tumor antigens; describe oncofetal antigens.

**10.** Appreciate the concept of cancer immunoediting and its three phases.

**11.** Evaluate the contribution of T cells, NK cells, macrophages, dendritic cells, and B cells to tumor immunity.

**12.** List the different ways tumors can camouflage themselves to evade immune defenses.

**13.** Describe the advantages of immunotherapy over other forms of cancer therapy; distinguish between specific and nonspecific immunotherapy; describe the use of monoclonal antibodies.

All cells of the body are descendants of ancestral precursor stem cells. Cells must proliferate and differentiate to mature. This process leads to specialized cells with new characteristics and functions. In adulthood, the process reaches a balance between multiplication and differentiation. Normally, this process is carefully regulated, but sometimes a cell escapes the strict controls and starts multiplying continuously. Eventually many immature, dividing cells are produced and form a cancer. The qualities of proliferation and differentiation are essentially all that distinguishes a normal cell from a cancer cell. *Cancer is a disorder of cell division*. Metaphorically, cancer is a disorganized and, in the end, a disastrous attempt by some cells to return to their freewheeling days of fetal life. This behavior does not escape the immune system's attention, in fact, as early as 1863 Rudolf Virchow noted that the immune system sent leukocyte emissaries to infiltrate tumors, which he believed represented a host attempt to eradicate cancer cells.

Roughly 45 years later, at the turn of the 20th century, Paul Ehrlich stated that the science of immunology might have a bearing on curing cancer (he called tumors "aberrant germs"). Because of the specificity of the immune system, a tumor should be destroyed immunologically without destruction of normal tissue—a concept that is at the heart of immunotherapy (discussed later). In cancer, the neoplastic cells that result from the transformation of normal body cells escaping intrinsic controls have become immunogenically altered self-cells that are now exposed to extrinsic controls; they are recognized as foreign by the immune system—a process called *immunosurveillance*. If immunologic responses are started, the cancer cells may be destroyed. These responses may occur frequently throughout life, but in a cancer patient they are often ineffective, even though they have tumor-specific lymphocytes in circulation, in draining lymph nodes, and *in situ*. Detectable tumors may represent rare occasions when cancer cells escape destruction due to selection of tumor-cell variants that display reduced immunogenicities or when the immune response has become ineffective in rejecting cancerous cells as they arise because of tumor-induced suppressive mechanisms.

This chapter discusses the characteristics of cancer cells and how our immune system can counterattack by recognizing cancer cells' markers. Immune cells also eliminate many tumors before they gain a foothold. Several different mechanisms that may explain how tumors evade immunologic destruction and the different aspects of cancer immunotherapy also are discussed.

# EARLY THEORIES ABOUT THE CONNECTIONS BETWEEN TUMOR GROWTH AND TUMOR IMMUNITY WERE SUPPORTED BY LATER STUDIES

The study of tumor immunology began at the turn of the 20th century. Early experiments involved transplanting tumors to non-tumor-bearing mice, where the grafted tumor would initially grow, then shrink, and eventually disappear. This result led to the erroneous conclusion that the tumor cures represented specific immune responses to tumor-specific antigens. However, inbred strains of mice were not available at that time. In the 1930s, Peter Gorer showed that the rejection of transplanted tumors follows the laws of transplantation (see Chapter 14). Because the recipient recognized foreign surface antigens on the donor's cells, the immune response to the grafted tumor was caused by allogeneic differences. This idea opened the door for studies on the major histocompatibility complex (MHC), but closed it (until the 1950s) for studies correlating the resistance of tumor growth and the immune system. If tumor antigens cause tumor rejection, then the immune system need only detect the antigens. The transfer of tumors between genetically identical animals demonstrated this claim. Transplanting a tumor from a rat to a mouse transfers not only unique tumor antigens but also transplantation antigens. What causes rejection? If a tumor transplant between two identical strain A mice leads to destruction of the tumor, then the rejection may be caused by the immune cells' recognition of unique tumor antigens.

The modern era of tumor immunology started in the 1950s with the work of Foley and of Prehn and Main, who found that mouse carcinogen-induced transplantable tumors could be immunogenic for their hosts. They inoculated mice with tumors, excised the tumors several days later, and then exposed these mice and tumor-naïve syngeneic mice to the same tumor cells; the results would be either that the tumor grows and kills the animal or that it grows and regresses. If these tumors are injected into allogeneic recipients, they are rejected as allografts. Figure 15-1 presents the experimental approach used by Prehn and Main to show tumor immunity to syngeneic tumors. This experimental approach showed that tumor rejection involved the hallmarks of adaptive immunity—specificity and memory. These results led to the reformulation by Thomas in 1959 of the theory of immune surveillance proposed by Paul Ehrlich in 1909. Nonetheless, subsequent experiments bred an era of skepticism because naturally induced (spontaneous) rodent tumors were found to be nonimmunogenic. It was not until experiments of the early 1980s, which showed that the inability of the host's immune system to reject tumors was not due to the lack of tumor immunogenicity—that is, the absence of tumor-rejection antigens—but the inability of the growing tumor to activate the immune system. Once the immune system was activated, it could reject the so-called nonimmunogenic tumor; however, it was not until the 1990s that studies using gene-targeting, transgenic mouse technologies, and the ability to produce blocking monoclonal antibodies to immune system components, that the relationship between innate and adaptive immunity and cancer became testable in unequivocal, molecularly defined murine models and lead to the validation of the cancer immunosurveillance concept (detailed later in the chapter).

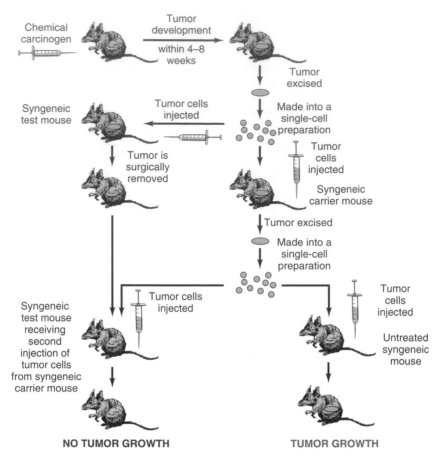

**FIGURE 15-1 Demonstration of immunity to syngeneic tumors.** Prehn and Main performed an adoptive transfer of chemically induced tumor cells to tumor-exposed and unexposed syngeneic mice to prove animals develop immunity against autochthonous tumors.

# WHILE CANCERS ARE MADE UP OF IMMORTAL CELLS, THEY USUALLY ARE NOT DEADLY UNTIL THEY MOVE

The physiology of normal mature tissues and organs is maintained by the generation of adequate cell numbers (no small task since the human body consists of roughly $10^{13}$ cells) to offset dying cells. The proliferation and differentiation of cells is tightly monitored and regulated by cell-cycle checkpoints to preserve constant numbers. Nuclear alterations of these cells, which lead to changes in signaling pathways that control homeostatic cell growth, cell survival, and cell death, perturb normal cellular functions and start the events in early carcinogenesis—the development of cancer. The cell-intrinsic characteristics associated with these cellular events include the ability for the cells to provide their own growth signals, ignore growth-inhibitory signals, evade apoptosis, induce ceaseless growth, support angiogenesis, and invade surrounding tissues. Cancer is not just a cell disease but also an organismal disease; therefore, an additional hallmark of cancer development has been proposed—the avoidance of innate and adaptive immune responses.

*Conversion of a normal, nondividing mature cell into one with uncontrollable growth leads to a* **tumor** (L., from *tumere*, to swell) *or* **neoplasm** (Gr., *neos*, new; *plasma*, thing formed). Some neoplasms, such as leukemias, do not form tumors. The terms *tumor, neoplasm,* and *cancer* refer to uncontrollable cellular growth and are therefore used interchangeably. *The term* **transformation** *signifies this conversion.* Tumors are either benign or malignant. Because malignant cancers can invade surrounding tissues, they present a greater danger. Ultimately, malignant cancers spread from their site of first appearance (the primary tumor) throughout the body (secondary tumors), but benign tumors do not.

The primary tumor is usually not the threat to the cancer patient. A cancer patient dies from the **malignancy** of a cancer. *The three principal characteristics of malignancy are (1) sustained cell division, (2) reversion of structure and metabolic activity to a more primitive or embryonic form (anaplasia),*[1] *and (3) cell migration* (**metastasis**). Continuous cancer cell multiplication spawns billions of similar cells, which constitute the tumor mass. In fact, tumor cells become immortal. They show a different shape and outer membrane, display new antigens recognized by the immune system, and rely to an unusual extent on anaerobic metabolism. Although uncontrollable cell division is common to both benign and malignant cancers, anaplasia and metastasis distinguish these two kinds of tumors.

A primary tumor can be either benign or malignant (Table 15-1). A **benign tumor**—a solid neoplasm—remains similar in structure to the tissue from which it was derived. A benign tumor grows slowly, by simple expansion, and remains encapsulated by a layer of connective tissue; its cell nuclei divide almost normally, with few chromosomal abnormalities—they are not cancerous. In contrast, a **malignant tumor** is usually atypical in tissue structure, grows rapidly, does not remain encapsulated, and displays many nuclear division and chromosomal abnormalities. Furthermore, a malignant tumor invades the surrounding normal tissue and sheds cells that can colonize new sites. This ability to invade surrounding tissue and colonize distant sites, known as *metastasis*, defines a solid malignant/invasive tumor or **cancer.** Cancer metastasis is a complex, long series of sequential, interrelated events involving the interaction between malignant cells from the primary tumor and the surrounding normal cells. A possible sequential scenario is listed in Table 15-2. Ninety percent of human cancer deaths are due to the effects of metastases.

Cancers can arise in most differentiated cells and are classified according to the cell in which they originate, leading to over 200 different forms of cancers (such as, hepatomas, cancers of liver cells [hepatocytes] or melanomas, cancers of pigment-producing

**TABLE 15-1 Difference between a Benign and Malignant Tumor**

| Benign tumor | Malignant tumor |
|---|---|
| Encapsulated | Nonencapsulated |
| Noninvasive | Invasive |
| Highly differentiate | Tendency toward de-differentiation |
| "Slow" growth | Usually rapid growth |
| Little or no anaplasia | Anaplasia to varying degrees |
| No metastases | May metastasize |

melanocytes). The different forms of cancers are classified into three groups according to the tissue they are derived from, but most of them fall into three general categories: carcinomas, sarcomas, and lymphomas/leukemias (see the *Glossary* for definitions of different types of cancers). **Carcinomas** are malignant tumors derived from epithelial cells, such as, skin or the lining of internal organs or glands. Carcinomas are the most common group of cancers (>80% of cancers), including breast, colon, lung, and prostate cancer. Roughly 9% of cancers in the United States are represented by **lymphomas** and **leukemias**, which are derived from hematopoietic stem cells in the bone marrow. Lymphomas begin in lymphocytes and tend to grow as tumor masses; some exceptions exist, for example, plasma cell neoplasms. Leukemias start in the bone marrow in lymphoid or myeloid lineages, proliferate as single cells, and release large numbers of abnormal blood cells into the bloodstream. The cancer with the lowest incidence (roughly 1%) in the United States is **sarcomas.** They are derived from mesodermal connective tissue (such as blood vessels, bone, cartilage, fat, and muscle).

## MINI SUMMARY

The connection between tumor growth and tumor immunity was made by experimental tumor transplants and by Ehrlich's 1909 proposal of immune surveillance. During the 1950s, the immunogenicity of tumors was demonstrated but it took until the 1990s to definitely validate the concept of immune surveillance.

Transformation is the change from a normal cell to a cancer cell. Tumors are classified as either benign or malignant. Benign tumors are slowly growing, localized, and noninvasive, while malignant tumors are rapidly growing and metastasize.

---

[1]Anaplasia means, "to form backward"; therefore, it suggests dedifferentiation, or the loss of functional and structural normal cell differentiation. However, some cancers can arise from individual cancer stem cells; therefore, the failure of differentiation of these tumor cells accounts for undifferentiated tumors.

**TABLE 15-2 Cancer Metastasis**

1. Primary tumor cells progressive grow, initially receiving nutrients by diffusion, and extend into surrounding tissues. As proliferation grows the tumor mass beyond 1–2 mm in diameter, extensive vascularization (*angiogenesis*) must occur.
2. Tumor cells then detach and penetrate the body cavities and vessels, such as lymphatics, venules, and capillaries.
3. Tumor cells detach from vessel wall and form either single-cell or aggregate emboli, which can interact with lymphocytes and platelets. Most circulating tumor cells are rapidly destroyed; ones that survive the circulation are arrested in organs (such as, metastatic breast cancer localizes mainly in the lung or bone marrow). They are trapped in the distant organ's capillary beds by adhering to capillary endothelial cells.
4. Traveling tumor cells reinvade tissue (*extravasation*) at the site of arrest.
5. They then manipulate the new microenvironment to promote tumor cell survival, vascularization (*angiogenesis*), and tumor growth in organ parenchyma.
6. This process is repeated until it is either stopped by treatment or the host dies.

---

Malignancy is characterized by sustained cell division, reversion of structure and metabolic activity to a less differentiated form, and cell migration. The general term cancer is usually applied to malignant tumors.

Cancers are grouped into three types, carcinomas, lymphomas and leukemias, and sarcomas, depending on their cell of origin.

---

# EVEN THOUGH ENVIRONMENTAL FACTORS ARE IDENTIFIABLE CAUSES OF CANCER, CANCERS ARE MAINLY A DYSFUNCTION OF GENES

Carcinogenesis is a complex process that arises when a cell acquires growth advantages through a multi-step accumulation of changes in gene function. The alterations in the cell's genetic material transform the cell into a cancer cell. These alterations may be due to environmental factors such as chemicals, radiation, and infection by tumorigenic viruses, which act as **carcinogens** (*cancer-causing agents*) by generating point mutations and/or chromosomal abnormalities. The etiologies (causes) of cancer can be divided into three general groups: (1) mutation in genes—the oncogenes—that promote cell growth and survival, (2) mutation in genes—the tumor suppressor genes—that inhibit cell growth and survival, and (3) alterations in microRNAs.

## Human Cancers Can Be Caused by Chemicals, Radiation, and Viruses

The precise causes of most cancers are unknown. However, clear connections exist between specific environmental factors and some cancers (cigarette smoke or asbestos and lung cancers, or some plastics and tumors in blood vessels). Chemical carcinogens act by mutating DNA[2]; a chemical's carcinogenic potency correlates with its ability to bind to DNA. Like most chemical carcinogens, radiation is mutagenic and causes cancers by inducing changes in DNA. Various types of radiation are capable of causing or enhancing cancer. Exposure to sunlight increases skin cancers (such as melanoma), and exposure to X rays or radioactive elements increases the danger of cancer in general.

Evidence also shows that infections by certain viruses cause some human cancers. Many DNA viruses (papillomaviruses, hepadnaviruses [Hepatitis B virus], and certain herpes viruses) and RNA viruses of the Hepacivirus and Retrovirus genus can cause cancer. Discussions of other viruses, such as polyomaviruses, adenoviruses, human endogenous retroviruses, and human mammary tumor virus, with potential roles in human cancers are beyond the scope of this text.

Certain DNA viruses are tumorigenic in their natural hosts; they include human papillomaviruses, which cause anogenital, cervical, and oral cancers; Hepatitis B virus, which causes hepatocellular carcinoma; Epstein-Barr virus, which causes Burkitt's lymphoma, nasopharyngeal carcinoma, and lymphomas; and human herpes virus 8 (also called *Kaposi's sarcoma-associated herpesvirus*), which causes Kaposi's sarcoma and primary effusion lymphoma.

*Retroviruses* are the most widely studied and were the first viruses to be shown to cause cancers. *Rous sarcoma* virus, first described in 1911 by Peyton Rous, is used as a model cancer-causing agent. Retroviruses are not lytic for their cellular host.

---

[2]*Mutagens* are substances that cause DNA mutations. Mutagens that cause cancer are called *carcinogens*.

Retroviruses mediate their effect by allowing the host cell to translate the viral gene for reverse transcriptase, which converts viral RNA into DNA, and then integrating this DNA into the host's genome. This process can lead to the transformation of a normal cell into a cancerous cell. Transformation occurs either because the viral gene products can change cell growth or because integration changes the expression of a cellular gene. Although retroviruses are associated with many animal tumors, only one human retrovirus, human T-cell leukemia virus (HTLV-1), is associated with human cancers (particularly adult T-cell leukemia). Another RNA virus that is associated with human cancer is hepatitis C virus (HCV); a persistent HCV infection can lead to hepatocellular carcinoma. Viruses are the cause of some 15 to 20% of all human cancers.

## Cancer Genes Derail Normal Cell Growth

Cancer results from mutations, rarely single genetic alterations, which lead to a step-wise accumulation of changes that disrupt normal cellular growth and development. These mutations occur in growth-promoting genes, growth-suppressing genes, and microRNA genes. The resulting genetic damage in the parental cancer cell is maintained such that it is an inheritable trait. Genes that aid cell growth and tumor formation are called *oncogenes*; mutation or overexpression is oncogenic. Genes that inhibit cell growth and tumor formation are called *tumor suppressor genes*; loss or inactivation is oncogenic. For roughly 30 years, it was thought that changes in oncogenes and/or tumor suppressor genes were the causes of tumorigenesis. The recent discovery of thousands of genes that produce nonprotein-coding RNA transcripts led to the detection of a well-defined group of tiny RNAs 21–22 nucleotides in length called *microRNAs*. MicroRNAs can act as oncogenes or tumor suppressor genes. Cancer arises from mutations in either genes that facilitate cellular proliferation and tumor formation or genes that inhibit these processes.

During cancer, mutations among both oncogenes and tumor suppressor genes are part of the malignant process. Because cancer is a dysfunction of genes arising from genetic damage of different sorts, cancer researchers are continually trying to identify cancer genes. The only known cancer genes are the *oncogenes of retroviruses*. These viral genes are called *viral oncogenes* or **v-*oncs***. Oncogenes are DNA elements involved in the malignant transformation of cells. The normal cellular counterparts to viral oncogenes are called **cellular oncogenes** (**c-*oncs***) or **proto-oncogenes** (*proto*, "to go before"). Viral oncogenes arise from genetic recombination between proto-oncogenes and slow retroviruses. Unlike acute transforming retroviruses, slow retroviruses are unable to transform cells *in vitro* or *in vivo*. The structures of viral and cellular oncogenes—v-*src* (for sarcoma-producing) and c-*src*, respectively—provided verification that v-*src* is a derivative of c-*src* and led to the realization that the virus can develop the ability to cause cancer.[3] Base sequences of c-*src* and v-*src* show that c-*src* sequences always contain introns, whereas v-*src* sequences never contain them. In general terms, tumor cells possess changed proto-oncogenes. The process of activation from proto-oncogene to oncogene status is involved in the genesis of cancer; it can include retroviral transduction or integration (see above), mutations, gene fusion, chromosomal translocation, and gene amplification.

There is mounting evidence that a class of small RNA molecules of 20–23 nucleotides in length called **microRNAs** also play a role in tumorigenesis by acting either as oncogenes or tumor suppressor genes. Unlike other genes involved in cancer, microRNAs do not encode proteins. The products of microRNAs are single-stranded RNAs of 20–23 nucleotides that negatively regulate gene expression. The microRNA strand can anneal to its complementary target messenger RNA (mRNA) nucleotide sequence, thereby blocking protein translation or causing degradation of the mRNA. MicroRNAs were initially identified in B-cell chronic lymphocytic leukemia; subsequently, differences in microRNA expression levels were found in many types of human cancers. In cancer cells, microRNA genes can be upregulated or downregulated. When microRNA genes are upregulated, they function as oncogenes by downregulating tumor suppressor genes. In contrast, when microRNA genes are downregulated, they function as tumor suppressor genes by downregulating oncogenes.

Cancer development is not limited to genetic changes; epigenetic alterations in gene expression that are not caused by changes in primary DNA

---

[3]The v-*src* oncogene of Rous sarcoma virus was the first (1976) oncogene detected in normal cell DNA. Bishop and Varmus found that the *src* gene was responsible for transforming a normal cell into a cancerous cell. The exciting part of this discovery was that the gene actually is derived from a normal gene present in chromosomes of all animals, including humans. Bishop and Varmus won the 1989 Nobel Prize in Physiology and Medicine for their discovery of cancer-causing genes called *oncogenes*.

sequence are known to cause tumorigenesis. Epigenetics changes in cancer pathophysiology suggest that non-mutational alterations in DNA can lead to differences in gene expression. These epigenetic changes may involve DNA methylation of cytosine bases and methylation or acetylation of amino acid residues in histones around which the chromosomal DNA is wrapped. Methylation is associated with gene silencing, that is, normally, oncogenes are silent because of DNA methylation; therefore, if there is loss of methylation, it could induce abnormal oncogene expression, leading to tumorigenesis. The epigenetic silencing of tumor suppressor genes plays a major role in cancer development.

### Oncogene-Associated Activities Established the Existence of a Genetic Component to Cancer

The earliest evidence for the connection between cancer and oncogenes resulted from studies of Burkitt's lymphoma. It arises from the translocation of the *myc* oncogene, on chromosome 8q24, to one of three loci on immunoglobulin (Ig) genes (chromosomes 14q, 22q, and 2p). The placement of *myc* in the Ig loci, which contain enhancer elements, activate the juxtaposed *myc* oncogene (Figure 15-2). All malignant lymphocytes carry this translocation.

Realization that one gene could cause transformation led to a search for oncogenes in cancers surgically excised from cancer patients. When DNA isolated from tumor cells was transferred into normal cells, the recipient cells turned cancerous. Transmission of cancer from tumor cells to normal cells was accomplished by gene transfer (*transfection*) using DNA as the vehicle. The DNA-mediated transformation was traced to a human homologue of the rat retroviral *ras* oncogene, which encoded a 21 kD protein called *p21*. p21 associates with the inner surface of the cell plasma membrane and regulates several specific phosphorylation events. Oncogenic *ras* genes differ from their normal c-*ras* alleles by showing reduced GTPase activity associated with p21; from 10 to 30% of human tumors have an activated *ras* gene. All of the *ras* genes studied to date show a significant correlation between transforming ability and decreased GTPase activity. This correlation suggests that the inherent GTPase activity of *ras* plays a pivotal role in its biologic function.

Another group of oncogenes were shown to regulate *programmed cell death* (also called *apoptosis*). The cloning and characterization of chromosomal breakpoints, associated with follicular lymphomas and some diffuse large B-cell lymphomas, show a placement of the *Bcl-2* oncogene to enhancer elements in the Ig heavy-chain locus, which leads to deregulation of *Bcl-2*. *Bcl-2*, an anti-apoptosis gene, encodes a cytoplasmic protein that localizes to the mitochrondria and increases cell survival by inhibiting apoptosis. Bcl-2's antiapoptotic activity is upregulated in many cancers.

The use of transgenic mice supported the connection between oncogenes and cancer, that is, by expressing an activated oncogene from a human tumor, these mice developed cancers that resembled their human counterparts.

### Even Though Oncogenes Are Cancer-Causing Genes and Proto-Oncogenes Are Not, They Both Function as Cell-Growth Regulators

More than 100 proto-oncogenes and oncogenes are known (some oncogenes are listed in Table 15-3), but their protein products (discussed below) operate through only four different mechanisms: (1) protein phosphorylation with tyrosine and threonine as the substrate amino acids (the involvement of the enzyme protein kinase), (2) regulation of metabolism by proteins that bind GTP, (3) modulation of gene expression by influencing the development of mRNA, and (4) involvement in the replication of DNA. Collectively, proto-oncogenes appear to regulate cellular replication and differentiation significantly. If we think of a web of interconnected systems, moving from the cell surface to the nucleus, being required to regulate cell proliferation, then the proto-oncogene-encoded products provide the controls acting at important points along the system.

Although native-form proto-oncogenes are unable to transform cells, three different, but not mutually exclusive, mechanisms have been proposed to account for the way genetic damage might induce oncogenic changes in a proto-oncogene or its product. (1) Genetic damage might cause a quantitative change that leads to a glut of an otherwise normal gene product. This possibility suggests that the intracellular concentration of a proto-oncogene product is important in determining the cellular phenotype. (2) Genetic damage might cause a qualitative change in constitutive activity. This change does not mean that the gene expression is any greater than its usual maximum, just that it cannot be regulated. (3) Genetic damage might cause a second kind of qualitative change. Mutations in the coding domain of a proto-oncogene might change the manner in which its protein product acts.

Oncogenes encode protein products that can be classified into six groups (Table 15-4): apoptosis regulators, chromatin remodelers, growth factors, growth factor receptors, signal transducers, and transcription

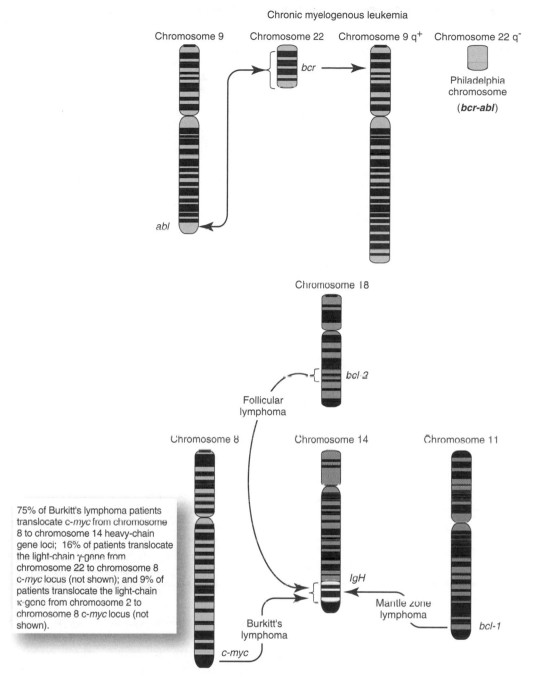

**FIGURE 15-2 Some cancers are associated with chromosomal translocations**. Several cancers exhibit translocations. For example, one of the most characterized translocations is designated t(9;22)(q34;q11), the Philadelphia chromosome, which is associated with chronic myelogenous leukemia (CML). Another translocation, t(14;18)(q32;q21), between chromosomes 14 and 18 leads to the overexpression of the *bcl-2* gene, which blocks apoptosis and is associated with follicular lymphoma development. It is a slow progressing, chronic B-cell lymphoma that results from transformation of B cells normally found in the center of lymph node follicles. An additional well-characterized translocation is the c-*myc* translocations associated with Burkitt's lymphoma; there are three variants, the most common is t(8;14)(q24;p32), then t(8;22)(q24;q11), followed by t(2;8)(p12;q24). Many mantle-zone lymphomas, B-cell lymphomas of the cells that surround the germinal center within a follicle, have associated translocations of the *bcl-1* gene from chromosome 11 to the Ig heavy-chain gene cluster on chromosome 14. This translocation causes over-expression of cyclin D1 protein, which normally promotes cell cycling advancement from $G_1$ to S phase, leading to cell division. Its over-expression induces increased mantle cell proliferation.

**TABLE 15-3** Some Oncogenes: The Cancers they Induce, Mechanism of Activation, and Proposed Functions

| Oncogene | Neoplasm | Activation mechanism | Proposed function(s) |
|---|---|---|---|
| *abl* | Chronic myelogenous leukemia | DNA rearrangement | Protein tyrosine kinase |
| *bcl-2* | B-cell lymphomas | Deregulated activity | Anti-apoptotic protein |
| *erb*A1 | Erythroblastosis | Deregulated activity | Transcription factor |
| *ets* | Erythroblastosis | Deregulated activity | Transcription factor |
| *fes* | Sarcoma | Constitutive activation | Protein tyrosine kinase |
| *fgr* | Sarcoma | Constitutive activation | Protein tyrosine kinase |
| *fms* | Sarcoma | Constitutive activation | Receptor for M-CSF |
| *fos* | Osteosarcoma | Deregulated activity | Transcription factor AP1 |
| Her-2/*neu* | Breast carcinoma, neuroblastoma | Point mutation/gene amplification | Protein related to EGF receptor |
| H-*ras* | Colon, lung, and pancreas | Point mutation | GTPase |
| K-*ras* | Acute myeloid leukemia, thyroid carcinoma | Point mutation | GTPase |
| *mos* | Sarcoma | Constitutive activation | Protein kinase |
| *myb* | Myeloblastosis | Deregulated activity | Transcription factor |
| *myc* | Carcinoma myelocytomatosis | Deregulated activity | Transcription factor |
| N-*ras* | Carcinoma, melanoma | Point mutation | GTPase |
| *raf* | Sarcoma | Constitutive activation | Protein kinase |
| *rel* | Lymphatic leukemia | Deregulated activity | Mutant NFκB |
| *ros* | Sarcoma | Constitutive activation | ? |
| *sis* | Fibrosarcoma/glioma | Constitutive production | B chain of PDGF |
| *ski* | Carcinoma | Deregulated activity | Transcription factor |
| *src* | Colon carcinoma | Constitutive activation | Protein tyrosine kinase |
| *yes* | Sarcoma | Constitutive activation | Protein tyrosine kinase |

**TABLE 15-4** Classes of Oncogene Products

| Products | Oncogene |
|---|---|
| Apoptosis regulators | *bcl-2* |
| Chromatin remodelers | *All1(mll)* |
| Growth factors | *sis, int2, Ks3* |
| Growth factor receptors | *fms, EGFR, neu, ros* |
| Signal transducers | *abl, fes, fgr, H-ras, K-ras, mos, N-ras, raf, src, yes* |
| Transcription factors | *ErbA1, fos, jun, myb, myc, rel, ski* |

factors. This oncogenic products list is by no means exhaustive or detailed, that is beyond the scope of this text. Examples of some products are mentioned below.

Some oncogenes do not induce or inhibit cellular proliferation but regulate programmed cell death (discussed earlier). Examples are *bcl-2* and *bcl-xl*, suppressors of apoptosis.

Chromatin is the complex of DNA and proteins that compose chromosomes; it packages DNA into a small enough volume to fit into a cell, it strengthens DNA for the rigors of mitosis and meiosis, and it serves to control gene expression. The changes in chromatin compaction affect gene expression, that is, the positioning of nucleosomes in histones leads to patterns of histone modification, which is an epigenetic mechanism that determines chromatin structure and its transcriptional competence. Chromatin remodeling plays a role in acute lymphoblastic leukemia (ALL) and chronic myelogenous leukemia (CML). Ninety-five percent of CML patients and 25–30% of adult patients and 2–10% of pediatric patients with ALL present with the chromosomal abnormality called *Philadelphia chromosome* (also called *Philadelphia translocation*) (see Figure 15-2).

Growth factors are proteins that can stimulate cellular proliferation and differentiation of specific target cells, such as vascular endothelial growth factor (VEGF) that stimulates blood vessel differentiation (angiogenesis) or platelet-derived growth factor (PDGF, the PDGF B chain is encoded by the *sis* oncogene) that is released during coagulation and stimulates fibroblasts to participate in wound healing. The constitutive activation of a growth factor gene can induce malignant transformation by causing cells to chronically produce growth factors thereby encouraging uncontrolled proliferation. This activation can also lead to loss of cell-cell adhesion and increased cell mobility associated with some tumors.

Growth factor receptors for epidermal growth factor (EGF), fibroblast growth factor (FGF), insulin-like growth factor, nerve growth factor, PDGF, and VEGF are altered in an assortment of human cancers. For example, the deletion of the ligand-binding portion of EGF receptor leads to constitutive activation of the receptor in the absence of the ligand, which causes deregulated signaling in several pathways. Similar mutations in other members of the EGF receptor family and the HER2/neu and kit receptors, lead to breast cancer, lung cancer, and gastrointestinal cancers.

Signal transducers include receptor tyrosine kinases, non-receptor protein tyrosine kinases (also called *cytoplasmic tyrosine kinases*), receptor serine/threonine kinases (also called *cytoplasmic serine/threonine kinases*), G-protein coupled receptors, and membrane-associated G-proteins (also called *regulatory GTPases*). These signal transducers become oncogenic if they carry activating mutations. Receptor tyrosine kinases (RTKs) are transmembrane receptors that have intrinsic enzymatic activity, which include those that are tyrosine kinases (such as EGF, FGF, insulin, and PDGF receptors), tyrosine phosphatases (such as CD45), guanylate cyclases (such as natriuretic peptide receptors), and serine/threonine kinases (such as TGF-β receptors). Other RKTs include fms, HER2/neu, and trk. Cancer can result when these receptors are constitutively turned on. Examples of non-receptor protein tyrosine kinases are abl (found in CML Philadelphia chromosome), lck (associated with CD4 and CD8 coreceptors of T cells), and src (the first identified oncogene and prototypal tyrosine kinase). Raf kinase, a serine/threonine kinase, is involved in most RTK signaling pathways. The *mas* gene encodes the angiotensin receptor, a G-protein coupled receptor; the *mas* gene was identified in a mammary carcinoma. The *ras* gene-encoded ras protein, a G-protein, is the most frequently associated altered gene in colorectal carcinomas. Other important G-proteins associated with cancer are the *nf1* gene, a tumor suppressor gene that encodes neurofibromin and the *bcr* gene-encoded protein. The *bcr* locus is translocated in the Philadelphia chromosome, which is observed with high frequency in CMLs and ALLs. The translocation is designated t(9;22)(q34;q11), which means parts of the two chromosomes 9 and 22 are exchanged; the *bcr* gene from chromosome 22 (region q11) is fused with part of the *abl* gene on chromosome 9 (region q34). The fused gene, *bcl-abl*, is constitutively active, induces a number of cycle-controlling enzymes that increase cell proliferation, and inhibits DNA repair, leading to genomic instability that may cause blast crisis, the terminal phase of CML.

Transcription factors are proteins that bind to specific portions of DNA and control the transfer of genetic information from DNA to RNA; they accomplish this transfer alone, or by interacting with other proteins in a complex, by increasing or preventing the presence of RNA polymerase. The myc protein is a transcription factor that regulates the expression of 15% of all genes by binding to enhancer sequences. The mutated form of *myc*, which causes persistent expression of myc, induces the unregulated expression of many genes that control cell proliferation and leads to the formation many different types of cancers. One example of *myc* overexpression is seen in Burkitt's lymphoma, it results from the chromosomal translocation of the c-*myc* gene from chromosome 8 to chromosome 14 (see Figure 15-2). Some tumors result from the fusion of two transcription factors; for example, the Fos transcription factor interacts with the Jun transcription factor to form the transcriptional regulatory complex AP1, which increases the expression of several genes that control cell proliferation.

### Are Oncogenes Villains or Accomplices in Tumor Progression?

The information presented so far about oncogenes may give the impression that the presence of an oncogene will transform a cell. However, cancer arises from a protracted, multistep, sequence of events, and each stage creates more phenotypic aberrations. The first event, **initiation**, involves the acquisition of the mutation. The second event, **promotion**, involves the expression of the mutation. Evidence suggests that oncogenes may fit into this scheme. For example, either the Harvey (H-ras) or the Kirsten (K-ras) viruses are enough to induce neoplastic transformation. While the activated c-*ras* genes transform some immortalized cell lines, they fail to transform primary cell lines. However, the cotransfection of primary cell lines with *ras* and *myc* leads to transformation. These data support the large body of evidence showing that most cancers are the result of two or more mutational events. As many as 10 distinct stepwise mutations may have to accumulate in a cell before it becomes cancerous (Figure 15-3). Although the precise mechanism or mechanisms of change are unknown, oncogenes and tumor suppressor genes constitute the final common pathway of all cancers.

### The Loss or Inactivation of the Oncogene's Mirror Image, the Tumor Suppressor Gene, Can Lead to Cancer

**Tumor suppressor genes** (or **anti-oncogenes**) influence cell proliferation, cell-cell communication,

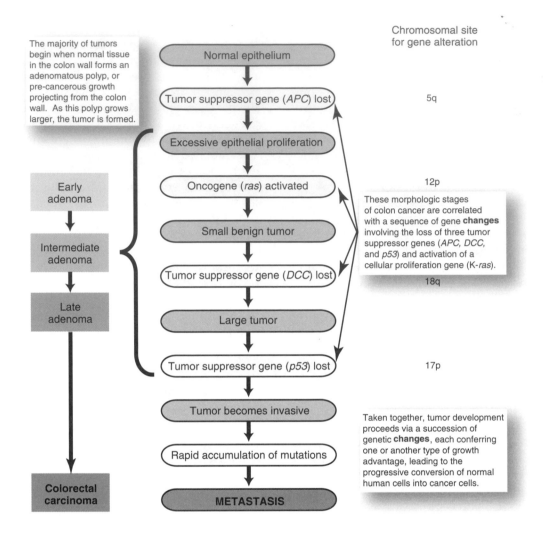

The majority of tumors begin when normal tissue in the colon wall forms an adenomatous polyp, or pre-cancerous growth projecting from the colon wall. As this polyp grows larger, the tumor is formed.

Chromosomal site for gene alteration

Normal epithelium

Tumor suppressor gene (*APC*) lost — 5q

Excessive epithelial proliferation

Early adenoma

Oncogene (*ras*) activated — 12p

These morphologic stages of colon cancer are correlated with a sequence of gene **changes** involving the loss of three tumor suppressor genes (*APC*, *DCC*, and *p53*) and activation of a cellular proliferation gene (K-*ras*).

Small benign tumor

Intermediate adenoma

Tumor suppressor gene (*DCC*) lost — 18q

Late adenoma

Large tumor

Tumor suppressor gene (*p53*) lost — 17p

Tumor becomes invasive

Taken together, tumor development proceeds via a succession of genetic **changes**, each conferring one or another type of growth advantage, leading to the progressive conversion of normal human cells into cancer cells.

Rapid accumulation of mutations

Colorectal carcinoma

METASTASIS

**The immune system can recognize these "changes."**

**FIGURE 15-3** Development of colorectal cancer: A multistep induction process.

and apoptosis. They are activated by cellular stress or DNA damage. Normally, tumor suppressor gene proteins would repress genes necessary for promoting cell cycling. Cell cycling is coupled with DNA integrity; damaged DNA prohibits the cell from dividing until the DNA is repaired. If the DNA cannot be repaired, the cell commits suicide, that is, it initiates apoptosis. When tumor suppressor genes become dysfunctional, tumors can arise because the tumor suppressor gene-encoded proteins can no longer dampen or repress the cell cycle or promote apoptosis. The tumor suppressor genes seem to be one of nature's successful approaches to protection against cancer.

Though few tumor-suppressor genes have been identified, the two best-characterized tumor sup-

pressor genes are the retinoblastoma gene (*Rb*) on chromosome 13 and the *p53* gene on chromosome 17. *Rb* and *p53* are nuclear genes; *Rb* is a suppressor of retinoblastoma, bone cancer, small-cell lung cancer, and breast cancer. *p53* is a suppressor of a wide range of cancers, there is a homozygous loss of p53 in 30–50% of breast cancers, 70% of colon cancers, and 50% of lung cancers. Mutations in *p53* are also present in leukemias, lymphomas, and sarcomas. Other tumor suppressor genes include *APC* (suppressor of adenomatous polyposis; involved in colon and stomach cancers), *BRCA1* and *BRCA2* (suppressors of breast and ovarian cancers), *DCC* (suppressor of colon carcinoma), *DPC4* (suppressor of pancreatic cancer), *NF1* (suppressor of neurofibromatosis; involved in cancers of the peripheral nervous system and myeloid leukemia), *NF2* (suppressor of brain cancers, such as meningioma and ependymoma), and *WT1* (suppressor of Wilm's tumor of the kidney). Tumor suppressor genes have been difficult to identify because they have a "negative phenotype": their effect is noticed only when they are absent or inactivated. Because tumor suppressor genes prevent tumors from arising, a cell becomes cancerous when these genes are absent or inactivated. Thus, activation of cellular oncogenes is not enough for the development of malignancy. Cancer also involves the loss or inactivation of two or more tumor suppressor genes, which presumably function normally to inhibit cell growth. In fact, point mutations in *p53* tumor suppressor genes are the most common genetic alterations identified with human cancers and are associated with many hereditary cancers.

Compelling evidence suggests that tumor suppressor gene loss and oncogene activation are equally important in the transformation of a normal cell to a cancerous one. A cell will become cancerous only if its growth is unchecked and its oncogene expression is uninhibited.

## MINI SUMMARY

Cancer is usually considered to be caused by carcinogens such as chemicals, radiation, and viruses. Mechanisms leading to cancer include alterations in (1) oncogenes; (2) tumor suppressor genes; and (3) microRNAs. The cancerous phenotype of a cell is stably inherited, which suggests that genetic changes are responsible for the loss of cellular growth control.

Oncogenes encode proteins that induce cellular transformation. Gene sequences similar to those of viral oncogenes are detected in normal cells. These normal (noncancerous) cellular genes are called cellular oncogenes or proto-oncogenes. The change from proto-oncogenes to oncogenes initiates the genesis of cancer. Mechanisms by which oncogene-encoded proteins act may include (1) protein phosphorylation by protein kinases, (2) regulation of metabolism by GTP-binding proteins, (3) modulation of gene expression by influencing the development of mRNA, and (4) involvement in the replication of DNA. Although the normal phenotype of an oncogene is cancer, the normal phenotype of a proto-oncogene is not. The conversion may be caused by (1) a quantitative change leading to a glut of an otherwise normal gene product, (2) a qualitative change in constitutive activity leading to an

unregulatable oncogene or its product, and (3) a second kind of qualitative change: mutations in the coding domain of a proto-oncogene may change the manner in which its protein product acts. Cancer also can result from the loss or inactivation of tumor suppressor genes that control cellular growth. Small nonprotein-coding RNAs, microRNAs, through their regulation of gene expression, are also involved in tumorigenesis. Thus, cancer arises from at least two genetic events: initiation and promotion. Epigenetic changes also play a role in carcinogenesis.

# GENETIC DYSREGULATION OF IMMUNE CELLS CAN LEAD TO IMMUNE SYSTEM NEOPLASMS

Immune system neoplasms (also called *hematological neoplasms*) are classified as lymphomas or leukemias. Lymphomas (originate in lymphocytes) present as solid tumors within lymph nodes, spleen, and thymus. Informally, lymphomas are generally characterized as Hodgkin's and non-Hodgkin's lymphomas. Leukemias (originate in lymphoid or myeloid lineages in the bone marrow) present as single cells in increased numbers in the blood or lymph. The World Health Organization (WHO), considered the authoritative standard, classifies the types of lymphomas and leukemias on the basis of cell origin (B cell *versus* T cell/NK cell) and differentiation stage (immature *versus* mature). According to the WHO classification, which is based on cell origin, lymphomas and leukemias are not separated if derived from the same malignant cell source. Table 15-5 outlines the WHO classification for lymphoid neoplasms.

Malignant hematological diseases can be generally grouped into lymphomas as mature B cell neoplasms, mature T cell and NK cell neoplasms, and Hodgkin's lymphoma, whereas leukemias are traditionally grouped as acute lymphoblastic leukemia (ALL), acute myelogenous leukemia (AML), chronic lymphoblastic leukemia (CLL), and chronic myelogenous leukemia (CML) (Table 15-6). ALLs are characterized by a rapid rise of immature cells and it is the most common type of leukemia in young children, whereas CLLs are distinguished by excessive build-up of mature cells and occur most often in adults over the age of 55. AMLs and CMLs occur more commonly in adults but AMLs are more common in men than women.

**TABLE 15-5** The WHO Classification of Lymphoid Neoplasms

**I. B cell neoplasms**
   a. Precursor B cell neoplasm
      1) Precursor B-lymphoblastic leukemia/lymphoma
   b. Mature (peripheral) B-cell neoplasms
      1) B-cell chronic lymphocytic leukemia/small lymphocytic lymphoma
      2) B-cell prolymphocytic leukemia
      3) Lymphoplasmacytic lymphoma
      4) Splenic marginal zone B-cell lymphoma
      5) Hairy cell leukemia
      6) Plasma cell myeloma/plasmacytoma
      7) Extranodal marginal zone B-cell lymphoma of MALT type
      8) Nodal marginal zone B-cell lymphoma (1/2 monocytoid B cells)
      9) Follicular lymphoma
     10) Mantle cell lymphoma
     11) Diffuse large B-cell lymphoma
        a) Mediastinal large B-cell lymphoma
        b) Primary effusion lymphoma
     12) Burkitt's lymphoma/Burkitt cell leukemia

**II. T cell and NK cell neoplasms**
   a. Precursor T-cell neoplasm
      1) Precursor T-lymphoblastic lymphoma/leukemia
   b. Mature (peripheral) T and NK cell neoplasms
      1) T-cell prolymphocytic leukemia
      2) T-cell granular lymphocytic leukemia
      3) Aggressive NK cell leukemia
      4) Adult T-cell lymphoma/leukemia (HTLV-1$^+$)
      5) Extranodal NK/T-cell lymphoma, nasal type
      6) Enteropathy-type T-cell lymphoma
      7) Hepatosplenic $\gamma\delta$ T-cell lymphoma
      8) Subcutaneous panniculitis-like T-cell lymphoma
      9) Mycosis fungoides/Sezary's syndrome
     10) Anaplastic large-cell lymphoma, T/null cell, primary cutaneous type
     11) Peripheral T-cell lymphoma, not otherwise characterized
     12) Angioimmunoblastic T-cell lymphoma
     13) Anaplastic large-cell lymphoma, T/null cell, primary systemic type

**III. Hodgkin's lymphoma (Hodgkin's disease)**
   a. Nodular lymphocyte-predominant Hodgkin's lymphoma
   b. Classical Hodgkin's lymphoma
      1) Nodular sclerosis
      2) Lymphocyte-rich classical
      3) Mixed cellularity
      4) Lymphocyte depleted

**TABLE 15-6** Four major types of leukemia

| Cell type | Onset | |
|---|---|---|
| | **Acute** | **Chronic** |
| Lymphobastic (also *called lymphocytic leukemia*) | Acute lymphoblastic leukemia (ALL) | Chronic lymphoblastic leukemia (CLL) |
| Myelogenous (also called *myeloid leukemia*) | Acute myelogenous leukemia (AML) | Chronic myelogenous leukemia (CML) |

Chromosomal translocations are a common cause of lymphoid neoplasms; they are uncommon in solid tumors. Early in the chapter, the association of Philadelphia chromosome with CML was discussed. Other translocations associated with cancers include: t(2;5)(p23;q35) in anaplastic large cell lymphoma; t(8;14)(q24;p32) (see Figure 15-2), t(8;22) (q24;q11), or t(2;8)(p12;q24) in Burkitt's lymphoma;

t(15;17)(q22;q12) in acute myelogenous leukemia; t(15;17)(q22;q21) in acute promyelocytic leukemia; and t(X;18)(p11.2;q11.2) in synovial sarcoma.

## MINI SUMMARY

Malignant hematological diseases are represented by lymphomas and leukemias, cancers of the immune system that are characterized by their cell of origin and stage of differentiation. Many of these diseases are associated with the translocation of proto-oncogenes. The juxtaposed genes are usually constitutively expressed, leading to dysregulation of cell growth and death.

# TUMORS ARE CHARACTERIZED BY THEIR ASSOCIATED ANTIGENS

As discussed in Chapter 4, antigens must satisfy certain standards to be considered immunogenic; tumor antigens fulfill these standards—the outcome is that tumor-bearing hosts can develop immune responses to tumors. Tumor cell immunogenicity is assessed using the following functional criteria: (1) re-exposure to the tumor leads to rejection; (2) *in vitro* tumor cells are sensitive to cell-mediated immune reactions of the host; and (3) tumors can induce tumor-specific antibodies in the host. Using these criteria, two types of tumor antigens are recognized: (1) **tumor-specific antigens (TSAs)**, which are detected only on tumor cells, and (2) **tumor-associated antigens (TAAs)**, which are found on both tumor cells and other types of tissues. TSAs are qualitatively different from those antigens expressed on their normal counterparts—they are unique to tumor cells. In contrast, TAAs are not unique to tumor cells; normal cells share them. The TSAs and TAAs frequently are called **tumor-specific** or **tumor-associated transplantation antigens (TSTAs or TATAs)**, respectively; these terms represent a functional definition used to show that the antigen in question can induce rejection of the tumor graft *in vivo* (Figure 15-4). Tumor cell-surface antigens are schematically represented in Figure 15-5. TSAs are the result of point mutations in genes encoding cytosolic proteins; at least 20 have been identified. These mutations cause single amino acid changes in proteins, the proteins are processed to peptides, and the novel peptides are displayed by self-MHC class I molecules on the tumor cell. These changed, or now foreign, peptides are recognized by $CD8^+$ cytotoxic T ($T_C$) cells and induce their cytotoxic effector functions (such as the unique human melanoma antigen, resulting from the point mutation of cyclin-dependent kinase [CDK4]).

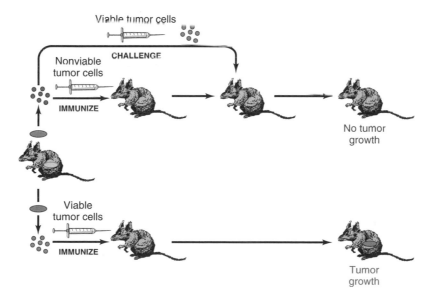

**FIGURE 15-4 Experimental demonstration of TATA.** TATA are demonstrated by transferring viable but nondividing (inhibited by irradiation or mitomycin-C) tumor cells from a tumor-bearing mouse to an immunized or unimmunized animal. The animal immunized with treated tumor cells fails to develop a tumor on exposure (challenge) to the untreated tumor cells.

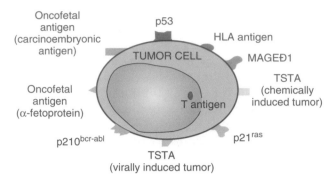

**FIGURE 15-5 Tumor-induced cell-surface antigens.** The cancerous transformation of cells leads to the expression of different cell-surface antigens. The chemically and virally induced tumors express TSTA but also are considered to be TSA (such as, MAGE-1, p21$^{ras}$, p210$^{bcr-abl}$, p53, and T antigen). In contrast, oncofetal antigens are considered to be TATA and TAA.

T$_C$ cells target tumor cells by recognizing tumor antigens that can be classified into tumor antigens that are (1) unique to tumor cells, but absent on normal counterparts; (2) common to both tumor cells and normal cells, which are masked on normal cells but become unmasked on tumor cells; (3) qualitatively similar to ones on normal cells but are over-expressed on tumor cells, and (4) expressed at high levels on tumor cells and normal developing fetal but not adult tissues.

## There Are Three Types of Experimental Tumors: Chemically and Physically Induced, Virally Induced, and Spontaneously Occurring

To study the host's immune response to tumors, three types of experimental tumors are used: (1) chemically and physically induced, (2) virally induced, and (3) spontaneously occurring. The etiology of the last type of tumor is usually undetermined and it is difficult to demonstrate the presence of TSAs because the host's effector response eliminates the tumor cells expressing high levels of TSAs and thereby selects for cells expressing low levels of TSAs. Chemically (such as methylcholanthrene) and physically (such as ultraviolet light) induced tumors provided initial evidence for TSAs. (Methylcholanthrene and ultraviolet light are carcinogens.) Cells from these tumors express unique antigens not shared by other comparable chemically or physically induced tumors, even when the tumors originate in the same animal. Tumor antigens for each tumor are antigenically unrelated; thus, the immune response to one does not protect against the other. The immunogenicity

of TSAs induced by chemicals is difficult to characterize because they can only be detected by T$_C$ cell-mediated killing. Characterization of chemically induced TSAs is accomplished by elution and purification of tumor peptides by high-pressure liquid chromatography or facilitating tumor antigen harvesting by increasing their expression through the transfection of cells with tumor cell cDNA-containing plasmids. The immunogenicity of virally induced tumors can be caused by the expression of either virally induced new antigens or viral antigens. In contrast to chemically induced tumors, the cellular antigens (TSAs) of virally caused tumors are shared by all tumors induced by the same virus, irrespective of the species. This similarity suggests a common mechanism of malignant transformation. The adoptive transfer of virus-specific lymphocytes to syngeneic recipients that are subsequently challenged with the same virally induced tumors leads to tumor rejection. With the introduction of hybridoma technology, highly specific monoclonal antibodies have been raised against cell-surface molecules of human and experimental malignancies.

## There Are Two General Types of Antigens Associated with Tumor Cells: Tumor-Specific and Tumor-Associated

As discussed above, two types of antigens are found on tumor cells: tumor-specific antigens (TSAs) and tumor-associated antigens (TAAs; such as, the inappropriate expression of embryonic gene-encoded oncofetal antigens or overexpression of normal protein) (Table 15-7).

Chemically induced or radiation-induced tumors display unique TSAs, even within the same animal. In contrast, virally induced tumors share TSA caused by the same virus, irrespective of the species in which the tumor grows. This sameness of cell-surface antigens is probably caused by viral products that serve as the target antigens. CD8$^+$ T$_C$ cells recognize TSAs in an MHC-restricted fashion. Thus, TSAs (discussed here and in the next two paragraphs) interact with MHC molecules of host accessory cells (macrophages or dendritic cells) to form the cell-surface antigen recognized by specific T$_C$ cells (and CD4$^+$ T$_H$ cells).

Another category of TSAs is the products of oncogenes activated by point mutations (such as p21$^{ras}$) or rearrangement of normal genes (such as p210$^{bcr-abl}$), both encode unique tumor antigens. Ten percent of human cancers are associated with mutations in p21$^{ras}$, while roughly 95% of chronic myelogenic leukemias are associated with translocation of *bcr-abl*.

**TABLE 15-7 Some Tumor Antigens Recognized by Human T Cells**

  **I.** Antigens encoded by specifically expressed tumor genes
    a. Oncogene products: *Ras* mutations in ~10% carcinomas
    b. Tumor suppressor gene products: mutated *p53* in ~50% of human tumors
  **II.** Antigens encoded by variant normal genes that have been altered by mutation
    a. Mutated proteins (such as cyclin-dependent kinase 4) in melanomas that are recognized by $T_C$ cells
  **III.** Antigens expressed only at certain stages of cellular differentiation
    a. Prostate-specific antigen (PSA)
    b. Differentiation antigens expressed by melanocytes and melanomas
    c. Oncofetal antigens: α fetoprotein and carcinoembryonic antigen
  **IV.** Antigens expressed only by certain differentiation lineages
    a. MAGE antigens in melanomas, breast carcinomas, and glioma tumors
    b. CD10 in B cell-derived lymphomas
  **V.** Antigens over-expressed in certain tumors
    a. HER-2/neu in breast and other carcinomas
    b. Tyrosinase in melanomas
  **VI.** Oncogenic virus-encoded antigens
    a. Human papilloma virus E6 and E7 proteins associated with cervical carcinomas
    b. Epstein-Barr virus NA-1 protein associated with EBV-associated lymphomas (Burkitts lymphoma) and nasopharyngeal carcinoma

Tumor antigens also can be the products of inactivated tumor suppressor genes. Mutations in the *p53* tumor suppressor gene are common in more than 50% of human cancers. Identified tumor antigens encoded by oncogenic viruses are simian virus (SV) 40 T antigen in rodents, human papilloma virus *E6* and *E7* gene products (human cervical carcinoma), and Epstein-Barr virus *EBNA-1* gene product (Hodgkin's and Burkitt's lymphomas and nasopharyngeal carcinoma).

Several types of TAAs have been described. Some tumor antigens are products of "silent" cellular genes not expressed in normal cells, for example, melanoma antigen 1 (MAGE-1, -2, and -3); therefore, these antigens are sometimes called *shared TSAs*. MAGE-1, and MAGE-2 and -3, are expressed in roughly 40% and 75%, respectively, of human melanomas and 25% of human breast carcinomas, glioma tumors, and head and neck carcinomas. (MAGE antigens are not expressed in any adult tissues except in the testes, where they are expressed on male germline cells. However male germline cells cannot express antigen to T cells because they lack HLA molecules.) Roughly 20% of identified tumor antigens are over-expressed in tumor cells as compared to their normal counterparts. Normal melanocytes express differentiation antigens, such as, tyrosinase and Melan-A/MART-1, whereas melanoma cells express increased levels of these antigens. Another differentiation antigen that is over-expressed is the oncoprotein HER-2/neu, which is receptor tyrosine kinase homologous to the epidermal growth factor receptor. This receptor is over-expressed in breast and ovarian cancers.

Tumor-associated antigens, such as **oncofetal antigens**, normally appear on the surface of embryonic cells and are reexpressed on the surface of some adult neoplastic cells. Expression of these fetal antigens in the adult is probably caused by derepression of fetal genes. The two best-characterized fetal antigens found on cancerous cells are α-*fetoprotein (AFP)* and *carcinoembryonic antigen (CEA)*. The former antigen, a 70-kD α-globulin glycoprotein, is secreted in large amounts primarily by hepatocarcinoma cells, while the latter antigen, a 180-kD highly glycosylated membrane protein, is produced by colonic adenocarcinomas. These antigens have no importance in antitumor immunity or cancer screening in the general population because such antigens develop not only in cancer but in other diseases as well. They are self-antigens expressed during development. They serve, however, as a diagnostic tool for tumor load and recurrence of metastases after therapy. In the fetus, AFP is found at milligram levels in the blood, but drops to nanogram levels in adults; however, it is elevated in the majority of liver cancer patients. CEA is expressed on gastrointestinal and liver cells in 2- to 6-month-old fetuses; however, roughly 90% of advanced colon cancer patients and 50% of early colon cancer patients have increased levels of CEA in their blood.

Numerous altered glycoprotein and glycolipid antigens are associated with most human and experimental tumors. These antigens are the result of underglycosylation of core proteins or lipid molecules. For example, mucin, encoded by the *MUC-1* gene, is a sequestered, fully glycosylated normal protein present in the ductal epithelium of the breast, pancreas, and ovary. Transformed ductal cells express underglycosylated mucin. Altered glycolipid tumor antigens, such as CA-125 and CA-19-9, are expressed on ovarian carcinomas.

# IMMUNE SURVEILLANCE REFINED, NOW CALLED IMMUNOEDITING, EXPLAINS HOW THE IMMUNE SYSTEM BOTH PROTECTS AGAINST, AND PROMOTES, CANCER DEVELOPMENT

Because the immune system recognizes tumors and demonstrates responsiveness to tumor-associated antigens, most evidence supports the concept of **immune surveillance**, which was proposed in its original form in the late 1950s. *The concept states that patrolling cells of the immune system provide continuing body-wide surveillance and eliminate cells that undergo cancerous transformation.* After years of debate because of the inability of scientists to prove immune surveillance in experimental animals, new evidence shows that the immune system is a crucial player in the outcome of cancer development. The controversy subsided because the paradoxical effects of immunity on cancer were explained: immunity does prevent cancer development (the concept is called *immunosurveillance*) but immunity also promotes cancer development—the latter is described as the *immunosculpting of the tumor* by the immune system. As immunity to a tumor continues, it exerts a selective pressure by eliminating immunogenic tumors, an *equilibrium* develops; however, if the immune system fails to completely destroy the tumor, the surviving tumor cell variants with reduced immunogenicity *escape* immune destruction. The combination of these events is now referred to as **cancer immunoediting**, a process comprised of three phases: elimination, equilibrium, and escape. *Elimination*, as originally described in cancer immune surveillance, is the phase where the immune system detects and eliminates tumor cells. As the process continues, *equilibrium* develops between the immune system and the developing tumor, where genetically unstable tumor cells accumulate changes that modulate the TSAs they display and the constant immune pressure eliminating susceptible tumor cells. The process

selects for tumor cell variants that can resist, avoid, or suppress antitumor effector functions. *Escape* refers to the variants that have overcome immune pressures. Failure to destroy all tumor cells leads to tumor cells with reduced immunogenicity emerging, which now in the absence of immunologic hindrance are capable of progressive growth.

Compelling experimental evidence from spontaneous and carcinogen-induced tumor development in molecularly defined murine models of immunodeficiency combined with clinical data from human cancer patients unequivocally demonstrated that cancer immunosurveillance functions as an effective antitumor mechanism. Table 15-8 lists some evidence for human immune surveillance and Table 15-9 lists the association between mouse immunodeficiencies and cancer incidence; immunodeficient mice are more susceptible to the development of spontaneous and carcinogen-induced tumors.

---

**MINI SUMMARY**

The immunogenicity of tumors is proved by (1) rejection of the homologous tumor on reexposure, (2) the *in vitro* sensitivity of tumor cells to the host's cellular immune reactions, and (3) the induction of tumor-specific antibodies by the host. These criteria distinguish tumor-specific antigens (TSA) and tumor-associated antigens (TAA). Immunity to tumors is studied using three types of experimental tumors: (1) chemically and physically induced, (2) virally induced, and (3) spontaneously occurring. The two types of antigens associated with tumor cells are TSAs (such as chemically, physically, and virally induced antigens and oncogene-derived proteins) and TAAs (such as oncofetal antigens). The incidence of cancer may be lower than expected because of immunoediting, which is divided into three phases: elimination, equilibrium, and escape.

---

# CELLULAR IMMUNITY AGAINST TUMORS INVOLVES DIFFERENT CELLS AND THEIR WEAPONS

When tumor cells invade healthy tissue, the immune system can counterattack. In animal studies and human cancers, antitumor immune responses are

**TABLE 15-8 Evidence that Favors Human Immunoediting**

Points in favor of elimination (immune surveillance)
1. Individuals that are immunosuppressed due to clinical syndromes characterized by either primary or secondary immune deficiencies or therapy to prevent transplant rejection can lead to an increased incidence of nonviral cancers than in age-matched immunocompetent control populations.
2. Cancer patients can develop spontaneous innate and adaptive immune responses to the tumors that they bear. The appearance of human infiltrating tumor-reactive T lymphocytes, NK cells, or NKT cells are associated with improved prognosis for a number of different tumor types.
3. Some malignancies spontaneously regress.

Points in favor of equilibrium
1. The equilibrium phase is supported by clinical evidence, for example, the immune system controls premalignant monoclonal gammopathy of undetermined significance (MGUS) cells but does not eliminate them, the MGUS cells eventually progress to multiple myeloma cells.

Points in favor of escape
1. The best-characterized phase is the escape phase, an example is when melanoma growth induces a tumor-specific immune response, even though the immune response is usually unable to eliminate tumors. How tumors escape is an active area of research, some of the escape/evasion mechanisms are discussed later in the chapter.

Principles that can be concluded from the above points
1. Both human (and animal) tumors are immunogenic to the host.
2. Immune surveillance is an important immune defense mechanism in preventing the establishment of potential tumors and is in part a T-cell-dependent activity.
3. All the components of the immune system evoked by foreign tissue antigens (such as grafted tissue and virally infected cells) are stimulated by tumor cells.

Question: Why do tumors escape/survive?
There is no clear-cut answer. What has been proposed is a steady-state scenario. Establishment of a tumor causes the tumor and host to act synergistically in favoring tumor growth. The tumor contributes by its antigen-producing abilities and the host, paradoxically, by its own highly active immune system.

detected, and include innate, antibody, and T cell-mediated immune responses. *At least five different immune cells play roles in tumor rejection: (1) T lymphocytes, (2) NK cells, (3) macrophages, (4) dendritic cells, and (4) B cells.* The basic properties of these cells are discussed in Chapter 2. Development of effector B- and T-cell functions are discussed in Chapter 10.

## Cytotoxic T Lymphocytes Are Specific Killers

An important function of mature CD8$^+$ T$_C$ cells is to destroy targets such as tumor cells from solid or dispersed tumors. This process is antigen-specific, requires cell contact, and does not injure the T$_C$ cell. Direct involvement of T cells during tumor immunity can be shown with the *Winn assay*, generally called a *mixed lymphocyte-tumor culture* (Figure 15-6). This experimental approach evaluates the ability of T cells from animals undergoing successful tumor rejection to lyse syngeneic tumor targets. Extrapolating results from a Winn assay to an *in vivo* situation should be done with caution because of the high T-cell to tumor-cell ratio and the small area of the *in vitro* environment.

Similar *in vitro* situations occur *in vivo*; in fact, tumor-specific T$_C$ cells that recognize tumor antigens in association with class I MHC molecules can be isolated from animals and humans with established cancers. Cells collected from the blood of a cancer patient, incubated with IL-2 *in vitro*, and adoptively transferred back into the patient are called **lymphokine-activated killer (LAK) cells**. They are a heterogenous population of cells, which include NK cells; however, they are not only NK cells because they can kill tumor cells resistance to NK cell-mediated killing. Tumor-infiltrating lymphocytes (TILS), discussed later in the context of immunotherapy, are mononuclear cells derived from the inflammatory infiltrate in human solid tumors. These infiltrates include T$_C$ cells that kill tumor cells from the tumor they were derived. Using their T-cell antigen receptor (TCR), CD8$^+$ T$_C$ cells can recognize and destroy tumor cells in an MHC-restricted manner by perforin/granzyme-, FasL–Fas-, or tumor necrosis factor (TNF)-related apoptosis-induced ligand

**TABLE 15-9 Development of Spontaneous and Carcinogen-induced Tumors in Immunodeficient Mice**

| Strain | Description | Phenotype | |
| --- | --- | --- | --- |
| | | Spontaneous tumors | Carcinogen-induced tumors |
| SCID | Lack T and B cells | 15% of the mice develop T cell lymphomas | Increased susceptibility to MCA-induced sarcomas |
| $Rag2^{-/-}$ | Lack T and B cells | 50% of mice develop intestinal adenomas, 35% adenocarcinoma of the intestine, and 15% of the lung | Increased susceptibility to MCA-induced sarcomas |
| $Rag2^{-/-}$ $Stat1^{-/-}$ | Lack T and B cells, type I and type II IFN signaling-deficient | Like $Rag2^{-/-}$ mice, 20% develop intestinal adenomas, but also 40% develop adenocarcinoma of the breast, 10% of the colon, 20% of the colon and breast | N.D. |
| $Stat1^{-/-}$ | Type I and type II IFN signaling-deficient | N.D. | Increased susceptibility to MCA-induced sarcomas |
| $Perforin^{-/-}$ | Lack perforin | Mice develop B cell lymphomas at 14–21 months of age | Increased susceptibility to MCA-induced sarcomas |
| $Ifng^{-/-}$ | Lack IFN-γ | Mice develop predominantly T cell lymphomas at 13–19 months of age | Increased susceptibility to MCA-induced sarcomas and N-methyl-N-nitrosourea-induced sarcomas |
| $Perforin^{-/-}$ $Ifng^{-/-}$ | Lack perforin and IFN-γ | Like perforin-deficient mice, they develop B cell lymphomas but at earlier onset | Increased susceptibility to MCA-induced sarcomas |
| $Trail^{-/-}$ | Lack TRAIL | 25% of mice develop lymphomas late in life | Increased susceptibility to MCA-induced sarcomas |
| $Lmp2^{-/-}$ | Defective class I MHC antigen presentation | 36% of the mice develop uterine neoplasms | N.D. |
| $Il-12p35^{-/-}$ | Lack IL-12 | N.D. | Increased susceptibility to MCA-induced sarcomas and N-methyl-N-nitrosourea-induced sarcomas |
| $IL23p19^{-/-}$ | Lack IL-23 | N.D. | Decreased susceptibility to DMBA/TPA-induced skin carcinogenesis |
| $IL-12p40^{-/-}$ | Lack IL-12 and IL-23 | N.D. | Increased susceptibility to MCA-induced sarcomas, decreased susceptibility to DMBA/TPA-induced skin carcinogenesis |
| $CD80^{-/-}$ $CD86^{-/-}$ | Lack CD80 and CD86 costimulatory molecules | N.D. | Increased susceptibility to UV-induced skin carcinogenesis |

Source: Adapted from J.B. Swann and M.J. Smyth. 2007. *J. Clin. Invest.* 117:1137. DMBA, 7,12-di-methylbenz[a]-anthracene; IFN, interferon; MCA, methycholanthrene; N.D., Not Determined; TPA, 12-O-tetradecanoyl-phorbol-13-acetate; TRAIL, TNF-related apoptosis-inducing ligand.

(TRAIL)-mediated apoptosis. They can indirectly limit tumor growth through their secretion of IFN-γ, which is anti-angiogenic. (CD8$^+$ T$_C$-cell-mediated killing is discussed in Chapter 10.) Despite T$_C$ cell specificity, their cell-mediated activity is limited because class I MHC molecule expression decreases in many tumors.

The role of CD4$^+$ T$_H$ cells in tumor immunity remains somewhat obscure when compared to T$_C$ cell antitumor activity. Tumor rejection requires a robust cell-mediated response, which necessitates the close collaboration between cells of the innate immune system, the dendritic cells, and cells of the adaptive immune system, CD4$^+$ T$_H$ cells and

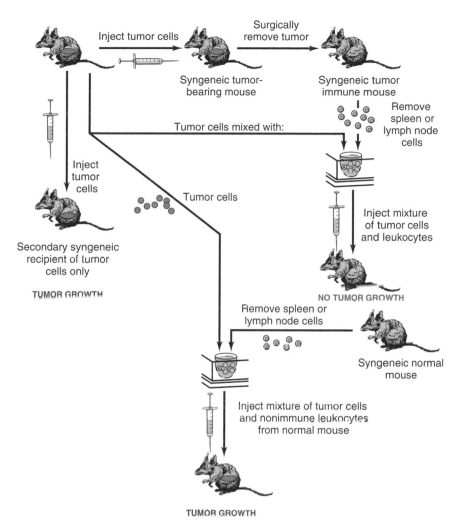

**FIGURE 15-6 The Winn assay.** This assay used to test the ability of leukocytes to inhibit tumor growth *in vivo*. Spleen or lymph node cells are removed from tumor-immunized mice and separated into T and B cells, NK cells, and macrophages. Different numbers of purified immune cells are mixed with a constant number of tumor cells and injected into normal mice, and the mice are observed for tumor growth. The cells of those animals that have antitumor immunity can kill the tumor cells *in vitro*, and no tumor grows in the injected host.

CD8$^+$ T$_C$ cells. CD4$^+$ T cells play a role in antitumor activities by enhancing and supporting the immune environment by cytokine secretion (such as TNF-$\alpha$ and IFN-$\gamma$), directly stimulating the development of T$_C$ cells through IL-2, TNF-$\alpha$, and IFN-$\gamma$ production, direct cytotoxic effect to the tumor itself through FasL expression, and orchestrating the recruitment and activation of innate immune cells through chemokine release.

Activated CD4$^+$ T$_H$1 cells recognize tumor-infiltrating macrophages in an MHC class II-dependent manner, converting interleukin-10 (IL-10)-producing, tumor-promoting M2 macrophages into IFN-$\gamma$-pro-ducing, tumor-inhibiting (depends on stage of tumor development) M1 macrophages. The M1 and M2 macrophage profiles (detailed in an upcoming section) are directly associated with T$_H$1 and T$_H$2 cell responses. Activated CD4$^+$ T$_H$1 cells can also release IFN-$\gamma$, which inhibits angiogenesis, increases tumor cell class I MHC molecule expression thereby facilitating T$_C$ cell-mediated killing of tumor cells, and activates macrophages to become tumoricidal. T$_H$2 cells can also be supportive by producing IL-4, which indirectly blocks neo-angiogenesis. Figure 15-7 depicts some roles for T-cell-produced cytokines in tumor cell destruction.

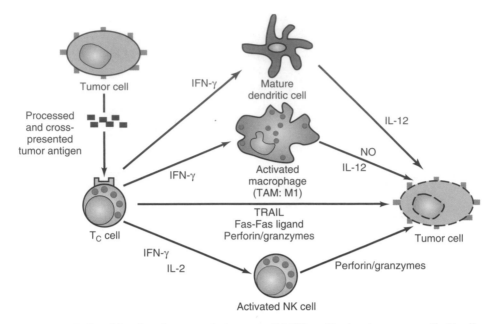

**FIGURE 15-7 Cytokine involvement in tumor cell killing.** During tumor growth, T cells are activated by tumor antigens that induce them to release cytokines. T cells release primarily IL-12 and IFN-γ. IFN-γ and IL-2 activates NK cells, which in turn kill tumor cells, while TRAIL, Fas-FasL, and perforin/granzymes allow $T_C$ cells to directly destroy tumor cells. IFN-γ attracts macrophages to the tumor site, keeps them there, and activates them. Activated macrophages either inhibit tumor cell proliferation or kill (nitric oxide [NO]) the tumor cells.

A chronic question that plagues tumor immunology is how do tumor cells stimulate tumor antigen-specific CD8+ $T_C$ cells? Most tumor cells are not professional antigen-presenting cells (APCs) (in particular, they lack costimulatory molecules); therefore, they cannot stimulate naïve T cells directly. To circumvent this hurdle, tumor antigens are probably scavenged, processed, and displayed by tissue-resident, immature dendritic cells in association with class I MHC molecules—the process is known as *cross-presentation* (see Chapter 10), which allows $T_C$ cells to recognize antigens that would normally be associated with class II MHC molecules. The APCs, as licensed dendritic cells express costimulatory molecules, would directly provide the signals required for the differentiation of naïve $T_C$ cells into antitumor-specific $T_C$ cells or the triad of APCs via their class II MHC molecules activate CD4+ T cells, which in turn activate CD8+ T cells.

Another recently characterized heterogeneous subset of T cells, the **NKT cells**, which share properties of both T cells and natural killer (NK) cells, are key players in innate and adaptive immune responses, including antitumor responses. NKT cells coexpress an αβ TCR, along with a variety of NK cell markers, such as, NK1.1; NKT T cells can be both NK1.1+ and NK1.1−. Like NK cells, NKT cells also express CD16 and CD56 and produce perforin and granzymes. NKT cells (also see Chapter 2) recognize the nonpolymorphic molecule called *CD1d* (see Chapter 7), like classical MHC molecules, they are antigen-presenting molecules but they bind self- and foreign lipids and glycolipids not peptides; therefore, they are called *CD1d-restricted T cells*. There are at least two subsets of NKT cells (Figure 15-8): type I NKT cells (also called *classical* or *invariant NKT [iNKT] cells*), which express an invariant TCR α chain (called *Vα14 receptor*); and type II NKT cells (also called *nonclassical* or *diverse NKT cells*), which express heterogeneous non-Vα14 receptors. Both subsets are CD1d-restricted but type I NKT cells are stimulated by the specific glycolipid ligand α-galactosylceramide (α-GalCer) and type II NKT cells are not. Once activated by dendritic cell CD1d-presented tumor-derived glycolipid, type I NKT cells produce large amounts of $T_H1$ cell (IL-2, IFN-γ, and TNF-α) and $T_H2$ cell (IL-4 and IL-13) cytokines; the rapid release of these cytokines promote or suppress different immune responses. α-GalCer-activated type I NKT cells rapidly produce large amounts of IFN-γ, which leads to activation of dendritic cells, NK cells, and $T_C$ cells. In addition,

Tumor Microenvironment

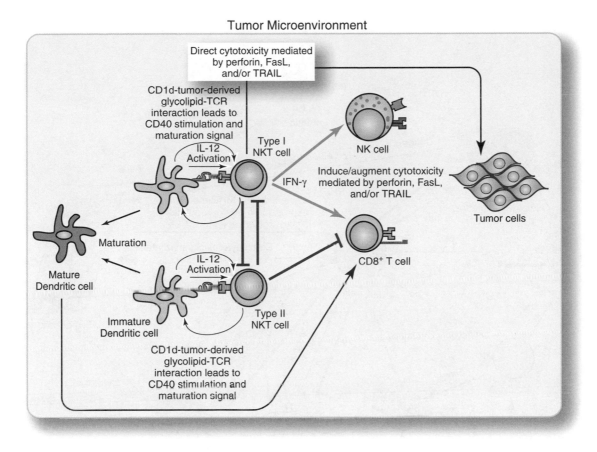

**FIGURE 15-8 Possible interactions in NKT cell-mediated antitumor activity.** Type I NKT cells (and type II NKT cells) recognize dendritic cell (DC) processed tumor glycolipids displayed by CD1d molecules. After activation, NKT cells upregulate CD40 ligand (CD40L), which stimulates DCs through CD40 to produce IL-12 and undergo maturation, which in turn induces NKT cells to turn out large amounts of IFN-γ, and mediate direct antitumor cytotoxic activity, through perforin/granzymes, Fas ligand–Fas interaction or TNF-α-related apoptosis-inducing ligand (TRAIL). The NKT cell-produced IFN-γ induces NK cell- and $T_C$ cell-mediated antitumor cytotoxicity. Mature, licensed DCs can activate $T_C$ cells. By unknown mechanisms, type II NKT cells downregulate type I NKT cell and $T_C$ cell activity. Red bars signify inhibitory activity. Green bars signify enhancing activity.

activated NKT cells mediated NK cell-like class I MHC molecule-independent antitumor cytotoxicity by three cell-death inducing mechanisms: perforin/granzyme, Fas ligand (FasL)–Fas, or TNF-related apoptosis-induced ligand (TRAIL). Experimental evidence suggests cross-regulation between the two subsets, type I NKT cells enhance antitumor responses, whereas type II NKT cells suppress antitumor responses; mechanisms are unknown.

## NK Cells Are Natural, Nonspecific Tumor Killers

The host contains a population of naturally occurring lymphocyte-like cells (they are not depleted in nude mice) that are cytotoxic to tumor cells. They induce apoptosis in tumor cells by releasing perforin and granzymes, FasL–Fas interaction, or TRAIL binding (Figure 15-9). Their cytotoxicity is considered "nonspecific" and non-MHC restricted; therefore, decreased class I MHC expression on tumor cells does not detract them, in fact, it induces them. Because of these characteristics, they are known as **natural killer (NK) cells**. They do not express T-cell antigen receptor, CD3, or surface immunoglobulin but do express CD16 (FcγRIII) and CD56. NK cells, part of the innate immune system, are considered important players in immune surveillance. They can eliminate spontaneously arising tumors. Until recently, this idea was difficult to prove because it was thought that NK cells do not require a period of stimulation, as do T- and B-cell immunity; however, the picture that

Tumor Microenvironment

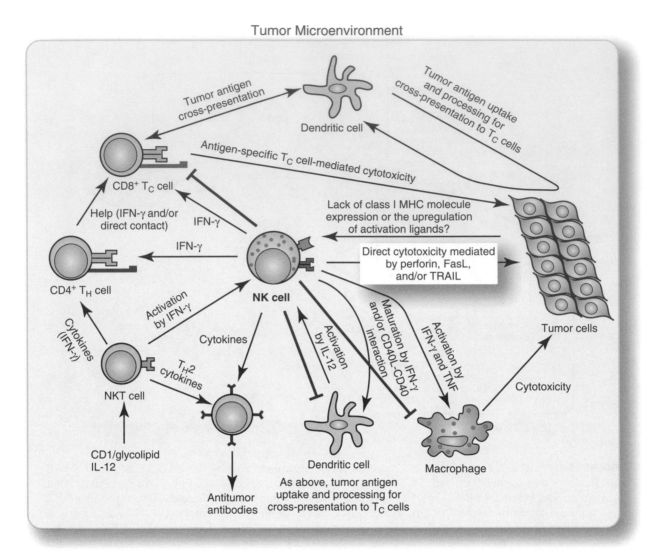

**FIGURE 15-9 Possible interactions in NK cell-mediated antitumor activity.** NK cells may recognize danger signals, such as a lack of class I MHC molecules or the upregulation of activation ligands, emanating from the tumor cells, which can lead to NK cell-mediated tumor cell death and regulation of the surrounding immune cells. Priming of NK cells by cytokines such as, type I interferons, IL-15, IL-12, and IL-18 from activated dendritic cells or macrophages, induces NK cells to boost dendritic cell and macrophage maturation and activation. In concert with $T_C$ cells, NK cells are the principal mediators of antitumor immunity. NK cells, during the process of lysing tumor cells, provide tumor antigens to dendritic cells, which can influence the development of adaptive B and T cell responses. Activated NK cells produce interferon-γ (IFN-γ), which activate $T_H$ and $T_C$ cell activity. This induces $T_H$ cells to proliferate and produce cytokines. Activated NKT cells also contribute to NK cell activation by their IFN-γ production. NK cells can negatively regulate immature dendritic cells and activated $T_H$ cells and macrophages by killing them (represented by red bars).

appears now is that NK cells acquire functionality through priming by dendritic cells. Nonetheless, NK cell importance is seen in *beige mice*, which have a mutation that causes defective lysosomal trafficking and corresponds to Chediak-Higashi syndrome in humans. The severely reduced NK cell function and phagocytosis is associated with an increase in certain types of cancer. NK cells kill on contact with

the tumor targets. A direct correlation exists between resistance to NK-cell killing *in vitro* and growth of a tumor *in vivo*. NK cells also are involved in host immunity to viral and microbial infections, as well as in the control of lymphoid and other hematopoietic cell populations. Mechanisms for NK cell recognition and killing of target cells are discussed in Chapters 2 and 10.

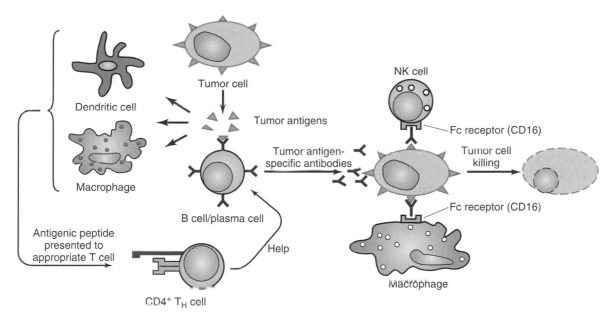

**FIGURE 15-10 Tumor immunity—Antibody-dependent cell-mediated cytotoxicity (ADCC).** The process of ADCC occurs when specific antibody binds to cell-surface antigens on tumor cells. NK cells or macrophages possessing Fc receptors bind to the Fc portion of the cell-associated antibodies, killing the cells.

Because NK cells express Fc receptors (CD16), they can bind to exposed Fc portions of antibody-coated tumor cells and cause **antibody-dependent cell-mediated cytotoxicity (ADCC)**, antigen specificity to tumor antigens is conferred by immunoglobulins (in this case by IgG), which bind to tumor cells. Immune cells with ADCC activity are NK cells and macrophages. Figure 15-10 illustrates ADCC (see Chapter 10 and Figure 10-24).

NK cells are regulated by cytokines (Figure 15-11). NK cells express receptors for IL-2 and the IFNs. NK cells proliferate in response to IL-2 without the requirement for activation by a primary stimulant such as an antigen or lectin. IL-2 may act as a recruitment molecule that amplifies the immune response to the target antigens. All three species of IFN augment NK-cell function. The type II IFN, IFN-γ, causes the NK cells to kill a broader range of

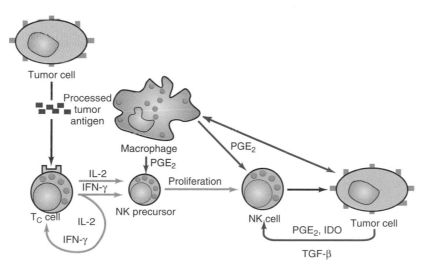

**FIGURE 15-11 The importance of cytokines in regulating NK-cell activity.** T cells regulate NK-cell activity through cytokines. These cytokines control NK-cell proliferation.

target cells with greater efficiency. The type I IFNs (IFN-α and IFN-β) do not increase binding efficiency but recruit nonlytic pre-NK cells to become cytolytic. A molecule important in downregulating NK-cell activity is prostaglandin $E_2$ ($PGE_2$), indoleamine 2,3-dioxygenase (IDO), and TGF-β, which can be secreted by macrophages and tumor cells.

## Macrophages Are Nonspecific Killers "Activated" to Pursue Tumor Cells but Are Subverted to Promote Tumor Initiation and Progression

As described in Chapter 3, innate immunity is one of the two members of the immunological "tag-team" of innate and adaptive immunity; both members may sometimes attack tumor cells. The hallmark characteristic of innate immunity is inflammation. The idea suggesting a link between cancer and inflammation is not a new one; in 1863 Rudolf Virchow noticed the infiltration of leukocytes in malignant tissues. Other early studies also noticed the development of malignant tumors at the sites of chronic inflammation and suggested links between cancer and inflammation. Evidence using transgenic mouse models has provided definitive proof of the connection. One of the key-infiltrating cells in inflammation is the macrophage—the "big eater" (see Chapters 2 and 3); therefore, it is not surprising they show up in tumors. Conventional wisdom would suggest that they are recruited to the tumor because they are capable of killing tumor cells. However, tumor cells protect themselves by reeducating macrophages to promote tumor onset and progression. In fact, the tumor microenvironment is immunosuppressive; the process of immunoediting would suggest selection for such an environment.

Leukocytes infiltrating tumors can represent up to 50% of the tumor mass, the majority of these cells correspond to lymphocytes and macrophages—T cell infiltration is correlated with a good prognosis, whereas macrophage infiltration is correlated with a poor prognosis. Blood circulating monocytes are selectively recruited to solid tumors by tumor-derived chemokines and other chemotactic molecules, such as CCL2, VEGF, and M-CSF, once monocytes infiltrate the tumor microenvironment, particularly the hypoxic areas, they differentiate into tissue resident macrophages called **tumor-associated macrophages (TAMs)** (Table 15-10). TAMs can be subclassified into subsets that contribute to neoplastic transformation in chronic inflammation sites where tumors develop called *M1 macrophages* and macrophages in established tumors called *M2 macrophages*, which support tumor growth, angiogenesis, and metastasis. The M1 and M2 profiles are associated with $T_H1$ and $T_H2$ cell responses, respectively. The M1 macrophages are proinflammatory, releasing inflammatory cytokines TNF-α, IL-1β, IL-12, and IL-23; and chemokines, such as CXCL9, CXCL10, and CXCL11; and reactive nitrogen intermediates and oxygen intermediates; therefore, they are considered microbicidal/tumoricidal macrophages. In contrast, M2 macrophages are polarized to the opposite extreme, they are poor APCs and support tumor growth, neoangiogenesis, and metastasis and suppress immune reactivity by responding to anti-inflammatory cytokines such as IL-4, IL-10, IL-13, and IL-21, apoptotic cells, and immune complexes. Immunosuppression is associated with the upregulation of IL-1α receptor, IL-10, and TGF-β production by tumors cells and macrophages. IL-10 production also favors the development of M2 macrophages and reduces

**TABLE 15-10 Tumor Promotional Activities of TAMs**

| Protumoral functions | Mediators |
|---|---|
| Growth factor production | IL-6, CXCL8, EGF, PDGF, and VEGF |
| Angiogenic factor production | CCL2, CXCL1, CXCL2, CXCL8, EGF, FGF, PDGF, TGF-β, and VEGF |
| Tissue remodeling | CCL2, MMP9, and TGF-β |
| Immune suppression | |
|    Immunosuppressive mediator production | IL-10, $PGE_2$, and TGF-β |
|    Lack of immunostimulatory mediator production | IL-12 |
|    Recruiting chemokine production | CCL18 (recruit naïve T cells), CCL17 and CCL22 (recruit $T_H2$ cells and $T_{reg}$ cells) |

EGF, epidermal growth factor; FGF, fibroblast growth factor; MMP9, matrix metallopeptidase 9; PDGF, platelet-derived growth factor; $PGE_2$, prostaglandin $E_2$; TGF-β, transforming growth factor-β; VEGF, vascular endothelial growth factor.

the differentiation of monocytes to dendritic cells and/or paralyzes dendritic cell functions. The TAMs found in malignant tumors are predominantly M2 macrophages.

Recent evidence suggests that the polarization of TAMs depends on the stage of tumor development, tumorigenic M1 macrophages localize to chronic inflammation sites where they predispose the tissue to tumor initiation. Subsequently, M1 macrophages shift to tumor-promoting M2 macrophages when the tumor is established. The connection between cancer and inflammation has moved from the cellular to the molecular level, providing strong evidence for the inflammation-link to carcinogenesis. The master switch, the transcription factor nuclear factor-kappa B (NF-κB), which controls the inflammatory repertoire of macrophages, regulates the shift in macrophage phenotype. Macrophage NF-κB activation correlates to the stage of tumor growth; it is activated during early stages of tumor initiation but is faulty in established tumors. Inhibition of NF-κB can revert the macrophages to the appropriate phenotype, ones that are directly tumoricidal through the production nitric oxide or indirectly through the production of IL-12, which promotes NK cell-mediated antitumor activity.

The ability of macrophages to migrate to specific sites, increase tissue remodeling, and induce angiogenesis is inherent in normal host development and mechanisms used in wound healing and inflammation. Tumors co-opt these macrophage activities for their own use; however, malignant tumors, due to intrinsic mutations, have lost positional identity so by chronically soliciting these activities, tumor cells continue to invade distant tissues.

The relationship between TAMs and tumor cells is complex. On the one hand, both TAMs and tumor cells produce reciprocal growth factors that lead to a symbiotic relationship. On the other hand, when activated, TAMs take on a M1 phenotype and can inhibit tumor growth and destroy tumor cells. Changes in this balance affect tumor growth.

## Dendritic Cells Are More Than Sentinels that Sense Tumor Cells and Alert Effector Cells; They Can Be Directly Tumoricidal

We saw in the preceding section that TAMs promote tumor growth and that M1 macrophages, in some cases, lead to tumor-disruptive inflammation. As described in Chapters 2 and 3, dendritic cells are the most potent, therefore called *professional*, APCs, specialized in the activation of naïve T lymphocytes;

this specialization suggests that they have the potential to activate or deactivate NK cells, NKT cells, tumor-specific T lymphocytes, and M1 macrophages, and thereby play an important role in immunosurveillance (Figure 15-12). Dendritic cells reside in all tissues, represent only 0.1–1.0% of the immune cells in different lymphoid and nonlymphoid tissues, and are composed of subsets with different functions. Nonactivated, immature dendritic cells maintain tolerance by presenting self-antigen to T cells in the absence of costimulation, whereas antigen-activated, mature dendritic cells present foreign antigen to T cells initiating adaptive immunity by inducing T cell proliferation and differentiation into effector $T_H$ cells and $T_C$ cells. As immature dendritic cells, they act as innate immunity's scavengers seizing invading pathogens and altered tissues, processing and transporting the associated antigen to the draining lymph nodes where they present it in association with MHC molecules to T cells and produce cytokines that influence the innate and adaptive arms of immunity. As they vehicle antigen to lymphoid organs, they mature from phagocytic cells to APCs, priming naïve T lymphocytes. The role of dendritic cells in the development of antitumor responses revolves around their ability to engulf dying tumor cells killed by NK cells and cross-presenting the tumor antigens to $T_C$ cells. Tumor-infiltrating dendritic cells exhibit an immature phenotype, whereas mature dendritic cells are found in the tumor-surrounding tissue. Dendritic cells are associated with leukocyte infiltrates of bladder, breast, colon, lung, pancreatic, and stomach carcinoma and correlated with a favorable prognosis. Nonetheless, tumor-infiltrating dendritic cells in many tumors are dysfunctional and may represent another immune evasion mechanism (discussed later). In addition to activating CD4$^+$ and CD8$^+$ T cells and cross-talking with NK cells, there is growing evidence that dendritic cells have direct tumoricidal activity; they are called *killer dendritic cells*.

## B Lymphocytes Are Indirect Killers Through Antibody Production

*In vitro* antitumor IgM and IgG antibodies exhibit complement-mediated killing, the *in vivo* relevance is debated. In fact, some evidence suggests that antitumor antibodies enhance tumor growth. It seems that in tumor resistance, humoral immunity is indirect. B cells produce tumor-specific antibodies that, in turn, activate other immune cells, such as NK cells (discussed earlier).

## Tumor Microenvironment

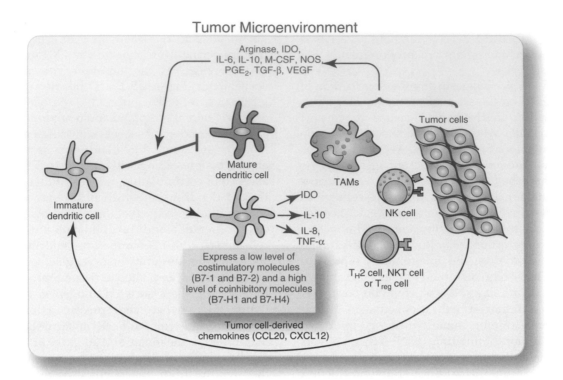

**FIGURE 15-12 Possible interactions in dendritic cell-mediated antitumor activity**. Dendritic cells are modulated at the tumor site by tumor cell- and immune cell-derived factors. Immature dendritic cells (tolerogenic stage) are recruited to the tumor and their differentiation and maturation is blocked by factors present in the tumor microenvironment. The resulting dendritic cells function as regulatory cells, reeducated by the tumor to become an important component of the immunosuppressive network in the tumor microenvironment.

---

### MINI SUMMARY

The immune cells responsible for tumor rejection include (1) T lymphocytes, (2) NK cells, (3) macrophages, (4) dendritic cells, and (5) B cells. $T_C$ cells can destroy tumor cells directly by perforin/granzyme-, FasL–Fas interaction-, or TRAIL-mediated killing. NK cells are involved in immune surveillance and mediate tumor cell death in mechanism similar to $T_C$ cells but in a nonMHC-restricted manner and requiring no prior sensitization. Activated macrophages should be principal participants in immune surveillance; however, tumors subvert them to predispose inflamed tissue to tumor initiation and promote tumor progression of established tumors. Dendritic cell's primary function in antitumor immune responses is engulfing tumor cells killed by NK cells and cross-presenting tumor antigens to $T_C$ cells. B cells are indirectly involved in tumor cell death. Their tumor-specific antibodies allow NK cells and macrophages, through their Fc receptors, to start ADCC.

## TUMORS CAMOUFLAGE THEMSELVES TO EVADE ANTITUMOR DEFENSES

Despite the impressive array of innate and adaptive immune cells and molecules that are activated by tumor antigens, neoplastic tissue eludes these mechanisms—the paradox that defines tumor immunology. How does the tumor escape destruction? Two generic possibilities can account for this paradox: generalized immunodeficiency (discussed in Chapter 16) associated with tumor-bearing or tumor cell modulatory abilities that hinder immune functions in the tumor microenvironment. The following paragraphs present some of the latter possibilities.

1. *"Sneaking through."* Tumor cell immunogenicity correlates with its survival against immunosurveillance, the more immunogenic the lower its survival, the less immunogenic greater its survival chances. Immunosurveillance places a

selective pressure on developing tumors. Because tumors are heterogenous and genetically unstable, the elimination of immunogenic tumor cells within the tumor mass by antitumor immune responses may lead to the outgrowth of tumor variants with reduced immunogenicity; this leads to "sneaking through." Under optimized conditions, a few isolated tumor-escape variants express too little antigen to stimulate the immune system or, and by the time the host's tumor immunity is adequate, the tumor burden is too large to reject. This situation may account for the times the immune surveillance mechanism fails and allows the growth of palpable clinical or experimental tumors.

2. *Antigenic modulation or shedding.* In the presence of immunity some antigens disappear from the cell surface of target tumors. This phenomenon is called *antigenic modulation* or *immunization-induced immune escape*. It involves the temporary loss of target antigens by either antigen shedding or internalization and redistribution within the cell membrane, with a change in immune cell reactivity but not a complete loss of tumor-specific antigens. The classic example is the modulation of TLa antigens from syngeneic TLa$^+$ leukemia cells in the presence of high titers of cytotoxic anti-TLa antibodies. Paradoxically, the animals that modulate TLa antigens do not destroy the tumor but succumb to it. If the tumor cells are harvested from the animal before death, they are not sensitive to antibody plus complement-mediated lysis and cannot adsorb the antibodies *in vitro*. Tumors are known to shed antigen that circulate in the blood. Antibodies produced against the circulating tumor antigens form antigen-antibody complexes that can restrict local effector cell activities.

3. *Modulation of class I MHC molecule expression.* T$_C$ cells recognize target tumor cells through tumor cell-derived peptide–class I MHC molecule complexes. Unfortunately, in many instances tumor growth decreases or alters class I MHC molecule expression, which prevents CD8$^+$ T$_C$ cell-mediated death of tumor cells. Transfection of class I MHC genes into murine tumors supports these results by showing that increased expression of class I molecules increases susceptibility to T$_C$ cell-mediated lysis. If the tumor loses expression of all class I molecules, they become more susceptible to NK cell-mediated lysis (see Chapters 2 and 10). However, if the tumor expresses one less class I molecule, they may be unrecognizable by specific T$_C$ cells.

4. *Altered APC activity.* Tumor-specific T$_C$ cells are dependent, in part, on T$_H$-cell help to differentiate. If APCs, due to abnormal TAP1/TAP2 function or altered β$_2$-microglobulin production, are unable to process and present tumor antigen to T$_H$ cells to activate them or to directly cross-present to T$_C$ cells, T$_C$-cell activity is minimal. Furthermore, tumor cells are poor APCs. They generally do not express class II and costimulatory (B7) molecules, making them unable to provide the signals for full T-cell activation. In fact, tumor cells acting as APCs lead to tolerance induction because of their lack of costimulatory molecules.

5. *Immunologic impairment.* Any natural (immune deficiency diseases; see Chapter 16) or artificial (immunosuppression to limit graft rejection) situation that changes the immune system enough to allow the tumor to elude immune defenses is called *immunologic impairment*. These situations suggest the presence of an immune surveillance mechanism; when the mechanism is changed, immune dysfunction arises and an increased incidence of certain cancers result.

6. *Inhibitory cells.* CD4$^+$CD25$^+$ T cells (called $T_{reg}$ cells; see Chapter 10) are a distinct lymphocyte lineage comprising 5–10% of all peripheral T cells, which regulate a variety of innate and adaptive immune cells and priming and effector phases of immune responses. According to their origin and suppressor activity, $T_{reg}$ cells are classified into two subsets: *natural* and *adaptive* (or *induced*) $T_{reg}$ cells. Natural $T_{reg}$ cells originate in the thymus following medium- to high-affinity interaction with TCR and self-antigen and suppress T-cell proliferation in a contact-dependent, cytokine-independent manner. They constitutively express CD25, cytotoxic T lymphocyte antigen 4 (CTLA-4), glucocorticoid-induced tumor necrosis factor receptor, OX40, and the lineage-specific transcription factor FOXP3. Adaptive $T_{reg}$ cells are generated in the presence of IL-10 or TGF-β and exert suppression through IL-10 and TGF-β production. $T_{reg}$ cells are a normal part of the immune regulatory system, but they seem to be in a heightened state of reactivity in tumor-bearing hosts; these T cells act as the tumor's allies. $T_{reg}$ cells need antigen-specific TCR triggering to become functional. They inhibit the development of specific effector antitumor responses (including the development of T$_C$ cells), but once activated, they indiscriminately suppress T cells regardless of their target. During tumor growth, the number of $T_{reg}$ cells increases, which favors unresponsiveness by the host's

immune cells against the tumor cells. $T_{reg}$ cells express CC-chemokine receptor 4 (CCR4), tumor cells produce significant amounts of CCL22 (the ligand for CCR4); therefore, $T_{reg}$ cells from the thymus, lymph nodes, bone marrow, and blood readily traffic to the tumor. Natural and adaptive $T_{reg}$ cell expansion results from proliferation of preexisting natural $T_{reg}$ cells and the conversion precursor adaptive $T_{reg}$ cells to newly derived adaptive $T_{reg}$ cells. The tumor has subverted guardian $T_{reg}$ cells that protect against overzealous immunity (autoimmune disease) to suppressors of necessary antitumor rejection responses. Nonspecific suppression during tumor growth also can be attributed to TAMs (discussed earlier) because they produce reactive oxygen species, TGF-β, and IL-10, which promotes T cell apoptosis. Abnormal dendritic cell differentiation during tumor growth leads to immature dendritic cells in the tumor microenvironment, which mirror TAM activities. Another recently described heterogeneous group of inhibitory cells are increased during tumor growth; they are called *myeloid-derived suppressor cells (MDSCs)*. They can inhibit antigen-specific CD4$^+$ and CD8$^+$ T cells through diverse mechanisms, including L-arginine metabolism, nitric oxide production, upregulation of reactive oxygen species, and IL-10 production. Induction of MDSCs is due to increased levels of tumor-derived granulocyte-macrophage colony-stimulating factor (GM-CSF) and VEGF production.

7. *Inhibitory ligands.* T cell activation requires a two-signal interaction with APCs; the first signal by the interaction of TCRs with antigenic peptide associated with APC MHC molecules, and the second signal provided by APC costimulatory molecules like the stimulatory B7 family members (CD80 and CD86) and others reacting with CD28 on T cells. B7 molecules not only provide positive signals, as described in the preceding scenario, but afford negative signals that control and suppress T-cell responses. The two B7 family members that negatively regulate immune responses are B7-H1 (also know as programmed death receptor ligand 1 [PD-L1] or CD273) and B7-H4. Tumor cells, stromal cells, and immune cells in the tumor microenvironment have upregulated expression of B7 inhibitory molecules, which inhibit tumor-specific T-cell immune responses. For example, tumor-compromised dendritic cells release IL-6 and IL-10, which induces expression of increased levels of B7-H4 on TAMs that, in turn, induces T-cell cycle arrest.

The dual signaling mechanism described above is naturally controlled by the competitive binding of CD80/CD86 on the APC with CTLA-4, a key negative regulator of adaptive immune responses, with CD28 on the T cell—an immune checkpoint, CD28–CTLA-4 binding, interrupts signal 2 and stops the activated T cell. This negative regulator maintains emergent immune responses at needed levels. In a tumor microenvironment, where the antitumor activated immune cells are unable to mediate tumor rejection, the host does not need to add insult to injury by inducing an inhibitor of already inhibited immune activity. Using inhibitors to inhibit negative regulators like CTLA-4 is an anticancer treatment strategy.

8. *Tolerance.* Although tumors are autochthonous transplants and have recognizable unique cell-surface neoantigens, our view of tumor cell antigens changed in the 1990s with the observation that most tumor antigens were not new antigens but rather tissue-differentiation antigens also expressed on their nontumor counterparts. Irrespective of the type of tumor antigens, tumor cells usually are not rejected by the host's activated immune system. This situation resembles immunologic tolerance; it was proven to be due to tolerance in experimental murine models and during the progression of human tumors. Experimental evidence suggests that tumor cell antigens are seen during ontogeny and that the host is unresponsive to these antigens in adulthood. What cell induces tolerance to tumor antigens, tumor cells alone or APCs? The answer is APCs but the decision leading to T-cell tolerance versus T-cell priming is influenced by the environment—inflammatory versus noninflammatory—in which dendritic cells capture antigen. In the absence of inflammatory signals, such as IL-12, type 1 IFNs, IFN-γ and CXCL14, and/or the presence of immunosuppressive mediators, such as IL-10, TGF-β, PGE$_2$ and VEGF, in the tumor microenvironment, it leads to an inhibition of dendritic cell maturation.

9. *Blocking factors.* Another widely studied evasion mechanism of tumors involves blocking factors. Sera of tumor-burdened patients can inhibit lymphocyte-mediated cytotoxicity *in vitro* as well as enhance tumor growth *in vivo*. Inhibition is caused by blocking factors which, when isolated from sera and characterized, were found to be antigen-antibody complexes. By binding to NK cells, these complexes can negate NK-cell-mediated cytotoxicity. When

antigen-antibody complexes bind to NK cells, these cells cannot recognize the tumor cells. Even though the blocking factors are found in the sera of tumor-bearing hosts, they must work in the immediate area of the primary tumor mass. Animals with tumors in one leg will reject limited numbers of the same tumor cells injected into the other leg. If blocking factors have worked throughout the body, they should block killing activity in the other leg.

10. *Tumor-derived factors.* Tumor cells can make products that abrogate tumor immunity (Figure 15-13). For example, prostaglandin $E_2$ decreases dendritic cell class I and II MHC molecule expression and inhibits $CD4^+$ $T_H$ cell cytokine production. Tumors also can make IL-10, which blocks dendritic cell priming of $T_C$ cells

and GM-CSF-induced chemotaxis of dendritic cells; GM-CSF, which promotes angiogenesis for tumor growth and acts as a chemoattractant for myeloid suppressor cells and immature dendritic cells; TGF-β, which inhibits T cell-mediated antitumor responses, promotes VEGF production by stromal cells, induces $T_{reg}$ cell intratumoral proliferation, and blocks the maturation of dendritic cells; indoleamine-2,3-dioxygenase (IDO), which hampers T cell function by tryptophan depletion and proapoptotic metabolite production; arginase, which impairs T-cell activation by downregulation of the TCR CD3ζ chain; and adenosine, which inhibits tumor antigen-specific $T_C$ cells. Tumors release soluble FasL, which binds to Fas on T cells inducing their apoptosis.

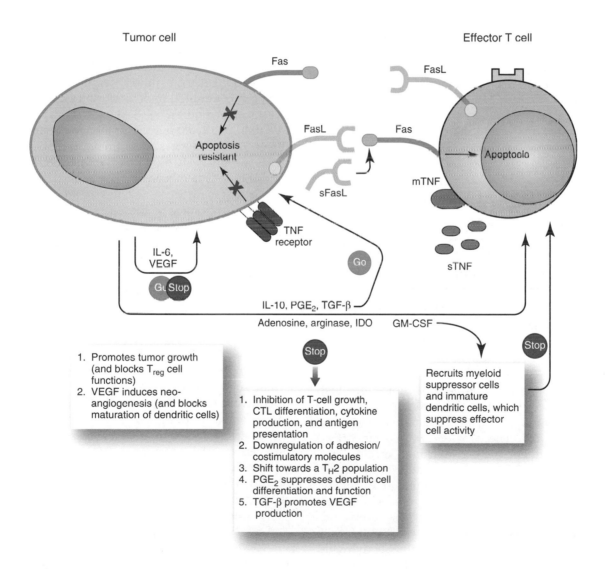

**FIGURE 15-13 Immune system avoidance through tumor camouflaging.** See text for details.

11. *Alterations in tumor cell signaling.* Not only do immune cells fail to mediate an effective anti-tumor immune response but they also promote tumor growth. What is the discordant crosstalk between tumor cells and immune cells that leads to such aberrant behavior? The signal transducer and activator of transcription 3 (STAT3) molecule is a culprit. Constitutively activated STAT3 is an important mediator of tumor-induced immunosuppression. Constitutive STAT3 activity in tumor cells promotes IL-10 and VEGF production, which are immunosuppressive and STAT3 activating. They also upregulate STAT3 signaling in immune cells, which turn out more immunosuppressive and growth-promoting molecules, such as IL-6, IL-10, TGF-$\beta$, and FoxP3. These factors, in turn, impair dendritic cell maturation (they remain tolerogenic), generate $T_{reg}$ cells, paralyze various effector immune cells, and promote growth and neoangiogenesis. The constitutive STAT3 activity in tumor cells and co-opted immune cells stalls the production of salutary molecules, including IL-12, TNF, IFN-$\beta$, IFN-$\gamma$, CCL5, CXCL10, CD40, CD80, CD86, and class II MHC molecules, which are indispensable to immune-mediated tumor rejection.

# IMMUNOTHERAPY INVOLVES FIGHTING CANCER BY USING OUR BUILT-IN PHARMACY OF MOLECULES AND CELLS

The two most widely used cancer therapies are surgery and radiation, but these treatments are effective only if the tumor is localized. Disseminated tumors are impossible to treat this way. Chemotherapy can react with cancer cells throughout the body and remains the treatment of choice for most advanced cancers, but most chemotherapeutic agents can injure normal cells; thus, their effectiveness is frequently limited. The problem with using drugs for cancer treatment is their toxicity. Cancer-killing doses are often poisonous to normal cells. Nontoxic doses, though, are not strong enough to kill many cancer cells. A case of "damned if you do and damned if you don't." To avoid these problems, immunotherapy is being attempted.

The immune system provides the body with defenses against cancer. When normal cells turn into tumor cells, some of their surface antigens change, existing ones increase in expression or new ones appear; however, in most cases the antigens are tissue-differentiation antigens expressed on normal cells, which suggests that tolerance is an obstacle in the development of antitumor immune rejection. Nonetheless, these antigens are flagged by $T_C$ cells, NK cells, macrophages, and dendritic cells. However, the tumor cells also are able to use the immune system to their own advantage. Factors released by the cancer cells not only subvert immune cells to not kill tumor cells but recruit them to augment tumor growth or stimulate the production of $T_{reg}$ cells, which together slow down the immune response against the cancer. *Efforts to attack tumor cells through the immune system,* **immunotherapy**, *center on stimulating or replenishing the antitumor elements of the patient's immune response, without further stimulating the suppressor mechanisms—use the immune system to reject cancer.* Immunotherapy uses the exquisite specificity of immune defenses. A great deal of research and many clinical studies are being done to exploit the immune system's inherent defenses against cancer.

Cancer, once an almost certain death sentence, has been commuted in 50% of the cases through the assistance of modern medical treatments and innovative therapy. Realizing the immense power they can direct against tumors in animals, tumor immunologists are intensely frustrated after trying to unlock the immune system's power in humans. A major difficulty in assessing the importance of immune defenses in tumor immunity is the enormous heterogeneity of the immune system and of known tumor types. Furthermore, as mentioned earlier, the tumor has an extensive arsenal that it can use to defend itself against the immune system. Each case of cancer in humans is different and responds to different treatments, depending on the features of the particular cancer and on genetic and environmental factors in the patient. The immune response may be augmenting rather than impeding tumor growth. In fact, the fulminant progress of tumors in the young lends strong support to the idea that immune stimulation is operative at certain stages of life and promotes rather than prevents tumor growth.

Despite these obvious differences among patients and cancers, there was once a tendency to consider immunologic factors in cancer as a single entity. This attitude has changed dramatically in light of all the new immunological approaches to treating cancer, which can be grouped into two forms: (1) specific and (2) nonspecific. **Specific immunotherapy** relies on vaccines of tumor cells or tumor cell fractions administered directly to the patient to augment or induce a host immune response to tumor antigens.

**Nonspecific immunotherapy** relies on the activation of immune responses that are not tumor-specific but inhibit tumor growth.

## Specific Immunotherapy Uses Tumor Vaccines or "Magic Bullets"

Preventative vaccines, based on induction of antiviral or antibacterial neutralizing antibodies, are the most successful biomedical treatment approaches known. Therapeutic tumor cell vaccines are a form of specific immunotherapy. However, their use is successful only when the host is made resistant before tumor challenge. Therapeutic vaccines are unsuccessful when immunotherapy is applied simultaneously with tumor cell inoculation. Nonetheless, several different approaches have been attempted to enhance the immunogenicity of tumor cells. They include immunizing with (1) virally infected tumor cells, (2) cell surface-changed tumor cells (by chemical or enzymatic means—for example, haptenization or antigenic modification), (3) tumor cell hybrids that express foreign antigens, and (4) modification of tumors by transfected cytokine or costimulator genes.

The fourth approach has received significant attention. Although tumor cells express TSAs and TAAs that are recognized by T cells, they are poor APCs because they do not provide the second signals needed for full T cell activation. Transfection of these tumor cells with constitutively expressed cytokines (IL-2, IL-4, TNF-α, IFN-γ, or GM-CSF) or costimulatory (B7) genes enhances the immunogenicity of the tumors, and on their reintroduction into the host can lead to tumor regression or rejection. Some tumor-derived cytokines induce nonspecific inflammatory responses that can drive the maturation and activation of dendritic cells thereby augmenting tumor-specific T-cell responses. B7-expressing tumor cells could *fully* activate tumor-specific T cells, leading to T-cell-mediated tumor rejection. A variation on this theme is to increase the expression of tumor antigens by linking *tumor antigen* genes to active promoters, transfecting the constructs into unmodified host tumors, and rechallenging the host with the transfected tumor cells. The flipside would be to engineer T cells expressing TCRs directed against TAAs. Anti-TAAs specific TCRs are cloned into a replication incompetent virus able to integrate into a patient's *ex vivo* cultures of T cells, following integration, the cells are expanded, and reinfused into the patient. A variation on a theme would be to harness the most potent APCs, the dendritic cells to activate anti-tumor cytotoxic responses through *ex vivo* loading (pulsed with an antigen or transfected with a viral vector)

or *in vivo* targeting (delivering antigen-complexed antibodies to specific surface receptors) of dendritic cells.

Monoclonal antibodies, a passive form of specific immunotherapy, have provided some solutions to the many problems of using immunotherapy to treat cancer. Currently, they are the most widely used form of cancer immunotherapy. Hybridomas can produce unlimited supplies of tumor antigen-specific monoclonal antibodies that can be used to detect, diagnose, and treat cancer. Even though, some cancer cells can undergo antigenic modulation, several therapeutic monoclonal antibodies are approved for human use by the Food and Drug Administration (FDA) (Table 15-11). Cancer therapeutic monoclonal antibodies are found in two forms, *naked monoclonal antibodies* are unmodified antibodies, that is, they do not have a drug, toxin, or radioactive material conjugated to them, whereas *conjugated monoclonal antibodies* have chemotherapeutics, toxins, or radioactive material attached to them to improve their efficacy. Naked monoclonal antibodies can act either as a red flag to mark tumor cells for destruction by the host immune system (Alemtuzumab or Rituximab) or to block functional receptors of cancer cells that are over-expressed (Bevacizumab, Cetuximab, Panitumumab, and Trastuzumab).

If the selectivity of monoclonal antibodies is combined with the killing power of cancer drugs, toxins, or radioactive substances their efficacy might be improved. The technical name for the agents that combine monoclonal antibodies with chemotherapeutic drugs, toxins, or radiolabeled particles are called **chemolabeled monoclonal antibodies** (antibody-paclitaxel conjugates), **immunotoxins** (Gemtuzumab ozogamicin), or **radiolabeled monoclonal antibodies** (Ibritumomab tiuxetan and Tositumomab), respectively. These are tumor-targeting drug-delivery systems that consist of a tumor recognition moiety, the monoclonal antibody to which cytotoxic drugs (or other compounds) are directly attached, or through a linker, to form a conjugate. The conjugate should be systemically nontoxic. Once antibody binds to the tumor cell, the cell "modulates," thereby internalizing the antibody along with the drug where it is cleaved to regenerate the active toxic drug; it is a microscopic version of the Trojan horse called a "magic bullet."

What toxins are used to kill tumor cells? Bacteria and plants are two sources of toxins. The two broad categories of toxins are those with two disulfide-linked polypeptide chains and those that are single-chained proteins. Examples of two-chained molecules are tetanus toxin, botulinum toxin, and

**TABLE 15-11** FDA Approved Therapeutic Monoclonal Antibodies used to Treat Cancer

| Antibody name | Trade name | Approval date | Target antigen | Treatment of |
|---|---|---|---|---|
| Alemtuzumab | Campath | 2001 | CD52 | Chronic lymphocytic leukemia |
| Bevacizumab | Avastin | 2004 2006 2008 | Vascular endothelial growth factor | Colorectal cancer in 2004; Non-small cell lung cancer in 2006; Advanced breast cancer in 2008 |
| Cetuximab | Erbitux | 2004 2006 | Epidermal growth factor receptor | Colorectal cancer in 2004; Head & neck cancers in 2006 |
| Gemtuzumab ozogamicin* | Mylotarg | 2000 | CD33 | Acute myelogenous leukemia (AML) |
| Ibritumomab tiuxetan* | Zevalin | 2002 | CD20 | Non-Hodgkin lymphoma (follicular lymphoma) |
| Panitumumab | Vectibix | 2004 | Epidermal growth factor receptor | Colorectal cancer |
| Rituximab | Rituxan | 1997 | CD20 | Non-Hodgkin lymphoma (follicular lymphoma) |
| Tositumomab* | Bexxar | 2003 | CD20 | Non-Hodgkin lymphoma (follicular lymphoma) |
| Trastuzumab | Herceptin | 1998 | Epidermal growth factor receptor 2 | Breast cancer |

*Conjugated monoclonal antibodies.

diphtheria toxin (examples of bacterial toxins), while ricin and gelouin are examples of double- and single-chain plant toxins, respectively. In toxins that have two chains, the B chain is responsible for recognizing receptors and aiding the transport of the toxic A chain across the cell membrane. Neither chain alone is toxic, and only on reaching the cytoplasm is the A chain toxic. Single-chain toxins are similar to the A chain of dipeptide toxins; that is, they must enter the cytoplasm before showing toxicity. Gemtuzumab ozogamicin is the only immunotoxin approved for treating human cancers (Figure 15-14); it is primarily used in the treatment of patients with relapsed acute myeloid leukemia. Gemtuzumab ozogamicin targets CD33, a sialic acid-dependent surface molecule commonly found on leukemic blast cells. The anti-CD33-specific monoclonal antibody, attached to the cytotoxic antitumor toxin calicheamicin (an antibiotic isolated from the soil microorganism *Micromonospora echinospora*), which works by binding to the minor groove of DNA causing double-strand DNA breaks that leads to apoptosis and cancer cell death. An FDA approved immunotoxin-like anti-cancer drug, where the antibody is replaced by a cytokine, is called *denileukin diftitox (Ontak)*. It is a fusion protein composed of amino acid sequences for diphtheria toxin fragments A and B followed by the sequence for IL-2, which is designed to deliver the toxin to cells expressing the IL-2 receptor. Denileukin diftitox is used to treat a rare type of skin lymphoma (cutaneous T cell lymphoma).

Radioimmunotherapy uses target cell-surface antigen-specific monoclonal antibodies conjugated to radioactive isotopes. Ibritumomab tiuxetan is a CD20-specific monoclonal antibody conjugated with tiuxetan, which chelates the beta emitter Yttrium-90. Another radiolabeled anti-CD20 monoclonal antibody is Tositumomab, which is covalently linked to the beta and gamma emitter Iodine-131. Both antibodies are used in the treatment of follicular lymphoma.

## Nonspecific Immunotherapy Works by Boosting Existing Host Mechanisms

The other category of cancer treatment is nonspecific immunotherapy. This kind of therapy involves efforts to attack cancer through the immune system by replenishing the patient's immune responses with **biologic response modifiers**. These modifiers, when administered, lead to direct inhibition of tumor growth (such as TNF), stimulation of general immune defenses (such as cytokines, or bacteria and bacterial extracts), or both (such as IFNs). Bacterial products that act as biologic response modifiers include Bacillus Calmette-Guerin (BCG) and attenuated forms of *Bacillus pertussis* or *Corynebacterium parvum*. Bacteria augment tumor immunity by activating macrophage-mediated antitumor responsiveness.

Another approach in nonspecific immunotherapy involves using the host's own built-in pharmacy of molecules. These biologic response modifiers are

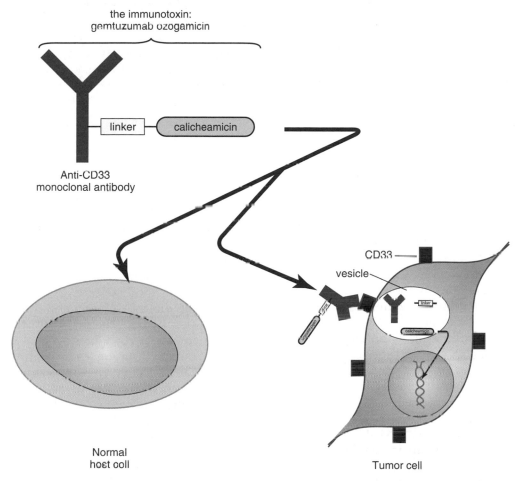

Calicheamicin alone can kill any cell once it enters; targeting it to only CD33+ leukemia blast cells is accomplished by attaching it to an anti-CD33-specific antibody.

**FIGURE 15-14 Immunotherapy using the immunotoxin gemtuzumab ozogamicin.** The basic strategy for gemtuzumab ozogamicin is simple. Calicheamicin can normally kill any cell it enters (normal or tumor cell), but it can easily be converted into a highly selective toxin by converting it into an immunotoxin. This conversion is done by covalently linking calicheamicin through an acid-labile linker to a humanized anti-CD33 monoclonal antibody molecule; the immunotoxin is called *gemtuzumab ozogamicin*. Under acidic conditions, the linker allows for rapid release of calicheamicin from its conjugate state. The immunotoxin through its high affinity and specificity for CD33 molecules, can bind to the target of choice, CD33-expressing tumor cells. Thus, calicheamicin can be targeted to any cell type, here a tumor cell. The immunotoxin is rapidly internalized into lysozomal vesicles, wherein the acidic pH facilitates the dissolution of the linker, releasing calicheamicin that attacks cellular DNA, cause cell death.

called *cytokines* (see Chapter 9). The most widely used cytokines are the IFNs and IL-2. The IFNs are a family of glycoproteins that have high antiviral activity and mediate profound effects on the immune system. Low doses of IFN-γ will increase antibody production and lymphocyte blastogenesis. In contrast, high doses of IFN-γ will inhibit both of these functions. Moderate to high doses can suppress delayed-type hypersensitivity, activate macrophages (increased phagocytosis and cytotoxicity), increase primed lymphocyte cytotoxicity, increase NK-cell activity, and augment the expression of class II MHC molecules on APCs. IFN-α can prolong or inhibit cell division in almost every cell system studied, increase NK-cell lytic potential, and increase class I MHC expression on different cell types. IFN-α is responsible for their clinical anticancer activity in renal carcinoma, melanomas, Kaposi's sarcoma, and hairy cell leukemias.

**Adoptive cell therapy** overlaps specific and nonspecific immunotherapy. In animal studies, the early use of IL-2 alone, then high-dose of IL-2 combined with tumor-bearing host immune lymphocytes grown *in vitro* with IL-2, and lastly high-dose of IL-2 combined with tumor-infiltrating lymphocytes spurred the development of adoptive cell therapy as a treatment modality for human cancer immunotherapy. Lymphocytes were collected from cancer patients and mixed with IL-2 *in vitro*. This *in vitro* mixing transformed some of the patient's own peripheral blood leukocytes into tumor-hungry cells called *LAK cells*. When LAK cells were reinfused along with IL-2 into cancer patients, the regression of several advanced metastatic cancers occurred. This protocol was further modified by obtaining immune cells that are 50 to 100 times more potent than LAK cells when used in adoptive cell immunotherapy. Immune cells that have infiltrated the tumor are harvested and expanded *in vitro* with IL-2 to numbers sufficient to cause regression of large metastatic tumors. The cells are called **tumor-infiltrating lymphocytes (TILs)**. The TILs, including NK cells and specific $T_C$ cells, are adoptively transferred in the presence of low levels of IL-2. The first demonstration of cancer regression using TILs in the adoptive cell therapy of patients with metastatic melanoma was reported in 1988. The procedure has been modified so that multiple cultures of autologous TILs are initiated from freshly excised tumor fragments, each incubated with IL-2, cultures are assayed for high antitumor reactivity, those with high reactivity are expanded to $>10^{10}$ cells, and reinfused into the cancer patient immediately following a lymphodepleting chemotherapy regimen. The patients also received IL-2 after TIL reinfusion. The high rate of cancer regression in these patients demonstrates the improved antitumor efficacy of this version adoptive cell therapy.

## MINI SUMMARY

Tumors develop within a host even though the host has immune cells to counteract tumors. The possibilities include (1) "sneaking through," (2) antigenic modulation or shedding, (3) modulation of class I MHC molecule expression, (4) altered APC activity, (5) immunologic impairment, (6) inhibitory cells, (7) inhibitory ligands, (8) tolerance, (9) blocking factors, (10) tumor-derived factors, and (11) alterations in tumor cell signaling. Two immunologic approaches (specific and nonspecific) are used to overcome tumor diversionary tactics. Specific immunotherapy relies on vaccines of tumor cells or tumor cell fractions, whereas nonspecific immunotherapy relies on the activation of non-tumor-specific and/or overlapping specific and nonspecific immune responses, such as, adoptive cell therapy.

# SUMMARY

The unrestrained or uncontrollable growth of cells leads to a **tumor** or **neoplasm**. Conversion of normal cells to cancer cells is called **transformation**. Transformation into abnormal cells leads to either **benign** or **malignant tumors**. The unrestrained proliferation of tumor cells at the primary site is not usually a threat to the cancer patient because the tumor may be in reach of local surgery. In benign tumors, the cells divide more frequently and do not invade the surrounding tissues. The malignant tumor has cells able to spread to alien sites such as the surrounding tissue or to distant sites through the circulatory or lymphatic systems. This property of invasiveness is called **metastasis**. The other two characteristics of malignancy are sustained cell multiplication and reversion of cellular structure and metabolic activity to a more primitive or embryonic form.

Three general mechanisms are thought to lead to cancer: (1) mutation in oncogenes; (2) mutation in tumor suppressor genes; and (3) alterations in microRNAs. Tumors can be induced by **carcinogens**. DNA viruses such as papovaviruses, adenoviruses, and certain herpes viruses can cause tumors. Viral transformation by RNA viruses is mediated by **oncogenes**. These viral genes are called **viral oncogenes** or **v-oncs**. Normal cellular genes with the potential to become oncogenes are called **cellular oncogenes** (**c-oncs**) or **proto-oncogenes**.

The presence of oncogenes is determined by the **transfection** of DNA from cancer cells to normal cells and later transformation of the normal cells. The first human oncogenes identified as responsible for transformation were the **ras genes**. Oncogene action, through encoded products, may involve four different mechanisms: (1) protein phosphorylation by protein kinases with tyrosine and threonine as the substrate amino acids, (2) regulation of metabolism by proteins that bind GTP, (3) modulation of gene expression by influencing the development of mRNA, and (4) involvement in the replication of DNA. Normally functioning proto-oncogenes do not cause cancer. Genetic damage may cause (1) a quantitative change leading to a glut of an otherwise normal gene product, (2) a qualitative change in constitutive activity, or (3) a qualitative change (such as a mutation) in the coding domain of a proto-oncogene that may change the manner in which its protein product acts. The most widely studied oncogene-encoded proteins are the *protein kinases*. Not only can oncogenes cause cancer, but also the loss or inactivation of *tumor suppressor genes*, the anti-oncogenes that inhibit cell growth and tumor formation, can lead to cancer.

At least two steps are required to induce cancer. They are *initiation*, the acquisition of a mutation, and *promotion*, the expression of the mutation.

Cell-surface antigens that induce tumor rejection are called *tumor antigens*. The criteria used to assess tumor immunogenicity include (1) the rejection of a tumor by a tumor-immunized animal on reexposure to the specific tumor, (2) *in vitro* killing of tumor cells by the host's immune cells, and (3) the appearance of tumor-specific antibodies in the tumor-burdened animal. *Tumor-specific antigens* (*TSA*) are unique to tumor cells, whereas *tumor-associated antigens* (*TAA*) are not unique to tumor cells and are found on other cells. Using these antigens to study the immunogenicity of tumors, tumors can be divided into three experimental types: chemically induced, virally induced, and spontaneously arising.

If spontaneously arising tumors are immunogenic, the immune system should play an important role in recognizing and destroying newly formed tumors. The immune cells involved in tumor rejection are T$_C$ cells, NK cells, macrophages, dendritic cells, and, indirectly, B cells (target cell-bound antibodies can interact with NK cells). T$_C$ cells can destroy tumor cells directly by *apoptosis* through *perforin-, FasL-, or TRAIL-mediated killing*. T$_C$ cells can also be indirectly involved in tumor cell killing by producing cytokines such as macrophage-activating factor (IFN-γ). Also, the host has *NK cells*. The lytic activity of NK cells is as described for T$_C$ cells. A similar type of cell is the *lymphokine-activated killer* (*LAK*) *cell* and its specific counterpart the *tumor-infiltrating lymphocyte* (*TIL*).

*Tumor-associated macrophages* (*TAMs*) are reeducated by tumors to secrete many products that favorably affect the initiation (*M1 macrophages*) and progression (*M2 macrophages*) of tumor growth. Dendritic cells, as the most potent antigen-presenting cells, can potentially present tumor antigens. They determine whether T cells become tolerant or are primed to tumor antigens. Antibody-mediated resistance to tumors is indirect because B cells produce tumor-specific antibodies that, in turn, activate other immune cells such as NK cells. NK cells mediate tumor killing through *antibody-dependent cell-mediated cytotoxicity* (*ADCC*).

Despite these defense mechanisms, cancers still occur. The possibilities for tumor camouflage include (1) "sneaking through," (2) antigenic modulation or shedding, (3) modulation of class I MHC molecule expression, (4) altered APC activity, (5) immunologic impairment, (6) inhibition by suppressor cells, (7) inhibitory ligands, (8) tolerance, (9) blocking factors, (10) tumor-derived factors, and (11) alterations in tumor cell signaling. Because tumors seem to be good at avoiding immunity, immunologists can use *specific* and *nonspecific immunotherapy* to counteract them. Specific immunotherapy relies on vaccines of tumor cells or tumor cell fractions administered directly to the patient to augment or induce the host immune response to TSA. In contrast, nonspecific immunotherapy relies on the activation of immune responses that are not tumor-specific yet still inhibit tumor growth. The most promising specific approaches have been the use of *chemolabeled monoclonal antibodies, immunotoxins,* and *radiolabeled monoclonal antibodies*. Nonspecific immunotherapy involves using *biologic response modifiers* administered to a patient. For example, TNFs can cause direct inhibition of tumor, some cytokines can stimulate general immune defenses, and molecules like IFN can do both. *Adoptive cell therapy* using TILs plus IL-2 is an effective treatment modality for patients with metastatic melanoma.

# SELF-EVALUATION

## RECALLING KEY TERMS

Adoptive cell therapy
Antibody-dependent cell-mediated cytotoxicity
  (ADCC)
Benign tumor
Biologic response modifiers
Cancer
Carcinogens
Cell adoptive therapy
Cellular oncogenes (c-*oncs*) (or proto-oncogenes)
Chemolabeled monoclonal antibodies
Immunoediting
    Elimination (Immune surveillance)
    Equilibrium
    Escape

## MULTIPLE-CHOICE QUESTIONS

*(An answer key is not provided, but the page[s] location of the answer is.)*

1. All of the following are naturally occurring components of the immune response to cancer cells except (a) the NK cell effect, (b) specific cellular immunity via lymphocytes, (c) blocking factors that interfere with the immunologic attack on tumor cells, (d) heightened ("turned on") general immune responsiveness, (e) macrophage killing of tumor cells, (f) none of these. *(See pages 505–513.)*

2. A form of cancer that is caused by a virus is (a) hepatoma, (b) Rous sarcoma, (c) ataxia telangiectasia, (d) all of these, (e) none of these. *(See page 493.)*

3. Which of the following factors favor tumor growth? (a) cellular immunity and cytotoxic antibodies, (b) cytotoxic antibodies and NK cells, (c) cellular immunity and activated macrophages and/or dendritic cells, (d) blocking factors, (e) none of these. *(See page 516.)*

4. Examples of cancer-associated antigens that probably arise from tissue dedifferentiation include (a) carcinoembryonic antigen, (b) α fetoprotein, (c) *a* and *b* are correct, (d) neither *a* nor *b* are correct, (e) none of these. *(See page 502.)*

5. To classify a tumor antigen as a oncofetal antigen, it must be present in regenerating cells or (a) in fetal or embryonic cells, (b) in plasma or serum, (c) in cells of endodermal origin, (d) in virus-transformed cells, (e) none of these. *(See page 503.)*

6. Tumor-specific transplantation antigens (TSTA) (a) are internal antigens, (b) are similar to T antigens, (c) really stands for timothy-stuart-thomas-allen antigen, (d) are surface antigens, (e) none of these. *(See pages 501 and 502.)*

7. A raised level of α-fetoprotein in the blood is associated with which of the following? (a) primary liver cancer, (b) secondary liver cancer, (c) viral hepatitis, (d) all of these, (e) none of these. *(See page 503.)*

8. A tumor-associated antigen present on the skin tumor cells of a mouse is also likely to be found on the skin tumor induced by which of the following? (a) a different chemical carcinogen in mice of the same strain, (b) the same chemical carcinogen in mice of different strains, (c) a different chemical carcinogen in mice of different strains, (d) a different oncogenic virus in mice of the same strain, (e) the same oncogenic virus in mice of different strains, (f) none of these. *(See page 502.)*

9. Tumor-specific antigens are unique to each tumor type. (a) true, (b) false. *(See pages 501 and 502.)*

10. The strongest evidence for the role of the immune system in preventing the establishment of tumors (immune surveillance) is (a) the markedly increased incidence of malignancies in persons with congenital or acquired immune deficiencies, (b) the hereditary pattern of malignancies, (c) the peak incidence of malignancies between the ages of 10 to 40, (d) the rapid transformation of normal cells into malignant cells in culture where the immune system is not available, (e) none of these. *(See page 504.)*

11. Theoretically, each of the following should be attempted in the immunotherapy of cancer except (a) using viable, unaltered tumor cells for specific immunization of the patient, (b) reducing the tumor burden to the lowest possible level by surgery, (c) using soluble tumor antigens to stimulate antibodies, (d) activating macrophages/dendritic cells and lymphocytes

by adjuvants such as BCG and *C. parvum*, (e) none of these. *(See pages 518–522.)*

12. In treating a cancer patient, you are asked to selectively destroy only the tumor cells. Which approach is probably best? (a) subject the patient to high doses of radiation (radiation therapy), (b) treat the patient with tumoricidal drugs (chemotherapy), (c) treat the patient with immunotoxins, (d) treat the patient with cytokines, (e) none of these. *(See pages 518–522.)*

13. Which of the following experiments suggests that tumor cells express tumor-specific transplantation antigens? (a) when a syngeneic mouse is injected with the tumor cells, accepts the tumor, and dies, (b) when a syngeneic mouse is injected with the tumor cells, rejects the tumor, and survives, (c) when an allogeneic mouse is injected with the tumor cells, rejects the tumor, and survives, (d) when an allogeneic mouse is injected with the tumor cells, accepts the tumor, and dies, (e) none of these. *(See pages 489 and 490.)*

14. One of the following is not a characteristic of natural killer (NK) cells. (a) they exhibit immunologic specificity and memory-like T cells, (b) they can kill tumor cells, (c) they are lymphocyte-like cells, (d) they are similar to cytotoxic T cells in mechanisms that mediate death of a target cell, (e) none of these. *(See pages 509–512.)*

15. Lymphokine-activated killer (LAK) cells destroy (a) allografts, (b) tumors, (c) virus-infected cells, (d) cells causing autoimmunity, (e) none of these. *(See pages 505 and 506.)*

16. Oncogenes are DNA elements involved in the malignant transformation of cells. (a) true, (b) false. *(See page 493.)*

17. Cellular oncogenes are also called (a) *v-oncs*, (b) oncogenes, (c) *c-oncs*, (d) proto-oncogenes, (e) *c* and *d* are correct, (f) none of these. *(See page 493.)*

18. Experimental approaches that have implicated proto-oncogenes in carcinogenesis include: (a) transduction and transfection, (b) transduction and recombination, (c) conjugation and transduction, (d) insertional mutagenesis and transduction, (e) none of these. *(See pages 493 and 494.)*

19. Proto-oncogenes are a family of (a) cell-growth regulators, (b) cell-growth inhibitors, (c) abnormal genes, (d) genes that do not encode proteins, (e) none of these. *(See page 493.)*

20. Tumor suppressor genes cause cancer by losing their ability to suppress oncogenes. (a) true, (b) false. *(See page 497.)*

## SHORT-ANSWER ESSAY QUESTIONS

1. Tumors and transplants are similar to one another, yet very different. Explain this fact in the context of what the immune system recognizes and the result of this recognition.

2. The qualities of proliferation and differentiation are essentially all that distinguishes a normal cell from a cancer cell. Explain.

3. How would you go about proving that the immune system provides immunity against tumors? Design an experiment using mice.

4. Distinguish between a benign tumor and a malignant tumor. Describe three characteristics of malignancy.

5. The causes of cancer can be divided into three groups; describe each and give an example of each.

6. What are carcinogens? Give two examples.

7. Distinguish between oncogenes and proto-oncogenes. The discovery of oncogenes established the existence of a genetic component to cancer. Design an experiment to show this.

8. More than 100 oncogenes have been isolated, yet only several different mechanisms for their activity are recognized. Describe these mechanisms.

9. How do oncogenes fit into the scheme of initiation and promotion in the cause of cancer?

10. What are tumor suppressor genes, and how do they work? Why have they been difficult to identify?

11. Distinguish between tumor-specific transplantation antigens (TSTA) and tumor associated transplantation antigens (TATA). Design an experiment to show TATA.

12. What are the main difference separating cell-surface antigens from chemically induced and virally induced cancers? Speculate on why this difference leads to difficulty in designing anticancer vaccines.

13. What are oncofetal antigens? Are they important in tumor immunity? If your answer is no, why?

14. What is cancer immunoediting? What is its connection to immune surveillance?

15. What immune cells play a role in tumor rejection? Briefly describe how each accomplishes this task. Include such things as cytokines, perforins, ADCC, and so on.

16. Cancers camouflage themselves to evade antitumor defenses. Pick three possible forms of camouflage that you think are most important,

describe them, and state why you think they are most important.

**17.** Surgery, radiation, and chemotherapy are the methods most widely used to treat cancer patients. What are the problems with this regimen, and how does/would immunotherapies overcome these problems. Distinguish between specific and nonspecific immunotherapy. What are immunotoxins?

## FURTHER READINGS

Allavena, P., A. Sica, G. Solinas, C. Porta, and A. Mantovani. 2008. The inflammatory micro-environment in tumor progression: The role of tumor-associated macrophages. *Crit. Rev. Oncol./Hematol.* 66:1–9.

Biswas, S.K., A. Sica, and C.L. Lewis. 2008. Plasticity of macrophage function during tumor progression: Regulation by distinct molecular mechanisms. *J. Immunol.* 180:2011–2017.

Blattman, J.N. and P.D. Greenberg. 2004. Cancer immunotherapy: A treatment for the masses. *Science* 305:200–205.

Chan, C.W., and F. Housseau. 2008. The 'kiss of death' by dendritic cells to cancer cells. *Cell Death Differ.* 15:58–69.

Drake, C.G., E. Jaffee, D.M. Pardoll. 2006. Mechanisms of immune evasion by tumors. *Adv. Immunol.* 90:51–81.

Frey, A.B., and N. Monu. 2008. Signaling defects in anti-tumor T cells. *Immunolog. Rev.* 222:192–205.

Gabrilovich, D. 2004. Mechanisms and functional significance of tumour-induced dendritic-cell defects. *Nat. Rev. Immunol.* 4:941–952.

Rabinovich, G.A., D. Gabrilovich, and E.M. Sotomayor. 2007. Immunosuppressive strategies that are mediated by tumor cells. *Annu. Rev. Immunol.* 25:267–296.

Hanahan, D., and R.A. Weinberg. 2000. The hallmarks of cancer. *Cell* 100:57–70.

Knutson, K.L., and M.L. Disis. 2005. Tumor antigen-specific T helper cells in cancer immunity and immunotherapy. *Cancer Immunol. Immunother.* 54:721–728.

Leen, A.M., C.M. Rooney, and A.E. Foster. 2007. Improving T cell therapy of cancer. *Annu. Rev. Immunol.* 25:243–265.

Long, E.O. 2007. Ready for prime time: NK cell priming by dendritic cells. *Immunity* 26:385–387.

Lucas, S., and P.G. Coulie. 2008. About human tumor antigens to be used in immunotherapy. *Semin. Immunol.* 20:301–307.

Pollard, J.W. 2004. Tumour-educated macrophages promote tumour progression and metastasis. *Nat. Rev. Cancer* 4:71–78.

Rabinovich, G.A., D. Gabrilovich, and E.M. Sotomayor. 2007. Immunosuppressive strategies that are mediated by tumor cells. *Annu. Rev. Immunol.* 25:267–296.

Rosenberg, S.A., N.P. Restifo, J.C. Yang, R.A. Morgan, and M.E. Dudley. 2008. Adoptive cell transfer: A clinical path to effective cancer immunotherapy. *Nat. Rev. Cancer* 8:299–308.

Schreiber, H. 2003. Tumor immunology. In *Fundamental Immunology*, 5th ed. W.E. Paul, ed. Philadelphia: Lippincott Williams & Wilkins. p. 1557–1592.

Seino, K-I, S. Motohashi, T. Fujisawa, T. Nakayama, and M. Taniguchi. 2006. Natural killer T cell-mediated antitumor immune responses and their clinical applications. *Cancer Sci.* 97:807–812.

Sica, A., and V. Bronte. 2007. Altered macrophage differentiation and immune dysfunction in tumor development. *J. Clin. Invest.* 117:1155–1166.

Smyth, M.J., G.P. Dunn, and R.D. Schreiber. 2006. Cancer immunosurveillance and immunoediting: The roles of immunity in suppressing tumor development and shaping tumor immunogenicity. *Adv. Immunol.* 90:1–50.

Stewart, T.J., K.M. Greeneltch, M.E.C. Lutsiak, and S.I. Abrams. 2007. Immunological responses can have both pro- and antitumor effects: Implications for immunotherapy. *Expert Rev. Mol. Med.* 9:1–20.

Stix, G. 2007. A malignant flame. *Sci. Amer.* 297:60–67.

Swann, J.B., and M.J. Smyth. 2007. Immune surveillance of tumors. *J. Clin. Invest.* 117:1137–1146.

Tacken, P.J., I.J.M. de Vries, R. Torensma, and C.G. Figdor. 2007. Dendritic-cell immunotherapy: From *ex vivo* loading to *in vivo* targeting. *Nat. Rev. Immunol.* 7:790–802.

Talmadge, J.E., M. Donkor, and E. Scholar. 2007. Inflammatory cell infiltration of tumors: Jekyll or Hyde. *Cancer Metastasis Rev.* 26:373–400.

Terbe, M., and J.A. Berzofsky. 2007. NKT cells in immunoregulation of tumor immunity: A new immunoregulatory axis. *Trends Immunol.* 28:491–496.

Vakkila, J. and M.T. Lotze. 2004. Inflammation and necrosis promote tumour growth. *Nat. Rev. Immunol.* 4:641–648.

de Visser, K.E., A, Eichten, L.M. Coussens. 2006. Paradoxical roles of the immune system during cancer development. *Nat. Rev. Cancer* 6:24–37.

Vivier, E., E. Tomasello, M. Baratin, T. Walzer, and S. Ugolini. 2008. *Nat. Immunol.* 9:503–510.

Yu, H., M. Kortylewski, D. Parrdoll. 2007. Crosstalk between cancer and immune cells: Role of STAT3 in the tumour microenvironment. *Nat. Rev. Immunol.* 7:41–51.

Zitvogel, L., A. Tesniere, and G. Kroemer. 2006. Cancer despite immunosurveillance: Immunoselection and immunosubversion. *Nat. Rev. Immunol.* 6:715–727.

Zou, W. 2005. Immunosuppressive networks in the tumour environment and their therapeutic relevance. *Nat. Rev. Cancer* 5:263–274.

Zou, W. 2006. Regulatory T cells, tumour immunity and immunotherapy. *Nat. Rev. Immunol.* 6:295–307.

Zou, W., and L. Chen. 2008. Inhibitory B7-family molecules in the tumour microenvironment. *Nat. Rev. Immunol.* 8:467–477.

# CHAPTER SIXTEEN

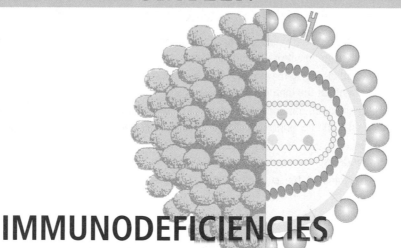

# IMMUNODEFICIENCIES

## CHAPTER OUTLINE

1. Primary immunodeficiency diseases are "real"-world models for identifying molecular components of the immune system.
   a. Primary immunodeficiencies are classified into several major categories.
   b. Primary immunodeficiency diseases have a strong genetic basis.
   c. Most laboratories can perform tests assessing for the presence of immunodeficiencies.
2. Primary immunodeficiency diseases: examples of naturally occurring immunosuppression.
   a. Immunodeficiency diseases involving only B cells.
   b. Immunodeficiency diseases involving only T cells.
   c. Immunodeficiency diseases involving both B and T cells.
   d. Immunodeficiency diseases involving innate immunity components.
   e. Immunodeficiency diseases involving complement components.
3. Secondary immunodeficiency diseases are exemplified by acquired immunodeficiency syndrome (AIDS).
   a. More than 25 years into the AIDS pandemic, HIV infection continues to exact a tremendous toll worldwide.
   b. The immunopathogenesis of AIDS is complex.
   c. The cause of AIDS is infection by the retrovirus HIV-1.
   d. The clinical course of HIV infection is divided into three phases.
   e. The comprehensive approach of education, prevention, diagnosis, and treatment only controls HIV infections.

The human immune system is continually confronted with antigenic challenges that are usually successfully met using synergistically acting components of innate and adaptive immune responses. The primary cellular lineages mediating these responses are lymphoid (NK cells and T and B cells) and myeloid (neutrophils, macrophages, and dendritic cells). Defects in any of one these cells, whether due to overzealous responses to self-constituents leading to autoimmunity (see Chapter 13) or their inability to defend against disease-causing organisms or cancer cells leading to **immunodeficiency**, the host faces dire consequences. The latter state, discussed here, in which the immune system's defense mechanisms are compromised or absent due to a genetic or developmental defect, is called a **primary immunodeficiency**. It is usually present at birth but may not manifest itself until later in life. Immunodeficiencies acquired due to the loss of immune function caused by external processes or diseases are called **secondary**, or **acquired, immunodeficiencies**. The most common secondary immunodeficiency is **acquired immunodeficiency syndrome** (**AIDS**) caused by human immunodeficiency virus 1 (HIV-1). It is discussed in the latter parts of the chapter. First, an introduction to primary immunodeficiency diseases including classification, genetic basis, and laboratory assessment, followed by discussion of common examples of the defined categories of primary immunodeficiency diseases.

# PRIMARY IMMUNODEFICIENCY DISEASES ARE "REAL"-WORLD MODELS FOR IDENTIFYING MOLECULAR COMPONENTS OF THE IMMUNE SYSTEM

Most primary immunodeficiencies are inherited monogenic disorders that affect innate or/and adaptive immune activities through altered expression and function of proteins that are involved in immune development, effector cell functions, signaling cascades, and maintenance of immune homeostasis. Thus, the hallmark of primary immunodeficiency diseases is susceptibility to infections. Studies, using immunological and molecular genetic approaches to determine infectious disease susceptibilities, have defined more than 200 primary immunodeficiency diseases and more than 100 disease-related genes. Most of these diseases are rare; the estimates of incidence range from 1 in 2 million for extremely rare conditions to 1 in 10,000 to 1 in 2000 live births for most others. The most frequently diagnosed primary immunodeficiency disease is IgA deficiency with an incidence of 1 in 333 live births. The most common primary immunodeficiency diseases are associated with the development of humoral immunity, representing more than 50% of cases, while roughly 10–20% of the cases include cellular immunity, or humoral and cellular immunity, or phagocyte disorders. Defects in the complement system only represent about 1–3% of cases. By default, using primary immunodeficiency diseases as natural models have their limitations, nonetheless they provide "real" world instructions to the consequences of molecular defects when compared to artificial challenges of immunodeficient mice.

## Primary Immunodeficiencies Are Classified into Several Major Categories

Most recently, the International Union of Immunological Societies and the World Health Organization define eight categories of primary immunodeficiency diseases: combined T cell and B cell immunodeficiencies; predominately antibody deficiencies; other well-defined immunodeficiency syndromes; diseases of immune dysregulation; congenital defects of phagocyte number, function, or both; defects in innate immunity; and autoinflammatory disorders.

Taken together, primary immunodeficiency diseases may involve distinct components of the immune system, such as, neutrophils, macrophages, dendritic cells, NK cells, complement proteins, and T and B lymphocytes, which in turn are generically classified into broad immunodeficiencies of humoral, cell-mediated, combined humoral and cell-mediated immunity, phagocyte function, complement pathway activities, and other well-defined primary immunodeficiency syndromes of uncertain molecular mechanism. Table 16-1 lists some examples of primary immunodeficiency diseases that will be discussed.

## Primary Immunodeficiency Diseases Have a Strong Genetic Basis

Primary immunodeficiency diseases are a genetically heterogeneous group of diseases. To date, roughly 120 distinct genes have been identified that lead to primary immunodeficiency diseases. In most cases, primary immunodeficiency diseases are secondary

**TABLE 16-1 Gene Defects, Associated Features, Inheritance for Some Primary Immunodeficiencies**

| Disease | Gene defect | Associated features | Inheritance |
|---|---|---|---|
| **B cell/Immunoglobulin deficiencies** | | | |
| X-linked agammaglobulinemia | Mutations in *btk* | No mature B cells; severe bacterial infections | XL |
| X-linked hyper-IgM syndrome | Mutations in *CD40L* | Decreased IgG and IgA | XL |
| Selective IgA immunodeficiency | Unknown | Low or no IgA | Variable |
| Common variable immunodeficiency | Unknown | Low IgG and IgA; variable IgM | Variable |
| **T cell deficiencies** | | | |
| 22q11 deletion syndrome | Contiguous gene defect in 90% affect thymic development | Thymic aplasia | AD |
| ZAP-70 deficiency | Defects in ZAP-70 signaling kinase | Defective TCR signaling; decreased $CD8^+$ T cells | AR |
| CD3γ or CD3ε deficiencies | Defect in TCR CD3γ and ε chains | T cells markedly decreased; serum Ig decreased | AR |
| CD3δ deficiency | Defect in TCR CD3δ chains | T cells markedly decreased; serum Ig decreased | AR |
| CD8 deficiency | Defects in CD8α chain | $CD8^+$ T cell absent | |
| **B and T cell deficiencies** | | | |
| Common γ chain deficiency | Defect in γ chain for IL-2, -4, -7, -9, -15, -21 | T cells and NK cells markedly decreased; serum Ig decreased | XL |
| ADA deficiency | Absent ADA | Elevated lymphotoxic metabolites | AR |
| PNP deficiency | Absent PNP | Elevated lymphotoxic metabolites | AR |

*(continued overleaf)*

**TABLE 16-1** (*Continued*)

| Disease | Gene defect | Associated features | Inheritance |
|---------|-------------|---------------------|-------------|
| RAG1/RAG2 deficiency | Complete defect of RAG 1 or 2 | Defective VDJ recombination; T cells and B cells markedly decreased; serum Ig decreased | AR |
| Omenn syndrome | Missense mutations in RAG1 and 2 genes | B cells normal or decreased; serum Ig decreased | AR |
| Artemis deficiency | Defect in Artemis DNA recombinase-repair protein | Defective VDJ recombination; T cells and B cells markedly decreased; serum Ig decreased | AR |
| JAK3 deficiency | Defective JAK3 signaling kinase | T cells markedly decreased; serum Ig decreased | AR |
| Wiskott-Aldrich syndrome | Mutations in *WAS* gene | Progressive decrease in T cells; decreased IgM; thrombocytopenia with small platelets | XL |
| Ataxia-telangiectasia | Mutation in *ATM* gene | Progressive decrease in T cells; decreased IgA, IgE, and IgG subclasses | AR |
| Bare lymphocyte syndrome | Mutations in *TAP1*, *TAP2* or *tapasin* genes (no class I MHC molecules); mutations in transcription factors for class II MHC molecules | Decreased CD8$^+$ T cells; Decreased CD4$^+$ T cells, serum Ig decreased | AR |
| Leukocyte adhesion deficiency | Mutations in *ITGB2* gene (type 1); mutations in FUCTI GDP-fucose transporter (type 2); mutations in Cal DAG-GEF1 (type 3) | Affects adherence, chemotaxis, endocytosis of N, M, L and NK, and T/NK cell cytotoxicity | AR |
| **Innate immunity deficiencies** | | | |
| NEMO syndrome | Mutations of *NEMO (IKBKG)*, a modulator of NF-kB activation | Affects L and M, lack of antibody response to polysaccharides | XL |
| IRAK-4 deficiency | Mutation of *IRAK4*, a component of the TLR signaling pathway | Affects L and M, bacterial infections | AR |
| WHIM syndrome | Gain-of-function mutations of *CXCR4*, the receptor for CXCL12 | Increased response of the CXCR4 to its ligand CXCL12 | AD |
| Chronic granulomatous disease | Mutations in *CYBB* and *CYBA* genes | Affects N and M, not oxidative burst for killing | XL and AR |
| Chediak-Higashi syndrome | Defects in *LYST* gene, impaired lysosomal trafficking | Low NK and T$_C$ cell activity | AR |
| IL-12 p40 deficiency | Mutation in *IL-12p40* subunit gene | Affects M, IL-12-dependent IFN-$\gamma$ production: susceptibility to *Mycobacteria* and *Salmonella* | AR |
| IL-12R $\beta$1 chain deficiency | Mutation in *IL-12R$\beta$1* gene | Affects L and NK, IL-12-dependent IFN-$\gamma$ production: susceptibility to *Mycobacteria* and *Salmonella* | AR |
| IFN-$\gamma$R 1 & IFN-$\gamma$R 2 deficiency | Mutation in *IFN-$\gamma$R1* and IFN-$\gamma$R2 genes | Affects M and L, IFN-$\gamma$ binding and signaling, susceptibility to *Mycobacteria* and *Salmonella* | AR and AD |
| STAT1 deficiency | Mutation in *STAT1*, controls IFN-$\alpha$/-$\beta$/-$\gamma$ signaling | Affects L and M; susceptibility to *Mycobacteria*, *Salmonella*, and viruses | AR |
| **Complement component deficiencies** | | | |
| See Figure 16-3 | | | All are AR |

Abbreviations: autosomal-dominant, AD; autosomal-recessive, AR; immunoglobulin, Ig; lymphocytes, L; monocytes/macrophages, M; natural killer, NK cells; neutrophils, N; X-linked, XL.

to inherited autosomal recessive, monogenic abnormalities. A few primary immunodeficiency diseases are X-linked recessive (such as Bruton's agammaglobulinemia). The genetic flaws that lead to primary immunodeficiency diseases can affect the production and function of proteins that participate in various biological activities, such as immune organ and cell development, effector-cell functions, signaling cascades, and maintenance of immune system hemostatsis. Uncovering the genetic defects creates a foundation from which target gene therapy may be possible.

## Most Laboratories Can Perform Tests Assessing for the Presence of Immunodeficiencies

The immunological workup for suspected primary immunodeficiency diseases includes an initial screening that accesses complete blood count and levels of serum IgG, IgM, and IgA (Figure 16-1). Other tests used are flow cytometry (see Figure 5-13) to quantify peripheral blood T cell, B cell, NK cell, and monocyte numbers, complement activity, T and B cell functional evaluations, and phagocyte function evaluations. Diagnostic criteria revolve around a blood count (cell number per μl) and immunoglobulin levels, followed by assessment for mutation in the suspected gene. The latter assessment is required for a definitive diagnosis of many primary immunodeficiency diseases.

### MINI SUMMARY

Primary immunodeficiency is the result of immune system defense mechanisms that are compromised or absent due to genetic or

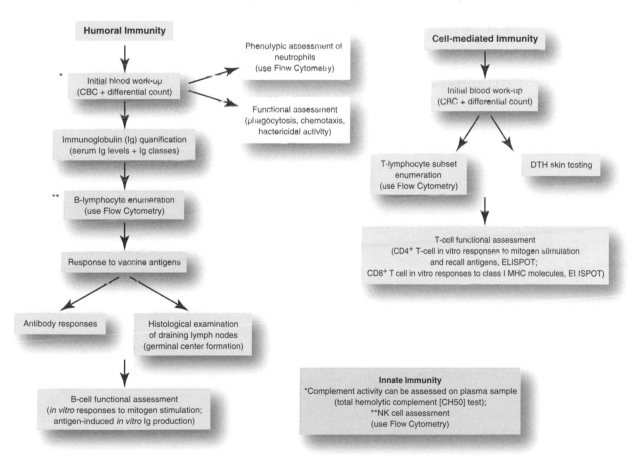

FIGURE 16-1 **Evaluation of humoral and cell-mediated immunity.** Schematic approaches are used to assess B- and T-cell numbers, products, and functions. Components of innate immune system can also be evaluated. Abbreviations: complete blood count, CBC; delayed-type hypersensitivity, DTH; enzyme-linked immunospot, ELISPOT.

developmental defects. More than 200 primary immunodeficiency diseases and about 120 disease-related genes are characterized. Primary immunodeficiency diseases are broadly defined as humoral, cell-mediated, combined humoral and cell-mediated, phagocyte function, and complement pathway activities; their distribution follows the same sequence with B-cell deficiencies with the highest frequency (50%) to complement component deficiencies with the lowest frequency (1–3%). Most primary immunodeficiency diseases are inherited autosomal recessive, monogenic disorders; a few are X-linked recessive. Initial screening tests for immunodeficiencies include complete blood count, assessment of serum immunoglobulin levels, quantification of peripheral blood immune cells, followed by functional tests and assessment for mutation.

# PRIMARY IMMUNODEFICIENCY DISEASES: EXAMPLES OF NATURALLY OCCURRING IMMUNOSUPPRESSION

Throughout the fetal, neonatal, and young adult stages of life, the individual undergoes progressive immunologic maturation. Primary immunodeficiency diseases are caused by either genetic or developmental factors, or both, may lead to abnormal maturation of the immune system and undue susceptibility to infection. Primary immunodeficiency may involve nearly complete failure to mature of either T or B cells, or both or defective components in innate immunity, and complement pathways. The result is a *naturally occurring immunosuppression*. Primary immunodeficiency diseases can affect humoral immunity, cell-mediated immunity, phagocytosis, or the complement system; examples of each are discussed (Figure 16-2).

## Immunodeficiency Diseases Involving Only B Cells

Primary immunodeficiency diseases involving B cells comprise a spectrum of disorders ranging from absence of all classes of immunoglobulins to a selective deficiency of one immunoglobulin class. The first such disease characterized at the genetic level was described by Bruton in 1952. **X-linked agammaglobulinemia** (also called **Bruton's agammaglobulinemia**) occurs in young boys (4 to 12 months) and is inherited as an X-linked recessive character. It is the most common of the agammaglobulinemias. The disease results from a defective Bruton tyrosine kinase gene called *btk*, which encodes a tyrosine kinase that regulates signaling pathways. The *btk* gene is required for intracellular signal transduction that occurs in bone marrow pre-B cells for development to B cells and plasma cells. All X-linked agammaglobulinemia patients have low or undetectable levels of btk mRNA and kinase activity. Little or no IgG and few circulating B cells are found in the blood; that is, IgM, IgA, and IgG are markedly reduced (there is less than 2 mg/ml of IgG) and plasma cells are absent from the bone marrow and lymph nodes. T cell numbers and functions are normal. These patients cannot cope with bacterial infections due to encapsulated bacteria such as *Streptococcus pneumonia*, *Haemophilus influenza*, *Neisseria meningitidis*, and *Mycoplasma* and *Pseudomonas* species, but are able to cope with viral infections. Prophylactic and long-term antibiotics and regular transfusions of human IgG enable them to live normal lives.

Other agammaglobulinemias include autosomal recessive, non-X-linked **hyper-IgM syndrome**, which is represented by defects in the nucleotide editing enzymes activation-induced cytidine deaminase and uracil nucleoside glycosylase. Defects in these enzymes, present only in germinal center B cells, cause disrupted B-cell development and antibody production. In fact, defects in these enzymes lead to malformed germinal centers and enlarged lymph nodes. Patients with hyper-IgM syndrome exhibit hypoagammaglobulinemia and have recurrent infections as seen with X-linked agammaglobulinemia patients. Another X-linked humoral deficiency is **X-linked hyper-IgM syndrome**, a disease where patients have normal B- and T-cell development but low levels of IgG and IgA and normal or elevated levels of IgM. Roughly 70% of patients with hyper-IgM syndrome are X-linked in inheritance. The disease results from a defect in the CD40 ligand (CD154) (see Chapter 8) on activated T cells, which cannot engage B-cell CD40 (the B cells are normal). The B cells cannot undergo isotype switching or somatic hypermutation. Male patients with X-linked hyper-IgM syndrome present with recurrent pyogenic infections, are exceptionally susceptible to *Pneumocystis carinii*, and are prone to neutropenia, autoimmune hemolytic anemia, and thrombocytopenic purpura. Long-term survival rate for these patients is poor, less than 30% of them survive beyond 25 years of age.

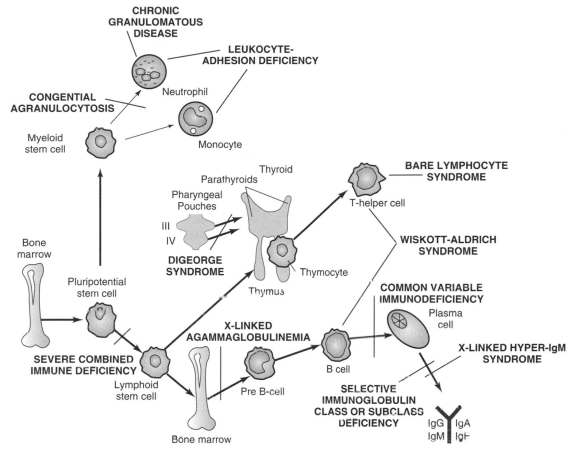

**FIGURE 16-2** Sites of developmental dysfunction in humoral, cell-mediated, and innate immunity immunodeficiencies.

Another category of less severe humoral primary immunodeficiency disorders is known as **selective IgA immunodeficiency**; it is the most common primary immunodeficiency disease. Only 30% of the patients with selective IgA immunodeficiency are prone to infections. It results from a defect in the interaction between T and B cells, which blocks B-cell development. The gene defect is unknown. This deficiency disease exhibits an imbalance mainly in IgA, but all combinations of globulin imbalance may be observed.

A similar type of immunodeficiency disease is **common variable immunodeficiency**, where there is variable reduction in multiple immunoglobulin isotypes (usually low IgG and IgA, variable IgM) caused by four monogenic defects, insufficiency of each encoded molecule disrupts B-cell maturation, function, and differentiation at a different stage. Common variable immunodeficiency typically affects adults; they are treated regularly with intravenously or subcutaneously administered purified human immunoglobulin, and antibiotic therapy.

The latter therapeutic approach is the mainstay for agammaglobulinemias and common variable immunodeficiency.

## Immunodeficiency Diseases Involving Only T Cells

Congenital immunodeficiency diseases involving T cells are rare. The diseases are caused by mutations in genes that are required for T-cell differentiation. At least 35 different human gene variants are known to cause monogenic severe T-cell immunodeficiency diseases. Based on the cellular function of the proteins encoded by these genes, they can be grouped into five categories: cytokine signaling, somatic recombination, T cell receptor (TCR) signaling, antigen presentation by class I and class II molecules, and basic cellular processes. In most cases, an associated defect in B-cell–mediated immunity occurs because complete immunity requires T cells. **22q11 deletion syndrome** (also called **DiGeorge syndrome** or congenital thymic hypoplasia) is caused by migration defects of neural crest-derived tissues and abnormal embryologic development of the thymus (the etiologic source of impaired immune responses) but many other parts of the body can be affected. The syndrome affects roughly 1 in 4000 live births and results from a microdeletion near the center of the long arm of chromosome 22 at the designated location q11.2. Cell-mediated immune responses are absent at birth. The number of peripheral T cells is severely decreased, and T-cell function in peripheral blood is absent. B cells are unaffected but T cell-dependent antibody function is absence in many patients. In fact, individuals with a 22q11 deletion can present with more than 200 symptoms. 22q11 deletion syndrome can be successfully treated with a thymus graft; there is no genetic treatment. Symptomatic antibiotic treatment is used to counter infections.

Another set of diseases associated with T-cell immunodeficiencies exhibit normal numbers of T cells but they are nonfunctional. The absence of T-cell immunity is caused by dysfunctional TCR signaling due to deficient expression of zeta-associated protein 70 (ZAP-70), p56 *lck*, CD3γ, CD3ε, and CD3δ. Antigenic peptide–MHC molecule interaction with the TCR initiates signal transduction through the CD3–ζ complex (see Chapters 8 and 10), which activate tyrosine kinases such as ZAP-70 and p56 *lck* that eventually lead to T-cell activation.

Defects in the ZAP-70–encoding gene (**ZAP-70 deficiency**), inherited in an autosomal recessive manner, leads to a combined immunodeficiency disease with markedly decreased numbers of CD8+ T cells, normal numbers of nonfunctional CD4+ T cells, normal B and NK cell numbers and functions, and normal serum immunoglobulin levels. The affected children have recurrent and opportunistic infections within the first year of life. ZAP-70 deficiency is fatal unless treated by bone marrow transplantation. Defects in the p56 *lck*-encoding gene (**p56 *lck* deficiency**) leads to a CD4+ T-cell lymphopenia and low serum immunoglobulin levels but normal B and NK cell numbers.

Rare immunodeficiency diseases are caused by mutations in the γ and ε CD3 subunits (**CD3γ and CD3ε deficiencies**), which are inherited in an autosomal recessive manner. The resultant disease is moderate to severe with normal numbers of circulating T cells that are markedly unresponsive to stimuli. In contrast to CD3γ and CD3ε deficiencies, **CD3δ deficiency** leads to a T-cell lymphopenia. **CD8 deficiency** also has been reported; it results from mutations in the *CD8α*-encoding gene. These individuals have normal immunoglobulin levels and NK cell function but recurrent infections.

There are no replacement therapies, such as used in agammaglobulinemias, for the cellular deficiencies. Treatment revolves around aggressive antibiotic treatment of infectious complications as they occur or preventative antibiotic treatment when appropriate.

## Immunodeficiency Diseases Involving Both B and T Cells

Very rarely, infants are born lacking all major immune defenses—absence of humoral and cell-mediated immunity; this third category of immunodeficiency diseases includes the disorders called **severe combined immunodeficiency diseases** (**SCIDs**). These infants are susceptible to overwhelming recurrent bacterial, fungal, and viral sinopulmonary and skin infections. SCID is a heterogenous group of primary immunodeficiencies that are the result of abnormal B- and T-cell development and function and in some cases the complete absence of functional lymphocytes—hence the name SCID.

The most common (about 50% of SCIDs patients) and prototypical SCID is **common γ (γ$_C$) chain deficiency**. It results from mutations in the γ$_C$ chain gene that encodes a chain shared by the cytokine receptors for IL-2, IL-4, IL-7, IL-9, IL-15, and IL-21. The defective γ$_C$ chain gene encodes either an abnormal or absent cytokine receptor; therefore, early lymphoid progenitor cells lacking the receptor are unresponsive to these cytokines that are essential to the normal development of T and B cells. This leads to markedly decreased numbers of circulating T cells and NK cells and normal or increased levels of circulating B cells that are dysfunctional. Common γ chain deficiency patients exhibit an X-linked recessive pattern of inheritance (thus, also called *X-linked SCID*); the defect maps to chromosome Xq13, which contains the defective IL-2 receptor γ gene.

The next most common of the X-linked autosomal recessive forms of SCIDs (accounts for roughly 20% of SCIDs cases) is caused by a deficiency in an enzyme, *adenosine deaminase (ADA)*, which catalyzes the deamination of adenosine and deoxyadenosine to inosine and 2'deoxyinosine. The lack of ADA leads to an accumulation of the toxic metabolites adenosine and deoxyadenosine that kills the developing lymphocytes. **ADA deficiency** patients present with similar symptoms as γ$_C$ chain deficiency patients; however, ADA deficiencies cause a more severe lymphopenia than other SCIDs but their NK cell numbers and function are normal. A rarer form of SCID is due to a deficiency in another enzyme, *purine nucleoside phosphorylase (PNP)*, which catalyzes the conversion of inosine to hypoxanthine and of guanosine to guanine. Again, the buildup of toxic metabolites kills the developing lymphocytes; there is a progressive decrease in circulating T cells, circulating B cells are normal in number. The SCID is called **PNP deficiency**.

Antigen receptor production requires the expression of protein encoded by the recombination activating genes, *RAG1* and *RAG2*, which control the somatic recombination of T and B cell receptor genes. Their absence or dysfunction leads to an inability to assemble receptor gene segments; therefore, receptors do not form, arresting the T and B cells at an immature stage of development. Mutations that cause a total absence of *RAG1* or *RAG2* gene product, **RAG1/RAG2 deficiency**, leads to SCID, whereas missense mutations on one allele that exhibit some recombinase activity cause **Omenn syndrome**. The latter disorder is characterized by autoimmune features that resemble graft-versus-host disease, where circulating T cells are present but have restricted heterogeneity, circulating B cells numbers are decreased, and serum immunoglobulin levels are decreased, except IgE is increased. Associated features include erythroderma, protracted diarrhea, eosinophilia, and heptosplenomegaly. These SCIDs are fatal unless corrected by bone marrow transplants.

Once the RAG1 and RAG2 recombinase enzymes cut DNA, the Artemis gene-encoded DNA recombinase-repair protein is responsible for repairing the DNA. If this protein is absent, cut DNA does not get repaired, leading to a SCID with a T and B cell deficiency but normal NK cell numbers. This SCID is called **Artemis deficiency** and presents a clinical and immunologic picture similar to RAG1/RAG2 deficiency. A trademark of Artemis deficiency is increased radiation sensitivity.

A non-X-linked autosomal recessive SCID called **Janus kinase 3 (JAK3) deficiency** is caused by mutations of the *JAK3* gene, which encodes the JAK3 protein, an intracellular tyrosine kinase that is a crucial signaling molecule associated with the $\gamma_C$ chain. The lack of JAK3 kinase activity impairs cytokine signaling as seen in $\gamma_C$ chain SCID, leading to an immunologic and clinical picture similar to $\gamma_C$ chain SCID. Abnormal JAK3 signaling by IL-2, IL-4, IL-7, IL-9, IL-15, and IL-21 causes an early and severe block in T and NK cell development and associated B cell dysfunction.

**Wiskott-Aldrich syndrome (WAS)** is another X-linked recessive disease in which cell-mediated immune reactions are absent and antibody responses are defective. A notable characteristic of the disease is an inability to respond to polysaccharide antigens because patients have low levels of serum IgM, whereas IgA and IgE levels are elevated, and IgG levels are normal. The earliest abnormality found in these patients is thrombocytopenia with small defective platelets. The disease results from various mutations in the gene on the short arm of the X chromosome encoding WAS protein (WASP), which is found only in lymphocytes and megakaryocytes. WASP is critical in maintaining cytoskeletal structure and function. WAS patients have recurrent infections of the ears and sinuses. They are treated with intravenous immunoglobulin and splenectomy to treat the thrombocytopenia; this results in a median life expectancy of 15 years. The disease X-linked thrombocytopenia is also due to WASP mutations. The collective incidence of WAS and X-linked thrombocytopenia is approximately 4–10 in 1 million live births.

Another devastating immunodeficiency disease is **ataxia-telangiectasia** (*ataxia* refers to the difficultly in walking; *telangiectasias* are small, red spider veins found on the surface of the cheeks and ears and in the corners of the patient's eyes), which results from a mutation in the ataxia-telangiectasia mutated (*ATM*) gene (leads to a disorder of cell check-point and DNA double-strand break repair). It is inherited in an autosomal recessive manner. Immunologic pathogenesis is manifested by thymic hypoplasia (progressive decrease in circulating T cells; circulating B cells are normal) and serum immunoglobulin deficiencies (80% of the patients have an IgA and $IgG_2$ and $IgG_4$ deficiency). Most patients present with recurrent respiratory bacterial infections and increased susceptibility to hematological cancers and to ionizing radiation; the latter is due to the inability to repair DNA and chromosomal instability. Ataxia-telangiectasia has an estimated incidence of 1 in 40,000 to 1 in 300,000 live births. The prognosis for ataxia-telangiectasia patients is poor; they usually die in their teens or early 20s. Gamma-globulin and antibiotic treatment is symptomatic and supportive.

**Bare lymphocyte syndrome type I** and **II** are autosomal recessive forms of SCID. It is a deficiency in either MHC class I (type I) or II (type II) gene expression. The defective expression of HLA class II molecules accounts for about 5% of SCIDs. The HLA class II defects, caused by mutations in transcription factors for class II molecules, cause a more severe immunodeficiency than that associated with HLA class I molecule defects. Human B cells, macrophages, and dendritic cells express little or no HLA-DP, -DQ, or -DR molecules and are unable to express these molecules when exposed to interferon-γ (IFN-γ). Circulating T and B cell levels are normal but $CD4^+$ T cell numbers are reduced; immunoglobulin levels are normal or decreased. The inability to express class II molecules leads to a failure to present antigen to CD4$^+$ T cells. Children with this disease are susceptible to bacterial, fungal, and viral infections beginning in the first year of life; most die by the age of 4 years from overwhelming recurrent infections. Bone marrow transplant is the only treatment. Bare lymphocyte syndrome type I is caused by mutated *transporter associated with antigen processing 1* and *2* (*TAP1* and *TAP2*) genes in the HLA (see Chapter 7). The mutated *TAP1* and *TAP2* genes lead to deficient expression of HLA class I molecules on cell surfaces. Bare lymphocyte syndrome type I is also caused by mutations in the *Tapasin* gene.

Defects in proteins mediating leukocyte rolling and adhesion describe a SCID-like disease called **leukocyte adhesion deficiency (LAD)**. LAD is separated into four types: LAD type 1, LAD type 2, LAD type 3, and LAD with Rac2 deficiency. LAD type 1 is caused by an autosomal recessively inherited deficiency of a 95-kD β-chain (CD18) structure. The β chain is linked noncovalently to each of three distinct α-chain types to form different cell-surface molecules (see Chapter 8): (1) LFA-1 (CD11a/CD18) on B, T, and NK cells; (2) complement receptor type 3 (CR3; also called *CD11b*) on eosinophils, neutrophils, monocytes, macrophages, and NK cells; and (3) CR4 (also called *CD11c*). Thus, the absence of LFA-1 leads to marked reduction of adhesion required for neutrophil chemotaxis, cell adherence, and reduced degradation functions during phagocytosis. The prognosis for all patients with these combined immunodeficiency diseases is poor because of their susceptibility to systemic bacterial and fungal infections, poor wound healing, scarring skin infections, and gingivitis. They usually succumb to overwhelming infections. LAD type 2 results from a defective carbohydrate fucosylation, leading to a lack of CD15s, sialyl-Lewis$^X$, the ligand for the E and P selectin molecules on endothelial cells. Patients with LAD type 2 present with clinical symptoms similar to LAD type 1. LAD type 3, a less well-characterized immunodeficiency, is due to defective regulatory GTPase called *Rap-1*, which mediates activation of β1-3 integrins. It leads to impaired adhesion of lymphocytes and NK cells. The clinical picture is similar to LAD type 1 plus additional bleeding propensity. The Rac2 deficiency results from mutations in the GTPase Rac2, which regulates NADPH oxidase and actin cytoskeleton. This GTPase plays an important role in regulating cytoskeleton reorganization, integrin formation, and cell adhesion; these activities are abnormal in Rac2 deficiency patients. The neutrophils exhibit abnormal chemotaxis, adherence, secretion of primary granules, and production of superoxide.

Purified human immunoglobulin replacement can be used to treat the antibody component of combined immunodeficiency but this therapy alone is insufficient. Bone marrow transplantation remains the only long-term hope for SCID patients. The combination of patient age at transplantation and donor type (identical versus haplioidentical versus nonidentical) drives the success rate, which ranges from 50% to almost 100%. The idea that SCID can be modified by gene therapy is appealing; the first success of *ex vivo* gene transfer and reinfusion of stem cells with a functional copy of the γ$_C$ gene has been reported. IFN-γ supplementation for single-gene defects in patients carrying IFN-γ and IL-12 receptor mutations in ADA deficiency or chronic granulomatous disease (discussed shortly) has been beneficial. These successes have led to gene replacement therapy for these two deficiency diseases; the clinical test results look promising. As with any treatment there are risks that need to be balanced against benefits, in two incidences reinfused treated cells uncontrollably proliferated causing leukemia in the SCID patients.

## Immunodeficiency Diseases Involving Innate Immunity Components

Primary immunodeficiency diseases associated with lymphoid lineage cells such as T and B cells affect adaptive immunity, whereas deficiency defects in myeloid lineage cells lead to dysfunctional innate immune responses. Deficiencies in innate immunity principally revolve around but are not limited to phagocytic cells such as neutrophils and monocytes/macrophages—dysfunctional phagocytic activities. There are also a few rare primary immunodeficiency diseases associated with innate immunity specifically called *innate immunity deficiencies*.

The innate immunity deficiencies include NF-κB essential modulator (NEMO) defect, inhibitor of κB (IκB) defect, IL-1 receptor-associated kinase 4 (IRAK-4) deficiency, and warts, hypogammaglobulinemia, infections, and myelokathexis (WHIM) syndrome. The transcription factor, NF-κB, plays a key role in regulating the immune response through the production of down-stream cytokines such as IL-1, IL-2, IL-6, IL-8, G-CSF, GM-CSF, and TNF-α. NF-κB activation is controlled by inhibitor of NF-κB (IκB), which is prevented from inactivating NF-κB by another molecule IκB kinase that degrades IκB, and thereby NF-κB remains active. A mutation in the γ chain of IκB kinase (called *NF-κB essential modulator* or *NEMO*) leads to an inhibition of NF-κB activity; the functional defect in the NF-κB signaling pathway in lymphocytes and monocytes results in the **NEMO**

**syndrome** (also called *ectodermal dysplasia associated immunodeficiency* [*EDA-ID*]). The NEMO syndrome is characterized by anhidrotic ectodermal dysplasia, lack of specific antibody responses to polysaccharide antigens, and mycobacterial infections. A number of patients with NEMO syndrome also exhibit deficient NK cell cytotoxicity. A gain-of-function mutation of IκB leads to impaired activation of NF-κB, which also causes the NEMO syndrome.

Many of the toll-like receptors (see Chapter 3) use the IRAK-4 signaling pathway in innate immunity. A mutation of the *IRAK4* gene encodes a faulty protein kinase, which disrupts lymphocyte and monocyte inflammatory responses leading to recurrent pyogenic bacterial infections—the **IRAK-4 deficiency**.

Another gain-of-function mutation, this time of CXCR4 (chemokine receptor for CXCL12 [also called *stem cell derived factor 1; SDF-1*]), causes a defect in innate immunity. The altered chemokine receptor CXCR4 has an increased response to its ligand CXCL12, which leads to retention of mature neutrophils in the bone marrow (myelokathexis), severe neutropenia, hypogammaglobulinemia, reduced B cell numbers, and treatment resistant warts due to human papilloma virus infection—the **WHIM syndrome**. Antibiotics, G-CSF, GM-CSF, and intravenous immunoglobulin administration are used to manage WHIM.

X-linked and autosomal forms of phagocyte (neutrophils, monocytes, and macrophages) disorders that cause primary immunodeficiencies have been described including chronic granulomatous disease, LAD (described earlier), Chediak-Higashi syndrome, and defects in the IFN-γ/IL-12 axis. **Chronic granulomatous disease** (CGD), whether the X-linked or autosomal recessive forms, is the prototypical phagocyte function disorder that presents in children and infrequently in adults. It affects roughly 1 in 200,000 individuals in the U.S. The functional defect underlying all CGDs is a deficiency of the respiratory burst, which normally allows the cell to generate superoxide and other reactive species that kill ingested microorganisms. A mutation of the enzyme nicotinamide adenine dinucleotide phosphate (NADPH) oxidase (also called *phagocyte NADPH oxidase* or *PHOX*) causes this defect. Defects in any one of the four subunits of PHOX (gp91phox, p22phox, p67phox, and p47phox) can cause CGD. Mutation in the *gp91phox*-encoding gene is the most common cause of CGD; it is the defect associated with X-linked CGD. Less-common mutations in *p22phox-*, *p67phox-*, and *p47phox*-encoding genes cause the autosomal recessive forms of CGD. Patients with CGD, usually diagnosed before the age of 5, present with recurrent bacterial infections, and have marked propensity for *Aspergillus* infections, which lead to granuloma formations in many organs. Early diagnosis and aggressive antibiotic therapy and IFN-γ treatment prevents infections; IFN-γ treatment is standard for CGD.

**Chediak-Higashi syndrome** is a rare autosomal recessive disorder characterized by partial oculocutaneous albinism, increased susceptibility to bacterial infections (especially to *Staphylococcus aureus*), and progressive neuropathy. Mutations of the lysosomal trafficking protein called *LYST* are responsibility for the defects associated with Chediak-Higashi syndrome. Phagocytic cells with this defective protein are unable to form phagolysosomes (the combination of lysosomes and phagosomes is dysfunctional), which leads to the inability of these cells to destroy phagocytosed bacteria. Chediak-Higashi syndrome patients have normal levels of circulating T and B cells and immunoglobulins; however, their NK cells and $T_C$ cells are dysfunctional. Most Chediak-Higashi syndrome patients develop fatal complications called *accelerated phase*, which results from unbridled T cell and macrophage activation throughout the body.

Defects in IFN-γ/IL-12 axis compromises the phagocyte's (monocytes/macrophages) ability to be activated to kill intracellular pathogens such as mycobacteria, listeria, and salmonella. IFN-γ is the main activator of macrophages and dendritic cells, which in turn release IL-12, the main stimulus of $T_H1$ cells to produce IFN-γ. The autosomal recessive deficiency of the IL-12 p40 subunit (**IL-12 p40 deficiency**) leads to mild intracellular infections because the lack of IL-12 production translates into decreased IFN-γ production. It mainly affects monocytes or macrophages. A similar clinical picture results from the autosomal recessive deficiency of the IL-12 receptor β1 chain (**IL-12R β1 chain deficiency**); however, it primarily affects lymphocytes and NK cells. Like IL-12 or IL-12 receptor deficiencies, defects in the IFN-γ receptor α or β chains (**IFN-γR 1 deficiency** and **IFN-γR 2 deficiency**, respectively) leads to mycobacterial and Salmonella infections and affects lymphocytes and monocytes/macrophages. Mutations leading to complete loss of either of the IFN-γ receptor α or β chains lead to severe infections, whereas partial defects cause mild disease. Defects in the transcription factor signal transducer of transcription 1 (STAT1), which transduces the IFN-γ–IFN-γ receptor binding signal, causes increased propensity for mycobacterial and Salmonella but not viral infections. It is called **STAT1 deficiency**.

## Immunodeficiency Diseases Involving Complement Components

The complement system participates in innate and adaptive immune responses (see Chapter 11). The complement components mediate *cell lysis, stimulation of an inflammatory response, opsonization* (augments phagocytosis), *removal of antigen-antibody (immune) complexes,* and *B-cell activation.* Deficiencies in all complement components have been reported except for factor B. Complement disorders are rare, when they occur as partial deficiencies they do not lead to increased susceptibility to infections; however, complete deficiencies predispose individuals to infections (mostly by *Neisseria*) and autoimmune diseases, in particular, immune complex diseases such as systemic lupus erythematosis. The latter diseases result from the disrupted clearance of immune complexes, which lead to increased susceptibility to autoimmune diseases. Some complement component deficiencies lead to noninfectious diseases, such as with hereditary angioedema, which is caused by C1 esterase inhibitor deficiency. Examples of the different complement deficiencies are listed in Figure 16-3.

### MINI SUMMARY

Primary immunodeficiency diseases are examples of naturally occurring immunosuppression. They can be categorized according to whether B cells (X-linked agammaglobulinemia, hyper-IgM syndrome, X-linked hyper IgM syndrome, selective IgA deficiency, and common variable immunodeficiency), T cells (22q11 deletion syndrome, ZAP-70 deficiency, p56 *lck* deficiency, and CD3γ, CD3ε, CD3δ, and CD8 deficiencies), or both (severe combined immunodeficiency diseases such as γC chain deficiency, ADA deficiency, PNA deficiency, RAG1/RAG2 deficiency, Omenn syndrome, Artemis deficiency, JAK3 deficiency, Wiskott-Aldrich syndrome, ataxia-telangiectasia, bare lymphocyte syndrome, and leukocyte adhesion deficiency) are affected. Immunodeficiency diseases are also associated with innate immunity components (NEMO sysndrome, IRAK-4 deficiency, WHIM syndrome, chronic granulomatous disease, Chediak-Higashi syndrome, IL-12 p40 deficiency, IL-12R β1 chain deficiency, IFN-γR 1 and IFN-γR 2 deficiency, and STAT1 deficiency) and complement components.

## SECONDARY IMMUNODEFICIENCY DISEASES ARE EXEMPLIFIED BY ACQUIRED IMMUNODEFICIENCY SYNDROME (AIDS)

Immunodeficiency diseases are also the result of environmental effects (such as cancer chemotherapy and immunosuppressive drug treatment after organ transplants) or diseases (such as leukemia, lymphoma, multiple myelomas, and chronic infections exemplified by AIDS); the resultant condition is known as **secondary,** or **acquired, immunodeficiency.**

AIDS, a set of symptoms and infections caused by infection by human immunodeficiency virus (HIV), is the most well known secondary immunodeficiency, principally because of its prevalence and its high mortality rate if untreated. AIDS is not the most prevalent cause of immunodeficiency worldwide, severe malnutrition is; however, it is beyond the scope of this text and only AIDS will be discussed.

### More Than 25 Years into the AIDS Pandemic, HIV Infection Continues to Exact a Tremendous Toll Worldwide

Starting in 1981, a new disease of unknown cause and high virulence (as high as 60%, in many cases 100%, mortality within 12–15+ years of diagnosis) had by December 2006 in the U.S., afflicted 982,498 people, killing roughly 60% of them. Even though reporting AIDS cases is mandatory, many states do not report HIV-infections that have not progressed to AIDS; therefore, the number of HIV-infected individuals is an estimate. In 2006, there were 36,828 AIDS diagnoses and 14,016 deaths of persons with AIDS, a death rate of 38% (the death rate has decreased over the last few years). It is a different story worldwide. As of December 2007 (Figure 16-4), the World Health Organization estimates that 30.8 million adults and 2.5 million children (under the age of 15) worldwide are infected with the HIV. It is estimated that more than 25 million people have died of AIDS. In 2007, there were 2.5 million AIDS diagnoses worldwide and 2.1 million deaths of persons with AIDS. The daily infection rate is roughly 6800 people and more than 5700 people die of AIDS each day. Sub-Saharian Africa is the most seriously affected region in the global AIDS epidemic, where AIDS is the leading

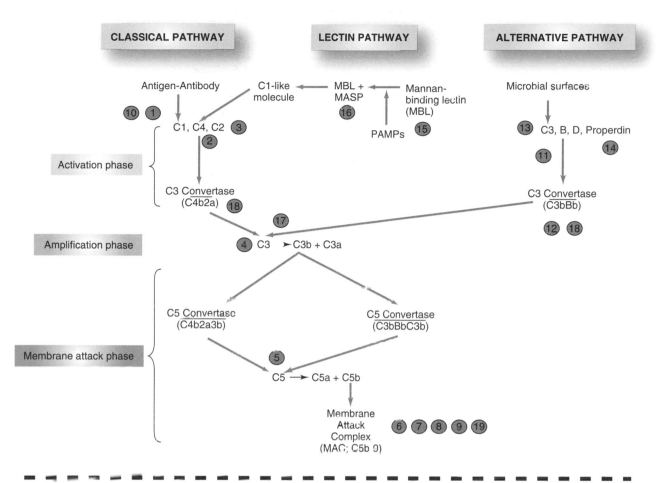

**Deficiencies**

1. C1q, C1r, C1s: Absent C hemolytic activity, defective MAC, abnormal dissolution of immune complexes = SLE-like syndrome, rheumatoid disease, infections
2. C4: Absent C hemolytic activity, defective MAC, abnormal dissolution of immune complexes, defective humoral immunity = SLE-like syndrome, rheumatoid disease, infections
3. C2: Absent C hemolytic activity, defective MAC, abnormal dissolution of immune complexes = SLE-like syndrome, pyogenic infections
4. C3: Absent C hemolytic activity, defective MAC, defective bactericidal activity, defective humoral immunity = recurrent pyogenic infections
5. C5: Absent C hemolytic activity, defective MAC, defective bactericidal activity = SLE, Neisserial infections
6. C6: Absent C hemolytic activity, defective MAC, detective bactericidal activity = SLE, Neisserial infections
7. C7: Absent C hemolytic activity, defective MAC, defective bactericidal activity = SLE, Neisserial infections
8. C8a & C8b chains: Absent C hemolytic activity, defective MAC, defective bactericidal activity = SLE, Neisserial infections
9. C9: Absent C hemolytic activity, defective MAC, defective bactericidal activity = Neisserial infections
10. C1 inhibitor: Spontaneous activation of the C pathway with consumption of C4/C2 = hereditary angioedema
11. Factor D: Absent C hemolytic activity by the alternative pathway = Neisserial infections
12. Factor H: Absent C hemolytic activity by the alternative pathway with consumption of C3 = Neisserial infections, renal disease (hemolytic-uremic syndrome)
13. Factor I: Spontaneous and continuous activation of C3 of the alternative pathway = recurrent pyogenic infections, glomerulonephritis, hemolytic-uremic syndrome
14. Properdin: Absent C hemolytic activity by the alternative pathway = Neisserial infections
15. MBL: Defective mannose recognition, defective hemolytic activity by the lectin pathway = pyogenic infections
16. MASP2: Defective hemolytic activity by the lectin pathway = SLE syndrome, pyogenic infections
17. CR3: Defective adherence and phagocytosis = skin ulers, infections
18. MCP: Decreased C3 binding = glomerulonephritis, hemolytic-uremic syndrome
19. MIRL: Erythrocytes are highly susceptible to C-mediated lysis = hemolytic anemia, thrombosis

**FIGURE 16-3 Complement deficiencies.** The three different complement (C) pathways and some associated deficiencies are shown. Most complement deficiencies lead to increased bacterial infections and rheumatic disorders due to abnormal clearance of immune complexes. The latter dysfunction causes the appearance of autoimmune diseases, particularly systemic lupus erythematosus (SLE). (See also Chapter 11, Figures 11-13 and 11-14) Abbreviations: CR3, complement receptor 3; MASP2, MBL-associated serine protease 2; MCP, membrane cofactor protein; and MIRL, membrane inhibitor of reactive lysis.

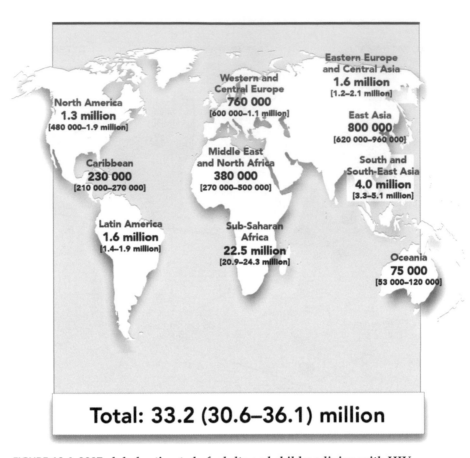

**FIGURE 16-4** 2007 global estimated of adults and children living with HIV.

cause of death (76% of all deaths); HIV infects approximately 22.5 million people. Unlike other regions of the world, 61% HIV-positive individuals in sub-Saharian Africa are women. Irrespective of the global region, the proportion of women with HIV infections or AIDS has increased significantly. In the U.S., the proportion of women among newly diagnosed HIV infections or AIDS increased from 15% before 1996 to 26% in 2006. The next most seriously affected region in the world is South and Southeast Asia, with roughly 4.9 million people living with HIV. Taken together, more than 90% of all individuals living with HIV reside in developing countries. This does not mean that other regions, such as North America and Western and Central Europe are not affected; they have increased numbers of HIV-infected individuals due to prolonged survival provided by aggressive antiretroviral therapy and new HIV diagnoses. Worldwide to date, the estimated total number of people infected with HIV since 1981 is 58 million, of whom 25 million have died.

Within a year of the first reported cases, the U.S. Centers for Disease Control and Prevention (CDC)

coined the term **acquired immunodeficiency syndrome (AIDS)** for this new disease. It can be defined by describing the combination of words used to make up its name: (1) *acquired* because victims did not inherit the disease; this form of disease contraction is a major difference between AIDS and the previously discussed primary immunodeficiency diseases; (2) *immunodeficiency* because the one disease characteristic AIDS victims have in common is a breakdown of their immune system; (3) *syndrome* because of the plethora of rare but ravaging diseases that take advantage of the body's collapsed defenses. HIV affects almost all organs of the body. AIDS is characterized by dramatic weight loss, fever, night sweats, swollen lymph nodes, increasingly frequent opportunistic infections[1] including a rare type of pneumonia caused by *Pneumocystis jirovecii* (originally known as *Pneumocystis carinii* pneumonia), and rare malignancies,

---

[1]Opportunistic infections are caused by common organisms that do not trouble people whose immune systems are healthy but that take advantage of the "opportunity" provided by an immune defense in disarray.

such as Kaposi's sarcoma, Burkitt's lymphoma, and cervical cancer caused by human papilloma virus. The CDC defines AIDS on the basis of clinical conditions associated with HIV infection and CD4+ T-cell counts. This definition allows a more accurate count of cases because a person with a CD4+ T-cell count under 200 cells per μl blood is probably severely ill but may not have any of the designated syndromes (Table 16-2). If an HIV-positive individual has a CD4+ T cell count below 200 per μl of blood (roughly 1100 cells per μl is normal) or 14% of all lymphocytes and/or an AIDS-defining disease that person has AIDS. This categorization stands even if antiretroviral treatment raises CD4+ T cell counts above 200/μl of blood or cures the AIDS-defining diseases.

In the U.S., AIDS increased to epidemic proportions within a year of the first reports. From June 1981 to August 1983, 2008 confirmed cases were reported, with 4 to 5 new cases occurring each day. By the end of 1985 there were roughly 14,000 cases, and as of December 2006 there were 982,498. Because of an incubation period ranging from a months to perhaps 20 years, there are probably many more asymptomatic carriers harboring the virus for every diagnosed case. It is suggested that individuals unaware of their HIV infection status account for 54–70% of all new sexually transmitted infections. Furthermore, those infected with HIV include people who do not belong to the defined high-risk groups

AIDS was first detected because of *marker diseases* (high incidence of known diseases). About 25 to 33% of early AIDS patients had a rare cancer,[2] and 50% had infections caused by *P. jirovecii*, with about 10% of the victims having both. AIDS is a contagious disease spread by intimate sexual contact, by exposure to infected blood or blood products, or from mother to child during pregnancy. HIV infection transmission requires contact with blood, milk, semen, salvia, or vaginal fluid from an infected individual. Sexual transmission of HIV occurs on contact between sexual fluids of one person with the genital, oral, or rectal mucous membranes of the other. The presence of other sexual transmitted diseases (STDs) increases the risk of HIV transmission and infection, because

they act as cofactors for HIV by disrupting the normal epithelial barrier through genital ulcerations and by the accumulation HIV-susceptible or HIV-infected pools of CD4+ T lymphocytes, macrophages, and dendritic cells in semen and vaginal secretions. Avoiding any activity that exposes broken or abraded skin or mucous membranes to fluids from an infected individual can reduce the risk of sexually transmitting HIV. The use of condoms is the most effective means to reduce the sexual transmission of HIV and other STDs. Exposure to blood-borne HIV is relevant to intravenous drug users, hemophiliacs, and blood transfusion or blood product recipients. Sharing of nonsterile syringes represents a major risk for HIV infection. This activity is responsible for roughly 30% of all newly diagnosed HIV infections in China, Eastern Europe, and North America. In developed countries, the risk of blood-transfusion recipients contracting HIV infections is exceedingly low. The majority of the world's population does not have access to safe blood or its products; therefore, between 5% and 10% of global HIV infections are due to transfusions of infected blood or blood products. Perinatal HIV transmission can occur during childbirth; without treatment the transmission from mother to child is 25%, with antiretroviral treatment it drops to 1%. Breastfeeding increases the risk of HIV transmission by approximately 4%. Figure 16-5 illustrates the latest (circa 2006) U.S. cases by transmission categories. The mode of HIV transmission varies depending on global regions: in sub-Saharan Africa heterosexual intercourse is the primary mode; in Eastern Europe and Central Asia use of nonsterile injecting drug paraphernalia is the primary mode; and in North America male-to-male sexual contact is the primary mode. Irrespective of the portal of entry of the HIV, the outcome is the same—immunosuppression, neuropsychiatric abnormalities, and death.

## The Immunopathogenesis of AIDS Is Complex

AIDS is a syndrome of immune dysregulation, dysfunction, and deficiency. The main target of HIV in the host is CD4+ T cells. Commonly, AIDS patients present a lymphopenia primarily affecting CD4+ $T_H$ cells—T cells are low in number, dysfunctional, and abnormal in composition; CD4+ T cells are depleted or missing and if present are function-less, although there seems to be little direct effect on CD8+ T cells, at least not in the early stage of infection. There is a severely reduced CD4:CD8 T-cell ratio, found in AIDS patients; healthy individuals have a ratio of roughly 2.

---

[2]Kaposi's sarcoma is a cancer of blood-vessel endothelial cells evidenced by purple to brown splotches of the skin but can affect other organs, such as the mouth, gastrointestinal tract, and lungs. Until 1979, it was a tumor rarely seen in North America and Europe, and it occurred mainly in patients aged 50 years or older. A γherpes virus called *Kaposi's sarcoma-associated herpes virus* causes Kaposi's sarcoma.

**TABLE 16-2** CDC Classification System for Diagnosis of HIV-Infected Individuals*

| CD4+ T-cell count categories | Clinical categories | | |
|---|---|---|---|
| | A | B | C |
| 1. ≥ 500 μl | A1 | B1 | C1 |
| 2. 200–499/ μl | A2 | B2 | C2 |
| 3. <200/μl | A3 | B3 | C3 |

**AIDS-defining clinical conditions**

*All categories in shaded darker yellow boxes are considered AIDS. For Category A diagnosis one or more of conditions listed below with documented HIV infection and conditions listed in Categories B and C must be absent. For Category B diagnosis one or more of conditions listed below with documented HIV infection and conditions listed in Category C must be absent.*

Category A:
• Asymptomatic HIV infection
• Acute primary HIV infection
• Persistent generalized lymphadenopathy

Category B:
• Bacillary angiomatosis
• Candidiasis, oropharyngeal (thrush)
• Candidiasis, vulvovaginal; persistent, frequent, or poorly responsive to therapy
• Cervical dysplasia (moderate or severe)/cervical carcinoma in situ
• Constitutional symptoms, such as fever (38.5°C) or diarrhea lasting greater than 1 month
• Hairy leukoplakia, oral
• Herpes zoster (shingles), involving at least two distinct episodes or more than one
• dermatome
• Idiopathic thrombocytopenic purpura
• Listeriosis
• Pelvic inflammatory disease, particularly if complicated by tubo-ovarian abscess
• Peripheral neuropathy

Category C:
• Candidiasis of bronchi, trachea, or lungs
• Candidiasis, esophageal
• Cervical cancer (invasive)
• Coccidioidomycosis, disseminated or extrapulmonary
• Cryptococcosis, extrapulmonary
• Cryptosporidiosis, chronic intestinal for longer than 1 month
• Cytomegalovirus disease (other than liver, spleen, or lymph nodes)
• Encephalopathy (HIV-related)
• Herpes simplex: chronic ulcer(s) (for more than 1 month); or bronchitis, pneumonitis, or esophagitis
• Histoplasmosis, disseminated or extrapulmonary
• Isosporiasis, chronic intestinal (for more than 1 month)
• Kaposi's sarcoma
• Lymphoma, Burkitt's, immunoblastic, or primary brain
• *Mycobacterium avium* complex
• *Mycobacterium*, other species, disseminated or extrapulmonary
• *Pneumocystis jirovecii* pneumonia (formerly called *Pneumocystis carinii* pneumonia)
• Pneumonia (recurrent)
• Progressive multifocal leukoencephalopathy
• *Salmonella* septicemia (recurrent)
• Toxoplasmosis of the brain
• Tuberculosis
• Wasting syndrome due to HIV

*Individuals greater than or equal to 13 years of age. *Source*: CDC MMWR 41:1–19 (1992).

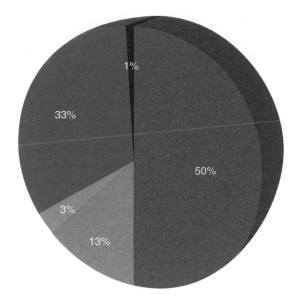

- ● Male-to-male sexual contact
- ● Injection drug use
- ● Male-to-male sexual contact and injection drug use
- ● High risk heterosexual contact
- ● Other: hemophilia, blood transfusion, perinatal

**FIGURE 16-5** U.S. 2006 transmission categories of adults and adolescents diagnosed with HIV/AIDS.

HIV is present early throughout the lymphoid system and its persistence is related to failure of the otherwise effective CD8$^+$ T-cell response against it (which destroys infected cells). Because CD4$^+$ T cells orchestrate the immune response (see Figure 2-6 in Chapter 2), any change in the CD4$^+$ T-cell profile, whether functional or loss through cell death, leads to increased susceptibility to multiple opportunistic infections and rare malignancies. The reason that CD4$^+$ T cells are the main targets of HIV is that the CD4 molecule and chemokine receptors act as specific receptors that bind with high affinity to the HIV's envelope glycoprotein gp120 and gp41 (discussed shortly). Other unwitting accomplices, such as brain cells, monocytes, macrophages, and dendritic cells also express CD4 molecules but in much lower numbers. In fact, monocytes and macrophages play a major role in the propagation and pathogenesis in the early stages of HIV infections. Monocytes are more refractory to the cytopathic effects of the virus—meaning that the virus can survive in these cells and thus be transported to different parts of the body, such as the brain and lung. The important implication is that monocytes/macrophages serve as a major reservoir for HIV in the body and are not dying in the process of disgorging new copies of the virus. Furthermore, even though macrophages have

inherent properties that allow HIV to persist in them in the absence or presence of drug therapy, they also can seek out anatomical refuges such as the central nervous system (CNS) where they are sheltered from drugs, immunity, or both.

The development of immunity revolves around having adequate numbers of correctly functioning CD4$^+$ T cells, the antithesis of immunity during HIV infection. The crippling of CD4$^+$ T cells by HIV is multifactorial. HIV induces T-cell lymphopenia (selective depletion of T cells) and function loss by several mechanisms. They include viral lysis of infected cells, T$_C$ cell-mediated killing of infected CD4$^+$ T cells or by antibody-dependent cytotoxicity (ADCC), HIV manipulation of apoptotic machinery (such as syncytia-dependent apoptosis, HIV-product–dependent apoptosis, activation-associated apoptosis, bystander killing, and HIV evasion of apoptosis), HIV impairs immunological synapses and enhances virological synapses, and autophagy induced by HIV Env protein in uninfected T cells.

The preceding paragraph strongly suggests that HIV manipulates the host cell's apoptotic machinery to ensure its spread in the hostile environment of the immune system. Apoptosis, a tightly regulated form of cell death, is necessary to maintain a steady lymphocyte population size despite the continuous arrival of new lymphocytes and homeostatic proliferation of existing cells. In addition, it is required during an immune response to eliminate unused activated antigen-specific T cells. Apoptosis (see Figure 10-23) occurs through an extrinsic pathway, which is mediated by binding of TNF-family death receptor ligands to their death receptors or an intrinsic pathway, which is mediated by internal sensors, such as bcl-2–related proteins that transmit signals to the mitochondria.

HIV-infected cells can connect with one another forming syncytia. The HIV envelope glycoprotein complex (gp120–gp41), *Env*, expressed on the plasma membrane of infected cells and bystander uninfected cells, can interact with a CD4 molecule and a suitable co-receptor to trigger cell-to-cell fusion; the resulting syncytia consequently undergo apoptosis.

In addition to Env, several other HIV-encoded products (detailed later in chapter) can trigger apoptosis in both infected and uninfected cells. *Vpr* alters the mitochondrial transmembrane potential causing release of cytochrome *c*, which leads to apoptosis. *Tat* suppresses bcl-2 (an inhibitor of apoptosis) activity and augments caspase-8 activity; the shift induces apoptosis. The binding of HIV gp120 to CD4 receptors on activated cells downregulates bcl-2; in turn, the mitochondria release cytochrome *c* inducing apoptosis. HIV-encoded protease can activate caspase-8, which can degrade bcl-2 causing apoptosis. HIV can also influence the extrinsic pathway in productively infected cells and in bystander cells. Cross-linking of CD4$^+$ T cells by gp120 activates the Fas receptor (CD95)–Fas ligand (FasL; CD178) pathway, and *Nef*-expressing T cells co-express FasL, thereby becoming potential killers of uninfected Fas-expressing T cells. Similarly, *Tat*, which is secreted by infected cells, upregulates Fas and FasL on uninfected cells and enhances their susceptibility to Fas-induced apoptosis. Macrophages can also mediate bystander T-cell killing; the ligation of macrophage chemokine receptors by HIV gp120 or their ligands induces cell-surface TNF expression, which triggers apoptosis of TNF receptor (R) 2-expressing CD8$^+$ T cells. Activated T cells, especially CD8$^+$ T cells, express Fas and high levels of FasL. Interestingly, here T cells also may kill each other via a so-called *fratricidal process*. This form of cell death is inhibited by overexpression of bcl-2. This may explain the killing of T cells from normal individuals by CD8$^+$ T cells from HIV-infected patients, that is, CD8$^+$ T cells from HIV-infected, but asymptomatic, individuals kill both syngeneic and allogeneic bystander CD4$^+$ T cells from either normal or HIV-infected individuals.

The activation-states of T cells from HIV-positive individuals affect the intrinsic and extrinsic pathways of apoptosis induction. When peripheral blood T cells from HIV-infected individuals are cultured in the absence of an exogenous stimulus, they undergo spontaneous apoptosis. This is associated with the downregulation of bcl-2 and is not limited to cell cultures. For example, activated cells from the lymph nodes and blood of HIV-infected patients express low levels of bcl-2, suggesting that spontaneous apoptosis of their T cells is primarily from immune activation by repeated virus antigen, or any other antigen, exposure. This chronic antigen exposure tips the balance in favor of pro-apoptotic bcl-2 molecules. HIV-infected individuals also have a compromised TNF–TNFR death pathway, which is again associated with the downregulation of bcl-2.

As mentioned above, CD4$^+$ T cells by upregulating FasL can become possible killers of activated Fas-expressing (Fas$^+$) cells, which are found in high numbers in HIV-infected individuals. This is confirmed *in vitro*, that is, activated FasL$^+$ CD4$^+$ T cells can kill Fas$^+$ CD8$^+$ T cells independent of antigen recognition. FasL$^+$ macrophages can also kill uninfected bystander Fas$^+$ T cells in an MHC-unrestricted and Fas/TNFR-dependent manner. HIV-specific T$_C$ cells are also potential killers of Fas$^+$ activated lymphocytes. For example, an MHC class-I-restricted, viral protein-specific T$_C$ cell from an HIV-infected individual is able to mediate both perforin- and Fas-dependent cytotoxic activities against either viral protein-presenting target cells or Fas-expressing cells, respectively. Therefore, some of the HIV-specific T$_C$ cells might be harmful to the immune system of an HIV-infected individual through the FasL-dependent destruction of uninfected Fas$^+$ T cells, which is induced by persistent HIV-driven immune stimulation. Even though virus-specific CD8$^+$ T cell effector function can be misdirected, development of this specificity can lead to an eventual failure of the CD8$^+$ T-cell compartment to kill virally infected cells. In fact, *T$_C$ cell escape*,[3] the evasion of HIV from T$_C$ cell-mediated responses, drives the evolution of HIV at the population level. Thus, T$_C$ cell escape is also a major obstacle to immune control of HIV.

Even though HIV targets CD4$^+$ T cells, the viral replication level in these cells is strongly linked to their activation state. In activated memory CD4$^+$ T cells, HIV readily undergoes multiple rounds of replication and the cells have a half-life of about two weeks, whereas resting T$_H$ cells are mostly refractory to productive infection; if they support a productive infect, they only have a half-life of two days. Even though HIV readily enters quiescent CD4$^+$ T cells, there are blocks throughout the life cycle of HIV that stop virus propagation when T cells are insufficiently activated. Despite these blocks, HIV infection does not require full T-cell activation, although the magnitude of viral replication is much higher in activated T cells. Taken together, it suggests that HIV can modulate the activation state of target CD4$^+$ T cells. Why? A rapidly killed cell would limit viral production; therefore, it behooves HIV to ensure the infected cell's survival at least until enough new virions are produced. The next paragraph suggests how HIV accomplishes this task.

As we saw, HIV uses several schemes to induce apoptosis in hostile immune effector cells; however, it avoids a similar fate for HIV-infected cells, at least until sufficiently high numbers of progeny virus are produced. HIV gene products also have anti-apoptotic activity. In fact, some of them have

---

[3]Viral-sequence variation caused by viral turnover ($\sim$10 $\times$ 10$^9$ new virions produced daily) and high mutation rate (viral reverse transcriptase is error-prone, leading to each new virion encoding approximately one new mutation) leads to loss of, or diminished, recognition of HIV by T$_C$ cells.

both pro-apoptotic and anti-apoptotic activity. Nef, gp120 and *Vpu* contribute to the downregulation of CD4 receptor expression by infected cells, thereby preventing gp120–CD4-mediated apoptosis. Nef downregulates class I MHC molecule expression and upregulates FasL expression by infected cells, which could block $T_C$ or NK cell-mediated cytolysis. *Vpr* expression inhibits apoptosis by causing the upregulation of bcl-2 and the downregulation of bax, a promoter of apoptosis. Tat promotes cell-cycle progression, inhibits apoptosis, and allows the cells to increase virus production. Counterintuitively, in lymph nodes from HIV-infected individuals, apoptosis is detected predominantly in uninfected bystander cells, such as apoptotic $CD8^+$ T cells, B cells, and dendritic cells. At the same time, productively infected cells are not apoptotic, suggesting that they are resistant to direct HIV-induced killing. Therefore, to ensure its spread, HIV travels through a minefield of apoptosis-prone activation, HIV product-dependent apoptosis, and the replication-unfavorable environment of resting cells, plus it must manipulate cellular apoptotic machinery to destroy the immune system, thereby favoring immune escape. In essence, the immune system may burn itself out and be unable to generate memory T cells because of the overactivation of effector ($T_H1$) cells, causing widespread apoptosis.

Dysfunction of the cell-mediated immunity against HIV due to these apoptotic mechanisms may trigger the inability to form a $T_H1$-type memory. Instead, cells that proliferate less in response to infection may survive. These are the $T_H2$-type cells that mediate weaker antibody-mediated responses. A $T_H2$-type memory may dominate and be less able to cope with the rapid HIV replication after the $T_H1$ cells die out. Interestingly, $T_H2$ cell lines are refractory to activation-induced T-cell death, and this correlates with decreased expression of Fas on these cells.

Besides apoptosis, HIV can weaken the ability of infected T cells to conjugate with antigen-presenting cells through the immunological synapse and to cluster TCRs and the tyrosine kinase Lck at the immunological synapse, leading to diminished signaling capacity. Despite this weakened interaction, the HIV-infected T cells still produce significant amounts of IL-2, which may stall apoptosis extending the cells life, and thereby increase the time to build up the viral load. While on the one hand HIV compromises anti-HIV immunity, in the same cell virus survival and propagation are facilitated by the conjugation of infected T cells with uninfected ones; this cell-to-cell fusion zone is called the *virological synapse*.

The exact contribution of B cells is obscure, but elevated IgG and IgA levels are seen. The most obvious sign of humoral dysfunction is an inability to mount an adequate IgM response to antigenic challenge. Normally, viruses are removed by opsonizing antibodies and complement; however, in the case of anti-HIV antibodies Fc receptor-positive cells, such as macrophages, could bind the complex and become infected. Also, virus variability leads to escape from neutralizing antibodies.

NK cells are a key to protection against viruses and tumor, so it is not surprising that they would attempt to control HIV infections. The number of circulating NK cells in AIDS patients is not significantly reduced, but their cytotoxic ability is diminished. This is surprising because HIV-infected cells downregulate class I MHC molecule expression. The catch is that HIV selectively downregulates cell-surface expression of HLA-A and HLA-B while preserving HLA-C and HLA-E molecule expression, thereby evading $T_C$ cell- or NK cell-mediated killing of HIV-infected cells. HIV viremia reduces NK-cell expression of various activating receptors while increasing the expression of inhibitory NK cell receptors (see Figure 10-24); antibody-dependent cell-mediated cytotoxicity (ADCC) mediated by NK cells is impaired in the later stages of HIV infection. During AIDS, NK cell secretion of CC chemokines (such as CCL3, CCL4, and CCL5) are inhibited, thereby their ability to block R5 virus (discussed shortly) entry is compromised. NK cell production of the proinflammatory cytokines IFN-γ, TNF, and GM-CSF is also inhibited, which causes faulty crosstalk between NK cells and dendritic cells ultimately leading to defective adaptive immune responses.

Dendritic cells –sentinel cells that capture and present antigen—play a pivotal role in marshalling immune responses through the generation and regulation of adaptive immunity; therefore, it is not unexpected that HIV has developed ways to exploit dendritic cells. HIV hijacks dendritic cells to promote viral dissemination by capturing and binding HIV, simply trafficking HIV through the cell, and transferring them to $CD4^+$ T cells in a process called *trans-infection*[4] or the infected dendritic cells transfer progeny virus

---

[4]Certain dendritic cells can capture and transfer HIV to target cells without themselves becoming infected by using concurrent distinct processes involving transfer across the cell-to-cell infectious/virological synapse or HIV-containing exosomes. Dendritic cell-specific intercellular adhesion molecule 3 (ICAM3)-grabbing nonintegrin (DC-SIGN) contributes in the formation of the virological synapse.

to CD4$^+$ T cells by a process called *cis-infection*.[5] These two processes can occur concurrently. HIV replication in dendritic cells is less productive and the infection frequency of dendritic cells is often 10- to 100-fold lower than that observed in CD4$^+$ T cells. HIV also interferes with antigen-presenting function by impairing the formation of the immunological synapse. Like macrophages, follicular dendritic cells act as reservoirs of HIV. Whether mature dendritic cells provide reservoirs for HIV remains to be determined but they seem to be refractory to the cytopathic effects of HIV.

Irrespective of how HIV depletes the immune system of CD4$^+$ T cells, the host's thymus continuously tries to replenish the ones lost; however, over time the regenerative capacity of the thymus succumbs to direct infection of its thymocytes. The immune system no longer has the tools to protect the host, leading to AIDS, and eventually the death of the host and the HIV source.

## The Cause of AIDS Is Infection by the Retrovirus HIV-1

Initially, it was naïvely thought that lifestyle was the cause. As soon as AIDS was recognized as an infectious disease, researchers began looking for an infectious agent as the most plausible cause. Several viruses or virus families were implicated at first, such as cytomegalovirus and herpes simplex virus, but an RNA retrovirus proved to be the culprit. It is a member of the genus Lentivirus, part of the family of retroviruses. The visna virus of sheep, equine infectious anemia virus, and feline immunodeficiency virus represent this family of viruses. These viruses and their human counterpart cause a slowly progressive and inevitably fatal disease in their hosts.

The etiologic agent in AIDS was isolated on its own in 1984 by Luc Montagnier[6] and his associates at the Institute Pasteur in France and shortly thereafter by Robert Gallo and his associates at the National Institutes of Health in the U.S. Immunologic analysis and the biologic properties of this retrovirus show that it is a member of the family of human T-cell leukemia viruses. It was originally called *human T-lymphotropic virus type III (HTLV-III)*, *lymphadenopathy-associated virus (LAV)*,

and *AIDS-associated retrovirus (ARV)*. It is now called **human immunodeficiency virus type 1**, or **HIV-1**. The number *1* distinguishes HIV-1 from HIV-2, which shares serologic reactivity and polynucleotide sequence homology with simian T lymphotropic virus (STLV)-III. STLV-III causes a disease in captive macaques but does not seem to be pathogenic for wild African green monkeys. HIV-2 has been isolated from West African patients with a clinical syndrome indistinguishable from HIV-1-induced AIDS. This second virus is endemic to West Africa and is less transmittable than HIV-1—so HIV-1 and HIV-2 infections are considered pandemic and endemic, respectively. As of 2006, >1% of the report cases of HIV diagnoses in West Africa are caused by HIV-2 and only 130 cases have been reported in the United States since 1987. HIV-1 primarily infects T cells. *The virus is especially tropic[7] to CD4$^+$ T cells, but any cells expressing CD4 are susceptible to HIV infection; in humans, these include monocytes, macrophages, dendritic cells, and microglia cells of the nervous system plus CD4$^+$ T cells.* However, initially HIV seems to preferentially infect macrophages on transmission of the virus, a selection for which determinants have yet to be elucidated. HIV-1 also invades brain cells, which accounts for the mental symptoms (dementia) that occur in the later stages of AIDS in at least 60% of AIDS patients. This is due to a metabolic encephalopathy induced by HIV infection and fueled by host- and viral-origin neurotoxins released from infected brain macrophages and microglia.

Unlike other identified retroviruses, HIV is roughly spherical. HIV-1 consists of (1) a dense cylindrical core of two copies of single-stranded genomic RNA that encodes 9 genes, (2) a capsid composed of copies of viral p24 that encloses the core RNA (3) group-specific antigen (gag) proteins and enzymes such as, reverses transcriptase, proteases, and integrase (4) a capsid-surrounding matrix composed of viral p17, (5) a viral envelope lipid bilayer derived from the host cell when the virion buds from the cell, and (6) host-derived proteins embedded in the viral envelope (Figure 16-6). The latter structures are 72 copies of a glycoprotein complex that protrude through the envelope of the virus. Each HIV glycoprotein complex, Env, consists of a cap made up of three molecules of the 120 kD glycoprotein gp120 and a stem made up of three molecules of the 41 kD transmembrane glycoprotein gp41 critical for HIV binding and fusion to CD4$^+$ cells. Gp120 does not contain a

---

[5]HIV-infected dendritic cells release virons by budding that in turn can infect CD4$^+$ T cells.

[6]Luc Montagnier shared the 2008 Nobel Prize with Francoise Barre-Sinoussi "for their discovery of HIV" and Harald zur Hausen "for his discovery of human papilloma viruses causing cervical cancer."

[7]It is the predilection of HIV to infect CD4-expressing cells.

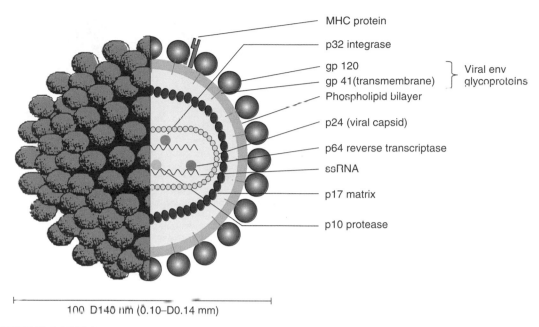

100 D140 nm (0.10–D0.14 mm)

**FIGURE 16-6** HIV-1 structure.

transmembrane domain, but remains bound by non-covalent interactions with gp41, which anchors the structure into the viral envelope—a trimeric structure of 3 gp120/gp41 pairs. HIV-1 differs from other retroviruses in its complex structure; it contains a minimum of nine genes, some of which are not found in other retroviruses (Figure 16-7). The nine genes of the HIV genome can be divided into three structural genes—*gag, pol,* and *env*—and six regulatory genes—*vif, vpr, tat, rev, vpu,* and *nef*. HIV replication is intimately associated with mechanisms that stimulate the growth of host T cells. For instance, in response to a viral infection, most individuals develop an immune response. For AIDS, the patient's immune response escalates viral activity, which also leads to increased immune activity—a vicious cycle of HIV infection and escalated viral activity in HIV-infected patients. How does having an immune response lead to elevated HIV production? DNA-binding proteins (or nuclear factors such as NF-κB) within the T cell bind to enhancer sequences of the cell's own DNA during activation (see Chapter 8). These enhancer sequences also are found in the HIV genome. Infected cells are induced by cytokines to produce DNA-binding proteins that normally interact with cellular DNA to speed transcription of cellular genes. Instead they bind to enhancer sites within the HIV genome. Once bound, the cellular proteins stimulate the production of new virus. Thus, the virus may remain in a dormant (latent or proviral) state in an infected

CD4+ T cell, but it is induced to replicate when the T cell itself is activated to replicate through interaction with cytokines. This common regulatory mechanism allows HIV to undermine the immune system and cause its collapse.

Chronologically, the first event in the infection of a cell by HIV-1 is the interaction by its high-affinity gp120 coat protein (envelope, or env) to the target cell's high-affinity receptor for the virus, the **CD4 molecule** (Figure 16-8). The specific HIV-1 envelope glycoprotein, or gp120, interaction with the CD4 molecule on CD4+ T cells or monocytes/macrophages and others is the first step, or *binding of virus to target cells*. CD4–HIV interaction along is crucial but not sufficient for virus entry and productive infection. An additional group of molecules on T cells and monocytes/macrophages, called *coreceptors* (initially called *fusin*), are required for HIV infection. These coreceptors are the chemokine receptors (see Chapter 9) CXCR4 on T cells and CCR5 on monocytes and macrophages, which coreceptor used (i.e., tropism) is determined by which gp120 variant (associated with the amino acid sequence in the V3 loop[8]) is expressed by HIV. T cell-tropic HIV uses CXCR4, the HIV coreceptor that

---

[8]It is the third variable (V3) region of the HIV envelope gp120 molecule. The amino-acid sequence in the V3 region determines whether the virus uses CXCR4 or CCR5 as its coreceptor.

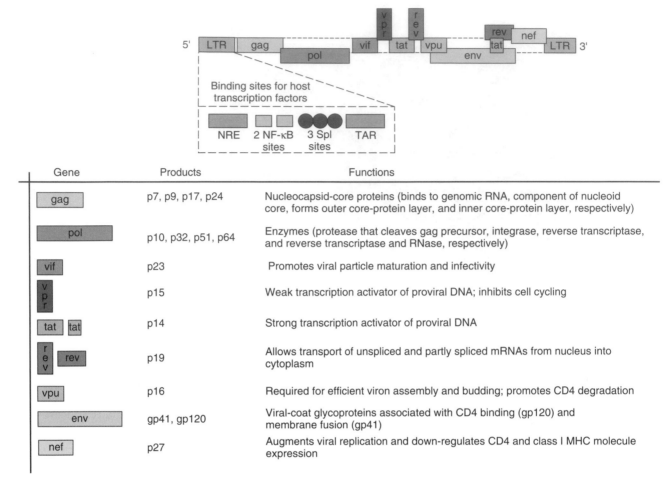

| Gene | Products | Functions |
|------|----------|-----------|
| gag | p7, p9, p17, p24 | Nucleocapsid-core proteins (binds to genomic RNA, component of nucleoid core, forms outer core-protein layer, and inner core-protein layer, respectively) |
| pol | p10, p32, p51, p64 | Enzymes (protease that cleaves gag precursor, integrase, reverse transcriptase, and reverse transcriptase and RNase, respectively) |
| vif | p23 | Promotes viral particle maturation and infectivity |
| vpr | p15 | Weak transcription activator of proviral DNA; inhibits cell cycling |
| tat tat | p14 | Strong transcription activator of proviral DNA |
| rev rev | p19 | Allows transport of unspliced and partly spliced mRNAs from nucleus into cytoplasm |
| vpu | p16 | Required for efficient viron assembly and budding; promotes CD4 degradation |
| env | gp41, gp120 | Viral-coat glycoproteins associated with CD4 binding (gp120) and membrane fusion (gp41) |
| nef | p27 | Augments viral replication and down-regulates CD4 and class I MHC molecule expression |

**FIGURE 16-7 HIV-1 genome.** HIV-1's entire complement of genes consists of three structural genes (common to all retroviruses) and six regulatory genes (several of which appear unique to HIV). The structural genes are *gag*, group-specific antigen; *pol*, polymerase; and *env*, envelope. The regulatory genes are *vif*, virion infectivity factor; *vpr*, viral protein R; *tat*, transactivator of transcription; *rev*, regulator of virion protein expression; *vpu*, virion productivity factor U; and *nef*, negative regulatory factor. As in all retroviruses, proviral DNA is flanked at both ends by identical segments called *long terminal repeats* (*LTR*). The LTRs contain regulatory sequences that serve as initiation sites for the transcription of viral genes. These regulatory sequences bind the cellular proteins NF-κB (at two sites) and Sp1 (at three sites) and thereby start transcription. The LTRs also contain sequences called *nef-responsive elements* (*NRE*) and *tat-responsive elements* (*TAR*), which interact with the HIV regulatory proteins *nef* and *tat*, respectively, leading to an increased rate of transcription. HIV-2 and SIV genomes are similar to HIV-1 except the *vpx* gene replaces the *vpu* gene in both of them.

is characteristically found late in infection, and needs high density of CD4 on the cell surface. The natural ligand for CXCR4 is CXCL12 (stromal-derived factor 1); it suppresses T cell-tropic HIV replication. Macrophage-tropic HIV uses CCR5, the HIV coreceptor that is characteristically associated with primary infection, and needs low density of CD4 on the cell surface. Macrophages and dendritic cells, which express low levels of CD4, and CD4+ T cells, express CCR5. The natural ligands for CCR5 are CCL3 (macrophage inflammatory protein 1 [MIP-1α]), CCL4 (MIP-1β), and CCL5 (regulated on activation, normal T-cell expressed and secreted

[RANTES]); they suppress macrophage-tropic HIV replication. The older terminology of T cell- and macrophage-tropic HIV variants, use CXCR4 and CCR5 as coreceptors, respectively, is now replaced with **R4** and **R5**; HIV variants that can bind both chemokine coreceptors are called **R5R4**. CCR5 is required to establish primary infection, which is supported in part by people with the CCR5 mutation Δ32-CCR5; these individuals are partially resistant to R5 virus because expression of the mutated receptor prevents viral fusion, leading to reduced infection. In individuals exposed to HIV by sexual contact, mucosal-associated macrophages and dendritic cells

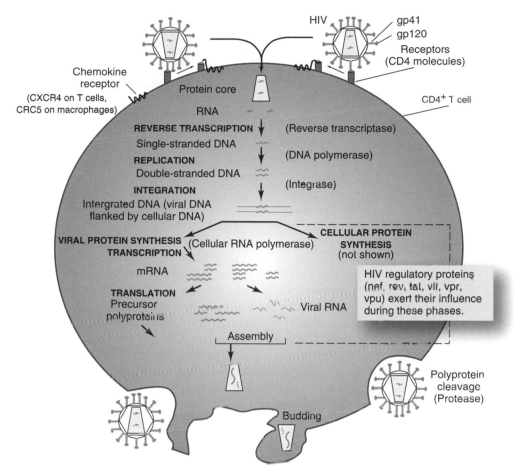

**FIGURE 16-8 The life cycle of HIV.** Free virus binds to and enters a susceptible host cell by a membrane receptor, the CD4 molecule. Once inside the cell, viral RNA separates from the capsid and undergoes reverse transcription into DNA. The double-stranded DNA is integrated into the host cell's DNA. The integrated viral DNA, or proviral DNA, is transcribed with the cellular DNA into mRNA once the cell is activated. The mRNA is translated into precursor polyproteins, which are assembled with the viral RNA into new viral particles. These particles bud from the cell surface, acquiring envelopes as they exit the cell. As free viruses, the polyproteins are cleaved by viral and cellular proteases into biologically active proteins.

become infected by R5 virus and provide reservoirs for the virus, because these cells are refractory to killing by HIV and can migrate to regional lymph nodes to present antigen to T cells—tropism changes as the HIV infection becomes systemic. As the infection progresses, tropism broadens because of mutations in the virus envelope protein V3 loop, this allows the virus to infect a broader repertoire of T cells. CCR5 is generally expressed by $T_H1$ memory cells and is upregulated after activation, which explains the early loss of HIV-specific CD4+ T cells. In contrast, naïve T cells predominantly express CXCR4. During infection, the population of virus evolves from the initial infecting strain to new variants that cause changes its predominant tropism from R5 to R4 in late disease. This tropism switch is often accompanied with a precipitous drop in CD4+ T cell numbers.

The ligation of viral gp120 subunits with CD4 causes gp120 to undergo conformational change that exposes its V3 loop and permits secondary binding to adjacent chemokine receptor. A resulting gp41 conformational change exposes gp41-associated fusion protein, which inserts into the T cell membrane; *this allows fusion of viral and cellular membranes*, leading to viral genome and associated viral protein entrance. Once the virus enters the target cell, it sheds its envelope coat and releases RNA into the cytoplasm.

Every time HIV creates progeny viruses, it must undergo the conversion of single-stranded RNA to DNA, which is an inherently sloppy procedure prone to errors that lead to mutations in the viral copy.

These mutations get inherited and as the progeny viruses copy themselves more mutations are added. Furthermore, if two HIV virions with different genetic sequences enter the same cell, they can swap RNA in a process called *recombination*, creating an entirely new virus variant.

The viral RNA then acts as a template for DNA production by the enzyme reverse transcriptase. Following viral replication, the DNA copy (provirus) of HIV-1 becomes either linear or circularized. The circularized HIV-1 DNA may either be integrated into the host chromosomal genome or remain unintegrated. After integration of proviral DNA, the infection may enter a latent phase, resuming the cycle if the infected cell is activated. Once the infected cell is activated, the viral DNA is transcribed to viral genomic RNA and mRNA and then translated into viral proteins. During the final phases of the HIV-1 life cycle, secondary processing of specific viral proteins occurs. Processing uses proteases and glycosylating enzymes; polyprotein precursor cleavage does not occur until after viral particles are released from the cell as virions[9] by viral budding, which damages the cell membrane and kills the infected cell. Infectious (mature) virions have cleaved (active) polyproteins, while noninfectious (immature) virions have uncleaved polyproteins. The infection continues by free infectious virions binding to uninfected cells or by uninfected CD4$^+$ T cells binding to gp120 expressed on infected cells, fusing, and HIV genomes passed between the fused cells. Fusion can lead to large, multinucleated giant cells or syncytia that die rapidly by apoptosis.

## The Clinical Course of HIV Infection Is Divided into Three Phases

Overall, HIV infection is allied with a progressive decrease in CD4$^+$ T cell count and an increase in viral load. These two characteristics combined with antibody production (progressing from an absence of HIV-specific antibody to its presence, which is called *serconversion*) allow for the creation of the clinical course of the HIV infection to be divided into three phases: acute, latent (or chronic), and AIDS (Figure 16-9).

Within two weeks of initial HIV infection, roughly 50% of patients present with flu-like symptoms (fever, sore throat, swollen lymph nodes, muscle pain, and malaise), while the other half remains asymptomatic. Thus, it is not surprising that this phase generally goes unnoticed. During the acute

phase, either type of patient has a significant increase in HIV in the peripheral blood (viremia) with millions of viruses per μl of blood, which is accompanied by a plummeting number of circulating CD4$^+$ T cells. The gut-associated lymphoid tissue (GALT) is also associated with high viremia, vigorous T-cell activation, and severe depletion of T cells, particularly memory CD4$^+$CCR5$^+$ T cells. The majority of CD4$^+$ T-cell loss occurs during the first few weeks of HIV infection, particularly in the GALT, its numbers remain depleted throughout the infection. Enough CD4$^+$ T cells remain in the GALT to initially counteract any translocation of normal gut flora.

The immune system "kicks-in" with the activation of CD8$^+$ T$_C$ cells, which kill HIV-infected cells, mainly CD4$^+$ T cells; therefore, the immune system is partially responsible for the reduction in CD4$^+$ T cells. Concomitantly, the patient produces detectable levels of HIV protein-specific antibodies, that is, the patient has *seroconverted*. The patient's CD4$^+$ T cell counts rebound but not to normal blood values. This suggests that antigen-presenting cells disseminated, and continue to disseminate, HIV throughout the body's lymphoid system. During the central portion of the acute phase, the patient is much more infectious.

The acute phase of HIV infection ends within a few months and is replaced by the latency phase of infection, a time when HIV wages covert activities, which is characterized by an absence of symptoms that may last 20 or more years. Early higher viral loads predict shorter latency. By all outward signs, the immune system has won the first round (the acute phase) of this three-round fight. To win the fight outright, it would have had to eradicate ("knockout") the virus instead of merely limit it. The blood picture suggests victory; virus levels in the blood are now low or undetectable, which would suggest that the immune system has recuperated. However, the opposite is true, instead there is a disconnect between the low number of infected circulating CD4$^+$ T cells and the continuing extend of T$_H$ cell dysfunction. This issue was resolved with the discovery that virus replication continues to be active but has moved to the lymph node compartment and that HIV has a preference to replicate in recently activated T cells whether by HIV or unrelated antigens—activated memory CD4$^+$ T cells can undergo several rounds of HIV replication, whereas naïve ("resting") T cells are refractory to productive infection. In fact, a generalized state of immune activation persists throughout the latent phase. Macrophage, perhaps also dendritic cell, reservoirs plus virus trapped in follicular dendritic cells leads to continuous presentation of viral

---

[9]A virion is a single virus particle—*a cell-free virus.*

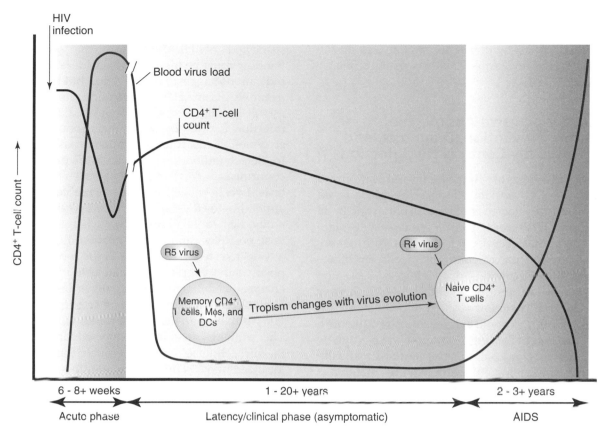

**FIGURE 16-9 Clinical course of untreated HIV infection.** A generalized graph depicting the relationship between viral load (number of HIV copies) and CD4+ T-cell counts over the course of an untreated HIV infection. A threshold of roughly 200 CD4+ T cells per μl of blood is reached where immune deficiency results that leads to opportunistic infections and ultimately death. Abbreviations: macrophages, Mφs; dendritic cells, DCs.

antigen to T and B cells, converting primary follicles to chronically stimulated secondary follicles with continual germinal centers causing hyperplasia and lymphadenopathy (swelling of lymph nodes), symptoms typical of the latent/chronic phase. Furthermore, HIV-specific activated T cells that are recruited to lymph nodes to respond to HIV antigens are highly susceptible to infection by HIV. Another pool of activated CD4+ T cells become fresh targets for HIV; the breakdown of the GALT seen in the acute phase eventual leads to systemic exposure of the immune system to normal gut flora-derived microbial antigens—development of non-HIV-specific activated T cells. Under these pressures, the T cell pool undergoes a slow, low rate of lysis, which eventually causes lymph node atrophy. Once the absolute peripheral blood CD4+ T cell count drops to 200 T cells per μl of blood, the patient becomes susceptible to AIDS-defining opportunistic infections and malignancies (see Table 16-2). Even though there are only low levels of HIV in the blood, these patients are still infectious.

When an HIV-infected person has a low CD4+ T-cell count, increase in viral load, impaired delayed-hypersensitivity reactions, and what physicians call an "AIDS-defining illness" or "opportunistic infection," that person has AIDS—the final phase of HIV infection. The patient may present with any number of life-threatening AIDS-defining diseases, the most common are *Pneumocystis jirovecii* pneumonia, candidiasis (thrush), toxoplasmosis, and cytomegalovirus infections, and an unusual cancer called *Kaposi's sarcoma* and others. Treatments are available for these conditions and most other opportunistic infections; however, at this stage of HIV infection called *AIDS*, the immune system is destroyed and these diseases establish themselves with fatal consequences. Dysfunctional, chronically activated immune cells over-produce proinflammatory cytokines, particularly IL-1 and TNF-α, causing cachexia (severe weight loss and muscle wasting). In the terminal stages of AIDS, HIV can attack cells besides immune cells, such as cells of the CNS. HIV-infected macrophages outside the CNS can cross the blood-brain barrier, leading to neurological problems. These patients begin to experience dementia, problems with balance, and an inability to move their legs and arms. Death is usually not far behind.

## The Comprehensive Approach of Education, Prevention, Diagnosis, and Treatment Only Controls HIV Infections

Significant resources are funneled into education and public awareness campaigns to teach people to avoid behaviors—unprotected contact with blood and body fluids from HIV-infected individuals—that place them at risk for HIV infection. Preventive interventions include the use of condoms, needle-exchange programs for intravenous drug abusers, screening blood and blood products, antiretroviral therapy to HIV-infected pregnant women and their infants, caesarian section to avoid passage through the birth canal, replacement feeding to avoid breastfeeding by infected mothers, and safety paraphernalia by health care workers. Immediate antiretroviral therapy is provided to individuals that are accidentally exposed to infected materials.

The CDC recommends that every American between the ages 13 and 64 be tested for HIV at least once and it should be made a standard part of medical care regardless of an individual's risk factors or HIV prevalence in the community. There are at least four FDA-approved rapid diagnostic tests

for HIV infection, which use whole blood, plasma, serum, or oral fluid. (When testing individuals suspected of HIV infection, the seroconversion window must be taken into consideration. If clinical indications suggest HIV infection but blood tests are negative, plasma HIV RNA testing should be done to establish diagnosis.) Confirmatory diagnosis of HIV infection is done by screening venous blood using enzyme-linked immunosorbent assay (ELISA)[10] to detect antibodies against HIV protein 24 and confirmed by Western blot analysis. Following rapid tests, two serologic tests are available which detect antibodies to HIV-1 (Figure 16-10). The ELISA detects antibodies to HIV proteins, usually p24. Because false positives can occur, a positive ELISA sample is always retested in duplicate. If the second test also is positive, the sample is then subjected to Western blot analysis, a method of choice when a definitive answer is needed. This assay also is a test for antibodies to HIV, but it contains a full range of HIV proteins. The proteins are electrophoresed and transferred to nitrocellulose paper. Because the proteins are localized into discrete bands,[11] antibodies specific for the proteins bind to the appropriate bands and create

---

[10] The mechanics of an ELISA test are discussed in detail in Chapter 5. The number of each glycoprotein (gp) and protein (p) tells its molecular weight in thousands of daltons.

[11] The mechanics of Western blotting are discussed in detail in Chapter 5.

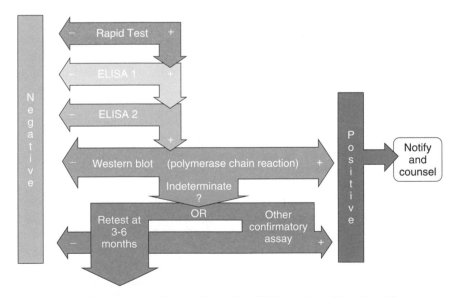

**FIGURE 16-10 Conventional algorithms for AIDS testing.** The algorithms may vary in the number of times tests are repeated, the kind of confirmatory assay used, and the types of tests used, but most follow this format.

black bands when the paper is stained. The Western blot assay gives a profile of the anti-HIV antibodies present in the serum being tested. The test is not without problems because the bands can be faint and difficult to read. Children as old as 18 months from HIV-infected mothers are tested using an HIV DNA polymerase chain reaction (PCR) test, because of passively acquired maternal antibodies in the child's blood. These antibodies could lead to a false-positive ELISA test, even if the child is uninfected.

In light of the viral etiology of AIDS, successful therapeutic intervention requires the prevention of viral replication within different cells of the body, including $CD4^+$ T cells, macrophages, dendritic cells, and cells of the CNS. Furthermore, therapy must completely clear HIV from infected individuals, which would require removal of all latently infected T cells. Anti-HIV therapy is recommended when the patient (older than 12 months) presents with AIDS-defining diseases, a $CD4^+$ T-cell count <350 cells per µl of blood, or has a viral load of >100,000 copies per ml of plasma. Because HIV is a retrovirus, the first promising target for intervention was reverse transcriptase. As is usually the case, however, a multifactorial approach to therapeutic intervention was required. Current treatments for AIDS are empirical; no cure for AIDS exists. Antiretroviral drugs (Table 16-3) of which more than 25 have been approved, have reduced the virus load, but cannot cure the infection and virus numbers increase if treatment is interrupted. Furthermore, HIV rapidly develops drug resistance. Current HIV infection treatment is drug-combination approach called **highly active antiretroviral therapy (HAART)**. The drug combination includes three drugs belonging to at least two classes of antiretroviral drugs; for example, typically, the "cocktail" contains two nucleoside analogue reverse transcriptase inhibitors plus either a protease inhibitor or a non-nucleoside reverse transcriptase inhibitor. HAART is successful in reducing HIV infections in individuals who have access to this therapy; however, patient adherence, drug toxicity, and drug resistance test the long-term efficacy of drugs. Because neither antiretroviral drugs nor the immune system are able to eliminate HIV infection, the only way to end the HIV pandemic is to develop a safe, accessible, and preventive vaccine. Traditional approaches for developing an AIDS vaccine are inadequate because the many peculiarities of HIV have turned out to be major obstacles (Table 16-4). In particular, as mentioned earlier, viral reverse transcriptase is extremely error prone, leading to each new virion encoding roughly one new mutation; therefore, within a few years of infection, the error frequency combined with a virus production rate exceeding $10^9$ virions per day, cause the virion diversity in an individual to be exceedingly large. An effective anti-HIV vaccine would have to be against thousands or more different viruses. In effect, the ideal vaccine would prevent infection from the wide spectrum of globally diverse HIV isolates—induce a sterilizing immunity (immunity in which no infection occurs, which has not been achieved with any vaccine) and protect against infection. To date, no HIV vaccine tested in humans has been able to induce the diverse expression of neutralizing antibodies needed to block HIV from infecting cells; therefore, the current goal is more along the lines of creating a vaccine, which induces immune responses that contain the virus, thereby slowing the progression to AIDS, and blunts the rate of transmission—that is, attenuate virus replication. The latter type of vaccine could be augmented with the use of microbicides (topically applied agents that prevent person-to-person HIV transmission). Whether these approaches will provide protection is unknown. Nonetheless, without antiretrovirus treatment (the case in developing regions of the world), the net median survival time after HIV infection is estimated to be 9 to 11 years depending on the HIV subtype. Once diagnosed with AIDS and left untreated, the median survival time ranges between 6 and 19 months.

---

**MINI SUMMARY**

Acquired immunodeficiency syndrome (AIDS) was first identified in 1981. It is characterized by immunosuppression leading to high susceptibility to opportunistic infections. AIDS patients become vulnerable to multiple infections. The CD4 molecule acts as a specific receptor for the binding of the HIV (therefore, the primary target cells are $CD4^+$ T cells), whereas fusion/entry into the cell is mediated by coreceptors, the chemokine receptors CCR5 and CXCR4. AIDS is caused by human immunodeficiency virus type 1 (HIV-1) or HIV-2 infection. There is no completely effective treatment or cure for AIDS.

# SUMMARY

Naturally occurring defects (*primary immunodeficiency diseases*) can reduce or negate the immune

**TABLE 16-3** The Current FDA-Approved Anti-HIV Drugs

| Generic name | Brand and other names |
|---|---|
| **Nucleoside reverse transcriptase inhibitors** _(These inhibitors are nucleoside analogues that HIV requires to make more copies of itself. When HIV uses them instead of normal nucleosides, reproduction of the virus is stalled.)_ | |
| Abacavir | Ziagen, ABC |
| *Abacavir, Lamivudine | Epizcom |
| *Abacavir, Lamivudine, Zidovudine | Trizivir |
| Didanosine | Videx,ddl, Videx EC |
| Emtricitabine | Emtriva, FTC, Coviracil |
| *Emtricitabine, Tenofovir DF | Truvada |
| Lamivudine | Epivir, 3TC |
| *Lamivudine, Zidovudine | Combivir |
| Stavudine | Zerit, d4T |
| Tenofovir DF | Viread, TDF |
| Zidovudine | Retrovir, AZT, ZDV |
| **Non-nucleoside reverse transcriptase inhibitors** _(These non-nucleoside analogues bind to and disable reverse transcriptase, an enzyme that HIV requires to make more copies of itself.)_ | |
| Delavirdine | Rescriptor, DLV |
| *Efavirenz | Sustiva, EFV |
| Etravirine | Intelence, Celsentri, TMC125 |
| Nevirpine | Viramune, NVP |
| **Protease inhibitors** _(These inhibitors disable protease, an enzyme that HIV requires to assemble itself.)_ | |
| Amprenavir | Agenerase, APV |
| Atazanavir | Reyataz, ATV |
| Darunavir | Prezista, TMC114 |
| Fosamprenavir | Lexiva, FPV |
| Indinavir | Crixivan, IDV |
| Lopinavir, Ritonavir | Laletra, LPV/r |
| Nelfinavir | Norvir, RTV |
| Saquinavir | Invirase, SQV |
| Tipranavir | Aptivus, TPV |
| **Entry/Fusion inhibitors** _(These inhibitors block HIV entry into cells.)_ | |
| Enfuvirtide | Fuzeon, T-20 |
| Maraviroc | Selzentry, MVC |
| **Integrase inhibitors** _(These inhibitors disable integrase, an enzyme that HIV uses to insert its viral genome into the infected cell's genome.)_ | |
| Raltegravir | Isentress |

*These drugs can also be found as fixed dose combination tablets, which contain two or more anti-HIV medications from one or more drug classes.

**TABLE 16-4 Approaches Used to Develop an AIDS Vaccine and Some Obstacles to Its Development**

1. Vaccine development
   a. Whole HIV vaccines
      1) Live attenuated HIV
      2) Inactivated HIV
   b. Live recombinant viruses
   c. HIV protein vaccines
      1) Synthetic HIV peptides
      2) HIV proteins
   d. HIV gene vaccines
      1) Naked DNA
      2) Viral vectors
      3) Bacterial vectors
2. Major obstacles in development
   The problem that overshadows the design and development of a successful AIDS vaccine is that, to date, no one knows exactly what constitutes an effective immune response against HIV. Even if we can solve this frustrating problem, we still have to overcome the following obstacles (it is not meant to be an exhaustive list):
   a. The virus infects, suppresses, and destroys the immune system.
   b. The virus's ability to change its surface antigens rapidly (antigenic drift), plus the antigens needed for protection remain undefined.
   c. The virus's ability to establish latent infections, hiding itself in resting cells by insinuating itself into a host cell's DNA.
   d. The virus's proficiency at covert cell-cell infection, thereby hiding itself from the patrolling immune system.
   e. The virus is transmitted as cell-free and cell-associated virus.
   f. The virus infects mainly through the genital tract; the majority of vaccines protect against infections by respiratory and gastrointestinal tract mucosa.
   g. The virus has no suitable animal model to tested for safety and efficacy before trials with human volunteers.

system's effectiveness with the same end result: increased susceptibility to infection. Immunodeficiency diseases can be grouped according to which immune cells are affected: B cells, T cells, or both. Defects affecting B cells may reflect the absence of B cells (*X-linked agammaglobulinemia* or *Bruton's agammaglobulinemia*) or the selective inability to produce one or more class of immunoglobulin (*hyper-IgM syndrome, X-linked hyper-IgM syndrome,* or *selective IgA immunodeficiency,* or *common variable immunodeficiency*). These individuals are more susceptible to bacterial infections and can be helped by antibiotics and gamma globulin administration. Defects affecting T cells are represented by such diseases as *22q11 deletion syndrome* (also called *DiGeorge syndrome;* absence of thymus and parathyroids). These patients may respond to thymus grafting. Other T-cell immunodeficiencies include *ZAP-70* or *p56 lck deficiency, CD3γ, CD3ε, CD3δ,* and *CD8α deficiencies. Severe combined immunodeficiency diseases (SCIDs)* result from defects affecting both B and T cells. These types of deficiency are exemplified by *common γ chain deficiency* (absence of T- or B-cell immunity), *adenosine deaminase (ADA)* or *purine nucleoside phosphorylase (PNP) deficiency* (toxic metabolite buildup that kills lymphocytes), *RAG1/RAG2 deficiency* (inability to assemble T-

and B-cell antigen receptor genes), *Wiskott-Aldrich syndrome* (platelet deficiency and absence of an antibody response to polysaccharide antigens), *ataxia-telangiectasia* (a combination of defects in T cells, IgA production, brain, and skin), and *leukocyte adhesion deficiency (LAD)* (inability of immune cells to interact with each other, or with antigen if antigen-presenting, because of adhesion defects in B, T, and NK cells). Immunodeficiencies associated with innate immunity include diseases such as *NEMO syndrome* (characterized by anhidrotic ectodermal dysplasia, lack of specific antibody production to polysaccharide antigens, and mycobacterial infections), *WHIM deficiency* (chemokine receptor dysfunction leading to neutropenia, reduced B cells, and increased infections by human papilloma viruses), **chronic granulomatous disease** (phagocyte inability to kill ingested microbes), *Chediak-Higashi syndrome* (phagocyte lysosomes cannot join with phagosomes leads to in ability to kill ingested microbes), and others. Complement deficiencies have been reported for almost all complement components, which cause increased susceptibility to infections and presentation of autoimmune diseases.

The most intensively studied immunodeficiency disease is *acquired immunodeficiency syndrome (AIDS)*. AIDS is caused by a retrovirus called *human immunodeficiency virus type 1 (HIV-1)* and *HIV-2*.

HIV-1 has a tropism for mainly CD4$^+$ T cells but any CD4$^+$ cells can be infected. AIDS, generally fatal, is a disease characterized by a defective immune system displaying a high rate of AIDS-defining infections caused by opportunistic microbes and the appearance of rare cancers. At this time, no completely effective treatment or cure for AIDS has been found.

# SELF-EVALUATION

## RECALLING KEY TERMS

22q11 deletion syndrome (DiGeorge syndrome)
Acquired immunodeficiency syndrome (AIDS)
CD3δ, CD3ε, CD3γ, and CD8α deficiencies
CD4 (HIV receptor)
Chediak-Higashi syndrome
Chronic granulomatous disease
Common variable immunodeficiency
Coreceptors (for HIV)
   CCR5
   CXCR4
Human immunodeficiency virus type 1 (or HIV-1)
Hyper-IgM syndrome
   X-linked hyper-IgM syndrome
IL-12 p40 deficiency
IL-12R β1 chain deficiency
Immunodeficiencies
   Primary
   Secondary
Interferon-γ receptor 1 (IFN-γR1) and IFN-γR2
   deficiency
IRAK-4 deficiency
Kaposi's sarcoma
NEMO syndrome
p56 *lck* deficiency
R5
Selective immunoglobulin immunodeficiency
   Selective IgA deficiency
Severe combined immunodeficiency diseases (SCIDs)
   Adenosine deaminase (ADA) deficiency
   Artemis deficiency
   Ataxia-telangiectasia
   Bare lymphocyte syndrome type I and II
   Common γ (γ$_C$) chain deficiency
   Janus kinase 3 (JAK3) deficiency
   Leukocyte adhesion deficiency (LAD)
   Omenn syndrome
   Purine nucleoside phosphorlylase (PNP) deficiency
   Recombination activating genes 1 & 2
      (RAG1/RAG2) deficiency
   Wiskott-Aldrich syndrome
STAT1 deficiency
WHIM syndrome

X4
X-linked agammaglobulinemia (Bruton's
   agammaglobulinemia)
ZAP-70 deficiency

## MULTIPLE-CHOICE QUESTIONS

*(An answer key is not provided, but the page[s] location of the answer is.)*

1. Which of the following infectious agents is most often seen in early AIDS patients? (a) *M. tuberculosis*, (b) *B. subtilis*, (c) *P. carinii*, (d) genital warts, (e) none of these. *(See pages 540 and 541.)*

2. Which of the following is not considered to be a combined B- and T-cell deficiency? (a) ataxia-telangiectasia, (b) common γ chain deficiency, (c) Wiskott-Aldrich syndrome, (d) X-linked agammaglobulinemia, (e) none of these. *(See pages 529 and 530.)*

3. The entry of HIV into CD4$^+$ T cells depends on the binding of which portion of the virus to the CD4 molecule? (a) core protein p25, (b) membrane protein gp120, (c) membrane protein gp42, (d) lipid bilayer, (e) none of these. *(See pages 547 and 548.)*

4. The human immunodeficiency disorder Wiskott-Aldrich syndrome involves primarily (a) macrophages, (b) stem cells, (c) T cells, (d) B cells, (e) T and B cells, (f) none of these. *(See page 535.)*

5. The human immunodeficiency disorder DiGeorge syndrome involves primarily (a) macrophages, (b) stem cells, (c) T cells, (d) B cells, (e) T and B cells, (f) none of these. *(See page 533.)*

6. The human immunodeficiency disorder X-linked agammaglobulinemia involves primarily (a) macrophages, (b) stem cells, (c) T cells, (d) B cells, (e) T and B cells, (f) none of these. *(See page 532.)*

7. Patients have AIDS when they (a) have more than 200 virions per μl of blood, (b) have <200 CD4$^+$ T cells per μl of blood, (c) have <200 CD4$^+$ T cells per μl of blood and an AIDS-defining illness, (d) become infected with HIV, (e) die of AIDS, (f) none of these. *(See page 551.)*

8. HIV may kill infected CD4$^+$ T cells by (a) replicating, budding, and damaging cells, (b) inducing cytotoxic T cells, (c) formation of syncytia, (d) induction of apoptosis, (e) all of the above. *(See pages 541–546.)*

9. The latency phase of HIV infection is characterized by (a) a good time to treat with antiretroviral

drugs, (b) no virions in the blood or lymph nodes, (c) no symptoms, (d) a steady-state between virus production and virus dead, (f) none of these. (*See pages 550 and 551.*)

**10.** Current antiretroviral therapy for HIV/AIDS interferes with all of the following except (a) reverse transcriptase, (b) protease, (c) integrase, (d) fusion, (e) opportunistic infections, (f) none of these. (*See pages 552 and 553.*)

**11.** All of the following are obstacles to the development of an HIV vaccine except (a) antigenic drift, (b) latent infections, (c) knowing what constitutes an effective immune response against HIV, (d) the inability to induce a sterilizing immunity, (e) access to excellent animal models, (f) none of these. (*See page 555.*)

## SHORT-ANSWER ESSAY QUESTIONS

**1.** Usually, what two different kinds of preparations are used to treat B-cell deficiencies?

**2.** Why would you consider HIV the ultimate (at least to date) immunosuppressive agent?

**3.** What is the extent and significance of the current AIDS epidemic in the U.S. and Sub-Saharian Africa? What differences are there in the distribution of cases within the population of these regions?

**4.** How does HIV replicate and cause damage to the immune system? Why may years elapse between HIV infection and AIDS development?

**5.** What secondary diseases are indicative of AIDS? Why?

**6.** One concern when testing for AIDS is maintaining a balance between tests that are too sensitive, yielding false positives, and tests that are too specific, yielding false negatives. Explain.

**7.** How is the multiplication of HIV retarded with antiretroviral drugs?

**8.** What problems are there in the development of an effective vaccine against AIDS?

## FURTHER READINGS

Buckley, R.H. 2003. Primary immunodeficiency diseases. In *Fundamental Immunology*, 5th ed. W.E. Paul, ed. Philadelphia: Lippincot Williams & Wilkins. p. 1557–1592.

Buckley, R.H. 2004. Molecular defects in human severe combined immunodeficiency and approaches to immune reconstitution. *Ann. Rev. Immunol.* 22:625–655.

Cavazzana-Calvo, M., C. Lagresle, S. Hacein-Bey-Abina, and A. Fischer. 2005. Gene therapy for severe combined immunodeficiency. *Annu. Rev. Med.* 56:585–602.

Cunningham-Rundles, C., and P.P. Ponda. 2005. Molecular defects in T- and B-cell primary immunodeficiency diseases. *Nat. Rev. Immunol.* 5:880–892.

Dybul, M., M. Connors, and A.S. Fauci. 2003. Immunology of HIV infection. In *Fundamental Immunology*, 5th ed. W.E. Paul, ed. Philadelphia: Lippincott Williams & Wilkins. p. 1285–1318.

Fackler, O.T., A. Alcover, and O. Schwartz. 2007. Modulation of the immunological synapse: A key to HIV-1 pathogenesis? *Nat. Rev. Immunol.* 7:310–317.

Fischer, A. 2007. Human primary immunodeficiency diseases. *Immunity* 27:835–845.

Geha, R.S., et al. 2007. Primary immunodeficiency diseases: An update from the International Union of Immunological Societies Primary Immunodeficiency Diseases Classification Committee. *J. Allergy Clin. Immunol.* 120:776–794.

Gonzalez-Scarano, F., and J. Martin-Garcia. 2004. The neuropathogenesis of AIDS. *Nat. Rev. Immunol.* 5:69–81.

Gougeon, M-L. 2003. Apoptosis as an HIV strategy to escape immune attack. *Nat. Rev. Immunol.* 3:392–404.

Haase, A.T. 2005. Perils at mucosal front lines for HIV and SIV and their hosts. *Nat. Rev. Immunol.* 5:783–792.

Hladik, F., and M.J. McElrath 2008. Setting the stage: Host invasion by HIV. *Nat. Rev. Immunol.* 8:447–457.

Kumar, A., S.S. Teuber, and M.E. Gershwin. 2006. Current perspectives on primary immunodeficiency diseases. *Clin. Develop. Immunol.* 13:223–259.

Lederman, M.M., R.E. Offord, and O. Hartley. 2006. Microbicides and other topical strategies to prevent vaginal transmission of HIV. *Nat. Rev. Immunol.* 6:371–382.

Levine, B., and V. Deretic. 2007. Unveiling the roles of autophagy in innate and adaptive immunity. *Nat. Rev. Immunol.* 7:767–777.

Letvin, N.L. 2005. Progress toward an HIV vaccine. *Annu. Rev. Med.* 56:213–223.

Letvin, N.L. 2006. Progress and obstacles in the development of an AIDS vaccine. *Nat. Rev. Immunol.* 6:930–939.

Lim, M.S., and K.S.J. Elenitoba-Johnson. 2004. The molecular pathology of primary immunodeficiencies. *J. Mol. Diagn.* 6:59–83.

Marodi, L., and L.D. Notarangelo. 2007. Immunological and genetic bases of new primary immunodeficiencies. *Nat. Rev. Immunol.* 7:851–861.

McMichael, A.J. 2006. HIV vaccines. *Annu. Rev. Immunol.* 24:227–255.

Peterlin, B.M., and D. Trono. 2003. Hide, shield and strike back: How HIV-infected cells avoid immune eradication. *Nat. Rev. Immunol.* 3:97–107.

# CHAPTER SEVENTEEN

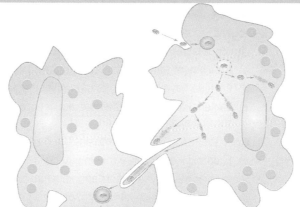

# IMMUNITY TO MICROBES

    d. Viruses are neutralized by antibodies or controlled and cleared by cell-mediated immunity.
       1) Innate and adaptive immunity are needed to eradicate viruses.
       2) Why are there annual concerns about influenza?.
    e. Pathogens can evade immune responses.
       1) Virulence factors can promote infection by bacteria or parasites.
          a) Attachment to tissue cells can initiate an infection.
          b) Bacteria have special types of motility that facilitate infections.
          c) Bacterial factors can either prevent or encourage phagocytic engulfment or allow intracellular survival and multiplication.
       2) Virulence factors such as exotoxins can damage the host.
          a) Endotoxins also play a role in pathogenicity.
       3) Some microbe-derived factors and -inherent properties are associated with virulence.
          a) Bacteria can inject detrimental proteins into a host cell.
          b) Microbes can undergo antigenic switching to avoid immune defenses.
          c) Cord factor of *M. tuberculosis* makes the organism virulent.
       4) Virulence factors produced by viruses facilitate their pathogenicity.
          a) Like bacteria, viruses need to attach to host cells to initiate infection.
          b) Some viruses constantly change their guises to avoid immune defenses.
          c) Some viruses can hide (latency) to avoid immune defenses.
       5) The body's own immune response to infection can contribute to pathogenicity.

**4.** Immunity to infectious microbes can be accomplished by active or passive immunization.

**5.** Vaccines for active immunization are developed using microbes or their products, and genetic engineering.

## OBJECTIVES

The reader should be able to:

**1.** Generally discuss how the body encounters pathogens; give examples.

**2.** Summarize how pathogens cause disease.

**3.** Distinguish between innate and adaptive immune responses.

**4.** Define humoral immunity and cell-mediated immunity; divide them into primary and secondary responses; define immunologic memory.

**5.** Discuss examples of immune responses to the four classes of microbial pathogens; describe how these microbes can evade the immune system.

**6.** Describe the nature of the material used for passive immunization.

**7.** Discuss the various types of vaccines and their advantages and disadvantages.

Our entire life is spent in contact with microorganisms. Many kinds of microbes normally inhabit the human body—harmlessly held in check by the body's defense mechanisms. If these mechanisms are weakened, however, some of these microorganisms can become opportunistic pathogens and cause disease. Other pathogenic microorganisms can invade the human body; whether a disease condition occurs depends on the outcome of the interaction between the microbe and the immune status of the host.

Worldwide, infectious diseases are the largest single cause of illness experienced each year. These diseases range from the common cold to much more serious illness such as discussed in Chapter 16, AIDS. Furthermore, infectious diseases are a common complication associated with therapy, such as immunosuppression for transplants, chemotherapy for cancer, and major surgical operations. In spite of the many antibiotics and other antimicrobial drugs, we are still beset by infectious diseases causing disability, death, and economic consequences. These drugs have not been able to eliminate infectious diseases—such as methicillin-resistant *Staphylococcus aureus* (MRSA) bacteria or Human Immunodeficiency Virus (HIV). Our immune system, in part, has to "take-up the slack." The most important function of the immune system is to protect against infectious diseases. On a day-to-day basis, the efficiency of the immune system is taken for granted; however, if the immune system is compromised we quickly recognize the serious consequences of an inadequate defense. The power of the immune system is impressive but the level of protection can be improved by vaccination (Table 17-1). In fact, as a tool for prevention, vaccination has led to the elimination or greatly reduced the incidence of many diseases, such as smallpox, diphtheria, pertussis, poliomyelitis, and tetanus. The continued study of vaccine prophylaxis holds the promise of controlling other diseases. The immune response to infectious diseases is not always protective; exposure to certain infectious agents can initiate or intensify certain types of pathological states, such as glomerulonephritis and rheumatic fever.

In the immunological world, innate immunity (see Chapter 3) is the most common and basic means of warding off disease. Most animals survive a hostile world of potential pathogens with only nonspecific innate resistance as their defense. Only vertebrate animals are capable of acquiring specific resistance. Thus, they are more efficient in combating infection. First, they use nonspecific resistance mechanisms, composed of internal and external barriers, which are immediately available, against invading parasites. Next, they rely on the mechanisms of specific immunity as reinforcement or, in the case of a persistent infection, as the ultimate means of resistance. If the combined effects of both innate immunity and adaptive immunity are unable to halt the spread of infection, the death of the host is invariably the final result.

The present chapter provides an introduction to the subject of immunity to microbes and obviously can only highlight the important features of a few selected pathogens and the diseases that they cause in humans. Discussions will include a brief introduction into what allows a microorganism to cause disease, the types of immune responses to infections, followed by the characteristics of immunity to representative examples of the four types of pathogens, bacteria, fungi, parasites, and viruses, and how they evade host defenses. A description of the immunization process with an emphasis on some current vaccines and their use ends the chapter.

# A MICROORGANISM CAPABLE OF CAUSING A DISEASE IS A PATHOGEN

Most microbially caused diseases are infectious diseases (an exception is food poisoning) and occur as the result of interactions between pathogenic microorganisms and the host. Most infectious diseases begin at some surface of the host, whether it is the external surfaces such as the skin and conjunctiva or internal surfaces such as the mucous membranes of the respiratory tract, intestine, or urogenital tract. Many pathogens can selectively attach to specific host surfaces. In most infectious diseases, the pathogen penetrates the body surface, gains access to the internal tissues, and remains either localized or is transported to some other body site. Pathogens can also cause generalized infections. Some pathogens grow extracellularly and cause damage to body cells by elaborating toxins. Others can grow in the cells of the host, causing severe disruption of normal physiological processes.

If a host is to recover from an infection, it must eradicate the pathogenic microorganisms. However, as a group, pathogens exhibit a vast array of weapons, termed *virulence factors*, which can combat the various host defense mechanisms. Thus, an infection represents a battle between the defenses mounted by the host and the armamentarium of virulence factors produced by the pathogen. The infection can prove lethal to the host; however, it is to the microbe's advantage

**TABLE 17-1** Vaccines Available in the United States for Use in Humans

| Vaccine | Type | Administration route |
|---|---|---|
| **Anthrax** | Formalin-inactivated cellular supernatant vaccine comprising the protective antigen (PA) component of the toxin | SC |
| Cholera | Killed bacteria of the Inaba and Ogawa serotypes | SC or ID |
| **DTP** | | IM |
| (D = Diphtheria) | Toxoid | |
| (T = Tetanus) | Toxoid | |
| (P = Pertussis) | Killed bacteria | |
| DTaP (Tdap) | | IM |
| (D = Diphtheria) | Toxoid | |
| (T = Tetanus) | Toxoid | |
| (P = Pertussis) | Acellullar (toxoid plus other cellular components) | |
| **Human papillomavirus (HPV; cervical cancer)** | Inactivated virus | IM |
| *Haemophilus influenzae* b | | |
| —Conjugate (HbCV) | Type b capsular polysaccharide conjugated to any of several immunogenic proteins | IM |
| **Hepatitis A virus** | Inactivated virus | IM |
| Hepatitis B (HBV) | | IM |
| —Plasma-derived | HBsAg particles extracted from blood of chronically ill persons | |
| —Recombinant DNA | HBsAg protein made by baker's yeast into which a plasmid containing the gene for HBsAg has been inserted | |
| **Influenza** | Inactivated virus or viral components | IM |
| Measles | Live attenuated virus | SC |
| **Meningococcal** | Capsular polysaccharides of serotypes A, C, X, Y, and W-135 | SC |
| MMR | | SC |
| (M = Measles) | Live attenuated virus | |
| (M = Mumps) | Live attenuated virus | |
| (R = Rubella) | Live attenuated virus | |
| **Mumps** | Live attenuated virus | SC |
| Poliomyelitis | | |
| —IPV; inactivated poliovirus vaccine | Inactivated viruses of all three serotypes | SC |
| —OPV; oral poliovirus vaccine | Live attenuated viruses of all 3 serotypes **(use discontinued in the U.S.)** | O |
| **Plague** | Killed bacteria | IM |
| Pneumococcal | | IM or SC |
| —Mainly for elderly persons | Capsular polysaccharides of the 23 most frequent serotypes | |
| —Heptavalent conjugate, for infants | Capsular polysaccharides of the 7 serotypes that cause 85% of invasive pneumococcal disease and 65% of pneumococcal otitis media in the U.S.; the polysaccharides are conjugated to an immunogenic protein | |
| **Rabies** | Inactivated virus | SC or ID |
| Rotavirus | Live attenuated viruses of the 4 serotypes that cause nearly all rotatvirus disease in the U.S. | O |
| **Rubella** | Live attenuated virus | SC |
| Tetanus | Toxoid | IM |
| Td or DT | | IM |
| (T = Tetanus) | Toxoid | |
| (D or d = Diphtheria) | Toxoid | |
| **Tuberculosis (BCG)** | Live attenuated bacteria | ID or SC |

**TABLE 17-1** (*Continued*)

| Vaccine | Type | Administration route |
|---|---|---|
| **Typhoid** | | |
| | Killed bacteria | SC |
| | Live attenuated bacteria | O |
| | Vi capsular polysaccharide | IM |
| **Vaccinia (smallpox)** | Live virus | PC |
| **Varicella (chickenpox)** | Live attenuated virus, Oka strain | SC |
| **Yellow fever** | Live attenuated virus | SC |
| **Zoster (shingles)** | Live attenuated virus | SC |

Abbreviations: intradermal, ID; intramuscular, IM; oral, O; percutaneous, PC; subcutaneous, SC.

that the battle be somewhat indecisive, that is, that the disease is not so severe as to kill the host, because this would diminish the pathogen's chance of survival. Host-microbe interactions can lead to chronic, long-lasting infections versus acute infections, having a short and relatively severe course. In some infectious diseases, the pathogen itself can be nonaggressive; most of the tissue damage is due to the body's overproduction of cytokines in response to the pathogen's presence in the tissues.

## The Pathogen's Disease-Causing Modus Operandi Is Complex

The ability of a microorganism to cause disease is called **pathogenicity**. When a microbe invades a host, that is, when it enters the body tissues and multiplies, it establishes an infection. Impairment of function in a susceptible host is called **disease**. Thus, a **pathogen** is any microorganism capable of causing disease; they include bacteria, fungi, parasites, and viruses.

The pathogenicity of a microorganism is influenced not only by the properties inherent in the microbe but also by the ability of the host to resist infection. Most members of the normal microbiota (also called *commensals*) of the human body do not ordinarily cause disease. However, they can cause infections if a person's defense mechanisms are compromised by another disease; prolonged antibiotic treatment; immunosuppressive therapy; or an abrasion, cut, or wound. Such microorganisms are called **opportunistic pathogens**. They are distinguished from **primary pathogens**, which can initiate disease even in healthy individuals.

Different strains of the same pathogenic species differ in their degree of pathogenicity, that is, their **virulence**. Microorganisms can range from highly virulent to avirulent depending on the number of organisms needed to cause the associated disease. Virulent strains of many pathogens, when repeatedly

cultured on laboratory media, grown *in vivo* in hosts other than their normal hosts, or genetically modified, can lose their virulence: such avirulent strains are called *attenuated strains* and are often used as vaccines to elicit immunity to various diseases. For instance, the live attenuated strains of poliovirus used in the Sabin vaccine for immunization against poliomyelitis can attach to the gastrointestinal tract just as the wild-type poliovirus does, but because of mutation in the genes encoding the viral surface proteins these attenuated strains have lost the ability to attach to cells of the central nervous system and thus do not cause the paralysis that is characteristic of poliomyelitis.

The properties of a microorganism that affect a microorganism's virulence are called **virulence factors**. The ability of a microorganism to make a particular virulence factor can be due to a chromosomal gene. However, in some instances, it is due to the process of **lysogenic conversion**. Bacteria can also gain virulence or show enhanced virulence by acquiring a plasmid that carries the gene for a toxin or other virulence factor. Examples of toxins or other virulence factors encoded by genes on phages or plasmids are listed in Table 17-2. The toxins, endotoxins or exotoxins (discussed later), can be pathogenic by various means. Endotoxins, such as lipopolysaccharide (LPS), are usually bacterial cell wall components, whereas exotoxins, such as tetanus or diphtheria toxins, are secreted by the bacteria.

On exposure to a microbe, the host either eliminates the organism or becomes infected. **Infection** is the invasion and multiplication of microorganisms in or on a host's tissues that leads to damage to the tissue. Infection can cause so little damage as to be clinically inapparent or it can result in overt clinical disease.

The four steps in the infection process are as follows: (1) adherence or attachment of the pathogen to some surface of the host (such as skin or mucous membranes); (2) penetration of the tissue surface

**TABLE 17-2** Some Toxins or Other Virulence Factors Mediated by Bacteriophages or Plasmids

| Bacterium | Toxin or other virulence factor |
| --- | --- |
| Lysogenic conversion | |
| *Corynebacterium diphtheriae* | Diphtheria toxin |
| *Vibrio cholerae* | Cholera toxin |
| *Clostridium botulinum* Types C and D | Botulinum toxin |
| *Clostridium novyi* Type A | Novyi type A toxin |
| *Streptococcus pyogenes* | Erythrogenic (scarlet fever) toxin |
| *Escherichia coli* | Verotoxin (Shiga-like toxin) |
| *Staphylococcus aureus* | Type A enterotoxin |
| Plasmids | |
| *Escherichia coli* | LT-1 and $ST_a$ enterotoxins |
| *Yersinia pestis* | A protein component of the antiphagocytic capsule |
| *Yersinia enterocolitica* | Adherence and invasion factors |
| *Shigella* species | Invasion factors |
| *Bacillus anthracis* | Anthrax toxin components and antiphagocytic capsule |

layer; (3) resistance toward host defenses (such as innate and adaptive immunity); and (4) damage to host tissue by the pathogen's virulence factors.

Some infections lead to only a minor amount of damage to the host, so minor that there are no detectable clinical symptoms of the infection; such infections care called **subclinical infections**. Other infections vary in their degree of damage, their location, and the number of microbial species involved (Table 17-3).

Although most microbially caused diseases are infections, some are not. An example of one that is not an infection is a type of food poisoning called *botulism* (caused by *Clostridium botulinum*), in which there is no invasion of the body by the causative microorganism. Another example is staphylococcal food poisoning, in which food containing a toxin produced by the bacterium *S. aureus* is consumed.

### MINI SUMMARY

The ability of a microorganism to cause disease is called pathogenicity. Unlike primary pathogens, opportunistic pathogens do not ordinarily cause disease but can do so after a person's defense mechanisms have been compromised. Virulence is the degree of pathogenicity of a strain. Strains can range from highly virulent to avirulent. Attenuated strains have lost their virulence and are often used as vaccines. The ability of a microorganism to make a particular virulence factor can be due to a chromosomal gene, a gene acquired from a

bacteriophage by lysogenic conversion, or a gene acquired from a plasmid.

Infection, the invasion and multiplication of microorganisms in or on a host's tissues that leads to damage to the tissue, involves four steps; adherence or attachment of the pathogen, penetration of the tissue surface layer, resistance toward host defenses, and damage to host tissue by the pathogen's virulence factors. Infections without clinical symptoms are subclinical infections. Other infections vary in their degree of damage, their location, and the number of microbial species involved. Some microbially caused diseases such as botulism and staphylococcal food poisoning are not infections.

## The Portals of Entry by Pathogenic Organisms Are Numerous

Microorganisms enter the body by various means. To do this they must penetrate the body's protective surfaces such as the skin and mucous membranes (see Chapter 3). Pathogens can penetrate body surfaces passively by wounds, the bite of an arthropod, or inhalation of an airborne microorganism. However, many pathogens possess the means to actively penetrate body surfaces such as the conjunctiva of the eye or the mucous membrane of the respiratory tract, oral cavity, intestinal tract, and genitourinary tract. For instance, the spirochetes that cause leptospirosis can be acquired if the conjunctiva comes into contact with water contaminated with the urine from infected domestic or wild animals.

**TABLE 17-3** Some Types of Infections

| Term | Definition | Example |
|---|---|---|
| Acute | Has a short and relatively severe course | Streptococcal pharyngitis ("strep throat") caused by *Streptococcus pyogenes* |
| Chronic | Has a long duration | Tuberculosis caused by *Mycobacterium tuberculosis* |
| Fulminating | Occurs suddenly and with severe intensity | Cerebrospinal meningitis caused by *Neisseria meningitides* |
| Localized | Is restricted to a limited area of the body | Urinary tract infection caused by *Escherichia coli* |
| Generalized | Affects many or all parts of the body | Typhoid fever, caused by *Salmonella typhi* |
| Mixed, or polymicrobial | Infection by more than one kind of microorganism | Gas gangrene, in which a combination of *Clostridium* species can occur |
| Primary | An initial localized infection that decreases resistance and thus paves the way for further invasion by the same microorganism or other microorganisms | Influenza, caused by an influenza virus |
| Secondary | Infection that is established after a primary infection has caused a decreased resistance | Pneumococcal pneumonia following influenza |

### Wounds Provide a Facilitated Entry for Pathogens

Passive penetration can occur when any mechanically caused wound or break in the skin or mucous membranes allows pathogens a direct access to the underlying tissues. For example, wounded soldiers can develop gas gangrene if the wound becomes contaminated by *C. perfringens* present in soil. Burns often become infected by *Pseudomonas aeruginosa* or other aerobic or facultatively anaerobic bacteria from the surrounding environment.

### Arthropod Bites Introduce the Arthropod's Contents Into the Host

Arthropods serve as **vectors** for pathogenic microorganisms. A vector is an organism, such as an insect, that transports a pathogenic microorganism. Some arthropods are *mechanical vectors*, merely transmitting pathogens that adhere to their mouthparts or legs. The common housefly, *Musca domestica*, is the classic example; it can become contaminated with pathogens from feces and transmit them to food or other objects. Diseases can include gastroenteritis and other intestinal diseases. In most arthropod-borne diseases, however, the arthropod serves as a *biological vector*, one in which the pathogen undergoes a period of growth or development within the arthropod, as in epidemic typhus or malaria.

Transmission to humans by biological vectors occurs by several means: (1) The salivary glands of the arthropod are infected and some of this saliva is transferred to the human during the bite. The transmission of malaria protozoa by mosquitoes is a classic example of this mode of infection. (2) All of the tissues and fluids of the arthropod are infected and if the arthropod is crushed on the skin, as by scratching, the microorganisms are released onto the skin and can be able to penetrate tiny abrasions or scratches. Alternatively, the microorganisms are excreted in the arthropod's feces as it takes its blood meal and, while scratching the bite, the human victim rubs the infected feces into the bite. This type of transmission occurs with human lice in epidemic typhus. (3) The microorganisms cause blockage of the arthropod's alimentary tract. As the arthropod takes its blood meal, the ingested blood acquires the microorganisms and is then regurgitated into the bite. This is the main type of transmission that occurs with rat fleas in bubonic plague.

### The Respiratory Tract Is One of the Primary Entrances for Pathogens

Humans can become infected by inhaling an aerosol—a spray of small and large droplets—that contains microorganisms. Inhaling infectious dust, that is, dust containing pathogenic microorganisms, can also infect humans. Aerosols and infectious dust are generated from human and environmental sources.

Microorganisms that cause respiratory infections occur in secretions from the nose and throat of infected individuals. When a person coughs or sneezes, an aerosol is expelled. The larger droplets (10 μm or more in diameter) can be inhaled by people nearby and trapped in the recipient's nose and nasopharynx. They can also settle onto clothing and other inanimate objects, which then act as sources of infection. Small droplets (1 to 4 μm in diameter) can be inhaled directly, but the water in these droplets tends to evaporate quickly and leave droplet nuclei—a residue of solid material, including microorganisms. Droplet nuclei that contain living microorganisms can remain suspended in air for hours or days and travel long distances.

Some microorganisms that cause respiratory infections, such as the measles virus, are unable to survive for long outside the body. Transmission of such microorganisms depends upon rapid airborne transfer of large droplets from one person to another, or by even more direct transfer, as by kissing. Other pathogenic microorganisms, such as *Mycobacterium tuberculosis*, can survive for long periods outside the body.

Some human infections result from inhaling airborne pathogens from an environmental source rather than from infected persons. For example, epidemics of Legionnaires' disease are attributed to aerosols generated from the contaminated water of air-conditioning equipment and from mist sprays used in grocery stores to keep vegetables fresh.

Some airborne pathogens inhabit soil and are not transmitted from person to person; instead, they are transmitted by inhaling dust arising from this soil. For instance, the fungus that causes histoplasmosis is usually acquired in this manner. Inhaling infectious dust derived from the excreta of animals can also lead to infections. For instance, inhaling dust from virus-contaminated rodent urine or feces is the major mode of transmission of hantaviruses.

### The Alimentary Tract Is the Other Primary Entrance for Pathogens

Pathogenic microorganisms can be present in inadequately cooked or improperly stored food, or in food subjected to poor sanitary conditions during its preparation. The two major categories of foodborne diseases caused by microorganisms are food poisoning and foodborne infections.

Food poisoning occurs when a microorganism produces a toxin in a food; when people consume the food, the ingested toxin causes diarrhea, vomiting, or other symptoms.

Foodborne infections occur when the pathogen is ingested, escapes destruction by the stomach acidity, and multiplies in the alimentary tract. Some pathogens such as *Helicobacter pylori*, the major cause of peptic ulcers in humans, can even infect the wall of the stomach. Foodborne infections are usually diseases of the intestine. In some intestinal infections, such as cholera, the bacterium is noninvasive; it merely attaches to the epithelial layer of the small intestine and secretes a toxin that causes the disease. Other intestinal pathogens are invasive, able to penetrate the intestinal wall and multiply there, causing inflammation and extensive damage. For example, in bacillary dysentery, *Shigella* bacteria penetrate into and kill epithelial cells of the colon, and then spread to adjacent epithelial cells, which are in turn killed. Infectious microorganisms are also acquired through the drinking of water that has been contaminated with fecal matter containing pathogens from humans or animals.

### Pathogens Can Use the Genitourinary Tracts to Enter the Host

In a healthy person, the kidney, urinary bladder, and ureters are free of microorganisms. Normally the mechanical removal of bacteria by the flushing action of urination is a major factor that prevents these bacteria from growing along the surfaces of the urinary tract. However, many opportunistic pathogens such as *Escherichia coli* can adhere to and colonize the mucous membranes of the lower portion of the urethra of both males and females.

Sexual intercourse can allow direct access of pathogenic organisms to the skin and mucous membranes of the genital tract if one of the sexual partners has a sexually transmitted disease. The following are some examples. During sexual contact, the HIV—the virus that causes AIDS—can gain entrance to the blood stream of an uninfected individual, male or female, because of microscopic breaks in the mucous membrane lining of the genital organs (see Chapter 16). In gonorrhea, *Neisseria gonorrhoeae* preferentially attaches to columnar epithelial cells but not squamous epithelial cells. Columnar epithelial cells line the urethra of males and females and the cervix in females. From an infected cervix the organism sometimes spread to other areas of a woman's genital tract, such as the fallopian tubes or the lining of the uterus, which can result in infertility. Eventually the organism can spread to other areas of the body that are far removed from the genital tract. In syphilis, *Treponema pallidum* initially binds to and penetrates the skin or mucous membranes of the genital organs, multiplies locally, invades the lymphatic and blood circulatory systems, and eventually becomes distributed throughout the entire body.

### Pathogens Can Passage from the Initial Site of Infection

In some infections the microorganism simply grows in the tissue in which it finds itself, causing a localized infection. An example is the type of infection caused by *S. aureus*, where the characteristic lesion is an **abscess**, that is, a walled-off cavity in the tissues containing the staphylococci, numerous white blood cells (that collectively form a pasty mass called **pus**), and dead, disintegrating tissue cells that have been killed by the toxins elaborated from the staphylococci.

In other infections, the organism does not remain localized but spreads directly through the tissues. An example is the anaerobe *C. perfringens*; as it begins to grow, the bacteria elaborate toxins that kill some of the surrounding healthy tissue. This dead tissue becomes anaerobic and supports the growth of more clostridia, which in turn elaborate more toxins that kill more tissue and allow the organisms to spread further.

*Pathogens Can Passage to the Lymphatic System.* Microorganisms present in tissues can be collected by lymphatic vessels. For instance, in erysipelas, a skin disease of the face caused by *Streptococcus pyogenes*, the painful lesions spread because the streptococci have invaded the lymphatic vessels of the subepidermal tissue.

*Pathogens Can Passage to the Blood Circulatory System.* From the initial site of entry into the body by passive or active means, a pathogenic microorganism can sometimes directly enter a blood capillary or venule and thereby gain access to the blood vascular system, causing a **bacteremia** (presence of bacteria in the blood). Alternatively, pathogenic organisms might first infect the lymphatic system and then pass to the blood circulatory system. A bacteremia can allow a pathogen to be carried to various parts of the body where it can cause localized infections. For instance, *N. meningitidis* initially present in the nasopharynx can reach the meninges (membranes that cover the brain and spinal cord) by means of transient bacteremia and cause severe meningitis.

Some pathogenic bacteria actively multiply in the bloodstream and produce toxic products—a condition known as **septicemia**. Septicemic infections range from chronic to acute. One of the most severe is anthrax, a disease of animals and sometimes humans, in which the number of *Bacillus anthracis* organisms often exceeds the number of erythrocytes in the blood. Septicemic infections often begin as localized infections that later become generalized.

## MINI SUMMARY

Pathogens can penetrate body surfaces passively or actively. Arthropods can serve as mechanical

or biological vectors for pathogens. Humans can become infected by inhaling airborne pathogens in aerosols and infectious dust generated from human sources or from environmental sources. Two major categories of foodborne diseases caused by microorganisms are food poisoning and foodborne infections. Some foodborne bacteria are noninvasive, as in cholera, whereas others are invasive, as in bacillary dysentery. Many opportunistic pathogens colonize the mucous membranes of the lower portion of the urethra. Sexual intercourse can allow direct access of pathogens to the genital tract. In some infections, the pathogen remains at the initial site of entry and causes a localized infection, such as an abscess. In other infections, the organism spreads directly through the tissues. Invading organisms can pass into lymphatic vessels, infect the nearest lymph node, and eventually reach the bloodstream.

# INNATE AND ADAPTIVE IMMUNITY PROVIDE PROTECTION AGAINST INFECTIOUS DISEASES

Vertebrate animals can manifest immunity in two ways, **innate** and **adaptive immunity**, which is mediated by nonspecific and specific components, respectively. The nonspecific components act as first line defenders by either using existing barriers or generalized eliminators that target a wide range of pathogens without specificity. In contrast, the specific components are the second-line defenders that use a set of specialized cells and molecules that adapt to each pathogen encounter and become activated. Activation leads to the expression of pathogen-specific effector functions that eliminate or neutralize the pathogens.

## Innate Immunity Provides External Frontline Defenses and Internal Cellular, Chemical, and Biological Defenses

**Innate**, also called *nonspecific, natural,* or *native resistance,* **immunity** is the sum of host defenses that *exist before,* and function independently of, any exposure to an invader such as a microbe; that is, *innate immunity has a broad specificity for different classes of microbes.* (Innate immunity will only be briefly discussed here; it is detailed in Chapter 3.)

Innate immunity serves as the first line of defense and includes both *external* and *internal* nonspecific responses. External defenses are present in those areas of the body exposed to the outside environment (the contact areas for pathogens). Internal defenses come into play after the pathogen has penetrated the external defenses. Taken together, the components of innate immunity are *preformed* (the components [such as cytotoxic cells, phagocytic cells, complement, and other molecules] are present before challenge); *standardized* (the response magnitude is consistent); *without memory* (the host does not realize it has been reexposed to the same invader); and *nonspecific* (innate immunity does not distinguish *between* invaders, that is, all invaders are foreign) (see Table 1-1). Nonetheless, it has a unique specificity for microbial structures characteristic of pathogens, which is different from the acquired immune system's specificity. The innate immune system is unable to *recognize* nonmicrobial molecules. (It can react to nonmicrobial molecules, that is, phagocytic cells internalizing some macromolecules.) Innate and adaptive immunity do not operate independently of each other; rather innate mechanisms reduce the workload for the immune system's specific defenses and keep infections in check until specific immunity can develop, and induce adaptive immune components (see below), while adaptive immunity supplements and augments the nonspecific defenses.

External defense mechanisms prevent penetration of pathogens into our tissues; they include intact skin and mucous membranes; tears; respiratory tract; alimentary tract; urogenital tract; and normal intestinal flora. Internal defense mechanisms come into play once a pathogen has entered our tissues; they include chemical/physiological barriers; natural killer (NK) cells; interferon (other cytokines); alternative complement pathway (and lectin pathway of complement activation); and detection of pathogens using germline-encoded receptors.

The innate system, present in all multicellular organisms, is the oldest host defense system. Complex multicellular organisms arose in the presence of rapidly dividing single-cell microbes. The multicellular organisms developed innate defense mechanisms to combat and protect themselves against the constant barrage of the more-rapidly-dividing single-cell invaders. The response had to be rapid and capable of distinguishing the invaders from self-tissues, so the innate system focused on so-called *pathogen-associated molecular patterns (PAMPs)* or *pattern recognition sequences*, that is, biologic patterns unique to and necessary for the survival of microorganisms; they are not found on mammalian cells.

One such pattern is the conserved bacterial lipid-A pattern in LPS, a component of the Gram-negative bacterial cell wall. LPS is necessary for microbial survival; thus, bacteria always express this marker (if they shed or alter their LPS in order to evade innate immunity, they are no longer viable). So common are these pattern recognition sequences that their identity is encoded into the germline DNA of multicellular organisms; our body has the inherent capacity to identify any organism that displays these patterns and to mount a rapid response to eliminate it. Soluble mediators (initiators of complement system) and the receptors on innate immune system cells (such as macrophages, dendritic cells, and neutrophils) that recognize pattern recognition sequences are called *pattern-recognition receptors*; they include *scavenger, LPS, nucleotide-binding oligomerization domain (NOD)*, and *Toll-like receptors (TLRs)* (see Table 3-1).

Because the innate immune system recognizes a limited number of antigens found exclusively in microbial pathogens, it deploys a limited number of receptors with specificity for conserved microbial structures. Recognition of these structures by the innate immune system induces costimulators, cytokines, and chemokines, which recruit and activate antigen-specific lymphocytes and initiate adaptive immune responses. So how does this connection work? The adaptive immune system recognizes virtually any antigen; it accomplishes this through the random generation of a highly diverse repertoire of antigen receptors. But the price of this diversity is the inability to distinguish foreign antigens from self-antigens. To distinguish between the two antigens, adaptive immune system cells (such as T lymphocytes) need *two signals* to become activated: (1) binding of foreign antigen, the first signal, and (2) binding of costimulators (costimulators are expressed on innate immune system cells that have reacted with PAMPs), the second signal.

Despite physical and chemical barriers, pathogens do gain entry to the bloodstream and other tissues. These attacks are met, and usually eliminated by specialized cells that ingest and degrade large particles, microorganisms, and even other cells. Phagocytosis is a specialized form of endocytosis where large particles, such as microorganisms and cell debris, are taken up in large endocytic vesicles (1–2 μm) called *phagosomes*. Phagosomes fuse with *lysosomes* to form *phagolysosomes*. These vesicles contain a number of acid hydrolases, as well as other molecules, which lead to degradation of the ingested material. All cells mediate endocytosis, but only monocyte/macrophages, dendritic cells, and neutrophils mediate phagocytosis.

When pathogens cross epithelial barriers and establish a local focus of infection, the host must mobilize its defenses and direct them to the site of pathogen growth. *Inflammation* describes a series of changes that occur at such sites in a few minutes to a few hours in response to tissue injury or introduction of a foreign substance. The hallmarks of inflammation include redness, swelling, heat, pain; increased blood flow to the site; increased vascular permeability; and influx of cells from the immune system. These changes all augment pathogen clearance.

## There Are Two Types of Adaptive Immunity

### Humoral Immunity Involves the Result of Antibody Production

*Humoral immunity* involves antibody secretion by plasma cells into the body's fluids or humors.[1] Antibodies can combine with and neutralize bacterial toxins, inhibit viral attachment to target cells, or coat bacteria to enhance phagocytosis. Antibodies do not remove or kill antigens by themselves; instead, they serve as the "search" elements of the immune response. Complement activation and opsonization are the "destroy" aspects of the antibody-mediated mission. Once an infection is overcome, antibody production

---

[1] The word *humoral* is derived from the medieval reference to the four fluids or "humors." In medieval times, the humors of the body included blood, phlegm, yellow bile (or choler), and black bile. These fluids were thought to decide a person's character and general health. Imbalances in the humors were believed to cause disease, personality flaws, and so on.

wanes because of influences wielded by regulatory cells, their cytokines, and antibodies themselves.

### The Primary Antibody Response Occurs on First Exposure to Antigen.

*A host's first exposure to a specific antigen leads to the appearance of specific serum antibody. This reaction is called the* **primary antibody response**. All immunogens can induce a primary antibody response. A latent period of 5 to 10 days, sometimes called *early-induced response*, occurs in which most antigens is rapidly catabolized. The kinetics of the antibody response can be divided into two general events: (1) *antigen elimination* (Figure 17-1) and (2) *antibody formation*. Note that serum antibody is not observed immediately in the circulation following antigen exposure. The duration of antigen elimination dictates when antibody will appear.

If an antigen is artificially introduced (intravenous injection), antigen elimination is divisible into three phases: *equilibration, nonimmune catabolism* (metabolic elimination), and *immune catabolism* (immune elimination). The equilibration phase begins within 10 min of injection, and due to antigen trapping more than 90% of the antigen is removed from circulation. During the first few hours, the antigen is present in the liver and lung, but the highest concentration is found in the spleen. (If the antigen were extravascular, it would be delivered to local lymph nodes.) Eventually an equilibration of antigen between the intravascular and extravascular compartments is reached. The second phase, nonimmune catabolism, lasts for 2 to 7 days and involves the gradual enzymatic breakdown, digestion, and removal of antigen. The enzymatic competence of the host determines the length of this phase. Any

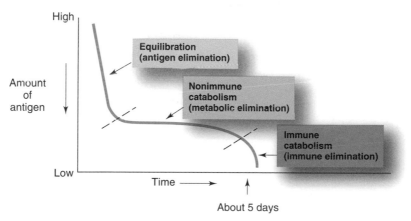

**FIGURE 17-1 Antigen elimination curve.** Antibody does not appear immediately after antigen exposure, nor is a host immediately immune to the antigen. A latent period occurs before these two events. The extent of the latent period depends on the antigen and the host species exposed to the antigen.

change or dysfunction in macrophage activities such as antigen processing and cytokine synthesis can significantly disrupt this phase. Complement activation is important in this phase (see Chapter 11). The third and last phase, immune catabolism, also removes antigen from circulation. Newly produced antibody rapidly combines with and coats the antigen, which leads to enhanced phagocytosis. Antigen-antibody complexes also are removed by the complement system. The rate of antigen removal during immune catabolism varies from species to species with a given antigen and from antigen to antigen in a given species.

Other parameters besides antigen elimination affect the length of time required before antibody is produced (see Table 4-1).

The production of antibody after first exposure to antigen follows a characteristic four-part sequence that collectively constitutes the primary antibody response (Figure 17-2). The response begins with a latent period of several days (highly variable, depending on the factors listed in Table 4-1) with no detectable antibody, followed by an exponential increase to a maximum titer. Antibody production eventually plateaus and declines over time.

The primary response results mainly in the production of IgM early in the response followed by some IgG. IgM is the main class of secreted antibody because resting naïve mature B cells express only IgM and IgD (IgD is not secreted).

Antigens on first exposure elicit IgM production rather than IgG production because the functional V-D-J gene joins 5' to the closest C-gene exon, Cμ (see Chapter 6). The IgM-producing B cells have not undergone somatic hypermutation; therefore, their IgM antibodies are of low affinity. However, class switching occurs soon after antigenic stimulation.

Increased antibody affinity is associated with IgG, and smaller doses of antigen seem to increase the affinity of IgG molecules. Hence the concentration of antigen required to stimulate a B cell is inversely related to the affinity of the antibody secreted by the resulting progeny plasma cells. This relationship means that a high antigen concentration usually elicits the production of low-affinity antibodies. As the primary response proceeds, antigen concentration declines. The result is higher average antibody affinity, which is especially evident during a secondary response. This process, called *affinity maturation* (see Chapter 6), results from both somatic mutations in antibody genes and selective activation of B-cell clones with membrane-associated, high-affinity antibody. Additionally, the **avidity** (the dissociation strength of antigen-antibody complexes) of antibodies increases with time.

***Immunologic Memory Distinguishes between the Primary and the Secondary Response.*** Two main characteristics of the immune response are *specificity* and *memory*. The first exposure to antigen (primary response) activates previously unstimulated B cells that have undergone few somatic mutations and thus express low-affinity immunoglobulin receptors. Whereas reexposure to the same antigen (secondary response) activates expanded clones of memory cells that have undergone extensive somatic mutation and thus express high-affinity immunoglobulin receptors. These memory cells also include helper T ($T_H$) cells that appear earlier than do memory B cells, suggesting their requirement in B-cell somatic hypermutation and isotype switching. *This process*, **immunologic memory**, *is the immediate recognition and response to a previously encountered antigen.* The host's response during the second exposure to a specific antigen is faster and greater in magnitude than the response during the first exposure. When antigens are recognized during rechallenge, memory cells ensure a much swifter immune response. Immunologic memory is the main difference between primary and secondary antibody and T-cell responses.

***The Secondary Antibody Response Occurs on Reexposure to the Antigen That Caused the Primary Antibody Response.*** Reexposure to antigen at some interval (7 to 10 days) after the first exposure elicits a faster response time (usually 1 to 3 days), a more rapid increase in antibody titer, and longer persistence of antibody synthesis (that is, a *shortened latent period, higher titer,* and *extended duration of detectable antibody*) (Table 17-4). *These are the characteristics of a* **secondary antibody response**, *also*

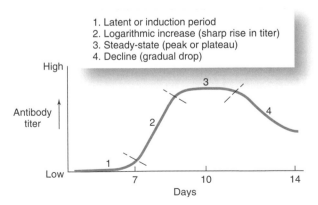

1. Latent or induction period
2. Logarithmic increase (sharp rise in titer)
3. Steady-state (peak or plateau)
4. Decline (gradual drop)

**FIGURE 17-2 Antibody titer following one injection of antigen.**

**TABLE 17-4** Comparison of Primary and Secondary Antibody Responses

| Parameter | Primary response | Secondary response |
| --- | --- | --- |
| Responding B cell | Naïve B cell | Memory B cell |
| Latent period | 5–10 days | 1–3 days |
| Peak antibody titer | Smaller | Larger |
| Persistence of antibody titer | Short | Long |
| Predominating antibody class | IgM | IgG |
| Antibody affinity | Lower average affinity | Affinity maturation occurs, leading to higher average affinity |
| Induced by | All immunogens | Only protein antigens, therefore T-cell-dependent |
| Dose of immunogen for immunization | High doses (optimal with the use of adjuvants) | Low doses (adjuvant not needed) |

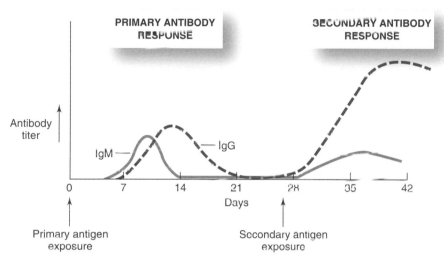

**FIGURE 17-3 Secondary antibody response.** Compared with the primary antibody response, the secondary antibody response appears much more quickly (1 to 2 days after exposure to the homologous antigen) and lasts longer (for months to years). The antibody titer attained is higher and consists mainly of IgG.

*called a* **booster response** (Figure 17-3). In contrast to the primary antibody response, only protein antigens induce a secondary antibody response. The heightened responsiveness is due to increased antibody affinity. The increased affinity occurs in the germinal centers, when B cells undergo somatic hypermutation and selection by antigen presented on follicular dendritic cells (see Chapters 2 and 10). The secondary antibody response can be increased by repeated immunizations until the physiologic limit of responsiveness is reached. The secondary response requires a lower antigen dose, produces primarily IgG rather than IgM (*class switching*), and involves *affinity maturation* (both topics are discussed in Chapter 6). If the interval between the two exposures is too short or too long, the secondary antibody response is reduced.

Nonetheless, the potential for a secondary response persists for many months to years in humans; long after detectable antibody titer has disappeared.

### Cell-Mediated Immunity Is the Destruction of Invaders Unreachable by Antibodies

*Cell-mediated immunity is specific immunity that dependents on the presence of sensitized T cells* and does not involve antibodies to mediate its protective activities. (Indirectly, antibodies can contribute through antibody-dependent cell-mediated cytotoxicity [ADCC; see Chapter 10].) Cell-mediated immunity helps protect the host against intracellular infectious agents. Once activated by macrophages that present antigen and release chemical regulators, T cells go to work. Some subpopulations of T cells synthesize and secrete their own chemical regulators that spur additional T-cell growth. Some of these regulators attract immune cells to the site of the infection or direct the activities of immune cells at the infection site. If the antigen replicates in macrophages, it leads to the activation of CD4$^+$ T$_H$1 cells. Some T cells become cytotoxic cells that destroy host cells infected by intracellular parasites. When the infection is brought under control, regulatory cells terminate the immune response. Collectively, cellular immunity involves (1) responses against infectious microorganisms, especially intracellular organisms; (2) the development of immunity to soluble protein antigens; (3) elements of autoimmune diseases; (4) delayed-type hypersensitivity; (5) reactions against transplanted tissues; and (6) reactions against tumors.

The chief instigators of cellular immunity are intracellular parasites such as bacteria, viruses, fungi, and protozoa. Because the growth of these microorganisms is not normally stopped when phagocytic cells internalize them, cell-mediated immunity supplies the additional means to destroy these microorganisms. These means include the accumulation and activation of macrophages at the site of infection. Once macrophages are activated, they can help stop the growth of the pathogen. For viral infections, CD8$^+$ T$_C$ cells recognize the virus-encoded antigen on the infected cell surface. The T$_C$ cells react with viral antigen in association with MHC-encoded class I molecules (whose structure and function are described in Chapters 7 and 8), leading to the destruction of the infected cell. Table 17-5 lists some of the intracellular pathogens of humans that need cellular responses for their killing.

The development of a primary and a secondary cell-mediated immune response follows the same timetable as for humoral immunity, and both cell-mediated and humoral immune responses generate memory cells. Secondary cellular immunity can be induced months to years after a primary exposure to antigen. Figure 17-4 shows primary and secondary cellular immune responses to grafted tissue. Note the similarities between humoral immunity (Figures 17-2 and 17-3) and cellular immunity (Figure 17-4).

---

**MINI SUMMARY**

The introduction of antigen, such as a pathogen, into a host starts sequential reactions that lead to the production of antibodies (humoral immunity) and to the mobilization of sensitized T cells (cellular immunity). The first exposure to antigen is called a primary response. The immune system responds much more rapidly when the same antigen enters the body again (a secondary response). This phenomenon is known as immunologic memory.

---

# FOR EFFECTIVE IMMUNITY AGAINST THE FOUR CLASSES OF MICROBIAL PATHOGENS, THE IMMUNE SYSTEM MUST AGGRESSIVELY APPLY ALL ITS RESOURCES

The immune system has evolved to protect us from infectious disease caused by the four major groups of pathogens. A small number of all microbes are considered human pathogens and most of them do not cause infections that lead to death of the host, but the disease sequelae of some them can leave their mark, such as arthritis and glomerulonephritis. The implication is that the immune system must wield its power wisely.

## Antibodies Primarily Mediate Anti-bacterial Immunity

Protection against bacteria is accomplished mainly by antibody development unless the bacterium can grow intracelluarly. In the latter scenario, delayed-type hypersensitivity comes into action. As discussed earlier, bacteria can enter the host by various routes. When bacteria enter the host, their numbers and level of virulence dictate the level of the host's counter

---

**TABLE 17-5 Intracellular Pathogens Requiring Cellular Immunity for Their Destruction**

1. Bacteria
   a. *Brucella abortus*
   b. *Listeria monocytogenes*
   c. *Mycobacterium tuberculosis*
   d. *Salmonella typhosa*
2. Fungi
   a. *Candida albicans*
   b. *Cryptococcus neoformans*
   c. *Histoplasma capsulatum*
3. Protozoa
   a. *Leishmania donovani*
   b. *Malarial plasmodia*
   c. *Toxoplasma gondii*
   d. *Trypanosoma cruzi*
4. All viruses

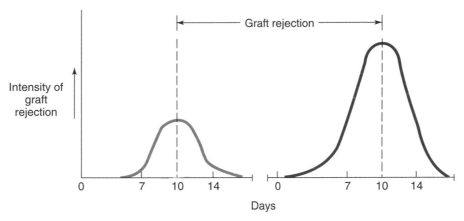

**FIGURE 17-4 Primary and secondary cell-mediated immune responses.** The time responses for the rejection of a foreign skin graft are similar to the primary and secondary antibody responses.

response. Few bacteria with low virulence may elicit surrounding tissue phagocytes, which internalize and eliminate them using innate immune defenses. Larger numbers of bacteria with greater virulence usually also elicit an adaptive response.

Infectious extracellular bacteria are usually pathogenic because they can cause a localized inflammation or because they produce toxins. The main anti-bacterial defenses against extracellular bacteria are antibodies produced by plasma cells in the draining lymph nodes or the submucosa of the respiratory or gastrointestinal tracts. These antibodies can mediate bacterial killing by antibody plus complement, opsonization, and phagocytosis or the neutralization of the bacterial toxins.

Some infectious intracellular bacteria are resistant to innate immune responses, but they activate NK cells, which can mediate early defense mechanism through cytokine release. Delayed-type hypersensitivity, a form of cell-mediated immunity, tends to be induced by these bacteria. $T_H1$ cells are induced to release interferon-γ (IFN-γ), which in turn activates macrophages to kill the internalized bacteria.

Other characteristics of pathogenic bacteria influence immune reactivity against them; these characteristics include whether the bacteria are Gram-positive or Gram-negative bacteria, mycobacteria, or spirochetes. Gram-positive bacteria have cell wall composed of a thick *peptidoglycan* layer outside the plasma membrane; the cell wall also contain carbohydrates, proteins, and teichoic acids. Even though teichoic acids are important immunogens associated with Gram-positive bacteria, the bacteria's thick layer protects them against classic complement-mediated lysis. Nonetheless, the specific antibody generated against Gram-positive bacteria leads to opsonization

and enhanced phagocytosis. The latter activities involve the action of IgM or IgG alone or in concert with C3b (see Chapter 11). The alternative complement system also may be activated. Although complement cannot directly lyse Gram-positive bacteria, its activation contributes opsonins and inflammatory mediators, which provide defenses against Gram-positive bacteria.

The cell-wall structure of Gram-negative bacteria is different from Gram-positive organisms; Gram-negative bacteria have a thin peptidoglycan layer between an outer and inner membrane. The outer membrane contains LPS, also called *endotoxin* (which refers to the lipid-A portion of LPS). LPS contains epitopes that are immunogenic. These immunogenic epitopes induce specific antibodies, which allow for the classification of many Gram-negative bacteria into different serotypes. Unlike Gram-positive bacteria, Gram-negative bacteria are sensitive to complement-mediated lysis, irrespective of the complement pathway that is initiated.

Endotoxin is toxic to humans. Endotoxins are associated with intact bacteria and are not secreted by living bacteria. After Gram-negative bacteria die (as when attacked by antibodies plus complement), endotoxins can be released in soluble form as the cells autolyze and the outer membrane of the cell breaks down. The harmful effects of endotoxins include the ability to cause high fever, hypotension (low blood pressure), disseminated blood clotting, and lethal shock. However, endotoxins do not act directly on the body to cause these effects, but instead act mainly by stimulating the body's macrophages to overproduce various substances. These substances include: cytokines such as tumor necrosis factor (TNF), interleukin (IL)-1, IL-6, and IL-8; toxic forms of oxygen, such as superoxide radicals, hydrogen peroxide, and nitric oxide; and lipids, such as prostaglandin $E_2$, thromboxane $A_2$, and platelet-activating factor. These substances can act independently, together, or in certain sequences to cause various effects.

The cell walls of mycobacteria are distinct from Gram-positive and Gram-negative bacteria; their cell walls contain high lipid content. Mycobacteria are slow-growing organisms. They induce strong antibody responses and cell-mediated responses; however, cell-mediated immunity predominates in the form of delayed-type hypersensitivity (see Chapter 12). The latter reaction revolves around the activation of macrophages by $T_H1$ cells. It is also the basis for the tuberculin test. The hypersensitivity reactions to mycobacteria may be the cause of the associated pathogenesis when infected with mycobacteria.

The fourth class of bacteria, spirochetes, is thin, fragile, helical bacteria that have cell walls different from Gram-positive, Gram-negative, or mycobacteria. The spirochete's outer membrane has few proteins. Nonetheless, they induced specific antibodies, which activate the classical complement system.

---

### MINI SUMMARY

The principal immune response to extracellular bacteria is the production of antibodies, which opsonize bacteria for enhanced phagocytosis, activate complement-mediated lysis, and neutralize toxin activity. In contrast, intracellular bacteria are handled by $T_H1$ cell-mediated delayed-type hypersensitivity responses.

---

## Innate Immunity Deals with Many Fungal Infections but Adaptive Immunity Develops

Although there are 75,000 scientifically identified species of fungi with some scientists suggesting there are millions, only about 50 of these are known to be pathogenic for humans. Of these, only a few are frank pathogens; most of them are opportunistic pathogens, that is, they cause disease only when the host's immune system is damaged. Over the last several decades, the opportunity for fungal infections has increased significantly because of the increasing population of immunocompromised hosts, such as HIV-infected individuals (see Chapter 16), transplant recipients, and chemotherapy of cancer patients. The opportunistic fungi can then grow unrestrained and cause systemic infections. Damage to the tissues is caused not by toxins but by development of allergic necrosis due to hypersensitivity of the host immune system to the fungi. Other pathogenic fungi are of exogenous origin, that is, coming from outside the body, such as from soil or bird droppings. The mortality associated with opportunistic fungal infections exceeds 50% and have been reported to reach 95% in bone-marrow recipients infected with *Aspergillus* species. Because fungi are eukaryotes, they share many of their biologic processes with humans, which are evidenced by the toxicity of antifungal drugs when used therapeutically. There are no antifungal vaccines.

Pathogenic fungi cause diseases called **mycoses**. Some pathogenic fungi have the ability to infect hair, nails, or the superficial layers of the skin. These fungi are called *dermatophytes* and the infections are referred to as dermatomycoses. Dermatomycoses are often called *ringworm* (the first disease showed to be of fungal origin, circa 1843) on the basis of an early mistaken notion that worms or lice caused the skin infections and also because the skin lesions are more or less circular with an inflamed border that gives a ring-like appearance. Other pathogenic fungi can invade the subcutaneous tissue (the tissue underlying the skin); these fungi cause infections called *subcutaneous mycoses*. Subcutaneous mycoses are far more serious than dermatomycoses and can lead to extensive tissue destruction. Still other fungi can invade the subcutaneous tissues or the lungs and then spread to other organs of the body where they become established and cause disease—often severe; these diseases are called *systemic mycoses*.

Many species of dermatophytes are known; some of the most common ones, and the infections they cause, are listed in Table 17-6. These species are differentiated on the basis of various morphological features, such as the size and shape of the asexual spores, pigmentation of the mycelium, and the occurrence of special hyphal structures and arrangements.

The correlation of a particular dermatophyte species with a characteristic disease is difficult because a single species can cause a variety of clinical symptoms. Furthermore, the same clinical disease can be caused by different species of dermatophytes. For these reasons, dermatologists often describe the infections by a terminology based on the part of the body involved. The first word used in this terminology is *tinea*, which means "small insect larva" and originated from the mistaken notion that these infections were caused by insects. For example, tinea capitis is ringworm of the scalp; tinea unguium, or onychomycosis, is ringworm of the nails; and tinea pedis is ringworm of the feet. The type of tinea pedis in which scaling between the toes

**TABLE 17-6 Common Dermatophytes**

| Groups of fungi | Species | Occurrence and disease |
|---|---|---|
| Epidermophyton | E. floccosum | Causes infections of the skin and nails on fingers and toes |
| Microsporum | M. audouinii | Causes epidemic ringworm of the scalp in children |
| | M. canis | Common cause of infection of skin and hair on cats, dogs, and other animals; causes tinea capitis in children |
| | M. gypseum | Occurs as a saprophyte in the soil and as a parasite on lower animals; occasionally found in ringworm of the scalp in children |
| Trichophyton | Gypseum subgroup | |
| | T. mentagrophytes | Primarily a parasite of the hair |
| | T. rubrum | Causes ringworm on many parts of the body; infects hair and scalp |
| | T. tonsurans | Infects hair and scalp |
| | Faviform subgroup | These fungi cause ringworm of the skin and scalp and glabrous skin in humans; T. verrucosum causes ringworm in cattle also |
| | T. schoenleinii | |
| | T. violaceum | |
| | T. ferrugineum | |
| | T. concentricum | |
| | T. verrucosum | |
| | Rosaceum subgroup | |
| | T. megnini | Causes ringworm of the human scalp |
| | T. gallinae | Causes an infection in chickens |
| Miscellaneous | Piedraia hortae | Causes an infection of the hair and scalp characterized by hard, black concretions; black piedra |
| | Trichosporon beigelii | Causes an infection similar to the above, except that the concretions are white; white piedra |
| | Malassezia furfur | Causes tinea versicolor, a generalized fungus infection of the skin covering the trunk and sometimes other areas of the body |
| | Candida species | Causes candidiasis of skin, mucous membranes, and nails |

occurs is often termed *athlete's foot*. Dermatophytes are unable to invade the living tissue below the outer keratinized layer, and dermatophyte infections, although annoying, are relatively mild infections and are not life-threatening.

The yeast *Candida albicans* is part of the normal flora of the mouth, gastrointestinal tract, and vagina; it is a harmless commensal—but it can be a treacherous guest! When we are healthy, *C. albicans* does not cause any disease symptoms. Its multiplication usually is suppressed by other normal flora organisms and by normal body defenses. However, it is a fair-weather friend. The moment our resistance is down, this treacherous guest turns on us and multiplies unchecked into large numbers. For example, some debilitating disease such as diabetes or AIDS, or an alteration of the normal microbial flora by broad-spectrum antibiotic therapy, can lead to uncontrolled growth of *C. albicans*. Individuals with primary immunodeficiency diseases associated with neutrophil dysfunction are at risk for *C. albicans* over growth and other fungal diseases.

Subcutaneous mycoses are more severe than dermatomycoses because the causative microorganisms can attack the living tissue below the skin. One example of a subcutaneous mycosis is mycetoma, a serious disease in which destruction of skin, subcutaneous tissue, connective tissue, muscle, and even bone can occur. Mycetoma is found mainly in the tropics and subtropics but is not limited to these areas. The causative agents are various soil fungi (or soil bacteria) that gain access to subcutaneous tissue through a wound. The fungal species include *Madurella grisea*, *Madurella mycetomatis*, *Pseudallescheria boydii*, and others. Infection usually occurs on a foot and begins with a small, painless papule. As the microorganism spreads through the tissues, multiple abscesses and cavities develop from which pus drains to the skin surface. This pus contains tiny granules 0.2–3.0 mm in diameter, composed of the fungal hyphae. Eventually the foot becomes a swollen, deformed mass of destroyed tissue and is subject to secondary infection by various bacterial pathogens. In advanced cases of mycetoma the foot might have to be amputated.

The fungi that cause the deep mycoses are important not only because the diseases they cause can be very serious, but also because the symptoms produced by some of them resemble tuberculosis or other diseases. Accurate diagnostic procedures are essential so that the most suitable treatment can be used. The principal causative agents of several systemic mycoses, their characteristics, and the characteristics of the infections they cause are given in Table 17-7. They are exemplified by airborne infections caused by environmental fungi such as *Histoplasma capsulatum* and *Cryptococcus neoformans*.

The immunological relationship between fungi and the infected host is unusual, that is, fungi have the ability to exist in different forms and switch between the forms during an infection. For example, some species of *Candida* grow in different forms, such as yeasts or hyphae, depending on infection site, whereas others, such as *Aspergillus* and *Fusarium* species are inhaled as unicellular conidia, which can transform into branching hyphae in the lungs. Hyphae growth is the invasive form that is associated with fatal infection. These transformations are driven by interactions between fungi and phagocytes and/or dendritic cells.

Innate immunity plays a major role in controlling fungal infections through its use of phagocytes (neutrophils and macrophages). As mentioned earlier,

### TABLE 17-7 Causative Agents of Systemic Mycoses

| Causative organism | Characteristics of the organism | Disease | Characteristics of the infection |
|---|---|---|---|
| *Blastomyces dermatitidis* | Dimorphic: grows as a mold at 25°C and as a yeast at 37°C. Habitat: unknown | Blastomycosis | The infection resembles pulmonary tuberculosis. It is characterized by tubercle-like lesions in the lungs, but the infection can spread to any organ. The disease occurs only in the U.S. and Canada, most commonly among rural males aged 30–50. Disseminated infections are often fatal, even with treatment. The organism is not spread from humans or other animals to humans. |
| *Paracoccidioides brasiliensis* | Dimorphic: grows as a mold at 25°C and as a yeast at 37°C. Habitat: presumably soil | Paracoccidi-oidomycosis | The infection occurs most frequently in South America. Clinically, it is similar to blastomycosis. Lesions are commonly found not only in the lungs but also in the mouth and intestinal tract and in the lymph nodes of the neck. |
| *Coccidioides immitis* | In the body, occurs as large spherules containing many endospores. In laboratory culture at 25°C and 37°C, grows as a mold and produces numerous arthrospores. Habitat: soil, | Coccidioido-mycosis | The arthrospores are highly infectious and occur in the soil of certain regions of the southwestern U.S. and Central and South America. The disease is usually a mild, transitory infection of the lungs. The rare (but often fatal) disseminated form usually involves the meninges, bones, and skin. |
| *Histoplasma capsulatum* | Dimorphic: grows as a mold at 25°C and as a yeast at 37°C. Habitat: soil, particularly soil containing bird or bat excrement | Histoplasmosis | After being inhaled, it is ingested by lung macrophages, in which it survives and multiplies. Pulmonary histoplasmosis can occur as an asymptomatic infection or with symptoms ranging from mild to severe. The infection can progress to the disseminated and potentially fatal form. |
| *Cryptococcus neoformans* | Budding yeast-like cells that are surrounded by a larger capsule. Habitat: soil, and also avian excrement, such as pigeon droppings | Cryptococcosis | The organism can infect any part of the body but usually starts in the lungs and spreads through the bloodstream. Infection of the brain and meninges usually causes death unless treated. Immunosuppressed persons, such as those with leukemia, Hodgkin's disease, or AIDS, are particularly susceptible to infection. The disease occurs worldwide. |

patients with neutropenia are highly susceptible to opportunistic fungal infections. The optimal control on fungal growth is mediated effector phagocytes through a combination of oxidative mechanisms (production of oxidizing agents, such as reactive oxygen and nitrogen intermediates) and degranulation and intracellular or extracellular release of effector molecules, including defensins and neutrophil cationic peptides, and iron sequestration (see Chapter 3). Because the fungal cell wall is composed of cross-linked polysaccharides, fungi are impervious to complement-mediated lysis; therefore, the protective efficacy of specific antibody production, even though it occurs, is questioned. (The absence of antibody in immunodeficient patients and the lack of increased susceptibility to fungal infections suggests little protective role for specific antibodies.) However, the other aspects of complement activation, such as opsonization are important. Nonetheless, many fungal cell wall components are important in the activation of the alternative and lectin pathways of complement, which play a significant role in the resolution of most fungal infections in healthy individuals. Mannose-binding protein binds specifically to terminal mannose residues, which are abundant on the surface of many fungi, such as C. albicans and some strains of C. neoformans and A. fumigatus and activate either the alternative or lectin pathway. Their activation leads to opsonization and phagocytosis. Surfactant proteins A and D, found on the mucosal surfaces of the lung and gastrointestinal tract, recognize similar microbial ligands as mannose-binding protein and act as opsonins, thereby facilitating phagocytosis in these tracts. Another group of cell-bound receptors, the complement receptor CR3 and the Toll-like receptors TLR2, TLR4, and TLR9 through MyD88 (see Table 3-1), induce host defenses to fungi, such as C. albicans, C. neoformans, and A. fumigatus. CR3, also called *CD11b/CD18*, ligation is a proficient means of engulfing opsonized fungi; however, it does not always lead to cellular activation. For example, H. capsulatum uses CR3 to gain entry into macrophages, where it survives, but not dendritic cells, where it is rapidly degraded. Whereas, C. albicans uses CR3 to enter dendritic cells, where it survives. Even though most fungi that infect humans induce IL-12 production, the preceding interactions inhibit IL-12 production, which has serious consequences on the development of adaptive immunity. The opposite occurs with ligation of mannose receptors. The first optimistic signs that specific antifungal immunity does develop is positive skin-reactivity testing, which suggests that fungal infections are common but the development of severe fungal diseases are rare, which

is consistent with the induction of adaptive immunity. Granuloma formation occurs in response to many fungal pathogens, a hallmark of cell-mediated immunity. The polarization to a $T_H1$ cell response, driven by macrophage- or dendritic cell-produced IL-12, is paramount for protective antifungal immunity. $T_H1$ cells, in turn, produce their signature cytokine, IFN-$\gamma$, to promote cell-mediated immunity a prime defender against fungal infections. Disseminated fungal infections tend to occur in patients who have a decreased level of cell-mediated immunity. For instance, AIDS patients are prone to develop the disseminated rather than the localized forms of histoplasmosis or coccidioidomycosis. Other chronic debilitating diseases such as tuberculosis, cancer, diabetes, and leukemia can also result in decreased resistance to fungal diseases.

## MINI SUMMARY

Dermatophytes infect hair, nails, or the superficial layers of the skin. Dermatomycoses include tinea capitis, tinea unguium, and tinea pedis. Dermatophytes are transmitted by direct contact with infected animals or people, or with inanimate objects contaminated with the fungi. Dermatophytes have the ability to digest keratin, which helps them spread through the skin. The multiplication of C. albicans usually is suppressed by other normal flora organisms and by normal body defenses, but some diseases or antibiotic therapy can lead to uncontrolled growth. Subcutaneous mycoses, such as mycetoma, are more severe than dermatomycoses because the causative microorganisms can attack the living tissue below the skin. The fungi that cause deep mycoses such as histoplasmosis can cause serious diseases and the symptoms produced by some of them resemble tuberculosis or other diseases. Fungal infections causing disease are rare in healthy individuals; however, they pose a great risk to immunocompromised individuals. Innate and adaptive immunity can control fungal infections.

## Parasites Elicit Both Innate and Adaptive Immune Responses

The eukaryotic pathogens, **parasites**, are represented by a complex group of single-celled protozoa and multicellular helminths. Protozoan and helminthic parasites varied greatly from one another in their structure, life cycles, and pathogenesis. Protozoa are unicellular organisms that often have several different life cycle stages with different appearances, diverse antigenic epitope expressions, and various growth locations in the host. In some of the development stages, protozoan reproduction is sexual, while in others it is asexual. Some protozoan parasites can live freely in the environment and in a host. Protozoa that live in human blood or tissues are transmitted to humans by arthropod vectors, such as the through the bite of a mosquito or sand flea. In the blood-borne stage of their life cycle, they are susceptible to specific antibodies, while intracellular, cell-mediated immunity is necessary. In contrast, the helminths (worms) are multicellular, macroscopic (ranging in size from 0.3 mm to 25 m long) organisms with specialized organs; they undergo sexual reproduction. In their adult form, they cannot multiply in humans; in humans, they must pass through stages and then undergo additional stages in one or more animals, or in soil or water. Helminths are large parasites that do not grow within cells. Some individuals may harbor a few helminthic parasites; therefore, the infestation remains subclinical and symptomless and does not induce a significant immune response. In many cases, there are repeated exposures, leading to massive infestation, and illness presents. If immunity is present antibodies mediate it. The majority of parasitic infections are chronic rather than acute infections. This supports the evidence that many parasites can evade the immune system and thereby establish chronic infections.

The human infectious protozoa are classified into four groups based on their mode of movement: (1) Sarcodina—the ameba (*Entamoeba*), (2) Mastigophora—the flagellates (*Giardia, Leishmania*), (3) Ciliophora—the ciliates (*Balantidium*), and (4) Sporozoa—organisms whose adult stage is not motile (*Plasmodium, Cryptosporidium*). The human infectious helminths (worms) are classified into three groups, which include: (1) Platyhelminths (flatworms)—the trematodes (flukes) and cestodes (tapeworms), (2) Acanthocephalins (thorny-headed worms)—the adult worms reside in the gastrointestinal tract, and (3) Nematodes (roundworms)—the adult worms can reside in the gastrointestinal tract, blood, lymphatic system or subcutaneous tissues. The larval (immature) states of worms can cause disease because of their ability to infect various body tissues.

Although more than 30,000 species of protozoa have been described, only a few (perhaps 70) cause disease in humans. Roughly 350 species of helminths have been isolated from humans. Those few parasites have engendered untold misery for millions of people, especially in the rural areas of tropical countries. One reason for the prevalence of parasitic infections is that their control is dependent on an increased standard of living, as manifested by improved sanitation and better education, nutrition, and medical care. Another reason is that no effective vaccine exists for any of these diseases.

In adapting to their hosts, protozoa, like other animal parasites, have evolved many life-cycle patterns. Whereas some species are parasitic during only one phase of their life cycle, others have adapted to more than one host during the different phases of their life cycle. The host in which a parasite reaches sexual maturity and reproduction is termed the *definitive host*. If no sexual reproduction occurs in the life cycle of a protozoan, such as a trypanosome or an amoeba, the host that is believed to be the most important is arbitrarily identified as the definitive host. An *intermediate host* is one in which the other stages of the life cycle occur. For example, for the malaria protozoa, the mosquito is the definitive host, and humans or other vertebrates are the intermediate hosts. An animal (or human) that is routinely infected with a parasite that can also infect humans is termed a *reservoir host*. The major human diseases caused by protozoa are summarized in Table 17-8. Only the protozoan disease malaria and the helminthic disease schistosomiasis are briefly discussed below.

The most important genus of sporozoans is *Plasmodium*, whose species cause malaria. **Malaria** is a disease that has been known from antiquity and has probably been the single greatest disease scourge of humanity. More than 50 species of *Plasmodium* cause malaria, but only four species cause malaria in humans (see Table 17-8); the rest attack several hundred other animal hosts. Malaria exemplifies the fact that biologists must understand the life cycle of a pathogenic protozoan in order to understand how the parasite causes disease. Knowing the life cycle can also help in finding potential ways to prevent the disease.

*Plasmodium* protozoa are transmitted to humans by mosquitoes of the genus *Anopheles*. The saliva of an infected *Anopheles* mosquito contains sporozoites, sickle-shaped infective forms of the protozoa. When the mosquito bites a human, the sporozoites are injected into the bloodstream of the victim and quickly reach the liver (Figure 17-5). There they divide asexually inside the liver cells and give rise to numerous round daughter cells called merozoites. As an infected liver cell disintegrates, the merozoites are released into the bloodstream, where they invade red blood cells. A merozoite develops inside a red blood cell to give rise to a trophozoite, the active feeding

**TABLE 17-8 Examples of Protozoa that Cause Human Diseases**

| Protozoan | Disease | Mode of transmission to humans | Definitive hosts | Intermediate hosts | Reservoir hosts |
|---|---|---|---|---|---|
| *Entamoeba histolytica* | Amoebiasis | Ingestion (mature cyst) | Humans | None | Humans |
| *Balantidium coli* | Balantidiasis | Ingestion (mature cyst) | Hogs, humans | None | Hogs, humans |
| *Giardia lamblia* | Giardiasis | Ingestion (mature cyst) | Humans | None | Humans |
| *Trichomonas vaginalis* | Vaginitis | Contact (flagellate) | Humans | None | Humans |
| *Trypanosoma rhodesiense, T. gambiense* | African sleeping sickness | Fly bite | Humans, animals | Tsetse flies (*Glossina* spp.) | Humans, animals |
| *T. cruzi* | Chagas' disease | Feces of bug | Animals, humans | Reduviid bugs | Armadillos, opossums |
| *Leishmania donovani* | Kala-azar | Fly bite | Humans, dogs | Sandflies (*Phlebotomus* spp.) | Dogs, humans |
| *L. tropica* | Cutaneous leishmaniasis | Fly bite | Humans, dogs | Sandflies | Dogs, humans |
| *L. brasiliensis* | Espundia (naso-oral/ mucocutaneous leishmaniasis) | Fly bite | Humans | Sandflies | Humans |
| *Plasmodium vivax* *P. falciparum* *P. ovale* *P. malariae* | Malaria | Mosquito bite | Anopheles mosquitoes | Humans | Humans |

stage. The trophozoite in turn divides asexually to produce more merozoites (see Figure 17-5). As the host red blood cell disintegrates, the merozoites are liberated to attack more red blood cells, producing more merozoites that attack more red blood cells, and so on (the erythrocytic cycle; see Figure 17-5).

Some of the merozoites that infect red blood cells develop into gametocytes. When an uninfected *Anopheles* mosquito bites a person with malaria, it ingests blood containing the gametocytes. In the stomach of the mosquito, the gametocytes develop into free male and female gametes—egg cells and whip-like sperm cells. After the sperm cell fertilizes an egg, the zygote passes to the outside of the mosquito's stomach lining, where it develops into an oocyst (see Figure 17-5). Sporozoites develop within the oocyst and, when mature, migrate to the mosquito's salivary glands, from which they can be injected by a mosquito bite into the bloodstream of a new victim to begin the cycle all over again.

The symptoms of malaria, which occur during the asexual erythrocytic cycle, are probably caused by release of a fever-inducing substance from the injured cells. The symptoms usually begin 10–16 days after infection by mosquitoes. The patient experiences bed-shaking chills followed by recurrent fevers, sweating, headache, and muscular pain. The cycles of fever vary according to the *Plasmodium* species causing the infection. The symptomatic periods usually last fewer than 6 hr. The spleen becomes enlarged and tender. Eventually the patient becomes weak and exhausted, and an anemia develops due to destruction of the red blood cells by the *Plasmodium* merozoites. The pattern of periodic illness interspersed with periods of well-being is characteristic of benign malaria, caused by *P. vivax, P. ovale,* and *P. malariae.* If not treated, benign malaria usually subsides spontaneously and recurs at a later date.

In patients with malignant falciparum malaria (caused by *P. falciparum*), the fever and symptoms are usually more persistent and also include tissue swelling in the brain and lungs and blockage of kidney activity. Malignant malaria has a high fatality rate if not treated promptly; this is due in part to the high rate of reproduction of the asexual form of the protozoan within red blood cells. The small veins and capillaries

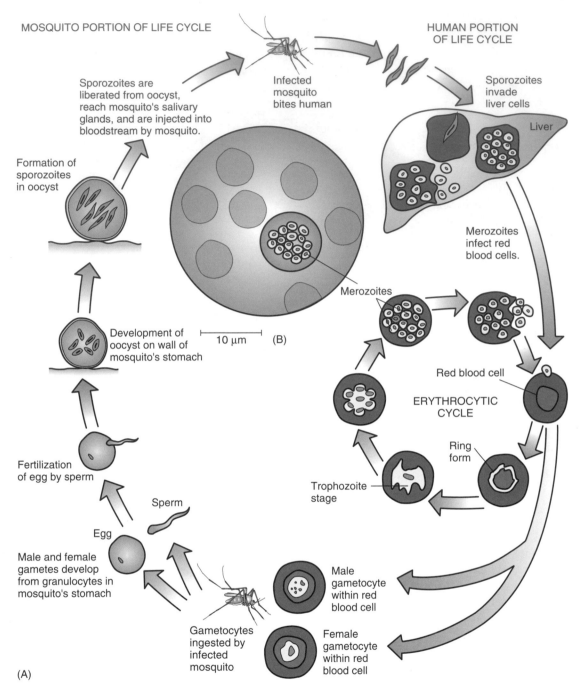

MOSQUITO PORTION OF LIFE CYCLE

HUMAN PORTION OF LIFE CYCLE

Sporozoites are liberated from oocyst, reach mosquito's salivary glands, and are injected into bloodstream by mosquito.

Infected mosquito bites human

Sporozoites invade liver cells

Liver

Formation of sporozoites in oocyst

Merozoites infect red blood cells.

10 μm (B)

Merozoites

Development of oocyst on wall of mosquito's stomach

Red blood cell

ERYTHROCYTIC CYCLE

Ring form

Fertilization of egg by sperm

Trophozoite stage

Sperm

Egg

Male and female gametes develop from granulocytes in mosquito's stomach

Male gametocyte within red blood cell

Gametocytes ingested by infected mosquito

Female gametocyte within red blood cell

(A)

**FIGURE 17-5** (A) **The life cycle of the malaria protozoan *Plasmodium*.** Step 1: Female *Anopheles* mosquito transmits sporozoites from its salivary glands when it bites a human. The sporozoites travel in human blood to the liver. Step 2: In the liver, the sporozoites multiply and become merozoites, which are shed into the bloodstream when the liver cells rupture. Step 3: The merozoites enter blood cells and become trophozoites, which feed and eventually form many more merozoites. Step 4: Merozoites are released by the rupture of the red blood cells, accompanied by chills, high fever (40°C), and sweating. They can then infect other red blood cells. Step 5: After several such asexual cycles, gametocytes (sexual stages) are produced. Step 6: Upon ingestion by a mosquito, the gametocytes form a zygote, which gives rise to more infective sporozoites in the salivary glands. These can then infect other people. (B) The "ring" stage of *Plasmodium falciparum*, seen as dark circular structures within red blood cells. At this stage, merozoites have become trophozoites upon invading the host's red blood cells. Wright's stain of a blood smear showing a red blood cell filled with merozoites of *Plasmodium vivax* just before disruption of the cells.

of the heart become clogged with parasitized red blood cells, and effective coronary blood flow and cardiac function are diminished.

On a global scale, malaria is one of the most common infectious diseases of humans. Malaria protozoa infect about 600 million people and kill 1–3 million every year. At present, the disease is widely distributed in Africa, Asia, and Latin America. In the United States, malaria has been associated mainly with the return of travelers, or the arrival of immigrants, from areas of the world where malaria is prevalent, particularly Nigeria, Mexico and other countries of Central America, and New Guinea. Malaria is rarely contracted within the United States itself.

It is likely that only mass immunization programs will permit the ultimate eradication of malaria. Unfortunately, no commercial vaccine is presently available against malaria, although some are under development. One of the difficulties is that, although the sporozoite and the merozoite forms of the parasite are free in the bloodstream, they are free for only a very short time. Antibodies have only a brief chance to attack them because malaria protozoa mainly live intracellularly. Nevertheless, three types of potential vaccines are currently being tested: (1) vaccines against sporozoite antigens, (2) vaccines against merozoite antigens, and (3) vaccines against antigens of gametocytes within mosquitoes. This third type is novel because the vaccines would not directly protect humans; instead, when the mosquito bites a vaccinated person, the ingested blood would contain antibodies that destroy the gametocytes within the insect, thus, helping to break the transmission cycle to humans.

Another group of important parasites are the *hemoflagellates*, flagellated protozoa that are transmitted to humans by the bites of infected bloodsucking arthropods. The group includes members of the genera *Leishmania* and *Trypanosoma*. These agents and the diseases they cause are listed in Table 17-9. *Leishmania* parasites live in the host's macrophage phagosomes. Individuals infected with the protozoan flagellate parasite *Leishmania major* either clear the parasite or die from the infection. In fact, this dichotomy of responses and the relevance to the $T_H1/T_H2$ balance arose from studies in the *L. major* mouse model. Most mouse genotypes are *L. major*-resistant and control the infection; however, certain strains, such as BALB/c mice are *L. major*-susceptible and fail to control the infection, which leads to progressive lesions and systemic disease. These mice are considered a model of non-healing forms of the human disease, such as kala-azar or diffuse cutaneous leishmaniasis. Mouse susceptibility or resistance to *L. major* infection correlates with the dominance of an IL-4–driven $T_H2$ response that causes disease or an IL-12–driven, IFN-γ–dominated $T_H1$ response that promotes parasite clearance, respectively. $T_H1$ cell-derived IFN-γ is required to activate infected macrophages for parasite killing.

The ability of trypanosomes to change their surface antigens and thus defeat the immune response of the body is discussed later in the chapter.

## MINI SUMMARY

Protozoa and multicellular helminths represent parasites, organisms that live in or on another organism and derive nourishment from it. Protozoan infections elicit both humoral and cell-mediated immune responses. As extracellular bacteria, the blood-borne stages of the protozoan life cycles are susceptible to antibodies; however, when they become intracellular, cell-mediated immunity is activated.

*Plasmodium* species cause malaria. *Plasmodium* sporozoites are transmitted to humans by *Anopheles* mosquitoes. In the liver, the sporozoites give rise to merozoites, which can invade red blood cells and become trophozoites. Some of the merozoites develop into gametocytes, which can be ingested by a mosquito. The gametocytes develop into male and female gametes; after a sperm cell fertilizes an egg, the zygote develops into an oocyst, in which sporozoites develop. The sporozoites migrate to the mosquito's salivary glands and can be injected into a human by a mosquito bite. The most severe form of malaria is malignant falciparum malaria. It is likely that only mass immunization programs will permit the ultimate eradication of malaria, but no vaccine is yet available.

The hemoflagellate group of protozoa includes *Leishmania* and *Trypanosoma*, which cause leishmaniasis and trypanosomiasis, respectively.

## Viruses Are Neutralized by Antibodies or Controlled and Cleared by Cell-Mediated Immunity

The term virus is a Latin word for "poison," an appropriate name, given the problems viruses can cause. Viruses are minute infectious agents, 10 to 100 times smaller than most bacterial cells, with an approximate size range of 20 to 300 nm. Viruses do not have

**TABLE 17-9** Pathogenic Protozoa of the Genera *Trypanosoma* and *Leishmania* and the Arthropod-Borne Diseases they Cause

| Protozoan and geographic distribution | Disease | Biological vector and animal reservoir | Arthropod-pathogen–human relationship |
|---|---|---|---|
| *Trypanosoma cruzi* (continental Latin America) | Chagas' disease | Reduviid bugs (*Triatoma* spp., *Panstrongylus* spp.) Reservoir: armadillos, opossums, dogs, cats, and other animals | Pathogen multiplies in hindgut of bug; humans infected by rubbing bug's feces into the bite |
| *Trypanosoma brucei* subspecies *gambiense* (west and central Africa) and *T. brucei* subspecies *rhodesiense* (east and central Africa) | African trypanosomiasis (sleeping sickness) | Tsetse flies (*Glossina* spp.) Reservoir: antelopes and other wild game animals in Africa | Pathogen multiplies in midgut and passes to salivary glands; humans are infected by bite |
| *Leishmania donovani* (China, India, Africa, Mediterranean area, continental Latin America) | Kala-azar | Sandflies (*Phlebotomus* spp.) Reservoir: wild rodents and other wild animals; dogs | Pathogen multiplies in midgut and reaches mouthparts of fly; humans infected through bite |
| *Leishmania tropica* and *L. major* (Mediterranean area to western India) | Cutaneous leishmaniasis | Same as above | Same as above |
| *Leishmania brasiliensis* (Mexico to northern Argentina) | Espundia (naso-oral/mucocutaneous leishmaniasis) | Same as above | Same as above |

the complex organization of cells and are structurally simply but come in many different shapes. They consist of a nucleic acid (either DNA or RNA that is either double-stranded or single-stranded) *genome* wrapped in a protein coat (*capsid*), and sometimes surrounded by a lipid *envelope* derived from the host cell's plasma membrane. The virus's outermost layer (capsid or envelope) projects protein receptors, which must bind to specific counter glycoproteins on host cell membranes before the virus can enter the target cell and begin its replicative cycle. Once the virus enters the cell, it must uncoat its capsid to release the nucleic acid and virally controlled cellular enzymes, plus viral enzymes sometimes replicate the viral nucleic acid, synthesize mRNA, and viral proteins. If it is a DNA virus, it replicates and assembles in the host cell nucleus, whereas a RNA virus replicates and assembles in the host cell cytoplasm. Virus subunits are self-assembled to make new virions. A single virion supplies all the information required by the cell to construct thousands to millions of copies of progeny virions. If they are enveloped virions, they exit the host cell by budding, thereby coating themselves with host cell membrane that displays virus receptors. In contrast, nonenveloped virions collect in the cell until it bursts, releasing virions to bind and infect other cells.

Incapable of independent growth in artificial media, viruses can replicate only in animal, plant, or microbial cells. Viruses are therefore referred to as **obligate intracellular parasites** and represent the ultimate in parasitism; they can "take over" the host cell's genetic machinery. The fact that viruses are obligate intracellular parasites does not mean that they necessarily cause overt disease. Some viruses cause latent or inapparent infections that never lead to clinical signs or symptoms. Others cause inapparent infections that later give rise to clinical disease; here, the link between the virus and the disease has often been difficult to establish. Still other viruses are frank pathogens, causing disease in humans, animals, insects, or plants; these viruses have naturally received the most attention. Some viruses that can cause human disease are strictly limited to human hosts; others are mainly pathogens of animals, and humans serve only as accidental hosts. Since viral diseases cannot be cured with chemotherapeutic agents, great emphasis is given to epidemiological and immunological methods by which viral infections can be prevented. For instance, such measures have totally eradicated smallpox, and many other viral diseases have been greatly reduced in incidence. The reduction in incidence of virus- (and bacterial) caused diseases in the U.S. is due primarily to childhood and adolescent immunization programs (Table 17-10). It is beyond the scope of this text to discuss all the attributes of viruses. Innate and adaptive immune responses to viruses are broadly discussed. A

**TABLE 17-10 Recommended 2008 Immunization Schedule for Children in the United States**

| Vaccines | Birth | 1 month | 2 months | 4 months | 6 months | 12 months | 15 months | 18 months | 19–23 months | 2–3 years | 4–6 years |
|---|---|---|---|---|---|---|---|---|---|---|---|
| Hepatitis | HepB | | | | | | | | | | |
| Rotavirus | | | | Rota | Rota | Rota | | | | | |
| Diphtheria, tetanus, pertussis | | | DTaP | DTaP | DTaP | | | | | | |
| *Haemophilus influenzae* type b | | | Hib | Hib | Hib | | | | | | |
| Pneumococcal | | | PCV | PCV | PCV | | | | | | |
| Inactivated poliovirus | | | IPV | IPV | | | | | | | |
| Influenza* | | | | | | | | | | | |
| Measles, mumps, rubella | | | | | | | | | | | |
| Varicella | | | | | | | | | | | |
| Hepatitis A** | | | | | | | | | | | |
| Meningococcal | | | | | | | | | | | |

Adapted from CDC Web site and approved by Advisory Committee on Immunization Practice, the American Academy of Pediatrics, and the American Academy of Family Physicians. Boxes in darkened yellow represent time ranges during when an immunization is recommended. Any doses not administered at the recommended times should be given at any subsequent visit.

*Initial dose of trivalent inactivated influenza vaccine should be given at a minimum age of 6 months, yearly thereafter.

**The Hepatitis A vaccine should be administered to all children aged 1 year. The two doses in the series should be administered at least 6 months apart.

section that introduces one viral pathogen, which continues to be a source of annual clinical disease, follows.

### Innate and Adaptive Immunity Are Needed to Eradicate Viruses

The induction of innate immune system components, the type I interferons (IFN-α and IFN-β; see Chapter 3) and NK cells are important early defenders against viral infections. IFN-α and -β (also called *viral IFNs*) are produced by leukocytes and fibroblasts, respectively; however, most types of cells can produce type I IFNs. Type I IFNs bind to their receptors on neighboring cells, which lead to the activation of a ribonuclease that degrades viral RNA and induces the production of a RNA-dependent protein kinase that inactivates protein synthesis, thereby blocking virus replication in infected cells (see Figure 3-16). NK cells produce IFN-γ, a type II IFN, and are responsive to the type I IFNs, which induce NK cell lytic activity making them more effective killers of virus-infected cells. Toll-like receptors (TLRs; see Chapter 3) recognize viral nucleotides, thereby inducing the vigorous production of type I IFNs and proinflammatory cytokines. Viral DNA is recognized by TLR9, single-stranded RNA by TLR7 and TLR8, and double-stranded RNA by TLR3. These interactions lead to the activation of nuclear factor-κB (NF-κB) and the production of type I IFNs. The importance of IFNs is illustrated by IFN-α/-β- or IFN-γ-receptor–knockout mice; they cannot mount effective antiviral responses. The IFN receptors have no enzymatic activity, but

they instigate a complex signaling pathway that eventually leads to the transcription of hundreds of IFN-stimulated genes. Despite the robust IFN response, viruses fight back minimizing the antiviral power of IFNs (discussed later). The early production of the proinflammatory cytokine IL-12 during a viral infection enhances NK cell activity. In turn, NK cells produce IFN-γ that activates macrophages and dendritic cells, which primes them to convey information that induces the adaptive immune system. As the infection continues and antibodies become available, NK cells can kill antibody-coated virus-infected cells by *antibody-dependent cell-mediated cytotoxicity (ADCC)*.[2] Some complement components can damage the envelope of some viruses, thereby providing protection against those viruses (see Chapter 11). Taken together, innate immunity slows and somewhat contains viral infections; the induction of innate immunity also initiates the adaptive immune response.

The adaptive immunity mediates resistance against viral infections with the production of specific neutralizing antibodies (humoral immunity), which contain the spread of viruses and cytotoxic T cells ($T_C$ cells; cell-mediated immunity), which control and clear viruses from the host. During the acute phase of viral infections, antiviral protein antibodies not only contain the spread of viruses but block virus attachment and entry into host

---

[2]Only enveloped viruses place their proteins on host cell membranes, which can be bound by antibodies.

cells (hence the name *neutralizing antibodies*). These antibodies are often specific for the serologic type of the virus. Most viruses, through their specific receptors, target the appropriate host cells by binding their counterpart cell-membrane molecules that leads to viral entry. The production of localized antibodies, such as secretory IgA, obstruct virus binding to mucosal epithelial cells that line the respiratory and gastrointestinal tracts, primary sites of viral entry into the host. For example, the use of oral attenuated polio vaccine, works by inducing mucosal immunity. Other examples of where the production of antiviral receptor antibodies plays a role in preventing infection of cells include Epstein-Barr virus (linked to mononucleosis and Burkitt's lymphoma) binding to CD21 on B cells, influenza virus (causes the flu) binding to sialic acid residues on cells, and rhinovirus (causes the common cold) binding to intercellular adhesion molecules (ICAMs). In addition to viral neutralization, specific IgM and IgG antibodies can opsonize virions, thereby promoting their clearance by Fc-receptor positive phagocytes. These antibodies also activate complement, which also opsonizes virions facilitating C3b-receptor–mediated phagocytosis and causing direct lysis of enveloped viruses. Previous infection or vaccine-induced humoral immunity protects individuals from infection but it cannot eliminate an established infection (such as in a latent infection). Neutralizing antibodies would also protect against reexposure by the same virus.

Cell-mediated immunity mediated by $T_C$ cells, which kill virus-infected cells, is paramount for the eradication of viruses residing within cells. $CD8^+$ $T_C$ and $CD4^+$ $T_H1$ cells composed the antiviral defense duet. $T_C$ cells recognize cytosolic viral antigens presented in association with class I MHC molecules expressed on all nucleated cells. Activated $T_H1$ cells produce IL-2 and IFN-$\gamma$. IL-2 (and costimulators on cross-presenting dendritic cells; see Chapter 10) acts indirectly by assisting the development of pre-$T_C$ cells into mature effector cells. IFN-$\gamma$ acts directly by inducing cells to prevent viral replication in infected cells. IL-2 and IFN-$\gamma$ activate NK cells early in the infection for efficient killing of virus-infected cells. Three to four days after infection, specific $T_C$ cell proliferation undergoes a significant increase that corresponds to the increase in antiviral activity, which peaks at 7–10 days, and then declines. The importance of $T_C$ cells is seen in individuals that are deficient in $T_C$ cells; they have increased susceptibility to viral infections (see Chapter 16). An exception to the latter scenario is when immunodeficient patients are infected with noncytopathic hepatitis B virus; they do not develop

the disease but become carriers of the virus and can transmit the disease to other individuals.

### Why Are There Annual Concerns About Influenza?

Epidemic **influenza**, or "flu," as it is commonly known, is characterized by nasal discharge, headache, muscle pains, sore throat, a marked weakness and exhaustion, and a tendency to develop secondary bacterial pneumonias. During the disease, the virus remains localized in the respiratory tract, where it kills ciliated epithelial cells. This killing effect might actually be due to $T_C$ lymphocytes that respond to the viral antigens on infected cells.

RNA viruses of the family Orthomyxoviridae cause influenza. There are three main antigenic types of the influenza virus, A, B, and C. Epidemics of influenza occur in cycles: those caused by type A influenza viruses commonly follow a 2- to 3-year cycle, while those caused by type B viruses have a 4- to 6-year cycle, cause less severe epidemics than type A viruses, and have not caused pandemics. Type C influenzas rarely, if ever, give rise to epidemics; they cause subclinical infections or small outbreaks of influenza among children. Influenza is primarily spread through aerosols created by coughs and sneezes.

In addition to epidemics, influenza can occur in pandemics, which are epidemics of worldwide proportions. Pandemics illustrate the enormous geographic range and the rapid spread that airborne diseases can achieve. Great pandemics of influenza have occurred at intervals of 10–30 years or even longer; they are caused by type A influenza virus strains. In 1918–1919 a strain of type A influenza virus caused the deadliest influenza pandemic on record, killing more than 20 million persons (it claimed about 650,000 persons in the U.S.).

Influenza type A viruses can infect birds, horses, people, pigs, and other animals, but wild birds are the natural hosts. Influenza viruses of type A are further classified into subtypes based on the spike-like projections, hemagglutinin (HA) and neuraminidase (NA) proteins, they possess. The HA proteins bind to sialic acid groups on the host cell's surface, which allows the virus to enter the host cell. The NA proteins are composed of neuraminidase, which cleaves sialic acid residues; thus, destroying the receptors for the HA proteins. This destruction of the receptors breaks the bond that holds new viral progeny to the infected cell and allows the progeny to become free to infect other cells, thereby spreading the infection within the respiratory tract. So far, 16 major subtypes of HA proteins (H1 to H13) and 9 subtypes of NA proteins (N1 to N9) have been identified in isolates from humans, animals, and birds. In influenza A viruses isolated from humans, only three of these HA proteins (H1, H2, and H3) and two types of NA proteins (N1 and N2) have been identified. HA and NA proteins can occur in different combinations to yield various subtypes of influenza A viruses. For instance, the strain that caused the worldwide human "Asian flu" epidemic in 1957 was of the A(H2N2) subtype, whereas the strain that caused the "Hong Kong flu" epidemic in 1968 was of the A(H3N2) subtype. During the 2000–2001 influenza season in the United States, influenza virus A (H1N1) strains predominated; however, approximately one fourth of the influenza virus isolates were influenza type B. Influenza type B viruses are usually found only in humans and are not classified according to subtypes as are type A viruses.

The H and N antigens of an influenza virus have practical importance because antibodies against them can prevent attachment of the virus to host cells. However, antibodies formed by a host population against one antigenic subtype of influenza A virus, for example, A(H2N2), do not protect against other subtypes that might develop by mutation, such as A(H3N2). Moreover, varieties having different antigenic properties can develop within a particular influenza virus subtype. For instance, during the 1990–1991 influenza season three antigenically distinct varieties of A(H3N2) viruses were isolated worldwide. New subtypes and new varieties of influenza A viruses are responsible for pandemics in populations that are immune to an older subtype or variety.

How do new influenza virus subtypes arise? The hallmark of influenza viruses is their variability. They undergo frequent changes in their surface antigens; therefore, immunity resulting from infection by one influenza virus does not fully protect against antigenic variants of the same influenza A virus subtype or other types. Consequently, influenza outbreaks occur every year. The antigenic variants result from changes in the HA and NA envelope proteins. The changes occur by two different mechanisms: antigenic drift and antigenic shift. **Antigenic drift** results from gradually occurring spontaneous point mutations in the HA and NA protein-encoding genes, which lead to minor changes in these proteins. **Antigenic shift** results from an abrupt, major change leading to an emergence of a completely new influenza A virus subtype with a novel HA antigen or a novel HA and NA antigen in humans, the new subtype was not currently circulating among people. The new A subtype may lead to the occurrence of a pandemic. Antigenic shift can occur in at least two ways: *re-assortment* and *direct transmission*. Type A influenza viruses occur naturally in a number of birds and mammals, as well as humans. When different subtypes infect the same animal host, genetic recombinants can occur; for instance, if a bird strain and a human strain both infect swine, such recombination can give rise to a more virulent human strain. When a type A strain appeared in 1998 in Hong Kong that killed four people and caused illness in several others, a genetic analysis showed that it was similar to a bird strain called *H5N1* that had earlier killed thousands of chickens. In this instance, however, no intermediate host was identified and apparently the bird strain was transmissible directly to humans. This threat caused public health authorities in Hong Kong to authorize the killing of 1.5 million chickens, thereby greatly reducing the chances of a pandemic.

Despite the development of antiviral drugs, vaccination remains the primary method of preventing and controlling influenza. Vaccination against influenza is accomplished by use of a trivalent vaccine that contains purified and formalin-inactivated virus from three viral strains, which are two influenza A virus subtypes and one influenza B strain. A person should be vaccinated each year because immunity is subtype-specific, and the vaccine consists of a mixture of several of the hemagglutinin subtypes most likely to cause infection that particular year.

### MINI SUMMARY

Viruses are obligate intracellular parasites. They are counteracted by innate immunity, through the production of IFNs and activation of NK cells, which buys time until adaptive immunity, through the production of neutralizing antibodies and activated $T_C$ cells reduces virus numbers and clears the virus by killing infected cells.

The only member of the orthomyxoviruses is the influenza virus, which has three main antigenic types, A, B, and C. Type A strains are divided into subtypes based on HA and NA proteins. Changes in these proteins are responsible for the antigenic variants of influenza virus. The variants are generated by antigenic drift and antigenic shift. The new subtypes and new varieties of influenza A viruses are responsible for pandemics in populations that are immune to an older subtype or variety. When different subtypes infect the same animal host, genetic recombinants can occur. Anti-influenza vaccines are the most effective way to prevent the flu.

# Pathogens Can Evade Immune Responses

## Virulence Factors Can Promote Infection by Bacteria or Parasites

Several categories of virulence factors that promote infection are associated with pathogenic microorganisms. These factors range from structural components of the pathogen to enzymes and other biochemical substances that allow survival and multiplication within the tissues of the patient.

***Attachment to Tissue Cells Can Initiate an Infection.*** As discussed earlier, attachment of pathogenic bacteria to host tissue cells is usually a prerequisite for establishing a bacterial infection. In fact, some pathogens have specific structures that facilitate their attachment to host cells. A few mechanisms for attachment are summarized below.

Many pathogenic bacteria have *adhesins*, special proteins that bind to complementary receptors on the host cell surface. Adhesins can be on the bacterial cell surface or at the tips of pili. The following are examples. (1) Adhesins are located on the tips of the pili of urogenic *E. coli* strains, strains that cause urinary tract infections. (2) F-HA, also called "filamentous protein" is located on the surface of *B. pertussis*, the causative agent of whooping cough. F-HA causes binding of the bacteria to the cilia of tracheal epithelial cells, allowing the bacteria to multiply there and produce pertussis toxin. (3) The pili of *N. gonorrhoeae* are responsible for specific attachment to nonciliated, columnar epithelial cells. In addition, pilin, the protein component of the *N. gonorrhoeae* pili, is highly variable, leading to antigen variation that allows the organism to evade neutralizing secretory IgA antibodies. (4) P1 protein, located at the differentiated tip of filamentous cells of *Mycoplasma pneumoniae*, binds to sialic acid (*N*-acetylneuraminic acid) on the surface of host cell membranes.

Some pathogenic bacteria adhere to tissue cells by means of fibronectin-binding proteins. Fibronectin is a plasma glycoprotein that readily sticks to the surface of mucosal cells. Some bacteria make cell wall proteins that bind to fibronectin and thereby attach the bacteria to the mucosal cells. For example, *S. pyogenes*, the cause of streptococcal sore throat, makes Protein F, which binds to fibronectin and is thought to be the main factor in binding of the streptococcus to epithelial cells of the throat.

Secretory IgA neutralizing antibodies specific for above-mentioned molecules prevent pathogen attachment to mucosal epithelial cells; however, certain pathogens including *Haemophilus influenzae*, *N. meningitidis*, and *N. gonorrhoeae* are known to produce enzymes that promote colonization and invasion. These enzymes are *IgA proteases* that destroy secretory IgA antibodies; thus, their destruction promotes colonization.

Lipases catalyze the hydrolysis of triglycerides (fats and oils) to fatty acids and glycerol. *S. aureus*, which causes infections of hair follicles, cuts, and surgical incisions, secretes lipases that attack fats and oils on the skin, in sebaceous secretions (part of innate immunity; see Chapter 3), and in blood plasma. This action is essential for *S. aureus* to invade cutaneous and subcutaneous tissues.

Urease is an important factor in establishing infection by *H. pylori*, the main cause of peptic ulcers. The bacterium makes a powerful urease that enables the organism to survive the high acidity in the stomach.

Several infectious bacteria, such as *C. neoformans*, *H. influenzae, N. meningitidis* (meningococcus), *S. mutans* (adheres to the surface of teeth and initiates dental caries), and *S. pneumoniae* (pneumococcus) make capsules (exocellular polysaccharides or polypeptides) that are extremely viscous, which permit the organisms to stick to surfaces and make them antiphagocytic. The latter property protects bacteria from ingestion by phagocytes. Capsules also have anticomplement activities. Polysaccharide capsules are weakly immunogenic and tend to induce low-affinity IgM antibodies. Infants, young children, and immunodeficient individuals are more susceptible to encapsulated organisms. Table 17-11 lists some bacteria that make antiphagocytic capsules.

***Bacteria Have Special Types of Motility that Facilitate Infections.*** Some pathogens such as *Shigella* species, *Listeria monocytogenes*, and enteroinvasive strains of *E. coli* not only survive and multiply within host cells but also can move within the cells and invade other cells by pushing the cytoplasmic membrane of one cell into another cell. This intracellular locomotion is not due to flagella. In fact, *Shigella* species are incapable of making flagella. Instead, intracellular locomotion depends on bacterial gene products that cause actin monomers in the host tissue cells to polymerize and form short fibrils. These fibrils become organized in the form of a "tail" at one end of the bacterium. The continuous formation of actin fibrils on the surface of the bacterium pushes the bacterium along at speeds of up to 1.5 μm per second. Because the bacteria move directly from one cell to another, they escape destruction by antibodies in the blood or tissue fluids (Figure 17-6).

**TABLE 17-11 Some Bacteria That Make Antiphagocytic Capsules**

| Bacterium | Type of capsule | Number of antigenic types of capsule |
|---|---|---|
| Streptococcus pneumoniae | Polysaccharide | >80 |
| Streptococcus pyogenes (some strains) | Polysaccharide (hyaluronic acid) | 1 |
| Haemophilus influenzae | Polysaccharide | 6 (a, b, c, d, e, f) |
| Yersinia pestis | Protein and polysaccharide | Fraction 1 (F-1) |
| Bacillus anthracis | Polypeptide (polymer of D-glutamic acid) | 1 |
| Neisseria meningitidis | Polysaccharide | 13 (A, B, C, D, X, Y, Z, $Z^1$, W-135, H, I, K, L) |

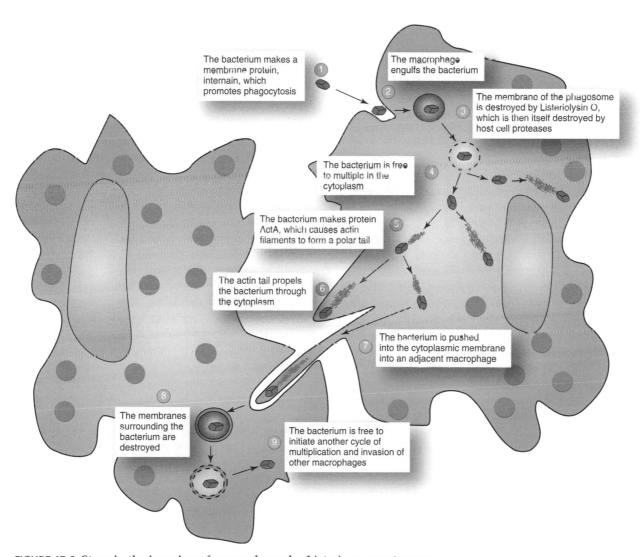

**FIGURE 17-6 Steps in the invasion of macrophages by *Listeria monocytogenes*.**

*Bacterial Factors Can Either Prevent or Encourage Phagocytic Engulfment or Allow Intracellular Survival and Multiplication.* As discussed earlier (see Table 17-11), many bacterial pathogens make capsules that prevent engulfment of the bacteria by phagocytes. Production of antibodies against the capsular antigens can overcome this antiphagocytic activity.

Some pathogens produce antiphagocytic surface proteins. For example, virulent strains of *S. pyogenes* possess short fibrils of protein called the *M protein* on the surface of the cell wall. The M protein is antiphagocytic by inhibiting activation of the alternate complement pathway. In this pathway, a component of complement called *C3b*, formed by cleavage of C3, normally accumulates on the surface of microorganisms, causing the microorganisms to bind to receptors for C3b on the surface of phagocytes. M proteins inhibit this process because of two properties: (1) an ability to bind complement factor H, which is an inhibitor of alternative pathway activation by inhibiting the cleavage of complement protein C3; and (2) an ability to bind the blood plasma protein, fibrinogen, which can then bind Factor H. The outermost tip of the M protein molecule, or N-terminal end, extends beyond the fibrinogen coating and is accessible to antibodies that could bind to it and act as opsonins to promote phagocytosis. However, the tip is hypervariable in its amino acid sequence—more than 70 different kinds of M protein have been described. Each strain of *S. pyogenes* has only one kind (and therefore only one antigenic type) of M protein.

Some bacteria prefer to multiply within host tissue cells. They can even induce a host cell to engulf the bacteria, regardless of whether or not the host cell is normally phagocytic. They do this by making certain bacterial surface proteins that cause rearrangement of the actin cytoskeleton of the host cell. The host cell develops projections, ruffles, or pits that enfold the bacterium and draw it in. The process culminates in the formation of a membrane-bounded vacuole that contains the bacterium. Examples include internalin proteins of *L. monocytogenes*, invasin proteins of *Yersinia enterocolitica*; and IpD, IpB, and IpC proteins of *Shigella* species.

Several kinds of virulence factors are instrumental in allowing pathogens to survive and multiply within macrophages. Some bacteria such as *L. monocytogenes* use an enzyme to destroy the phagosomal membrane—the membrane of the phagocytic vacuole. Destruction of this membrane allows the organisms to multiply freely in the host cell cytoplasm. Studies of the enzyme made by *L. monocytogenes*, listeriolysin O, explained why the enzyme does not also destroy the cytoplasmic membrane of the host cell, which would kill the host cell, the "home" of the bacterium, and subject the bacteria to destruction by antibodies. Listeriolysin O contains a 19-amino acid sequence that identifies it as a target for destruction by proteinases that are present in the host cell's cytoplasm; thus, the enzyme is protected from these cytoplasmic proteinases while it is within the phagosome, but after the phagosomal membrane is destroyed, the listeriolysin O is itself destroyed before it can kill the host cell.

How do intracellular pathogens survive within a phagosome? Some pathogenic bacteria, after being engulfed by a neutrophil or macrophage, have cell surface components that prevent lysosomes from fusing with the bacteria-containing phagosome; thus, the powerful hydrolytic enzymes contained within the lysosomes cannot be discharged into the phagosome and attack the bacteria. For example, sulfolipids in the cell wall of *M. tuberculosis* act in this manner.

Some bacteria can resist destruction by the acidic environment within phagosomes. Phagosomes containing microorganisms become acidified with a pH of 5.5 or less. The low pH occurs because the membrane of a phagosome acquires a proton-translocating ATPase, and the hydrolysis of ATP causes protons to pass into the phagosome. Some bacteria such as *Legionella* and *Mycobacterium* species can prevent this acidification. In most instances, the mechanism by which the prevention occurs is not known, but immunoelectron microscopy of macrophages infected with *M. avium* or *M. tuberculosis* show that the phagosomal membrane surrounding the bacilli lacks the proton-translocating ATPase.

When engulfed by a phagocyte, some bacteria are able to prevent the usual respiratory burst that otherwise would generate toxic forms of oxygen such as superoxide radicals, hydrogen peroxide, hydroxyl radicals, and nitric oxide. For instance, the cell wall lipids of *M. leprae* abrogate the oxidative respiratory burst and phagocytic ability of mouse bone marrow-derived macrophages. Other intracellular pathogens can survive by making enzymes such as superoxide dismutase, catalase, and peroxidases that protect against toxic forms of oxygen. Still other pathogens protect themselves by synthesizing cell surface polysaccharides that destroy toxic forms of oxygen.

## MINI SUMMARY

Attachment of pathogenic bacteria to host tissue cells is usually required for establishing a bacterial infection. Adherence factors can be adhesins, fibronectin-binding proteins, or exocellular polysaccharides. IgA proteases can promote colonization of mucous membranes. Lipases can aid the invasiveness of skin staphylococci. Some pathogens can move within tissue cells and invade other cells by means of actin fibrils on the surface of the bacterium that push the bacterium. Many bacterial pathogens make capsules or surface proteins that prevent engulfment of the bacteria by phagocytes. Pathogenic bacteria can induce a host cell to engulf them by making certain bacterial surface proteins that cause rearrangement of the actin cytoskeleton of the host cell. Survival within tissue cells can be aided by destruction of the phagosomal membrane, prevention of lysosomal fusion with the phagosome, and prevention of the acidification of the phagosome.

### Virulence Factors Such as Exotoxins Can Damage the Host

Microbial virulence factors that directly damage or kill host tissue cells are poisonous substances called **microbial toxins**. The many kinds of microbial toxins act in many different ways and vary in their potency, that is, their degree of toxicity, some being much more potent than others.

Exotoxins are toxic proteins secreted by living microorganisms (although a few, such as tetanus toxin, are exceptions because they accumulate within the microbial cells and are released only when the cells disintegrate). Examples of the classic exotoxins are botulinum toxin, tetanus toxin, diphtheria toxin, cholera toxin, and pertussis toxin. They have the following features:

1. They have a high toxicity.
2. They exhibit heat lability: They are easily destroyed by boiling.
3. They are highly effective in stimulating an animal to make antibodies (antitoxin) against the toxin. However, the toxoid form of the toxin (toxin that has been modified so that it is no longer toxic but still retains its immunogenic properties) must be used for immunizing animals since the toxins are so potent and lethal.
4. Their toxicity can be neutralized by antitoxin.
5. Each has a unique mechanism of action.

Examples of other types of exotoxins are Streptolysin O of *S. pyogenes*, α toxin of *C. perfringens*, and the Panton-Valentine leucocidin of *S. aureus*. Much larger amounts of these are required to kill an animal compared to the classic exotoxins.

Exotoxins are often divided into various categories based on the site of the damage that they cause or the kind of cells that are affected. Botulinum and tetanus toxins affect nerve tissue and are termed *neurotoxins*. The toxin made by *Vibrio cholerae* affects the intestinal tract and is termed an *enterotoxin* (from the Greek word *enteron*, meaning "intestine"). Diphtheria toxin kills several different kinds of cells and is thus termed a *cytotoxin*. Some cytotoxins kill leucocytes and hence are known as *leucocidins*. Others cause the lysis of red blood cells and therefore are termed *hemolysins*.

Exotoxins lose their toxicity when treated with formaldehyde, although their antigenic properties are retained. In this form, they are called *toxoids* and have the ability to stimulate the production of *antitoxins* (antibodies that react with toxins and neutralize their toxicity) in the body of the host animal. This is important in the protection of susceptible hosts from diseases caused by bacteria that produce exotoxins. For instance, toxoids are widely used as vaccines for immunization against diphtheria and tetanus. There are four combination vaccines used to prevent diphtheria, tetanus, and pertussis: DTaP, Tdap, DT, and Td.[3]

Many exotoxins consist of two parts, an A part and a B part. Sometimes A and B occur as different portions of a single protein molecule and are later separated when the molecule is "nicked" by a protease. In other exotoxins, the A and B portions are separate molecules that are subunits of the toxin.

Just as adherence of microorganisms to tissue cells is an important first step in the process of infection, an initial binding of exotoxins to tissue cells is an important first step in their toxic activity. The binding is usually accomplished by the B part of the toxin, whereas the A part has the enzymatic activity of the toxin. Moreover, the B part is responsible for translocating the A part across the host cell membrane into the cytoplasm.

---

[3]Upper-case letters denote full-strength doses of diphtheria (D) and tetanus (T) toxoids and pertussis (P) vaccine. Lower-case "d" and "p" denote reduced doses of diphtheria and pertussis used in the adolescent/adult-formulations. The "a" in DTaP and Tdap stands for "acellular," meaning that the pertussis component contains only a part of the pertussis organism (from CDC).

The mechanism of action of several classic exotoxins is known. In some exotoxins, the A part of the toxin catalyzes a reaction known as ADP ribosylation. Examples of exotoxins that cause ADP ribosylation include diphtheria toxin, cholera toxin, and pertussis toxin. The mechanism of action of diphtheria toxin and pertussis toxin are briefly discussed below.

The product of gene *tox* in *Corynebacterium diphtheriae* is a single protein molecule (Figure 17-7). After being made and secreted by *C. diphtheriae* in the throat, diphtheria toxin becomes "nicked": a protease normally occurring in the tissues cleaves the peptide bond that links the A and B fragments. However, the A and B fragments are still linked by a disulfide bond between a cysteine residue on the A fragment and a cysteine residue on the B fragment.

The toxin is then taken into a tissue cell by receptor-mediated endocytosis. The toxin's B fragment binds to a cell surface receptor called *heparin-binding epidermal growth factor (HB-EGF)*, a hormone that occurs on the surface of many different types of cells in the human body. The toxin is carried to one of many "coated pits," where the plasma membrane invaginates and pinches off to form an endosome. The acidic environment within the endosome causes the B fragment's hydrophobic region to insert itself into the endosomal membrane, allowing the A chain to cross the membrane. Then glutathione reduces the disulfide bond linking the A and B fragments.

After the A fragment is released into the cytoplasm, it catalyzes elongation factor 2 (EF-2), the elongation factor required for translocation of polypeptidyl-*t*RNA from acceptor to donor site on the eukaryotic ribosome. The ADP ribosylation of EF-2 leads to inactivation of EF-2 and thus inhibition of protein synthesis by the eukaryotic cell. Eventually the cell dies. In diphtheria, much of the toxin is absorbed into the body and can cause fatal damage to the heart and nervous system. Alternatively, the patient can die from suffocation due to a tough pseudomembrane that forms in the throat and blocks the trachea.

Pertussis toxin (PTx), made by *B. pertussis*, the causative agent of whooping cough, is composed of six subunits, representing five different kinds: one S1, one S2, one S3, two S4, and one S5. Subunit S1 acts as the A part and has ADP-ribosylating activity. The complex [S2 + S4]-S5-[S3 + S4] functions as the B part of the toxin to bind the toxin to a receptor on the epithelial cells of the trachea, or windpipe, of the patient. It also facilitates passage of the S1 subunit across the endosomal membrane. The S1 subunit causes an increase in the level of cAMP in tissue cells, which interferes with the normal inhibitory regulation of adenylate cyclase.

Tetanus toxin acts on the proteins of synaptic vesicles in the axons of certain neurons, specifically, inhibitory neurons, in the central nervous system. An understanding of the effects of the toxin requires an understanding of how muscular movements occur in the body. Such movements usually involve a cooperative action between two muscles, in which one muscle opposes the other. If both muscles were to contract at the same time, no movement would be possible, because one muscle would counteract the other. Normally, however, one muscle is prevented from contracting because an inhibitory transmitter is secreted by inhibitory neurons in the central nervous system. This inhibitor inactivates the nerve cells controlling the opposing muscle. Tetanus toxin prevents the secretion of the inhibitory transmitter; thus opposing sets of muscles contract simultaneously and in an uncontrollable fashion. The contractions lead to rigid muscular spasms that can be powerful enough to break bones and tear tissue. Death usually results from respiratory failure brought on by an inability of the patient to control the diaphragm and muscles of the chest involved in breathing. Effective toxoid vaccines are available for diphtheria, pertussis, and tetanus toxins.

*B. anthracis* produces systemic shock and death in susceptible animals by means of its exotoxin. Recent studies indicate that macrophages are the main target of the anthrax toxin, and that the symptoms of anthrax may result primarily from the effects of high levels of macrophage-produced cytokines, particularly IL-1. Anthrax toxin consists of three proteins: protective antigen (PA), edema factor (EF), and lethal factor (LF). None of the three is lethal alone but the proteins are lethal in certain combinations: EF + PA + LF = lethal; EF + PA = not lethal; PA + LF = lethal; and EF + LF = not lethal.

The PA binds to a receptor on the surface of the host cell and is cleaved by proteases located on the host cell membrane to expose a binding site for LF and EF. Following proteolytic activation on the host cell surface, the PA forms a membrane-inserting heptamer that somehow allows passage of the EF and LF into the cytoplasm. The EF is an adenylate cyclase and the LF is a zinc metallopeptidase. The LF acts on the mitogen-activated protein kinase (MAPK) signal transduction pathway that occurs in eukaryotic cells, an evolutionary conserved pathway that controls eukaryotic cell proliferation and differentiation. The enzyme MAPK kinase is an important component of the MAPK pathway and must be phosphorylated to be active. Another protein, MAPKK1, is the enzyme

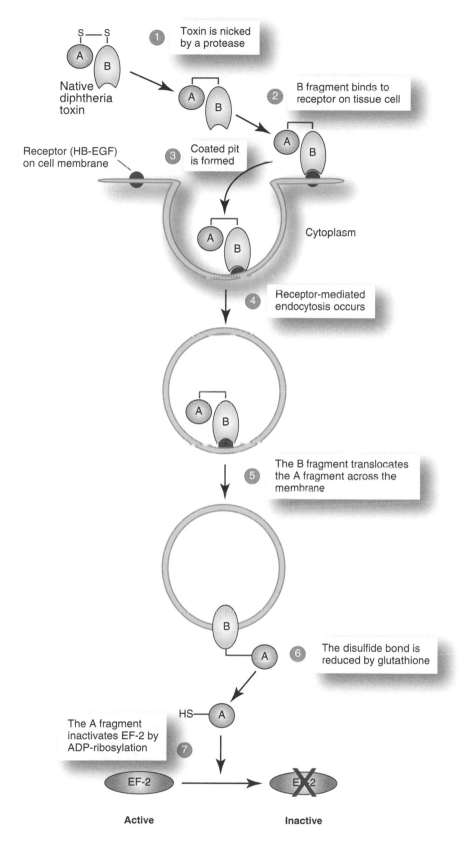

**FIGURE 17-7** Steps in the binding, penetration, and action of diphtheria toxin on throat cells.

that phosphorylates, and thus activates, the MAPK kinase. LF cleaves the amino terminus of MAPKK1 and renders it inactive, thereby stopping signaling along the pathway.

A cell-free anthrax vaccine as been developed that is protective against invasive disease, but is currently only recommended for high-risk populations. Presently, it is mainly given to military personnel. A cell-free filtrate of *B. anthracis* culture that contains no dead or live bacteria is formalin-treated. The filtrate contains a mix of cellular products including the protective antigen (PA) component of the toxin.

Many bacterial pathogens produce exotoxins that disrupt the structure of host cell membranes. These factors include *hemolysins* and *leucocidins*. Hemolysins are substances that attack red blood cells and produce visible changes on blood-agar plates. Colonies of certain hemolytic bacteria are surrounded by a clear, colorless zone where the red blood cells have been lysed completely. This is called *β hemolysis*. Other types of bacteria can reduce the hemoglobin in red cells to methemoglobin. The result is a greenish zone around the colonies called *α hemolysis*. In regard to mechanism of action, there are two major kinds of β hemolysins: catalytic hemolysins and pore-forming hemolysins. Catalytic hemolysins are phospholipases that attack the phospholipids in the membrane lipid bilayer. Pore-forming hemolysins are crescent- or doughnut-shaped oligomers that insert themselves into membranes, forming pores through which hemoglobin and other cytoplasmic components leak out. In the body, hemolysins probably do not contribute much to disease by destroying red blood cells but they usually exhibit other, more serious activities. For instance, many are leukocidins, substances that kill phagocytes.

An example of a hemolysin that is a phospholipase is the α toxin of *C. perfringens*. This hemolysin is a lecithinase that destroys not only red cells but also blood platelets and leukocytes and is the major cause of muscle death in gas gangrene. The β hemolysin of *S. aureus* is another example of a phospholipase. An example of an oligomeric, pore-forming hemolysin is streptolysin O (SLO), made by *Streptococcus pyogenes*. It is oxygen-labile and causes β hemolysis on blood agar plates only if the plates are incubated anaerobically or if the colonies are subsurface. Streptolysin S (SLS) is similar to SLO but is oxygen stable. Examples of oxygen-labile hemolysins similar to SLO include the listeriolysin O of *L. monocytogenes* and the theta (θ) toxin of *C. perfringens*.

Many leukocidins are hemolysins, such as SLO and SLS, but one that is not is the Panton-Valentine leucocidin of *S. aureus*. It consists of two proteins, S and F, which act together. The S component binds to ganglioside $G_{M1}$ on the surface of phagocytes. The binding causes activation of a phospholipase that damages the membrane of the phagocyte and creates pores through which potassium ions are lost from the cell. The F component binds to the membrane with the aid of the S component, but its mode of action is not well understood.

Some exotoxins are superantigens. As discussed in Chapter 8, a superantigen is a molecule that binds to T-cell receptors that contain a specific $V_β$ region (outside the antigen-binding cleft), regardless of either the other components of the receptor or the major histocompatibility complex context of the antigen. Superantigens cause a tremendous overproduction of cytokines, which can lead to symptoms of toxic shock syndrome. This serious syndrome includes high fever, exhaustion, red rash, decreased blood pressure, and other symptoms of multiorgan failure. Examples include the toxic shock syndrome toxin one (TSST-1) of *S. aureus* and the streptococcal pyrogenic exotoxin (SPE) A of *S. pyogenes*.

Some superantigens are enterotoxins that cause food poisoning, such as the enterotoxins of *S. aureus* and *C. perfringens*. The symptoms include nausea, vomiting, and/or diarrhea, but usually not fever. In staphylococcal food poisoning, it is proposed that the symptoms are due to the uptake of tiny amounts of these enterotoxins by cells of the alimentary tract, which can lead to the generation of inflammatory chemical mediators such as prostaglandin $E_2$ and leukotriene $B_4$. Ultimately, the vomiting and nausea are due to activation of the medullary "vomiting center" in the brain stem.

Other exotoxins have been described that have distinctive mechanisms of action. Most are enzymes that damage host tissue by acting on specific substrates. The following few paragraphs describes several of these virulence factors.

Although the pertussis exotoxin indirectly causes increased host cell adenylate cyclase activity, *B. pertussis* secretes an adenylate cyclase that can enter a host cell and be activated to produce cAMP from host cell ATP. This secreted adenylate cyclase is also a hemolysin that produces pores in red blood cell membranes.

Elastase is an enzyme that destroys elastin, a protein that allows lung tissue to be able to expand and contract. *P. aeruginosa*, which often causes lung infections in cystic fibrosis patients, makes two proteins, LasA and LasB, which act synergistically as an elastase. The elastase activity is thought to aid the establishment of infection by *P. aeruginosa* by damaging lung tissue. Elastin also occurs in the walls of blood vessels, and elastase can contribute to hemorrhaging in the lungs. Elastase not only can destroy elastin but also can inactivate the C3a and C5a components of complement (see Chapter 11).

The tracheal cytotoxin (TCT) of *B. pertussis* contributes to whooping cough. Normally it is difficult for a pathogen to colonize the trachea because the mucus layer overlying the epithelium traps bacteria and moves upward toward the mouth, where the bacteria are swallowed and destroyed by stomach acidity. The movement of the mucus layer is accomplished by the coordinated beating of cilia on the epithelial cells. The TCT of *B. pertussis* overcomes this bacteria-clearing action by damaging the ciliated cells of the trachea and preventing the growth of new cells. The toxin is thought to generate the cytokine IL-1, which in turn induces enzymatic production of nitric oxide (NO). The NO is toxic to the epithelial cells.

***Endotoxins Also Play a Role in Pathogenicity.*** The term endotoxin refers to the lipid A portion of the LPS components of the outer membrane of Gram-negative bacteria. Endotoxins are associated with intact bacteria and are not secreted by living bacteria. After Gram-negative bacteria die (as when attacked by antibodies plus complement), endotoxins can be released in soluble form as the cells autolyze and the outer membrane of the cell breaks down. Endotoxins have the following general features.

1. They have a low toxicity. It takes far more endotoxin than a classic exotoxin to kill a laboratory animal.
2. They exhibit heat stability. Endotoxins can resist autoclaving at 121°C for several hours.
3. The toxoid form of an endotoxin cannot be made.
4. All endotoxins have a similar mode of action and cause similar effects.

The harmful effects of endotoxins include the ability to cause high fever, hypotension (low blood pressure), disseminated blood clotting, and lethal shock. However, endotoxins do not act directly on the body to cause these effects, but instead act mainly by stimulating the body's macrophages to overproduce various substances. These substances include:

1. Cytokines, such as TNF, IL-1, IL-6, and IL-8.
2. Toxic forms of oxygen, such as superoxide radicals, hydrogen peroxide, and nitric oxide.
3. Lipids, such as prostaglandin $E_2$, thromboxane $A_2$, and platelet-activating factor.

These substances can act independently, together, or in certain sequences to cause various effects.

## MINI SUMMARY

Exotoxins are toxic proteins that are secreted by living microorganisms. They have a high toxicity, are heat-labile, can be made into toxoids, stimulate antibody production, can be neutralized by antitoxin, and have highly specific mechanisms of action.

Many exotoxins consist of an A part and a B part. The A part has the enzymatic activity whereas the B part binds the toxin to the tissue cell and translocated the A part across the tissue cell membrane into the cytoplasm. The A portion of diphtheria toxin and pertussis toxin catalyzes ADP ribosylation, and thus inactivation, of specific essential tissue cell proteins. Tetanus toxin prevents secretion of inhibitory transmitter in the central nervous system and causes rigid muscular spasms. Vaccines are available for diphtheria, tetanus, and pertussis toxins. Anthrax toxin is tripartite, and the PA portion has the binding and translocating activity. A vaccine for anthrax is also available.

Some hemolysins act by destroying membrane phospholipids, whereas others are pore-forming hemolysins. Superantigens such as TSST-1 cause overproduction of cytokines by binding to T-cell receptors that contain a specific $V_\beta$ region, regardless of either the other components of the receptor or the major histocompatibility complex context of the antigen.

In contrast to exotoxins, endotoxins have low toxicity, are heat stable, cannot be made into toxoids, are not neutralized by antibodies, and have similar modes of action.

### Some Microbe-Derived Factors and -Inherent Properties Are Associated with Virulence

Many virulence factors are not conventional exotoxins or endotoxins but have unique and unusual ways of overcoming the defense mechanisms of the body. Some of these virulence factors have only recently been discovered. The following section describes a few of these factors.

***Bacteria Can Inject Detrimental Proteins into a Host Cell.*** Most proteins exported from bacterial cells use the secA system; however, some protein virulence factors made by pathogenic bacteria are exported in an entirely different way, by the type III protein secretion system. These proteins are not released into the surrounding medium but instead are directly injected into the tissue cell by the bacterium. One example is the protein YopE, which is injected directly into phagocytes by *Yersinia* species. It kills the phagocyte by paralyzing its actin cytoskeleton. *Yersinia* species also produce protein YopP, which induces apoptosis. Like YopE, YopP seems to act after being injected into macrophages.

*Microbes Can Undergo Antigenic Switching to Avoid Immune Defenses.* The antigens on the surface of an invasive pathogen are the main targets of the host's immune responses to an infection because antibodies can readily come into contact with them (in contrast to antigens in the cytoplasm). If a pathogen can change its surface antigens during an infection, it can foil the body's immune system. The immune response against one set of antigens will no longer work if the pathogen now makes a different set of antigens. The best examples of how this happens are relapsing fever and trypanosomiasis.

Relapsing fever is caused by species of *Borrelia* (other than those that cause Lyme disease) that are transmitted to humans by infected lice or ticks. The disease begins with a primary febrile attack phase. The patient develops a high fever, shaking chills, headache, muscle pain, pain in joints of arms, legs, and back, nausea, vomiting, chest pain, coughing, weakness, and lethargy. This phase lasts for 3 to 6 days, after which the symptoms disappear and the patient enters an afebrile period that lasts 5–10 days. Then the first relapse occurs, and all the symptoms that happened earlier occur again. The relapse is followed by an afebrile period, then by a second relapse, and so forth. There can be up to nine relapses.

The borrelias are numerous in blood during the febrile periods, but few are present during the afebrile periods, when the organisms leave the blood and invade other tissue, such as, brain tissue. The body's main defense against the borrelias is the production of borrelicidal antibodies, and the disappearance of the spirochetes from the blood coincides with the production of these antibodies. When a relapse occurs, the spirochetes return to the blood and are again present in large numbers. However, the surface antigens, or *variable major proteins (VMP)*, on the spirochete's outer membrane change with each relapse; thus, the previous antibody response will not be effective against the new antigens (Figure 17-8).

How does this antigenic switching occur? The genes for the VMPs are located on linear plasmids in the *Borrelia* cells. Some of these linear plasmids contain "silent" (unexpressed) copies of the structural VMP genes, silent because they have no promoter. Other plasmids have an expression locus with the promoter. Antigenic switching occurs when different silent genes recombine with the expression locus (see Figure 17-8). Work with *Borrelia hermsii* suggests that there can be up to 26 different surface antigens. Eventually the antibodies become effective when the borrelia runs out of its antigenic changes, and if the patient has managed to live through the relapses.

Chronic African sleeping sickness is caused by the flagellated protozoan *Trypanosoma brucei gambiense*, which is transmitted by the bite of the tsetse fly. In this disease, which can last for months or years, the patient becomes progressively more lethargic and sleepy and eventually sleeps continuously. If not treated, the patient will probably die of either malnutrition or secondary infections. The invasive and the bloodstream forms of *T. brucei* are covered with a dense surface coat called a *variant-specific glycoprotein (VSG)*. Although a trypanosome has up to a thousand genes for different VSG proteins, only one gene is expressed at a given time. However, the VSG can undergo *antigenic switching* and can change hundreds of times during an infection. The mechanism of switching is somewhat similar to that in *Borrelia*: a duplicative transposition of a silent VSG gene into one of the telomeric VSG expression sites of the trypanosome leads to the replacement of the previously expressed VSG gene.

*Cord Factor of M. tuberculosis Makes the Organism Virulent.* Cord factor is composed of one molecule of the disaccharide trehalose and two molecules of mycolic acid. Strains of *M. tuberculosis* that have it in their cells grow in serpentine cable-like arrangements (cords). Strains that do not form cords are not virulent. The role of cord factor in virulence can be related to the following properties:

1. It is toxic to leukocytes and to mice.
2. It increases the susceptibility of animals to the endotoxins of Gram-negative bacteria.
3. It disrupts mitochondria, decreasing respiration and oxidative phosphorylation in tissue cells.
4. Injection of cord factor mixed with oil into mice by intraperitoneal injection causes a wasting disease and ultimately death. Intravenous injection causes granulomatous lesions in the lungs of mice, with the appearance of tubercles indistinguishable from those caused by active infection with virulent whole cells of *M. tuberculosis*.

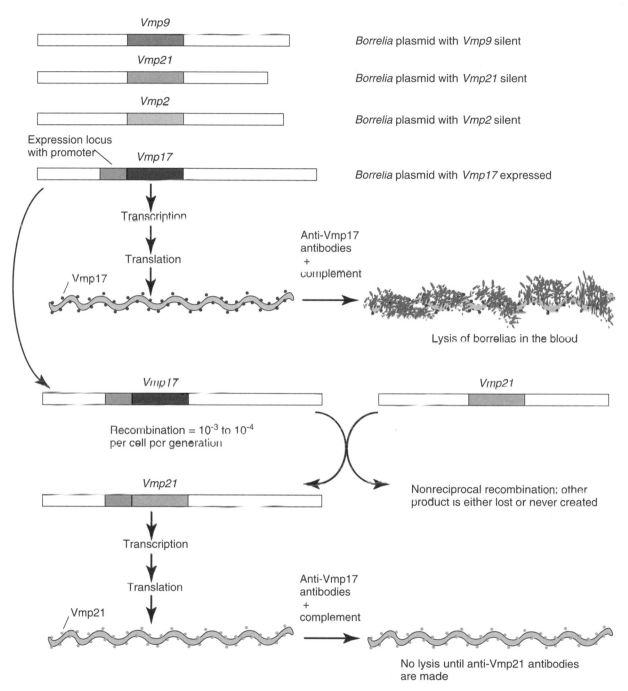

**FIGURE 17-8 Basis of the antigenic switching in the variable major proteins (VMPs) in the *Borrelia* species that cause relapsing fever.** By a recombination process, silent genes for VMPs on linear plasmids can acquire the expression locus needed for their transcription into mRNA.

**MINI SUMMARY**

Many virulence factors are not conventional toxins. Some protein virulence factors such as the YopE and YopF of *Yersinia* species are exported by the Type III protein secretion system and are injected directly into the tissue cell by the bacterium. In relapsing fever, the *borrelia* changes its surface antigens with each relapse, thereby avoiding destruction by antibodies. A similar kind of antigenic switching occurs in chronic African sleeping sickness, in which the variable surface antigen on the trypanosome can change hundreds of times during an infection. Cord factor made by *M. tuberculosis* is toxic to leukocytes, disrupts mitochondria, and causes a wasting disease in mice.

### Virulence Factors Produced by Viruses Facilitate Their Pathogenicity

Viruses do not produce toxins, as do bacteria. Most of the damage to tissue cells in a virus infection is due to the intracellular replication of the virus. The virus subverts the genetic control of the cell's metabolism to turn the cell into a virus-producing factory.

***Like Bacteria, Viruses Need to Attach to Host Cells to Initiate Infection.*** Viruses do have one thing in common with bacterial pathogens, the necessity for mechanisms of attachment to the host cell. Each kind of virus has surface proteins or glycoproteins specific for host cell receptors.

The capsid of HIV is surrounded by a lipid envelope studded with a glycoprotein called *gp120/gp41 complex* (see Chapter 16). This complex allows the virus to attach to a receptor called *CD4* mainly on the surface of CD4$^+$ T$_H$ cells—the commander-in-chief cells of the immune system. However, CD4 alone is not sufficient for attachment and entry. A host cell protein called *CCR5* acts as a co-receptor for HIV variants that predominate in the early stages of infection, and another protein called *CXCR4* acts as a co-receptor for variants that predominate during later stages of infection. The co-receptors aid the penetration of the virus into host cells.

The helical nucleocapsid of an influenza virus is wound up to form a rounded mass and is covered by a lipid envelope from which protein spikes project (discussed earlier). These spikes are hemagglutinins (HA proteins), so named because they allow attachment of the virus to red blood cells and other host cells. Also, projecting from the lipid envelope are mushroom-shaped protrusions composed of neuraminidase (NA proteins). This enzyme can degrade the protective mucus layers of mucous membranes; this degradation allows attachment of the virus to the underlying tissue cells. The spike-like proteins are the targets for neutralizing antibodies induced by flu vaccine.

A protein on the surface of polioviruses seems to be critical for attachment of the virus to lipid- and glycoprotein-containing receptors on host cells. The attachment is specific for cells of the intestinal tract and the central nervous system, and subsequent infection of the latter can lead to paralysis. It is interesting that the attenuated strains of poliovirus used in the Sabin vaccine for immunization against poliomyelitis can attach to the gastrointestinal tract as the wild-type poliovirus does; however, because of mutation in the genes for the viral surface proteins, these attenuated strains have lost the ability to attach to cells of the central nervous system and thus do not cause the paralysis that is characteristic of poliomyelitis.

***Some Viruses Constantly Change Their Guises to Avoid Immune Defenses.*** The kind of antigenic switching based on genetic recombination that occurs in some bacterial and protozoan pathogens during an infection does not occur in viruses. However, some viruses can give rise to antigenic variants during an infection because the mechanism for replication of their genetic material is highly error prone. For instance, the reverse transcriptase of HIV-1, which synthesizes DNA complementary to the viral RNA, tends to make mistakes, there is no "proofreading" mechanism as occurs in normal DNA synthesis. Thus, HIV-1 rapidly mutates during infection, and the mutations lead to variants that can escape the immune defenses of the body. In fact, the sloppiness of the viral replication is so great that the genome of each progeny virion probably differs in at least one position from the original infecting virus' genome.

Rhinoviruses are the most frequent causes of the common cold, the most prevalent of all human infections. Antibodies appear in response to a rhinovirus infection, including secretary IgA antibodies in respiratory tract secretions. Such antibodies should protect against subsequent infections, yet a person can have several colds each year. The reason is that there are at least 115 immunologically distinct types of rhinoviruses, and immunity against one type does not prevent infection by another type. No vaccine exists for prevention of the common cold because so many antigenic types would have to be included in the vaccine.

Antigenic variation, even though it is a main strategy used by RNA viruses to evade host antiviral immune defenses, is a passive activity—random mutations lead to an overwhelming number of different virus antigenic profiles. Large DNA viruses, such as poxviruses and herpesviruses, also take an active role in developing guises to avoid antiviral immune responses; they encode molecules that mimic host cytokines, chemokines, and their receptors. These mimetics, in turn, may inactivate inflammatory cytokines or redirect the immune response. Viruses that infect leukocytes might use cytokine pathways to dictate when the host needs to proliferate, to migrate, or control its homeostasis to enhance viral replication.

As discussed earlier, IFNs have some of the most potent antiviral and immunomodulatory properties of any host molecules. So it is not surprising that viruses encode mechanisms to counteract host IFN responses and to ensure efficient viral replication. These mechanisms include: jamming of IFN induction/expression, substituting host IFN receptors with viral decoy IFN receptors, disturbing intracellular IFN signaling pathways, and directly downregulating the level of IFN-stimulating gene expression.

***Some Viruses Can Hide (Latency) to Avoid Immune Defenses.*** Some viruses have the ability to evade body defenses by "disappearing" after the initial infection and then reappearing months or even years later. HIV and the herpesviruses are two examples.

HIV becomes latent by integrating its genetic material into the host cell genome. After entering a host cell, the viral reverse transcriptase synthesizes a single strand of DNA that is complementary to the viral RNA. The single-stranded DNA is converted to double-stranded DNA, which is then integrated into the host cell's own DNA. In this integrated form, the virus is dormant and causes no damage to the infected cell. However, at some later date the virus becomes activated from its dormant state and directs the synthesis of new viral RNA and viral proteins, which are assembled into numerous viral progeny. HIV latency is one of the obstacles in developing an AIDS vaccine (see Chapter 16).

In herpesvirus infections, after the primary lesions disappear the virus becomes latent, but the viral DNA is not integrated into the host cell genome and the mechanism of the latency is not yet understood. HSV-1, which causes cold sores and fever blisters, and HSV-2, which causes genital herpes, travel along sensory nerves to the spinal ganglia, where they remain. During latency of HSV-1, transcription of a particular region of the HSV genome produces RNAs called *latency-associated transcripts (LAT)*; however, these transcripts are not essential for the latency. The latent virus can be

reactivated periodically by environmental factors such as heat or cold, by hormonal or emotional disturbances, or by other stimuli; it then travels down the nerves to infect cells in the skin and mucous membranes. Similarly, after a case of chickenpox (varicella), the varicella-zoster virus (VZV) becomes latent in sensory ganglia but later can emerge to cause a severe painful neuralgia called *"shingles."* The licensed zoster vaccine is a lyophilized preparation of a live, attenuated strain of VZV, the same strain used in the varicella vaccines (the potency of the two vaccines are different). Zoster vaccine is shown to be partially efficacious at preventing zoster, at reducing the severity and duration of pain, and at preventing postherpetic neuralgia among those developing zoster. Cytomegalovirus, which causes congenital infections and a mononucleosis-like disease, becomes latent in mononuclear cells, but no viral protein or RNA synthesis occurs in the latent form. Epstein-Barr virus, the cause of mononucleosis, becomes latent in B lymphocytes and nasopharyngeal cells; the latency depends on synthesis of several proteins, but their exact role is not yet clear.

**MINI SUMMARY**

Viruses have mechanisms of attachment to the host cell. HIV has a gp120/gp41 complex that allows attachment to the CD4 receptor on CD4+ cells. Influenza viruses have HA proteins that allow attachment to tissue cells. Polioviruses have surface proteins that allow attachment to intestinal and nerve cells. Some viruses, such as HIV-1, can give rise to antigenic variants during an infection because the mechanism for replication of their genetic material is highly error prone and there is no proofreading mechanism. Many large DNA viruses make molecules that mimic cytokines, chemokines and their receptors. Other viral-counteracting strategies can block and interfere with the IFN pathway. Some viruses such as HIV and herpesviruses have the ability to evade body defenses by becoming latent after the initial infection; they can reappear months or even years later. In some instances, as in HIV infections, latency occurs because the viral DNA becomes integrated into the host cell's DNA. The exact mechanism of the latency in herpesvirus infections is not known.

### The Body's Own Immune Response to Infection Can Contribute to Pathogenicity

In some infections the body's response to the presence of the pathogen can cause much or most of the damage, while the pathogen itself assumes the role of a bystander. This pattern occurs in several infections including tuberculosis, leprosy, listeriosis, brucellosis, and tularemia. The bacterial agents of these infections are mainly intracellular—they live inside macrophages. The body's main defense against them is cell-mediated immunity, since antibodies do not penetrate macrophages. In these infections the characteristic lesion is the *granuloma*, a small nodule composed of concentric layers of macrophages surrounded by a mantle of $T_H1$ cells.

The paradigm of a granulomatous infection is tuberculosis, in which the granulomas are called *tubercles*. Tuberculosis demonstrates that granuloma formation can be either beneficial or disastrous, depending on the body's response to the infection.

Pulmonary tuberculosis begins when *M. tuberculosis* lodges within an air sac in the lungs. The bacteria are rapidly engulfed by alveolar macrophages and multiply slowly within these phagocytes. The first evidence of infection is development of a delayed-type hypersensitivity to the bacteria after about a month. This hypersensitivity can be detected by the *tuberculin test* (see Chapter 12), in which an extract of proteins from *M. tuberculosis* is injected into the skin. A reddening that occurs in 72 hours indicates a positive test.

Some of the mycobacterial cell proteins are processed by the macrophages and appear on the surface as a class II MHC molecule-peptide complexes. This complex is present to specific $CD4^+$ $T_H1$ cell and, which induces the macrophages to secrete IL-1β, IL-8, and IL-12. IL-8 attracts more T cells to the site of infection, IL-1β causes the T-cells to proliferate, and IL-12 stimulates the differentiation of uncommitted (naïve) $CD4^+$ $T_H$ cells to become $CD4^+$ $T_H1$ cells, which direct cell-mediated immune responses, rather than $CD4^+$ $T_H2$ cells, which direct humoral immune responses.

The T cells activated by IL-1β secrete IFN-γ, which attracts more macrophages to the site of infection. It also serves to activate macrophages so that they have more lysosomes and hydrolytic enzymes. The activated macrophages usually cannot kill *M. tuberculosis*, but they do prevent the mycobacteria from actively multiplying. The T cells also secrete *migration inhibition factor*, which renders macrophages incapable of migrating away from the site of infection. A small pearl-gray granuloma forms, with mycobacteria in the middle (inside macrophages), concentric layers of macrophages around the bacteria, and an outer mantle of T cells.

Cell-mediated immunity usually keeps the infection from developing further and the infection remains subclinical in about 10 percent of *M. tuberculosis* infections. However, if a person's immune system is compromised by factors such as malnutrition, alcoholism, immunosuppressive agents, AIDS, old age, or other factors, then cell-mediated immunity can not succeed in arresting the growth of the mycobacteria and the disease progresses into *clinical tuberculosis*.

A slowly progressive disease, clinical tuberculosis can take months to kill a patient. As more tubercles develop, they become larger and some of the macrophages inside die and fuse together to form an amorphous cheese-like mass. The tissue cell death is probably due to overproduction of IL-1β and TNF-α, which mycobacteria and mycobacterial proteins cause to be released from macrophages. Lack of oxygen (there is no circulation within a tubercle) and toxic mycobacterial lipids such as cord factor might also contribute to death of macrophages.

The initial tubercle becomes larger and more tubercles form. Eventually they fuse together to form areas of dead tissue in the lung that are now large enough to be seen by a chest x-ray. The area of damage in the lungs expands and the patient begins to exhibit clinical symptoms of tuberculosis—night sweats, fever, chills, and weight loss. These symptoms are thought to be mediated mainly by overproduction of cytokines, especially IL-1β and TNF-α. Eventually the wall of a bronchus is eroded; this erosion allows mycobacteria to spill into the bronchus, and acid-fast bacilli begin to appear in the sputum. Eventually the mycobacteria enter the blood capillaries of the lung and become distributed throughout the body. Thousands of tubercles develop everywhere and cause fatal damage to vital organs.

The nature of granuloma formation in diseases other than tuberculosis has not been so well studied and may not occur in the same manner, particularly since mycobacteria have an unusual chemical composition compared with other bacteria (mycolic acids, cord factor, sulfolipids, etc.). However, there are certain general aspects found in all granulomatous diseases:

1. The structure of granulomas is similar from one disease to another even though the causative microorganism varies.
2. Activated macrophages within a granuloma can halt bacterial multiplication and sometimes even kill the bacteria.
3. Granuloma formation is a two-edged sword, it can prevent an infection from progressing beyond the subclinical stage, or it can lead to extensive tissue damage and death of the patient.

The current vaccine for tuberculosis disease consists of the attenuated strain of *M. bovis* called *Bacille Calmette-Guérin* or *BCG*. BCG vaccine is used in many countries, but it is not generally recommended in the United States. BCG vaccination is effective against extrapulmonary tuberculosis but questionable against pulmonary tuberculosis. It may also cause a false-positive tuberculin skin test; therefore, the combination of vaccine inconsistencies and the inability to monitor for tuberculosis after vaccination has precluded its use in the U.S.

## MINI SUMMARY

In some bacterial infections, the body's response to the presence of the pathogen can cause much or most of the damage. The body's main defense against these bacteria is cell-mediated immunity and the characteristic lesion is the granuloma. In tuberculosis, the first evidence of infection is development of delayed-type hypersensitivity. Then, as specific $T_H1$ cells interact with antigen-presenting macrophages, the macrophages secrete cytokines that cause proliferation of the T cells. The $T_H1$ cells in turn secrete IFN-$\gamma$ that causes macrophages to become activated macrophages, which usually are able to prevent multiplication of the bacteria. However, overproduction of IL-1$\beta$ and TNF-$\alpha$, lack of oxygen within a tubercle, and toxic factors made by the bacteria, can lead to tissue cell death and progressive clinical disease.

# IMMUNITY TO INFECTIOUS MICROBES CAN BE ACCOMPLISHED BY ACTIVE OR PASSIVE IMMUNIZATION

As discussed in Chapter 1, humoral and cell-mediated adaptive immunity can each be further divided into immunity induced in the host or passively transferred from an immune host (see Figure 1-3)—that is, immunization, the exposure process by which the host develops immunity, can be achieved by either by active or passive **immunization. Active immunity** is induced in the host itself, acquired gradually (5 to 14 days after antigen exposure), lasts for years (perhaps life-long; called *immunologic memory*), and is highly protective. **Passive immunity** is immediate because antibodies or lymphocytes are acquired

from an immune host, lasts for days to months, has low to moderate protective effectiveness, and does not develop memory in the recipient. Both active and passive immunity are often further subdivided depending on how the immunity was introduced, that is, natural or artificial forms. It is natural, when immunity occurs through a nondeliberate, direct contact with an infectious microbe. In contrast, it is artificial, when immunity occurs through a deliberate contact, such as by administration of a *vaccine* (called *vaccination*; discussed shortly). In active immunity, an individual has acquired immunity mediated by antibodies or sensitized T cells formed by that individual. If an individual is exposed to an infectious microbe naturally through the environment, rather than by immunization with a vaccine (discussed below), that individual acquires the natural rather than the artificial form of active immunity, which leads to a primary response and immunologic memory. In passive immunity, an individual has acquired immunity mediated by antibodies or sensitized T cells formed in another individual or animal. Artificial, passive acquired immunity occurs when preformed antibodies (such as gamma globulin injections for hepatitis; called *passive transfer*) or immune cells (called *adoptive transfer*) are given to a nonimmune individual. Passive immunization is warranted when there is a high risk of infection, insufficient time to develop an immune response, or to restore immunity when there is an immunodeficiency. Passive immunization is routinely given to individuals exposed to microorganisms that cause acute respiratory failure (caused by respiratory syncytial virus), botulism, diphtheria, hepatitis A and B, measles, rabies, or tetanus or to black widow spider bites or snakebites. Thus, specific adaptive immunity is acquired either passively or actively and by natural or artificial means (see Figure 1-3).

Passive and active immunizations are not without risks. The passive transfer of preformed antibody produced in another species, such as a horse, into a human recipient can induce an antibody response against the foreign protein's (the horse antibodies') antigenic isotypic determinants. Some recipients can produce IgE anti-horse antibodies, which bind to mast cells and if complexed with the passive antibodies can cause mast-cell degranulation, instigating systemic anaphylaxis (see Chapter 12). In contrast, other recipients can produce IgG and IgM anti-horse antibodies, which can lead to complement-activating immune complex formation, instigating type III hypersensitivity reactions. In the case of restoring humoral immunity in immunodeficiency or immunosuppressed patients (receiving a transplant or undergoing chemotherapy for cancer treatment) with human immunoglobulins, the recipient can develop anti-allotypic antibodies. The response mediated by anti-allotypic determinants is not as intense as those mediated by an anti-isotypic determinant response. Hazards associated with active immunization using vaccines will be mentioned later.

---

### MINI SUMMARY

Adaptive immunity can be divided into active and passive immunity, each of which is further subdivided into natural and artificial forms. Active immunity is the specific resistance to disease acquired by individuals as a result of their own reactions to pathogenic microorganisms or to the products of such organisms. In contrast, passive immunity is immunity produced by receiving blood or serum containing antibodies.

---

# VACCINES FOR ACTIVE IMMUNIZATION ARE DEVELOPED USING MICROBES OR THEIR PRODUCTS, AND GENETIC ENGINEERING

Natural antigens are everywhere. They are in the water we drink, the air we breathe, and the food we eat. Most are harmless and are merely a part of the organic material of which all life is made. But when you are exposed to a significant amount of these antigens in such a way that the immune system is stimulated, an immune response occurs. The most common source of natural antigens is the microbial world—because, as mentioned earlier, microbes can actively invade our bodies, grow rapidly to produce high numbers of organisms, and express epitopes that are foreign to the immune system. Therefore most immune responses are generated against microbial antigens as a result of natural exposure during the progress of disease (for example, the common cold).

In cases where microorganisms are virulent and likely to cause life-threatening disease, it is best to help the host acquire specific immunity before the disease is encountered. Therefore special preparations of microorganisms have been developed to deliberately immunize the population, in a sense exposing

people to an "artificial antigen." Prevention of infectious diseases by immunization is one of the greatest achievements of medical science. The most important substances used for immunization are vaccines (see Table 17-1). A **vaccine** is an immunogen-containing substance that, on introduction (called *vaccination* or *immunization*) into an animal or individual, stimulates active immunity for future protection against infection by the appropriate organism (Figure 17-9 and see Table 17-1). In contrast, a **toxoid**, which is also a vaccine, is a toxin that has been changed to eliminate its toxicity but still act as an immunogen. Certain bacteria, such as those species associated with botulism, cholera, diphtheria, or tetanus, manifest disease through toxin production. Their treated toxins, toxoids, induce antibodies that can neutralize the native toxins. Diphtheria and tetanus toxoid are components of the whole-cell pertussis DTP (diphtheria toxoid, tetanus toxoids, and killed *Pertussis* bacteria) vaccine. Concerns about safety prompted the development of more purified (acellular) pertussis vaccines (DTaP); it is associated with a lower frequency of adverse events and is effective in preventing pertussis disease. Toxoids are not without risks; they can provoke local hypersensitivity reactions. Booster immunizations of tetanus toxoid are administered with attention to the nature of the injury and immunization history. Adolescents and adults have increased hypersensitivity to diphtheria toxoid; therefore, they receive smaller doses than children. Taken together, **vaccination** is the process of using vaccines to do harmlessly what the body does after recovering from a disease—establish resistance.

Even though vaccinations are one the best ways to prevent infections, they are not 100% effective. As with any exposure to an antigen, some small percentage of individuals will respond inadequately to provide sufficient protection. Because most vaccinated individuals are effectively immunized, the transmission of communicable disease is interrupted in the population; therefore, the susceptible individual has little chance of becoming infected. This is an important principle in epidemiology, known as **herd immunity**; an entire population can be protected by the immunization of most individuals. If the number of people that do not get vaccinated increases or the vaccinations are infective, herd immunity is jeopardized, leading to increased infections.

The experimental foundation of vaccination occurred a little over 200 years ago. As described in Chapter 1, the English physician Edward Jenner built on the concept of *variolation*, in which individuals were deliberately exposed through inhalation or small cuts in the skin to dried crusts of smallpox

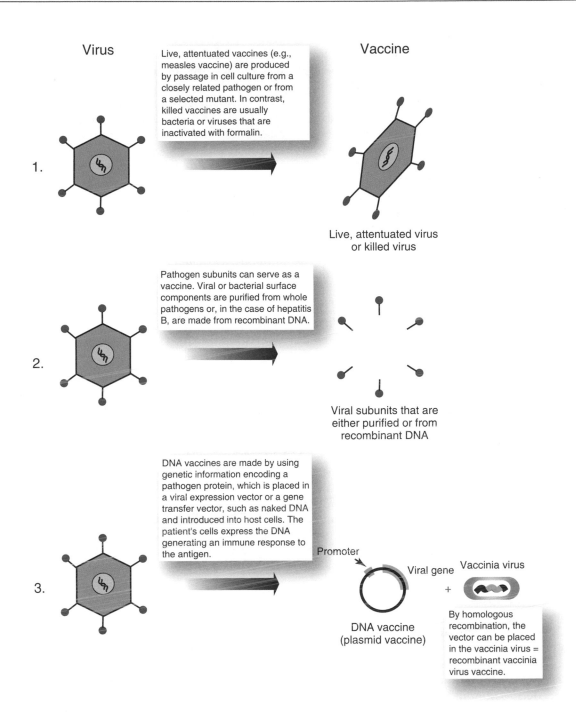

**FIGURE 17-9  Examples of some vaccines.**

pustules. The practice of variolation ceased with the success and acceptance of Jenner's work. Jenner recognized that milkmaids who had contracted cowpox were not susceptible to smallpox. He introduced the safer method of inoculation with cowpox lesion material, which contained the cowpox virus *vaccinia*, a non-fatal virus that also induced immunity to smallpox. This was the beginning of vaccinations, which eventually led to the worldwide eradication of smallpox in 1979. Building on Jenner's early work, Louis Pasteur, working on the attenuation of chicken cholera, first used the word vaccine (from the Latin word *vacca*, meaning "cow") in honor of the work by Edward Jenner on cowpox inoculation. Pasteur attenuated other organisms, such as the anthrax-causing organism *B. anthracis* and rabies virus for their use as vaccines. Other diseases have been targeted for eradication by vaccination. In 1988, the World Health Organization targeted polio for eradication by 2000, the mark was missed but eradication is close.

In active immunization, the vaccine induces the host's own immune system to provide protection against the pathogen. Vaccines provide immunogenic epitopes that induce a specific primary immune response by stimulating antibody formation and often T-cell sensitization. Subsequent exposure to the infectious agent will lead to a secondary response with a greater immunity. The goal for any vaccine series is lifelong protection; however, some vaccines require boosters later in life. The three main traditional vaccines are produced from:

1. inactivated (killed) bacteria or viruses or antigenic subunits of these agents (called *inactivated vaccines*) (see Figure 17-9),
2. live, attenuated (weakened) bacteria or viruses (called *live, attenuated vaccines*) (see Figure 17-9), or
3. inactivated toxins from the disease-causing agent (called *toxoids*; see earlier paragraph).

**Inactivated (killed) vaccines** are produced by killing the disease-causing organism with heat and/or chemicals (such as formaldehyde). The Salk polio vaccine is an example of an inactivated vaccine, which is developed by treating virus cultures with formaldehyde, killing the virus so that it cannot replicate—it no longer is infectious. A mixture of three poliovirus serotypes is used to generate good protection against all common types of polio. Protection is mediated by neutralizing antibodies that block the ability of poliovirus to infect host cells. Inactivated vaccines are stable, safe, and cannot revert to the virulent form; however, immunity to most inactivated vaccines stimulates a weak immune response and must be given several times (boosters). For example, in the case of the Salk polio vaccine, the virus cannot multiply, and large numbers of virions are needed to stimulate immunity, plus the vaccine induces only humoral immunity; therefore, the vaccine must be repeatedly injected to maintain immunity, which makes it expensive to administer. The flu shot and vaccines for cholera, hepatitis A, and plague are inactivated vaccines (see Table 17-1). The disadvantage of the influenza vaccine is that the flu viruses mutate rapidly; therefore, new antigen specificities must be added to each year's vaccine. Inactivated vaccines are not without side effects, for example, the killed *Bordetella pertussis* bacteria in the DTP vaccine was associated with serious side effects, such as encephalopathy in the infant.

However, the benefits greatly overshadowed any of the immunization risks; therefore, the killed vaccine was replaced by an acellular vaccine (called *DTaP*), which contained pertussis toxoid and other antigenic components, such as filamentous hemagglutinin and fimbriae. The DTaP vaccine has fewer side effects but the efficacy remains the same as the DTP vaccine.

**Live attenuated (avirulent) vaccines** are produced by growing the disease-causing organism under special laboratory conditions that cause it to lose its virulence. Live vaccines required special handling and storage to maintain potency; however, in contrast to inactivated vaccines, they produce both antibody-mediated and cell-mediated immunity and usually require only one boost. Most live vaccines are injected but some are given orally, such as the Sabin polio vaccine, or intranasally such as a new influenza vaccine (FluMist) that shows promise in preventing the flu. The advantages of an attenuated Sabin polio vaccine is that it contains an infectious virus; therefore, it can replicate, fewer virus needs to be administered, and humoral and cell-mediated immunity with memory is induced. The latter activity results because the antigen, the virus, is in its natural conformation. There is one caution in using live vaccines—there is a remote chance that the organism may revert to a virulent form. For this reason people with compromised immune systems are usually not given live virus vaccines (such as measles, mumps, oral polio, rubella, and bacille Calmette-Guérin). Vaccination recommendations for polio have changed because the incidence of vaccine-acquired polio is higher than naturally acquired polio; therefore, the inactivated polio vaccine is now the recommended vaccine in the U.S. Live, attenuated vaccine administration to pregnant women is avoided because of potential harm to the fetus. The vaccines for measles, mumps, polio, rubella, and yellow fever are produced from live, attenuated organisms (see Table 17-1).

New technologies are being used to improve traditional vaccines. These new second-generation vaccines are made using powerful techniques such as recombinant genetic engineering. The new second-generation vaccines are produced from:

1. pieces of an infectious agent (called *subunit vaccines*) (see Figure 17-9),
2. bacterial carbohydrates that are conjugated to proteins (called *conjugate vaccines*),
3. identified microbial immunogenic epitopes that are synthesized using recombinant DNA technology (called *recombinant antigen vaccines*),

4. microbial antigen-encoding genes that are introduced into noncytopathic viruses (called *recombinant vector vaccines*), or
5. plasmid DNA encoding immunogenic proteins (called *DNA vaccines*) (see Figure 17-9).

**Subunit vaccines** can be developed from purified immunogenic fragments, derived from infectious microorganisms, to avoid side effects caused by whole organisms. These vaccines are made by breaking down the actual infectious organism, or they can be made in the laboratory using recombinant engineering techniques, that is, placing a protein gene that encodes the target immunogenic protein in another virus. The non-infectious carrier virus expresses the protein. There are three general forms of subunit vaccines, inactivated exotoxins or toxoids, capsular polysaccharides, and recombinant protein antigens. These vaccines are used to protect against *S. pneumoniae* induced pneumonia and against a type of meningitis (see Table 17-1).

Subunit vaccine effectiveness is improved when they are administered with adjuvants (see Table 4-2). Adjuvants slow the release of antigen, thereby chronically stimulating the immune system; they bind macrophage and dendritic cell TLRs inducing the production of inflammatory cytokines and activate antigen-presenting cells to express B7 molecules. All of these activities stimulate immune responsiveness. The pertussis toxoid in acellular DPT vaccine acts as an adjuvant.

**Conjugate vaccines** protect against bacteria that use special polysaccharide-outer coats to disguise themselves, that is, protect themselves from phagocytosis, which leads to an inability to activate $T_H$ cells. Protective immunity requires opsonizing antibodies but infants activate B cells in a thymus-independent manner (see Chapter 10), leading to the production of IgM antibodies but no affinity maturation, class switching, or memory response. The immature immune systems of infants and younger children have difficulty recognizing these bacteria. If proteins from a second type of organism, one recognized by an immature immune system, such as tetanus or diphtheria toxoid, are linked to the outer coats of the stealthy disease-causing organisms it induces immunity against the disease agent. Conjugate vaccines are available to protect against bacterial meningitis caused by *H. influenzae* type b (Hib).

A variation of conjugate vaccines, called **peptide vaccines**, target immunostimulatory peptides for presentation to the immune system. Because peptides have no native structure, they are unable to bind the pattern recognition receptors on phagocytic cells that promote pathogen uptake. To enhance the immunogenicity of peptides, they are treated with detergent to integrate protein antigens into protein micelles, liposomes (lipid vesicles), and immune stimulatory complexes (ISCOMs). These antigen delivery systems have powerful immunostimulating activity (act as adjuvants). Mixing the antigenic proteins in detergent and subsequently removing the detergent forms protein micelles. These micelles orient the hydrophilic proteins to the outside, whereas the hydrophobic proteins are oriented inwards. Liposomes, or vesicles, are spherical entities composed of a phospholipid bilayer shell with an aqueous core. Sizes range from 50 nm to several micrometers. Mixing antigenic proteins with a phospholipid suspension under conditions that allow lipid bilayer formation produces liposomes. For vaccine delivery, an antigen can be encapsulated in the liposome core, buried within the lipid bilayer, or adsorbed on the surface for presentation to antigen presenting cells. ISCOMs are spherical, micellar cage-like structures, typically 40 nm in diameter, that are comprised of protein antigen, cholesterol, phospholipid, and the saponin adjuvant Quil A. They are prepared by mixing protein with detergent and Quil A. The matrix that is formed traps the hydrophobic membrane protein antigens through apolar interactions. ISCOM-based vaccines promote both antibody and cellular immune responses in a variety of experimental animal models.

**Recombinant antigen vaccines** are made by taking genes encoding surface antigens from viral, bacterial, and protozoan pathogens and cloning them into bacterial, yeast, or mammalian expression systems, and the expressed antigens used for vaccine development. The first such vaccine approved for human use, is the hepatitis B vaccine. It was produced by cloning the gene encoding the major surface antigen of hepatitis B virus in yeast cells.

**Recombinant vector vaccines** use a vector, or carrier, that is an attenuated virus or bacterium into which harmless genes that encode major antigens from another disease-causing organism can be inserted. The antigen-expressing vector may be used as the vaccine or purified peptides of the antigen may be used as a subunit vaccine. The large vaccinia virus, causative agent of cowpox, has ample room to accept additional genes; thus, it is used to make recombinant vector vaccines. A close relative of vaccinia, canarypox virus, is also being engineered to act as a vector. It has an advantage over vaccinia because it is avirulent even in immunocompromised individuals. The advantages of recombinant vector vaccines is that they do not contain antigens that elicit no immune responses or antigens that elicit damaging responses and the antigens that are used would keep their native conformation, thereby elicit a complete immune response. A current disadvantage is the development cost associated with locating the desired gene, cloning it, and assuring efficient expression. No recombinant viral vector vaccines are licensed for general use in the United States.

In the newest method of vaccination under experimentation, **DNA vaccines**, plasmid DNA encoding immunogenic proteins is inoculated directly into the recipient's muscles. The muscle cells and surrounding dendritic cells take up the DNA and the encoded antigen is expressed in association with class I MHC molecules or as soluble, secreted protein, which is collected, processed, and present in association with class II MHC molecules, leading to cell-mediated and antibody-mediated immunity, respectively. The stimulation of both arms of immunity usually requires live attenuated vaccines. The prolonged expression of the antigen generates significant immunologic memory. A drawback that precludes the universal application of DNA vaccines is that only protein antigens can be encoded; for example, certain vaccines, such as those for pneumococcal and meningococcal infections, use polysaccharide antigens. The administration of DNA vaccines as been improved with the use of DNA-coated microscopic gold beads delivered by an air gun (called a *gene gun*). DNA vaccines for Ebola, herpesvirus, influenza, and malaria have been tested in humans.

Scientists are pursuing many promising new strategies in vaccine development and administration. A few examples include exposing mucosal membranes to vaccines, which produces an immune response in a less-stressful and better-targeted manner; using microspheres containing antigen, which allows release of small doses of vaccine over extended periods of time as the microspheres dissolve; advances in the use of nanotechnology to deliver vaccines are underway; and creating edible vaccines by genetically engineering plants like potatoes and bananas to incorporate synthetic antigens, which will produce protective immunity when eaten.

### MINI SUMMARY

Humoral and cell-mediated immunity can be divided into active and passive forms. Substances used for immunization include vaccines and toxoids. Vaccination refers to administration of any vaccine or toxoid that induces active immunization. Currently used vaccines in humans, including inactivated, attenuated, toxoid, subunit, and conjugate vaccines. Proteins derived from microorganisms make better vaccines. Polysaccharides derived from microorganisms are conjugated with proteins to enhance their immunogenicity. Experimental vaccines include recombinant vector vaccines and DNA vaccines. Recombinant vectors include avirulent bacteria and viruses, which are engineered to carry and express genes from infectious microbes. The encoded proteins induce cell-mediated immunity. Plasmid DNA encoding pathogen protein antigens can be administered by a gene gun to induce humoral and cell-mediated immunity.

## SUMMARY

Microbes that can cause an **infection**, the colonization of the host by the parasitic organism leading to a state of disease, are *pathogens*. Infections are *subclinical*, that is, there are no detectable clinical symptoms of disease. The quality or ability of the pathogen to cause pathological changes or *disease*, that is, impair function of a susceptible host, is called *pathogenicity*. Pathogens that take advantage of an immune compromised individual are called *opportunistic pathogens*, while *primary pathogens* initiate disease in healthy hosts. The degree of pathogenicity is known as *virulence*. Microorganisms can range from highly virulent to avirulent; the properties that affect a microorganism's virulence are known as *virulence factors*.

Pathogens can penetrate body surfaces passively or actively. Once pathogens enter the host, they can remain at the site of entry, such as *S. aureus*, and form an *abscess*, which contains *pus* or they can move throughout the host using the lymphatic or circulatory systems. When microbes are present in the blood, it is known as a *bacteremia*. If the organisms actively multiply in the blood, it is called a *septicemia*. The entrance by pathogens into a host induces nonspecific resistance referred to as *innate immunity*; these are the general mechanisms inherited as the build-in structure and function of each host. Its counterpart resistance is *adaptive immunity*, which is highly specific for antigenic structures recognized by B and T lymphocytes and is divided into *humoral* and *cell-mediated immunity*.

The development of adaptive immunity follows a set sequence of events. These events are highly *specific* and lead to antigen removal and, later, *immunologic memory* for the antigen. Exposure to antigen does not lead to an immediate appearance of specific antibody. Antibody production can be divided into two general events: *antigen elimination* and *antibody formation*. Antigen elimination involves three phases: (1) *equilibration*, (2) *nonimmune catabolism*, and (3) *immune catabolism*. The chemical and physical nature of the antigen, use of adjuvants, dosages, frequency of exposure, route of injection, and the genetic constitution of the host affect these phases. During the host's first exposure to an antigen, a *primary antibody response* occurs. The primary antibody response can be divided into four phases: (1) *induction period*, (2) *logarithmic increase in titer*, (3) *steady state*, and (4) *decline*. If a host has a second exposure to the homologous antigen, a *secondary antibody response* occurs, characterized by a shortened induction period, a higher titer, and extended duration of detectable antibody with higher *avidity*. The cell-mediated immune response follows the same sequence, except T cells mediate the immunity.

Intact innate immunity, which includes physical barriers, alternative and lectin complement pathways, phagocytic cells, and NK cells, is the first line of defense against pathogens. Humoral immunity by antibodies mediates protection against extracellular bacteria by opsonizing bacteria, activating the classical complement system, and neutralizing toxins. *Mycoses*, fungal diseases, are rarely severe in normal, healthy individuals; however, to immunodeficiency patients they pose a major threat. Both innate and adaptive immunity are induced by fungal infections. Protozoa and helminths represent *parasites*. Protozoa in the blood-borne stages of their life cycles are sensitive to specific antibodies, whereas in their intracellular phases cell-mediated is required. Viruses are *obligate intracellular parasites* that are targeted in innate immunity by Toll-like receptors, complement, and NK cells and by both arms of adaptive immunity; in humoral immunity, they are neutralized by antibodies and in cell-mediated immunity, they are controlled and cleared.

Pathogens invoke various strategies to avoid immune defenses, including adherence to tissue cells, enzymes that promote colonization and invasion, neutralization of acidity, special types of motility, factors that either prevent or encourage engulfment by phagocytes, factors allowing intracellular survival and multiplication, *microbial toxins* (exotoxins and endotoxins), injections of proteins into host cells, undergoing antigen switching, production of cord factor, attachment factors, rapid mutations, and latency phases. Some of these strategies elicit immune responses that increase the pathogenicity of the microbe, such as infection by *M. tuberculosis*.

Adaptive immunity against infectious diseases may be achieved by *active* or *passive immunization*. Active immunity may result from previous infections or from vaccinations, which lead to long-term protection with memory. In contrast, passive immunity is caused by transfer of preformed antibodies, which leads to short-term protection without memory. Immunization by *vaccines*, an immunogen-containing substance that on administration (called *vaccination* or *immunization*) into an individual, stimulates active immunity against future infection by the appropriate pathogen.

Three types of vaccine are currently used in prevention of human diseases; they include live attenuated (avirulent) microbes, inactivated (killed) microbes, and purified macromolecules, such *toxoids* (also called *inactivated exotoxins*), *subunit vaccines*, and *conjugate vaccines*. Experiment vaccines include *recombinant vector vaccines* and *DNA vaccines*. Vaccines are not 100% effective due changes such as rapid mutation, *antigenic drift*, and *antigenic shift*; however, herd immunity is in place as long as vaccinations continue.

# SELF-EVALUATION

## RECALLING KEY TERMS

**Abscess**
**Antigenic drift**
**Antigenic shift**
**Avidity**
**Bacteremia**
**Disease**
**Herd immunity**
**Immunity**
   Active
   **Cell-mediated**
   **Humoral**
   **Innate**
   **Passive**
**Immunization**
**Immunologic memory**
**Infection**
   **Subclinical**
**Lysogenic conversion**
**Malaria**
**Mycoses**
**Pathogen**
   **Opportunistic**
   **Primary**
**Parasite**

Obligate intracellular parasites
Pathogenicity
Primary antibody response
Pus
Secondary antibody response (booster response)
Septicemia
Vaccines
  Conjugated
  DNA
  Inactived
  Live, attenuated
  Peptide
  Recombinant vector
  Subunit
  Toxoid
Vectors
Virulence
  Factors

## MULTIPLE-CHOICE QUESTIONS

*(An answer key is not provided, but the page[s] location of the answer is.)*

1. While IgG is the predominant class formed in the primary response, IgM predominates in the secondary response. (a) true, (b) false. *(See page 570.)*

2. The second portion of the antigen elimination curve (a) may be shortened with the use of adjuvant, (b) is the same for low or high molecular weight antigens, (c) occurs during the same approximate time as antibody appearance, (d) is the same as the third portion in animals tolerant to the antigen, (e) none of these. *(See pages 569 and 570.)*

3. Compared to the primary antibody response, the secondary antibody response is characterized by (a) increasing of the lag phase, (b) lowering of the threshold dose of immunogen, (c) a lower rate of antibody production, (d) shorter persistence of antibody synthesis, (e) none of these. *(See pages 570 and 571.)*

4. Immunologic memory is provided by persisting (a) mature cytotoxic T cells, (b) IgM antibodies, (c) IgG antibodies, (d) memory cells activated to effector cells by rechallenging with previous antigen, (e) none of these. *(See page 571.)*

5. Pathogens can evade immune detection by all the following except (a) binding the IgM's Fc region to block complement activation, (b) altering their antigenic profile, (c) releasing anti-IgA proteases, (d) living in host cells, (e) none of these. *(See pages 564–567.)*

6. Latent viruses in host cells avoid elimination by (a) macrophages or neutrophils, (b) opsonizing antibodies, (c) neutralizing antibodies, (d) cytotoxic T lymphocytes, (e) antibody-dependent cell-mediated cytotoxicity, (f) none of these. *(See pages 581–584.)*

7. Superantigens (a) induce a "super" immune response against the pathogen that induced them, (b) fit into the T-cell antigen receptor's binding site, (c) induce CD8$^+$ T cells to produce cytokines that are immunosuppressive, (d) can lead to symptoms of toxic shock syndrome, (e) none of these. *(See page 592.)*

8. You can develop an antiviral recombinant DNA vaccine by expressing the virus DNA in (a) a genetic variant of the same virus, (b) an adjuvant, (c) polysaccharide-coated molecule, (d) a less virulent bacterial or viral vector, (e) an ISCOM, (f) none of these. *(See pages 603 and 604.)*

9. An advantage of giving passive immunization is that it provides (a) longterm immunity, (b) cell-mediated immunity, (c) faster protection, (d) a safer immunization, (e) none of these. *(See page 599.)*

10. The advantages of Sabin oral polio vaccine over the Salk killed polio vaccine is all except that it (a) induces both antibody- and cell-mediated immunity, (b) is less expensive to administer, (c) induces the formation of neutralizing antibodies, (d) can be administered to immunocompromised individuals (e) is none of these. *(See page 602.)*

11. Passive immunization to a bacterial toxin would be recommended if (a) the individual exhibits immunity to the toxoid, (b) the individual exhibits no immunity to the toxin, (c) the individual exhibits both immunity to the toxin and the toxoid, (d) the individual received the toxoid the day before toxin exposure, (e) it is none of these. *(See page 599.)*

12. Immune stimulatory complexes (ISCOMs) (a) are attenuated vaccines, (b) do not contain an adjuvant, (c) induce only humoral immunity, (d) are self-replicating vectors, (e) transport peptide vaccines into the antigen-presenting cell's cytoplasm for presentation in association with class I MHC molecules, (f) are none of these. *(See page 603.)*

13. DNA vaccines include all the following except that they (a) can be used in a "gene gun," (b) induce both humoral and cell-mediated immunity, (c) augment immunity against polysaccharide antigens, (d) induce only cell-mediated immunity, (e) are none of these. *(See page 604.)*

## SHORT-ANSWER ESSAY QUESTIONS

1. Explain the difference between the following: (a) pathogenicity vs. virulence; (b) opportunistic pathogen vs. primary pathogen; (c) virulent strain vs. attenuated strain; (d) clinical infection vs. subclinical infection; (e) acute infection vs. chronic infection.

2. By what routes might a pathogenic bacterium that enters the body through a cut gain access to the patient's bloodstream?

3. What do we mean by a primary and a secondary immune response? What characteristics usually distinguish the two responses?

4. Briefly discuss the antigen elimination curve. What things affect the shape of the curve, and how does this affect antibody production?

5. Briefly describe the four phases of a primary antibody response.

6. When comparing the primary and secondary antibody responses, three things change during the secondary antibody response. What are they, and which one would you consider the most important and why?

7. By what means can arthropods transmit pathogenic microorganisms to a human?

8. How do the following promote colonization and invasion of tissue? (a) IgA proteases; (b) urease; (c) sheathed flagella; (d) the M protein of *Streptococcus pyogenes*.

9. Contrast the properties of exotoxins with those of endotoxins.

10. In relapsing fever, what accounts for the occurrence of the repeated relapses?

11. Explain how the following contribute to pathogenicity: (a) the gp120/gp41 complex of HIV; (b) the H and N proteins of influenza viruses; (c) the error-prone reverse transcriptase of HIV.

12. Why is cell-mediated immunity regarded as a two-edged sword in infections such as tuberculosis?

13. For immunization against poliomyelitis, what are advantages and disadvantages of the Salk vaccine? Of the Sabin vaccine? Why has use of the Sabin vaccine been discontinued most incidences?

14. Why is it difficult to devise a vaccine against the common cold? Against HIV? Against malaria?

## FURTHER READINGS

The November 2007 issue of *Nat. Immunol.* 8:1141–1193 contains several articles that deal with pathogenesis and immunology.

Akira, S., S. Uematsu, and O. Takeuchi. 2006. Pathogen recognition and innate immunity. *Cell* 124:783–801.

Alcami, A. 2003. Viral mimicry of cytokines, chemokines and their receptors. *Nat. Rev. Immunol.* 3:36–50.

Anthony, R.M., L.I. Rutitzky, J.F. Urban Jr., M.J. Stadecker, and W.C. Gause. 2007. Protective immune mechanism in helminth infections. *Nat. Rev. Immunol.* 7:975–987.

Doherty, P.C., S.J. Turner, R.G. Webby, and P.G. Thomas. 2006. Influenza and the challenge for immunology. *Nat. Immunol.* 7:449–455.

Donnelly, J.J., B. Wahren, and M.A. Liu. 2005. DNA vaccines: Progress and challenges. *J. Immunol.* 175:633–639.

Ertl, H.C.J. 2003. Viral immunology. In *Fundamental Immunology*, 5th ed. W.E. Paul, ed. Philadelphia: Lippincott Williams & Wilkins. p. 1201–1228.

Gruenberg, J., and F.G. van der Goot. 2006. Mechanism of pathogen entry through the endosomal compartment. *Nat. Rev. Immunol.* 7:495–504.

Holt, P.G., D.H. Strickland, M.E. Wikström, and F.L. Jahnsen. 2008. Regulation of immunological homeostasis in the respiratory tract *Nat. Rev. Immunol.* 8:142–152.

Katze, M.G., Y. He, and M. Gale, Jr. 2002. Viruses and interferon: A fight for supremacy. *Nat. Rev. Immunol.* 2:675–687.

Kaufmann, S.H.E. 2003. Immunity to intracellular bacteria. In *Fundamental Immunology*, 5th ed. W.E. Paul, ed. Philadelphia: Lippincott Williams & Wilkins. p. 1229–1262.

Kaufmann, S.H.E. 2006. Envisioning future strategies for vaccination against tuberculosis. *Nat. Rev. Immunol.* 6:699–704.

Kersten, G.F.H., and D.J.A. Crommelin. 2003. Liposomes and ISCOMs. *Vaccine* 21:915–920.

Kumagai, Y., O. Takeuchi, and S. Akira. 2008. Pathogen recognition by innate receptors. *J. Infect. Chemother.* 14:86–92.

Mazmanian, S.K., and D.L. Kasper. 2006. The love–hate relationship between bacterial polysaccharides and the host immune system. *Nat. Rev. Immunol.* 6:849–858.

Nahm, M.H., M.A. Apicella, and D.E. Briles. 2003. Immunity to extracellular bacteria. In *Fundamental Immunology*, 5th ed. W.E. Paul, ed. Philadelphia: Lippincott Williams & Wilkins. p. 1263–1284.

Nossal, G.J.V. 2003. Vaccines. In *Fundamental Immunology*, 5th ed. W.E. Paul, ed. Philadelphia: Lippincott Williams & Wilkins. p. 1319–1370.

Pamer, E.G. 2004. Immune responses to *Listeria monocytogenes*. *Nat. Rev. Immunol.* 4:812–823.

Romani, L. 2004. Immunity to fungal infections. *Nat. Rev. Immunol.* 4:1–13.

Rook, G.A.W., K. Dheda, and A. Zumla. 2005. Immune responses to tuberculosis in developing countries: Implications for new vaccines. *Nat. Rev. Immunol.* 5:661–667.

Rosenberg, C.M., and B.B. Finlay. 2003. Phagocyte sabotage: Disruption of macrophage signaling by bacterial pathogens. *Nat. Rev. Immunol.* 4:385–396.

Sacks, D., and N. Noben-Trauth. 2002. The immunology of susceptibility and resistance to *Leishmania major* in mice. *Nat. Rev. Immunol.* 2:845–858.

Sher, A., T.A. Wynn, and D.L. Sacks. 2003. The immune response to parasites. In *Fundamental Immunology*, 5th ed. W.E. Paul, ed. Philadelphia: Lippincott Williams & Wilkins. p. 1171–1200.

Steveson, M.M. and E.M. Roley. 2004. Innate immunity in malaria. *Nat. Rev. Immunol.* 4:169–180.

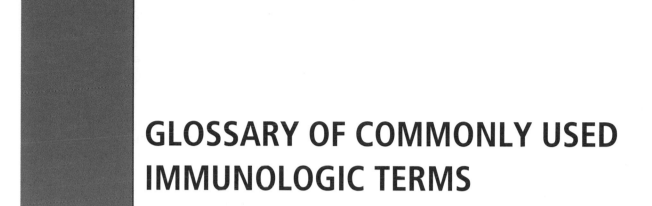

# GLOSSARY OF COMMONLY USED IMMUNOLOGIC TERMS

## A

**ABO blood group:** Human red blood cells (RBCs) are divided into four phenotypes depending on whether they express A, B, AB, or O antigens. These glycosphingolipid antigens, found on RBCs and endothelial cells, can differ between individuals and act as alloantigens during mismatched blood transfusions and hyperacute allograft rejections.

**Abscess:** A localized collection of pus in a cavity formed by tissue disintegration. See also Pus.

**Abzyme:** A monoclonal antibody with catalytic activity.

**Absorption:** An immunological procedure used to remove antigens or antibodies from a mixture. For example, absorption can be accomplished by adding antigen and then removing the antigen-antibody complex.

**Accessibility:** A feature of immunogenicity. Antigenic determinants must be at the surface of molecules to come in contact with antibodies.

**Accessory cells:** Non-lymphoid cells usually of the monocyte and macrophage, or dendritic cell, lineage that cooperate with T cells in the generation of immune responses to protein antigens.

**Accessory molecules:** Lymphocyte cell-surface molecules other than the T cell receptor complex involved in lymphocyte adhesion, T-cell activation, and T-cell migration.

**Acquired immunodeficiency syndrome (AIDS):** The late stage of an often sexual transmitted disease, caused by a retrovirus called *human immunodeficiency virus 1 (HIV-1)*. AIDS is a disease characterized by a defective immune system (centered around decreasing numbers of CD4+ T cells), which leads to opportunistic infections, wasting, malignancies, and encephalopathy, and is generally fatal. See also Human immunodeficiency virus.

**Acquired immunity:** See Adaptive immunity.

**Actinomycin D:** An antibiotic that acts as an immunosuppressant by inhibiting DNA-associated synthesis of RNA. See also Mitomycin C and Puromycin.

**Activated macrophages:** Macrophages that have augmented functions, such as heightened phagocytic ability, due to the action of mediators released by antigen-stimulated T cells.

**Activation-induced cell death (AICD):** The activation of lymphocytes leads to normal eventual apoptotic cell death, that is, activated lymphocytes have inherent programs that make them prone to apoptosis. AICD ensures the rapid removal of effector cells after their antigen-induced clonal expansion, for example, the pathway used by T cell suicide through upregulation of Fas ligand that binds to the death receptor Fas. Dysfunctional AICD is associated with lymphoproliferative autoimmune disorders.

**Activation-induced cytidine deaminase (AID):** A germinal center B cell-specific enzyme required for somatic hypermutation and class-switch recombination of immunoglobulin genes. In class-switch recombination, it deaminates cytidine residues in DNA converting them to uridine residues. The G–U mismatch can then be processed to introduce gaps or nicks on opposite strands of the switch (S)-region DNA. Staggered ends-processing by exonucleases can lead to blunt double-stranded breaks that can then be ligated to similarly created breaks on downstream S-region DNA to complete class-switch recombination.

**Activation phase:** The acquired immune response phase that follows the recognition phase and involves the proliferation of lymphocytes and their differentiation into effector cells. See also Recognition phase and Effector phase.

**Activation protein-1 (AP-1):** A DNA-binding transcription factor family that is composed of dimers of proteins, which bind to one another through a shared structural motif called a *leucine zipper*. The Fos and Jun combination protein is the best described AP-1 factor. AP-1 is important in transcriptional regulation of many immune cell genes (e.g., cytokine genes).

**Active immunity:** Protection (adaptive immunity) developed by an individual through an immune response mediated by his or her own antibodies or sensitized T cells following stimulation with antigen. This is in contrast to passive immunity, where an individual receives antibodies or lymphocytes from another individual that was actively immunized.

**Acute graft rejection:** Acute graft rejection refers to the speed with which a graft such as a kidney is rejected. Usually, the rejection occurs within two weeks of implantation and is due to prior exposure to the donor's transplantation antigens.

**Acute lymphocytic leukemia (ALL):** An aggressive, undifferentiated form of lymphoid malignancy derived from progenitor cells that can give rise to T and B cell lineages. Most leukemias exhibit partial differentiation toward the B cell lineage (called *B-ALL*), a few show features of T cells (called *T-ALL*).

**Acute myelogenous leukemia (AML):** A cancer of myeloid cell lineage, where the proliferating cells usually are in the blood.

**Acute phase proteins:** Serum proteins, mostly synthesized in the liver, that rapidly appear at the start of inflammatory responses. They include C-reactive protein that binds the C-protein of *Pneumococcus* species and facilitates phagocytosis. Mannose-binding protein, serum amyloid A, and fibrinogen are other examples of acute phase proteins. Inflammatory cytokines such as interleukin-6 (IL-6) and tumor necrosis factor (TNF) upregulate acute phase protein production. Acute phase proteins can

be mediators of inflammatory reactions by acting as soluble pattern recognition receptors. See Acute phase response.

**Acute phase response:** Shortly after the start of many infections, there is the rapid production of certain serum proteins (acute phase proteins) by liver cells that provide early innate defense.

**Adapter proteins:** They are proteins, involved in lymphocyte signal transduction pathways that serve as bridge molecules for the recruitment of other signaling molecules. Adapter proteins, during lymphocyte activation, may be phosphorylated on tyrosine residues allowing them to bind other Src homology-2 (SH2) domain-containing proteins. AP-1 proteins involved in T-cell activation include Grb-2, LAT, and SLP-76. See also Src homology-2 (SH2) domain.

**Adaptive immunity:** Immunity that develops due to an exposure (or infection) to a foreign substance or organism (an immunogen) and adapts to the infection. It is mediated by B cells (humoral immunity) and T cells (cell-mediated immunity) that exhibit specificity, memory (may last decades), and diversity. Also called *acquire immunity* or *specific immunity*. This is in contrast to innate immunity, which does not exhibit specificity and memory. See also Innate immunity.

**ADCC:** See Antibody-dependent cell-mediated cytotoxicity.

**Addressins:** Molecules expressed on endothelial cells that bind to ligands on lymphocytes called *homing receptors* (or *selectins*) and direct organ-specific lymphocyte homing; for example, gut-homing T cells express the integrin α4β7 that binds to mucosal addressin cell adhesion molecule-1 (MAdCAM) expressed in Peyer's patches in the intestinal wall. In contrast, lymph node-homing T cells express L-selectin (CD62L) that binds to the CD34 addressin molecules on high endothelial venules in lymph nodes.

**Adenocarcinoma:** A cancer of glandular tissue. See also Carcinoma.

**Adenoids:** They are mucosal-associated lymphoid tissues located in the nasal cavity.

**Adenosine deaminase deficiency:** An enzyme defect that leads to an accumulation of toxic nucleosides and nucleotides, which leads to the death of most developing thymic lymphocytes. It is a cause of severe combined immunodeficiency (SCID).

**Adenosine diphosphate (ADP) ribosylation:** It is the posttranslational modification of proteins by the addition of one or more ADP nucleotides and ribose moieties. This process occurs in cell signaling and the control of many cell activities, such as DNA repair and apoptosis. The bacterial toxins, cholera and pertussis toxins, mediate their activity through ADP-ribosylation. For example, cholera toxin acts on G proteins, which causes the release of large amounts of fluid from the small intestine.

**Adhesion molecule:** A cell surface molecule that promotes adhesive interactions with other cells or extracellular matrix (such as, selectins, integrins, and members of the immunoglobulin superfamily). They play a major role in lymphocyte migration and activation in innate and adaptive immune responses.

**Adjuvant:** A substance injected with an antigen (or better described as an immunogen) that nonspecifically enhances T-cell activation to that immunogen by promoting the accumulation and activation of accessory cells (costimulator expression and cytokine production) at the site of immunogen exposure—increases immunity in general to that immunogen. See also Complete Freund's adjuvant and Incomplete Freund's adjuvant.

**Adoptive transfer:** The transfer of lymphoid cells from an immune donor to a nonimmune recipient.

**Adsorption:** The nonspecific attachment of soluble substances to the surface of some insoluble matrix, such as cells or inert particles.

**Afferent lymphatic vessels:** They drain fluid from tissues and transport macrophages and dendritic cells from infection sites to the lymph nodes.

**Affinity:** The association constant (K liters mole$^{-1}$) of an antibody toward an antigen, measured at equilibrium. It refers to the binding strength and stability between an antibody-combining site and an antigenic determinant.

**Affinity maturation:** The phenomenon by which the average affinity of antibody (usually IgG) increases during an immune response or in the secondary antibody response. Affinity maturation is the result of somatic mutation of immunoglobulin variable-region genes, followed by the selection of higher affinity variants in the germinal center, leading to survival of B cells producing the highest affinity antibodies. Selection is a competitive process in which B cells compete with free antibody to capture decreasing antigen amounts.

**Agglutination:** A secondary antigen-antibody interaction involving the combination of particulate (insoluble) antigen with specific antibody, leading to clumping of the particles.

**Agonist:** A molecule that binds to a receptor and induces it to function.

**Agonist peptides:** Peptides that mimic cognate antigen, which activates specific T cells, causing them to proliferate and to make cytokines.

**Agretope:** The part of an MHC class I or II molecule that associates with the foreign antigen when antigen is processed and presented by an antigen-presenting cell. The derivation is taken from *a*ntigen *re*cognition.

**AID:** See Activation-induced cytidine deaminase.

**AIDS:** See Acquired immunodeficiency syndrome.

**AIRE:** See Autoimmune regulator.

**Alkylating agents:** Immunosuppressive drugs that affect mainly DNA synthesis. They are effective in the inductive phase or throughout the immune response.

**Allele:** An alternate form of a gene that controls a particular characteristic present at a chromosomal locus. Thus, one allele is expressed per haploid genome, leading to intraspecies variance at a particular gene locus. If an individual is heterozygous at a locus, they have two different alleles each on a different pair of chromosomes; one allele is inherited from the mother, the other from the father.

**Allelic exclusion:** The phenotypic expression of a single allele in cells with two different alleles for that locus (heterozygous cells). For example, a B cell has six gene pools, the maternal and the paternal κ, λ, and heavy-chain antibody gene pools. Thus, the B cell must determine whether to express maternal or paternal light and heavy chains, and whether to express κ or λ light chains. Allelic exclusion also involves the T cell receptor β chain but not α chain; therefore, some T cells can express two different T cell receptor types. The process that prevents the production of two different chains is known as allelic exclusion.

**Allergen:** Any substance (an antigen) capable of inducing an allergic response in atopic individuals. Allergens are noninfectious protein molecules, such as house dust mites, plant pollens, and animal danders, or chemicals bond to proteins that induce the formation of IgE antibodies.

**Allergic asthma:** It is the result of bronchial tree constriction due to an allergic reaction to inhaled allergens.

**Allergic conjunctivitis:** An allergic reaction in the lining of the eye (conjunctiva) in sensitized individuals exposed to allergens.

**Allergic rhinitis:** An allergic reaction, also called *hay fever*, in the nasal mucosa that causes a runny nose, sneezing, and tears.

**Allergy:** An immediate hypersensitivity state acquired through exposure to a specific allergen; for example, pollens lead to hay fever. See Atopy, Immediate hypersensitivity, and Type I hypersensitivity.

**Alloantigens:** Different (allelic) forms of an antigen encoded by the same gene locus in all genetically different individuals of a species, such as histocompatibility antigens, A and B blood group antigens, and Rh antigens.

**Allogeneic:** A term used to describe genetically dissimilar individuals within the same species.

**Allograft:** The transplanting of a graft from a donor to a recipient that is genetically dissimilar but within the same species.

**Alloreactivity:** The responsiveness is due to 1 to 3% of T cells (or antibodies) reacting to allo-major histocompatibility complex molecules (i.e., alloantigens).

**Allotypes:** Antibody variants defined by genetically determined antigenic determinants that vary in different members of the same species. In other words, allotypes are products encoded by one allele of a given antibody gene. So allotypes are present in only some members of a species. Allotypic determinants are represented by the Gm and Am markers on the heavy chains of human IgG and IgA molecules, respectively. On the human κ light chain, they are represented by Km determinants.

**Allotypic determinants:** Define antibodies called *allotypes* and are encoded by genes that have several alleles. They are present in the antibodies of some members of a species. See also Allotypes.

**Alpha-fetoprotein:** A tumor-associated antigen that is called an *oncofetal antigen* because it associated with normal fetal tissue and cancerous adult tissue. Antibodies to this protein are used to follow the progression of tumor growth in patients.

**Altered peptide ligands:** Peptides that have altered T cell receptor contact residues, which elicit responses different that caused by the native peptide. These ligands may have importance in the regulation of T-cell activation in physiologic, pathologic, or therapeutic settings.

**Altered self:** The concept describes the binding of foreign (nonself) peptide to an MHC molecule, which creates an MHC-peptide complex that is different from any found in the individual's normal cells.

**Alternative complement pathway:** The activation of the complement system by direct stimulation of the third component of complement (C3) without activation of the first three components (C1, C4, and C2). Usually, antibody molecules are not required for activation of the alternative pathway; instead, molecules or bacterial surfaces directly. See Complement system for a description of the classical pathway of complement activation. See also Lectin pathway of complement activation.

**Alternatively activated macrophages:** Macrophages induced by the T-helper 2 (T$_H$2) cytokines interleukin-4 (IL-4) and IL-13, which leads to a cellular phenotype involved in humoral immunity and repair. They are also called *M2* or *Type-2 macrophages*. They are distinct from classically induced (i.e., by interferon-γ) macrophages. See Macrophage activation.

**Alums:** Compounds of aluminum that precipitate proteins. Alums can be used with proteins to form a tissue deposit that has an adjuvant effect.

**Am determinant:** An allotypic determinant found on the heavy chain of human IgA.

**Aminopterin:** A folic acid analog that inhibits DNA synthesis. It is used in cancer chemotherapy.

**Amplification phase:** The second phase of activation of the classical complement pathway, amplification phase involves the cleavage of C3 into 1000s of molecules that amplify the overall immune response to an antigen. See also Activation phase, Membrane attack phase, and Complement system.

**Anamnestic response (memory):** A heightened responsiveness following a second exposure of an antigen to an immune animal; a secondary immune response. Anamnesis is taken from the Greek for a recalling or nonforgetting.

**Anaphylactic shock:** Shock occurring during systemic anaphylaxis. See Systemic (generalized) anaphylaxis.

**Anaphylatoxin inactivator:** The plasma enzyme carboxypeptidase N. It inactivates the anaphylatoxins C4a and C3a and decreases the activity of C5a.

**Anaphylatoxins:** A group of mediators involved in inflammation that are produced and released in serum during complement activation (derived from the third [C3a] and fifth [C5a] components of complement). These components interact with their counterpart receptors on various cell types. Anaphylatoxins cause mast cells to release histamine, leading to vasodilation, edema, and smooth muscle contraction. These effects are similar to those seen in Type I immediate hypersensitivity reactions.

**Anaphylaxis:** An acute immediate hypersensitivity reaction following a second or subsequent exposure to an allergen. Anaphylaxis can be localized or systemic. Systemic anaphylaxis is the most dire form of allergy and can lead to anaphylactic shock and death.

**Anaplasia:** A loss of ability of cells to differentiation (they dedifferentiate), loss of their orientation to one another and to their axial framework and blood vessels. The combination of anaplasia and metastasis is the major contributor to the malignancy of cancer.

**Anchor residues:** The peptide amino acid residues whose side chains fit into the peptide-binding cleft pockets of class I MHC molecules. The side chains bind to complementary MHC molecule amino acid residues and thereby serve to anchor the peptide in the MHC molecule cleft. Each class I MHC molecule has different patterns of anchor residues thereby allowing it some binding specificity. Class II MHC molecule anchor residues are less obvious for specific peptide binding.

**Anergy:** In clinical practice, an absence of immune reactions in supposedly sensitized individuals. Anergy is seen in advanced cases of *Mycobacterium tuberculosis* infections; the tuberculin test is negative. Lymphocyte anergy, also called *clonal anergy*, is the absence of T and B cell reactivity to antigens; this is a mechanism for maintaining peripheral immunologic tolerance to self-antigens. Anergy can result from incomplete activation signals mediated by low-affinity T cell receptor interactions or a lack of costimulation.

**Anergic T cells:** T cells that are unable to undergo proliferation, secretion of inflammatory cytokines or other functions in response to antigens.

**Angiogenesis:** The formation of new blood vessels from existing blood vessels by proteins that are elaborated by cells of the innate and adaptive immune system. It is frequently associated with inflammation and tumor development.

**Ankylosing spondylitis:** It is a member of a group of inflammatory joint diseases, called *autoimmune spondyloarthropathies*, associated with the expression of the HLA class I molecule HLA-B27. It is a chronic, painful degenerative inflammatory arthritis that targets the spine and sacroiliac joints.

**Annexin-V staining:** Annexin V binds to phosphatidylserine, which is normally located on the plasma membrane's inner layer, but which flips to the outer layer during apoptosis and thus used as an indicator of apoptosis.

**Antagonist:** A molecule that binds to a receptor and prevents it from functioning.

**Antagonist peptide:** A variant peptide ligand, which binds to a T cell receptor, in which one or two T cell receptor contact residues have been changed, leading to the delivery of negative signals to specific T cells thus inhibiting responses to native peptides.

**Antibiotics:** Antimicrobial agents. Some of them have immunosuppressive activity.

**Antibody:** A glycoprotein molecule (also called an *immunoglobulin*) produced by plasma cells in response to stimulation by antigen and capable of specific combination with the antigen that induced its formation. All antibodies are immunoglobulins. Their structural unit is composed of two identical light chains and two identical heavy chains. The amino-terminal variable regions of the light and heavy chains form the antigen-binding sites. Individuals have millions of different antibodies, each with a specific unique antigen-binding site. The COOH-terminal constant regions of the heavy chains functionally interact with other immune system molecules, leading to different effector function. The effector functions of soluble antibodies include neutralizing antigens, activating complement, inducing allergies, passage across placenta, and promoting leukocyte-dependent destruction of microbes. See also Immunoglobulin.

**Antibody affinity:** The strength of antigen-antibody bonds between one epitope and an individual antibody's antigen-binding site.

**Antibody-dependent cell-mediated cytotoxicity (ADCC):** A form of cytotoxicity in which Fcγ receptor III (CD16)-bearing natural killer (NK) cells recognize and kill antibody-coated target cells by interacting with the Fc portion of the target-bound antibody. The interaction initiates a signaling cascade that leads to the release of cytotoxic granules, which induce apoptosis of the antibody-coated target cells. The target-bound antibody is usually IgG. Macrophages and neutrophils are also capable of mediating ADCC.

**Antibody excess zone:** The first part of the precipitin curve, where the lattice has a high ratio of antibody to antigen. If there is free antigen, the precipitate formed is less than maximum. See also Antigen excess zone, Equivalence zone, and Zone phenomenon.

**Antibody feedback:** The mechanism that inhibits antibody formation by secreted IgG antibodies when antigen-antibody complexes simultaneously engage B-cell membrane immunoglobulin and Fcγ receptors, which transduce inhibitory signals inside the B cell.

**Antibody fragments:** See Fab fragment, F(ab')$_2$ fragment, and Fc fragment.

**Antibody (or T cell receptor) repertoire:** It is the total variety of antibodies (or T cell antigen receptors) of an individual.

**Antibody-secreting cells:** Cells that encompasses both plasmablasts, which proliferate, and plasma cells, which do not proliferate. It is a term generally used when both cell types are present. See also Plasmablasts and Plasma cells.

**Antibody subclasses:** Isotypic heavy-chain determinants that define differences within the antibody class (e.g., IgG1, IgG2, IgG3, and IgG4, and IgA1 and IgA2). See also Immunoglobulin subclasses.

**Antibody valence:** See Valence.

**Antigen:** Any molecule that binds specifically to an antibody or T cell receptor—word initially derived from the ability to *generate anti*bodies. The definition is arbitrary, since specific responsiveness is a property of the host, not of the antigen. All classes of molecules can bind to antibodies. In contrast, protein-derived peptides complexed with MHC molecules can bind to T cell receptors. It also is described as a substance that elicits a specific immune response when introduced into the body. See also Immunogen.

**Antigen-antibody complexes:** See Immune complex.

**Antigen 2:** A protein in strains of mice discovered by Peter Gorer. It is found only in some strains and is correlated with graft rejection. See also H-2.

**Antigen-binding site (or antibody combining site):** The surface of the antibody molecule that makes physical contact with an epitope of an antigen. This site is composed of six hypervariable loops (also called *complementarity-determining regions [CDRs]*), three from the light-chain variable region and three from the heavy-chain variable region. See also Complementarity-determining regions (CDRs) and Hypervariable regions.

**Antigen display libraries:** These libraries include the cDNA clones of expression vectors and bacteriophage libraries that encode random peptide sequences, which are used to identify specific antibody targets.

**Antigen excess zone:** The last part of the precipitin curve, where the lattice has a lower ratio of antibody to antigen than in the equivalence zone. Once the ratio falls below a threshold, the lattice is soluble. Because there is free antigen, the precipitate does not reach maximum. See also Antibody excess zone, Equivalence zone, and Zone phenomenon.

**Antigenic determinant (epitope):** A small, restricted site on an antigen molecule that induces immunity, that is a site to which antibody or the T cell antigen receptor-peptide-MHC complex can specifically bind.

**Antigenic drift:** The result of spontaneous point mutations in pathogen genes that causes structural differences in surface antigens, leading to strain differences. This leads to the year-to-year differences in influenza strains.

**Antigenic peptides:** Protein antigen fragments that bind to MHC molecules; class I MHC molecules accommodate 8–9 amino acid-long peptides, whereas class II MHC molecules accommodate 13–18 amino

acid-long peptides. These peptide-MHC complexes are recognized by the T cell receptor and can induce immune responses.

**Antigenic shift:** The process whereby influenza viruses reassort their segmented genomes with one another and thereby change their surface antigens radically. The new viruses resulting from this process are the cause of influenza pandemics.

**Antigenic variation:** A mechanism whereby many pathogens evade adaptive immune responses by displaying new antigens that are not recognized by antibodies or T cells elicited in earlier infections.

**Antigen presentation:** The event that follows antigen-processing whereby the antigen is presented to lymphocytes in a form they can recognize. The cells that perform this function are called *antigen-presenting cells* (*APCs;* usually thought of as macrophages or dendritic cells and B cells), but any nucleated cell may serve as an APC. If antigen is presented to T cells, it is associated with class I or II MHC molecules.

**Antigen-presenting cells (APCs):** Usually a variety of lymphoid cells that carry/present antigenic peptides in the context of class II MHC molecules and deliver co-stimulatory signals that can stimulate lymphocytes. Professional APCs are represented by macrophages, dendritic cells, and B cells. Nonprofessional APCs present peptide for short periods of time; they include thymic epithelial cells and vascular endothelial cells.

**Antigen processing:** The series of antigen degradation events that occur between exposure to an antigen and eventual antibody production or T-cell activity. Usually thought of as the interaction of antigen with antigen-presenting cells (APCs) that leads to the degradation of the antigen via two pathways yielding antigen-derived peptides, which are displayed in MHC molecules on APCs and altered self-cells (target cells) to T cells.

**Antigenic modulation:** The disappearance of antigenic determinants from cells when in the presence of specific antibody.

**Antigenic site mobility:** The mobility of antigenic determinants contributes to the immunogenicity and antigenicity of proteins.

**Antigenicity:** The potential of an antigen to react with the specific antibodies or T cell receptor/MHC complexes it induces. The terms *antigen* and *antigenicity* versus *immunogen* and *immunogenicity* are generally used interchangeably. See also Immunogenicity.

**Antigen-specific:** A phrase to describe interactions confined to antibodies and cells that bind an appropriate antigen.

**Anti-idiotopes (AB$_2$):** Antibodies that react with the idiotopes of other antibodies.

**Anti-metabolic agents:** Immunosuppressive drugs that cause faulty cell metabolism.

**Anti-immunoglobulin antibodies:** Antibodies produced against immunoglobulin constant regions that are used for detecting bound antibodies in immunoassays and in characterizing antibodies. There are three levels of anti-immunoglobulin antibodies: anti-isotype antibodies that are made in a different species against markers in the constant region; anti-allotype antibodies that are made in the same species against allotypic markers in the constant region; and anti-idiotype antibodies that are made against unique determinants in the variable of a single antibody.

**Antiserum (plural: antisera):** Serum, the fluid portion of clotted blood, from any animal or individual that contains antibodies against a particular antigen.

**Antitoxins:** Antibodies that neutralize the effects of toxins.

**AP-1:** A family of transcription factors that participate in lymphocyte activation. See Activation protein-1 (AP-1).

**APCs:** See Antigen-presenting cells.

**Aplastic anemia:** Bone marrow stem cells fail to form, leading to a cease in formation of all blood elements. It can be treated by bone marrow transplantation.

**Apoptosis:** The morphologic changes associated with programmed cell death. These include decreased cell volume, membrane blebbing, condensation of chromatin, and degradation of the DNA into multiples of <180 base pair fragments, which causes the cell to break up into many membrane-bound apoptotic bodies that are phagocytosed without inducing inflammation, unlike necrosis, which leads to damage of surrounding cells. Apoptosis is important in lymphocyte development, control of lymphocyte response to antigens, and maintenance of tolerance to self-antigens. See also Programmed cell death.

**Apoptosome:** An apoptotic protein complex that forms when mitochondrial cytochrome $c$ is released and interacts with the cytosolic protein apoptotic-protease-activating factor 1 (APAF1), which recruits pro-caspase-9. This interaction leads to the activation of caspase-9 and the formation of a caspase-3–activation complex, leading to cell death.

**Appendix:** A gut-associated lymphoid tissue located at the start of the colon.

**Arginase:** An enzyme that converts L-arginine into L-ornithine and urea.

**Arthus reaction:** A local inflammatory reaction characterized by necrosis, occurring a few hours after intradermal inoculation of antigen into an animal previously immunized to the same antigen. The immunized animal has high titers of precipitating IgG antibodies. It is an example of a Type III hypersensitivity.

**Ascites:** The effusion of serious fluids into the peritoneal cavity, caused by tumor cells growing in the peritoneal cavity. Hybridomas grown in the peritoneal cavity of mice produce ascites containing high concentrations of monoclonal antibody.

**Association constant (K):** The mathematical representation of the affinity between antigen and antibody, which measures the extent of a reversible association between antigen and antibody at equilibrium. Association constant is represented by the reaction: $Ag + Ab \rightarrow \, <-Ag - Ab$ and the equation $K = [Ag - Ab]/[Ag][Ab]$

**Associate recognition:** A hypothesis for T cell recognition of foreign antigens. T cells recognize processed antigen, that is, antigen that has bound to an MHC molecule; the resulting combination is recognized by T cells. See also Altered self.

**Ataxia-telangiectasia:** An immunodeficiency disease characterized by multiple disorganized blood vessels. It involves both T and B cells with thymic hypoplasia and serum immunoglobulin deficiency. The immunodeficiency results from the lack of a protein called *ATM* that contains a kinase important in signaling of double-stranded DNA breaks, and thus leading to problems in proliferation of lymphocytes.

**Atopy:** It means "strange disease" and was invented to describe a genetic tendency to develop Type I IgE-mediated immediate hypersensitivity states (allergy) such as hay fever and allergic asthma.

**Attenuated vaccine:** A vaccine composed of living infectious organisms that exhibit low virulence. Such organisms stimulate active protective immunity but are unable to cause serious disease.

**Attenuation of virulence:** Elimination or reduction of disease-causing potential.

**Autoantibodies:** Antibodies that are formed against self-antigens.

**Autoantigens (self-antigens):** Antigens that make up the normal constituents of the body and that can stimulate an immune response in the same individual in autoimmune disease.

**Autochthonous:** Designates self-constituents that arise within an individual, such as a tumor, which is an autochthonous transplant.

**Autocoupling haptens:** A group of haptens that can spontaneously couple to a carrier, such as the breakdown products of penicillin.

**Autocrine (factor):** The manner in which a cell produces a factor that acts on itself, such as the interleukin-2 (IL-2) molecule does by acting on the same CD4$^+$ T cell that make it; thus, IL-2 is an autocrine T cell growth factor that stimulates mitosis of the T cell that produced it.

**Autograft:** A graft between genetically identical individuals within the same species. For example, an autograft can occur between identical twins or inbred animals, or can even simply be the transplanting of tissue from one location to another on the same individual.

**Autoimmune hemolytic anemia:** An autoantibody-mediated disease. The low levels of red blood cells (anemia) results from the binding of autoantibodies to red blood cell surface antigens, leading to lysis of the red blood cells.

**Autoimmune polyendocrinopathy-candidiasis ectodermal dystrophy (APECED):** A rare human autoimmune syndrome also called *Autoimmune Polyendocrinopathy Syndrome type 1 (APS-1)*, which is characterized by various autoimmune diseases, the most common are hypoparathyroidism, primary adrenocortical failure, and chronic mucocutaneous candidiasis. It is caused by mutations in the APECED gene that encodes autoimmune regulator (AIRE). See Autoimmune regulator.

**Autoimmune regulator (AIRE):** Autoimmune regulator (AIRE) is a protein that is primarily expressed in the thymus, mostly by medullary epithelial cells and at much lower levels by dendritic cells. It regulates the ectopic expression of a range of genes that encode peripheral-tissue self-antigens. This expression allows maturing thymocytes to become tolerant of peripheral-tissue self-antigens, thereby reducing the incidence of autoimmune diseases.

**Autoimmune thrombocytopenic purpura:** This disease results from the reaction of antibodies against platelets. When antibody binds to the platelets, Fc receptor and complement receptor-bearing cells take-up the platelets, causing a drop in platelet counts that leads to bleeding (purpura).

**Autoimmunity:** Immunity to one's own body constituents that occurs when mechanisms of self-tolerance fail.

**Autologous:** Cells or tissues derived from the same individual.

**Autophagy:** A catabolic process that literally means, "to digest oneself"; it involves the sequestration and degradation of a cell's own components through a lysosomal pathway. The cell performs these activities to recycle nutrients, remodel and dispose of unwanted cytoplasmic constituents. Autophagy is also important in immunological control of bacterial, parasitic, and viral infections.

**Autoradiography:** A method used to locate radio-isotope-labeled materials, which have been separated in gels or are present in blots. The location of the radiolabeled material is determined by overlaying the test material with a photographic film.

**Autoreactive lymphocytes:** Cells that can react with autoantigens, sometimes leading to an autoimmune reaction.

**Autosomal:** Not on the X and Y (sex) chromosomes.

**Autosomes:** Chromosomes other than the X and Y sex chromosomes.

**Average affinity:** The average strength of antigen-antibody bonds. See Average intrinsic association constant.

**Average intrinsic association constant ($K_0$):** A measure of average affinity. See Average affinity.

**Avidity:** A measurement of the binding strength of an antiserum toward a complex antigen. The avidity depends on the affinity of the various antibodies present in the antiserum. Thus, it is a composite description of the overall antigen-antibody interaction. Avidity depends on both on the valency and the affinity of interactions. T cell receptor avidity is determined by the direct binding affinities of multiple cell-bound T cell receptor molecules for peptide-MHC complexes.

**Azathioprine (Imuran):** A purine antimetabolite that preferentially suppresses antibody responses. It is also used to prevent allograft rejection. See also 6-Mercaptopurine.

## B

**B7-1 (CD80):** A costimulatory protein ligand for CD28 and an inhibitory ligand when it interacts with CTLA-4. B7-1 is expressed on dendritic cells, activated macrophages, and activated B cells. See also CTLA-4.

**B7-2 (CD86):** A costimulatory protein ligand for CD28 and an inhibitory ligand when it interacts with CTLA-4. B7-2 is expressed on dendritic cells, activated macrophages, and activated B cells. See also CTLA-4.

**B cells (B lymphocytes):** Lymphocytes derived from the bone marrow in mammals, and in fowls, from the bursa of Fabricius. B cells express surface antibodies (immunoglobulins) that act as receptors for specific antigens. B cells play the major role in humoral immunity because after interaction with antigen and other lymphoid cells or their factors, B cells proliferate and differentiate into antibody-forming cells, called *plasma cells*. The plasma cells produce antibody molecules with the same specificity as their B cell surface-bound antibody counterparts.

**B-1 cells (also called *CD5 B cells*):** A Mac-1 (CD11b) and CD5-expressing population of B lymphocytes whose immunoglobulin receptors are generated by somatic recombination but have limited diversity. B-1 cells seem to be specific for bacterial associated polysaccharide and lipid antigens. They produce IgM antibodies, called *natural antibodies*, against bacteria common in the environment; these antibodies have a low affinity and broad specificity, which provide protection for microbes that penetrate epithelial barriers. B-1 cells also recognize self-components. B-1 cells may be self-renewing and found mainly in the peritoneal and pleural cavities. They do not depend on MHC class II-mediated T-cell help.

**B-2 cells (also called *conventional B cells*):** The main population of B lymphocytes that express B220 and CD23 but do not express CD5 or Mac-1, that arise from stem cells in the bone marrow, and secrete antibody of high affinity and specificity within the secondary lymphoid organs.

**B-cell activation factor (BAFF):** BAFF is a member of the tumor necrosis factor family, which is a survival factor for B cell maturation at a critical immune checkpoint. Overproduction of BAFF can lead to autoimmunity.

**B-cell coreceptor:** A three-protein complex, including CR2 (also called *CD21*), CD19, and TAPA-1 (CD81), that is associated with the B-cell receptor complex. The B-cell coreceptor amplifies the activation signal induced by cross-linking of B-cell receptors (i.e., immunoglobulins) by microbial antigen. See also B-cell receptor complex.

**B-cell mitogens:** They are substances that cause B cells to proliferate, irrespective of their antigen specificity.

**B-cell receptor complex:** The complex formed by the association of two invariant signal-transducing Ig-α/Ig-β molecules (also called *CD79a* and *CD79b*, respectively) with a membrane-bound immunoglobulin molecule. It is essential in B cell signal transduction.

**B-cell-specific activator protein (BSAP):** A *Pax-5* gene encoded transcription factor that is important in early and later stages of B-cell development.

**B-cell tyrosine kinase (Btk):** A Src family tyrosine kinase that plays an essential role in B-cell maturation. X-linked agammaglobulinemia, a disease characterized by failure of B cells to mature beyond the pre-B cell stage, is caused by mutations in the gene encoding Btk.

**Bacteremia:** A condition in which bacteria are present in the bloodstream.

**BAFF:** See B-cell activation factor.

**BALT:** See Bronchial-associated lymphoid tissue.

**Bare lymphocyte syndrome:** An autosomal recessive form of severe combined immunodeficiency disease. It is a deficiency in major histocompatibility class II gene expression. The inability to express class II molecules leads to a failure to present antigen to CD4$^+$ T cells.

**Basement membrane:** A specialized form of extracellular matrix that consists of a number glycoproteins that separates epithelia from underlying supporting tissues. Different organs have different compositions of basement membrane.

**Basophils:** A multinucleated leukocyte with granules containing acid glycoproteins that binds basic dyes leading to a blue color. When these granules release their contents, anaphylactic reactions may result. They express high-affinity Fc receptors for IgE. Bone marrow-derived basophils can be considered the circulating version of mast cells. They are recruited into tissue that contains allergen responsible for immediate hypersensitivity reactions.

**Bb:** It is the large active component of complement factor B. Bb is produced when bound C3b captures factor B and is cleaved by factor D. The resulting Bb remains attached to C3b and thereby becomes the serine protease component of the alternative complement pathway C3 convertase.

**Backcross:** The mating of an F$_1$ animal with one of its parents.

**BCG:** *Bacillus Calmette-Guerin* (BCG) is an attenuated strain of the tuberculosis organism found in cattle. It is used now as a living attenuated vaccine against the human form of tuberculosis.

**Bcl-2 family (B-cell-lymphoma-2 family):** Mitochondrial proteins encode by the *bcl-2* or *Bcl-xl* genes that protect cells from apoptosis by binding to the mitochondrial membrane. When the levels of either Bcl-2 or Bcl-xl are increased, a cell is more resistant to cell death.

**Beige mouse:** The beige (bg) mutant mouse lacks natural killer (NK) cells and has impaired macrophage mobility and chemotaxis.

**Bence-Jones protein:** Free monoclonal immunoglobulin light chains found in the urine of patients with multiple myeloma. They were one of the first sources of homogenous preparations of immunoglobulin light chains used in characterization studies. Bence-Jones protein has an unusual temperature sensitivity profile: it precipitates when the urine is heated at 60°C, and redissolves at higher temperatures.

**Benign tumors:** Tumors that lack the capacity to invade surrounding normal tissues (opposite of malignant). See Malignant tumor.

**β procedure:** A precipitin test, also called the *Ramon procedure*, in which the tubes contain the same amount of antigen to which serial dilutions of antibody are added. The results are expressed as a titer of the highest dilution (or smallest amount) of antibody that will cause precipitation with a given amount of antigen.

**β sheet (β barrel or β sandwich):** It is one of the fundamental structural building blocks of proteins. It is composed of adjacent, extended strands of amino acids (the β strands) that are bonded together by amide and carbonyl groups. β sheets can be parallel or antiparallel. All immunoglobulin domains are constructed of antiparallel β-sheet structures; also called the *immunoglobulin-fold*.

**$\beta_2$-microglobulin:** A non-MHC (human chromosome 15, mouse chromosome 2) gene-encoded polypeptide of 11,600 molecular weight that is associated with class I MHC molecules. It is invariant among all class I MHC molecules and is structurally homologous to an immunoglobulin domain. In the absence of $\beta_2$-microglobulin, MHC class II molecules are structurally unstable.

**Biogenic amines:** See Vasoactive amines.

**Biologic response modifiers:** In cancer immunotherapy, products that lead to direct inhibition of tumor growth, stimulation of general immune defenses, or both. In general, they are molecules that are clinical modulators of inflammation, immunity, and hematopoiesis.

**Biotin:** It is a small (mw 244) molecule (a vitamin essential for fat synthesis) that can be coupled to antibodies (or any protein molecule), a target for detection by fluorescently or enzymatically labeled avidin or streptavidin. See Streptavidin.

**Bispecific antibodies:** Hybrid antibodies that are either produced by chemically cross-linking to two different antibodies or by fusing hybridomas that make two different monoclonal antibodies in which each of two antigen-binding sites is specific for separate antigenic determinants.

**Blast cell:** A cell, usually large, undergoing division and containing high amounts of RNA in the cytoplasm and actively synthesizing DNA. For example, the stage of T or B cells between resting cells and effector cells following antigen stimulation.

**Blastogenesis:** The generation of blast cells following exposure to antigen or mitogen (also called *blast transformation*).

**Blocking antibodies:** Antibodies that inhibit the access to an antigenic determinant with its appropriate soluble or cellular receptor.

**Blood group antigens:** Chemical markers on the surface of red blood cells. These markers distinguish the red blood cells of one individual from those of another individual.

**Blood typing:** Before administering a blood transfusion, the donor and recipient blood is characterized to determine whether they have the same ABO and Rh blood group antigens.

**Bloom's syndrome:** It is a disease caused by mutations in a DNA helicase, which leads to low T-cell numbers, reduced antibody levels, increased respiratory infections, and cancer.

**B-lymphocyte chemokine (BLC):** A CXC chemokine that attracts B cells and activated T cells into peripheral lymphoid tissue follicles by binding to the CXCR5 receptor.

**B-lymphocyte stimulator (BLyS):** A TNF family cytokine that is secreted by T cells and plays a role in germinal center and plasma cell formation, and maybe dendritic cell maturation.

**Blotting:** Following the separation of proteins in a polyacrylamide gel, the proteins are transferred onto nitrocellulose. The blotted proteins are then identified by immunochemical means. See Immunoblotting.

**BLyS:** See B-lymphocyte stimulator (BLyS).

**Bone marrow:** It is the site for the generation of cellular elements of the blood (hematopoiesis), including monocytes, polymorphonuclear leukocytes, platelets, and red blood cells. It is also the site of B-cell development and the source for stem cells that migrate to the thymus and give rise to T cells.

**Bone marrow chimeras:** Blends of normally incompatible tissues. Chimeras are animals containing cells from two genetically different parents.

**Bone marrow-derived cells:** These lymphoid cells populate one of the lymphoid organs, originate in the bone marrow, and are not influenced by the thymus. All lymphoid cells originate in the bone marrow. It also is the site of B-cell maturation.

**Bone marrow transplantation:** The transplanting of bone marrow into a recipient. The transplant contains stem cells, which give rise to all blood cells including lymphocytes. It is clinically performed to remedy malignancies and hematopoietic disorders.

**Booster immunization:** A readministration of antigen after a primary immunization to increase antibody titers.

**Bovine:** Material derived from a cow.

**Bradykinin:** A kinin that is involved in inflammatory reactions. Kinins are generated following tissue injury. Of the kinins, bradykinin is the most important and is involved in vasodilation, smooth muscle contraction, and increased vascular permeability.

**Brambell receptor (FcRB):** An FcR with a class I MHC molecule-like structure that transports IgG across epithelia.

**5-Bromodeoxyuridine:** A pyrimidine antimetabolite (i.e., a thymidine analogue that is incorporated into DNA during DNA replication) used mainly to depress antibody formation and tumor growth and, to a lesser extent, cellular immunity. See also Cytosine arabinoside and 5-Fluorouracil.

**Bronchial-associated lymphoid tissue (BALT):** The lymphoid cells and tissues in the respiratory tract that are important in the induction of immune responses of inhaled antigens and respiratory infections.

**Bronchocarcinoma:** A cancer of the lungs, which arises from the bronchus. See also Carcinoma.

**Bruton's agammaglobulinemia:** See X-linked agammaglobulinemia.

**Burkitt's lymphoma:** A malignant B-cell cancer that is associated with a reciprocal chromosomal translocation of immunoglobulin gene loci and the chromosome 8 cellular c-myc gene. In many instances, Epstein-Barr virus causes it.

**Bursa of Fabricius:** A lymphoepithelial hindgut organ located in the cloaca of birds, responsible for the maturation of B cells. There is no anatomical equivalent in humans; the human bone marrow seems to be its functional counterpart. Bursectomy, removal of the bursa of Fabricius, leads to the inability of birds to develop antibodies.

**Bystander lysis:** Occurs when cells near to a site of complement activation are lysed because complement components are deposited on them.

# C

**C (constant) genes:** The antibody or T cell receptor constant (C)-region genes, located downstream (3′) of the V, (D), and J genes, that encode the constant regions of an antibody heavy or light chain and T cell receptor $\alpha\beta$ or $\gamma\delta$ chains.

**C1:** The first component in the complement cascade. In activation of the classical pathway, the first event is the noncovalent binding of C1 (specifically the C1q molecules) to sites on the Fc region of two adjacent IgG antigen and single IgM-antigen complexed antibodies.

**C1 inhibitor (C1-INH):** Controls the classical pathway to complement activation by combining with the active site on activated C1r, destroying its protease activity and so preventing C1s from cleaving C4 and C2. C1-INH deficiency causes the disease angioneurotic edema.

**C1q, C1r, C1s:** Noncovalently bound glycoproteins that form C1 in serum.

**C2:** The third component in the complement cascade of the classical pathway. When it becomes activated, it splits into C2a and C2b.

**C2a, C2b:** The two molecules resulting from the cleavage of C2. C2a binds to C4b, forming C4b2a (C3 convertase).

**C3:** The third component of the complement system, and the pivotal molecule in both the classical complement pathway, the alternative pathway, and the lectin pathway. It is responsible for the amplification phase of complement activation. See also Complement system, Alternative pathway, Amplification phase, and Lectin pathway of complement activation.

**C3a, C3b:** The two main molecules resulting from the cleavage of C3. C3a is an anaphylatoxin. Some C3b is deposited on the membrane of the target cell, where it serves as a site for attachment of phagocytic cells and as an opsonin. Other C3b becomes associated with C4b2a (C3 convertase) to form C4b2a3b (C5 convertase).

**C3b/C4b receptor (CR1; CD35):** A regulatory protein that mediates the homeostatic maintenance of complement activation on cells.

**C3 convertase:** An enzyme of the complement system that cleaves C3 into C3a and C3b. In the classical complement pathway, it is formed from a membrane-bound C4b molecule complexed with C2b. In the alternative complement pathway, it uses a homologous C3 convertase, a membrane-bound C3b complexed with Bb. Both convertases catalyze the deposition of many C3b molecules, leading to opsonization of coated organisms.

**C3dg:** A breakdown product of C3b that remains attached to the microbe's surface, where it can bind to the complement receptor CR2 (CD21).

**C4:** The second component in the complement cascade of the classical pathway. When it becomes activated, it splits into C4a and C4b. See C4a, C4b.

**C4a, C4b:** The two molecules resulting from the cleavage of C4. C4a has anaphylatoxin activity. C4b attaches to the surface of the target cell near the antigen-antibody-C1 complex and acts as an anchor for C2a.

**C4-binding protein (C4-bp):** A regulatory protein that mediates the homeostatic maintenance of complement activation in plasma.

**C5:** The fifth component in the complement cascade of the classical pathway. When it is activated, the membrane attack complex starts to form.

**C5a, C5b:** The two molecules resulting from the cleavage of C5. C5a has anaphylatoxin activity and chemotactic activity. C5b starts the assemble of C6 to C9 (membrane attack complex) by acting as an anchor for C6.

**C5 convertase:** An enzyme of the complement system that cleaves C5 into C5a and C5b.

**C5a receptor:** A receptor that binds to the C5a complement fragment, which couples to heterotrimeric G protein.

**C6 to C9:** The sixth to ninth components in the complement cascade of the classical and alternative pathway. One molecule each of C6, C7, C8 unite with 10–16 C9 molecules to form the membrane attack complex.

**Cachexia:** Severe weight loss, muscle wasting, and debility caused by prolonged disease, mediated through neuroimmunoendrocrine interactions.

**Calcineurin:** A cytosolic serine/threonine phosphatase that has a role in signaling through the T cell receptor (TCR). It is activated by calcium signals generated through TCR-antigen binding, which initiates dephosphorylation of the transcription nuclear factor of activated T cells (NFAT) leading to activation of NFAT. The immunosuppressive drugs cyclosporin A and FK506 (tacrolimus) complex with immunophilins that bind and inactivate calcineurin, leading to suppressed T-cell responses.

**Calnexin:** The first molecular chaperone (a molecule that facilitates the folding of polypeptides) involved in class I MHC molecule assembly (and other immunoglobulin superfamily proteins). It associates with the free class I $\alpha$ chain and promotes its folding. When $\beta_2$-microglobulin associates with the $\alpha$ chain, calnexin is released and the $\alpha$ chain-$\beta_2$-microglobulin complex associates with the chaperones calreticulin and tapasin. Tapasin (TAP-associated protein) brings the TAP molecule close to the class I molecule and allows it to acquire an antigenic peptide.

**Calreticulin:** See Calnexin.

**CAMs:** See Cell-adhesion molecules.

**Cancer:** A malignant tumor.

**Cancer stem cells:** A small population of undifferentiated cancer cells that give rise to differentiated cancer cells. The stem cells may account for the relapse of conventional cancer treatment.

**Capping:** The movement to, and accumulation of, cell surface antigens at one pole of a cell after the antigens are cross-linked by specific antibody. Capping seems to precede internalization of the "patch" of antigen-antibody complexes.

**Carcinoembryonic antigen (CEA; CD66):** A tumor-associated antigen that is called an *oncofetal antigen* because it associated with normal fetal tissue and cancerous adult tissue (such as the colon, pancreas, stomach, and breast). Serum levels increase during these cancers. The serum levels are used to monitor the persistence and recurrence of cancer after treatment.

**Carcinogen:** Any biological (e.g., some viruses), chemical (e.g., methylcholanthrene), or physical (e.g., irradiation) means/substance capable of causing cancer.

**Carcinoma:** A tumor originating in epithelial cells, such as the skin and the lining of the digestive or respiratory tract. More than 80% of cancers are carcinomas.

**Carrier effect:** To obtain a secondary immune response to a hapten, the animal must be immunized with the homologous hapten-carrier conjugate. This phenomenon provides evidence for the cooperation between T and B cells specific for different determinants on the same antigen.

**Carrier molecule:** A macromolecule to which a hapten has been conjugated, rendering the hapten immunogenic or capable of stimulating an immune response.

**Caseation necrosis:** This type of necrosis is seen in tuberculosis, where death of tissue results in an appearance that resembles cottage cheese.

**Caspases:** The term is derived from *c*ysteine, *asp*artate, and prote*ase* because it is a family of intracellular cysteine proteases that cleaves after aspartate residues. These proteases are important in the chain of reactions that lead to apoptosis. The lymphocyte caspases are activated either by mitochondrial permeability changes in growth factor-deprived cells or by signals from death receptors in the plasma membrane. Caspases can be divided into proinflammatory caspases 1, 4, 5, and 11, which cleave and activate proinflammatory cytokines, and proapoptotic caspases, which cleave and activate proapoptotic substrates. Proapoptotic caspases comprise initiator caspases 2, 8, and 9, which, in turn, cleave and activate effector caspases 3, 6, and 7. Caspases 2, 8, and 9 is activated after DNA damage, after death receptor ligation, and after apoptosome activation, respectively. Caspases 3, 6, and 7 are important in the dismantling of cellular structures.

**Catalytic antibodies:** They bind their specific antigen, chemically change it, and then release it.

**Cathepsins:** They are broad specificity thiol and aspartyl proteases that are the most abundant endosomal proteases in antigen-presenting cells. They mediate the generation of exogenous antigen peptide fragments that associated with class II MHC molecules

**C-C subgroup:** The largest chemokine subgroup in which a disulfide bond links adjacent cysteines. See also Chemokines.

**CD molecules:** See Cluster of differentiation molecules.

**CD1:** They are a family of nonMHC-encoded class I-like molecules involved in antigen presentation; however, they do not present peptides but lipids or glycolipids to some T cells (such as $\gamma\delta$ T cells). They are molecules capable of presenting nonpeptide antigens to some T cells. There are a group of CD1-restricted cells called *NKT cells*.

**CD2 (LFA-2):** A member of the Ig-gene superfamily, it enhances antigen-specific functions by acting as a cell adhesion molecule that binds to CD58 (LFA-3). It was formerly called *lymphocyte function-associated antigen-2 (LFA-2)*.

**CD3 complex:** A polypeptide complex containing three dimers (a $\gamma\epsilon$ heterodimer, a $\epsilon\delta$ heterodimer, and either a $\zeta\zeta$ homodimer or a $\zeta\eta$ heterodimer) that is closely associated with the human T cell receptor and functions in signal transduction. CD3 $\zeta\zeta$ heterodimer has ITAMs, which become phosphorylated after T cell receptor binding to antigen/MHC, allowing it to bind tyrosine kinases thereby initiating a cascade of activation steps. It is essential in TCR signal transduction and in the cell-surface expression of the TCR. See also ITAMs, ZAP-70, Zeta ($\zeta$) chain.

**CD4:** A member of the Ig-gene superfamily. It defines T-cell functional responses by acting as a coreceptor on class II MHC-restricted T cells. Generally, helper T cells are CD4$^+$. It is also the receptor for human immunodeficiency virus (HIV).

**CD4$^+$CD25$^+$ regulatory T (T$_{reg}$) cell:** A specialized CD4$^+$ T-cell subset that can suppress other T cell responses. These "classic" regulatory T cells are CD4$^+$CD25$^+$FOXP3$^+$ T cells. They are characterized by IL-2 receptor $\alpha$-chain (CD25) expression and some activation markers. The FOXP3 transcription factor is specifically expressed by these cells and contributes to their suppressor activity—FOXP3 is a master regulator of T$_{reg}$ cells. T$_{reg}$ cells constitutively express, and are functionally associated with, CTLA-4. Dysfunctional T$_{reg}$ cells or their absence leads to with severe autoimmunity. During tumor growth, T$_{reg}$ cells are induced and proliferate, which leads to suppressed anti-tumor immunity. See also Regulatory T (T$_{reg}$) cells.

**CD5 B cells:** See B-1 cells.

**CD8:** A member of the Ig-gene superfamily. It defines T-cell functional responses by acting as a coreceptor on class I MHC-restricted T cells. Generally, cytotoxic T cells are CD8$^+$.

**CD8$\alpha\alpha^+$ intestinal epithelial lymphocyte:** A type of T cell that is found in the intestinal epithelium, which expresses the homodimer of CD8$\alpha$, rather than the CD8$\alpha\beta$ heterodimer that is expressed by conventional lymph nodes CD8$^+$ T cells. They may be self-reactive T cells that have regulatory properties. See also IELs.

**CD11aCD18 (lymphocyte function-associated antigen-1 [LFA-1]):** A member of the integrin family. It is needed for B-cell responses, T-cell-mediated killing, T$_H$-cell responses, natural killing, antibody-dependent cell-mediated cytotoxicity by macrophages, and adherence of leukocytes to endothelial cells.

**CD28:** A T-cell accessory molecule that is expressed by resting and activated T cells. It is the surface component of a signal transduction pathway that regulates cytokine production. Its ligand is the induced costimulatory molecules B7-1 (CD80) or B7-2 (CD86) usually found on antigen-presenting cells.

**CD40 (and CD40L):** A constitutive accessory molecule that is present on B cells, macrophages, dendritic cells, and endothelial cells. The CD40 ligand (CD154) is an inducible molecule expressed on activated T cells. Their interaction provides an activation signal to B cells, macrophages, dendritic cells, and endothelial cells, leading to a variety of immune and inflammatory responses including immunoglobulin class switching, memory B cell development, and germinal center formation. It is a member of the tumor necrosis factor receptor superfamily. A defect in the CD40L gene leads to an inability to undergo immunoglobulin class switching and is associated with hyper-IgM syndrome.

**CD44:** A T-cell accessory molecule involved in cell-cell adhesion and T-cell activation. It binds hyaluronan on endothelial cells and extrcellular matrix.

**CD45:** A T-cell accessory molecule present on T and B cells, granulocytes, and monocytes. Its function as a tyrosine phosphatase makes it important in B and T cell antigen receptor-mediated signaling.

**CD54:** See ICAM-1.

**CD58 (LFA-3):** A member of the Ig-gene superfamily, it is the ligand of CD2. The interaction between them promotes cell-cell adhesion.

**CD59:** A regulatory protein that mediates the homeostatic maintenance of complement activation on cells. It binds to C9 and thereby inhibits the formation of the membrane attack complex (MAC).

**CD80 and CD86:** B-cell activation molecules (also called *B7-1* and *B7-2*, respectively) that provides a costimulatory signal for activation or inhibition of T cells as a consequence of binding to the T cell ligands CD28 and CTLA-4 (CD152), respectively. They are type I membrane proteins that are immunoglobulin superfamily members, which are expressed by antigen-presenting cells. Binding of these proteins with CTLA-4 negatively regulates T-cell activation and decreases the immune response.

**cDNA library:** A set of DNA fragments prepared on mRNA templates obtained from an appropriate cell type.

**CDRs:** See Complementarity-determining regions.

**Cell-adhesion molecules (CAMs):** A group of cell-surface molecules that promote cell-cell adhesion; they are represented by four groups: immunoglobulin superfamily, integrins, selectins, and mucin-like proteins.

**Cell cycle:** The process of cell division can be separated into four phases: G1, S, G2, and M. The DNA of the cell replicates during the S phase, and the cell divides in the M (mitotic) phase.

**Cell line:** A population of cultured normal cells or tumor cells that have undergone transformation.

**Cell-mediated immunity:** Adaptive immunity mediated by specific T lymphocytes. Cell-mediated immunity involves reactions such as delayed-type hypersensitivity to the tuberculosis-causing organism, graft rejection, killing of virus-infected cells, and tumor immunity.

**Cell-mediated lymphocytolysis:** An *in vitro* test for cell-mediated immunity (mediated by cytotoxic T cells) in which a mixed lymphocyte reaction (MLR) is followed by killing of target cells that are used to stimulate allogeneic cells during an MLR.

**Cellular oncogenes (c-oncs) (or proto-oncogenes):** Normal cellular counterparts to viral oncogenes. They control cell growth. See Viral oncogenes.

**Centamorgan:** It represents a map unit or unit of physical distance on a chromosome. It is equivalent to a 1% frequency of recombination between closely linked genes.

**Central-memory T cells:** They are long-lived memory T cells (and B cells) that home to secondary lymphoid organs, are heterogeneous, lack immediate effector functions that are characteristic of plasma cells or effector T cells, and are responsible for secondary or chronic responses to antigen. The memory T cells express L-selectin and CC-chemokine receptor 7 (CCR7) and secrete interleukin (IL)-2 but not interferon-$\gamma$ or IL-4, on restimulation, they rapidly differentiate into cytokine-producing effector cells in lymphoid organs. See also Memory cells and Effector-memory T cells.

**Central tolerance:** The form of self-tolerance induced in central lymphoid organs (bone marrow and thymus) due to immature self-reactive lymphocytes recognizing self-antigens, which leads to either further rearrangement of antigen receptors or their death/deletion by apoptosis. See also Immunologic tolerance and Peripheral tolerance.

**Centroblasts:** They are large; rapidly dividing B cells found in the dark zones of germinal centers, and are probably undergoing somatic hypermutation. Plasma cells and memory B cells are derived from centroblasts.

**Centrocytes:** A small nonproliferating B cells found in the light zone of a germinal center. They are derived from centroblasts and may mature to plasma cells, memory B cells, or undergo apoptosis depending their interaction with antigen.

**Cervical carcinoma:** A cancer of the uterine cervix. See also Carcinoma.

**Chain association:** A mechanism for generating diversity in building light-chain and heavy-chain antibody genes and T cell receptor chain genes. i.e., any light chain can randomly associate with any heavy chain. See also Combinatorial freedom of gene segments and Multiplicity of V, D, and J germline gene segments.

**Challenge:** A term generally used to describe the administration of antigen and specifically used to describe any procedure, which induces an immune response *in vivo* or *in vitro*.

**Chaperones:** Proteins, such as, heat-shock proteins, which assist in protein folding.

**Chediak-Higashi syndrome:** A rare autosomal recessive Immunodeficiency disease caused by a defect in the lysosomal granules of macrophages and neutrophils, as well as the granules of NK cells and cytotoxic T cells. These patients have difficulty coping with pyogenic bacterial infections.

**Chemokine receptors:** Five families of cell-surface chemokine receptors that transduce signals stimulating the migration of leukocytes and expression of integrins. These families of receptors have seven-transmembrane α-helical, G-protein-linked molecules.

**Chemokines:** A large group of low molecular-weight cytokines that mediates leukocyte chemotaxis, regulates leukocyte migration from the blood to tissues, and controls the expression of leukocyte integrins. See also Integrin family. Chemokines play a major role in inflammatory reactions. Chemokines are subdivided into four families, the C-C, C-X-C, C, and C-X$_3$-C chemokines, depending on the first two cysteine locations in their protein sequence.

**Chemotaxis:** The increased directional migration of cells to a site across a concentration gradient.

**Chimeras:** Animals that contain cells from two genetically different parents (each parent has a different genotype). The recipient provides an environment where the two different cells survive with each other. Most experimental chimeras are produced by lethally irradiating an animal and reconstituting it with allogeneic bone marrow cells and mature immune cells. SCID-human mice are examples of chimeras.

**Chlorambucil:** An alkylating agent used as an immunosuppressive drug. It destroys lymphoid tissue within a few hours.

**Chromatids:** They are the two spiral filaments that make up a chromosome, which separate during cell division, each going to a different pole of the dividing cell.

**Chromatography:** A variety of techniques used to separate proteins; the techniques are based on the differential movement through an adsorbent, usually a column, by some substance.

**Chromium release assay:** An *in vitro* method that measures the death of a cell by detecting the release of intracellular $^{51}$Cr into the surrounding medium.

**Chromosomal translocations:** Most lymphoid tumors and many other types of tumors are marked by breakage and rejoining of the segment to different chromosomes. These breaks are frequent in lymphomas and leukemias.

**Chronic graft rejection:** Rejection of a graft that occurs over an extended period (years), usually after immunosuppressive therapy is stopped. It results from fibrosis and loss of normal organ structures and is mediated by antibodies and T cells. Arteriosclerotic lesions result from chronic delayed-type hypersensitivity reactions in the blood vessel walls, induced by T-cell cytokine production that encourages proliferation of endothelial cells and intimal smooth muscle cells, which eventually leads to vessel occlusion and organ death. It is the immune system's normal immune response to foreign transplantation antigens.

**Chronic granulomatous disease (GRD):** A rare inherited immunodeficiency disease that is characterized by recurrent intracellular bacterial and fungal infections, leading to chronic cell-mediated immune responses and granuloma formations. GRD is caused by a defect in the gene encoding a phagocyte oxidase enzyme component, which neutrophils and macrophages need to kill intracellular microbes.

**Chronic lymphocytic leukemias (CLLs):** They are B-cell cancers found in the blood. Most of these B cells express CD5 and unmutated V genes; thus, they are thought to arise from B-1 cells.

**c-*kit* ligand (stem cell factor):** A protein needed for hematopoiesis, T-cell development in the thymus, and mast cell development. It is produced in membrane-bound and soluble forms by stromal cells in the bone marrow and thymus, and binds to c-*kit* tyrosine kinase membrane receptor on pluripotent stem cells.

**Circulating dendritic cells (also called *veiled cells*):** Dendritic cells that are migrating to lymph nodes, carrying antigen, and there activate T helper cells. See also Veiled cells.

**Cis:** In immunogenetics, it is the phenomenon of using genetic material from only one chromosome.

**Cis-regulatory elements:** DNA sequences that are located next to or within transcribed genes, which either increase (enhancers) or decrease (repressor or silencer) gene transcription. These elements work by recruiting trans-acting transcriptional activators or repressor proteins.

**Cistron:** A term used to describe a gene, when the gene is specified as a hereditary unit of function.

**Clade:** See Human immunodeficiency virus (HIV).

**Class I molecules:** Histocompatibility or transplantation cell-surface proteins encoded in humans by the HLA complex A, B, and C loci and in mice by the H-2 complex K, D, and L loci. These molecules are found on all nucleated cells and consist of an MHC-encoded $\alpha$ chain associated noncovalently with a nonMHC-encoded $\beta_2$-microglobulin. Class I molecules present cytosolic antigen-derived peptides to CD8$^+$ T cells. See also Major histocompatibility complex (MHC) molecule.

**Class II molecules:** The histocompatibility cell-surface proteins encoded in humans by the HLA complex DP, DQ, and DR loci and in mice by the H-2 complex I and E loci. These molecules are found primarily on immune cells called *antigen-presenting cells* (*APCs*; such as B cells, macrophages, and dendritic cells) and allow them to interact or communicate with one another by presenting peptides derived from extracellular protein antigens that are internalized into phagocytic or endocytic vesicles to CD4$^+$ T cells. See also Major histocompatibility complex (MHC) molecule.

**Class II transactivator (CIITA):** A non-DNA-binding transcriptional activator that is a member of a family of structurally related proteins, such as nucleotide-binding oligomerization domain (NOD)-protein family and the CATERPILLER (caspase-recruitment domain (CARD) transcription enhancer. CIITA is a master control factor for the expression of MHC class II molecules. It alone provides the tissue specificity for the expression of MHC class II molecules, the accessory molecules invariant chain, and HLA-DM. It is one of several defective genes in bare lymphocyte syndrome; cells express no class II molecules.

**Class III molecules:** The class III molecules are complement components encoded in humans by the HLA complex C4, C2, Bf loci and in mice by the H-2 complex S loci.

**Class I regions:** They include the B, C, and A regions of the HLA complex and the K, D, and L regions located at opposite ends of the H-2 complex. They encode class I MHC molecules.

**Class I restriction:** CD8$^+$ T cells recognize foreign antigen-derived peptide only in association with class I MHC molecules.

**Class II-associated invariant (Ii) chain peptide (CLIP):** A fragment of the degraded Ii chain that occupies the class II MHC molecule peptide-binding groove, preventing premature binding of the antigenic peptide. It is removed by the action of the HLA-DM molecule before the antigen-binding cleft becomes accessible to exogenously internalized peptides. See also Invariant (Ii) chain and MIIC.

**Class II restriction:** CD4$^+$ T cells recognize foreign antigen-derived peptide only in association with class II MHC molecules.

**Class II vesicle (CIIV):** An organelle found in murine B cells that is important in the class II MHC pathway of antigen presentation. It is similar to the class II MHC compartment (MIIC). The CIIV contains all the components needed for the formation of antigen-derived peptide complexes and class II molecules, i.e., enzymes that degrade invariant chains, class II molecules, HLA-DM, and protein antigens. See also MIIC.

**Class (isotype)-switch recombination:** During an antibody response, B cells can switch the class of antibody produced (from IgM to IgG, IgA or IgE) thereby having a different effector function without changing antigen specificity. This is accomplished by class-switch recombination, which exchanges the initially expressed H chain C-region (C$\mu$) exons for an alternative set of downstream H chain C-region exons, such as C$\gamma$, C$\alpha$ or C$\epsilon$. Each 5' side of H chain C-region genes, except C$\delta$, is preceded by DNA sequences called *switch (S) regions*. The recombination event between two S regions, leads to the intervening sequences, including C$\mu$, being deleted. As a result, the VDJ exon is juxtaposed with a different downstream H chain C-region gene.

**Classical complement pathway:** Complement activation that is initiated by antigen-antibody complexes that involves plasma proteins C1–C9 that act in a sequential cascade, the intermediate components of the cascade enhance phagocytosis and adaptive immune responses, and eventually components 5–9 lead to the membrane attack complex. The latter complex kills extracellular pathogens by "punching" holes in their membrane, leading to osmotic death. See also Alternative complement pathway and Lectin pathway of complement activation.

**CLIP:** See Class II-associated invariant (Ii) chain peptide.

**Clodronate-loaded liposome:** A dichloromethylene diphosphonate-containing liposome, which is ingested by macrophages, leading to cell death.

**Clonal anergy:** A mechanism inducing peripheral immunologic tolerance. Autoreactive T and B cells that have escaped central tolerance are kept in a state of unresponsiveness by being stimulated through their antigen receptors in the absence of costimulatory signals—they are functionally silent. Once cells are anergy, they cannot respond to their cognate antigens under optimal conditions of stimulation. The breakdown of this mechanism can lead to autoimmune disease. See also Immunologic tolerance, Central tolerance, and Peripheral tolerance.

**Clonal deletion:** A mechanism primarily inducing central immunologic tolerance. The mechanism involves deletion of immature self-reactive B cells, in the bone marrow, and immature T cells, in the thymus, that strongly recognizes self-antigen. The breakdown of this mechanism can lead to autoimmune disease. See also Immunologic tolerance, Central tolerance, and Peripheral tolerance.

**Clonal exhaustion:** By repeated exposure to antigen, antigen-specific T cells are continually activated, such as during chronic viral infection, until the pool of mature cells becomes exhausted; they are not deleted, but persist in a nonfunctional state for extended periods of time.

**Clonal expansion:** The antigen-induced proliferation of antigen-specific lymphocytes that precedes their differentiation into effector cells. It is an essential step in the development of adaptive immunity—going from few cells to the many that are required to combat the pathogen that induced the response.

**Clonal restriction:** Only identical daughter cells within a clone react with their specific antigen.

**Clonal selection:** A fundamental tenet of adaptive immunity predicts that a normal individual carries a repertoire of lymphoid cell clones of capable of reacting with all possible antigenic determinants. When an antigen enters, it picks out (selects) the correct clone of B or T cells, the cells of the clone in turn proliferate and differentiate into antibody-producing cells or effector T cells that eliminate the eliciting antigen, and memory cells to sustain immunity. Throughout life self-reactive clones are eliminated, or are suppressed, or both—an individual's antigen-specific lymphocytes are self-tolerant.

**Clone:** A family of cells derived from a single progenitor or ancestor; thus, these cells are genetically identical.

**Cloning:** The processing of growing a population of cells from a single cell. Cloning can be done in two ways: (i) by limiting dilution cloning, that is, diluting a cell population until a single cell remains and then culturing it; or (ii) by cloning in soft agar which inhibits cell movement; thus colonies that have developed around a single cell can be removed by micromanipulation and cultured.

**Clonotype:** The gene product produced by members of a single clone.

**Clonotypic:** A feature that is unique to individual cells or members of a clone.

**Cluster of differentiation (CD) molecules:** A nomenclature to standardize the characterization of cell surface molecules expressed on various cell types of the immune system that are designated cluster of differentiation or CD. For example, the two functionally distinct subsets of T cells express either the antigen CD4 or CD8. The CD4$^+$ and CD8$^+$ cells can assume helper and cytotoxic functions, respectively. To date, about 340 CD molecules have been described.

**c-myc:** A cellular proto-oncogene that encodes a nuclear factor important in cell cycle regulation. When c-*myc* is translocated into immunoglobulin gene loci, it leads to B-cell malignancies.

**Coagulation system:** A proteolytic cascade of plasma enzymes that leads to blood clotting when blood vessels are damaged.

**Coding joints:** The sequence of nucleotides at the union point between DNA double-stranded breaks that are joined during V(D)J rearrangement to form rearranged immunoglobulin and T cell receptor genes. The joining sequences *code for* protein. In contrast, the signal joints instruct/signal to cut DNA strands at the recombination signal sequences. See also Recombination signal sequences (RSSs) and Signal joints.

**Codominant:** The equal expression of both alleles at one locus in heterozygotes.

**Cognate interactions:** They are cell-cell interactions between B and T cells that are specific for the same antigen.

**Cold antibody autoimmune hemolytic anemia:** A form of anemia characterized by high titers of autoagglutinating IgM antibodies that react optimally at 4°C. The disease can be idiopathic or secondary to infections or lymphomas. See also Warm antibody autoimmune hemolytic anemia.

**Cold antibodies:** Antibodies that are detected at higher titers and function better at temperatures below 37°C (also called *cold agglutinins*).

**Collectins:** A protein family, which includes mannose-binding lectin (MBL) that is characterized by the presence of a collagen-like domain and a lectin domain. Collectins mediate innate immune mechanisms by acting as microbial pattern recognition receptors that activate the complement system by binding to C1q. See also Mannose-binding lectin (MBL) and Pattern recognition receptors.

**Colony-stimulating factors (CSF):** Molecules (such as c-*kit* ligand, interleukin-3, interleukin-7, granulocyte-macrophage CSF, and macrophage CSF) that induce proliferation and differentiation of certain cell types.

**Colostrum:** The first milk secreted after giving birth; it is rich in antibodies.

**Combinatorial diversity:** There are two mechanisms that contribute the diversity of antigen receptors generated by gene combination: gene segments are joined in many different combinations and two different receptor chains (light and heavy chains in immunoglobulins; and α and β or γ and δ chains in T cell receptors) are combined to make antigen-binding sites.

**Combinatorial freedom of gene segments:** A mechanism for generating antibody and T cell receptor diversity using V, D, and J germline segments. These segments can randomly combine during somatic DNA recombination, which leads to a huge number of different combinations each one encoding a unique receptor. See also Chain association and Multiplicity of V, D, and J germline gene segments.

**Combinatorial joining:** The joining of V-J or V-D-J segments of DNA during somatic recombination of DNA, leading to new variable-region genes each one encoding a unique receptor. Joining leads to the formation of antibodies and T cell receptors during the development of B cells and T cells, respectively.

**Commensalism:** A relationship between members of different species living in proximity in which one organism benefits from the association but the other neither benefits nor is harmed.

**Commensals:** The normal flora microbes represent them; they benefit from the association with the host, but the host is not adversely affected. See Commensalism.

**Committed cells:** Lymphocytes sensitized to a specific antigen.

**Common γ chain (γ$_c$):** It is transmembrane polypeptide chain (CD132) that is present in Type I cytokine receptors. γ$_c$ was initially described as one of the interleukin-2 (IL-2) receptor chains. It is shared by the class I cytokine receptor IL-2 subgroup (including receptors for IL-2, IL-4, IL-7, IL-9, IL-15 and IL-21). It plays a role in the intracellular signaling mediated by these receptors. Humans with X-linked severe combined immunodeficiency have mutated γ$_c$.

**Common lymphoid progenitors:** Pluripotent hematopoietic stem-derived stem cells that give rise to all lymphocytes.

**Common variable immunodeficiency:** A little understood common pathogenesis exhibiting deficiency in antibody production. MHC genes seem to play a role in this immunodeficiency.

**Complement:** Nonimmunoglobulin plasma proteins that are sequentially (protein cascade) activated by antigen-antibody complexes, microbial surfaces, and plasma lectins, which cause irreversible damage to the membranes of target cells. They are also active in host defense mechanisms, involving both innate and adaptive immunity. There are three complement system activation pathways: the classical complement pathway, the alternative complement pathway, and the lectin pathway. See also Complement system.

**Complement-fixing antibodies:** During the human classical complement pathway cascade, only IgM and the IgG subclasses IgG1 and IgG3 readily fix or activate complement, whereas IgG2 is less effective. The IgG4 subclass and other classes of immunoglobulins do not fix complement or activate the classical complement pathway.

**Complement receptor one (CR1; also called CD35):** A receptor on erythrocytes, neutrophils, monocytes, macrophages, B lymphocytes, and a subpopulation of T lymphocytes binding C3b/C4b. It functions in opsonization and immune complex clearance.

**Complement receptor two (CR2; also called CD21):** A receptor on B cells, dendritic cells, and cervix and nasopharynx epithelium that binds C3d, C3bi, C3d,g and, more weakly, C3b. It functions in B-cell activation; it also is the receptor for Epstein-Barr virus.

**Complement receptor three (CR3; also called CD11b/CD18):** A receptor on neutrophils, monocytes, macrophages, and human NK cells that binds iC3b and C3d, thereby enhances phagocytosis of iC3b-coated particles.

**Complement system:** A series of nine plasma proteins that are activated through three pathways: the classical complement pathway (activated by antigen-antibody complexes), the alternative complement pathway (activated by microbe surfaces), and the lectin pathway (activated by lectins attached carbohydrate patterns on bacteria). Irrespective of pathway, components react in a sequential cascade, and play a major role in the destruction of foreign substances and lysis of cellular elements.

**Complementarity-determining regions (CDRs):** The most variable, short segments of the variable region of an antibody (light and heavy chains) and T cell receptor that form the antigen-binding site. There are three CDRs (CDR1, CDR2, and CDR3) present in the variable region of each antigen receptor chain and six CDRs in an intact antibody or T cell receptor. These segments form loop structures that together create a complementary site to the 3-D structure of the bound antigen. The CDRs are also known as the hypervariable regions.

**Complete Freund's adjuvant:** A commonly used adjuvant composed of a water-in-oil emulsion, containing a detergent and heat killed *M. tuberculosis*, which forms an antigen depot at the site of injection. See Adjuvant and Incomplete Freund's adjuvant.

**Con A:** See Concanavalin A.

**Concanavalin A (Con A):** A lectin from jack beans that acts as a mitogen for T cells.

**Confocal fluorescent microscopy:** The use of optics to produce images at high resolution by having two fluorescent light origins that come together only at one plane of a thicker section.

**Conformational determinants:** Protein epitopes composed of amino acids that are close together in the 3-D protein structure but far apart in the amino acid sequence. They are also called *discontinuous determinants* or *epitopes*.

**Congenic mice:** A line of mice possessing identical or nearly identical genotypes with other inbred strains except for a single substitution at one histocompatibility locus of a foreign allele—the allelic differences do not lead to an antigen that can elicit an immunological response when tissue is transplanted from one strain to another. The foreign allele is introduced by backcrossing an $F_1$ to a parent strain and selecting at each generation for heterozygosity at a specified locus. A minimum of 20 backcrosses is made, followed by intercrosses, and then homozygous mice are selected to start the line.

**Conjugate vaccines:** Vaccines that are made from capsular polysaccharides bound to immunogenic proteins, e.g., *H. influenzae* type b vaccine

**Connective tissue mast cell (CTMC):** The principal tissue fixed mast cell population, or ubiquitous cells that are susceptible to sodium cromoglycate. See also Mast cells.

**Constant (C) gene segments:** One of the three or four gene segments in humans that encodes C portion of antibody light (or T cell α and γ chains) and the heavy (or T cell β and δ chains) chains, respectively. See also Joining (J) gene segments and Variable (V) gene segments.

**Constant region:** The carboxyl-terminal end of either a light or heavy chain of an antibody molecule or T cell receptor chain that contains homology regions or domains. The region is so-called because the amino acid sequence is the same among different clones. The constant region of an antibody is responsible for its biological effector functions.

**Contact sensitivity:** A skin reaction seen in a sensitized individual after secondary skin contact with the offending allergen—a "sensitizer" hapten or antigen. It is also known as contact dermatitis. Poison ivy is an example of contact hypersensitivity. Once a dendritic cell acquires the allergen, it migrates to lymph nodes to prime contact-antigen-specific T cells.

**Contact-sensitizing agent:** A substance that leads to a local inflammation to the substance following repeated cutaneous or subcutaneous exposure.

**Continuous antigenic determinants:** Epitopes in which amino acid residues that make up the determinants are part of the primary sequence of the polypeptide. These epitopes are located in the flexible regions of the immunogen.

**Coombs test:** A test that determines antibody binding to red blood cells. Antibody-coated red blood cells agglutinate when exposed to an anti-immunoglobulin antibody. It is an important test in the detection of nonagglutinating antibodies against red blood cells produced during Rh incompatibility pregnancies.

**Copolymer:** Usually a linear polymer of two different amino acids in a specific ratio.

**Coreceptor:** A lymphocyte receptor that binds to its counterpart simultaneously as membrane immunoglobulin or T cell receptor binds the antigen, which delivers signals required for lymphocyte activation. CD4 and CD8 are coreceptors that bind to the nonpolymorphic domains of class II and I MHC molecules, respectively, while the T cell receptor binds to the polymorphic residues of the MHC molecules and the bound peptide. The complement receptor two (CR2; CD21) is a B cell coreceptor that binds to complement-coated antigen at the same time membrane immunoglobulin binds an antigen epitope.

**Cortex:** One of the two main compartments in the lobules of the thymus. It makes up 85 to 90% of the thymus. It is also a major part of lymph nodes.

**Costimulatory signal:** Optimal stimulation of T-cell and B-cell proliferation requires two signals. Signal one is transduced through T cell antigen receptors. Signal two is generically referred to as costimulation (it can be in the form of a soluble or membrane-bound molecule); several receptors on T cells mediate costimulation, mainly constitutively expressed CD28 that ligates with induced B7 on antigen-presenting cells or altered self-cells. Another T cell molecule is inducible T cell costimulator (ICOS). Likewise, to activate B cells, a signal is provided eventually by B cell CD40 interaction with CD40 ligand on activated T helper cells. Cytokines can act as costimulatory molecules.

**Countercurrent immunoelectrophoresis:** A technique related to immunodiffusion, but the antigens and antibodies are forced toward each other by an electrical field.

**Cowpox:** It is the disease caused by vaccinia virus. Edward Jenner used it to vaccinate against smallpox, which is caused by variola virus.

**CpG nucleotides:** They are unmethylated cytidine-guanine sequences and certain flanking nucleotides found in bacterial DNA that has adjuvant properties in the human immune system. These motifs are suppressed in mammalian DNA. Unmethylated CpG seems to have importance in the efficacy of DNA vaccines and induce innate immune responses through interaction with the Toll-like receptor 9, activating a signaling cascade that leads to the production of proinflammatory cytokines.

**CR1:** See Complement receptor one (CR1; also called *CD35*).

**CR2:** See Complement receptor two (CR2; also called *CD21*).

**CR3:** See Complement receptor three (CR3; also called *CD11b/CD18*).

**C-reactive protein (CRP):** A member of the pentraxin family of plasma proteins (an acute phase response protein) involved in innate immune responses to bacteria. It binds to phosphorycholine, which is a constituent of C-polysaccharide of the capsule of pneumococcal bacteria, hence its name. It binds to bacteria opsonizing them for uptake by phagocytes. CRP is a soluble pattern recognition receptor that does not bind to mammalian tissues.

**Crohn's disease:** An inflammatory autoimmune disease of the digestive system, therefore it is classified as an inflammatory bowel disease. It usually is found in the colon and terminal ileum and is thought to be caused by an abnormal T cell-mediated response to gut commensal bacteria.

**Crossed immunoelectrophoresis:** In the first step, or first dimension antigens. are separated according to charge by applying an electrical field. In the second

step, the antigens are electrophoresed at right angles to the first dimension. The areas under the precipitin arcs are proportional to the antigen concentration.

**Cross-matching:** A process of avoiding graft rejection by matching the donor and recipient's tissue. They are matched for ABO blood group antigens and for as many MHC class I and class II antigens as possible.

**Crossover:** A mechanism for recombination between genes on a chromosome. Crossing over is a breakage and repair mechanism of homologous DNA strands during meiosis. That is, part of one DNA strand derived from one parent is passed on to the gamete, with the remainder from the other parent.

**Cross-priming (or cross-presentation):** A mechanism whereby professional antigen-presenting cells (APCs) like dendritic cells take up extracellular antigen and prime (or activate) antigen-naïve CD8$^+$ cytotoxic T (T$_C$) cells. This happens when professional APCs internalizes an infected cell and the associated antigens are processed and presented in association with class I MHC molecules to CD8$^+$ T$_C$ cells—typically APCs would present extracellular antigens via class II MHC molecules. Cross-presentation is in the initiation of immune responses to viruses that do not infect APCs.

**Cross-reaction:** The reaction of a specific antibody (or T cell) with an antigen other than the one that induced its production. It occurs if two different antigens share an identical epitope or if receptors specific for one epitope also bind to an unrelated epitope possessing similar chemical characteristics.

**Cross-reactive idiotypes:** The idiotypes that occur on different antibodies, leading to cross-reactions with anti-idiotypic antibodies. These cross-reactive idiotypes may be found on antibodies that are for the same antigen or for different antigens.

**Cross-talk:** It is the bidirectional delivery of information and signals between two cell types. The conveyance of signals is mediated by cell–cell contact or by soluble factors, such as cytokines. The receipt of signals by each cell population affects its functions.

**Cross-tolerance:** It is observed when the addition of a Toll-like receptor (TLR) receptor ligand induces tolerance to a rechallenge with the ligand used for priming.

**Csk:** See C-terminal Src kinase.

**C-terminal Src kinase:** A constitutively active protein in lymphocytes that phosphorylates the C-terminal tyrosine of Src-family tyrosine kinases and thereby activates them.

**C-type lectins:** A large group of receptor proteins that bind carbohydrates in a $Ca^{2+}$-dependent manner using highly conserved carbohydrate recognition domains (CRD), which contain calcium-binding pockets that are essential for carbohydrate ligand binding. These lectins share a characteristic double-loop structure connected by two conserved disulfide bonds. C-type lectins are either secreted as soluble proteins or produced as transmembrane proteins that are present on self-antigens and pathogens.

**CTLA-4 (cytotoxic T-lymphocyte-associated protein 4; CD152):** An inhibitory ligand for B7-1 and B7-2 on antigen-presenting cells, i.e., engagement of CTLA-4 with B7 leads to an inhibitory signal to T cells, which includes cell cycle arrest and reduced cytokine production. CTLA-4 is expressed only on activated T cells. $CD4^+CD25^+$ T regulatory cells constitutively express CTLA-4. Mutations in the CTLA-4 gene are associated with autoimmune diseases, such as, insulin-dependent diabetes mellitus, Graves' disease, Hashimoto thyroiditis, celiac disease, systemic lupus erythematosus, and thyroid-associated orbitopathy.

**CTMC:** See Connective tissue mast cell.

**Cutaneous lymphocyte antigen:** A human lymphocyte-surface molecule that is involved in lymphocyte homing to the skin.

**Cutaneous T-cell lymphoma:** A malignant growth of T cells that home to the skin.

**C-X-C subgroup:** A chemokine subgroup in which a disulfide bond between cysteines is separated by a different amino acid (X). See also Chemokines.

**Cyclophosphamide:** A DNA alkylating drug frequently used as an immunosuppressant and anti-cancer drug.

**Cyclosporin A:** An antibiotic that acts as an immunosuppressant. It is not lymphocytic and has no antimitotic activity. It is selective for T helper cells and specifically inhibits transcription of the interleukin-2 gene through the binding of a cytosolic protein called *cyclophilin* (also called *immunophilin*). This complex binds to and inhibits the phosphatase calcineurin, which inhibits activation and nuclear translocation of the transcription factor NFAT. It is used to prevent transplanted organ rejection. See also Calcineurin and NFAT and FK506.

**Cytokines:** Low molecular weight proteins (such as monokines, lymphokines, and interleukins) produced by leukocytes and other cells that can affect target cells through binding their specific cytokine receptors. This binding initiates new activities in lymphocytes and other immune cells, such as proliferation, differentiation, or death. See also Chemokines.

**Cytokine-specific subunit:** A polypeptide chain of a multimeric cytokine receptor that is responsible for the specificity of the receptor for a particular cytokine.

**Cytophilic antibody:** Antibody (mostly IgG) having a propensity to bind to cells, usually macrophages.

**Cytophilins (also called *immunophilins*):** They are cytoplasmic proteins that bind the drugs cyclosporin A and FK506 (tacrolimus). This drug-cytophilin complex binds calcineurin, which prevents T-cell activation.

**Cytosine arabinoside:** A pyrimidine antimetabolite used mainly to depress antibody formation and tumor growth and, to a lesser extent, cellular immunity. See also 5-Bromodeoxyuridine and 5-Fluorouracil.

**Cytotoxic T lymphocytes (CTLs):** Effector cells of cell-mediated immunity, i.e., T lymphocytes, that can lyse allogeneic cells or virally infected cells following engagement by their T cell antigen receptor. CTLs express the coreceptor CD8 and recognize antigenic peptides that are presented by class I MHC molecules.

**Cytotoxins:** Cytotoxic T cell-derived proteins (e.g., perforin and granzymes) that participate in the destruction of target cells. See also Perforin and Granzymes.

**Cytotropic antibody:** Antibody (generally IgE) having a propensity to bind to mast cells and basophils, leading to immediate hypersensitivity reactions. See also Immediate hypersensitivity and Type I hypersensitivity.

# D

**D genes:** See Diversity (D) gene segments.

**D region:** One of the six regions of the murine H-2 map. It contains genes encoding class I molecules. See H-2 map.

**Danger signals:** They are host-cell damage triggers. These signals induce the activation of antigen-presenting cells usually by interacting with their Toll-like receptors and other pattern recognition receptors, which promotes the development of innate and adaptive immune responses. Endogenous danger signals are produced when cells are damaged, release of DNA and proteins, or inflammatory molecules and cytokines (e.g., interferon-$\gamma$) or other mediators, such as nitric oxide, leading to immune responses against the pathogen.

**Dark zone:** The portion of the germinal center that contains rapid cell proliferation by B cell-like cells called *centroblasts*.

**DC-SIGN (dendritic cell-specific ICAM-3 grabbing nonintegrin; CD209):** A ligand expressed only on dendritic cells that binds with high-affinity to ICAM-3. See also ICAM-3.

**Dean-Webb (α) procedure:** A precipitin test in which the tubes contain constant amounts of antibody with varying dilutions of antigen added. The titer is the highest dilution (or smallest amount) of antigen that will cause precipitation with a given amount of antibody.

**Death domains:** Originally defined as areas of proteins encoded by genes involved in programmed cell death; they are now known to be involved in protein-protein interactions that are involved signaling and apoptosis.

**Death receptors:** A family of cell-surface receptors that can mediate cell death following ligand-induced binding; they include tumor-necrosis-factor (TNF) receptor 1, CD95 (also called *FAS*) and two receptors for TNF-related apoptosis-inducing ligand (TRAILR1 and TRAILR2).

**Decay-accelerating factor (DAF):** A membrane glycoprotein of 70,000 molecular weight that binds C4b2a and C3bBb. It accelerates the decay of both the classical and the alternative pathway C3 convertases.

**Defensins:** Positively charged antimicrobial peptides that are 25–35 amino acid residues-long and rich in cysteine. They participate in innate immunity and are found in the skin, in neutrophil and macrophage granules, and act as broad-spectrum antibiotics killing many different bacteria and fungi. Proinflammatory cytokines interleukin-1 and tumor necrosis factor increase defensin synthesis. Some defensins are chemotactic for leukocytes.

**Degenerate binding specificity:** The type of antigen-derived peptide binding exhibited by MHC class I and class II molecules, i.e., each MHC allele-encoded molecule can bind numerous peptides of different amino acid sequences.

**Degranulation:** After cross-linking of two adjacent IgE molecules on the surface of a mast cell or basophil, the cell's granules fuse with the plasma membrane and release their contents (histamine and heparin) into the surrounding tissue. This activity is typically of a Type I hypersensitivity.

**Delayed-type hypersensitivity (DTH):** A cell-mediated immunity that is mediated by T cells and activated macrophages and takes 24 to 72 hours to reach its peak after challenge of an immune (sensitized) individual. Contact dermatitis, seen following contact with the leaves of the poison ivy plant, is an example of delayed-type hypersensitivity. See also Type IV hypersensitivity.

**Dendritic cells:** A group of professional antigen-presenting cells (APCs) that possess long processes, which interdigitate between lymphoid cells of lymphoid tissue, skin, and squamous epithelium. Dendritic cells are sentinel cells of innate immunity that bridge innate with adaptive immunity by acting as APCs to antigen naïve T cells and thus are important in the initiation of adaptive immune responses to protein antigens. The follicular dendritic cells (FDCs) present antigen to B cells; their processes bind antigen and retain it for extended periods of time, may play a role in B cell memory. FDCs are a lineage distinct from class II MHC molecule-expressing dendritic cells. See also Follicular dendritic cells (FDCs).

**Dendritic epidermal T cells:** A specialized class of mouse γδ T cells that all have the same γδ T cell receptor. Their function is unknown.

**Desensitization:** A procedure used to temporally suppress immediate hypersensitivity reactions by repeated injections of increasing amounts of the offending allergen. Protective mechanisms include production of IgG-blocking antibodies.

**Desetope:** The part of the antigen that binds to the MHC molecule. How the desetope binds to the antigen determines how the antigen is presented to the T cell; thus its name: *de*termination *se*lection.

**Determinant-selection model:** It states that the genetic unresponsiveness of some hosts is due to the failure of some major histocompatibility molecules to bind certain antigen-derived peptides.

**Determinant spreading:** The *de novo* activation of autoreactive T cells by intracellular antigen "spilling," which leads to the generation of autoreactive T cells and antibodies to other local molecules.

**Diacylglycerol (DAG):** During antigen activation of lymphocytes, the membrane-bound signaling molecule DAG is generated by phospholipase C-γ (PLCγ1)-mediated hydrolysis of the plasma membrane phospholipid phosphatidylinositol 4,5-bisphospate (PIP$_2$). DAG's main function is to activate protein kinase C, which participates in the generation of active transcription factors. See also Protein kinase C (PKC).

**Diapedesis:** The movement of leukocytes out of the bloodstream through the capillary endothelium by squeezing through the junctions between adjacent endothelial cells and moving into the surrounding tissue.

**Differentiation antigens:** Cell surface determinants that are used as immunologic markers, because they occur on certain lineages of immune cells at a particular stage of development.

**DiGeorge syndrome:** An immunodeficiency disease due to the congenital absence of the thymus, leading to thymic hypoplasia with low numbers of functional T cells.

**Direct agglutination reaction:** The agglutination of microorganisms, red blood cells, or other substances directly by specific antibody.

**Direct antigen presentation:** In transplantation reactions, the presentation of unprocessed allogeneic MHC molecules by graft cells to recipient T cells, which lead to their activation. This activation is the result of a cross-reaction caused by a T cell receptor recognizing foreign MHC molecules plus foreign peptide rather than self-MHC molecules and foreign peptide. See also Indirect antigen presentation.

**Direct fluorescent antibody method:** An immunofluorescence staining technique in which the fluorescently labeled antibody has specificity for the antigen to be detected. See also Indirect fluorescent antibody method.

**Discontinuous (conformational) determinants:** These epitopes are composed of amino acids that are distant from one another on a polypeptide backbone. The separated regions are brought into close proximity when the molecule folds, as happens with some of the determinants on lysozyme.

**Disease:** The impairment of function in a susceptible host.

**Disulfide bonds:** In antibodies, the chemical S-S bonds between sulfhydryl-containing amino acids that bind between heavy and light chains and within heavy and light chains.

**Diversity (D) gene segments:** These roughly 50 base pairs long coding sequences are situated between the variable region V and J segments of immunoglobulin heavy chains and T cell receptor β and δ chains. Random recombination with J and V segments contributes to the diversity of the antigen receptor repertoire.

**Dizygotic:** An organism that is derived from two separate fusions of sperm and ova.

**DM molecules:** See HLA-DM.

**DNA-binding proteins (or nuclear factors [NF]):** Trans-regulators that control immunoglobulin gene expression. See also Enhancers and Promoters.

**DNA-dependent kinase:** An enzyme that is part of protein complex that binds to the hairpin ends of double-stranded breaks in DNA. Its catalytic subunit is needed for VDJ recombination. A defect in this enzyme leads to severe combined immunodeficiency in mice (SCID mice) because these mice cannot rearrange their B and T cell receptor genes.

**DNA microarrays:** A system of placing a different DNA on a small part of a microchip and using them to assess RNA expression in normal and malignant cells.

**DNA transfection:** The introduction of DNA into mammalian cells, leading to expression of the DNA as if it were part of the cells' own genome.

**DNA vaccine:** A vaccine composed of a bacterial plasmid containing cDNA that encodes a protein antigen. The plasmid infected antigen-presenting cells (or any host cell) express immunogenic peptides that elicit specific responses.

**DNP (dinitrophenyl):** DNP is a commonly used hapten.

**Domains (homology regions):** Regions both in antibodies (heavy or light chains) and class I and II molecules that have a coherent tertiary structure.

**Dominant-negative protein:** A defective protein that retains interaction capabilities thereby distorting or competing with normal proteins.

**Double-negative (DN) thymocytes:** A thymic T-cell development stage were the differentiating cell does not express the T cell receptor nor CD4 or CD8 molecules.

**Double-positive (DP) thymocytes:** A thymic T-cell development stage were the differentiating cell does express a pre-T cell receptor and both CD4 and CD8 molecules. These cells are subject to selection processes. The survivors of these selection processes mature to single-positive T cells, expressing either CD4 or CD8.

**DR antigens:** The human counterpart to mouse MHC class II (I-A and I-E) molecules, which are expressed primarily on B cells and other antigen-presenting cells, e.g., macrophages and dendritic cells.

**Draining lymph node:** Any lymph node that is downstream of an infection site and thus receives antigens from the site by the lymphatic system.

**Drug-induced autoimmune hemolytic anemia:** Different drugs cause autoimmunity by four different mechanisms: (1) immune complex formation, (2) drug adsorption to red cell membranes, (3) modification of red cell membranes, and (4) idiopathic means.

**Dysgammaglobulinemia:** An immunodeficiency disease involving B cells. It shows an imbalance in IgA production, but all combinations of immunoglobulin imbalance may occur.

**Dysplasia:** A loss in individual cell uniformity and loss in their orientation, resulting from developmental changes in cell growth, shape, and organization. It is often found as a precursor to cancer, occurring mainly in epithelia.

# E

**E2A:** It is crucial in lymphoid progenitor commitment to the B-cell and T-cell lineages. A transcription factor that is essential for early events in B-cell development. It is required for the expression of recombination-activating genes (RAGs) and λ5 component of the pre-B-cell receptor. It is also important in the initial stages of T-cell development.

**E-selectins:** A molecule expressed on vascular endothelium that guides effector cells into sites of infection. See also Selectins.

**Early B-cell factor (EBF):** A transcription factor that is essential for B-cell development. It is required for the expression of recombination-activating genes (RAGs). See also Recombination-activating genes (RAGs).

**Ectopic lymphoid structures:** Organized aggregates of lymphocytic cells that form in chronic inflammation sites, which are segregated into B- and T-cell-rich zones, dendritic cells (DCs), germinal centers with follicular DC networks, and specialized endothelia. These structures are also called the *tertiary immune system.*

**Eczema:** A common childhood skin disease of unknown etiology.

**Edema:** The noticeable accumulation of serous fluid in tissue spaces.

**Effector cells:** A term used to describe any immune cell that mediates a function, such as helper activity, suppression, cytotoxicity, or even antibody production.

**Effector-memory T cells:** They are the plasma cells or the memory T cells (the latter cells lack L-selectin and CCR7 expression) that home to the bone marrow and secrete antibodies or home to peripheral inflamed tissues, respectively, and mediate immediate protection against antigen challenge. These memory T cells can also rapidly produce cytokines, such as interferon-γ or interleukin-4.

**Effector phase:** The acquired immune response phase that follows the recognition phase and activation phase, where foreign antigen is either inactivated or destroyed, for example by antibody-dependent complement activation or activated cytotoxic T cells. See also Activation phase and Recognition phase.

**Efferent lymphatics:** Leukocytes within the lymph nodes migrate across the node, enter the medulla, and exit the node through the efferent lymphatics; they carry lymph out of the lymph nodes.

**Electrophoresis:** The movement of charged particles suspended in a medium under the influence of an applied electric field. Electrophoresis is a technique of separating materials.

**ELISA:** See Enzyme-linked immunosorbent assay (ELISA).

**ELISPOT assay:** An ELISA variation in which cells are placed over antibodies attached to a plastic surface. The antibodies trap the cells' products, which are assessed by using an enzyme-tagged antibody that cleaves a colorless substrate, generating a localized colored spot. It enumerates specific CD4$^+$ and CD8$^+$ T cells that secrete a particular cytokine (often interferon-γ).

**Embryonic stem (ES) cells:** Mouse embryonic stem cells that growth continuously in culture and that retain their ability to give rise to all cell lineages. Tissue cultured ES cells can be genetically manipulated and inserted into mouse blastocysts to generate mutant mouse lines. Typically, genes in ES cells are deleted by homologous recombination and the mutant ES cells are used to generate gene knockout mice. They have been used to clone sheep and who knows what else.

**Endocrine:** The secretion of regulatory molecules like cytokines that move from producer cell to target cell by the blood stream.

**Endocytosis:** The internalization process mediate by all cells (immune and nonimmune) where they ingest extracellular fluids, macromolecules, or particles by surrounding them with a small portion of plasma membrane, which invaginates and pinches off to form an intracellular macromolecule-containing vesicle. Endocytosis is often used synonymously with pinocytosis. See also Pinocytosis.

**Endogenous:** Originating within the cell.

**Endogenous pyrogens:** These are cytokines that induce an increase in body temperature. In contrast to an exogenous substance such as gram-negative bacterial endotoxin that induces fever by triggering endogenous pyrogen production.

**Endosome:** An intracellular membrane-bound vesicle that internalizes extracellular protein during antigen processing. Endosomes have an acid pH and contain enzymes that degrade proteins into peptides that bind to class II MHC molecules.

**Endotoxin:** The lipopolysaccharide derived from the cell walls of Gram-negative bacteria; it is toxic and pyrogenic when injected *in vivo*. Nonetheless, it stimulates innate immune responses, such as cytokine secretion, macrophage activation, and leukocyte adhesion molecule expression on endothelium. Some endotoxins can act as superantigens. Gram-negative bacteria-induced sepsis results from endotoxin released into the bloodstream.

**Enhancers:** One of the two types of cis-regulators that control receptor (e.g., immunoglobulins) gene expression. More generally, they are regulatory nucleotide sequences in a gene that are located some distance either upstream or downstream of the promoter, which bind transcription factors, and increase the activity of the promoter. See also DNA-binding proteins.

**Envelope glycoprotein (Env):** A retrovirus-encoded membrane glycoprotein that is expressed on the infected cell's plasma membrane and on the virus particle's host cell-derived membrane coat. Envs are usually required for viral infectivity. HIV's Env proteins include gp120 and gp41, which bind to human T cell CD4 and chemokine receptors, and mediate fusion of the T cell and viral membranes, respectively.

**Enzyme-linked immunosorbent assay (ELISA):** The visualization of a primary antigen-antibody interaction by using an enzyme-labeled second antibody specific for the primary antibody. If the primary antibody binds the antigen, the secondary labeled antibody binds the first antibody (sandwich), and when the substrate for the enzyme is added, a resulting color change can be measured. The greater the color intensity, the more antigen bound.

**Eosinophils:** Phagocytic cells that make up 2–5% of the blood leukocytes that express large numbers of FcεRI receptors for IgE. They are found in the late-phase reaction of Type I hypersensitivities. Eosinophils contain granules composed of a basic protein and histaminase. The basic protein is released by exocytosis, leading to damage to some pathogens. The histaminase can downregulate inflammatory reactions. Eosinophils are cells involved in the protection against parasites, such as helminths.

**Eotaxin-1 (CCL11), -2 (CCL24) and -3 (CCL26):** They are CC chemokines that act specifically on eosinophils.

**Epigenetic:** An inheritable influence on gene or chromosome function, which is not accompanied by change in DNA sequence; such as, mammalian X-chromosome inactivation, centromere inactivation, and imprinting.

**Epithelioid cells:** Cells derived from macrophages, which contain fewer phagosomes and are found in granulomas. They appear as large flattened cells with large amounts of endoplasmic reticulum.

**Epithelium:** A diverse group of tissues that covers or lines nearly all body surfaces, cavities and tubes. It functions as an interface between different biological compartments. Epithelial layers provide physical protection and containment, and also mediate organ-specific transport properties.

**Epitope:** See Antigenic determinant.

**Epitope spreading:** Irrespective of the original antigenic stimulus, such as bacteria or viruses, the specificity of the immune response spreads to include self-epitopes—that is, epitopes other than the ones that initiated the immune response. This "spreading" occurs during tissue damage associated with inflammatory responses and leads to the priming of self-reactive T and/or B lymphocytes, in spite of the specificity of the initial insult.

**Epstein-Barr virus (EBV):** A double-stranded DNA virus of the herpesvirus family that causes infectious mononucleosis and is associated with nasopharyngeal carcinoma and some β-cell malignancies. EBV infects B cells and some epithelial cells by binding to CD21 (CR2).

**Equilibrium constant:** In antibody-antigen systems, a measure of equilibrium expressed by the association constant.

**Equilibrium dialysis:** A technique for measuring the affinity of antibody-combining sites for antigenic determinants.

**Equivalence:** The ratio of antigen and antibody concentrations leading to maximum precipitation.

**Equivalence zone:** The middle of the precipitin curve, where the lattice has a lower ratio of antibody to antigen than in the antibody excess zone. All antigen and antibody are in the lattice. The precipitate is at its maximum. See also Antibody excess zone, Antigen excess zone, and Zone phenomenon.

**Erp57:** A chaperone molecule that helps load peptide onto MHC class I molecules in the endoplasmic reticulum.

**Erythema:** The redness that results from localized capillary dilation, usually due to local inflammatory reactions.

**Erythroblastosis fetalis:** A condition characterized by the presence of erythroblasts in the blood of the newborn. This Type II (antibody-mediated cytotoxicity) hypersensitivity results from maternal antibodies directed against fetal Rh antigens. See Hemolytic disease of the newborn.

**Erythropoietin (EPO):** A cytokine that induces progenitor cells to become erythrocytes.

**Etiology:** The study of the origins of disease.

**Exocytosis:** The process by which cells release molecules contained in membrane-bound vesicles when the vesicle fuses with the plasma membrane.

**Exogenous:** Originating outside the cell.

**Exon:** A continuous segment of a gene (DNA) whose transcribed sequence is retained in mRNA and thereby encodes protein.

**Exosomes:** Small lipid bi-layer vesicles that contain cytosol and are secreted by dendritic cells and tumor cells. They contain antigen–MHC complexes and heat-shock protein 70 and 90, which could be cross-presented by dendritic cells to activate T lymphocytes.

**Experimental allergic encephalomyelitis (EAE):** An experimental model for human multiple sclerosis. It is an inflammatory autoimmune disease of the central nervous system that develops in mice after immunizing with neural antigens (such as the component of the myelin sheath called *myelin basic protein*). The disease is mediated by CD4$^+$ T cells and leads to a paralytic disease with inflammation and demyelination in the brain and spinal cord.

**Extracellular matrix (ECM):** A complex, three-dimensional network of large macromolecules that provides contextual information and an architectural scaffold for cellular adhesion and migration.

**Extravasation:** The movement of leukocytes through a blood vessel wall into the surrounding tissue, particularly at a site of inflammation.

**Exudate:** The accumulation of blood cells and fluid that is present at a site of inflammation.

# F

**F$_1$ generation:** The first generation of offspring after a particular mating.

**F$_2$ generation:** The second generation of offspring after a particular mating.

**Fab fragment:** The *f*ragment *a*ntigen *b*inding (Fab) is derived by papain hydrolysis of antibodies. The Fab fragment of human IgG (about 45 kD) contains a light chain disulfide-linked to the amino-terminal half of the contiguous heavy chain (that is, the Fc fragment). Each antibody molecule has two Fab fragments. Each Fab fragment has one antigen-combining site. Fab can bind with only one epitope; thus, it cannot form a precipitate.

**Fab′ fragments:** Two Fab-like fragments yielded on reduction by the F(ab′)$_2$ fragment.

**F(ab′)$_2$ fragment:** The fragment obtained after pepsin treatment of a human IgG antibody molecule, with a molecular weight of about 90,000. This fragment consists of that part of the antibody molecule that is on the amino-terminal side of the pepsin cleavage site. Thus, the F(ab′)$_2$ fragment is composed of both Fab fragments and a short piece (the hinge region) of the Fc fragment. The fragment can act as a divalent antibody molecule, but does not exhibit biological effector functions such as complement fixation and passage across the placenta.

**FACS:** See Fluorescence activated cell sorter or Flow cytometry.

**Factor B:** A component of the alternative pathway of complement activation, which on complexing with C3b is cleaved by factor D to form the alternative pathway C3 convertase.

**Factor D:** A serine esterase of the alternative pathway to complement activation, which cleaves factor B when the latter is complexed to C3b to form C3bB.

**Factor H:** A plasma polypeptide that binds fluid phase and membrane-bound C3b and thereby increases the susceptibility of C3b to cleavage by Factor I. Thus, Factor H controls the classical and alternative pathways to complement activation.

**Factor I:** Controls complement activation by enzymatically cleaving C3b to C3bi.

**Fas (CD95):** A cell-surface protein of the TNF receptor family that is expressed on T cells and many other cells that interacts with the Fas ligand and initiates a signaling cascade leading to apoptosis of the cell. Killing of T cells via Fas-Fas ligand association, called *activated-induced cell death*, is important in the maintenance of self-tolerance. Mutations in the *Fas* gene lead to systemic autoimmune diseases. See Fas ligand.

**Fas ligand (CD178):** A cell-surface protein of the TNF receptor family that is expressed on activated T cells. It is a death factor that binds to its receptor, Fas, on the target cell to induce apoptosis. Mutations in the *Fas ligand* gene lead to systemic autoimmune diseases. See Apoptosis and Fas (CD95).

**Fc fragment:** The fragment crystallizable (Fc) that is derived by papain hydrolysis of antibody molecules. The Fc fragment of human IgG has a molecular weight of 50,000 and consists of the carboxyl-terminal half of two heavy chains linked by disulfide bridges. It bears the sites for complement fixation and most of the carbohydrate portion of the antibody.

**Fc receptors (FcRs):** A receptor present on B cells, macrophages, and NK cells for the Fc region of an IgG antibody molecule (there are FcRs specific IgE and IgA). The macrophage FcR mediates opsonization, while the B cell FcRs control antibody production. NK cell FcRs mediated ADCC. There are three well-defined FcRs for IgG: FcγRI (CD64) is a high affinity IgG receptor on macrophages and neutrophils that binds monomeric IgG; FcγRII (CD32; there are A, B, and C forms, they are products of different but homologous genes) is a low-affinity IgG receptor on macrophages, neutrophils, eosinophils, platelets, and B cells that facilitates phagocytosis, and on B cells control antibody production; and FcγRIII (CD16) is a low-affinity IgG receptor on macrophages, neutrophils, and NK cells that facilitates phagocytosis, and in NK cells is an activation molecule. There are two FcRs for IgE: the high-affinity FcεRI expressed on mast cells and basophils that initiates immediate hypersensitivity reactions and FcεRII (CD23) that has an immunoregulatory role. Another FcR, which is specific for IgA, FcαR (CD89), is expressed on eosinophils, monocytes, neutrophils, and some dendritic cells; function is unknown.

**Fibrosarcoma:** A cancer originating from connective tissue. See also Sarcoma.

**First-set rejection:** Transplanted tissues are treated by the immune system as most foreign antigens; there is specificity and memory. The first exposure to transplanted tissue (allograft) will induce an immune response, leading to the rejection of the graft in 10–14 days, a primary immune response.

**FK506 (also called *tacrolimus*):** An immunosuppressive drug (a metabolite of the fungus *Streptomyces tsukubaensis*) used in the prevention of allograft rejection; it functions by blocking T-cell cytokine gene transcription. Its mode of action is similar to that of cyclosporine A. FK506 and cyclosporine A are the most commonly use immunosuppressants in organ transplantation. See also Cyclosporine A.

**Flow cytometry:** A method used to analyze the phenotype of cell populations. The instrument is called a *flow cytometer*, which detects fluorescence on individual cells within a mixture of cells and reports the number of cells expressing the molecule tagged by the fluorescent probe. The cell suspensions are incubated with fluorescently labeled antibodies and the amount of label bound to individual cells in the cell mixture is measured by passing the cells one at a time through a laser beam of light.

**FLT-3 ligand:** A cytokine that stimulates large numbers of dendritic cells to emigrate from the bone marrow to the peripheral tissues.

**Fluorescein:** A yellow dye used to label antibodies for fluorescence methods.

**Fluorescence:** A substance is activated by light of a given wavelength and emits light of a different wavelength. The latter light is detected and used in fluorescence methods.

**Fluorescence-activated cell sorter (FACS):** A flow cytometer, called *fluorescence-activated cell sorter (FACS)*, is modified to separate cells that are tagged

with an antibody specific for a cell marker, which is fluorescently labeled. See Flow cytometry.

**Fluorescence quenching:** The reduction in fluorescence following the binding of antibody with antigen. The amino acids in the antigen-binding site of the antibody emit light at a certain wavelength when excited by ultraviolet light; the inclusion of a hapten (antigenic determinant) into the binding site absorbs the light, quenching the fluorescence.

**Fluorochromes:** Organic dyes that emit absorbed light at characteristic wavelengths. They are used in the fluorescent antibody technique.

**5-Fluorouracil:** A pyrimidine antimetabolite used mainly to depress antibody formation and tumor growth and, to a lesser extent, cellular immunity. See also 5-Bromodeoxyuridine and Cytosine arabinoside.

**FMS-like tyrosine kinase 3 ligand:** A cytokine that promotes the *in vitro* growth of dendritic cells.

**Folic acid analogs:** Antimetabolites. They are derivatives of folic acid involved in one-carbon transfer reactions required for DNA synthesis.

**Follicles:** See Primary follicles.

**Follicular B cells:** As B cells end their development in the bone marrow and move to the periphery; they are considered immature B cells ($IgM^{high}IgD^{-/low}$), these B-cells seed the spleen and lymph nodes. Once there, they further differentiate through several transitional stages, eventually becoming recirculating, mature B cells ($IgM^{med}IgD^{med}CD21^{med}CD23^{med}$), which populate the follicles of the spleen and lymph nodes—thus called *follicular B cells*. They represent roughly 90% of mature spleen B cells; the marginal-zone B cells represent the remaining 10%. Follicular B cells are primarily responsible for creating humoral immune responses to protein antigens and with T-cell help; they form germinal centers. See Marginal-zone B cells.

**Follicular B helper T ($T_{FH}$) cells:** B cells require T-cell help for high-affinity antibody responses and B-cell memory. A discrete $CD4^+$, CXC-chemokine receptor 5 (CXCR5)-expressing follicular population of T cells mediates this help. Their homing preferences and helper function are distinct; $T_{FH}$ cells differ from $T_H1$ and $T_H2$ cells and thus are called *follicular B helper T ($T_{FH}$) cells*.

**Follicular dendritic cells (FDCs):** Stromal cells with extensive cell-surface processes that are located in spleen and lymph node follicles. FDCs do not internalize antigens but, because they express Fc and C3 receptors and CD40 ligand and have long cytoplasmic processes, they can bind intact antigen-antibody-complement complexes and present them to B cells. Because FDCs can retain intact antigen on their surface for extended periods of time, they may play a role in the selection of memory B cells during germinal center reactions. They do not express class II MHC molecules; thus, they are a lineage distinct from class II-expressing dendritic cells.

**Forbidden clones:** These clones were proposed by Burnet to explain that autoreactive immune cells are forbidden to react with self-constituents by being clonally deleted during ontogeny (now known as central tolerance; it occurs throughout life). It is also now known that we have autoreactive immune cells but they are usually in an inactive state.

**Fragmentin:** The enzymes present in cytotoxic T cells' granules that induce DNA fragmentation. See also Granzymes.

**Framework residues:** The four intervening sequences between the complementarity-determining regions (CDRs) are regions of restricted variability; that is, there is little difference in amino acid sequence between chains. The invariant segments make up the framework resides of both light and heavy antibody chains, which comprise approximately 80–85% of the total variable region.

**Fratricide:** A type of cell killing, which is seen during HIV infections, in which one of a group of similar cells kills another member or members of the group.

**Freund's adjuvant:** The most widely used adjuvant. There are two types: Complete Freund's adjuvant is a water-in-oil emulsion containing heat-killed mycobacteria; it is used with antigens to enhance their immunogenicity. Incomplete Freund's adjuvant does not contain mycobacteria.

**Fv:** See Single-chain Fv.

# G

**G proteins:** They are heterodimeric proteins that are important in many signaling pathways; they are active when their guanine-binding site is occupied by GTP and inactive when bound with GDP. GTP-bound G proteins activate a variety of cellular enzymes involved in different signaling cascades. The trimeric GPT-binding proteins are associated with cytoplasmic tails of many cell surface receptors, for example, chemokine receptors. Soluble G proteins like Rac and Ras are recruited into signaling pathways by adapter proteins. See also Adapter proteins.

**G protein-coupled receptor family:** A diverse family of hormone receptors for lipid inflammatory mediators and chemokines that use associated trimeric G proteins for intracellular signaling.

**GALT:** See Gut-associated lymphoid tissue.

*GATA-2* **gene:** A gene encoding a transcription factor that is essential for the development of erythroid, lymphoid, and myeloid lineages.

**Gamete:** The specialized cells (sperm and ova) combining in sexual reproduction to form the zygote, the beginning of a new individual.

**γδ T cells:** These mostly CD4⁻CD8⁻ (sometimes CD8αα⁺) T cells express the T cell receptor (TCR) composed of an γ-subunit and a δ-subunit (γδ-TCR) *versus* other T cells that express a TCR composed of a α-subunit and a β-subunit (αβ-TCR). The γδ TCR-expressing T cells are less abundant (1–5% in blood; 25–60% in gut [present in the intestinal epithelium as intraepithelial lymphocytes]) and the ligands for these receptors are not peptides associated with classical MHC molecules; they can bind protein and nonprotein. They are not MHC restricted. The αβ TCR-expressing T cells mainly recognize antigenic peptides bound to conventional class I or class II MHC molecules. Their function is unknown; they may mediate innate immune responses of the mucosal immune system. See also T cell receptor and T lymphocytes.

**Gamma globulins:** Serum proteins that have gamma electrophoretic mobility and make up most immunoglobulins and antibodies.

**GEF:** See Guanine-nucleotide exchange factor.

**Gene conversion:** A process whereby recombination occurs between two homologous genes in which a localized segment from one gene is replaced by the homologous segment from another gene. This is the main way immunoglobulin receptor diversity is generated in birds and rabbits, i.e., a homologous inactive V gene segments exchange short sequences with an active, rearranged V-region gene.

**Gene targeting (or gene knockout):** It is a technique used to specifically disrupt a gene. It involves homologous recombination in embryonic stem cells, which are then injected into blastocysts of mice.

**Gene therapy:** An approach used to correct a genetic defect by the introduction of a normal gene into bone marrow cells or other cell types. It also can be called *somatic gene therapy* because it does not affect the individual's germline cells.

**Genetic immunization:** A novel approach to induce adaptive immunity by injecting plasmid DNA encoding a protein of interest into muscle. By yet unknown mechanisms, the protein is expressed and elicits antibody and T-cell responses.

**Gene gun:** A device that uses compressed helium to shoot 1–2 μm in diameter DNA-coated gold beads into recipient cells.

**Generation of receptor diversity:** The process leading to the production of a large number (perhaps infinite) of antibodies or T cell receptors due to the generation of variable (V) regions. There are several mechanisms that contribute to the generation of diversity: (i) the number of germline V genes for antibody light chains and heavy chains or T cell receptor chains, (ii) recombination between V, D, and J genes with varied combinations of antibody light and heavy chains or T cell receptor chains, (iii) junctional diversity, (iv) insertion of N and P regions, and (v) somatic hypermutation of antibody receptors.

**Genetic restriction:** The term used to describe the phenomenon of lymphocytes and antigen-presenting cells cooperating effectively only when they share particular haplotypes.

**Genome:** The complete set of genetic material contained in the haploid assortment of chromosomes in a cell.

**Genome-stability genes:** Genes that control cell-cycle progression and/or DNA repair, which permit for the continuance of genome stability.

**Genotype:** The genetic constitution of an individual inherited from parents; the genotype is not necessarily all expressed in that individual.

**Germinal centers:** A region of metabolically active B lymphocytes within the primary follicles of lymph nodes, the spleen, or mucosal lymphoid tissue where B-cell activation, proliferation, and differentiation occurs following T cell-dependent antigenic stimulation. With the appearance of germinal centers, the follicles are called *secondary follicles*. B-cell somatic mutation, selection, and affinity maturation also occur in the germinal centers. B cells with receptors that cannot bind antigen die by apoptosis, whereas those that can bind antigen with high affinity are positively selected to exit the germinal center. This leads to the production of memory B cells and plasma cells that produce high-affinity antibody.

**Germline:** The genetic material passed from parents to offspring by the gametes (egg and sperm). In antibody and T cell receptor diversity, all the genetic information (genes) is contained in the genetic heritage (egg and sperm) or in immature lymphocytes. In developing B and T cells, the germline DNA is modified by somatic recombination to form functional immunoglobulin or T cell receptor genes.

**Germline theory:** The theory proposing that all genes encoding immunoglobulins are present in the germinal cells (eggs and sperm). The opposite theory is the somatic theory. See Somatic theory.

**Giant cells:** Large, multinucleated cells often found in granulomas. They may be derived from the fusion of epithelioid cells or macrophages.

**GLD mice:** They have a naturally occurring mutation of Fas ligand, which causes a generalized lymphoproliferative disease. See also LPR mice.

**Glomerulonephritis:** An inflammation of kidney glomeruli often initiated by deposition of circulating antigen-antibody complexes in the glomerular basement membrane or antibodies that bind to glomeruli-expressed antigen. The antibodies can activate complement and phagocytes.

**GlyCAM-1 (glycosylation-dependent cell-adhesion molecule 1):** A mucin-like molecule expressed on high endothelial venules (HEVs) of lymph nodes and Peyer's patches, which acts as a ligand for L-selectin (CD62L) expressed on antigen-naïve lymphocytes. It directs these lymphocytes to leave the blood and enter the lymphoid tissues.

**Glycosylation:** The process of adding carbohydrate groups.

**Gm:** An allotypic determinant found on the heavy chain of human IgG. See Allotypic determinants.

**Goblet cell:** A differentiated epithelial cell associated with mucous membranes that secretes mucus.

**Golgi:** A collection of tubular-like structures found in the cytoplasm of cells involved in the secretion of proteins.

**Goodpasture's syndrome:** An autoimmune disease characterized by autoantibodies against basement membrane (associated with kidney glomeri and lung alveoli) or type IV collagen, leading to extensive vasculitis, and rapid death.

**gp:** The abbreviation for glycoprotein.

**gp41:** Glycoprotein 41 is embedded in HIV's outer envelope and anchors gp120. It is important in HIV infection of CD4$^+$ T cells because it facilitates the fusion of viral and cell membranes. See also Human immunodeficiency virus (HIV).

**gp120:** Glycoprotein 120 is one of the proteins that forms the outer envelope of HIV. The gp120 molecules project from the membrane and bind to CD4 molecules on T helper cells. See also Human immunodeficiency virus (HIV).

**Graft arteriosclerosis:** The occlusion of grafted blood vessels due to the growth of intimal smooth muscle, probably caused by the chronic immune response to vessel wall alloantigens. It occurs within six months to a year or more later after transplantation and leads to the chronic rejection of vascularized grafted organs.

**Graft rejection:** A T cell-mediated immune reaction elicited by the grafting of genetically dissimilar tissue to a recipient. The outcome of the reaction is the destruction and rejection of the transplanted tissue.

**Graft-versus-host reaction:** A disease that results from the transfer of bone marrow-containing functionally mature T lymphocytes into an immunoincompetent genetically dissimilar individual. In other words, the graft is rejecting the host.

**Granulocyte:** Any cell of the granulocytic leukocyte series (containing cytoplasmic granules), such as eosinophils, neutrophils, or basophils.

**Granuloma:** A localized accumulation of densely packed lymphoid cells, such as macrophages (sometimes fusing to form giant cells), epitheloid cells (modified macrophages), lymphocytes, and plasma cells. This accumulation of cells leads to blockage of waste removal and nutrient influx, leading to tissue death (granuloma). Granulomas are often seen in tuberculosis.

**Granzymes:** A collection of serine protease enzymes (also called *fragmentins*) found in the granules of cytotoxic T cells and NK cells that enter target cells by a receptor-mediated endocytic pathway, cleave and activate intracellular caspases, and initiate apoptosis. See also Fragmentins.

**Graves' disease:** An antibody-mediated autoimmune disorder. Unlike other autoimmune disorders, it results directly from autoantibodies that stimulate thyroid cellular activity by displaying thyroid-stimulating hormone binding, leading to overproduction of thyroid hormone. Thus, it is also called *hyperthyroidism*.

**Guanine-nucleotide exchange factors (GEFs):** Proteins that can remove bound GDP from small G proteins, which allow GTP to bind and activate the G protein.

**Gut-associated lymphoid tissues (GALT):** The lymphoid tissues that are associated with the gastrointestinal tract, e.g., palatine tonsils, Peyer's patches, appendix, and layers of intraepithelial lymphocytes (IELs). They contain conventional and unconventional lymphocytes and specialized antigen-presenting cells. See intraepithelial lymphocytes (IELS).

**Gut lamina propria:** The mucosal tissue layer directly under the mucosal epithelial cell surface of the gastrointestinal tract, in which immune cells for mucosal immunity reside.

# H

**H substance:** The core/precursor carbohydrate of the ABO blood cell antigens.

**H-2 complex:** The MHC of the mouse. The genetic locus encoding class I and class II molecules that are important in graft rejection and immune responses in the mouse. See Antigen 2.

**H-2 congenic mice (congenic resistant mice):** Mice that are identical throughout their entire genomes except for a selected locus or closely linked loci that prevent the exchange of a graft. They are used to follow the effects of one against a constant genetic background.

**H-2 map:** The linear sequence of the H-2 complex. It can be divided into six regions, each encoding different molecules mediating immunologic functions: K, I, S, D, L, and Tla;Qa, from left to right.

**H-2K, H-2D, and H-2L:** The regions of the H-2 complex of the mouse that encode class I molecules. These molecules are classically thought of as transplantation antigens. Class I molecules present antigen-derived peptide to CD8$^+$ cytotoxic T cells.

**H-2I:** The region of the H-2 complex that encodes class II molecules (formally called *Ia molecules*), which are found on antigen-presenting cells such as B cells, macrophages, and dendritic cells. Class II molecules present antigen-derived peptide thereby allowing immune cells to communicate with each other.

**H-2S:** The region of the H-2 complex of the mouse that encodes class III molecules. These molecules are classically thought of as some of the complement components (such as C2, B, C4, and Slp).

**Haplotype:** The particular collection of alleles present on a single chromosome; often used to describe MHC genes. The haplotype is the group of closely linked genes of a single chromosome that are inherited from one parent and encode particular phenotypes.

**Hapten:** A small chemical that can combine with specific antibody, but cannot initiate an immune response unless it is bound to a larger "carrier" molecule. In other words, a hapten is antigenic but not immunogenic by itself. It is functionally equivalent to an epitope.

**Hashimoto's thyroiditis:** An organ-specific, cell-mediated and antibody-mediated autoimmune disease—an inflammation of the thyroid. Thyroid enlargement characterized by epithelial changes and lymphoid hyperplasia due to an inflammatory lymphocytic infiltrate, leading to a decrease in thyroid activity (hypothyroiditism). The target antigens are thyroglobulin and thyroperoxidase.

**Heat-shock proteins (HSPs):** A family of proteins that function in the assembly, transport, and folding of cellular proteins. HSPs increase in concentration as a response to heat and other stress in cells, which can then become targeted by an immune response.

**Heavy (H) chain (of antibody):** A long polypeptide chain of amino acids present in all antibodies. In humans, the IgG and IgM H chains have molecular weights of 50,000 and 70,000, respectively. The H chain is divided into an amino-terminal variable region (Fab portion) and a carboxyl-terminal constant region (Fc portion). It can also be divided into one variable domain and three or four constant domains. There are two H chains per antibody molecule, each connected by disulfide bridges to a light chain and to the other H chain. The H chain bears the antigenic determinants that distinguish the five antibody classes (or isotypes) each with their unique functional activity.

**Helminth:** A parasitic worm. Infection by this worm often elicits $T_H2$ cell responses characterized by eosinophil-rich inflammatory infiltrates and IgE production.

**Helper T ($T_H$) cell:** A subset of T lymphocytes that cooperate (through CD28 and CD40L expression and cytokine secretion) with macrophages, dendritic cells, and B cells to augment/induce antibody production or with other T cells to augment/induce cell-mediated immunity. The helper T cell phenotype is usually $CD4^+$. See also T helper cells and T lymphocytes.

**Hemagglutination:** The agglutination of red blood cells.

**Hematopoiesis:** The transition from a pluripotent hematopoietic stem cell in the bone marrow to a mature blood cell.

**Hemolytic disease of the newborn:** A disease that results from a mother's IgG antibodies crossing the placenta and destroying the fetus's red cells. The $Rh^-$ mother becomes sensitized during birth of the first child if the fetus's $Rh^+$ red cells enter the mother's circulation. The mother produces anti-Rh antibodies that are of the IgG class. These antibodies can cross the placenta during subsequent pregnancies, destroy fetal red cells, and lead to the disease state.

**Hemolytic (Jerne) plaque assay:** An *in vitro* method used to detect and enumerate antibody-producing cells. It involves the incorporation of spleen cells sensitized to sheep red blood cells (SRBC), SRBC, and complement into agarose. Wherever an antibody-producing cell comes in contact with the antigen SRBC, an antigen-antibody complex is formed and complement is fixed, resulting in a zone of lysis (plaque).

**Hepatocarcinoma:** A cancer of the liver. See also Carcinoma.

**Heptamer-nonamer and the spacer 12/23 rule:** Governs the joining of separate V-J or D-J and V to D-J gene segments on the DNA strand when antibody light or heavy chains or T cell receptor chains are synthesized. Heptamers are seven-nucleotide and nonamers are nine-nucleotide conserved recombination signal sequences (RSSs), respectively, that flank all rearranging gene segments. Heptamers and nonamers are separated by either 12 or 23 nucleotides. The RSSs are targeted by site-specific RAG-1 and RAG-2 recombinases that join the segments. Following the 12/23 rule, a RSS with a 12 bp-spacer (RSS-1) can combine only with a RSS with a 23 bp-spacer (RSS-2).

**Herd immunity:** The protection afford individuals in a population that have no protective immunity against a pathogen because the majority of the population is resistant to the pathogen.

**Hereditary angioedema:** An autosomal dominant deficiency of C1 complement inhibitor that leads to localized edema. See C1 inhibitor (C1-INH).

**Heteroantigen (xenoantigen):** An antigen derived from one species that can induce an immune response in another species, such as a bacterial vaccine injected into an individual.

**Heterologous antigen:** An antigen other than the one used to induce the immune response. For example, if bovine serum albumin (BSA) induces the immunity and we test the reactivity of anti-BSA antibodies with rat serum albumin (RSA), the RSA is the heterologous antigen. See Homologous antigen for its opposite counterpart.

**Heteronuclear RNA (hnRNA):** The fraction of large, heterogeneously-sized nuclear RNA that contains the primary transcripts of the DNA for antibodies before processing to form mRNA. In other words, the hnRNA contains the gene segments containing the recombined V-J (light chain) or the V-D-J (heavy chain) region and the C region that are transcribed into RNA. These segments still contain the intron between the J and C genes and thus are called the *primary transcript*.

**Heterophile antigen:** An antigen that is distributed on many different cells of many different species, such as an antigen that can be found on human red blood cells, bacteria, fish, etc. It is responsible for cross-reactions during testing of different antibodies.

**HEV:** See High endothelial venules.

**High endothelial venules (HEVs):** An area of capillary venules (small veins that join capillaries to larger veins) composed of plump, cuboidal (high) cells that have receptors, corresponding to ligands on some lymphocytes, which cause lymphocytes to migrate into the lymph nodes. HEVs are found in the paracortex of lymph nodes and tonsils and in the interfollicular areas of Peyer's patches but not in the spleen.

**High zone tolerance:** Tolerance can be induced by using high doses of antigen that tolerizes primarily B cells.

**Highly active antiretroviral therapy (HAART):** A combination therapy for HIV infection that consists of two types of reverse transcriptase inhibitors and one viral protease inhibitor. Multidrug-resistant patients are given another class of antiretroviral agent, a fusion inhibitor (enfuvirtide), which blocks the entry of HIV to cells.

**Hinge region:** The area in the constant (C) region of an antibody heavy chain between the first and second C-region domains (or Fab and Fc regions). It is often rich in cysteine and proline residues. The hinge portion of the chain allows for flexibility within the molecule. It is the site of pepsin cleavage into F(ab')$_2$ and Fc fragments.

**Histamine:** A vasoactive amine (also called a *biogenic amine*) released from granules within mast cells and basophils that causes vasodilation and smooth muscle contraction. It is the major mediator in immediate hypersensitivity reactions.

**Histocompatibility:** The sharing of transplantation antigens between two individuals.

**Histocompatibility antigen 2 (H-2) complex:** The MHC of the mouse. The genes of the H-2 complex encode the major transplantation (class I) molecules found on somatic cells, the class II genes (formerly called *immune-associated [Ia] genes*) that encode class II surface molecules on antigen-presenting cells, allowing immune cells to interact, thereby controlling the immune response. These latter genes were also called *immune response (Ir) genes*.

**Histocompatibility antigen H-Y:** It is a protein encoded on the Y chromosome; thus, female T cells respond to H-Y-derived peptides and so H-Y is a male-specific histocompatibility antigen.

**Histocompatibility genes:** The genes that encode surface antigens that induce graft rejection. The MHC is the most important loci for these genes; however, the MHC contains genes that have other important roles in the immune response.

**Histocytes:** Macrophages that are fixed in tissues.

**Histotope:** The part of the class I or II MHC molecule that is recognized in association with foreign antigen by the T cell antigen receptor.

**HLA complex:** The human leukocyte antigen (HLA) complex is the MHC of humans. Like the H-2 complex of mice, the HLA complex contains the genes that encode the major transplantation (class I) molecules found on somatic cells, the genes that encode class II surface molecules on antigen-presenting cells, allowing immune cells to interact, thereby controlling the immune response. These latter genes were also called *immune response (Ir) genes*.

**HLA-A, -B, and −C:** The loci of the human HLA complex that encode class I molecules (traditionally called *transplantation antigens*), which are expressed on all nucleated cells that present antigen-derived peptide to CD8$^+$ cytotoxic T cells.

**HLA-D:** The loci of the human HLA complex that encode class II molecules, composed of three loci called *DP*, *DQ*, and *DR*. Class II molecules are expressed on antigen-presenting cells, e.g., B cells, macrophages, and dendritic cells.

**HLA-DM:** The loci of the human HLA complex that encode class II-like molecules, which are involved in loading peptides onto class II molecules. The HLA-DM molecule is found in the MIIC endosomal compartment and facilitates removal of the CLIP peptide and the binding of antigen-derived peptides to class II MHC molecules. See also CLIP.

**HIV:** See Human immunodeficiency virus.

**Hodgkin's disease:** An immune system cancer characterized by the appearance of large cells called *Reed-Sternberg cells*, which are derived from mutated B-lineage cells. The disease exists in two forms: Hodgkin's lymphoma and nodular sclerosis.

**Holes-in-the-repertoire model:** States that the major histocompatibility complex influences the immune response by shaping the repertoire of functional T cells. T cells do not have the "matching" T cell receptors (the "holes") for an antigen-MHC molecule complex.

**Homeostasis:** The maintenance of a constant number and diverse repertoire of lymphocytes by the adaptive immune system. It is achieved by several regulated pathways of lymphocyte inactivation and death.

**Homing:** The differential migration of leukocytes to particular organs or tissues.

**Homing receptors:** Receptors that direct the differential migration (homing) of leukocytes to particular lymphoid and inflamed tissues. Homing receptors (also called *selectins*) bind ligands (addressins) on endothelial cells in particular lymphoid or inflamed tissue vascular beds. See also Selectins and Addressins.

**Homocytotropic antibodies:** IgE molecules whose binding is species-specific.

**Homologous antigen:** An antigen that can be classified according to its relationship to the substance that induced the immune response. Hence, the homologous antigen is the one that induced the immunity. For example, if an animal is immunized with bovine serum albumin (BSA), the resulting antibodies are specific for BSA. If one tests the reactivity of these antibodies with BSA, one is using the homologous antigen. See Heterologous antigen for its opposite counterpart.

**Homologous recombination:** The disruption of cellular genes with copies of the gene into which erroneous sequences have been inserted. The introduction of these exogenous DNA fragments into cells, leads to the selective recombination with the cellular gene through the remaining regions of sequence homology, replacing the functional gene with the nonfunctional one.

**Homopolymer:** Usually a linear polymer of repeating units of one amino acid.

**Horror autotoxicus:** A concept proposed by Paul Ehrlich around 1900 that immune responses against self-tissue are incompatible with life. That is, even though self-constituents are immunogenic in other individuals, they are not to ourselves, unless there is an autoimmune response.

**Human immunodeficiency virus (HIV):** The name given a retrovirus that belongs to the genus Lentivirus in the family *Retroviridae* that causes acquired immunodeficiency syndrome (AIDS) by infecting CD4-expressing T cells, macrophages, and dendritic cells, and leads to a chronic progressive destruction of the immune system and susceptibility to a range of opportunistic infections and cancers. HIV is divided into two strains: HIV-1 and HIV-2. HIV-1 is responsible for most infections worldwide. HIV-2 is endemic to West Africa. HIV-1 is genetically variable; because of its viral sequences it is divided into three groups named M, N, and O. HIV-1 group M, which has evolved in humans to form at least 11 genetic subtypes, also called *clades*, designated by letters from A to K. HIV-1 can also be divided into two groups depending on how they gain enter to target cells: R5 HIV, if they use CC-chemokine receptor 5 (CCR5) on macrophages as the coreceptor or R4 HIV, if they use CXC-chemokine receptor 4 (CXCR4) on T cells as the coreceptor. See also Acquired immunodeficiency syndrome.

**Human leukocyte antigen (HLA):** Definable major histocompatibility complex (MHC) molecules in humans that constitute the human counterpart of the mouse H-2 complex. They were initially describes as antibody-induced transplantation or alloantigens on leukocytes. See HLA complex.

**Humanized antibody:** A monoclonal antibody encoded by a recombinant hybrid gene that contains the antigen-binding region amino acids of a different species within the framework of a human antibody.

**Humoral immunity:** Adaptive immunity mediated by specific antibodies, produced by B cell-derived plasma cells, that are found in the blood and tissue fluids of the body.

**H-Y antigen:** A histocompatibility antigen encoded on the male Y chromosome. If tissue from a male mouse is transferred to a female mouse of the same strain, a graft rejection of the tissue can result. Rejection does not occur if a graft is transferred from a female mouse to a male mouse of the same strain. See also Histocompatibility antigen H-Y.

**Hybrid, chimeric, or recombinant monoclonal antibodies:** The novel, tailor-made monoclonal antibodies produced by transfection. See Transfection.

**Hybridoma:** Cell lines created by the *in vitro* fusing of lymphocytes and tumor cells, such as B cells and myeloma cells to generate hybridomas producing monoclonal antibodies. T cell hybridomas are created by fusing antigen-specific T cells with a T-cell tumor line.

**Hydrophilic:** If a compound is hydrophilic, it is soluble in water. Compounds that are hydrophilic bind water on the exterior surfaces of proteins and membranes.

**Hydrophobicity:** The general abhorrence of water; thus, if a molecule is hydrophobic it does not readily absorb water. The molecule lacks polar groups and therefore is insoluble in water. Hydrophobicity occurs because hydrophobic groups are pushed to the interior of protein molecules or membranes, away from water.

**Hyperacute graft rejection:** The speed with which an allograft such as the kidney is rejected. In this case, the rejection occurs within minutes of the transplant and is due to the presence of high titers of preformed antibodies to the donor's endothelial antigens, such as, blood group antigens that activate the complement system and cause thrombotic occlusion in graft blood vessels.

**Hyperplasia:** A reversible increase in the size of an organ due to increased number of cells; for example, the splenomegaly that can result after an infection.

**Hypersensitivity:** The state, existing in a previously immunized (sensitized) individual, that leads to tissue damage due to an exaggerated and inappropriate immune response on subsequent exposure to the antigen (allergen); for example, a form of allergy called *hay fever*.

**Hypervariable regions (loops):** Short segments, within the variable regions of antibody or T cell receptor molecules, of extreme variability that form loop structures that contact antigenic determinants. There are three hypervariable regions, also called *complementarity-determining regions (CDRs)*, in antibody heavy and light chains and in T cell receptor $\alpha$ and $\beta$ chains. Also see Complementarity-determining regions (CDRs).

**Hyposensitivity:** A reaction that occurs when repeated small doses of an allergen are given to reduce hypersensitivity. See also Desensitization.

**Hypoxanthine-aminopterin-thymidine (HAT) medium:** Used in the production of hybridomas. It allows selection for only myeloma-spleen cell fusion.

**Hypoxia:** Low oxygen levels in the tissue; also found in many areas of advanced cancers and is associated with poor prognosis.

# I

**I region:** That portion of the H-2 complex of mice containing genes that control immune responses by encoding class II MHC molecules.

**I-A subregion:** A subregion of the murine H-2 complex that encodes class II MHC molecules.

**ICAMs:** See Intercellular adhesion molecules.

**ICAM-1 (intercellular adhesion molecule-1; CD54):** A member of the Ig-gene superfamily, which is induced on endothelial cells by infection. It is important in local inflammations. Like ICAM-2, it is a ligand for CD11aCD18. See CD11aCD18.

**ICAM-2 (intercellular adhesion molecule-2; CD102):** A member of the Ig-gene superfamily, which is expressed at low levels on endothelial cells. Like ICAM-1, it is a ligand for CD11aCD18. See CD11aCD18.

**ICAM-3 (intercellular adhesion molecule-3; CD50):** A member of the Ig-gene superfamily, which is only expressed on leukocytes. It is a ligand with high affinity for DC-SIGN (it also binds CD11aCD18), which suggests its importance in adhesion between T cells and dendritic cells. See also DC-SIGN.

**Iatrogenic disease:** A disease caused by the activity of a physician, such as transfusion of incompatible blood.

**Iccosomes (immune-complex-coated bodies):** They are beaded cytoplasmic particles coated with immune complexes present on the extensions of follicular dendritic cells. They may act as long-term repositories for antigen; as they bud off, B cells may internalize them (giving themselves a re-exposure to antigen). See also Follicular dendritic cells (FCDs).

**ICOS:** See Inducible T-cell costimulator.

**Idiopathic:** A disease of unknown cause; for example, the autoimmune hemolytic disease idiopathic (autoimmune) thrombocytopenic purpura.

**Idiotope:** An antigenic determinant (epitope) on an idiotype formed by one or more of the hypervariable regions. Idiotopes may be recognized as foreign because they are present in amounts too low to induce tolerance.

**Idiotypes (Ab$_1$):** The variants defined by antigenic determinants localized in the variable portion of Igs and T cell receptors. The antigenic determinants are generated by the antigen-combining site of an immunoglobulin (Ig) or T cell receptor. The idiotypic determinants represent the uniqueness of each Ig or T cell receptor. Thus, for every unique antigenic determinant there is a specific antibody or T cell receptor having a unique idiotype.

**Idiotype networks:** See Network theory.

**Idiotypic determinants:** Used to classify antibodies or T cell receptors into idiotypes. They are common to antibodies or T cell receptors with specificity for the same foreign antigenic determinants. See also Idiotypes (Ab$_1$).

**IELs:** See Intraepithelial lymphocytes (IELs).

**Ikaros:** A gene that encodes a family of zinc-finger transcription factors, which is essential for the development of all lymphoid lineages. Ikaros-deficient mice lack all B cells, NK cells and fetal T cells, and have severely reduced numbers of T cells and dendritic cells after birth. It also is required for the development of lymph nodes and Peyer's patches.

**Immature B lymphocyte:** A B cell that is IgM$^+$ and IgD$^-$, which does not proliferate or differentiate in response to antigens. In fact, antigen reactivity induces apoptosis or functional unresponsiveness of these cells. Self-antigen-specific bone marrow-resident immature B cells are negatively selected by encounter with these antigens and do not complete their maturation.

**Immediate hypersensitivity:** A detrimental immune response to an allergen that occurs within seconds to minutes after the second exposure to the allergen. It results from the cross-linking of mast cell or basophil Fc receptor-bound IgE, which initiates the release of mediators that cause increase vascular permeability, vasodilation, bronchial and visceral smooth muscle contraction, and local inflammation. See also Type I hypersensitivity.

**Immune adherence:** An agglutination-like reaction between a cell bearing the C3b molecules and another cell that has a receptor for C3b, such as a macrophage. This interaction facilitates phagocytosis.

**Immune clearance:** The rapid removal of antigen-antibody complexes from the blood.

**Immune complex:** A complex of antigen-antibody molecules that can vary greatly in size. These complexes initiate humoral immunity effector mechanisms such as complement activation and FcR-mediated phagocyte activation. The deposition of immune complexes in blood vessels or kidney glomeruli can lead to inflammation and disease called *immune complex disease.*

**Immune deviation:** Antigen-induced polarization of an immune response to one dominated by either $T_H1$ or $T_H2$ cells.

**Immune precipitation:** Precipitation that occurs when antigen and antibody combine in solution and form a visible aggregate.

**Immune-privileged sites:** These are body areas with a decreased immune reactivity to foreign antigens, such as tissue grafts. These areas include the brain, eye, testis, and uterus.

**Immune response:** In a vertebrate host, the production of specific cells and molecules directed against the foreign invader.

**Immune response (Ir) genes:** An older term used to describe the class II MHC genes, which control the immune response's intensity to a particular antigen—the ability or inability of expressed class II molecules to bind antigenic peptides, thereby control the immune response.

**Immune stimulatory complexes (ISCOMs):** They are antigens held within a lipid matrix (lipid micelles) that act as adjuvants. These complexes mimic endogenous antigen; therefore, they are taken up by dendritic cells, processed by the cytosolic pathway, and presented with class I MHC molecules to initiate cell-mediated immune response.

**Immune surveillance:** Immunological protection that is provided by the immune system to continually recognize and destroy tumor cells, which constantly arise throughout life. The resulting immune effector cells are stimulated by immune recognition of either stress ligands or unique antigens expressed on tumor cells.

**Immune (Type II) interferon:** See Interferon-γ.

**Immunity:** The state of being resistant (immune) to an antigen, either as an intact trait (innate immunity) or by previous exposure (adaptive immunity).

**Immunization:** The exposure process by which the host develops immunity. See Active immunity and Passive Immunity.

**Immunoadsorption:** The process by which antibody or antigen is removed from a sample through the adsorption to a solid-phase system.

**Immunoblotting:** Once proteins have been blotted, they are identified by incubating the blot with a primary radiolabeled or enzyme-labeled antibody (antibody specific for antigen). The labeled antibody binds to the blotted antigens whose location is detected by using autoradiography or enzyme staining. Generally the primary antibody is not labeled, but is detected by using a secondary radiolabeled or enzyme-labeled antibody (anti-antibody). Also called *Western blotting.*

**Immunocompetent:** A functionally mature lymphocyte that can recognize antigen and is capable of mediating an immune response.

**Immunodeficiency:** Any inherited or acquired deficiency in an immune response, which could be caused by defects in phagocytosis, humoral immunity or cell-mediated immunity. The combination of the latter two defects leads to combined immune deficiencies.

**Immunodominance:** The fact that some amino acid residues within a determinant, or epitopes within a complex mixture (such as a whole virus) are more important immunologically than others, i.e., they are preferentially recognized or reacted against during an immune response.

**Immunodominant:** That portion of an epitope contributing most to the binding energy.

**Immunodominant epitope:** A linear amino acid sequence epitope of a multideterminant protein antigen for which most of an individual's responding T cells are specific. Immunodominant epitopes correspond to the proteolytically generated peptides within antigen-presenting cells that bind most avidly to MHC molecules and are the mostly likely to stimulate T cells.

**Immunoelectrophoresis:** A two-step technique: (1) molecules are separated by their charge; and (2) immunodiffusion of the antigens that leads to precipitin arcs.

**Immunoenhancement:** Reinforcement of the immune system to increase the antibody or cell-mediated immune response against antigens. See Immunosuppression.

**Immunofluorescence:** A histochemical technique in which antibody is conjugated to a fluorescent dye (fluorochrome) and used to detect and localize antigen by observation of the pattern of fluorescence in an ultraviolet microscope.

**Immunogen:** A substance which on introduction into the body stimulates an active immune response. An easy way to think of an immunogen versus an antigen is: all immunogens are antigens, but not all antigens are immunogens. See also Antigen.

**Immunogenicity:** The potential to induce humoral or cell-mediated immunity. In this context, the substance inducing the immune response is called an *immunogen*. See also Antigenicity.

**Immunogenic tumor:** Tumor immunogenicity is defined by its ability to enhance antitumor immune responses after irradiation and subcutaneous vaccination into tumor-naïve mice. Tumors can be divided into highly immunogenic or less immunogenic; the former allows for 100% protection of vaccinated hosts, whereas the less immunogenic tumors lead to poorer immune response with roughly 50% or less of the hosts succumbing to live tumor challenge after immunization.

**Immunoglobulin (Ig):** Any globulin protein composed of two light and two heavy chains linked by disulfide bonds. All antibodies are immunoglobulins. They can either be membrane bound or soluble molecules. See Antibody.

**Immunoglobulin (Ig)α/Igβ (CD79a & CD79b):** The disulfide-linked, surface transmembrane molecules Igα and Igβ noncovalently flank each immunoglobulin (Igα/Igβ-immunoglobulin), which contain ITAMs that transduce early activation signals to the B cell following antigen ligation. See also B-cell-receptor complex.

**Immunoglobulin class:** A subdivision of immunoglobulin molecules based on unique antigenic determinants in the constant regions of their heavy chains. These determinants divide the human immunoglobulins into five classes, designated IgG, IgA, IgM, IgD, and IgE, each associated with different immunologic effector functions. See also Antibody subclasses and Immunoglobulin subclasses.

**Immunoglobulin domains:** On the antibody chain, a tandem series of repeating homology units roughly 110 amino acid residues long, which fold independently into a compact 3-D globular structural motif. All proteins with this structural motif belong to the Ig-gene superfamily. See Immunoglobulin (Ig)-gene superfamily.

**Immunoglobulin fold:** The characteristic domain structure in immunoglobulins that consists of roughly 110 amino acid domain folded into two β-pleated sheets, each containing three or four antiparallel strands, and are stabilized by an intrachain disulfide bridge. See Immunoglobulin (Ig)-gene superfamily.

**Immunoglobulin subclass:** A subdivision of the immunoglobulin into subclasses based on unique antigenic determinants in the constant regions of their heavy chains. For example, these determinants divide the human IgG class into four subclasses, designated IgG1, IgG2, IgG3, and IgG4 and the human IgA class into two subclasses, designated IgA1 and IgA2.

**Immunoglobulin (Ig)-gene superfamily:** A group of related genes that encode immunoglobulins and other cell surface markers, such as class I and II MHC molecules, T cell receptor, CD4 and CD8 molecules. The encoded-structures contain the characteristic immunoglobulin-fold domains, which consists of 7–9 β-strands and often are involved in protein-protein interactions.

**Immunologic ignorance:** A form of self-tolerance where both reactive lymphocytes and their targets are present but autoimmune disease does not occur.

**Immunologic memory:** The phenomenon whereby the immune system of a host responds faster and more powerfully to an antigen on subsequent exposures. It leads to a heightened secondary immune response. See also Anamnestic response.

**Immunologic synapse:** The supra-molecular "bulls-eye-like" contact area that is established between a T cell and an antigen-presenting cell (APC) bearing the MHC molecule-peptide complex recognized by the T cell antigen receptor (TCR). At the center of the synapse, adhesion is mediated through binding of the TCR to the APC's MHC molecule-peptide complex. Peripherally, this complex is stabilized through additional interactions—for example, between LFA1 and ICAM1. Taken together, it involves adhesion molecules, as well as antigen receptors and cytokine receptors.

**Immunologic tolerance:** The specific lack of immune responsiveness conferred on a host by inactivation or death of self-antigen-specific lymphocytes. The response to all other antigens is normal. Self-tolerance is a normal feature of the adaptive immune system, which is mediated at two levels: central tolerance and peripheral tolerance. See also Central tolerance and Peripheral tolerance.

**Immunologically privileged sites:** Areas of the body that allow for the survival of allogenic tissues, areas like the brain and anterior chamber of the eye.

**Immunology:** The science that studies the structure and functioning of the immune system.

**Immunophilins (also called *cyclophilins*):** Isomerases that bind the immunosuppressive drugs cyclosporin-A, FK506 (tacrolimus), and rapamycin.

**Immunopotency:** The ability of a specific region of an antigen molecule to serve as an antigenic determinant and thereby induces of an immune response.

**Immunoreceptor tyrosine-based activation motifs (ITAMs):** They are conserved segments, composed of (D/E)XXYXX(L/I)X6–8YXX(L/I), where X denotes any amino acid, found in the intracytoplasmic tails of ζ and CD3 proteins, Igα/Igβ (CD79a/CD79b), NK cell receptors and in several immunoglobulin Fc receptors that are targets for phosphorylation by tyrosine kinases, allowing them to interact with cytosolic enzymes. When the ITAM-containing receptors bind their ligands, the ITAMs' tyrosine residues become phosphorylated and form docking sites for other molecules mediating cell-activating signal transduction pathways, triggering a cascade of intracellular events that leads to cellular activation. See also ZAP-70.

**Immunoreceptor tyrosine-based inhibitory motifs (ITIMs):** They are a six amino acid motifs found in the cytoplasmic tails of various immune system inhibitory receptors, such as the NK cell killer cell immunoglobulin-like receptor (KIR), CTLA-4 on T cells, and FcγRIIB and CD22 on B cells. During ligation of these receptors, ITIMs become phosphorylated on their tyrosine residues and form a tyrosine phosphatase-docking site, which in turn inhibits other signal transduction pathways. The prototype six amino-acid ITIM sequence is (Ile/Val/Leu/Ser)-Xaa-Tyr-Xaa Xaa-(Leu/Val).

**Immunoscnescence:** The decreased immune system function with age, exemplified by the decreased number of naïve T cells as thymic function decreases.

**Immunosuppression:** The suppression of innate or adaptive immune responsiveness by external agents, such as drugs or irradiation.

**Immunotherapy:** Efforts to attack tumor cells through the immune system, which focus on stimulating or replenishing antitumor elements of the patient's immune response without further stimulating the suppressor cells.

**Immunotoxins:** Agents that combine two activities: selectivity of monoclonal antibodies and the killing power of cellular toxins, such as ricin or diphtheria toxin. The antibodies target the toxins to the appropriate cancer cells without damaging the surrounding normal cells.

**Imprecise DNA rearrangement:** One of the methods used to increase receptor diversity. It is also known as flexible or imprecise recombination. See Insertion of random N (nucleotide) regions, N-addition, P-addition, and Junctional diversity.

**Inbred mice:** Mice produced by sequential, repeated brother-sister matings for as many as 20 generations. This inbreeding leads to a strain with all chromosomes having identical sets, except the sex chromosomes. In other words, the strain is homozygous for all chromosomes, producing identical homozygous progeny. If the progeny loci are of either parental homozygous genotype with no heterozygous loci, the progeny are then defined as inbred.

**Incidence:** The occurrence rate of some event, such as, the number of people who get a disease divide by a total given population per unit of time. Incidence is contrasted with prevalence. See Prevalence.

**Incomplete antibodies:** Antibodies that are structurally correct but functionally "incomplete." They can bind antigen, but the binding does not lead to precipitation or agglutination of the antigen.

**Incomplete Freund's adjuvant:** A commonly used adjuvant composed of a water-in-oil emulsion and a detergent that forms an antigen depot at the site of injection. See also Adjuvant and Complete Freund's adjuvant.

**Indirect agglutination (passive agglutination):** The agglutination of red blood cells or particles to which antibody have been conjugated.

**Indirect antigen presentation:** In transplantation reactions, the presentation of allogeneic donor MHC molecules by recipient antigen-presenting cells (APCs) in a mechanism similar to presentation of microbial antigens. The recipient's APCs process the allogeneic protein and the derived peptides are presented in association with the recipient's (self) MHC molecules to host T cells. Indirect antigen presentation is in contrast to direct antigen presentation. See Direct antigen presentation.

**Indirect fluorescent antibody method:** An immunofluorescence staining technique in which antibody with specificity for the desired antigen is unlabeled and a second, fluorescently labeled antibody with specificity for the first antibody is then added to the mixture. See also Direct fluorescent antibody method.

**Indoleamine 2,3-dioxygenase (IDO):** It is an intracellular enzyme that catalyzes the oxidative catabolism of tryptophan. If the latter molecule is in insufficient amounts in the cell, it can lead to T cell anergy and apoptosis.

**Inducible NO synthase (iNOS):** iNOS is expressed by macrophages and other cell types. It can be induced by many different stimuli to activate nitric oxide (NO) synthesis. It is an important mechanism in host resistance to intracellular infection.

**Inducible T-cell costimulator (ICOS):** A CD28-related protein that is induced on activated T cells ($T_H2 > T_H1$) and enhances their response; its ligand is the nonB7 molecule ICOS ligand (also called *B7-H2*), which is expressed on professional antigen-presenting cells, fibroblasts, epithelial cells, and endothelial cells. See also Costimulatory signal.

**Induration:** A localized inflammatory reaction, during which the area becomes hardened, such as the tuberculin skin reaction for tuberculosis.

**Infection:** A pathological condition due to the growth of microorganisms in a host.

**Infectious mononucleosis:** It results from infection by Epstein-Barr virus and consists of fever, malaise, and swollen lymph nodes.

**Infectious synapse:** The cell-cell contact zone (also called *virologic synapse*) between CD4$^+$ T cells and dendritic cells that facilitates HIV transmission by locally concentrating virus and viral receptors.

**Inflammasome:** A molecular complex composed of several proteins that, on assembly, cleave prointerleukin-1, leading to active interleukin-1.

**Inflammation:** A complex response of the innate immune system that results from tissue injury and involves increased blood supply to the site of injury, increased capillary permeability, and movement of leukocytes from the capillaries into the surrounding site. It leads to protection against infection and tissue repair. The flipside is it can also cause tissue damage and disease. Adaptive immune responses can promote inflammation. Inflammation can be either acute (appears quickly and is transient) or chronic (occurs with persistent infections and autoimmune diseases).

**Initiation:** The first event in the development of a cancer, involving acquisition of the mutation. See also Promotion.

**Innate immunity:** The collection of nonspecific and phylogenetically ancient defenses of a host that exist before, and function independently of, any exposure to foreign antigen. The immunity individuals have by being the individuals they are—it is the inborn first line of defense against infection, which does not involve memory. Innate immunity includes physical and chemical barriers, phagocytic cells, natural killer (NK) cells, cytokines, and the complement system. It uses a limited number of cellular and soluble receptors that recognize common patterns in microorganisms. See also Adaptive immunity.

**Innocent bystander cells:** Cells that are destroyed during immune reactivity directed toward other cells.

**Inositol 1,4,5-triphosphate (IP$_3$):** A cytoplasmic signaling molecule, which is activated during lymphocyte antigen binding. It is generated by phospholipase C-mediated hydrolysis of the membrane phospholipid PIP$_2$. IP$_3$'s main function is to release intracellular stores of Ca$^{2+}$ from membrane-bound compartments like the endoplasmic reticulum. See also Phospholipase C (PLC).

**Insertion of random N (nontemplated) nucleotide regions:** One of the methods used in junctional diversity to increase antibody and T cell receptor diversity. It is the random addition, mediated by the enzyme terminal deoxyribonucleotidyl transferase, of up to 20 nucleotides between V, D, and J segments during immunoglobulin or T cell receptor rearrangement. See also Imprecise DNA rearrangement and Junctional diversity.

**Insertional mutagenesis:** An experimental approach implicating proto-oncogenes in carcinogenesis. These studies suggest that integration of viral DNA may be mutagenic both directly and indirectly.

**Instructive theories of antibody formation:** Early theories of antibody formation proposing that immune cells have no specificity for antigen and that, when these cells come in contact with antigen, the antigen "instructs" the cell what antibody to make. In other words, the antigen acts as a template for the antibody to mold around. These theories were also called *template theories*.

**Insulin-dependent diabetes mellitus (IDDM; type 1 diabetes):** A cell-mediated autoimmune disease caused by destruction of insulin-producing β cells of the islets of Langerhans in the pancreas, characterized by a lack of insulin, which leads to high levels of glucose in the blood (hyperglycemia). T cells and antibodies are implicated in the disease.

**Integrin family:** A family of cell surface receptors that are transmembrane glycoproteins consisting of noncovalent heterodimers (two subunits, α and β). Each subunit has a small C-terminal intracellular domain and a large extracellular domain. The extracellular domain interacts with a wide variety of ligands such as extracellular matrix glycoproteins, complement, and other cells, while the intracellular domain interacts with the cytoskeleton. The integrins are physiologically important because they participate in cell-cell and cell-matrix adhesion including hemostasis, wound healing, and immune and non-immune defense mechanisms. There are two main integrin subfamilies; members of each family express a conserved β chain ($β_1$, or CD29, and $β_2$, or CD18) associated with different α chains. Members of the integrin family include fibronectin receptor, LFA-1, Mac-1, and the VLA antigens.

**Interallelic conversion:** A genetic recombination between two alleles of a locus in which one allele segment is replaced with the homologous segment from the other. This is the mechanism that generates new HLA class I and II alleles.

**Intercellular adhesion molecules (ICAMs):** They are cell-surface ligands for integrins (or adhesion molecule) found on leukocytes that are important in the binding of lymphocytes and leukocytes to certain cells. ICAMs are members of the immunoglobulin superfamily. See also ICAM-1, -2, and -3 and Integrin family.

**Interdigitating dendritic cells:** A potent antigen-presenting cell population, rich in MHC class II molecules that is found in blood, the paracortex of lymph nodes and the spleen, and the thymic medulla. As immature cells in the peripheral (highly phagocytic and express low levels of class II and costimulatory molecules), they internalize antigen in the periphery, migrate to lymph node and spleen paracortical regions becoming mature nonphagocytic cells expressing high levels of class II and costimulatory molecules thereby allowing them to interact with T cells.

**Interfacial (ring) test:** A precipitation test used to detect antigens antibodies. Antiserum in test tubes is overlaid with antigen of increasing concentration. Antigen and antibody react at the interface of the two solutions, forming a visible band or ring with a cloudy appearance.

**Interferon-γ (IFN-γ):** An interferon produced by CD4$^+$ T$_H$1 cells, CD8$^+$ T cells, and NK cells that regulates other immune cells; it is best known as a macrophage-activating agent in both innate immune responses and adaptive immune responses. It is also called *type II* or *immune interferon*. Type I interferons are represented by IFN-α and IFN-β. See also Type I interferons.

**Interleukin-1 (IL-1):** A factor, derived mainly from activated macrophages but many nonlymphoid cells also make it. It has a major role in mediating host inflammatory responses in innate immunity. It also promotes T-cell proliferation following antigen stimulation. There are two forms of IL-1: IL-1α and IL-1β, which bind to the same receptors and have the same biological effects. These effects include induction of: endothelial cell adhesion molecules, endothelial cell and macrophage chemokine production, acute phase proteins by the liver, and fever.

**Interleukin-1 (IL-1) receptor antagonist (IL-1ra):** A mononuclear phagocyte produced natural inhibitor

of IL-1, which is structurally homologous to IL-1. It binds to IL-1 receptors thereby blocking IL-1-mediated proinflammatory activity but IL-1ra itself is biologically inactivate.

**Interleukin-2 (IL-2):** A helper T cell-derived factor that allows other T cells to continue the immune response in an autocrine manner following antigen stimulation and that promotes long-term growth (proliferation) of T cells in culture, and stimulates the proliferation and effector functions of NK cells and B cells. It also mediates apoptosis of activated T cells; the process is called *activation-induced cell death (AICD)*. See Activation-induced cell death (AICD).

**Interleukin-3 (IL-3):** A CD4$^+$ T cell-derived cytokine, which promotes the expansion of immature bone marrow progenitors of mature blood cells; thus, it is considered to be one of the colony-stimulating factors.

**Interleukin-4 (IL-4):** A T$_H$2 CD4$^+$ T cell-derived cytokine required for B-cell proliferation and differentiation, IgE production by B cells, induction of differentiation of T$_H$2 cells from antigen naïve CD4$^+$ precursors, and suppression of interferon-γ-dependent macrophage functions. It is also a mast cell growth factor.

**Interleukin-5 (IL-5):** A T$_H$2 CD4$^+$ T cell-derived cytokine inducing differentiation of B cells and eosinophils (also recruits them to the site of antigen deposition), and activates mast cells.

**Interleukin-6 (IL-6):** A T cell-derived cytokine (but many other cells can produce it) that induces the proliferation of IL-4 stimulated thymocytes, expression of the acute phase protein (hepatocyte-stimulating factor) and others, antiviral activity (interferon-β$_2$), B-cell differentiation, and stimulation of IgG secretion, etc. Macrophages also are an important source of IL-6.

**Interleukin-7 (IL-7):** An important growth factor for the development of immature B and T cells and the proliferation of T cells that have exited the thymus. IL-7 triggers the expression of its receptor, which is composed of IL-7 α-chain (CD127) and a common g-chain (CD132).

**Interleukin-10 (IL-10):** A T$_H$2 cell- and macrophage-derived factor that inhibits activated macrophages thereby maintaining balance of innate and cell-mediated immune responses.

**Interleukin-12 (IL-12):** A macrophage and dendritic cell-derived factor that serves as a mediator of innate immunity and inducer of cell-mediated immunity. It has a broad array of biological activities. IL-12 activates NK cells and causes them and T cells to make interferon-γ, which enhances NK cell and cytotoxic T cell-mediated cytolytic activity, and promotes the development of $T_H1$ cells. Lymphocyte responses to IL-12 are mediated by the activator of transcription protein STAT4. Nitric oxide synthase 2A (NOS2A/NOS2) is required for the signaling process of IL-12 in innate immunity. See also STAT.

**Interleukin-17 (IL-17; also called IL-17A):** It is the founding member of the IL-17 family (IL-17B, IL-17C, IL-17D, IL-17E [also called *IL-25*], and IL-17F). It is produced by a recently described group of CD4+ T cells called *$T_H17$ cells*. IL-17, through the induction of many proinflammatory cytokines, mediates host defense against extracellular pathogens and is linked to excessive inflammation and autoimmune reactions.

**Interleukin-18 (IL-18):** A macrophage-derived proinflammatory cytokine that functions together with IL-12 as an inducer of cell-mediated immunity. IL-18 synergizes with IL-12 to stimulate interferon-$\gamma$ production by NK cells and T cells. IL-18 is structurally similar to IL-1 but not functionally. IL-18 and IL-12 inhibit B cell IL-4-dependent IgE and IgG1 production, and enhance IgG2a production. IL-18 binding protein (IL-18BP) interacts with IL-18, and negatively regulates IL-18's biological activity.

**Interleukins:** A generic name given to molecules secreted by lymphoid cells allowing them to communicate with each other. See also Interleukin-1, Interleukin-2, Interleukin-3, etc (there are interleukins 1 through 35 . . .).

**Internal image of the antigen:** The determinant on an antibody molecule that resembles an antigenic determinant of a foreign antigen and to which antibodies or T cell antigen receptors can bind. This is an essential part of the network theory, that the immune system has internal images of antigens before exposure to them. See also Network theory.

**Interstitial dendritic cells:** The dendritic cells that populate the gastrointestinal tract, heart, kidney, liver, and lungs.

**Interstitial fluid:** Fluid that is found in spaces between cells.

**Intestinal epithelium:** A primary lymphoid tissue that represents a site for thymus-independent T-cell development and positive and negative selection. In adults, it is a major site for T-lymphopoiesis and contains a large collection of T cells. It contains roughly 90% CD3+ T cells, 20–80% $\gamma\delta$ T cells, and the $\gamma\delta$ T cells and CD8$\alpha\alpha$+ $\alpha\beta$ T cells are of extrathymic origin.

**Intraepithelial lymphocytes (IELs):** T cells that express the $\gamma\delta$ T cell receptor of limited antigen diversity as well as the CD8$\alpha\alpha$ homodimer. IELs are found in the epidermis of the skin and the mucosal epithelia. Some of these lymphocytes

recognize microbial-derived glycolipids associated with the CD1 molecules (nonpolymorphic MHC-like molecules) expressed on intestinal epithelia, which leads to cytokine release, activated macrophages, and killing of infected cells. They are considered part of innate immunity. (Conventional CD8+ T cells express the CD8$\alpha\beta$ heterodimer.)

**Intrinsic binding reaction:** An equation that expresses the reaction of an epitope with an antigen-binding site: Ag + Ab ==><== [Ag - Ab].

**Intron:** A segment of a gene (DNA) between exons whose transcribed sequence is removed by splicing during the formation of mRNA; thus it cannot encode protein.

**Invariant (Ii) chain (also called *CD74*):** An early component of the class II MHC molecule that exhibits no genetic polymorphism; the Ii chain binds to and stabilizes the class II molecule structure before it acquires an antigenic peptide. It prevents loading of class II MHC molecule peptide-binding sites with peptides in the endoplasmic reticulum, forcing the peptides to associate with class I MHC molecules. The Ii chain also drives newly synthesize class II molecules to the MIIC, where antigen-derived peptide is loaded on the class II molecules.

**In vitro:** Literally means "in glass"; generally used to refer to experiments involving cells or tissues cultured outside the body.

**In vivo:** Literally means "within the living body"; generally used to refer to experiments carried out in a living animal.

**I-region-associated (Ia) antigens:** Synonymous with class II MHC molecules that are encoded by the I region of the murine H-2 complex; hence, the old name I-region-associated (Ia) antigens.

**Irradiation chimera:** A lethally X-irradiated animal that is reconstituted with lymphoid cells transferred from another donor. Thus, cells from genetically dissimilar individuals coexist in one body (chimerism).

**Ischemia:** A deficiency in blood supply due to obstructed blood vessels, which leads to injury to the surrounding tissue or organ.

**ISCOMs:** See Immune stimulatory complexes.

**Isoagglutinins:** The naturally occurring antibodies, such as the antibodies humans form against blood group antigens.

**Isoantigen:** An antigen found when the individual is the source of the antigen and the individual that responds to it is genetically identical (for example, in humans, identical twins; in animals, inbred strains of mice). Isoantigens are similar to autoantigens.

**Isograft:** A tissue or organ graft between genetically identical individuals.

**Isotypes:** Isotypes are antibody variants defined by antigenic determinants found in antibody heavy and light chain constant regions. Isotypic determinants are encoded by a gene that is carried by and expressed in each member of the species. In other words, isotypes are present in all members of a species. These determinants distinguish a given class or subclass or between types of light chains. For example, five classes (or isotypes) of heavy chains have been identified; they are designated by the Greek symbols, gamma ($\gamma$), alpha ($\alpha$), mu ($\mu$), delta ($\delta$), and epsilon ($\varepsilon$). The isotype establishes the effector mechanisms associated with their binding of antigens. The $\gamma$ and $\alpha$ classes are further divided into four and two subclasses, respectively. Antibodies are named according to which isotype they express; if they bear $\gamma$, for example, they are called *IgG*. There are two light chain isotypes, kappa ($\kappa$) and lambda ($\lambda$).

**Isotypic determinants:** The heavy-chain antigenic determinants within the constant region that define the antibody class of a species.

**ITAMs:** See Immunoreceptor tyrosine-based activation motifs.

**ITIMs:** See Immunoreceptor tyrosine-based inhibitory motifs.

# J

**JAK-STAT signaling pathway:** A cytokine-initiated signaling pathway that occurs when cytokines bind to type I and II cytokine receptors. The pathway starts with the activation of Janus kinase (JAK) tyrosine kinases, followed by JAK-mediated tyrosine phosphorylation of the cytoplasmic tails of cytokine receptors, binding of signal transducers and activators of transcription (STATs) to the phosphorylated receptor chains, phosphorylation of the STATs by JAK-mediated tyrosine, dimerization and nuclear translocation of the STATs, and STAT binding to target gene regulatory regions causing transcriptional activation of those genes. See also Signal transducer and activator of transcription (STAT) and Janus kinases (JAK kinases).

**Janus kinases (JAK kinases):** A family of four tyrosine kinases (JAK1, JAK2, JAK3 and TYK2) with a common domain structure that permanently associate with the cytoplasmic tails of certain cytokine receptors for cytokines such as interleukin-2 (IL-2), IL-4, IL-12, interferon-$\gamma$, and others. Jak kinases phosphorylate STATs, and stimulate other signaling responses. See JAK-STAT signaling pathway. See also STAT.

**Joining (J) gene segments:** Short coding sequences (about 50 base pairs long) found in the variable regions of all immunoglobulin light and heavy chains and T cell receptor chains. They recombine with V or D then V segments during lymphocyte development, leading to VJ or VDJ recombined DNA that encodes the antigen-binding site V regions. The random association of different J segments contributes to the antigen receptor repertoire diversity. See also Constant (C) gene segments and Variable (V) gene segments.

**Joining:** The linking of exons or DNA segments of somatic cell genes that are separated by introns or non-translating DNA segments in the germline cells.

**Joining (J) chain:** A short polypeptide, produced by plasma cells, with a molecular weight of 35,000 found in polymeric antibodies, such as IgM and IgA; it joins (J) monomeric molecules together. The disulfide linkage is between J chain and carboxyl-terminal cysteines of IgM and IgA heavy chains. The polymerization of IgM and IgA is required for their binding to the polymeric-immunoglobulin receptor and transport through epithelia. See Poly-Ig receptor.

**Jones-Mote reaction:** A reaction also called *cutaneous basophil hypersensitivity* appearing 24 hours after skin challenge with the offending allergen. The site of reaction is infiltrated with large numbers of basophils.

**Junctional diversity (or flexibility):** A mechanism for increasing antibody and T cell receptor diversity using random addition or removal of nucleotide sequences at junctions of V, D, and J gene segments.

# K

**K region:** One of the six regions of the H-2 map. It contains genes encoding class I molecules. See H-2 map.

**Kaposi's sarcoma:** A malignant cancer of blood-vessel endothelial cells, which is characterized by multiple bluish nodules in the skin. It occurred in about 25 to 30% of the early AIDS patients. Kaposi's sarcoma is associated with Kaposi's sarcoma-associated herpesvirus (human herpesvirus 8) infection.

**Kappa ($\kappa$) chains:** One group of antibody light chains characterized by their particular constant-domain amino acid sequence. It can combine with any of the different heavy-chain isotypes. See also Lambda ($\lambda$) chains.

**Karyotype:** The collection of chromosomes in a cell.

**Keyhole limpet hemocyanin (KLH):** A substance obtained from mollusks that is a strong T-dependent antigen and often is used in hapten-carrier conjugates.

**Killed virus vaccines:** Viral particle-containing vaccines, where the viruses have been killed by heat, chemicals or radiation. It typically induces antibody-mediated protection.

**Killer activatory receptors (KARs):** NK cell or cytotoxic T cells express these cell-surface receptors, which activate killing by these cells.

**Killer cell immunoglobulin-like receptors (KIRs):** NK cell receptors that recognize class I MHC molecules and delivery inhibitory signals, thereby preventing activation of NK cell-mediated cytotoxicity. Ligation of these receptors ensure that NK cells do not kill normal host cells expressing class I MHC molecules while permitting killing of virus-infected (or tumor) cells in which class I MHC molecule expression is suppressed. KIRs contain ITIMs in their cytoplasmic tails that initiate inhibitory signaling pathways. See Immunoreceptor tyrosine-based inhibition motifs (ITIMs).

**Kinin system:** Tissue damage triggers an enzymatic cascade of plasma proteins, leading to the production of inflammatory mediators such as the vasoactive peptide bradykinin.

**Kinins:** Small molecules released during an anaphylactic reaction that induce dilation of blood vessels and contraction of smooth muscle.

**KIT:** A receptor protein tyrosine kinase, expressed by stem cells and most other hematopoietic stem cells. KIT binds to stem-cell factor (SCF), which also called *KIT ligand*.

**KLH:** See Keyhole limpet hemocyanin.

**Km (Inv) determinant:** An allotypic determinant found on the κ light chains of human antibodies.

**Knockout mice:** Transgenic mice with a targeted disruption of a gene into the genome of a mouse embryonic stem cell by homologous recombination techniques. The result is the replaced mutant allele leads to an animal lacking a functional gene product, such as interleukin-2. See Transgenic mice.

**Kupffer cells:** Phagocytes (macrophages) that line the hepatic sinusoids in the liver.

# L

**L-selectin (CD62L):** A cell adhesion molecule expressed on most circulating lymphocytes, including naïve T cell that guides their exit from the blood into peripheral lymphoid tissues by binding to GlyCAM-1 and CD34 on high endothelial venules in the lymph nodes. See also Selectins.

**L region:** One of the six regions of the H-2 map. It contains genes encoding class I molecules. See H-2 map.

**LAK cells:** See Lymphokine-activated killer cells.

**Lambda (λ) chains:** Antibody light chains characterized by their particular constant-domain amino acid sequence. The λ chain can combine with any of the different heavy chain isotypes. See also Kappa (κ) chain.

**λ5:** During B-cell development, it associated with Vpre-B to form the surrogate light chain of the pre-B-cell receptor. See also Pre-B-cell, Pre-B-cell receptor, surrogate light chain, and Vpre-B.

**Lamellipodium:** A projection protruding from the anterior region of a cell, which is formed in response to a chemokine and propels a migrating cell forward.

**Lamina propria:** The connective tissue that underlies the gastrointestinal mucosa epithelium. It contains macrophages, dendritic cells, T cells, and B cells and is traversed by blood and lymphatic vessels.

**Langerhans' cells:** Immature bone-marrow-derived phagocytic dendritic cells, which are found in the epidermis of skin and certain mucosae. They can pick up antigen through toll-like receptors and carry it to the regional lymph nodes, where they mature into highly effective antigen-presenting cells (now nonphagocytic cells expressing high levels of class II and costimulatory molecules) and efficiently present antigen to naïve T cells. In the skin, they are known as veiled cells when they are moving to the lymph nodes and in the lymph nodes as lymph node dendritic cells.

**Large granular lymphocytes (LGL):** A population of human peripheral blood cells with lymphocyte-like morphologic characteristics that contain azurophilic granules. These cells exhibit NK cell activity. It is another name for NK cells.

**LAT:** See Linker of activation in T cells.

**Latency:** A characteristic of viruses that enter the cell but do not replicate; once the virus is reactivated and replicates, it causes disease.

**Late phase reaction of allergy:** A visible reaction to an allergen occurring 2 to 4 hr after some Type I immediate hypersensitivity reactions, peaking 6–9 hours after allergen exposure and resolving by 24–48 hours. It is characterized by edema and erythema resulting from an inflammatory infiltrate of eosinophils, basophils, neutrophils, and $T_H2$ lymphocytes. In the lungs, the reactions are characterized by airway narrowing and mucus hypersecretion.

**Lck:** A Src family nonreceptor tyrosine kinase that associates with the cytoplasmic tails of T cell CD4 and CD8 molecules. It is involved in the early signaling events of antigen-induced T cell activation. Lck works through the tyrosine phosphorylation of the cytoplasmic tails of CD3 and ζ proteins of the T cell receptor complex.

**LCMV:** See Lymphocytic choriomeningitis virus.

**LD antigens:** See Lymphocyte-defined antigens.

**LE cells:** Neutrophils or macrophages that have internalized lymphocytic nuclear material complexed with antibodies (LE factor). These cells are found in patients with the autoimmune disease systemic lupus erythematosus (SLE). See also Systemic lupus erythematosus (SLE).

**LE factor:** The anti-nuclear autoantibodies complexed with lymphocytic nuclear material during systemic lupus erythematosus (SLE). See also Systemic lupus erythematosus (SLE).

**Leader (L) sequence:** An exon that precedes each V-gene segment of B cell or T cell antigen receptors and encodes a leader polypeptide that is required for translation of, for example, an antibody molecule across the membrane of the endoplasmic reticulum. Once the antibody crosses the membrane, the leader sequence is removed.

**Lectins:** Substances that are derived from plants and bind to animal cell surfaces. Lectins are commonly thought of as mitogens. See Con A (Concanavalin A) and PHA (Phytohemagglutinin).

**Lectin pathway of complement activation:** A pathway of complement activation in the absence of antibodies that is initiated by the binding of serum protein mannose-binding lectin (MBL) to mannose-containing components of microbial cell walls. The binding of MBL, which is structural similar to C1q and like C1q, activates the C1r-C1s enzyme complex. The remaining steps are similar to the classical pathway of complement activation. See also Mannose-binding lectin (MBL).

**Lentiviruses:** A genus of slow growing viruses of the retroviruse family such as the human immunodeficiency virus, HIV-1 and simian immunodeficiency virus (SIV), that causes disease after a long incubation time.

**Leprosy:** A *M. leprae*-induced disease of usually either the lepromatus form, which is characterized by significant growth of leprosy bacilli, high levels of antibody production but no cell-mediated immunity or the tuberculoid form, which is characterized by low numbers of leprosy bacilli, minimal antibody production, and high levels of cell-mediated immunity.

**Lethal hit:** A term to describe the events that lead to irreversible damage to a target cell when a cytotoxic T cell binds to it. The lethal hit events include cytotoxic T-cell granule exocytosis, perforin polymerization in the target cell membranes, and entry of calcium ions and apoptosis-inducing granzymes into the target cell cytoplasm.

**Leucine-rich-repeat (LRR) domain:** A domain that mediates the detection of microbial-derived ligands. The LRR domains are associated with Toll-like receptors and NOD1 and NOD2 proteins. The domain consists of leucine-rich amino acid strands forming a peptide loop. The loops are found as tandem repeats that, together, form a coil and contain constant sequences, as well as variable residues for each ligand.

**Leukemia:** A cancer that originates in a class of hematopoietic cells; they can be lymphocytic, myelocytic, and monocytic. It is characterized by large numbers of proliferating malignant cells in the blood or lymph.

**Leukocyte:** Literally means "white cell," a general term to describe any lymphoid and myeloid cell.

**Leukocyte-adhesion deficiency (LAD):** An inherited immunodeficiency disease that is caused by defective expression of the leukocyte adhesion molecules; therefore, leukocytes are unable to migrate into sites of inflammation. LAD I is due to mutations in the CD18 protein-encoding gene, which is part of the $\beta_2$ integrins. LAD II is due to mutations in the gene encoding the enzyme responsible for synthesis of leukocyte ligands that bind endothelial selectins.

**Leukocyte common antigen (LCA):** An antigen expressed on all leukocytes. It is also called CD45, a protein tyrosine phosphatase that has several forms. It counteracts Csk-mediated prevention of the activation of Src-family kinases.

**Leukocyte receptor complex (LRC):** A group of genes that are located adjacent to one another on human chromosome 19, which encode a family of proteins including natural killer cell immunoglobulin-like receptors (KIRs), leukocyte immunoglobulin-like receptors (LIRs) and FcαRI. See also Killer cell immunoglobulin-like receptors (KIRs).

**Leukocytosis:** The increased number of leukocytes seen in the blood during acute infection.

**Leukopenia:** Reduction in the number of circulating leukocytes.

**Leukotrienes:** A collection of arachidonic acid metabolites (leukotriene $C_4$ [$LTC_4$], $LTD_4$, and $LTE_4$) produced by the lipoxygenase pathway that has pharmacological effects, particularly in immediate hypersensitivity reactions. Leukotrienes bind to specific smooth muscle receptors and cause prolonged bronchoconstriction. Collectively, they were also called *slow-reacting substance of anaphylaxis (SRS-A)*.

**LFA-1:** See Lymphocyte function-associated antigen 1 (LFA-1).

**LFA-2:** See Lymphocyte function-associated antigen 1 (LFA-2).

**LFA-3:** See Lymphocyte function-associated antigen 3 (LFA-3).

**LICOS:** The ligand for ICOS; also called B7-H2. ICOS is a CD28-related protein that is induced on activated T cells. The ligand is expressed on activated B cells, dendritic cells, and monocytes. See also Inducible T-cell costimulator (ICOS).

**Ligand:** A linking, or binding, molecule recognized by a receptor, such as an antigen, a cytokine, a chemokine, an adhesion molecule, etc. with its appropriate receptor.

**Light (L) chain:** For example, an antibody polypeptide chain, of fewer amino acids than a heavy chain, with a molecular weight of 22,000, present in all antibodies. The L chain can be divided into a amino-terminal variable region and a carboxyl-terminal constant region. There are two L chains per antibody molecule, one connected by disulfide bridges to each heavy chain. There are two types of L chains, kappa ($\kappa$) and lambda ($\lambda$). Molecules other than antibodies can have smaller polypeptide chains that are also designated L chains.

**Light zone:** The portion of the germinal center that contains many follicular dendritic cells.

**Limiting dilution analysis:** An *in vitro* method used to determine the number of antigen-specific clones of immune cells. An initial concentration of cells is diluted until there is, theoretically, only one cell in the culture; this cell grows out to a clone of cells.

**Line:** A group of cells that are grown up from an initially heterogeneous population. Lines are rarely monoclonal.

**Linkage (linked genes):** A condition in which two or more genes are in close proximity on a single chromosome and are inherited together.

**Linkage disequilibrium:** An unexpected association of linked genes (see Linkage) that is found in a population with greater frequency than predicted simply by the product of their individual genes. It is the difference between the frequency observed for a particular allelic combination and that expected from individual allelic frequencies. (For example, certain allelic combinations occur more frequently in HLA haplotypes than predicted by random combination; 16% and 9% of individuals in a population have HLA-A1 and HLA-B8, respectively, expected frequency [0.16 × 0.09] is 1.4%. However, this combination is found in 8.8% of the population.)

**Linker of activation in T cells (LAT):** The cytoplasmic adapter protein with several tyrosines that become phosphorylated by the tyrosine kinase ZAP-70. It mediates signaling events in T-cell activation.

**Lipid rafts:** Micro-aggregates of cholesterol and sphingolipid-enriched membrane detergent-resistant microdomains, which function as platforms for membrane and cytosolic signaling molecules, which are concentrated in these rafts (such as, Lyn).

**Lipopolysaccharides:** Molecules that have lipid linked to polysaccharide. Substances that are derived from Gram-negative bacteria that have a variety of functions, such as acting as an adjuvant and as a mitogen to B cells. They are equivalent to endotoxin. See Endotoxin.

**Liposomes:** A spherical particle that is formed by a lipid bilayer that encloses an aqueous compartment; it facilitates vaccine delivery.

**LMP-2 and LMP-7:** They are the two catalytic subunits of the proteasome, the organelle that degrades cytosolic proteins into peptides that associate with class I MHC molecules during antigen processing and presentation. Both subunits are encoded by the MHC and are upregulated by interferon-$\gamma$.

**Locus (plural loci):** The specific position of a gene on a chromosome that encodes a single polypeptide chain; also, the DNA at that position. The use of locus is sometimes restricted to mean regions of DNA that are expressed. In brief, it is the place on a chromosome where a specific gene is located—an address for the gene.

**Long-term nonprogressors:** Long-lived HIV-1-infected humans who typically have levels of blood viral RNA of less than 1000 copies per ml.

**Low responder mice:** Certain inbred mice respond to antigen with the production of low levels of antibody. This level of immune response is genetically controlled by the class II region of the H-2 complex.

**Low zone tolerance:** Doses of antigen that are much lower than immunogenic doses can tolerize animals. The mechanism responsible for this phenomenon is thought to involve the induction of suppressor cells.

**LPR:** See Lymphoproliferative gene.

**LPS-binding protein (LBP):** Bacterial lipopolysaccharide (LPS) has to first be bound by the serum protein LPS-binding protein (LBP) before it can interact with CD14; the LPS:LBP is found on macrophages. LBP functions by transferring LPS monomers to a high-affinity LPS receptor CD14. Another component of the LPS receptor complex is MD-2, a small adapter protein required for LPS recognition by Toll-like receptor 4 (TLR4). LBP, CD14, and MD-2 are part of TLR4, which functions as the signal-transducing receptor for LPS. See also Toll-like receptors (TLRs).

**LRR domain:** See Leucine-rich-repeat domain.

**Lymph:** Interstitial fluid derived from blood plasma that circulates through the lymphatic system and contains molecules and leukocytes.

**Lymph nodes:** Small, pea-sized organs distributed widely throughout the body but frequently localized in groups that drain a particular area of the body. For example, the inguinal and axillary lymph nodes drain the groin and arm pit regions, respectively. The lymph nodes are filters set across the lymphatic system and are composed mostly of lymphoid cells.

**Lymphadenopathy:** It is the enlargement of lymph nodes.

**Lymphatic system:** A vessel system covering the entire body that conveys lymph. This system is responsible for draining tissues and returning the plasma-derived fluids to the blood, the routing of antigen from the periphery to the lymph nodes, and the recirculation of lymphocytes and dendritic cells.

**Lymphoblast:** A proliferating lymphocyte, which increases its rate of RNA and protein synthesis.

**Lymphocytes:** Spherical cells (7–12 µm in diameter) with a large, round nucleus surrounded by a small amount of cytoplasm. They are associated with all aspects of specific immunity. Lymphocytes are the principal constituents of lymphoid tissue.

**Lymphocyte-defined (LD) antigens:** The cell-surface allogeneic antigens that provoke a proliferative response in T cells. They are the antigens responsible for the MLR reaction.

**Lymphocyte function-associated antigen 1 (LFA-1 or CD11aCD18):** A $\beta_2$ integrin (or adhesion molecule) found on most leukocytes that participates in cell-cell interactions during T cell help, during killing by both NK cells and cytotoxic T cells, and in adhesion of leukocytes to endothelia.

**Lymphocyte function-associated antigen 2 (LFA-2 or CD2):** An integrin in the immunoglobulin superfamily that binds LFA-3 (CD58) and is expressed on T cells, thymocytes, and NK cells.

**Lymphocyte function-associated antigen 3 (LFA-3 or CD58):** An integrin (or adhesion molecule) in the immunoglobulin superfamily found on most leukocytes that acts as the ligand for CD2.

**Lymphocyte function-associated antigen 1 (LFA-1) deficiency:** An immunodeficiency disease involving both T and B cells. It is characterized by leukocyte adhesion deficiency, abnormal phagocytic cell chemotaxis, cell adherence, and reduced degradation function during phagocytosis.

**Lymphocyte migration:** Lymphocyte movement from the blood stream into peripheral tissues.

**Lymphocyte recirculation:** It is the continuous movement of lymphocytes by the blood stream and lymphatics, between the spleen, lymph nodes, and other lymphoid tissues, and if activated, to peripheral inflammatory sites.

**Lymphocytic choriomeningitis virus (LCMV):** A virus that causes meningitis in mice and occasionally in humans.

**Lymphoepithelial organ:** An organ created by the migration of lymphocytes from bone marrow into the epithelial rudiment during embryogenesis.

**Lymphoid follicles:** The areas within lymph nodes and the spleen that are rich with B cells. It is the site of antigen-induced B cell proliferation and differentiation. During T cell-dependent antibody responses to proteins, follicles form germinal centers. See also Germinal centers.

**Lymphoid organs:** The tissues of the lymphoid (immune) system. They include the bone marrow, thymus, lymph nodes, spleen, and mucosa-associated lymphoid system (MALT). They are concerned with the growth, development, and deployment of lymphocytes.

**Lymphoid tissues:** The body tissues in which the lymphocyte is the predominant cell. Lymphoid tissues include the spleen, lymph nodes, thymus, tonsils, adenoids, and circulating lymph.

**Lymphokine-activated killer (LAK) cells:** NK cells that are activated *ex vivo* with interleukin-2 and when administered to a cancer patient are killers of tumor cells in the absence of MHC restriction.

**Lymphokines:** A generic name given to molecules secreted by antigen-stimulated lymphoid cells that can affect other lymphoid and nonlymphoid cells. See also Cytokines.

**Lymphoma:** A cancer of lymphoid tissue.

**Lymphopenia:** A deficiency of blood circulating lymphocytes.

**Lymphoproliferative gene (LPR):** A gene found in the LPR strain of mice that is involved in the generation of autoimmune reactions. LPR mice are naturally occurring mutants expressing a deletion of the *Fas* gene.

**Lymphosarcoma:** A cancer involving lymph nodes. See also Sarcoma.

**Lymphotoxin (LT, TNF-β):** A T cell-derived molecule that is cytotoxic for tumor cells, has proinflammatory effects by activating endothelial cells and neutrophils, and is critical in the normal development of lymphoid organs. It is also called *tumor necrosis factor-β*. See also Tumor necrosis factor.

**Lysogenic conversion:** The conversion of a bacterium to a phage-producing cell.

**Lysosome:** A cytoplasmic acidic organelle abundant in phagocytic cells that contains hydrolytic enzymes. These enzymes remain inactive until release during intracellular digestion following phagocytosis or endocytosis. Lysosomes are involved in the class II pathway of antigen processing and presentation.

**Lysozyme:** An enzyme found in tears, saliva, and nasal secretions lysing chiefly gram-positive cocci. It splits the muramic acid β(1-4)-N-acetylglucosamine linkage in the cell walls of the appropriate bacteria.

**Lytic granules:** Granules that contain perforin and granzymes and are characteristic of mature cytotoxic T cells and NK cells. See also Granzymes and Perforin.

# M

**M (microfold or membrane) cells:** A group of specialized epithelial cells of the nasopharynx-associated lymphoid tissues, the intestinal mucosa, and the urogential tract, which deliver antigen, using transepithelial vesicular transport, from the cell's lumen side to the intraepithelial lymphocytes of the sub-epithelial lymphoid tissues of the nasopharynx-associated lymphoid tissues and Peyer's patches. Their morphological features facilitate the uptake of antigen. They do not process the antigens, but deliver intact antigens and microorganisms through basolateral long protrusions that make direct contact with the macrophages and dendritic cells underneath.

**MIIC endosomes:** A subset of endosomes found in macrophages and B cells that are rich in class II MHC molecules. They are important in antigen processing and antigen presentation by the class II pathway. These endosomes contain all the components needed for the formation of peptide-class MHC molecule complexes, including the enzymes that degrade protein antigens, class II MHC molecules, invariant chain, and HLA-DM.

**Mac-1:** A surface molecule found on macrophages and NK cells that is identical to the C3bi receptor (CR3; CD11b).

**Macroglobulins:** Glycoprotein molecules with molecular weights greater than 200,000.

**Macrophages:** Any of the diverse group of mononuclear phagocytic leukocytes (not including granulocytes) characterized by the capacity to engulf (phagocytizing) and destroy foreign substances. They play a pivotal role in nonspecific (removal of foreign material) and specific immunity (processing and presenting antigen to T cells). Macrophages can be activated by microbial products such as lipopolysaccharide and by T cells products such as interferon-γ. Activated macrophages can kill bacteria, present antigen-derived peptides to T cells, and secrete numerous proinflammatory cytokines. See also Phagocytic cell.

**Macrophage-activating factor (MAF):** MAF increases the killing capacity of macrophages. Interferon-γ can be an MAF.

**Macrophage activation:** The enhanced state of antimicrobial or antitumor activity following macrophage stimulation by cytokines (e.g., interferon-γ), certain complement components, bacteria, etc. The these "classically" activated macrophages have greater phagocytic ability, secrete more enzymes, produce more superoxide, express greater numbers of Fc and C3b receptors, and present antigen-derived peptides to T cells. Classically activated (i.e., induced with $T_H1$ cell-derived interferon-γ) macrophages are also called *M1 macrophages* or *Type 1 macrophages*. They have an important role in cell-mediated immune responses and produce IL-12 and TNF-α. See also Alternatively activated macrophages.

**MAdCAM-1:** See Mucosal cell adhesion molecule-1.

**Major basic protein:** A component of eosinophil granules that is released on eosinophil activation, which acts on mast cells to cause their degranulation.

**Major histocompatibility complex (MHC):** A region on human chromosome 6 (mouse chromosome 17) that contains a large number of highly polymorphic genes. These genes encode surface molecules that display antigen-derived peptide to T cells, leading to an immune response. The MHC also contains genes that encode molecules needed for antigen processing and cytokine and complement production.

**Major histocompatibility complex (MHC) molecule:** The MHC genes encode heterodimeric membrane proteins that serve as display molecules for antigen-derived peptides. This MHC molecule-peptide complex is recognized by T cells. There are two structural distinct MHC molecules: (1) Class I MHC molecules that are displayed on all nucleated cells, bind cytosolic antigen-derived peptides (intracellular/endogenous antigens, such as viruses), and are recognized by CD8+ T cells. (2) Class II MHC molecules that are displayed on antigen-presenting cells, bind endosomal antigen-derived peptides (extracellular/exogenous antigens, such as bacteria), and are recognized by CD4+ T cells. See also Class I and Class II molecules.

**Malaria:** It is a disease transmitted to vertebrate hosts by the bite of female *Anopheles* mosquitoes that are infected with protozoan parasites of the genus *Plasmodium*.

**Malignancy:** A condition characterized by sustained cell division, anaplasia, and cell migration.

**Malignant tumor:** A tumor that is usually atypical in tissue structure, grows rapidly, does not remain encapsulated, and displays many nuclear division and chromosomal abnormalities. It also invades surrounding normal tissue and sheds cells that can colonize new sites.

**MALT:** See Mucosa-associated lymphoid tissue (MALT).

**Mannose receptor:** A carbohydrate-binding receptor expressed on macrophages that binds microbial mannose and fucose residues and thereby mediates their phagocytosis. It is a pattern recognition receptor.

**Mannose-binding lectin (MBL):** An acute-phase plasma protein that binds to bacterial cell wall mannose residues and thereby acts as an opsonin by promoting macrophage-mediated phagocytosis of the organism. Through the macrophage's expression of surface receptors for C1q, which can bind MBL, macrophages mediate uptake of opsonized organisms. It is also known as mannose-binding protein. It is a soluble pattern recognition receptor.

**Mantle zone:** The secondary follicle zone that surrounds the germinal center and contains naïve IgM$^+$ IgD$^+$ resting B cells.

**MAP kinases:** See Mitogen-activated protein (MAP) kinase cascade.

**Marginal-zone B cells:** Exiting bone marrow-derived immature B cells (IgM$^{high}$IgD$^{-/low}$) enter the periphery, where they seed the spleen, differentiate through several transitional stages, and become a static, mature B-cell subset IgM$^{high}$IgD$^{-/low}$ CD21$^{high}$CD23$^{-/low}$) that localizes in the marginal zone of the spleen, which is located at the white pulp border. Marginal-zone B cells represent roughly 10% of mature splenic B cells and are found only in the spleen. Their positioning in the marginal zone allows them to initiate a rapid and strong antibody response to blood-borne pathogens. See also Follicular B cells.

**Marginal zone of spleen:** The specialized region that surrounds the B-cell follicles in periarteriolar lymphatic sheath (PALS). It is primarily composed of B cells and marginal zone macrophages and dendritic cells that can present T-independent antigens (such as polysaccharide antigens) to the B cells or the antigens may be transported to the follicles.

**Margination:** It is the accumulation of lymphocytes at blood vessel walls during the early stages of inflammation.

**MASP-1 and -2:** They are MBL-associated serine proteases of the mannose-binding protein pathway of complement activation that bind to mannose-binding protein and cleave C4 as do C1r and C1s in the classical pathway. See also Lectin pathway of complement activation.

**Mast cells:** Tissue cells containing granules filled with mediators that cause the harmful effects seen with Type I (immediate) hypersensitivity reactions. They also express high-affinity Fc receptors for IgE. The allergen-induced cross-linking of adjacent mast cell-bound IgE causes the mast cell to release of their granule contents, as well as start new synthesis and release of other mediators.

**Mature B cell:** An IgM- and IgD-expressing, functionally mature antigen-naïve B cell that is exiting the bone marrow to populate peripheral lymphoid organs, principally the spleen where they complete their maturation.

**Medulla:** The central region of an organ. For example, it is one of the two main compartments that are found in the lobules of the thymus. It makes up about 10 to 15% of the thymus. There also is a medulla region in the lymph nodes. See also Cortex.

**Megakaryocyte:** A leukocyte that produces platelets by cytoplasmic budding.

**Membrane attack complex (MAC):** The C5b-9 complex of either the classical, alternative or lectin complement activation sequence responsible for lysis of target cells. See also Membrane attack phase.

**Membrane attack phase:** The third and final phase of complement activation, which involves the last five components of complement (C5 through C9) and which can lead to lysis of a target cell.

**Membrane-bound immunoglobulin (mIg):** The form of antibody that is attached to the B cell as a transmembrane protein, such as, the antigen-specific antibody molecules on the surface of a B cell. A mature B cell expresses both IgM and IgD mIgs. There are also B cells with membrane-bound IgA, ligation with rechallenge antigen activates a memory B cell response, leading to the production of IgA.

**Membrane cofactor protein (MCP or CD46):** A host-cell membrane regulatory protein along with factor I that cleaves C3b to its inactive iC3b derivative, preventing C3 convertase formation, that is, it mediates the homeostatic maintenance of complement activation on cells.

**Membrane (M) exon:** Each antibody heavy chain, constant-region gene has one or more associated coding segments called *M exons*. They encode for an approximately 40 amino-acid-long sequence at the carboxyl-terminal end of the membrane-bound forms of heavy chains. Thus, they provide the hydrophobic tail for attachment to the membrane.

**Membrane ruffling:** A rapid reorganization of the plasma membrane and the actin cytoskeleton. It often precedes the formation of a lamellipodium. See also Lamellipodium.

**Memory cells:** Functionally defined T or B cells that are responsible for recalling specific immunological memory after a primary exposure to antigen and thereby mediate rapid and enhanced responses to second and subsequent exposures to the same antigen. See also Central-memory cells and Effector-memory cells.

**6-Mercaptopurine:** A purine antimetabolite that preferentially suppresses antibody responses. It is also used to prevent allograft rejection. See also Azathioprine.

**Mesangial cells:** Kidney macrophages.

**Metastasis:** The migration and secondary growth of malignant cells away from the site of the primary tumor.

**Methotrexate (amethopterin):** A folic acid analog that inhibits DNA synthesis. When used in cancer chemotherapy, it causes temporary remission of certain leukemias. It is also used to inhibit graft-versus-host reactions in bone marrow transplant recipients and widely used in the treatment of more severe rheumatoid arthritis.

**MHC:** See Major histocompatibility complex.

**MHC class Ib:** MHC gene-encoded molecules that are not as polymorphic as MHC class I and class II molecules and present a limited set of antigen-derived peptides. Some class Ib molecules like CD1 bind lipids. See also CD1.

**MHC class I tetramers:** Biotinylated MHC molecules contain a specific peptide in the binding groove and tetramerized with a fluorescently labeled streptavidin molecule. Tetramers bind to T cells that express T cell receptors specific for the cognate peptide.

**MHC restriction:** The process whereby the MHC controls interactions between immune cells. It involves the recognition of foreign antigen in association with class I or II MHC molecules. The reactions that are considered to be MHC-restricted are: (1) antigen presentation by B cells, dendritic cells, or macrophages to T cells, (2) T and B cell cooperation, and (3) cytotoxic T-cell interactions with target cells.

**Microfold cells:** See M cells.

**Microglial cells:** Phagocytic cells (macrophages) found in the parenchyma of the central nervous system. They are brain-resident macrophages that express CD4 and chemokine receptors.

**MIF:** See Migration inhibition factor.

**Migration inhibition factor (MIF):** A T cell-derived factor (cytokine) that inhibits the migration of macrophages away from the site of antigen deposition.

**MIIC endosome:** The MHC class II compartment (MIIC) is an acidic endosomal compartment where antigenic peptides become associated with class II molecules. In the MIIC, the Ii chain is degraded leaving CLIP bound to the class II molecule. Using HLA-DM, CLIP is replaced by the antigenic peptide, leading to the peptide-class II molecule complex moving to the cell surface. See also CLIP and Invariant (Ii) chain.

**Mimetope:** An epitope that structurally resembles another epitope.

**Missing-self hypothesis:** A hypothesis proposing that natural killer cells can recognize and attack cells that do not express class I MHC molecules; the target cells are "missing self." A backup system of immune surveillance to patrol for cells infected with viruses that downregulate class I MHC molecule expression to evade detection by cytotoxic T lymphocytes.

**Mitogen:** Any agent that induces mitosis in lymphoid cells, such as concanavalin A (Con A) and lipopolysaccharide (LPS), which are polyclonal stimulators of T and B cells, respectively, and various superantigens can act as mitogens.

**Mitogen-activated protein (MAP) kinase cascade:** A signal transduction cascade that is initiated by the active form of the Ras protein. The sequential cascade involves the activation of three serine/threonine kinases; the last is the MAP kinase. It phosphorylates and activates other enzymes or transcription factors. This cascade is one of the several signal pathways activated by antigen ligation of the T cell receptor.

**Mitomycin C:** An antibiotic that acts as an immunosuppressant by inhibiting DNA replication. See also Actinomycin D and Puromycin.

**Mixed lymphocyte reaction (MLR):** An *in vitro* reaction for cell-mediated immunity (a T cell-mediated reaction) in which leukocytes or lymphocytes from two genetically dissimilar individuals are mixed and cultured together for 4–5 days. The greater the histoincompatibility is between the two individuals, the greater the T-cell proliferation.

**MLR:** See Mixed lymphocyte reaction.

**Molecular mimicry:** The antigenic similarity between a pathogen antigen and a host's cell antigen, which leads to the induction of antibodies or T cells that act against the pathogen but also cross-react with the self-antigen triggering an autoimmune reaction.

**Monoblasts:** Progenitors of the monocytes found in bone marrow.

**Monoclonal:** Derived from a single cell.

**Monoclonal antibodies:** Antibodies that are produced by a single clone of cells. The resultant antibody molecules are identical in all aspects, such as affinity, binding specificity, isotype, allotype, idiotype, etc.

**Monocytes:** Immature macrophages found in the blood. They differentiate into macrophages once they leave the bloodstream.

**Monocyte chemoattractant protein 1–4 (MCP1-4):** A group of chemokines (CCL2, CCL8, CCL7 and CCL13 [MCP1—MCP4, respectively]) produced by activated T cells that attracts monocytes and macrophages into an infection site. These chemokines also suppress the production of IL-12 by macrophages.

**Monokines:** Macrophage-derived substances that affect other immune cells (or nonimmune cells). See also Cytokines.

**Monomer:** A term used to represent the basic unit of an antibody, that is, a structure composed of two light chains and two heavy chains.

**Mononuclear phagocyte system:** The name for a diffuse system of mononuclear phagocytic cells derived from the bone marrow, located in the reticular connective tissue framework of lymph nodes, spleen, and liver.

**MRL.lpr mouse:** A mutant strain of mouse that develops autoimmunity; specifically, the *lpr* gene produces T cell proliferation and is used as a model for rheumatoid arthritis. See also Lymphoproliferative gene (LPR).

**Mucins:** A group of heavily glycosylated serine- or threonine-rich proteins, such as, CD34 and GlyCAM-1 on endothelial cells that are ligands for selectins. See Selectins.

**Mucosa:** It is the mucus-secreting epithelia that line the intestinal, respiratory, and urogential tracts. The eye conjunctiva and mammary glands are also considered in this category.

**Mucosa-associated lymphoid tissue (MALT):** A group of anatomically well-organized unencapsulated lymphoid tissues (adenoids, tonsils, Peyer's patches) that are found in submucosal areas of the gastrointestinal, respiratory, and urogenital tracts. The MALT contains lymphocytes and accessory cells.

**Mucosal cell adhesion molecule-1 (MAdCAM-1):** A mucosal addressin that is recognized by the lymphocyte surface proteins called *L-selectin* (*CD62L*) and *VLA-4* (*CD49d*). The interaction between these adhesion molecules mediates specific homing of lymphocytes to mucosal tissues. See also Very late antigen (VLA) molecules.

**Mucosal immune system:** Nonencapsulated clusters of lymphoid tissue with immune function. Their structural components are the mucosa-associated lymphoid tissue (MALT). See Mucosa-associated lymphoid tissue (MALT).

**Mucosal mast cells (MMC):** Mast cells that are found in the lung and gut.

**Multinuclear giant cells:** Groups of cells that form by the fusion of infected and uninfected macrophages and microglia. The fusion is mediated by HIV envelope proteins expressed on the surface of infected cells with CD4 and chemokine receptors on uninfected cells. Multinuclear giant cells are the hallmark of HIV neuropathology.

**Multiple myeloma:** A form of cancer, characterized by the proliferation of malignant antibody-forming cells (cancerous plasma cells) in the bone marrow. This form of cancer provided the first sources of large amounts of homogeneous antibody or parts of antibodies, which were used in the early characterization studies of antibody molecules.

**Multiple sclerosis (MS):** An antibody-mediated, chronic progressive autoimmune disease of the central nervous system. It is characterized by patches of demyelination in the central nervous system and lymphocyte infiltration into the brain. It is one of the most common causes of neurologic disease in Western countries.

**Multiplicity of V, D, and J germline gene segments:** A mechanism for generating antibody and T cell receptor diversity. The number of gene segments inherited from our parents, which can randomly recombine to generate large numbers of unique genes encoding antigen-specific receptors. See also Chain association and Combinatorial freedom of gene segments.

**Muramyl peptides:** Peptidoglycan fragments from Gram-negative bacteria that play a role in the generation of the immune response to Gram-negative bacterial infection.

**Murine:** Material derived from a mouse.

**Myasthenia gravis:** An antibody-mediated autoimmune disease characterized by muscular weakness and excessive fatigue. It is due to antiacetylcholine receptor antibodies that cause the reduction in the number of acetylcholine receptors or their blockage, which help trigger muscle contraction.

**Myeloid dendritic cells:** A subset of dendritic cells that are CD11c$^+$HLA-DR$^+$ mononuclear cells with a monocytoid appearance. In humans, these cells may differentiate from myeloid precursors (e.g., monocytes and macrophages).

**Myeloid suppressor cells:** A cell population composed of mature and immature myeloid cells, which develop during an inflammatory response. They negatively affect T cells through direct interaction and secreted components, leading to the downregulation of $\zeta$-chain expression and impairment of T cell function.

**Myeloid stem cell:** A cell that gives rise to the myeloid lineage of cells, such as macrophages and granulocytes.

**Myelomas:** Plasma cell tumors resident in bone marrow.

**Myelopoiesis:** The production granulocytes and monocytes in the bone marrow.

# N

**N-addition:** Untemplated nucleotides inserted by terminal deoxynucleotidyl transferase at the junction of V- or J- with D-gene segments (CDR3 junctions). They are inserted between V$_H$ and D$_H$ or between D$_H$ and J$_H$ segments as part of the joining process in generating functional immunoglobulin and T cell receptor genes. N-regions are encoded in the germline DNA.

**Naïve lymphocyte:** A mature T or B cell that has not encounter antigen, nor is it the progeny of an antigen-stimulated mature T or B cell. Once stimulated by antigen, they differentiate into effector lymphocytes, such as plasma cells or helper T or cytotoxic T cells. Naïve lymphocytes have surface markers that are distinct from activated lymphocytes.

**Natural killer (NK) cells:** A group of Fc receptor-bearing cytotoxic cells, distinct from B or T cells, which has the inherent ability to kill virally infected cells and some tumor cells without prior immunization. They are important cells in innate immunity. NK cells do not express antigen receptors like antibodies or T cell receptors, are potent producers of interferon-$\gamma$, tumor-necrosis factor, granulocyte-macrophage colony-stimulating factor, and chemokines. Their activation is balance between the combination of stimulatory and inhibitory receptors; inhibitory receptors recognize self-MHC molecules. NK cells can also destroy targets coated with IgG antibody by a process called *antibody-dependent cellular cytotoxicity (ADCC)*. ADCC is mediated by the Fc receptor (CD16) complex on NK cells. See Antibody-dependent cell-mediated cytotoxicity or ADCC.

**Natural-killer group 2, member D (NKG2D):** A lectin-type activating receptor that is expressed on the surface of NK cells, NKT cells, $\gamma\delta$ T cells and some cytolytic CD8$^+$ $\alpha\beta$ T cells. NKG2D ligands are HLA-E and MHC-class-I polypeptide-related sequence A (MICA) and MICB in humans, which are expressed at the surface of infected, stressed or transformed cells. NKG2D is also expressed in mice and rats.

**Natural-killer T cells (NKT cells):** Lymphocytes that have some of the characteristics of T cells; that is they express a semi-variant $\alpha\beta$ T cell receptor, as well as characteristics of NK cells (i.e., NK cell receptors). They exhibit rapid effector functions without need for priming and clonal expansion—they are cells that place themselves at the interface between innate and adaptive immunity. NKT cells do not interact with class I or II MHC molecules but with MHC-like molecules called *CD1*. The antigens associated with CD1 molecules, at least in mice, are $\alpha$-galactoceramide and glycerol-phosphatidylinositol. They can kill CD1-expressing targets. Once NKT cells are triggered, they are characterized by cytolytic activity and rapid production of cytokines (including interferon-$\gamma$ and interleukin-4) that support antibody production, inflammation, and the development of cytotoxic T cells. See also CD1.

**Natural selection:** A theory proposed by Niels Jerne stating that during embryonic life, the host may synthesize small amounts of specific antibody against the antigenic repertoire. When these natural, cell-bound antibodies interact with the right antigens, the resulting cell-antibody-antigen complexes localize within the body and act as models for the synthesis of identical antibodies.

**Naturally occurring antibodies (isoagglutinins):** Antibodies of the IgM class formed by humans against the blood group antigens they do not express.

**Necrosis:** The morphologic changes accompanying cell death frequently induced by toxic injury, hypoxia, or stress leading to the release of large amounts of intracellular components into the surrounding tissues, causing disruption and atrophy of tissue. Unlike apoptosis, which does not lead to damage of surrounding cells. Necrosis usually occurs together with inflammation.

**Negative thymic selection:** Responsible for clonal deletion of autoreactive T cells (tolerance induction). Negative selection of thymocytes involves high-avidity binding of a thymocyte to self-MHC molecules with bound self-peptide on thymic medullary epithelial or dendritic cells, which leads to thymocyte apoptosis. See also Positive selection.

**Neoantigens:** Nonself antigens that appear spontaneously on the surface of cells, usually during tumor growth.

**Neonatal Fc receptor (FcRn):** An IgG-specific Fc receptor that transports maternal IgG across the placenta and the neonatal intestinal epithelium. The FcRn is similar a class I MHC molecule. The adult form of this receptor protects plasma IgG antibodies from catabolism.

**Neoplasm:** Any new or abnormal growth, such as a tumor or a cancer.

**Network theory:** A theory proposed by Neils Jerne that there normally exists at equilibrium (no antigen stimulation) a network of idiotypic antibodies and anti-idiotypic antibodies (or T cell receptors). The disruption of this equilibrium by antigen exposure and the host's effort to restore equilibrium can lead to an immune response.

**Neutralizing antibodies:** Antibodies that inhibit (neutralize) virus infectivity and toxin toxicity by blocking their entry into cells by blocking receptors on the cells or the virus or toxin.

**Neutrophils:** Phagocytic cells, expressing Fc and C3 receptors, found in the circulation, that make up about 70% of leukocytes. Neutrophils remain in the circulation for only 48 hours before moving into tissues due to chemotactic stimuli. They phagocytize material, but unlike macrophages will die after the encounter. They are also called *polymorphonuclear leukocytes, PMNs*. They are an important cell in the late phase response of Type I hypersensitivities.

**Neutrophil chemotactic factor (NCF):** The old common name for the chemokine CXCL8 (IL-8). It is a major mediator attracting neutrophils to the site of inflammation; it does this by activating neutrophil chemokine receptors CXCR1 and CXCR2.

**Nezelof's syndrome:** An immunodeficiency disease involving T cells. The thymus is missing, causing absence of T-cell immunity. There are also various degrees of B-cell deficiency.

***N*-formylmethionine:** An amino acid that initiates all bacterial proteins and no mammalian proteins except those found in the mitochondria. It serves as a signal to the innate immune system of infection. Neutrophils express specific receptors for *N*-formylmethionine-containing proteins, their ligation leads to neutrophil activation.

**NFAT:** See Nuclear factor of activated T cells.

**NF-κB (nuclear factor-κB):** A family of transcription factors composed of protein homodimers homologous to c-Rel protein that existing in many types of cells. They are important in proinflammatory and anti-apoptotic responses. See Transcription factor.

**NIP (4-hydroxy,5-iodo,3-nitrophenylacetyl):** A commonly used iodine-containing hapten.

**Nitric oxide:** A biological effector molecule that is important in intercellular signaling and has microbiocidal function.

**Nitric oxide synthase (iNOS):** An enzyme that catalyzes the conversion of L-arginine and NADPH to nitric oxide, L-citrulline, and NADP.

**Nitrogen mustard:** An alkylating immunosuppressant. Too toxic for oral administration, it is infrequently used.

**NK cells:** See Natural killer cells.

**NOD:** See Nucleotide-binding oligomerization domain.

**Nonhomologous end joining (NHEJ):** It is the joining of broken DNA ends without depending on extended homology; it is important in repairing DNA-strand breakage during somatic DNA recombination for antigen receptor diversity. Components of this pathway include the DNA–end-binding proteins Ku70 and Ku80, the endonuclease ARTEMIS, X-ray repair cross-complementing protein 4 (XRCC4), DNA ligase IV, and the catalytic subunit of DNA-dependent protein kinase (DNA-PKs).

**Nonimmune hemagglutination inhibition test:** The use of a standard amount of red blood cells to test the amount of virus needed to agglutinate red blood cells. The titer is the highest dilution of antibody that inhibits hemagglutination.

**Non-obese diabetic (NOD) mice:** A mouse strain that develops autoimmune diabetes that closely resembles human type 1 diabetes. CD4$^+$ T cells recognize target antigens of unknown identity on pancreatic islet cells leading to disease.

**Nonproductive rearrangement:** Immunoglobulin or T cell receptor gene rearrangements in which gene segments are joined out of sequence, leading to triple-reading frames that are not preserved for translation.

**Nonresponder:** An animal that is unable to respond to an immunogen, usually because it lacks the appropriate immune response genes (i.e., genes that encode class II molecules).

**Nonsequential antigenic determinants (or epitopes):** Protein epitopes composed of amino acids that are close together in the 3-D protein structure but far apart in the primary amino acid sequence. See Conformational determinants.

**Nonspecific immunotherapy:** Cancer immunotherapy based on activation of immune responses that are not tumor-specific but inhibit tumor growth. See also Specific immunotherapy.

**Notch1:** Notch1 is a member of a highly conserved family (there are four members, Notch1–4) of transmembrane receptors that regulates cell-fate choices in many cell lineages. Signaling through the transmembrane protein Notch1 is necessary during the earliest steps of T-cell development. The interactions between Notch receptor-expressing thymocytes and Notch ligand-expressing thymic stromal cells drive progenitor cells to commit to the T cell lineage rather than the B cell lineage.

**NP (4-hydroxy,3-nitrophenylacetyl):** A commonly used hapten that partially cross-reacts with NIP.

**Nuclear factor of activated T cells (NFAT):** The NFAT family of transcription factors includes five members (NFAT1–5); they are needed for the expression of interleukin-2 (IL-2), IL-4, tumor necrosis factor (TNF), and other cytokine genes. NFAT1, NFAT2, and NFAT4 are expressed in T cells. Activation by $Ca^{2+}$-calmodulin-dependent, calcineurin-mediated phosphorylation of cytoplasmic NFAT permits NFAT translocation to the nucleus, where it binds to consensus binding sequences in the regulatory regions of IL-2, IL-4, TNF, and other cytokine genes. This binding is usually in association with the transcription factor AP-1.

**Nucleotide-binding oligomerization domain (NOD) proteins:** NOD proteins are involved in innate immune recognition systems, for example, NOD1 and NOD2 mediate the recognition of specific microbial components derived from bacterial peptidoglycan. Other NOD proteins are implicated in the induction of nuclear factor-κB activity and in the activation of caspases.

**Nude mouse:** A hairless mouse that is genetically athymic (has no thymus) and thus has a marked deficiency in functional T cells.

**Null cells:** Lymphoid cells that express neither B cell nor T cell markers, such as NK cells.

**Nurse cells:** Thymic dendritic cells that are surrounded by thymocytes. Nurse cells may be important in the development of the T cell repertoire.

# O

**Obese chicken:** This strain of chicken develops autoimmune thyroiditis and thus is used as a model for Hashimoto's disease.

**Oncofetal antigens:** Tumor-associated antigens that normally appear on the surface of embryonic (fetal) cells and are reexpressed on the surface of some adult neoplastic cells. They are a diagnostic tool for tumor load and recurrence of metastases after therapy. Alpha-fetoprotein and carcinoembryonic antigen (CEA) are examples of two oncofetal antigens expressed by certain carcinomas, and also found in the blood of some cancer patients.

**Oncogenes:** Genes present in most cells, which, if altered through excessive activity or a mutant product, cause the cell to move closer to becoming cancerous. Oncogenes that are introduced into cells by certain retroviruses are called *v-onc*, while their normal cell counterparts are called *proto-oncogenes* or *c-onc* (for cellular oncogenes).

**Oncogenesis:** The development of a neoplasm or malignancy.

**Oncogenic:** Capable of causing cancer.

**Ontogeny:** The developmental history of an individual organism within a group of animals, such as the first class of immunoglobulin to appear during embryogenesis. Compare Phylogeny.

**Opportunistic pathogen:** A microbe that is normally not pathogenic and causes disease only in immune-compromised individuals such as AIDS patients.

**Opsonins:** Substances, such as antibodies (IgG) and complement activation products (C4b, C3b, iC3b, C3dg, and C3d), capable of enhancing phagocytosis by attaching to the surface of microbes that are recognized by neutrophil and macrophage surface receptors.

**Opsonization:** A process whereby phagocytosis is enhanced by the deposition of opsonins on the antigen.

**Oral tolerance:** The suppression of immune responses to orally administered antigens mediated by anergic T cells or by the production of the suppressive cytokine transforming growth factor-β Oral tolerance prevents immune reactivity to food antigens and the intestinal normal microbiota.

**Organ:** An anatomically discrete collection of tissues that are integrated to perform specific functions.

**Organ-specific autoimmune diseases:** One of the two types of autoimmune disease See also Systemic autoimmune diseases.

**Osteoblasts:** They are highly specialized mesenchymal cells that are responsible for synthesis, deposition, and mineralization of bone extracellular matrix. Osteoblasts are important in the development of all bones.

**Osteoclasts:** Large, multinucleate cells, derived from monocyte/macrophage family members that arise from hematopoietic stem cells and maintain bone during homeostasis and remodeling. They are bone marrow macrophages that can resorb bone.

**Osteosarcoma:** A cancer of the bone, also called *osteogenic sarcoma*. See also Sarcoma.

**Ouchterlony method:** A protein diffusion method using double diffusion in two dimensions. It provides an estimate of the lowest number of antigen-antibody systems present.

# P

**p53:** *p*53 gene encoded tumor suppressor is found to be mutated in roughly 50% of all human cancers. It is a transcription factor that is activated by damage to DNA, anoxia, and expression of certain oncogenes. p53-activated genes regulate cell-cycle arrest, apoptosis, cell senescence and DNA repair.

**P-addition:** The process of nucleotide addition from cleaved hairpin loops formed by the junction of V-D or D-J gene segments during immunoglobulin or T cell receptor gene rearrangements that contribute to junctional diversity of antigen receptors. See also Palindrome (P).

**P-selectins:** Like E-selectin, it is a molecule expressed on vascular endothelium that guides effector cells into sites of infection. See also Selectins.

**Palindrome (P):** A term used in molecular biology to describe a self-complementary stretch of DNA that when read from the 5' to the 3' end displays an equivalent sequence whether read forward or backward or from the left or the right.

**PAMPs:** See Pathogen-associated molecular patterns (PAMPs).

**Panning:** Purified lymphocytes can be isolated from mixtures of cells by using plastic plates coated with either antigen or antibody. The cells are applied (panning) to the coated plates, the nonadherent cells are washed off, and the adherent cells are eluted. It is a positive selection method.

**Parabiosis:** The union of two individuals or animals during pregnancy so there is a crossing of the circulation by anastomosis of blood vessels.

**Paracortical:** It is the area between the cortex and medulla, generally called the *deep cortex* of lymph nodes, which contains most of the lymph node T cells.

**Paracrine:** The manner in which a cell can produce a factor that acts on other cells, such as the interleukin-1 molecule.

**Parallel sets of idiotopes:** Antibodies that share an idiotype but are directed against different antigenic determinants.

**Parasite:** An organism that lives in or on another organism and derives nourishment from it.

**Paratope:** The part of an antibody molecule or cell receptor that makes contact with an antigenic determinant (epitope).

**Parenteral:** The administration of antigen into the body by any route other than through the alimentary canal.

**Paroxysmal nocturnal hemoglobinuria:** A disease resulting from a defect in complement regulatory proteins; it is characterized by episodes of spontaneous hemolysis during complement activation.

**Partial agonist:** It is a variant peptide of a T cell receptor that induces some T-cell functional responses (may stimulate some cytokines or reduced levels of them) or responses totally different from what the unaltered peptide would induce. Synthetic peptides are usually partial agonists in which only one or two T cell receptor contact residues have been changed.

**Passenger leukocytes:** Leukocytes carried by the donor's graft tissue. These cells are considered important because they express class I and II MHC antigens, which can sensitize the recipient's T helper cells. This reaction is not localized because these passenger cells can move out into the recipient's lymphatic system.

**Passive cutaneous anaphylaxis (PCA):** An *in vivo* test used to detect cell-bound IgE in experimental animals injected intradermally with antibody and subsequently injected intravenously with the appropriate antigen and a dye.

**Passive hemagglutination:** Indirect agglutination in which soluble antigens are passively adsorbed or chemically coupled to particles or "carriers," especially red blood cells.

**Passive hemagglutination inhibition:** A result of inhibition of agglutination of antigen-tagged red blood cells. Inhibition occurs because free antigen competes with the bound antigen.

**Passive immunity:** Protection (adaptive immunity) provided by the transfer of antibodies acquired from another immune individual or animal. Their protective activity lasts for 2–3 weeks before it wanes due to catabolic breakdown.

**Passive transfer:** The transfer of immunity from one individual or animal to another using serum.

**Pathogen:** A microorganism that causes disease. This ability is called *pathogenicity*.

**Pattern recognition receptors:** Receptors that recognize pattern recognition sequence structures that are shared by different microorganisms but not found on human tissues. Signaling through these receptors leads to the production of proinflammatory cytokines, chemokines, and the expression of antigen-presenting cell (APC) costimulatory molecules. Costimulatory molecules, together with APC antigenic peptide presentation, couples innate immune recognition of pathogens with the induction of adaptive immune responses. CD14 receptors and mannose receptors on macrophages are examples of pattern recognition receptors; they can bind to bacterial endotoxin and microbial glycoproteins and glycolipids, respectively, leading to macrophage activation. Other examples of pattern recognition receptors are Toll-like receptors, which are activated by various microbial products, such as bacterial lipopolysaccharides, hypomethylated DNA, flagellin, and double-stranded RNA. See also Pattern recognition sequences and Toll-like receptors (TLRs).

**Pathogen-associated molecular patterns (PAMPs):** Molecular patterns found on, and shared by, pathogens (microbes in generally) but are not found on mammalian cells. PAMP examples include mannosylated and polymannosylated compounds that bind the mannose receptor, and various microbial products, such as lipopolysaccharide, hypomethylated DNA, flagellin, and double-stranded RNA that bind Toll-like receptors. PAMP interaction with pattern recognition receptors can initiate innate immunity. See also Pattern recognition receptors.

**Pax-5 gene:** The gene that encodes the protein called *B-cell-specific activator protein*, which is an essential transcription factor for B-cell development.

**PCA:** See Passive cutaneous anaphylaxis.

**PD-1:** See Programmed cell death 1.

**PEC:** See Peritoneal exudate cells.

**PECAM-1 (CD31):** A cell-adhesion molecule that is found on lymphocytes and on endothelial cells; the interactions between CD31 enable lymphocytes to exit blood vessels and enter tissues.

**PEG:** See Polyethylene glycol.

**Pentadecacatechol:** The chemical substance derived from poison ivy plant leaves that can cause Type IV delayed-type hypersensitivity reactions (contact dermatitis) on sensitized individuals.

**Pentraxins:** A family of acute-phase plasma proteins that contain five identical subunits. They are secreted pattern recognition receptors. The acute phase molecule C-reactive protein belongs to this family.

**Peptide-binding cleft:** The peptide-binding portion of an MHC molecule that contains the peptide, which is presented to T cells. It is composed of paired α-helices walls resting on a floor of an eight-stranded β-pleated sheet. The cleft contains the polymorphic amino acid residues that vary among different MHC alleles.

**Perforin:** A secreted protein, similar to the ninth component of complement, that supports the cytotoxic function of granzymes in target cells. Once internalized by the target cells, it disrupts the endosomal membrane and mediates transport of granzymes in the cytoplasm, usually leading to apoptosis. Cytotoxic T cells and NK cells contain granules full of perforin. (If target cells are exposed to high concentrations of perforin, it leads to dead by osmotic lysis, a form of necrosis.)

**Perforin-mediated killing:** A mechanism of $T_C$ cell- and NK cell-mediated killing. It involves delivery of the lethal hit by $T_C$ cell- or NK cell-derived cytoplasmic granules to the intercellular space at the site of contact between the $T_C$ cell or the NK cell and the target cell, which leads to apoptosis of the target cell. Another proposed mechanism suggests that perforin creates pores in the target-cell membrane, and granzymes, which are delivered to the target cell membrane with perforin, then diffuse into the target cell.

**Periarteriolar lymphoid sheath (PALS):** The PALS, located in the spleen, contains most of the lymphoid tissue. It is also called the *white pulp*. The T cells are located round the small arterioles, composed of two-thirds $CD4^+$ T cells and one-third $CD8^+$ T cells, while the B cells are further out. The B cells may be found in the primary or secondary follicles.

**Peripheral tolerance:** The unresponsiveness to self-antigens that is present in peripheral tissues (not the thymus and bone marrow; the latter are involved in central tolerance)—the lack of responsiveness of mature lymphocytes. It is induced by the recognition of antigens without adequate levels of costimulators needed for lymphocyte activation or by continual and repeated stimulation by these self-antigens or by the actions of regulatory T cells. It controls potentially self-reactive lymphocytes that have escaped central tolerance. See also Central tolerance.

**Peritoneal exudate cells (PEC):** Cells that are induced into the peritoneal cavity by various inflammatory agents, such as macrophages elicited into the peritoneal cavity with thioglycollate.

**Peritoneum:** The membrane that lines the abdominal cavity.

**Peyer's patches:** Nodules of lymphoid tissues located in the submucosa (lamina propria) of the small intestine where immune responses to ingested antigens may be initiated. They consist of a dome area, a B-cell follicle area that contains mostly B lymphocytes (precursors of IgA-producing cells), plasma cells, germinal centers, and a thymus-dependent (or interfollicular T cell) area. High endothelial venules are present mainly in the interfollicular areas.

**PGE$_2$:** See Prostaglandins.

**PHA:** See Phytohemagglutinin.

**Phage display library:** Bacteriophages that display antibodies; they can be created by cloning immunoglobulin V-region genes in to them; the antigen-binding domains on the phage's surface form the library. Because antigen-binding phage can be replicated in bacteria, they are used as antibodies. This technique allows the development of novel antibodies of any specificity.

**Phagocytic cells (phagocytes):** Cells that are able to internalize material and digest it. Examples of phagocytes are macrophages and neutrophils. See also Macrophages.

**Phagocytosis:** The engulfment ("cell-eating") and enclosing of large particles ($\geq 1.0$ μm in diameter) in phagosomes, which subsequently mature into phagolysosomes, by phagocytic cells (such as macrophages and neutrophils) in a receptor-, actin-, and energy-dependent manner. See also Phagosome and Phagolysosome.

**Phagolysosome:** A cellular organelle within phagocytic cells resulting from the fusion of a lysosome and a phagosome.

**Phagosome:** An intracellular vesicle of phagocytic cells (macrophages and neutrophils) that is formed during the process of phagocytosis by the invagination of the cell membrane around the material being internalized.

**Phenotype:** The outward, visible expression of the genetic constitution (see Genotype) of an organism, such as blue eyes.

**Phosphatase:** An enzyme, such as CD45, that removes phosphate groups from amino acid side-chains of proteins. For example, CD45 regulates the activity of various signal transduction molecules and transcription factors.

**Phosphatidylinositol biphosphate (PIP$_2$):** Phospholipase C-γ cleaves membrane-associated PIP$_2$ to release the signal molecules diacylglycerol (DAG) and inositol trisphosphate (IP$_3$).

**Phosphatidylserine:** A plasma membrane lipid whose exposure to the outer side correlates with apoptosis of the cell and promotes its uptake by phagocytic cells.

**Phospholipase A$_2$:** A membrane-associated enzyme releasing arachidonic acid from membrane phospholipid. The arachidonic acid acts as the initial substrate for the cyclooxygenase and lipoxygenase pathways, leading to the formation of prostaglandins and leukotrienes, respectively.

**Phospholipase Cγ (PLCγ):** An enzyme, activated in lymphocytes by receptor-antigen ligation, which catalyzes hydrolysis of the membrane phospholipid PIP$_2$ to generate the signaling molecules, IP$_3$ and DAG. See also Inositol 1,4,5-triphosphate (IP$_3$) and Diacylglycerol (DAG).

**Phylogeny:** The developmental history of a group of animals. Compare Ontogeny.

**Phytohemagglutinin (PHA):** A plant carbohydrate-binding protein, or lectin, derived from kidney beans that is a mitogen for T cells.

**Pinocytosis:** The engulfment of liquids ("cell-drinking") or very small particles by phagocytic cells, a form of endocytosis. Also called fluid-phase endocytosis.

**P-K reaction:** See Prausnitz-Kustner reaction.

**Peptide–MHC tetramers:** Engineered recombinant MHC molecules can be made to express the antigen-derived peptides in their peptide-binding groove. Tetrameric complexes are generated by biotinylation, followed by incubation with fluorescently labeled streptavidin. These complexes can be used to stain T cells that express the corresponding T cell receptors (TCRs). The intensity of tetramer staining correlates with TCR affinity.

**PKR kinase:** During viral infections, a serine-threonine kinase is activated by type I interferons IFN-α and IFN-β and phosphorylates eukaryotic protein synthesis initiation factor 2 (eIF-2) blocking translation, thereby inhibiting viral replication.

**Plaque-forming cells:** Antibody-producing cells capable of forming a plaque in the hemolytic plaque assay (see Hemolytic [Jerne] plaque assay).

**Plasma:** The fluid derived from uncoagulated blood (fibrinogen is not converted to fibrin) after removing the cells.

**Plasmablast:** A dividing antibody-secreting cell of the B-cell lineage with migratory potential that will mature into a plasma cell.

**Plasma cells:** A nondividing, terminally differentiated antibody-producing cells, which have distinct trafficking patterns that depend on their site of induction. IgA-producing plasma cells mainly arise in gut mucosal lymphoid tissues or the upper respiratory/digestive tract and have trafficking patterns that relate to their site of induction. In contrast, IgG-producing plasma cells primarily traffic to the bone marrow or inflammatory sites irrespective of their site of induction.

**Plasmacytoid dendritic cells (pDCs):** pDCs, immature DCs, that have the morphological appearance of B-lineage antibody-producing plasma cells, including the presence of rough endoplasmic reticulum; however, they do not produce immunoglobulin, lack most B-lineage markers, selectively express toll-like receptors (TLR) -7 and -9, and circulate as precursor cells in the blood or reside as immature cells in primary and secondary lymphoid tissues. The hematopoietic lymphoid pathway generates pDCs, which secrete large amounts of type I interferons (IFN-α and IFN-β) in response to viral infections. They express high levels of class II MHC molecules and CD123 (IL-3 receptor α-chain) but lack the expression of CD11c (human pDC is HLA-DR$^+$CD11c$^-$). pDCs are also called *interferon-producing cells*.

**Plasmacytoma:** The cancerous growth of plasma cells, and the cause of multiple myeloma in humans.

**Platelets:** They are small cell fragments in the blood that are derived from megakaryocytes and important in blood clotting.

**Platelet-activating factor (PAF):** A lipid mediator produced by basophils, mast cells, neutrophils, and macrophages that causes the release of mediators from platelets, leading to increased vascular permeability and smooth muscle contraction.

**Pluripotent hematopoietic stem cells:** The common ancestral cells for all blood cells.

**P-nucleotides:** The palindromic nucleotides that are found at V-region gene segment junctions of rearranged antigen receptors. They are an inverse repeat of the sequence found in the adjacent gene segment's end. P-nucleotides are generated from a hairpin intermediate during recombination.

**Poison ivy:** A plant whose leaves contain pentadecacatechol; a chemical that causes contact dermatitis in sensitive individuals.

**Pokeweed mitogen (PWM):** A lectin derived from the pokeweed (*Phytolacca americana*) that is a mitogen for both B and T cells.

**Polyclonal:** In antibody-producing cells, a number of different antigen-specific cells (many clones or polyclonal) producing a heterogenous mixture of antibodies.

**Polyclonal activators:** Substances that activate lymphocyte populations irrespective of their antigen specificity, such as Con A, PHA, anti-CD3 antibodies, and bacterial superantigens, which are polyclonal activators of T cells, or LPS, a polyclonal activator of B cells.

**Polyethylene glycol (PEG):** A substance used as a fusing reagent for the production of hybrids, such as the fusing of plasma cells and myeloma cells to form hybridomas secreting monoclonal antibodies.

**Polygenic:** A gene complex such as the MHC that contains several loci encoding proteins of identical function.

**Polymers:** Molecules that are composed of more than one repeating unit.

**Poly-Ig receptor:** An Fc receptor for polymeric IgA and IgM that is expressed on the basolateral surface of many mucosal epithelial cells and functions to transport IgA and IgM across epithelia.

**Polymerase chain reaction (PCR):** A method of copying and amplifying specific DNA sequences that is widely used as a preparative and analytical technique in all branches of molecular biology. PCR involves the use of short oligonucleotide primers complementary to the sequences at the end of the DNA to be amplified. The reaction involves repeated cycles of melting, annealing, and synthesis of DNA.

**Polymorphism of the MHC:** The large number of variants (alleles) seen in different individuals at the same gene locus and the molecules they encode. The MHC diversity within a species results from this polymorphism. There are roughly 300 A alleles, 560 B alleles, and 150 C alleles for human HLA class I molecules; the class II molecules are equally polymorphic (600 alleles). There are roughly 55 K alleles and 60 D alleles for mouse H-2 class I molecules.

**Polymorphonuclear leukocyte (PMN):** A phagocytic cell, also called a *neutrophil*, characterized by segmented nucleus and a high concentration of granules that are filled with enzymes. PMNs are the most abundant circulating blood leukocyte and the main cell involved in inflammatory reactions against bacteria. See also Neutrophils.

**Positive thymic selection:** Responsible for major histocompatibility restriction of antigen recognition. Positive selection of thymocytes that bind with low affinity to self-MHC molecules rescues them from apoptosis. In contrast, thymocytes that do not bind self-MHC molecules die by default. Positive selection ensures that CD4$^+$ and CD8$^+$ T cells are specific for foreign peptide associated with class II or class I MHC molecules, respectively.

**Postcapillary venules:** The blood vessels constructed of a layer of specialized endothelial cells, which allow lymphocytes to migrate across from the blood into the lymph nodes.

**Postvaccinal (allergic) encephalomyelitis:** A cell-mediated autoimmune disease following infectious diseases or immunization against them, characterized by demyelination of nerve sheaths.

**PPD:** See Purified protein derivative.

**Prausnitz-Kustner (P-K) reaction:** A passive transfer test used to detect antigen-specific cell-bound IgE by injecting antigen into a site, which had previously received serum from a possible sensitized individual.

**Pre-B cell (precursor B cell):** These bone marrow B cells, which follow the pro-B-cell stage of B-cell development, produce cytoplasmic μ heavy chains and express the pre-B-cell receptor. Cells are defined as $CD19^+$ cytoplasmic $IgM^+$ and are found only in hematopoietic tissues. See also the Pre-B-cell receptor and Pro-B-cell.

**Pre-B cell receptor:** The Igα/Igβ chain-membrane-bound immunoglobulin complex that consists of a μ heavy chain bound to the surrogate light chain Vpre-B/λ5. See Vpre-B and λ5.

**Pre-cytotoxic T cell:** A mature, antigen naïve $CD8^+$ T cell that cannot mediate effector functions, however, on activation by antigen and costimulators will differentiate into a T cell capable of lysing target cells and secreting cytokines.

**Pre-T cell:** A thymocyte that is characterized by expression of the T cell receptor β chain, but not the α chain or CD4 or CD8 molecules. The β chain is found on the surface of the thymocyte as part of the pre-T cell receptor. See Pre-T cell receptor.

**Pre-T cell receptor:** It is the receptor expressed on the surface of a pre-T cell that is composed of the β chain and an invariant pre-Tα protein. This complex associates with CD3 and ζ molecules to form the pre-T cell receptor complex. This complex delivers signals that drive further proliferation and antigen receptor gene rearrangements.

**Pre-Tα:** An invariant protein that associates with the T cell receptor β chain in pre-T cells to form the pre-T cell receptor.

**Precipitation:** A secondary antigen-antibody reaction involving the combination of soluble antigen with specific antibody, leading to the formation of an insoluble aggregate.

**Prevalence:** It is the number of individuals within a population affected with a particular condition or disease at a given time. Prevalence is contrasted with incidence. See Incidence.

**Primary follicles:** Tightly packed aggregates of B lymphocytes found in the cortex of lymph nodes or the white pulp of the spleen. This region is also composed of follicular dendritic cells. After antigenic stimulation primary follicles develop germinal centers and are called *secondary follicles.*

**Primary immune response:** The immune response following the first exposure to an antigen. In general, the primary immune response appears more slowly, is less protective, and does not last as long as the secondary immune response. See also the Secondary immune response (booster response).

**Primary lymphoid organs:** Lymphoid organs that are responsible for the maturation of functional immune cells in the absence of antigens, such as the thymus, bone marrow, and bursa of Fabricius.

**Primary pathogen:** In contrast to opportunistic pathogen, they can initiate disease even in healthy individuals. See Opportunistic pathogen.

**Primary transcript:** The direct transcript of genomic DNA that still contains introns before their excision to produce mRNA.

**Prime:** To give an initial exposure to antigen.

**Prime-boost vaccine:** When the initial application of vaccine is insufficient, it is followed by the same vaccine or different vaccine preparations to enhance the overall immune response. The initial exposure to a particular antigen diverts the antibody response to shared epitopes of the second antigen after exposure.

**Private specificities:** The MHC molecules unique to a given haplotype.

**Privileged sites:** The sites that lack good lymphatic drainage and thus, if they receive transplanted tissue, are isolated from the recipient's immune system—the graft survives. Examples of privileged sites are the hamster's cheek pouch, the anterior chamber of the eye, testes, and the brain.

**Privileged tissues:** Allogeneic tissues that induce only a weak, if any, allograft response in the recipient. Examples of privileged tissues are the cornea and cartilage.

**Pro-B cell (progenitor B cell):** During B-cell development in the bone marrow, it is the earliest recognizable cell of the B-cell lineage. Pro-B cells do not secrete antibody but can be distinguished from other cells by their expression B cell lineage-restricted cell-surface molecules such as CD10 and CD19. They are characterized by incomplete immunoglobulin-heavy-chain rearrangements.

**Prodrug:** A latent form of a drug that once introduced into the body is activated by metabolism or other chemical transformation.

**Productive rearrangement:** Immunoglobulin or T cell receptor gene rearrangements in which gene segments are joined in sequence to produce VJ or VDJ coding sequences that can be translated.

**Progenitor cells:** Cells that loose their capacity for self-renewal and become committed to the generation of a particular cell lineage.

**Programmed cell death:** Programmed cell death is also known as apoptosis. The release of mitochondrial cytochrome c into the cytoplasm, activation of caspase-9, and initiation of the apoptotic pathway characterize this form of apoptosis. It results from the lack of necessary survival stimuli such as growth factors or costimulators. See also Apoptosis.

**Programmed cell death 1 (PD-1; also called CD279):** A surface receptor that is inducibly expressed on $CD4^+$ and $CD8^+$ T cells, B cells, NK cells, and activated monocytes, which binds to two ligands, PD-L1 (CD274) and PD-L2 (CD273). PD-L1 is constitutively expressed on T cells, B cells, NK cells, dendritic cells, macrophages, and epithelial cells, whereas PD-L2 is inducibly expressed on dendritic cells and macrophages. PD-1–PD-L interactions control the induction and maintenance of peripheral T cell tolerance and the extend T cell proliferation in response to infections.

**Promonocytes:** Immature monocytes derived from monoblasts.

**Promoters:** One of the two types of cis-regulators that promotes initiation of immunoglobulin and T cell receptor gene expression in a specific direction. They are short DNA sequences that are immediately 5′ (roughly 200 bp upstream) to the gene's transcription start site where proteins bind that initiate RNA transcription in a specific direction. See Enhancers. See also DNA-binding proteins.

**Promotion:** The second event in the development of cancer, involving expression of the genetic mutation. See also Initiation.

**Properdin:** A component of the alternative pathway to complement activation that is converted from an inactive form to an active form during activation of the pathway. It complexes with C3b and stabilizes the alternative pathway C3 convertase.

**Properdin system:** Another name for the alternative pathway to complement activation. See Alternative pathway.

**Prostaglandins:** A variety of pharmacologically active derivatives of arachidonic acid, which results from the breakdown action of cyclooxygenase. They cause increased vascular permeability, smooth muscle contraction, and bronchial constriction. Activated mast cells produce prostaglandin $D_2$, which constricts smooth muscle and acts as a vasodilator. They are important mediators of Type I (immediate) hypersensitivity.

**Pro-T cell:** A thymic cortex thymocyte that is a recent arrival from the bone marrow, which does not express T cell receptors, CD3, ζ chains, or CD4 or CD8 molecules. These cells are also called *double-negative thymocytes*.

**Proteasome:** A large multiunit protease complex found in the cytoplasm and nucleus of most cells that degrades cytosolic proteins. Proteins covalently bound to ubiquitin are targeted for proteasomal degradation. The resulting peptides bind to class I MHC molecules.

**Protectin (CD59):** It is a cell-surface molecule that protects host cells from complement-mediated damage by inhibiting the binding of C8 and C9 to the C5b,6,7 complex, thus blocking the formation of the membrane-attack complex.

**Protein A:** It is a cell wall component of Staphylococci that binds to the Fc portion of IgG molecules in most species. It is used to purify IgG antibodies

**Protein kinase C:** A cellular enzyme activated by $Ca^{2+}$ that is involved in the activation of cells. It mediates the phosphorylation of serine and threonine residues and thereby propagates various signal transduction pathways leading to activation of transcription factors. Antigen receptor ligation in B and T cells leads to PKC activation by DAG. See Diacylglycerol (DAG).

**Protein tyrosine kinases (PTKs):** Enzymes that mediate phosphorylation of tyrosines in proteins, which promotes phosphotyrosine-dependent protein-protein interactions. Many PTKs play an important role in numerous signal transduction pathways in immune cells.

**Proto-oncogenes:** Genes that control the induction, modulation, and proliferation of normal cells. The recombination or translocation of proto-oncogenes with viral nucleic acid can transform them into oncogenes. See also Oncogenes.

**Provirus:** The integration of a DNA copy of the retroviral genome into the host cell genome, from which viral genes are transcribed, leading to reproduction of the viral genome. Thus, a provirus represents the latent form of a virus that exists in a cell without harming the cell or producing new virions until it is activated. For example, HIV by remaining in a provirus form, it is inaccessible to the immune system.

**Pseudogenes:** Genes that have similar structures to other genes but are incapable of being expressed, such as the Jκ3 gene in the mouse.

**Pseudopodia:** Membrane protrusions associated with phagocytic cells.

**Psoriasis:** A chronic skin disorder that affects roughly 1–2% of the population. The skin exhibits red scaly thickened patches with silvery scales. These scales are usually found on the elbows, knees, lower back, and scalp. Some evidence suggests a T cell-mediated pathogenesis, when T cells migrate into the skin and release tumor necrosis factor-α, which leads to inflammation and subsequent rapid skin cell production.

**Public specificities:** The MHC molecules not restricted to a given haplotype.

**Pulmonary surfactant A and D:** Protein members of the pentraxin family that function in the acute-phase response. See also Pentraxins.

**Purified antigen (subunit) vaccine:** A vaccine composed of purified microbial antigens or subunits, such as, diphtheria and tetanus toxoids, pneumococcus and *Haemophilus influenzae* polysaccharides vaccines, and hepatitis B and influenza virus vaccines. Purified antigen (subunit) vaccines may stimulate antibody and helper T cell responses, but they do not stimulate cytotoxic T cell responses.

**Purified protein derivative (PPD):** A soluble fraction obtained by precipitation of tuberculin by trichloroacetic acid. Tuberculin is found in the culture supernatant of *M. tuberculosis* and is used as a test antigen in the tuberculin test for tuberculosis.

**Purine analogs:** Antimetabolites. Their synthetic forms appear to block a stage of lymphocyte differentiation. They are used as immunosuppressants.

**Purine nucleotide phosphorylase deficiency:** An enzyme important in purine metabolism. Its deficiency leads to severe combined immunodeficiency. This results from the accumulation of purine nucleosides that are toxic to T cells, causing the immunodeficiency.

**Puromycin:** An antibiotic that acts as an immunosuppressant by inhibiting protein synthesis. See also Actinomycin D and Mitomycin C.

**Pus:** A whitish, pasty mass consisting of cell debris and dead neutrophil mixture that is present in wounds infected with extracellular encapsulated bacteria.

**PWM:** See Pokeweed mitogen.

**Pyrimidine analogs:** Antimetabolites that compete with enzymes involved in nucleotide synthesis or substitute for natural bases in nucleic acids.

**Pyrogen:** A fever-causing molecule released by activated leukocytes during an infection. Microbial product-induced cytokines such as tumor necrosis factor, which can increase the set point for body temperature, leading to fever.

**Pyogenic:** The ability, by bacteria such as staphylococci and streptococci, to cause pus production during an inflammatory response rich in neutrophils.

**Pyogenic bacteria:** They are extracellular encapsulated bacteria that are difficult to ingest by phagocytes and often produce pus at the site of infection.

## Q

**Qa locus:** A locus found in the murine H-2 complex mapping between the D and TL locus. It encodes for Qa antigens found on helper T cells.

**Quiescent:** Inactive or at rest.

## R

**R5 virus:** An HIV-1 strain that uses CC-chemokine receptor 5 (CCR5) as the coreceptor to enter target cells. See also Human immunodeficiency virus (HIV).

**Radioimmunoassay (RIA):** A competitive immunological procedure for measuring very low concentrations of antigens (or antibodies) by using radioactively labeled antigens as competitors.

**Rac:** During early T-cell activation events, Rac, a guanine nucleotide-binding protein is activated by the GDP GTP exchange factor Vav. The GTP-Vac complex triggers a three-step protein kinase cascade that leads to the activation of the stress-activated protein (SAP) kinase, c-Jun N-terminal kinase (JNK), and p38 kinase.

**RAG:** See Recombination activation genes.

**Rapamycin:** An immunosuppressive drug produced by *Streptomyces hygroscopicus*, which blocks the translation of mRNAs encoding cell-cycle regulators and controls progression from the $G_1$ to S phase of the cell cycle.

**Ras:** A member of the 21-Kd guanine nucleotide-binding protein family that has intrinsic GTPase activity. It is involved in many different signal transduction pathways of various cell types. In T-cell activation, tyrosine-phosphorylated adapter proteins recruit Ras to the plasma membrane, where it is activated by GDP-GTP exchange factors, then initiates the MAP kinase cascade, leading to *fos* gene expression, and assembly of the AP-1 transcription factor. Mutated *ras* genes are associated with cancer development.

**Reactive lysis:** If the fluid phase of the C5b67 complex is deposited on a cell, it may lyse the cell without earlier complement components.

**Reactive nitrogen intermediates (RNIs):** Highly bactericidal compounds formed by the combination of nitrogen and oxygen by neutrophils and macrophages.

**Reactive oxygen intermediates (ROIs):** Highly bactericidal compounds such as superoxide ($O_2^-$), hydroxyl radicals ($OH^-$), and hydrogen peroxide ($H_2O_2$) that are formed in the phagosome lumen following the respiratory burst of neutrophils and macrophages. They can damage intracellular targets, such as DNA, carbohydrates or proteins.

**Reagin:** An antiquated term for IgE antibody.

**Receptor-associated tyrosine kinase:** Lymphocyte antigen receptors are associated with these Src family kinases that bind to receptor tails through their SH2 domains.

**Receptor editing:** A process by which some bone marrow-residing immature B cells that recognize self-antigens are induced to change their immunoglobulin specificities. The editing involves the reactivation of *RAG genes*, additional light chain VJ recombinations, leading to new light chain synthesis that allows the cell to express a nonself-reactive immunoglobulin receptor. It also occurs in the T cell receptor α chain, but it is less well described.

**Receptor-mediated endocytosis:** The internalization of molecules bound to cell-surface receptors into cellular endosomes; B-cell internalization via immunoglobulin-bound antigen is an example of this process.

**Recessive lethal genes:** These genes encode proteins that are required for growth of the host; a defect in both copies leads to death of the host.

**Recognition phase:** The initial phase of an acquire immune response during which antigen-specific lymphocytes bind to antigens. The recognition phase usually takes place in secondary lymphoid organs such as lymph nodes and the spleen. See also Activation phase and Effector phase.

**Recognition signals (sequences):** Germline DNA recombination sequences that help control all DNA rearrangements. See also Recombination signal sequences (RSSs).

**Recombinant antibodies:** Also called *hybrid* or *chimeric monoclonal antibodies*. By using DNA that expresses the desired product and introducing it into an appropriate cell, one can custom-make antibodies. These antibodies can include molecules with enzyme genes fused to them (use in immunoassays in place of secondary antibodies), or the gene for the Fab portion of an antibody can be attached to a toxin gene (directs toxin to specific site). See also DNA transfection.

**Recombinant strains:** Animals produced by crossing two inbred strains. An $F_1$ animal that has undergone rearrangement of genetic information during meiosis (recombination) consisting of crossover and recombination of parts of two chromosomes, so that the affected chromosome has different haplotypes at each end. Thus, these animals can be used to determine the region of a chromosome that is responsible for specific immunologic characteristics.

**Recombinant inbred strains:** The crossing of two inbred strains of mice (AA x BB) leads to a heterozygous (AB) $F_1$ offspring. If one crosses the $F_1$ strains and then inbreeds the offspring ($F_2$), recombinant inbred strains are produced. The result is a strain of mice that have identical sets of chromosomes but the chromosomes are randomly of either the A or the B type. Thus, these recombinant inbred strains are used to identify which chromosomes carry the genes for each immunologic characteristic.

**Recombination:** The process by which the gene segments (exons) for either antibodies or T cell receptors are brought together and joined. Recombination depends on sequences of amino acids that flank each V, D, and J gene segment. These sequences are enzymatically cut and respliced, excising the intervening noncoding gene segments (introns). This process contributes to the generation of diversity of antibodies and T cell receptors. See also Generation of diversity.

**Recombination-activating genes 1 and 2 (RAG-1 and RAG-2):** Two linked genes, RAG-1 and RAG-2, that encode lymphocyte-specific proteins needed for immunoglobulin or T cell receptor gene segment rearrangement in the assembly of a function receptor gene. The RAG-encoded proteins are the lymphocyte-specific components of V-D-J recombinase, are expressed in developing B and T cells, and by binding to the recombination recognition sequences drive DNA recombination events that form functional B and T cell receptors.

**Recombination signal sequences (RSSs):** Highly conserved heptamer and nonamer nucleotide sequences that flank each germline V, D, and J gene segment, which constitute the recognition sites for the RAG-1/RAG-2–encoded V[D]J recombinase proteins and serve as signals for the gene rearrangement process of immunoglobulin and T cell receptor production. They always consist of a heptamer-12 bp spacer-nonamer complex (RSS-1) or heptamer-23 bp spacer-nonamer complex (RSS-2).

The heptamer is immediately adjacent to the V, D, J coding sequences. Joining only occurs between a RSS-1 and a RSS-2—the 12/23 rule. See also Heptamer-nonamer and 12/23 spacer rule.

**Red pulp:** The blood-filtering portion of the spleen composed primarily of red blood cells distributed within a network of splenic cords and venous sinuses lined with macrophages, dendritic cells, sparse lymphocytes, and plasma cells. Its main function is to destroy senescent erythrocytes.

**Region:** In immunogenetics, a segment of a chromosome serving as the locus for at least one defined gene, such as the K, I, S, D, and L regions of the murine H-2 complex or the D, B, C, and A regions of the HLA complex.

**Regulatory genes:** They control the quantitative expression of certain structural genes.

**Regulatory T ($T_{reg}$) cells:** The classic regulatory T cells are $CD4^+CD25^+FOXP3^+$. They functionally suppress an immune response by influencing the activity of another cell type. At least three phenotypically distinct regulatory T-cell populations exist. The forkhead box transcription factor Foxp3 is highly expressed and regulates $T_{reg}$ cell development and function. It serves as the best marker to identify $T_{reg}$ cells. $T_{reg}$ cells constitutively express CTLA-4. The primary role of $T_{reg}$ cells is to maintain self-tolerance. In the mouse, $T_{reg}$ cells comprise roughly 5–10% of the total population of $CD4^+$ T cells. See also $CD4^+CD25^+$ regulatory T ($T_{reg}$) cell.

**Replicon-based DNA vaccine:** A vaccine that is based on DNA molecules that autonomously replicate, such as plasmids and phage.

**Respiratory burst:** Shortly after phagocytosis, phagocytes undergo a burst of activity in which there is rapid oxygen consumption, leading to the production of reactive oxygen intermediates that are toxic to ingested microorganisms. See also Reactive oxygen intermediates (ROIs).

**Reticular cells:** They are the major stromal cells in the bone marrow.

**Retrovirus:** A group of viruses containing RNA as their genetic material that uses the enzyme reverse transcriptase to transcribe RNA to DNA, which may become integrated into the host cell nuclear DNA.

**Rev protein:** It is a product of the HIV *rev* gene, which promotes passage of viral RNA from the nucleus to the cytoplasm during HIV replication.

**Reverse passive hemagglutination:** A hemagglutination test in which antibodies rather than antigens are absorbed to red blood cells. The titer is the least amount of antigen that leads to agglutination.

**Reverse transcriptase:** A retrovirus (such as HIV) -encoded enzyme that synthesizes a DNA copy of the viral genome from an RNA template. Reverse transcriptase also is a widely used reagent for cloning complementary DNAs encoding genes of interest from mRNA.

**Reverse transcriptase polymerase chain reaction (RT-PCR):** A version of the PCR used to amplify a cDNA of a gene of interest. RNA is isolated from the cell expressing the gene, reverse transcriptase is used to synthesize cDNAs, and the resulting DNA of interest is amplified by conventional PCR.

**RGYW motifs:** The RGYW nucleotide sequence is considered a location where mutations are preferentially inserted during somatic hypermutation. (R denotes A [adenosine] or G [guanosine], Y denotes C [cytidine] or T [thymidine], W denotes A or T). See also Somatic hypermutation.

**Rh blood group:** Human red blood cells can be divided into two groups depending on whether they express the Rh antigen (RhD). Eighty-five percent of the population expresses the D antigen ($Rh^+$), and the remaining 15% do not ($Rh^-$).

**Rheumatic fever:** An antibody-mediated autoimmune collagen vascular disease following group A streptococcal pharyngitis. It occurs most commonly in children aged 5 to 15 years. Cardiac involvement is the most serious sign of the disease.

**Rheumatoid arthritis (RA):** An autoimmune disease exemplified by inflammation and deterioration of the joints. The joints are infiltrated by $CD4^+$ T cells, activated B cells, and plasma cells and proinflammatory cytokines, such as interleukin-1 and tumor necrosis factor-α.

**Rheumatoid factor:** Anti-immunoglobulin antibody (usually IgM) directed against IgG and found in the serum of some patients with rheumatoid arthritis.

**Rhodamine:** A dye used to label antibodies for fluorescence methods. See also Fluorescein.

**RIA:** See Radioimmunoassay.

**Ribosome:** A cytoplasmic organelle that serves as the site for amino acid incorporation during the synthesis of protein.

**RNA interference:** It is a technique to inhibit or decrease the expression of a specific target gene with short oligonucleotides that are complementary to the sequence of the gene mRNA.

**RNAse protection assay:** A method used to detect and quantify mRNA copies of particular genes. The method is based on the hybridization of the mRNA to radiolabeled RNA probes and the digestion of unhybridized RNA by RNAse. The created double-stranded RNAs are resistant to RNAse degradation and are of a particular size as determined by the probe's length. The double-stranded RNAs can be isolated by gel electrophoresis and detected and quantified by autoradiography.

**RNA splicing:** The removal from primary RNA transcripts of intronic DNA-transcribed sequences and the connecting of exon-transcribed sequences to generate an mRNA.

**RNIs:** See Reactive nitrogen intermediates (RNIs).

**ROIs:** See Reactive oxygen intermediates (ROIs).

# S

**S region:** The chromosomal region located between the I and D regions of the murine H-2 complex that encodes complement proteins. Also, the S region is a segment of a gene that plays a role in antibody class switching. See S-S recombination.

**Sarcoma:** A malignant tumor of mesodermal origin, such as connective tissues, bones, or muscle.

**Scatchard equation:** A formula used to determine antibody affinity:

$$R/c = nK - rK$$

where $r$ equals the moles of hapten bound per mole of antibody, $c$ equals free hapten concentration at equilibrium, $n$ equals antibody valence (number of combining sites), and $K$ equals the association constant. The equation states that the curve that represents $r/c$ values as a function of $r$ is a straight line. Thus, the data are usually plotted according to Scatchard as $r/c$ against $r$. Since this equation results in a straight line, the intercept of the line on the abscissa (the point where $r/c = 0$) is equal to $n$ ($n$ corresponds to the number of antibody combining sites, that is, antibody valence). The intercept of the line with the ordinate is equal to $nK$. The slope of the equation equals the reciprocal of the association constant $(-K)$. In fact, in haptenic excess (high free hapten concentration) close to saturation of the antibody combining site, represented in the equation as $c$, the $r/c$ ratio approaches zero; therefore $r$ is almost equal to $n$, because in the equation $r/c = nK - rK$.

**Scavenger receptors:** A cell surface receptor family that is expressed on macrophages, dendritic cells, endothelial cells, and other, which mediate endocytosis of oxidized or acetylated low-density lipoprotein particles and also bind to and mediate the phagocytosis of a variety of microbes and apoptotic cells. They are considered pattern recognition receptors. See also Pattern recognition receptors.

**SCID:** See Severe combined immunodeficiency diseases.

**SCID mouse:** An immunodeficient (lacks B and T cells) mouse strain resulting from an early block in maturation from bone marrow precursors. Homozygous SCID mice carry a mutation in the gene that encodes the catalytic subunit of an enzyme DNA-dependent protein kinase (DNA-PKs) component that is needed for double-stranded DNA break repair. This enzyme deficiency leads to abnormal joining of immunoglobulin and T cell receptor gene segments during recombination, which leads to a failure to express antigen receptors.

**Second set rejection:** Transplanted tissues are treated by the immune system as most foreign antigens; there is specificity and memory. If the recipient's immune system is exposed to the transplanted tissue for a second time, the rejection response is accelerated. This accelerated secondary reaction is called *second set rejection*.

**Second signal:** Lymphocyte activation requires two signals, the first is antigen binding to its receptor; the second signal (also called *costimulatory signal*) consists of a number of cell-surface ligand-receptor interactions and cytokine-cytokine receptor interactions.

**Secondary immune response (booster response):** It is the immune response following the second exposure to an antigen. In general, the secondary immune response appears more quickly, is more protective, and lasts longer than the primary immune response. See also Primary immune response.

**Secondary follicles:** In the cortex of the lymph nodes, a bull's-eye-like structure of concentrically packed, activated, dividing B cells that make up a germinal center. See Primary follicles. See also Germinal center.

**Secondary lymphoid-tissue chemokine (SLC):** A chemokine (CCL21) constitutively produced by lymphatic vessels (e.g., high endothelial venules [HEVs]) that attracts T and B cells and dendritic cells (DCs) to draining lymph nodes. The immune cells bind to CCL21 with CCR7. In addition to directing antigen-activated DCs to the draining lymph nodes, along with CCL19, CCL21 provides further maturation signals, which complete the DC-maturation process. The mature DCs localize within the lymph node T-cell regions and drive T-cell activation.

**Secondary lymphoid organs:** Filters set across the lymphatic system (lymph nodes) or the circulatory system (spleen). These organs are responsible for concentrating the antigen for interaction with immune cells. In other words, the secondary lymphoid organs are important in antigen-dependent differentiation of immune cells.

**Secretory component:** A 70,000 molecular weight protein fragment of the poly-Ig receptor produced by epithelial cells and attached to a dimer of IgA. It facilitates the passage of IgA through cells and also inhibits the effects of degradative enzymes.

**Segmental flexibility:** The ability of the two Fab portions of antibodies to move relative to one another on antigen binding.

**Segregation:** It is the distribution of genes among gametes such that two alleles must segregate. If segregation with another allele occurs more often than expected, it is called *linkage*.

**Selectins:** A group of three separate but closely related cell-adhesion molecules (CAMs) present on leukocytes (L-selectin [CD62L], activated endothelium (E-selectin [CD62E]), and on platelets and activated endothelium (P-selectin [CD62P]) that bind to mucin-like CAMs (e.g., CD34, GlyCAM-1, and PSGL-1 [P-selectin glycoprotein ligand; CD162])—the binding between leukocytes and endothelium directs leukocyte recirculation and promotes leukocyte activation. The selectins are a single-chain glycoprotein with a similar modular structure that includes an extracellular calcium-dependent lectin domain. See also GlyCAM-1 and Integrins.

**Selective immunoglobulin (Ig) deficiency:** A group of Ig deficiencies characterized by the lack of only one or a few Ig classes or subclasses. The most common is an IgA deficiency, followed by IgG2 and IgG3 deficiencies. These patients may be more susceptible to bacterial infections.

**Self-antigens:** A host's own cell markers/antigens. During lymphocyte development via central and peripheral tolerance, those lymphocytes that react against self-antigens undergo apoptosis.

**Self-peptides:** A host's self-antigen-derived peptides. Without infection, these peptides occupy the peptide-binding sites of cell-surface MHC molecules.

**Self-tolerance:** The phenomenon whereby an individual's own tissues are tolerated (see *Horror autotoxicus*). If there is a breakdown in this tolerance, autoimmune disease can result. Self-tolerance may occur because of clonal deletion of autoreactive lymphocytes, anergy, or through maintenance by regulatory T cells of autoreactive cells, or both. See also Central tolerance, Immunologic tolerance, and Peripheral tolerance.

**Sensitization:** Increased reactivity on the first exposure to an allergen.

**Sensitized cell:** An immune cell that has been exposed to specific antigen.

**Sepsis:** It is the infection of bloodstream that is usually serious and can be fatal. If the infection is due to gram-negative organisms, it can trigger septic shock via the release of tumor necrosis factor-α (TNF-α).

**Septic shock:** Often a fatal complication of severe gram-negative bacterial infections with spread to the blood (sepsis), leading to vascular collapse, disseminated intravascular coagulation, metabolic disturbances, cardiac dysfunction, and death. These effects result from bacterial lipopolysaccharide (LPS) and cytokines such as interleukin-1 (IL-1), tumor necrosis factor-α, and IL-12. Septic shock is also called *toxic* or *endotoxic shock*.

**Septicemia:** A systemic disease caused by the invasion and multiplication of pathogenic microorganisms in the blood stream.

**Sequence motif:** A nucleotide or amino acid pattern shared by different genes or proteins that often have similar functions.

**Sequential determinants:** Antigenic determinants whose specificity is determined by the sequence of subunits within the epitope rather than the three-dimensional structure of the epitope. However, one must remember that the sequence of subunits dictates the conformation or shape of the determinant.

**Seroconversion:** The first detection of antibodies in the serum specific for microorganisms in response to immunization or during the course of an infection, that is, an infected individual converts from an antibody-negative state to an antibody-positive state.

**Serologically defined (SD) antigens:** Any MHC molecules that are defined by their ability to induce, and react with, the appropriate antibodies.

**Serology:** The science that deals with the *in vitro* interactions of antibodies and antigens.

**Serotonin:** A molecule with a molecular weight of 176 that is present in mast cells (only some species) and in platelets; it contributes to immediate hypersensitivity reactions.

**Serpins:** A family of serine-protease inhibitors, which includes cathepsin G, neutrophil elastase, and proteinase 3. Serpins are involved in neutrophil-mediated killing of microbes. Microbial killing is accomplished in phagolysosomes; azurophil granules contribute to the intracellular degradation of microorganisms. Azurophil granules are defined by their high content of serpins and other bactericidal molecules.

**Serum:** Contrasted to plasma, serum is the liquid part of coagulated (fibrinogen is converted to fibrin) blood; the remaining cells and fibrin have been removed.

**Serum amyloid A:** During an infection and inflammatory reactions, this acute phase protein significantly increases in the serum due interleukin-1- and tumor necrosis factor-induced synthesis by the liver. Serum amyloid A induces leukocyte chemotaxis, phagocytosis, and adhesion to endothelial cells.

**Serum sickness:** An adverse reaction to foreign antigen that occurs because of the injection of large doses of a protein antigen into the blood, characterized by the deposition of antigen-antibody complexes in the blood vessels of kidneys and joints. These complexes lead to complement activation and leukocyte recruitment, leading to glomerulonephritis and arthritis. Serum sickness is an example of a Type III (immune complex-mediated) hypersensitivity.

**Severe-combined immunodeficiency diseases (SCID):** A group of diseases in which the patient exhibits a leukopenia and lack of humoral and cell-mediated immune responses due to the absence of B and T cells. As the name implies, the condition is quite serious and death is likely.

**Sex-limited protein (Slp):** A nonfunctional variant of the fourth component of complement.

**Shocking dose:** The second exposure to an allergen, at which time sensitization is noticed.

**Side-chain theory:** A theory proposed by Paul Ehrlich stating that a population of cells expresses a large number of special preformed side chains (we now know them as immunoglobulins) complementary with parts of the antigen. This complementarity allows specific interaction.

**Signal joint:** In V(D)J immunoglobulin or T cell receptor gene rearrangement, the sequence formed by the union of recombination signal sequences (RSSs). See Recombination signal sequences (RSSs) and Coding joint.

**Signal peptide:** The amino-terminal end (or leader sequence) of a newly synthesized polypeptide that allows it to enter the endoplasmic reticulum, at which time the signal peptide is cleaved away.

**Signal-transducing subunit:** A polypeptide chain of a multimeric cytokine receptor that, on binding the cytokine, activates the cytokine-mediated signal-transduction pathway.

**Signal transducer and activator of transcription (STAT):** A family of proteins that function as signaling molecules and transcription factors that bind to the phosphorylated tyrosine residues at their SH2 domains of type I and type II cytokine receptors and thereby play a role in signal transductions by many cytokines. STATs are found in cell cytoplasm as inactive monomers. They are recruited to the cytoplasmic tails of cross-linked cytokine receptors, are tyrosine-phosphorylated by JAKs, the phosphorylated STATs dimerize, and move to the nucleus. In the nucleus, they bind to specific sequences in the promoter regions of genes and stimulate their transcription, i.e., they act as transcription factors. See also JAK-STAT signaling pathway.

**Signal transduction:** A process whereby cells notice changes in their environment; for example, in lymphocytes it is the process of going from antigen exposure to development of adaptive immunity.

**Silencers:** DNA elements that suppress promoter and/or enhancer activity in a position- and orientation-independent manner.

**Simian immunodeficiency virus (SIV):** They are different HIV-related Lentiviruses isolated from non-human primates. SIV-infected rhesus macaques are an experimental model for HIV-1 infected humans. See also Human immunodeficiency virus (HIV).

**Single-chain variable-domain antibody fragment (Fv):** An antibody fragment, constructed by genetic engineering, that is composed of a heavy-chain V-region linked by a stretch of synthetic peptide to a light-chain V-region.

**Single-positive thymocyte:** A thymocyte found in the medulla of the thymus that expresses either CD4 or CD8 but not both. These thymocytes have matured from double-positive thymocytes are ready to exit the thymus.

**Skin test (for allergy):** Testing whether allergen-specific IgE is present in an individual by introducing minute amounts of allergen into the epidermis by a prick or scratch. If IgE is present, it induces the degranulation of mast cells, leading to a wheal-and-flare reaction; its size is used as a measure of allergen sensitivity in that individual.

**SLC:** See Secondary lymphoid-tissue chemokine.

**SLE:** See Systemic lupus erythematosus.

**Slow-reacting substance of anaphylaxis (SRS-A):** Pharmacologically active, 400 molecular weight, acidic lipoprotein that has a protractive constrictive effect on smooth muscle, especially bronchial muscle. SRS-A is slow reacting compared to histamine, hence its name. It is now known to be composed of three leukotrienes (LT), $LTC_4$, $LTD_4$, and $LDE_4$. See Leukotrienes.

**Slp:** See Sex-limited protein.

**Small G proteins:** They are monomeric G proteins that are intracellular signaling molecules. They are molecules like Ras that bind to GTP in their active form and hydrolyze it to its inactive GDP form.

**SOCS:** See Suppressors of cytokine signaling (SOCS).

**Somatic:** The body cells, not the germline cells.

**Somatic hypermutation:** A mechanism used to increase antibody diversity and antigen-binding affinity by introducing point mutations into rearranged immunoglobulin variable-region genes during activation and proliferation of germinal center B cells (centroblasts). These mutations lead to increased affinity of antibodies for their specific antigen, imparting a selective advantage to those B cells, and thus leading to affinity maturation of the antibody response. It can also lead to loss of nonself antigen recognition and the generation of a self-reactive B-cell receptor. See also RGYW motifs.

**Somatic recombination:** The recombination of DNA that leads to the formation of functional genes, which are formed during B and T lymphocyte development, and encode the variable regions of antigen receptors. The process involves using the inherited, or germline, separated DNA segments that are brought together by enzymatic deletion of intervening sequences and religation. The rearrangements are not passed from generation to generation. The process is also called *somatic rearrangement*.

**Somatic theory:** The theory that antibody diversity is generated by a somatic genetic change of a few inherited germline variable (V)-region gene segments during differentiation of B-cell precursors to mature B cells. The opposite theory is the germline theory. See Germline theory.

**Southern blot:** A technique in which DNA fragments are separated according to size by electrophoresis, reacted, and developed by hybridization with a radiolabeled nucleic acid probe. The location of the hybridized DNA fragments is determined by autoradiography of the dried gels.

**SP-40,40:** A regulatory protein that mediates the homeostatic maintenance of complement activation in plasma.

**S-protein:** The primary inhibitor of the membrane attack complex. By binding the complex, the S-protein prevents its attachment to the cell surface.

**Specific immunotherapy:** Cancer immunotherapy that relies on vaccines of tumor cells or tumor cell functions administered directly to the patient to increase or induce a host immune response to tumor-specific antigen. See also Nonspecific immunotherapy.

**Specificity:** A term defining the selective reaction occurring between an antigen and its corresponding

antibody-combining site (on free or surface antibody) or the T cell receptor. It is the cardinal feature of the adaptive immune system.

**Spectratyping:** A method to define certain DNA gene segment types that give a repetitive three-nucleotide spacing, i.e., one codon.

**Spleen:** A solid, encapsulated, deep red-colored organ in the abdominal cavity, composed mainly of lymphocytes and macrophages. The spleen is a filter set across the circulatory system and is an important site of antibody production.

**Splenomegaly:** An increase in spleen size seen after infections and some types of tumor growth. Splenomegaly is used as an index for graft-versus-host reactions.

**Splicing:** The process of removing the introns between the J and C exons of the primary hnRNA transcript. The excision of the precise introns and recombining to form the mRNA is determined by specific base sequences that flank the exons. The base sequences are called *donor* and *acceptor junctions*. The "cutting and pasting" leads to mRNA containing a polyadenylated tail. The precise function of the poly-A tail is unknown, but it seems to help subsequent RNA processing and the export of the mature RNA out of the nucleus.

**Src homology-2 (SH2) domain:** A 3-D 100-amino acid residue domain structure present in many signaling proteins that permits noncovalent interactions with other proteins by binding to phosphotyrosines. Each SH2 domain has a unique binding specificity that is determined by the amino acid residues adjacent to the target protein phosphotyrosines. Several proteins involved in B and T cell early signaling events interact with one another through SH2 domains, including the kinases of the Src and Syk (spleen tyrosine kinase).

**Src homology-3 (SH3) domain:** A 3-D 60-amino acid residue domain structure present in many signaling proteins that mediates protein-protein binding. SH3 domains bind to proline residues and cooperate with the SH2 domains of the protein.

**SRS-A:** See Slow reacting substance of anaphylaxis.

**S-S recombination:** A type of DNA rearrangement leading to class switching. The constant region of a μ chain of an antibody is replaced by another constant-heavy region while the variable-heavy region remains the same. The specific regions within the introns that contain frequent recombination sites include tandem repetitive sequences. The nucleotide sequence of these regions is called the *S region*. See S region.

**Staphylococcal enterotoxins:** These toxins are associated with food poisoning. They are also know to stimulate the many T cells that express particular $V_\beta$-containing T cell receptors, which bind to MHC class II molecule enterotoxin-associated complexes; they are therefore called *superantigens*.

**STAT:** See Signal transducer and activator of transcription.

**Steady state:** The state of a healthy host's immune system, that is, a host free of infections or inflammatory stimuli.

**Stem cells:** Immature or precursor cells from which all mature cells arise; for example, bone marrow stem cells are the precursor for any type of immune cell.

**Stem cell factor:** A transmembrane protein that is expressed on bone marrow stromal cells, which binds to the signaling molecule on stem cells called *c-kit*.

**Sterilizing immunity:** An immune response, which leads to the complete removal of the pathogen.

**Streptavidin:** A bacterial protein produced by *Streptomyces avidinii* that has high affinity and specificity for biotin. It can be tagged with fluorescent dyes and used in many immunologic assays to detect antibodies and other molecules labeled with biotin. See Biotin.

**Stroma:** An organ compartment that serves as the connective tissue framework; it includes fibroblasts, immune cells, and fat cells.

**Stromal cells:** Usually nonhematopoietic cells that form the framework of organs and support the growth and differentiation of hematopoietic cells by expressing various molecules, which support adhesion, proliferation and survival of distinct cell subsets. In the bone marrow, they include reticular cells, endothelial cells, and macrophages.

**Structural genes:** Genes that determine the primary structure of proteins, that is, the amino acid sequence of polypeptide chains.

**Subclinical:** Pertaining to an infection so minor that there is no detectable clinical signs or symptoms of the infection. See Infection.

**Subregions:** Areas of related loci within regions of the major histocompatibility complex.

**Subtractive hybridization:** A method that was initially used to isolate T cell receptor mRNA from all other mRNAs in the T cell.

**Subtypes of HIV-1:** These are genetically related clusters of HIV-1, which are also called *clades* and do not fall into specific categories based on their neutralizing antibody susceptibility. See Human immunodeficiency virus (HIV).

**Subunit vaccine:** A vaccine that encodes only portions of a pathogen.

**Superantigens:** Molecules that engage all T cell receptors containing a specific $V_\beta$ region, regardless of either the other components of the receptor or the major histocompatibility complex context of the antigen. Superantigens are presented to T cells by the nonpolymorphic regions of class II MHC molecules. Some Staphylococcal enterotoxins are superantigens, which by activating many T cells leads to massive amounts of cytokine production and a clinical syndrome similar to septic shock. Some virus-derived antigens can also act as superantigens. Superantigens can stimulate 2–20% of all T cells. Superantigen-induced stimulation does not induce an adaptive immune response specific for the pathogen.

**Suppressor macrophages:** In some experimental systems, macrophages can nonspecifically inhibit immune responses. The mechanisms of action are unknown.

**Suppressors of cytokine signaling (SOCS):** SOCS are a family of intracellular proteins, which regulator immune cell cytokine responses. The SOCS regulate signal transduction via a negative-feedback loop, which extinguishes signal transduction by interacting with cytokine receptor signal proteins—they are negative-feedback inhibitors of cytokine signal transduction.

**Surrogate light chain:** A complex of two nonvariable proteins, the Vpre-B chain and the $\lambda$5 chain, that associates with immunoglobulin $\mu$ heavy chains during the pre-B cell stage of development to form the pre-B cell receptor. The V pre-B chain is homologous to a light chain variable region and the $\lambda$5 chain, which is covalently attached to the $\mu$ chain by a disulfide bond. See also Pre-B-cell receptor. See also $\lambda$5, Pre-B-cell, Pre-B-cell receptor, and Vpre-B.

**Swiss-type agammaglobulinemia:** An immunodeficiency disease involving both B and T cells. The thymus, T-cell immunity, and B-cell immunity are absent.

**Switch:** In immunology, the change in antibody heavy-chain synthesis within a single B cell, such as synthesis from the $\mu$ to the $\gamma$ chain. The variable regions of the antibody molecule are not affected by heavy-chain switching.

**Switch recombination:** A molecular mechanism of DNA rearrangement that mediates immunoglobulin isotype (class) switching. A rearranged VDJ gene segment of an antigen-induced B cell recombines with a C gene and the intervening C gene is deleted. The DNA rearrangements in switch recombination are initiated by CD40 ligation and cytokine induction.

**Switch (S) regions:** Regions located in the introns at the 5' end of each immunoglobulin heavy chain C locus. The nucleotide sequences of these regions are the S regions.

**Synapsis:** The noncovalent juxtaposition of two nonadjacent DNA stretches.

**Syncytia:** Multinucleated giant cells that are formed by the fusion of HIV-infected cells expressing HIV-encoded envelope glycoproteins (gp120-gp41 complex) and uninfected cells expressing the CD4 coreceptor. The resulting syncytia undergo apoptosis.

**Syngeneic:** The genetic relationship between identical twins or inbred strains of animals that are of the same sex.

**Synovial fluid:** The fluid that accumulates in the joints of rheumatoid arthritis patients.

**Systemic autoimmune diseases:** One of the two types of autoimmune diseases. A systemic form may develop after an initial organ has been affected. See also Organ-specific autoimmune diseases.

**Systemic (generalized) anaphylaxis:** The most severe form of Type I (immediate) hypersensitivity. See Type I (immediate) hypersensitivity.

**Systemic inflammatory response syndrome (SIRS):** Patients with disseminated bacterial infections exhibit changes that in its mild form consists of neutrophila, fever, and a rise in acute phase proteins in the blood. Bacterial products like LPS and cytokines produced by the innate immune system stimulate this syndrome. In severe cases of SIRS, patients exhibit disseminated intravascular coagulation, respiratory distress, and septic shock.

**Systemic lupus erythematosus (SLE):** A chronic systemic autoimmune disease primarily of women, characterized by skin rashes, glomerulonephritis, arthritis, and blood disorders. These individuals have many different types of autoantibodies, particularly antinuclear antibodies (DNA, RNA or proteins associated with nucleic acids). Many of the manifestations associated with SLE are caused by the deposition of autoantibodies that form immune complexes in small blood vessels, especially in the kidney.

# T

**T-cell clone:** A group of cells derived from a single progenitor T cell.

**T-cell hybrids:** These cells are the result of fusing antigen-specific T cells with a T-cell lymphoma. The hybrid T cells express the T cell receptor of the specific parental T cell and are grown in culture like lymphoma cells.

**T-cell lines:** T-cell cultures that are grown by repeated stimulation with antigen and antigen-presenting cells. When single T cells from these cultures are propagated, they lead to cloned T-cell lines or T-cell clones.

**T cell receptor (TCR) complex:** The complex of TCR and the invariant CD3 and $\zeta$ chains. The latter group of molecules are involved in signal transduction of TCR-MHC-peptide interacting T cells.

**T cell receptors (TCR) (for antigen):** The TCR is a disulfide-linked glycoprotein heterodimer, consisting of $\alpha$ and $\beta$ (or $\gamma$ and $\delta$) chains, with molecular weights of 50,000 and 40,000 in humans. The TCR recognizes foreign antigen-derived peptide and MHC molecule simultaneously. The most common TCR is the $\alpha\beta$ combination expressed on both CD4$^+$ and CD8$^+$ T cells. The $\gamma\delta$ TCR is expressed by a T-cell subset found mostly in epithelial barrier tissues. It does not recognize peptides bond to polymorphic MHC molecules. See also $\gamma\delta$ T cells and T lymphocytes.

**T delayed-type hypersensitivity (TD) cells:** The old name for a group of CD4$^+$ T cells (T$_H$1 cells) that is responsible for bringing macrophages to the site of a Type IV (delayed-type) hypersensitivity reaction. See also Type IV (delayed-type) hypersensitivity.

**T lymphocytes (T cells):** Precommitted lymphocytes from the bone marrow that enter the thymus, briefly reside there, and leave as mature functional T cells, hence the name thymus-derived or T lymphocytes. T cells are involved directly in cell-mediated immunity as effectors or indirectly in humoral and cell-mediated immunity as regulatory cells. T cells express antigen receptors that can only recognized antigen-derived peptides associated with MHC molecules. There are two functional subsets of T cells: CD4$^+$ helper T cells and CD8$^+$ cytotoxic T cells that recognize antigenic peptides in association class II and class I MHC molecules, respectively. There are subsets of the latter to groups of T cells. T cells can also be divided into $\alpha\beta$ TCR- or $\gamma\delta$ TCR-expressing T cells. See also T cell receptor (TCR), $\gamma\delta$ T cells, T-helper 1 (T$_H$1) cells, T-helper 2 (T$_H$2) cells, and T helper 17 (T$_H$17) cells.

**Tac antigen:** Named after the antibody that recognized an "activation antigen" on T cells, hence the name "T-activated" (Tac) antigen. It is now known that the Tac antigen is the high-affinity $\alpha$-chain of the interleukin-2 receptor (also designated as CD25).

**TACI:** See Transmembrane activator and CAML-interactor.

**Tail pieces:** Additional amino acid residues on the heavy chains of IgM and IgA that permit these immunoglobulins to interact with like antibodies and form multimeric molecules.

**TAP:** See Transporters associated with antigen processing (TAP).

**Tapasin (TAP-associated protein):** It brings TAP close to class I MHC molecules and allows the class I molecules to acquire antigenic peptides. See also Transporters associated with antigen processing (TAP).

**Tandem alleles:** Closely linked gene loci that encode the same type of protein molecule; thus the variants are present within the same haplotype.

**Target cells:** Immune effector functions are assayed by measuring the changes caused in "target cells." The target cells can be B cells activated to produce antibodies, macrophages activated to kill bacteria, or labeled cells that are killed by cytotoxic T cells.

**Tat:** A product of the HIV tat gene. It is produced by activated latently infected cells, once produced it binds to an transcription enhancer in the provirus's long terminal repeat, which leads to proviral genome transcription.

**TATA box:** A highly conserved DNA sequence (consensus TATAA), 25–35 bases upstream of the RNA start site, which is found in the promoter of many rapidly transcribed cellular and viral genes.

**T-bet:** A member of the T-box transcription factor family, which is the master switch in T helper 1 ($T_H1$) cell development. It drives $T_H1$ cell development by regulating interleukin-12 receptor expression, blocking signals that encourage $T_H2$ cell development, and promoting interferon-$\gamma$ production.

**$T_{DH}$ cells:** Older name for $CD4^+$ $T_H1$ cells that mediate delayed-type hypersensitivity. See also Type IV (delayed-type) hypersensitivity.

**TdT:** See Terminal deoxynucleotidyl transferase.

**Tec kinase:** It is part of the src-like kinase family, which is involved in lymphocyte antigen receptor-binding activation by linking to and activating PLC-$\gamma$.

**Teleologic:** In immunology, a term used to suggest that a cell, molecule or activity has some function or purpose.

**Telomerase:** An enzyme that is responsible for the unchecked growth of cancer cells. The telomerase gene is strongly repressed in normal somatic cells but reactivated in cancer cells. Telomerase works on telomeres, which are DNA sequences (TTAGGG in all vertebrates) found at the ends of eukaryotic chromosomes that maintain the fidelity of genetic

information during replication. As cells replicate, their telomeres get shorter and shorter; a sufficiently short telomere signals the cell to stop dividing. In cancer cells, the telomerase, a ribonucleic protein, synthesizes telomeric DNA on chromosome ends—they can keep dividing.

**Teratocarcinoma:** A malignant germ-cell tumor arising from the ovary or testis, which is composed of embryonal carcinoma cells.

**Terminal deoxynucleotidyl transferase (TdT):** A surface enzyme found on immature lymphocytes but not on mature lymphocytes, which inserts nontemplated or N-nucleotides into the junctions between immunoglobulin and T cell receptor V-region gene segments (i.e., adds nucleotides to the free 3' end of DNA breaks). This activity contributes greatly to junctional diversity in antigen-receptor V regions.

**Terpolymer:** Usually a linear polymer of three different amino acids in a specific ratio.

**Tetraparental chimeras:** Animals that arise from the artificial fusion of two blastocysts at the 4- and 8-cell stage. Thus, they are considered to be allogeneic chimeras consisting of a mixture of genetically pure parental cells that are mutually tolerant to one another.

**T-helper 0 ($T_H0$) cells:** Precursors of T helper 1 ($T_H1$) cells and $T_H2$ cells that have the capacity to become $T_H1$ cells and/or $T_H2$ cells. $T_H0$ cells produce interferon-$\gamma$ and interleukin-4 (IL-4).

**T-helper 1 ($T_H1$) cells:** A functional subset of helper T cells that direct cellular immune, or $T_H1$, responses by secreting distinct cytokines, such as interferon-$\gamma$ that activate macrophages and T cells and downregulate $T_H2$ responses.

**T-helper 2 ($T_H2$) cells:** A functional subset of helper T cells that direct humoral immune, or $T_H2$, responses by secreting distinct cytokines, such as IL-4, IL-10, and IL-13 that stimulates IgE production and downregulates $T_H1$ responses.

**T-helper 3 ($T_H3$) cells:** A unique group of regulatory T cells that produce mainly transforming growth factor-$\beta$ (TGF-$\beta$) when stimulated by antigen. They are associated with mucosal immunity to antigens presented orally—they were originally thought to induce/control oral tolerance. Current evidence suggests they should be called inducible regulatory T cells that proliferate in the periphery.

**T-helper 17 ($T_H17$) cells:** $T_H17$ cells are a recently discovered subset of IL-17-producing $CD4^+$ $T_H$ cells, which have an important role at the interface between innate and adaptive immune responses.

They regulate granulopoiesis, host defense against extracellular pathogens, and contribute to the development of autoimmune disease. Naïve CD4$^+$ T cells differentiate into IL-17-producing cells distinct from that of T$_H$1- and T$_H$2-cell differentiation pathway—IL-17-producing CD4$^+$ T$_H$ cells represent a distinct inflammatory T$_H$-cell lineage; their generation involves IL-6, IL-21, and IL-23 as well as the transcription factors retinoic-acid-receptor-related orphan receptor-γt (RORγt) and signal transducer and activator of transcription 3 (STAT3).

**T regulatory type I (T$_{reg}$1) cells:** A CD4$^+$ regulatory T cells that secret high amounts of IL-10 and that down-regulate T$_H$1 and T$_H$2 cells by a contact-independent manner mediated by soluble IL-10 and TGF-β.

**Therapeutic index:** The most effective dose of a drug. It is the ration of the lethal dose to the effective dose.

**Thoracic duct:** The main lymphatic vessel that collects lymph and thereby returns recirculating lymphocytes from the lymphatic system to the blood by draining into the left subclavian vein.

**Thrombocytopenia:** A condition of low numbers of platelets in the blood that can lead to bleeding.

**Thrombocytopenic purpura:** The autoimmune form of thrombocytopenia, caused by increased platelet destruction primarily following coating of platelets with antibody. The antigen stimulus for the disease is unknown.

**Thromboxanes (Txs):** Like prostaglandins, Txs are produced by the action of cyclooxygenase on arachidonic acid and have effects similar to prostaglandins.

**Thymectomy:** The removal of the thymus.

**Thymic epithelial cells:** The cells that line, and are distributed throughout the thymus, are important in driving T-cell maturation. They secrete interleukin-7 and express high levels of class II MHC molecules that are used in the process of positive selection. See Positive selection.

**Thymic hormones:** Low molecular weight molecules that seem to be produced by the thymic epithelial cells and that play a role in the differentiation and development of T cells within the thymus. See Thymopoietin and Thymosin.

**Thymic involution:** The age-dependent decrease in thymic epithelial volume that leads to decreased production of T cells.

**Thymic selection:** The process whereby the thymus confers, through thymic epithelium or nurse cells, on the T cells the ability to recognize antigen with particular MHC products. In other words, T cells maturing in the thymus recognize only antigen on cells, which have the same haplotype as that thymus. See also Positive selection and Negative selection.

**Thymocytes:** Any lymphocytes residing in the thymus. They may or may not be functionally competent T cells.

**Thymoma:** A tumor of the thymus. Often used as the tumor cell partner with a T cell in the construction of a T cell hybridoma.

**Thymopoietin:** A 5562 molecular weight hormone produced by the epithelial cells of the thymus that regulates early T cell differentiation and proliferation.

**Thymosin:** A 3108 molecular weight hormone produced by the epithelial cells of the thymus that regulates late-stage T cell differentiation.

**Thymus:** A primary lymphoid organ of major importance in the ontogeny of immune capability. If the thymus is removed during the fetal or neonatal stage of development, the host does not develop functional cell-mediated or complete humoral responses. In other words, it is the organ responsible for the maturation of T cells. Its weight and absolute T-cell production rate increases until puberty. The thymus then begins involution; its size is reduced and replaced with fibrous and fat tissue but remains functional throughout life.

**Thymus (T)-dependent antigen:** An immunogen that requires T-cell involvement for a successful immune response.

**Thymus (T)-dependent area** A region of the lymph nodes (deep cortex) or spleen (periarteriolar sheath) that contains mostly T cells and atrophies after thymectomy.

**Thymus (T)-independent antigen:** An immunogen, such as polysaccharides and lipids that does not require T$_H$ cell involvement for a successful antibody response. T-independent antigens usually contain many identical epitopes that can cross-link B cell membrane immunoglobulins and thereby activate the B cells. Antibody responses to T-independent antigens show little or no isotype switching or affinity maturation because T$_H$ cell-derived signals mediate these activities. T-independent antigens can be subdivided into two groups, *type 1 antigens* and *type 2 antigens*, according to their degree of independence from T cells and their physiochemical properties. Type 1 antigens, such as bacterial lipopolysaccharide (LPS), can activate B cells in a polyclonal fashion (that is, all B cells are activated irrespective of their antigen specificity). Type 2 antigens contain multiple identical epitopes, which cross-link B-cell receptors, are not polyclonal, and induce mainly IgM antibodies.

**Thymus (T)-independent area:** A region of the lymph nodes (follicles of superficial cortex) that contains mostly B cells and does not atrophy after thymectomy.

**Tight junctions:** Dynamic protein structures, found in the skin and mucous membrane, which seal neighboring cells together to prevent paracellular traffic of macromolecules and microorganisms.

**TILs:** See Tumor-infiltrating lymphocytes.

**Tingible-body macrophages:** Germinal center macrophages that phagocytose the large numbers of apoptotic B cells during a germinal center response.

**TIR:** See Toll/interleukin-1 (IL-1) receptor (TIR) superfamily.

**Tissue:** A homogenous structure composed of an organized collection of cells with similar morphology and function.

**Tissue macrophages:** Mature end-cell macrophages. They are heterogeneous in structure.

**Titer:** A term used to describe the relative strength of antiserum. That is, the highest dilution of antiserum that results in a positive test (precipitation, agglutination, etc.).

**TL (thymic-leukemia) antigen:** A cell-surface antigen expressed on murine prothymocytes with a $TL^+$ gene, but the TL antigen is lost during thymic maturation (mature T cells do not express the TL antigen).

**Tla;Qa region:** One of the six regions of the H-2 map. It contains genes encoding class I MHC-like molecules.

**TLRs:** See Toll-like receptors (TLRs).

**TNF:** See Tumor necrosis factor-$\alpha$.

**Tolerance:** It is the acquisition of a specific nonresponsiveness to a molecule recognized by the adaptive immune system, as a result of inactivation or death of antigen-specific lymphocytes.

**Tolerization:** It describes a lack of immune system responsiveness to exogenous antigens, which is normally created by experimental manipulation, such as in organ transplantation, when the recipient's body is forced to accept an allograft.

**Tolerogen:** An otherwise immunogenic substance that, because of its chemical composition, dose, or route of introduction, induces immunological tolerance rather than immunity.

**Toll pathway:** It is considered one of the oldest signal pathways that activates the transcription factor NF-$\kappa$B through inhibition of I$\kappa$B.

**Toll/interleukin-1 (IL-1) receptor (TIR) superfamily:** This superfamily is divided into two main subgroups: the IL-1 receptors and the Toll-like receptors (TLRs). All members of this superfamily signal via a similar conserved TIR domain in the receptor's cytosolic region, which activates common signaling pathways, that lead to the activation of the transcription factor nuclear factor-$\kappa$B (NF-$\kappa$B) and stress-activated protein kinases. See also Toll-like receptors (TLRs).

**Toll-like receptors (TLRs):** Phagocytes and others (mostly on cells that are involved in innate or adaptive resistance to pathogens) express these cell-surface receptors, which signal macrophage and dendritic cell activation in response to microbial products like endotoxin during innate immune responses. These receptors share structural homology and signal transduction pathways with interleukin-1 receptors (see TIR). TLR proteins represent a conserved family of innate immune recognition receptors. TLRs are homologous to the Toll-receptor gene family in Drosophila; they have important roles in embryogenesis and defense against infection. TLRs recognize pathogen-associated molecular patterns (PAMPs), which are conserved between and shared by many microbial pathogens. Once the cells bind PAMPs, they mediate innate immunity and inflammatory responses, which in turn modulate adaptive immune responses. Eleven TLRs have been characterized.

**Tonsils:** They are large aggregates of lymphoid cells found on either side of the pharynx that is part of the mucosal- or gut-associated immune system.

**Toxic shock syndrome:** A systemic reaction caused by massive productions of $CD4^+$ T cell-derived cytokines initiated by *S. aureus* secretion of the bacterial superantigen toxic shock syndrome toxin-1 (TSST-1).

**Toxoid:** A bacterial toxin that has been altered (chemically or physically) so that it is no longer toxic (eliminates its toxicity, which then equals an attenuated toxin) but still remains an immunogen.

**TRAFs:** See Tumor necrosis factor (TNF) receptor-associated factors (TRAFs).

**Trait:** A genetically determined characteristic that is detectable and passed from one generation to another in a predictable manner. A trait can be either a specific molecule or a functional activity conferred by such a molecule.

**Trans:** In immunogenetics, the phenomenon of using genetic material from both chromosomes.

**Transcription:** The synthesis of RNA from a DNA template.

**Transcription factor:** A molecule that binds to DNA sequences in the enhancer or promoter regions of a gene and activates transcription of that gene. See also DNA-binding proteins.

**Transcytosis:** The transport of material across a membrane by uptake on one side into a vesicle, which is sorted through the Golgi network, and conveyed to the opposite site of the cell. For example, the movement of polymeric IgA and IgM antibodies across epithelial layers mediated by poly-Ig receptors.

**Transduction:** An experimental approach to carcinogenesis suggesting that recombination events between viral oncogenes and cellular DNA can "implant" cellular genes in the final genome. The implanted proto-oncogenes may become oncogenic in their new location.

**Transfection:** Recombinant DNA techniques used to produce new cells called *transfectomas*. See also Hybrid, chimeric, recombinant monoclonal antibodies.

**Transfectomas:** Cells produced by transfection.

**Transformation:** Conversion of a normal, nondividing mature cell into one with uncontrollable growth—a cancer cell.

**Transforming growth factor-β (TGF-β):** A cytokine that may limit an immune response. Actually a family of molecules, it seems to be made by all cells. It helps to transform neoplastic cells and may spur tumor-mediated immunosuppression. On the positive side, it stimulates fibrosis and tissue repair and may help limit immune cell function while promoting extracellular matrix formation, i.e., it regulates the duration of inflammatory responses. It also mediates immunoglobulin class-switching to IgA production.

**Transfusion reaction:** The reaction that can occur if mismatched blood is given to a recipient, for example, if the donor and recipient have different ABO blood groups. The recipient's naturally occurring antibodies against the donor's red cell antigens will induce complement activation and lysis of the infused red cells.

**Transgene:** A cloned foreign gene present in a plant or animal. The process of introducing this gene is called *transgenesis*.

**Transgenic mice:** Mice carrying a transgene that has incorporated into germline cells so it can be passaged to progeny. See also Knockout mice.

**Translation:** The synthesis of a peptide chain with individual amino acids to form a protein molecule; that is, going from RNA to protein.

**Translocation:** The process whereby one piece of one chromosome is abnormally linked to another chromosome, some cancers have chromosomal translocations.

**Transmembrane activator and CAML-interactor (TACI):** TNF-receptor family member found on B cells, dendritic cells, and T cells. It is one of the receptors for BLyS, probably an important signal receptor for BLyS. See B-lymphocyte stimulator (BLyS).

**Transplant (graft):** Tissues, cells, or organs transferred from one part of the body to another or from one individual to another.

**Transplantation (or grafting):** The placement of tissue from a donor to a recipient (exception is an autograft). Unless perfectly matched for histocompatibility antigens, the recipient will mount an immune response. See Allograft, Autograft, Isograft, and Xenograft.

**Transplantation laws:** These laws state that for grafts to be accepted the donor and recipient must share certain histocompatibility antigens. If the donor (A) and recipient (B) mice share identical histocompatibility antigens, the graft survives. If B does not share the antigens with A, a B graft is rejected by A and vice-versa. The $(A \times B)F_1$ will accept either A or B grafts because it has both the A and B antigens, but the A or B mouse will not accept $(A \times B)F_1$ grafts because it lacks either the A or the B antigens.

**Transplantation immunity:** An immune response to cell-surface or transplantation antigens.

**Transporters associated with antigen processing (TAP):** MHC-encoded proteins (TAP-1 and TAP-2) present in the rough endoplasmic reticulum (RER) membrane that mediates active transport of peptides from the cytosol into the RER lumen where they bind to class I MHC molecules. TAPs are heterodimeric proteins composed of TAP-1 and TAP-2 polypeptides.

**Triple response:** Erythema, edema, and wheal-and-flare, the reactions to skin testing for atopic conditions.

**Trophoblast cells:** They are the earliest extra-embryonic cells to differentiate from mammalian embryo cells, which surround the fetus throughout gestation and are in direct contact with maternal tissues.

**Tubercles:** Granulomas occurring in tuberculosis. See Granulomas.

**Tuberculin:** The crude protein material contained in the spent medium of *M. tuberculosis* cultures, which had been used for skin testing for tuberculosis; we now use PPD. See PPD.

**Tuberculin skin reaction:** The classic delayed-type hypersensitivity reaction described by Koch. He found that in tuberculosis patients, subcutaneous exposure to tuberculin caused a generalized illness and an inflammation reaction at the site of inoculation.

**Tuberculosis:** A chronic disease exhibiting Type IV (delayed-type) hypersensitivity caused by *Mycobacterium tuberculosis*. See Type IV (delayed-type) hypersensitivity.

**Tumor:** A mass of new tissue growing independently of its surroundings that has no physiological function. See also Neoplasm.

**Tumor-associated antigen (TAA):** Surface antigens that are not unique to tumor cells.

**Tumor-associated transplantation antigen (TATA):** Another name for tumor-associated antigen. It indicates that the antigen in question can induce rejection of the tumor graft *in vivo*.

**Tumor-infiltrating lymphocytes (TILs):** A tumor *in situ* heterogeneous population of T lymphocytes that are obtained from the tumor bed, which can be activated and expanded *ex vivo* with interleukin-2 (IL-2). They are a diverse group of cells with different antigen specificities, avidities, and functional characteristics. Adoptive therapy with TILs requires coadministration of high-doses of IL-2, which can be accompanied by significant morbidity.

**Tumor necrosis factor-α (TNF-α):** A multifunctional proinflammatory cytokine that is produced by activated macrophages, which is apoptotic for some types of tumor cells. More importantly, it stimulates the recruitment of neutrophils and monocytes to infection sites and their activation to kill microbes. TNF-α also promotes apoptosis of target cells, stimulates expression of new adhesion molecules on vascular endothelial cells, and induces macrophages and endothelial cells to secrete chemokines. It mediates these activities by binding to its receptors TNFR1 and TNFBR. (Lymphotoxin, or TNF-β, has identical biologic effects as TNF-α but is produced by T cells.)

**Tumor necrosis factor (TNF) receptors:** TNF receptors for TNF-α and TNF-β are present on most cell types. There two types of TNF receptors: TNF-RI and TNF-RII. Most biological effects of TNF are mediated through TNF-RI. TNF receptors belong to a family of receptors with homologous cysteine-rich extracellular motifs, members include Fas and CD40.

**Tumor necrosis factor (TNF) receptor-associated factors (TRAFs):** A family of adapter molecules that interact with various receptors of the TNF receptor family, such as TNF-RII, lymphotoxin-β receptor, and CD40. Each of these receptors contains a cytoplasmic motif that allows the binding of different TRAFs, the bound TRAFs lead to activation of the transcription factors AP-1 and NF-κB.

**Tumor-specific antigen (TSA):** An antigen, usually a cell-surface histocompatibility antigen, gained by the tumor and unique to the tumor (sometimes incorrectly called *tumor-associated antigen*).

**Tumor-specific transplantation antigen (TSTA):** An antigen, usually a cell-surface histocompatibility antigen, gained by the tumor that can initiate an immune rejection when the tumor is transplanted.

**Tumor-suppressor genes:** Genes, also called *anti-oncogenes*, which encode products that block excessive cell proliferation.

**TUNEL assay:** An assay that identifies *in situ* apoptotic cells through the characteristic fragmentation of their DNA during the internucleosomal cleavage. TUNEL is an abbreviation for TdT-dependent dUTP-biotin nick end labeling.

**Two-signal hypothesis:** A proven model that states lymphocyte activation requires two distinct signals: the first is antigen and the second is either microbial products or components of innate responses to microbes. The first signal ensures specificity and the second signal ensures that immune responses are induced when needed. The second signal is called *costimulation* and involves ligation of molecules on antigen-presenting cells, such as B7 proteins, and CD28 on T cells.

**Type I cytokine receptors:** A cytokine family of receptors, characterized by four conserved cysteines (C-C-C-C) and the membrane proximal WS motif (the conserved sequence of Trp-Ser-X-Trp-Ser [W-S-X-W-S]) in their extracellular domains (X = a nonconserved aa) that bind cytokines that fold into four α-helical strands. The family includes receptors for interleukin (IL)-2–IL-7, IL-9–IL-13, IL-15, granulocyte-macrophage (GM) colony-stimulating factor (CSF), and G-CSF. Some of these receptors contain a ligand-binding chain and one or more signal-transducing chains but all have the same structural motif. There are three subfamilies (members share signal-transducing chain): IL-2 (share γ chain [CD132]), IL-6 (share gp130), and GM-CSF (share β chain [CD131]). Type I family of receptors is dimerized by cytokine ligation, and they signal through JAK-STAT pathways. See also Common γ chain.

**Type I interferons (IFN-α & IFN-β):** A cytokine family composed of several structurally related IFN-α proteins and a single IFN-β protein with potent anti-viral activity. Mononuclear phagocytes produce IFN-α; many cells produce IFN-β, including fibroblasts. Both IFNs bind to the same cell-surface receptor where they could inhibit viral replication, increase NK cell-mediated lytic activity, increase class I MHC molecule expression on virally infected cells, and stimulate the development of $T_H1$ cells.

**Type I (immediate) hypersensitivity:** An immediate hypersensitivity mediated by antibodies, primarily IgE. It involves the secondary exposure to an offending allergen that binds to mast cell-fixed IgE. The allergen cross-links two adjacent IgE molecules, leading to degranulation of the mast cells with a release of preformed vasoactive mediators such as histamine and newly formed mediators such as prostaglandins. These mediators cause the symptoms of Type I hypersensitivity, which are manifested within seconds to minutes after secondary exposure. The Type I reaction is exemplified by allergic asthma, hay fever, food allergies, etc.

**Type I and II membrane proteins:** They are proteins that span the membrane only once and are classified into type I if their N-terminus is found in the extracellular/lumenal space or type II if their N-terminus is found in the cytosol.

**Type II (antibody-mediated cytotoxic) hypersensitivity:** A hypersensitivity mediated by antibodies (not IgE) and is also called *antibody-mediated hypersensitivity*. The Type II reaction involves antibody responses to surface antigens, particularly on red blood cells. An example of a Type II hypersensitivity is hemolytic disease of the newborn. The implicated antibodies can also activate NK cells to destroy sensitized cells via antibody-dependent cell-mediated cytotoxicity (ADCC). The autoimmune diseases Myasthenia gravis and Graves' disease are examples of Type II hypersensitivity.

**Type II cytokine receptors:** They are similar to class I cytokine receptors, but do not contain the WS motif. The ligands for these receptors are: interferon (IFN)-α, -β, and -γ (other IFNs); and the IL-10 family of cytokines.

**Type III (immune complex-mediated) hypersensitivity:** Another antibody-mediated hypersensitivity that is also called *immune complex-mediated hypersensitivity*. Type III reactions are due to the deposition of antigen-antibody complexes in tissues and blood vessels. These complexes activate complement, which can destroy the surrounding tissue directly or indirectly by attracting to the site of complex deposition neutrophils that release hydrolytic enzymes, causing local damage. Certain autoimmune diseases, such as, Systemic lupus erythematosus and Rheumatoid arthritis are exemplified by Type III hypersensitivities.

**Type IV (delayed-type) hypersensitivity:** This hypersensitivity is not mediated by antibodies, but is mediated by sensitized T cells releasing lymphokines, attracting macrophages to the site, and activating them. Once the macrophages arrive, they begin to cause tissue damage that may develop into a chronic granulomatous reaction if antigen persists. Also called *delayed-type hypersensitivity* because, following secondary exposure to the offending antigen, the manifestations of the interaction do not appear for more than 24 hours. The reaction to chronic infections such as with *M. tuberculous* is the classical example of a Type IV hypersensitivity reaction. See also Contact hypersensitivity.

**Tyrosine kinase:** It is an enzyme that specifically phosphorylates protein tyrosine residues, which is critical to the activation of T and B cells. Blk, Fyn, Lyn, and Syk tyrosine kinases are important to B-cell activation. Lck, Fyn, and ZAP-70 are important to T-cell activation.

## U

**Ubiquitination:** The covalent linkage of several ubiquitin molecules to a protein, causing the ubiquitinated protein to be targeted for proteolytic degradation by proteasomes. This is a critical step in the class I MHC molecule pathway of antigen processing and presentation.

**Uropod:** A posterior structure formed on a migrating leukocyte, which is enriched with intercellular adhesion molecule 1 (ICAM-1) or CD44.

**Urticaria:** A Type I (immediate) hypersensitivity reaction involving localized transient swelling of the skin that is caused by fluid and plasma protein leakage from small vessels in the dermis.

**Unprimed:** An animal or cell that has never had contact with or responded to a given antigen.

## V

**V3 region (of HIV gp120):** It is the third variable (V3) region of the HIV envelope gp120 molecule. The amino-acid sequence in the V3 region determines whether the virus uses CXCR4 or CCR5 as its coreceptor. See also Human Immunodeficiency virus (HIV).

**V(D)J recombinase:** The collection of enzymes that together mediate the somatic recombination events during B and T cell development, which cause the joining of gene segments into a rearranged V(D)J unit to form a functional receptor gene. Some enzymes are lymphocyte-specific, such as RAG-1 and RAG-2, while others are ubiquitous DNA repair enzymes.

**Vaccination:** The process of intentionally eliciting adaptive active immunity in an individual by administration of a vaccine.

**Vaccine:** An immunogen-containing substance, which on introduction into an animal or individual creates active immunity for future protection against infection by the appropriate organism.

**Valence:** The number of antigen-binding sites that are on molecules such as an immunoglobulins or T cell receptors. Immunoglobulins are either bivalent (an IgG antibody has two sites) or multivalent (an IgM molecule has ten sites), whereas T cell receptors are univalent.

**Vaccinia:** It is a cowpox virus that was the first effective vaccine used for immunity against the human smallpox virus.

**Variable (V) gene segments:** The DNA segments that encode amino-terminus amino acids of the variable (V) domains of immunoglobulin heavy and light chains and the T cell receptor $\alpha$, $\beta$, $\gamma$, and $\delta$ chains. The number of V genes recombining with D and/or J gene segments and then C genes dictate antibody and T cell receptor diversity.

**Variable (V) regions:** The amino-terminal end of either a light or heavy chain of an antibody molecule or a T cell receptor chain that contains variable domains. The regions are so-called because the amino acid sequences are variable between every clone of lymphocytes. These regions determine the configuration of the antibody- and T cell receptor-combining sites, allowing for specific interaction with their appropriate antigenic determinants. These regions are responsible for the diversity of antibody and T-cell responses.

**Variola:** The name given to both the smallpox virus and the disease it causes, smallpox.

**Variolation:** The inoculation of a healthy recipient with virus of unattenuated smallpox (variola) in crusts or exudates from smallpox lesions.

**Vascular addressins:** Tissue-specific adhesion molecules that direct the extravasation of different circulating lymphocyte populations into particular lymphoid organs.

**Vasoactive amines:** Substances such as histamine that are released from mast cells and basophils following exposure of a sensitized individual to the offending allergen. Vasoactive amines cause vasodilation and smooth muscle contraction.

**Vasodilation:** The dilation of blood vessels, caused by smooth muscle contractants such as histamine that act on the smooth muscle of the vessel walls, producing increase blood flow. Vasodilation is normally associated with inflammatory reactions.

**Vector:** An agent, such as an insect, capable mechanically or biologically transferring a pathogen from one organism to another (or virus in the case of recombinant vector vaccine).

**Veiled cells:** Cells circulating in the lymph that develop into dendritic cells and localize in the T cell-dependent areas of the secondary lymphoid organs; dendritic cell processes wrap around themselves producing a veiled appearance.

**Very late activation (VLA) molecules:** They are important in cell-cell adhesion of T cells to mucosal cell adhesion molecules. VLA-1 and -2 were initially described on T cells 2 to 4 weeks after *in vitro* antigen stimulation; thus, the name "very late antigen" molecules. VLA molecules are members of the $\beta_1$ (CD29)-containing integrin family; they include VLA-1 ($\alpha_1\beta_1$ [CD49aCD29]) to VLA-6 ($\alpha_6\beta_1$ [CD49fCD29]). VLA-4 ($\alpha_4\beta_1$ [CD49dCD29]) is a key molecule in the homing of T cells to sites of inflammation. See also Integrins.

**Vesicles:** They are small membrane-bound compartments found in the cytosol of cells.

**Viral oncogenes (v-oncs):** Oncogenes of the retroviruses, the only known cancer genes. They arise from genetic recombination between proto-oncogenes and slow retroviruses. See Cellular oncogenes.

**Virions:** The complete form of viruses, which is the form that can spread from cell to cell or human to human.

**Virological synapse:** The cell-cell contact zone between CD4$^+$ T cells and dendritic cells, or between CD4$^+$ T cells, which eases HIV transmission by locally concentrating virus and viral receptors. Contrast immunologic synapse. See Immunologic synapse.

**Virulence:** The degree of pathogenicity exhibited by a strain of microorganisms.

**Virulence factors:** The properties of a microorganism that affect a microorganism's virulence. See Virulence.

**Vitiligo:** A depigmenting skin disorder caused by the destruction of melanocytes that produce cutaneous pigments.

**Vpre-B:** A polypeptide chain, which is homologous to a V region, that associates with $\lambda$5, which is homologous to a $\lambda$ light chain, to form the surrogate light chain of the pre-B-cell receptor. See also $\lambda$5, pre-B-cell receptor, and Surrogate light chain.

# W

**Warm agglutinins:** They are antibodies that react with red blood cells at 37°C. See also Cold antibodies.

**Warm antibody autoimmune hemolytic anemia:** The most common form of autoimmune anemia, characterized by antibodies on red blood cells. Major symptoms are anemia, fever, jaundice, splenomegaly associated with hemolysis, and congestive heart failure. See also Cold antibody autoimmune hemolytic anemia.

**Western blotting:** See Immunoblotting.

**Wheal and flare reaction:** A localized short-term, circumscribed, elevated and red area at the surface of the skin resulting from an immediate hypersensitivity reaction. The wheal results from increased vascular permeability (swelling of the skin) and the flare (surrounding redness) results from increased local blood flow. Both manifestations result from mediators such as histamine released from activated dermal mast cells.

**White pulp:** See Periarteriolar lymphoid sheath (PALS).

**Wiskott-Aldrich syndrome:** An X-linked immunodeficiency disease involving both T and B cells. Cell-mediated immunity is absent and antibody responses are defective. Patients cannot respond to polysaccharide antigens because of their low levels of serum IgM. Patients with this disease have a defective gene that encodes a cytosolic protein (Wiskott-Aldrich syndrome protein [WASP]) involved signaling cascades and control of the actin cytoskeleton. The disease is characterized by thrombocytopenia with small plates, eczema, recurrent infections, and increased incidence of autoimmune disorders and malignancies.

**Wu and Kabat plot:** A plot to describe the amino acid variability between protein molecules.

# X

**X4 virus:** An HIV-1 strain that uses CXC-chemokine receptor 4 (CXCR4) as the coreceptor to enter target cells. See also Human immunodeficiency virus (HIV).

**Xenogeneic:** A term used to describe the relationship between genetically dissimilar individuals within different species.

**Xenograft:** A organ or tissue graft between members of two different species, such as from a pig to a human.

**X-linked agammaglobulinemia:** A disease in young boys inherited as an X-linked recessive character. It is an immunodeficiency that is characterized by a block in early B-cell maturation (mutations or deletions in the gene encoding Btk, an enzyme involved in signal transduction of developing B cells) and the lack of serum immunoglobulins; thus, these patients have normal T-cell function and cell-mediated immunity to viruses but do not exhibit antibody responses. Because of the lack of antibodies, they have great difficulty coping with bacterial infections.

**X-linked hyper-IgM syndrome:** A rare immunodeficiency disorder caused by mutations in the helper T cell CD40 ligand gene that is characterized by failure in B cell heavy chain isotype switching and development of cell-mediated immunity. These patients produce IgM but not other antibody isotypes, they do not develop germinal centers, they do not exhibit somatic mutation, and they do not develop memory B cells. They have great difficulty coping with pyogenic bacterial infections.

**X-linked lymphoproliferative syndrome:** A rare immunodeficiency that results from mutations in the SH2-domain containing gene 1A (SH2D1A). Boys who develop this immunodeficiency have overwhelming Epstein-Barr virus infections, which can lead to lymphoma or hypogammaglobulinemia.

**X-linked severe combined immunodeficiency (XSCID):** A immunodeficiency disease caused by inherited mutations in the common $\gamma$ chain of interleukin (IL)-2, IL-4, IL-7, IL-9, and IL-15; thus, it impairs the chain's ability to transduce signals from the receptor to intracellular proteins.

**X-irradiation:** A means of immunosuppressing the immune response. B cells and helper T cells are more susceptible than other T cells; however, very high doses will destroy all lymphocytes and even stem cells.

# Z

**ZAP-70 (zeta [$\zeta$]-associated protein of 70 kD):** A 70,000 molecular weight polypeptide of the Src family that becomes an active tyrosine kinase when it binds to the ITAMs of the T cell's CD3$\zeta$ chain and undergoes phosphorylation, and in turn phosphorylates adapter proteins that recruit other components of the signaling pathway.

**$\zeta$ chain:** A T cell-expressed transmembrane protein that is part of the T cell receptor complex, which contains ITAMs in its cytoplasmic tail. It binds to ZAP-70 during T-cell activation.

**Zone phenomenon:** Variation in the ratio of antibody to antigen leads to different levels of lattice formation and thus to different amounts of precipitates. The precipitation reaction is divided into three zones. See Antibody excess zone, Antigen excess zone, and Equivalence zone.

**Zymosan:** An insoluble yeast cell-wall polysaccharide that can trigger the alternative pathway of complement activation.

# APPENDIX: HUMAN CLUSTER OF DIFFERENTIATION (CD) MOLECULES

## HUMAN CLUSTER OF DIFFERENTIATION (CD) MOLECULES

| Cluster designation | Synonym | Cellular expression | Function |
|---|---|---|---|
| CD1d1** | Ly-38 | Leukocytes, intestinal epithelia | Presentation of nonpeptide (lipids and glycolipids) to some T cells; ligand for NKT cells |
| CD1a | R4, HTA1 | Cortical thymocytes, DCs, Langerhans cells, | Presentation of nonpeptide (lipids and glycolipids) to some T cells |
| CD1b | R1 | Same as CD1a | Same as CD1a |
| CD1c | M241, R7 | Cortical thymocytes, DCs, Langerhans cells, B cells | Same as CD1a |
| CD1d | R3 | Cortical thymocytes, DCs, Langerhans cells, intestinal epithelial cells | Same as CD1a |
| CD1e | R2 | Cortical thymocytes, DCs, Langerhans cells, intestinal epithelia | Same as CD1a |
| CD2 | T11, LFA-2 (CD58 receptor), sheep red blood cell receptor | T cells, thymocytes, NK cells | Adhesion molecule (binds to CD58, CD48, CD59) involved in T cell activation, and CTL- and NK cell-mediated lysis |
| CD2R | T11-3 | Activated T cells | Activation-dependent form of CD2 |
| CD3γ, CD3δ | T3, Leu-4 | Thymocytes, T cells | Required for TCR expression and its signal transduction |
| CD3ε | T3, Leu-4 | Thymocytes, T cells | Required for TCR expression and its signal transduction |
| CD3γ | T3, Leu-4 | Thymocytes, T cells | Required for TCR expression and its signal transduction |
| CD4 | T4, L3T4, Leu-3 | Helper T-cell subset, thymocytes, monocytes, MΦs | Coreceptor for class II MHC molecule-restricted T cell activation, differentiation marker of T cell development, HIV receptor |
| CD5 | T1, Leu-1, Lyb-1, Lyt-1 | T cells, thymocytes, B cell subset | Signal molecule that binds to CD72 |
| CD6 | T12 | T cells, thymocytes, B cell subset | An adhesion molecule for thymic endothelial cells, a T cell activation molecule, binds CD166 |

*Immunology: Understanding the Immune System, Second Edition*, by Klaus D. Elgert
Copyright © 2009 John Wiley & Sons, Inc.

## HUMAN CLUSTER OF DIFFERENTIATION (CD) MOLECULES *(Continued)*

| Cluster designation | Synonym | Cellular expression | Function |
|---|---|---|---|
| CD7 | Fc μ receptor (FcμR), gp40 | Subset of T cells, NK cells | Signaling, T cell costimulation |
| CD8a | T8, Leu-2, Lyt-2 | Cytotoxic T-cell subset, thymocyte subset | Coreceptor for class I MHC molecule-restricted T cell activation, differentiation marker of T cell development |
| CD8b | T8, Leu-2, Lyt-2 | Same as CD8α | Same as CD8α |
| CD9 | DRAP-27, MRP-1 | Pre-B and immature B cells, activated B cells, eosinophils, basophils, endothelial cells, epithelial cells, | Modulation of cell adhesion and migration, platelet activation |
| CD10 | Common acute lymphoblastic leukemia antigen (CALLA) | Germinal left B cells, lymphocyte progenitor cells, granulocytes | Metalloproteinase, regulates B cell growth |
| CD11a | LFA-1α chain, αL-integrin chain | All leukocytes | Cell-cell adhesion (binds ICAM-1 [CD54], ICAM-2 [CD102], and ICAM-3 [CD50]) |
| CD11b | Mac-1, αM-integrin chain, CR3 (iC3b receptor), Mo1 | Monocytes, MΦs, granulocytes, NK cells, B cells, DCs | Phagocytosis of iC3b-coated particles, adhesion of neutrophils and monocytes with endothelium (binds CD54) and extracellular matrix proteins, chemotaxis, apoptosis |
| CD11c | p150,95, αX-integrin chain, Leu-M5, CR4 α chain | Monocytes, MΦs, T cell subset, granulocytes, NK cells, DCs | Cell adhesion |
| CDw12* | Myeloid antigen | Granulocytes, monocytes | Unknown |
| CD13 | LAP1, aminopeptidase N | Granulocytes, monocytes | An aminopeptidase that trims peptides bound to class II MHC molecules, cleaves MIP-1 chemokine to alter target specificity, coronavirus receptor |
| CD14 | Leu-M3, Mo2, LPS receptor | Monocytes, MΦs, granulocytes, epidermal Langerhans cells | LPS and LPS-binding protein receptor, required LPS-mediated activation of MΦs; binds LPS-binding protein and apoptotic cells |
| CD15 | Lewis-x | Neutrophils, eosinophils, monocytes | Adhesion |
| CD15s | Sialyl Lewis-x | Leukocytes, endothelium | Adhesion of leukocytes to endothelial cells, binds to CD62E and P selectins |
| CD15u | Sulphated CD15 | Myeloid subset | Adhesion |
| CD16a | FcγRIIIA | MΦs, NK cells | Low-affinity Fcγ receptor, activation of NK cells, ADCC |
| CD16b | FcγRIIIB | Neutrophils | Synergy with FcRγII (CD32) in immune complex-mediated activation of neutrophils |
| CDw17 | Lactosylceramide | Granulocytes, monocytes, platelets | Lactosyl ceramide |
| CD18 | β chain of CD11a, b, and c, β2 integrin subunit | Leukocytes | See CD11a, CD11b, CD11c |
| CD19 | Leu-12, B4 | Most B cells | B cell activation, forms coreceptor with CD21 and CD81 complex that synergizes with signals from B cell antigen receptor complex ligation |
| CD20 | Leu-16, B1 | B cells, T cell subset | B cell activation |
| CD21 | C3d receptor (CR2), B2 | Mature B cells, follicular DCs | Receptor for complement fragment C3d, forms coreceptor complex with CD19 and CD81 for B cell signaling, receptor for Epstein-Barr virus |
| CD22 | Lyb8, BL-CAM | B cells | Adhesion molecule involved in regulation of B cell activation, cross-regulation with CD19 |
| CD23 | FcεRIIb, low-affinity IgE receptor | Activated B cells, eosinophils, platelets | IgE synthesis regulation, IL-4-induced low affinity Fcε receptor, trigger for monokine (TNF, IL-1, IL-6, and GM-CSF) release |

| Cluster designation | Synonym | Cellular expression | Function |
|---|---|---|---|
| CD24 | Heat stable antigen (HAS), BA-1 | Erythrocytes, thymocytes, myeloid cells | Binds P-selectin |
| CD25 | Tac, IL-2 receptor α chain, p55 | Activated T cells, B cells, and MΦs | α subunit of the IL-2 receptor, binds IL-2 |
| CD26 | Ta1, depeptidyl-peptidase IV | Activated T and B cells, MΦs, NK cells | T cell activation costimulatory molecule, serine peptidase |
| CD27 | S152, T14 | Most T cells, activated T cells, memory B cells, NK cells | Binds CD70 thereby mediating costimulatory signals for T and B cell activation |
| CD28 | T44, Tp44 | Most T cells, thymocytes, and plasma cells | A receptor for costimulatory molecules B7-1 (CD80) and B7-2 (CD86), T cell costimulation |
| CD29 | β$_1$-integrin subunit, β chain of VLA molecules, platelet GPIIa | Leukocytes | Leukocyte adhesion to endothelium and extracellular matrix (see also CD49) |
| CD30 | Ki-1 | Activated T and B cells, NK cells, monocytes | Involved in activation-induced cell death of CD8$^+$ T cells; binds to CD153 on neutrophils, activated T cells, and MΦs |
| CD31 | Platelet GPIIa, PECAM-1 | Granulocytes, monocytes, MΦs, B cells, platelets, endothelial cells | Adhesion molecule involved leukocyte diapedesis |
| CD32 | FcγRIIA, FcγRIIB, FcγRIIC | Neutrophils, monocytes, MΦs, B cells, eosinophils | Fc receptor for antigen-antibody complexed IgG molecules, binds C-reactive protein, involved in phagocytosis, ADCC, an inhibitory signal for activation signals initiated by the B cell antigen receptor |
| CD33 | Sialoadhesin, MY9 | Myeloid precursors, monocytes | Binds sialic acid, adhesion |
| CD34 | MY10, mucosialin | Hematopoietic progenitor cells, HEV endothelial cells | Cell-cell adhesion, binds L-selectin (CD62L) |
| CD35 | CR1, C3b receptor, type 1 complement receptor | Granulocytes, monocytes, B cells, erythrocytes, follicular DCs | Regulates complement activation, binds C3b and C4b, promotes phagocytosis of C3b- and C4b-coated particles |
| CD36 | GpIV, platelet GPIIIb | Monocytes, MΦs, platelets, endothelial cells | Scavenger receptor for lipoprotein, for platelet adhesion, for phagocytosis of apoptotic cells |
| CD37 | gp52-40 | B cells, some T cells and myeloid cells | Signal transduction, forms complexes with CD53, CD81, CD82, and class II MHC molecules |
| CD38 | T10, Leu-17 | Activated B and T cells, plasma cells | NAD glycohydrolase, ADP ribosyl cyclase, ADP ribose hydrolase |
| CD39 | gp80, E-ATPDase | B cells, monocytes | Regulation of platelet aggregation and thrombosis, an ectoenzyme with ADPase and ATPase activities |
| CD40 | gp50, TNFRSF | B cells, MΦs, DCs, endothelial cells | Binds to CD40L (CD154), role in T cell dependent activation of B cells, MΦs, DCs, and endothelial cells |
| CD41 | GPIIb, αIIb integrin chain | Platelets, megakaryocytes | Binds fibrinogen and fibronectin, platelet aggregation and activation |
| CD42a | Platelet gpIX | Platelets, megakaryocytes | Platelet adhesion, binds thrombin |
| CD42b | Platelet gpIbα | Platelets, megakaryocytes | See CD42a |
| CD42c | gpIbβ | Platelets, megakaryocytes | See CD42a |
| CD42d | GPV | Platelets, megakaryocytes | See CD42a |
| CD43 | Leukosialin, sialophorin | Leukocytes (except circulating B cells) | Adhesive and anti-adhesive functions |
| CD44 | H-CAM, Pgp-1, Hermes | Leukocytes, erythrocytes | Binds hyaluronan, involved in leukocyte adhesion to endothelial cells and extracellular matrix, leukocyte aggregation |

## HUMAN CLUSTER OF DIFFERENTIATION (CD) MOLECULES *(Continued)*

| Cluster designation | Synonym | Cellular expression | Function |
|---|---|---|---|
| CD45 | T200, leukocyte common antigen (LCA) | Hematopoietic cells | A tyrosine phosphatase that plays a critical role in B and T cell receptor signaling |
| CD45RA | Leu-18, restricted T200, restricted LCA, 2H4 | Naïve T cells, B cells, monocytes | See CD45 |
| CD45RB | Restricted T200 | T cell subset, B cells | See CD45 |
| CD45RC** | Restricted epitope of CD45 | B cells, T cell subset | See CD45 |
| CD45RO | Restricted T200, UCHL1, gp180 | Memory T cells, subset of B cells, monocytes, MΦs | See CD45 |
| CD46 | Membrane cofactor protein (MCP) | Leukocytes, fibroblasts, epithelial cells | Regulation of complement activation |
| CD47 | IAP | Hematopoietic cells, epithelium, endothelium, fibroblasts | Leukocyte adhesion, migration, activation |
| CD47R | Rh-associated protein, integrin-associated protein (IAP) | Broad | Adhesion molecule, thrombospondin receptor |
| CD48 | Blast-1, OX-45 | Leukocytes | Receptor for mouse CD2 |
| CD49a | VLA-1, $\alpha_1$ integrin chain | Activated T cells, monocytes | Leukocyte adhesion to extracellular matrix; binds collagen, laminin |
| CD49b | VLA-2, $\alpha_2$ integrin chain, platelet GPIa | Platelets, monocytes, some B cells, and activated T cells, | Leukocyte adhesion to extracellular matrix; binds collagen, laminin |
| CD49c | VLA-3, $\alpha_3$ integrin chain | T cells, some B cells, monocytes | Leukocyte adhesion to extracellular matrix; binds collagen, laminin, fibronectin |
| CD49d | VLA-4, $\alpha_4$ integrin chain | Monocytes, T cells, B cells | Leukocyte adhesion to extracellular matrix and endothelial cells, CD49dCD29 binds to VCAM-1, collagens, and fibronectin, CD49d$(\alpha_4)\beta_7$ binds to MadCam-1 |
| CD49e | VLA-5, $\alpha_5$ integrin chain | T cells, monocytes, platelets, and some B cells | Adhesion to extracellular matrix, binds to fibronectin |
| CD49f | VLA-6, $\alpha_6$ integrin chain | Platelets, megakaryocytes, activated T cells, monocytes | Adhesion to extracellular matrix, binds to fibronectin |
| CD50 | Intercellular adhesion molecule-3 (ICAM-3) | Leukocytes, some endothelium | Adhesion, binds CD11aCD18 |
| CD51 | $\alpha_V$ integrin subunit, vitronectin receptor $\alpha$ chain | Platelets, megakaryocytes | Adhesion, binds vitronectin and fibronectin |
| CD52 | Campath-1 | Thymocytes, lymphocytes, MΦs | Unknown |
| CD53 | OX44 | Leukocytes | Signal transduction |
| CD54 | Intercellular adhesion molecule-1 (ICAM-1) | B cells, T cells, monocytes, endothelial cells | Cell-cell adhesion, ligand for CD11aCD18 (LFA-1) and CD11bCD18 (Mac-1), receptor for rhinovirus |
| CD55 | Decay accelerating factor (DAF) | Broad | Regulation of complement activation; binds C3b and C4b |
| CD56 | Leu-19, NKH-1, isoform of neural cell adhesion molecule (N-CAM) | NK cells, B and T cell subset, brain | Adhesion |
| CD57 | HNK-1, Leu-7 | NK cells, T cell subset, monocytes | Adhesion |
| CD58 | LFA-3 | Broad | Leukocyte adhesion, T cell costimulation, binds CD2 |
| CD59 | Ly6c, membrane inhibitor of reactive lysis (MIRL) | Broad | Binds C9 and inhibits complement MAC formation |

| Cluster designation | Synonym | Cellular expression | Function |
|---|---|---|---|
| CD60a | GD3 | Carbohydrate structures | Costimulation |
| CD60b | 9-O-acetyl-GD3 | Subset of T cells, activated B cells | |
| CD60c | 7-O-acetyl-GD3 | Subset of T cells | |
| CD61 | $\beta_3$ integrin subunit, vitronectin receptor $\beta$ chain | Platelets, megakaryocytes, leukocytes, endothelial cells | See CD41, CD51 |
| CD62E | E-selectin, endothelial cell leukocyte adhesion molecule-1 (ELAM-1) | Endothelial cells | Leukocyte-endothelial cell adhesion |
| CD62L | L-selectin, leukocyte adhesion molecule-1 (LAM-1), MEL-14 | B and T cells, monocytes, granulocytes, some NK cells | Leukocyte-endothelial cell adhesion, homing of antigen-naïve T cells to lymph nodes |
| CD62P | P-selectin, GMP-140, LECAM-3, PADGEM | Platelets, endothelial cells | Leukocyte-endothelial cell adhesion, platelets; binds CD162 (PSGL-1) |
| CD63 | Platelet activation antigen, lysosomal membrane-associated glycoprotein-1 (LAMP-1) | Activated platelets; monocytes, MΦs | Lysosomal membrane protein, moves to cell surface after activation |
| CD64 | FcγRI | Monocytes, MΦs, activated neutrophils | High-affinity Fcγ receptor; it has a role phagocytosis, macrophage activation, ADCC |
| CD65 | Ceramide, VIM-2 | Granulocytes, monocyte subset, myeloid leukemias | Unknown |
| CD65s | VIM-2 | Granulocytes, monocyte subset, myeloid leukemias | Phagocytosis |
| CD66a | Biliary glycoprotein (BGP) | Granulocytes, epithelial cells | Cell adhesion |
| CD66b | CD67, CGM6 | Granulocytes | Cell adhesion, neutrophil activation |
| CD66c | NCA | Neutrophils, colon carcinoma | Cell adhesion |
| CD66d | CGM1 | Neutrophils | Neutrophil activation |
| CD66e | Carcinoembryonic antigen (CEA) | Colon epithelial cells | Cell adhesion, clinical marker of colon cancer burden |
| CD66f | Pregnancy-specific glycoprotein (PSG) | Placental syncytiotropoblasts, fetal liver | Immune regulation, protects fetus from maternal immune system |
| CD67 | Now CD66b | See CD66b | See CD66b |
| CD68 | Macrosialin | Monocytes, MΦs, DCs, granulocytes, activated T cells, B cell subset | Unknown |
| CD69 | Activation inducer molecule (AIM) | Activated T cells, B cells, MΦs, NK cells, neutrophils, eosinophils, platelets, Langerhans cells | Signal transduction in different cell types |
| CD70 | CD27-ligand, Ki-24 antigen | Activated T and B cells | Provides costimulatory signals for B and T cell activation, binds CD27 |
| CD71 | T9, transferrin receptor | Proliferating cells, activated B and T cells, MΦs | Transferrin receptor, role in iron metabolism, cell growth |
| CD72 | Lyb-2 (mouse) | B cells | Ligand for CD5 and CD100 |
| CD73 | Ecto 5′-nucleotidase | T and B cell subsets, germinal left follicular DCs | Signal transduction in T cells |
| CD74 | Class II MHC invariant (γ) chain, I$_i$ | B cells, monocytes, MΦs; other class II MHC molecule-expressing cells | Associates with and drives intracellular sorting of newly synthesized class II MHC molecules |
| CD75 | Lactosamines | Mature sIg+ B cells, germinal left B cells of lymphoid secondary follicle, small subpopulation of peripheral blood T cells, erythrocytes | Adhesion, binds CD22 |

## HUMAN CLUSTER OF DIFFERENTIATION (CD) MOLECULES *(Continued)*

| Cluster designation | Synonym | Cellular expression | Function |
|---|---|---|---|
| CD75s | Alpha-2,6-sialylated lactosamines | B cell subset, T cell subset | Unknown |
| CD76 | Not assigned | | |
| CD77 | Pk blood group antigen | Germinal left B cells | Apoptosis |
| CD78 | Not assigned | | |
| CD79a | MB-1, Igα | B cells | Required for cell-surface expression of and signal transduction by the B cell antigen receptor complex |
| CD79b | B29, Igβ | B cells | Required for cell-surface expression of and signal transduction by the B cell antigen receptor complex |
| CD80 | B7-1, BB1 | DCs, activated B cells and MΦs | Costimulator for T cell activation, ligand for CD28 and CD152 (CTLA-4) |
| CD81 | Target for antiproliferative antigen-1 (TAPA-1) | B cells, hematopoietic cells | B cell activation; forms B cell coreceptor complex with CD19 and CD21, which costimulatory signals in combination with B cell antigen receptor complex |
| CD82 | R2, IA4, 4F9 | On activated/differentiated hematopoietic cells; upregulated in T cells by activation | Signal transduction |
| CD83 | HB15 | Germinal left B cells, activated T cells, DCs, Langerhans cells | Regulates immune response |
| CDw84 | CDw84 | B cells, monocytes, MΦs, platelets, T cell subset | Unknown |
| CD85 | ILT/LIR (leukocyte immunoglobulin-like receptor) family | DCs, B cells, plasma cells, monocytes, T cell subset | Play a role in T-cell activation in peripheral blood |
| CD86 | B7-2 | B cells, monocytes, DCs, some T cells | Costimulator for T cell activation, ligand for CD28 and CD152 (CTLA-4) |
| CD87 | Urokinase plasminogen activator receptor (uPAR) | Monocytes, T cells, NK cells, neutrophils, endothelial cells | Receptor for urokinase plasminogen activator, role in inflammatory cell adhesion and migration |
| CD88 | C5a receptor | Granulocytes, DCs, mast cells | Receptor complement component C5a, role in complement-induced inflammation |
| CD89 | Fcα receptor (FcαR), IgA receptor | Granulocytes, monocytes, MΦs, T cells, NK cells | Binds IgA, mediates IgA-dependent cellular cytotoxicity |
| CD90 | Thy-1 | Mouse thymocytes and peripheral T cells, neurons (all species); human CD34$^+$ hematopoietic subset | Marker for mouse T cells, function unknown; hematopoietic stem cell and neuron differentiation |
| CD91 | α$_2$-Macroglobulin receptor, low-density lipoprotein receptor-related protein (LRP) | Monocytes and MΦs | Binds low-density lipoproteins |
| CDw92 | GR9 | Neutrophils, monocytes, platelets, myeloid cells | Unknown |
| CD93 | GR11 | Neutrophils, monocytes, endothelial cells | Unknown |
| CD94 | Kp43, KIR | NK cells, CD8$^+$ T cell subset | CD94/KNG2 complex functions as an NK cell killer inhibitory receptor, binds HLA-E class I MHC molecule |
| CD95 | APO-1, Fas | Multiple cell types | Binds to Fas ligand, mediates signals leading to apoptosis |

| Cluster designation | Synonym | Cellular expression | Function |
|---|---|---|---|
| CD96 | T cell activation-increased late expression (TACTILE) | Activated T cells and NK cells | Adhesion of activated T cells and NK cells |
| CD97 | BL-KDD/F12 | Activated B cells, activated T cells, monocytes/MΦs, DCs, granulocyte | Neutrophil migration |
| CD98 | 4F2, FRP-1 | Broad reactivity on activated and transformed cells, not hematopoietic specific, and found at lower levels on quiescent cells | Involved in the regulation of cellular activation |
| CD99 | E2, MIC2 | Broad | T cell activation, adhesion |
| CD99R | E2 | T, NK, and myeloid cells | Isoform of CD99 |
| CD100 | BB18, A8 | Hematopoietic cells, increased expression after T-cell activation, expressed on germinal left B cells | Increases PMA, CD3 and CD2 induced T-cell proliferation, increases CD45 induced T cell adhesion, induces B cell homotypic adhesion, down-regulates B cell expression of CD23; CD72 ligand |
| CD101 | P126, V7 | Granulocytes, monocytes, DCs, activated T cells | T cell activation |
| CD102 | Intercellular adhesion molecule-2 (ICAM-2) | Lymphocytes, monocytes, vascular endothelial cells | CD11aCD18 (LFA-1) ligand, cell-cell adhesion |
| CD103 | HML-1, $\alpha_\varepsilon$ integrin subunit | Intraepithelial lymphocytes, other cell types | Binds E-cadherin, role in T cell homing to mucosa |
| CD104 | $\beta_2$ integrin subunit | Epithelial cells, thymocytes | Adhesion, binds laminin |
| CD105 | Endoglin | Endothelial cells, activated MΦs | Binds TGF-β, regulates cellular responses to TGF-β |
| CD106 | VCAM-1, INCAM-110 | Activated endothelial cells, MΦs, follicular DCs, marrow stromal cells | Adhesion; CD49dCD29 (VLA-4) integrin receptor, role in lymphocyte trafficking, activation, role in hematopoiesis |
| CD107a | LAMP-1 | Activated platelets, T cells, endothelium, and neutrophils | Function unknown, lysosomal protein translocated to cell surface after activation, possible role in adhesion |
| CD107b | LAMP-2 | Activated platelets, T cells, endothelium, and neutrophils | Function unknown, lysosomal protein translocated to cell surface after activation, possible role in adhesion |
| CD108 | GR2 | Lymphocytes, erythrocytes | Unknown |
| CD109 | 8A3, 7D1, platelet activation factor | Activated T cells, platelets, endothelial cells | Unknown |
| CD110 | MPL, TPO receptor | Hematopoietic stem and progenitor cells, megakaryocyte progenitors, megakaryocytes, platelets | Upon binding of thrombopoietin to CD110 megakaryocyte proliferation and differentiation is induced and stem cells are protected from apoptosis |
| CD111 | PPR1/Nectin1 | Myeloid cells | Intercellular adhesion molecule |
| CD112 | PRR2 | Myeloid cells | Intercellular adhesion molecule; low-efficiency receptor for some Herpes simplex virus mutants |
| CDw113 | PVRL3, Nectin3 | Testis, placenta | Adhesion molecule that interacts with afadin |
| CD114 | G-CSF receptor | Granulocytes, monocytes, endothelial cells, hematopoietic cells | Binds G-CSF and mediates its effects |
| CD115 | M-CSF receptor, c-*fms* | Monocytes, MΦs, hematopoietic cells | Binds M-CSF and mediates its effects |
| CD116 | GM-CSF receptor α chain | Myeloid cells and their hematopoietic precursors | Binds GM-CSF and mediates its effects |
| CD117 | c-*kit*, stem cell factor receptor | Hematopoietic stem and progenitor cells, tissue mast cells | Binds c-kit ligand (stem cell factor) and mediates its effects |

## HUMAN CLUSTER OF DIFFERENTIATION (CD) MOLECULES *(Continued)*

| Cluster designation | Synonym | Cellular expression | Function |
|---|---|---|---|
| CD118 | LIFR | Epithelial cells in adult and embryo | Membrane-bound involved in signal transduction, soluble form inhibits activity of LIF |
| CDw119 | IFN-γ receptor | Monocytes, MΦs, DCs, B cells, endothelial and epithelial cells | Binds IFN-γ and mediates its effects |
| CD120a | TNF receptor type I | Broad | Binds TNF-α and TNF-β and mediates their effects |
| CD120b | TNF receptor type II | Broad | Binds TNF-α and TNF-β and mediates their effects |
| CD121a | Type 1 IL-1 receptor | Broad | Binds IL-1α and IL-1β and mediates their effects |
| CDw121b | Type 2 IL-1 receptor | B cells | A decoy receptor that binds IL-1α and IL-1β but does not mediate biologic effects |
| CD122 | IL-2 receptor β chain | NK cells, T cells, B cells, monocytes, MΦs | Binding and signaling component of IL-2 and IL-15 receptors, mediates biologic effects of IL-2 and IL-15 on T cells and NK cells |
| CDw123 | IL-3 receptor α chain | Bone marrow stem cells, monocytes, MΦs, megakaryocytes | Binds IL-3 and, in association with CDw131, mediates IL-3 biologic effects |
| CD124 | IL-4 receptor α chain | B and T cells, hematopoietic precursor cells, endothelium | Cytokine binding subunit of IL-4 and IL-13 receptor |
| CDw125 | IL-5 receptor α chain | Basophils, eosinophils, activated B cells | Binds IL-5 and, in association with CDw131, mediates IL-5 biologic effects |
| CD126 | IL-6 receptor α chain | Activated B cells, plasma cells, most leukocytes | Binds IL-6 and, in association with CDw130, mediates IL-6 biologic effects |
| CD127 | IL-7 receptor α chain | Bone marrow lymphoid precursors, T cells | Binds IL-7 and, in association with CD132, mediates IL-6 biologic effects |
| CDw128A | See CD181 | | |
| CDw128B | See CD182 | | |
| CD129 | Not yet assigned | | |
| CD130 | IL-6 receptor (R) β chain, IL-11 R β chain, oncostatin-M R β chain, leukemia inhibitory factor (LIF) receptor β, gp130 | Broad | IL-6, IL-11, oncostatin-M, and LIF receptor signaling function |
| CD131 | Common β chain for IL-3, IL-5, GM-CSF receptors | Myeloid cells and their progenitors, early B cells | IL-3, IL-5, and GM-CSF receptor signaling function |
| CD132 | Common γ chain for IL-2, IL-4, IL-7, IL-9, IL-15 receptors | T cells, B cells, NK cells, monocytes, MΦs, neutrophils | Some of the signaling functions of IL-2, IL-4, IL-7, IL-9, and IL-15 receptors |
| CD133 | AC133 | Stem/progenitor cells | Unknown |
| CD134 | OX40 | Activated T cells | Binds OX40 ligand, costimulatory signaling in T cells |
| CD135 | FMS-like tyrosine kinase 3 (Flt3), Flk2, STK-1 | Myeloid and B cell progenitor cells | Growth factor receptor involved in hematopoiesis |
| CDw136 | Macrophage stimulating protein receptor (MSP-R) | Epithelial cells from various tissues | Binds growth factors: MSP and hepatocyte growth factor-like protein; role in cell migration and growth |
| CDw137 | 4-1BB, induced by lymphocyte activation (ILA) | T cells, B cells, monocytes, epithelial cells | Costimulation of T cells, binds a ligand on B cells and MΦs |
| CD138 | Syndecan-1 | B cells | Receptor for ECM, cell morphology |
| CD139 | Cat 13, 4G9/BU30 | B cells, monocytes, granulocytes | Unknown |

| Cluster designation | Synonym | Cellular expression | Function |
|---|---|---|---|
| CD140a | Platelet-derived growth factor receptor α (PDGF Rα) | Broad | In association with CD140b, binds and mediates biologic effect of PDGF |
| CD140b | PDGF Rβ | Broad | In association with CD140ab, binds and mediates biologic effect of PDGF |
| CD141 | Fetomodulin, thrombomodulin | Endothelium | Regulation of coagulation |
| CD142 | Coagulation factor III, thromboplastin, tissue factor (TF) | Activated endothelial cells, epithelial cells and stromal cells in various tissues | Binds factor VIIa to form an enzyme that initiates the blood clotting cascade, regulates factor VIIa serine protease activity |
| CD143 | Angiotensin-converting enzyme (ACE) | Endothelial cells, epithelial cells, neurons, activated MΦs, some T cells | A peptidyl dipeptide hydrolase involved in metabolism of the vasoactive peptides angiotensin II and bradykinin |
| CD144 | VE-cadherin | Endothelial cells | Organizes endothelial cell adherent junction, which controls cell-cell adhesion, permeability, and migration |
| CDw145 | | Endothelial cells | Unknown |
| CD146 | MCAM, MelCAM, MUC18, S-endo | Endothelial cells, smooth muscle, subset of activated T cells | Adhesion |
| CD147 | Neurothelin, basigin | Endothelial cells, leukocytes, platelets, erythrocytes | Adhesion |
| CD148 | HPTP-η, p260 phosphatase | Granulocytes, monocytes, DCs, T cells, nerve cells, fibroblasts | Tyrosine phosphatase R Type II |
| CDw149 | New designation is CD47R | | |
| CD150 | Signaling lymphocyte activation molecule (SLAM), IPO-3 | Thymocytes, activated lymphocytes, DCs, endothelial cells | Binds itself as a self-ligand, regulation of B cell-T cell interactions and proliferative signals in B cells |
| CD151 | PETA-3, SFA-1 | Platelets, epithelial cells, megakaryocytes, endothelium | Adhesion |
| CD152 | Cytotoxic T lymphocyte-associated protein-4 (CTLA-4) | Activated T cells | Inhibitory signalling in T cells, binds APC CD80 (B7-1) and CD86 (B7-2) |
| CD153 | CD30 ligand | Activated T cells, thymocytes, resting B cells, granulocytes | Role in activation-induced cell death of CD8+ T cells, binds to CD30 |
| CD154 | CD40 ligand, T-BAM, TNF-related activation protein (TRAP), gp39 | Activated CD4+ T cells | Activates B cells, MΦs, and endothelial cells; ligand for CD40 |
| CD155 | Polio virus receptor (PVR) | Broad | Cell migration and adhesion, polio virus receptor |
| CD156a | ADAM-8, MS2 | Monocytes, neutrophils | Leukocyte extravasation |
| CD156b | TACE/ADAM17 | Broad | Adhesion structures |
| CDw156c | ADAM10 | Broad | Proteolytic cleavage of cell-surface molecules |
| CD157 | BST-1, MO-5 | Monocytes, granulocytes, B and T progenitor cells, bone marrow stromal cells | Pre-B cell growth |
| CD158a | p58.1, killer cell immunoglobulin (Ig)-like receptors (KIR) family (also called killer cell inhibitory receptors) | NK cells, T cell subset | KIR ligation by target cell HLA class I molecules inhibits NK cell activation |
| CD158b | p58.2, KIR family molecule | NK cells, T cell subset | KIR ligation by target cell HLA class I molecules inhibits NK cell activation |

## HUMAN CLUSTER OF DIFFERENTIATION (CD) MOLECULES *(Continued)*

| Cluster designation | Synonym | Cellular expression | Function |
|---|---|---|---|
| CD159a | NKG2A | NK cells, T cell subset | Associates with CD94, NK cell receptor |
| CD159c | NKG2C | NK cells | Associates with MHC class I HLA-E molecules, forms heterodimer with CD94 |
| CD160 | BY55, NK1, NK28 | Peripheral blood NK cells and CD8 T lymphocytes with cytolytic effector activity | Cross-linking CD160 with certain mAb triggers costimulatory signals in CD8 T lymphocytes |
| CD161 | NKRP-1 | NK cells, T cell subset | Role in NK cell activation |
| CD162 | PSGL-1 | T cells, monocytes, granulocytes, B cell subset | Mediates rolling of leukocytes on activated endothelium, on activated platelets, and on other leukocytes at inflammatory sites |
| CD162R | PEN5, selectin P ligand | Myeloid cells, activated T cells | High-affinity counter-receptor for P-selectin on myeloid cells and stimulated T cells, role in the tethering of these cells to activated platelets or endothelia expressing P-selectin |
| CD163 | M130 | Monocytes, MΦs | Endocytosis |
| CD164 | MGC-24 | Hematopoietic progenitor cells | Hematopoietic stem cell-stromal cell interaction |
| CD165 | gp37/AD2 | Thymocytes, thymic epithelial cells, mature lymphocytes, monocytes, platelets | Adhesion between thymocytes and thymic epithelial cells |
| CD166 | Activated leukocyte cell adhesion molecule (ALCAM) | Activated T cells, activated monocytes, endothelial cells, fibroblasts | Adhesion molecule that binds CD6 |
| CD167a | Discoidin domain receptor (DDR1) | Epithelial cells | Adhesion, a receptor tyrosine kinase (RTK), activated by various types of collagen |
| CD168 | Hyaluronan-mediated motility receptor (RHAMM) | Broad | Adhesion, mediates migration, transformation, and metastatic spread of murine fibroblasts; in humans, expressed as an intracellular protein in breast cancer cells |
| CD169 | Sialoadhesin | Subpopulation of tissue MΦs | Adhesion, cell-cell interactions |
| CD170 | Sialic acid-binding immunoglobulin-like lectin-5 (Siglec-5) | Hematopoietic cells, MΦs, neutrophils | Adhesion structure, mediates protein-carbohydrate interactions |
| CD171 | L1 | Epithelial cells, some cells of lymphoid and myelomonocytic origin | Adhesion structure, mediates cell-cell interaction, costimulatory molecule in T-cell activation |
| CD172a | Signal regulatory protein, α type, 1 (SIRPα) | Broad | Adhesion, complexes with CD47 |
| CD172b | SIRPβ | Monocytes and DCs | Adhesion structure, ligand for receptor tyrosine kinases (RTKs) signaling that regulates the growth of many cell types. |
| CD172g | SIRPγ | Broad | Binds with CD47 |
| CD173 | Blood group H type 2 | Erythrocytes, stem cell subset, platelets | Carbohydrate structures |
| CD174 | Lewis y | Stem cell subset, epithelium | Carbohydrate structures |
| CD175 | Tn | Stem cell subset | Carbohydrate structures |
| CD175s | Sialyl-Tn | Erythroblasts | Carbohydrate structures |
| CD176 | TF | Stem cell subset | Carbohydrate structures |
| CD177 | NB1 | Neutrophil subset | |
| CD178 | Fas ligand | Activated splenocytes, thymocytes, T cells | Interaction of FAS (CD95) with its ligand is critical in triggering apoptosis of some types of cells such as lymphocytes. |

| Cluster designation | Synonym | Cellular expression | Function |
|---|---|---|---|
| CD179a | Vpre-B | B cells | Associates with CD179b to form a surrogate light chain, it is a component of the preB cell receptor that plays a critical role in early B cell differentiation |
| CD179b | Lambda 5 | B cells | See CD179a |
| CD180 | RP105/Bgp95, LY64 | B cells | Chemokine receptor, regulates B cell recognition of lipopolysaccharide |
| CD181 | CXCR1, IL-8 receptor $\alpha$ | Neutrophils, basophils, mast cells, T cell subsets | Binds IL-8 and mediates its effects |
| CD182 | CXCR2, IL-8 receptor $\beta$ | Neutrophils, mast cells | Binds IL-8 and mediates its effects |
| CD183 | Chemokine (C-X-C) receptor 3 (CXCR3) | Activated T cells, eosinophils, NK cells, | Regulate the trafficking of immune cells during hematopoiesis and inflammatory responses; enhancement of $T_H1$ response |
| CD184 | Chemokine (C-X-C) receptor 4 (CXCR4) (fusin), HIV-1 coreceptor | T cells, B cell, neutrophils, some tissue cells | Chemokine receptor, attract and activate neutrophils, required for HIV-1 fusion to cell |
| CD185 | CXCR5 | Mature B cells | Associates with chemokine BLC, function in B cell differentiation, activation of mature B cells |
| CDw186 | CXCR6 | Activated T cells | Receptor for CXCL16 and coreceptor for SIV, strains of HIV-2 and m-tropic HIV-1 |
| CD191 | CCR1, MIP-1$\alpha$R, RANTES-R | T cells, monocytes, stem cell subset | Bind C-C type chemokines and transduces signal by increasing intracellular calcium ions |
| CD192 | CCR2, MCP-1-R | Activated NK cells and mononuclear phagocytes, T cell subset, B cells, endothelia | Binds MCP-1, MCP-3 and MCP-4, alternative receptor with CD4 for HIV-1 infection |
| CD193 | CCR3 | Eosinophils, lower expression in neutrophils and monocytes, T cell subset | Binds eotaxin, eotaxin-3, MCP-3, MCP-4, RANTES and MIP-1$\delta$, alternative receptor with CD4 for HIV-1 infection |
| CD195 | CCR5 | Monocytes, T cells | Chemokine receptor, role in granulocyte lineage proliferation and differentiation, coreceptor for HIV |
| CD197 | CCR7 | T cell subset, DCs | MIP-2$\beta$ receptor, drive cellular migration patterns that are important for effective immune responses |
| CDw198 | CCR8 | T cells, high expression in $T_H2$, NK, and monocytes | Role in allergic inflammation; alternative coreceptor with CD4 for HIV infection |
| CDw199 | CCR9 | Subset of memory T cells, lamina propria mononuclear cells | Binds SCYA25/TECK; alternative coreceptor with CD4 for HIV infection |
| CD200 | OX2 | Thymocytes, brain tissues | Inhibition of immune response |
| CD201 | Endothelial protein C receptor (EPCR) | Endothelial cells | Activated protein C receptor |
| CD202b | Tie2 (Tek) | Endothelial cells | Ligand is angiopoietin-1, role in endothelial cell-smooth muscle cell communication in venous morphogenesis |
| CD203c | NPP3/PDNP3 | Myeloid cells, basophils, mast cells, uterus tissue | A multi-functional ectoenzyme involved in the clearance of extracellular nucleotides |
| CD204 | Macrophage scavenger receptor | Myeloid cells | Mediates binding, internalization, and processing of a wide range of negatively charged macromolecules |

## HUMAN CLUSTER OF DIFFERENTIATION (CD) MOLECULES *(Continued)*

| Cluster designation | Synonym | Cellular expression | Function |
|---|---|---|---|
| CD205 | DEC205 | DCs | Endocytosis of antigen |
| CD206 | Macrophage mannose receptor | DCs, activated MΦs | Bind high-mannose structures on pathogenic viruses, bacteria, and fungi that leads to neutralization by phagocytic Engulfment |
| CD207 | Langerin | DCs | Binding by langerin leads to internalization of antigen into Birbeck granules and possibly access to the class I pathway |
| CD208 | DC-LAMP | Activated DCs | Unknown |
| CD209 | Dendritic cell-specific ICAM3-grabbing nonintegrin (DC-SIGN), HIV GP120-binding protein | DCs, resting T cells | Mediates transient adhesion with T cells, role in the CD4-independent association of HIV with cells |
| CDw210 | IL-10 receptor | Leukocytes | Binds IL-10 and mediates its effects |
| CD212 | IL-12 receptor β1 | T cells, NK cells | Binds IL-12 and mediates its effects, promotes CMI to intracellular pathogens by inducing $T_H1$ cell responses and IFN-$\gamma$ production |
| CD213a1 | IL-13 receptor α1 | Broad | Binds IL-13 and mediates its effects; it is also a necessary component for IL-4-induced signal transduction in type II IL-4 receptor system |
| CD213a2 | IL-13 receptor α2 | Broad | See CD213a1 |
| CDw217 | IL-17 receptor | Stimulated T cells | Binds IL-17 and mediates its effects |
| CDw218a | IL-18 receptor α | T, NK, and DCs | Binds IL-18 and leads to the activation of NF-κB |
| CDw218b | IL-18 receptor β | T, NK, and DCs | Forms heterodimeric receptor with IL-18Rα to enhance IL-18 binding |
| CD220 | Insulin receptor | | Binding of insulin to the insulin receptor stimulates glucose uptake |
| CD221 | Insulin-like growth factor 1 receptor precursor (IGF1 R) | | It has tyrosine kinase activity, role in transformation events, highly overexpressed in most malignant tissues where it functions as an anti-apoptotic agent by enhancing cell survival |
| CD222 | Mannose-6-phosphate receptor, insulin-like growth factor 2 receptor (IGF2 receptor) | Broad | Sorts newly synthesized lysosomal enzymes bearing M6P to lysosomes, it internalizes IGF-II, internalizes or sorts lysosomal enzymes and other M6P-containing proteins (e.g., latent TGF-β) as well as regulation of TGF-β activity |
| CD223 | Lymphocyte-activation gene 3 (LAG-3) | Activated T cells and NK cells | An MHC class II ligand |
| CD224 | Gamma-glutamyl transferase | Broad | Involved in absorption and secretion |
| CD225 | Leu13 | | Involved in cell growth |
| CD226 | DNAM-1 (PTA1) | NK cells, platelets, monocytes, subset of T cells | Mediates adhesion to an unknown ligand |
| CD227 | MUC.1 | Most glandular and ductal epithelial cells and some hematopoietic cell lineages | Cell surface protection, modulation of adhesion and signaling in response to specific ligands |

| Cluster designation | Synonym | Cellular expression | Function |
|---|---|---|---|
| CD228 | Melanotransferrin (MTf) | Human melanomas, brain | Brain iron homeostasis |
| CD229 | Ly9 | T cells | Adhesion between T cells and accessory cells |
| CD230 | Prion protein | Broad | Unknown |
| CD231 | T-cell acute lymphoblastic leukemia associated antigen 1 (TALLA-1) | T-cell acute lymphoblastic leukemia, neuroblastoma cells and normal brain neuron | Marker for T cell lymphoblastic leukemia |
| CD232 | Virus-encoded semaphorin protein receptor (VESP R) | Monocytes | An immune modulator during virus infection |
| CD233 | Band 3 | Erythroid cells | Mediates exchange of chloride and bicarbonate across the phospholipid bilayer, plays a central role in respiration of carbon dioxide |
| CD234 | Fy-glycoprotein, duffy antigen receptor for chemokines (DARC) | Erythroid cells | Receptor for IL-8, it acts as an intracellular sink to modulate the level of these proinflammatory molecules |
| CD235a | Glycophorin A | Erythroid cells | Unknown |
| CD235b | Glycophorin B | Erythroid cells | Unknown |
| CD235ab | Glycophorin A/B crossreactive mabs | Erythroid cells | Unknown |
| CD236 | Glycophorin C/D | Erythroid cells | Unknown |
| CD236R | Glycophorin C | Erythroid cells | Plays an important role in regulating the mechanical stability of red cells |
| CD238 | Kell blood group antigen | Erythroid cells | A zinc endopeptidase that yields endothelin-3, a potent bioactive peptide |
| CD239 | B-cell adhesion molecule (B-CAM) | Erythroid cells | Role in cell-cell, cell-matrix adhesion, signal transduction |
| CD240CE | Rhesus system C and E polypeptides (Rh30CE) | Erythroid cells | Unknown |
| CD240D | Rh blood group D antigen (RHD) Rh30D | Erythroid cells | Unknown |
| CD241 | Rhesus blood group-associated glycoprotein (RhAg) | Erythroid cells | Transport or channel function in the erythrocyte membrane |
| CD242 | Intercellular adhesion molecule 4 (ICAM-4) | Erythroid cells | Binds leukocyte-specific integrins |
| CD243 | MDR-1 | Stem/progenitor cells | Ion pump |
| CD244 | 2B4 | NK cells | Modulates NK cell cytokine production, cytolytic function and extravasation |
| CD245 | p220/240 | T cell subset | Signal transduction, costimulation |
| CD246 | Anaplastic lymphoma kinase | T cells | Plays an important role in the development of the brain and exerts its effects on specific neurons in the nervous system |
| CD247 | Zeta ($\zeta$) chain | T cells, NK cells | Signaling component of TCR complex and CD16 (Fc$\gamma$RIII) |
| CD248 | TEM1, Endosialin | Endothelial tissue, stromal fibroblasts | May function in tumor progression and angiogenesis |
| CD249 | Aminopeptidase | Epithelium, endothelium | Plays a role in the rennin-angiotensin system |
| CD252 | OX-40L | Activated B cells | T cell costimulation |
| CD253 | TRAIL | Activated T cells, NK cells, many tissues | Apoptosis |

## HUMAN CLUSTER OF DIFFERENTIATION (CD) MOLECULES *(Continued)*

| Cluster designation | Synonym | Cellular expression | Function |
|---|---|---|---|
| CD254 | TRANCE | Lymph node and bone marrow stroma, activated T cells | Enhances DC to stimulate naïve T cell proliferation, T-B cell interaction, bone development |
| CD255 | Reserved for TWEAK | | |
| CD256 | APRIL | Monocytes, MΦs | Promotes T and B cell proliferation |
| CD257 | BLyS, BAFF | Activated monocytes, dendritic cells | B cell growth factor and costimulator of Ig production |
| CD258 | LIGHT, HVEM-L | Activated T cells, immature DCs, activated monocytes | Binds LTBR to stimulate T cell proliferation, receptor for HVEM, apoptosis |
| CD261 | TRAIL-R1, DR4 | Activated T cells, PBLs | Contains death domain that mediates apoptosis via FADD and caspase-8, binds to TRAIL (CD253) |
| CD262 | TRAIL-R2, DR5 | Broad, PBLs | Contains death domain that mediates apoptosis via FADD and caspase-8, binds to TRAIL (CD253) |
| CD263 | TRAIL-R3, DcR1 | PBLs | Receptor for TRAIL but lacks death domain, inhibits TRAIL-induced apoptosis |
| CD264 | TRAIL-R4 | PBLs | Binds TRAIL but contains truncated death domain, inhibits TRAIL-induced apoptosis |
| CD265 | RANK | Broad | Binding of TRANCE mediates osteoclastogenesis and T cell-DC interactions |
| CD266 | TWEAK-R | Heart, placenta, and kidney | May play a role in cell-matrix interactions |
| CD267 | TACI | B cells, activated T cells | Binds BAFF and APRIL |
| CD268 | BAFFR | B cells, resting T cells, PBLs | Binding of BLyS promotes survival of mature B cells |
| CD269 | BCMA | Mature B cells | APRIL and BAFF receptor, B cell survival and proliferation |
| CD271 | NGFR | Neurons | Tumor suppressor mediates survival and death |
| CD272 | BTLA | Activated T cells, B cells, remains on $T_H1$ cells | HVEM receptor, inhibitory response |
| CD273 | B7DC | DC subset, monocytes, MΦs | PD-1 receptor, costimulation or suppression of T cell proliferation |
| CD274 | B7-H1 | Leukocytes, broad | PD-1 receptor, costimulation of lymphocytes |
| CD275 | B7-H2, ICOSL | B cells, DCs, monocytes | Costimulation promotes proliferation and cytokine production |
| CD276 | B7-H3 | In vitro cultures of DCs and monocytes, activated T cells | Costimulation of T cell activation and proliferation |
| CD277 | BT3.1 | T, B, and NK cells, monocytes, DCs, endothelium, CD34$^+$ cells | T cell activation |
| CD278 | ICOS | Activated T cells, $T_H2$ cells | Binds ICOS-L, costimulatory, T cell activation and proliferation |
| CD279 | PD1 | Activated T and B cells | B7-H1 and B7-DC receptor, autoimmune disease and peripheral tolerance |
| CD280 | ENDO180 | Chondrocytes, fibroblasts, endothelium, MΦs | Mannose receptor, collagen matrix remodeling and endocytic recyling |
| CD281 | TLR1 | Low levels in PBMCs, monocytes and possibly DCs | Innate immunity, regulates TLR2 function |
| CD282 | TLR2 | Monocytes, neutrophils, upregulated in MΦs | Interacts with dsRNA, pattern recognition in response to bacterial lipoproteins, innate immunity |
| CD283 | TLR3 | Derived monocyte DCs | Interacts with dsRNA, innate immunity |

| Cluster designation | Synonym | Cellular expression | Function |
|---|---|---|---|
| CD284 | TLR4 | PMBCs | Interacts with dsRNA, innate immunity |
| CD289 | TLR9 | In vitro derived DC | Reacts with CpG-DNA, innate immunity |
| CD292 | BMPR1A | Bone progenitor | BMP 2 and 4 receptor, bone development |
| CDw293 | BMPR1B | Bone progenitor | BMP receptor, bone development |
| CD294 | CRTH2 | $T_H2$ cells, eosinophils, basophils | Binds $PGD_2$, stimulatory effects on $T_H2$ cells, role in allergic inflammation |
| CD295 | LeptinR | Broad | Adipose metabolism |
| CD296 | ART1 | Heart and skeletal muscle, peripheral T cells, NK subset | Modifies integrins during differentiation, ADP ribosylation of target proteins |
| CD297 | ART4 | Erythoid, activated monocytes | ADP ribosylation of target proteins |
| CD298 | $Na^+/K^+$-ATPase $\beta3$ subunit | Broad | Transport of Na and K ions across membranes |
| CD299 | DC-SIGN-related | Endothelial subset | Binds ICAM-3, HIV-1 gp120 |
| CD300a | CMRF35H | NK cells, monocytes, neutrophils, T and B subsets | Unknown |
| CD300c | CMRF35A | Monocytes, neutrophils, T and B subsets | Unknown |
| CD300e | CMRF35L | Monocytes, M$\phi$s, DC subset | Unknown |
| CD301 | MGL | Immature DCs | Binds Tn antigen, uptake of glycosylated antigens |
| CD302 | DCL1 | Some myeloid and Hodgkin's cell lines | A fusion protein in Hodgkin's lymphoma with DEC-205 |
| CD303 | BDCA2 | Plasmacytoid DCs | Inhibit IFN-$\alpha$ production |
| CD304 | BDCA4 | Neurons, $CD4^+$ $CD25^+$ Treg cells, DCs, endothelial and tumor cells | Interacts with VEGF165 and semaphorins |
| CD305 | LAIR1 | NK cells, B cells, T cells, monocytes | Inhibitory receptor on NK and T cells |
| CD306 | LAIR2 | T cells, monocytes | Inhibits cellular activation and inflammation |
| CD307 | IRTA2 | B cell subset, B lymphoma | Implicated in B cell development |
| CD309 | VEGFR2 | Endothelial cells, angiogenic precursor cells | Binds VEGF, regulates adhesion and cell signaling |
| CD312 | EMR2 | Monocytes, M$\Phi$s, monocyte DCs | Predicted cell adhesion and migration for phagocytosis |
| CD314 | NKG2D, KLR | NK cells, $CD8^+$ activated cells, $NK1.1^+$ T cells, some myeloid cells | Binds MHC class I, MICA, MICB, engagement activates cytolysis and cytokine production, costimulatory |
| CD315 | CD9P1 | B cell subset, activated monocytes | Associates with CD9 and CD81 |
| CD316 | EWI2 | B and T cells, low on NK cells | Associates with CD9 and CD81; involved in cell migration |
| CD317 | BST2 | B, T, and NK cells, monocytes, DCs, fibroblast cell lines, myeloma | Pre-B cell growth, over expression multiple myeloma |
| CD318 | CDCP1 | Subset of $CD34^+$ HSCs, tumors | Cell adhesion with ECM |
| CD319 | CRACC | T, B, and NK cell subset, NK cells, upregulated in DCs | Regulates T and NK cells |
| CD320 | 8D6A | Follicular DCs, germinal lefts | Stimulates B cell proliferation, in tumor formation |
| CD321 | JAM1 | Platelet receptor, epithelia and endothelia, platelets | Tight junctions |
| CD322 | JAM2 | HEV, other endothelia | Cell adhesion, role in the process of lymphocyte homing to secondary lymphoid organs |
| CD324 | E-Cadherin | Non-neural epithelia | Cell adhesion, homotypic interaction and binds $\alpha E/\beta7$ |

## HUMAN CLUSTER OF DIFFERENTIATION (CD) MOLECULES *(Continued)*

| Cluster designation | Synonym | Cellular expression | Function |
|---|---|---|---|
| CDw325 | N-Cadherin | Brain, skeletal and cardiac muscle | Cell adhesion, involved in neuronal recognition mechanism |
| CD326 | Ep-CAM | Most epithelial cell membranes | May function as growth factor receptor |
| CDw327 | SIGLEC6 | Placenta, spleen, B cells | Sialic-acid dependent adhesion, membrane-bound and secreted forms |
| CDw328 | SIGLEC7 | Resting and activated NK cells, placenta, liver, spleen, lower in granulocytes and monocytes | Sialic-acid dependent adhesion, may inhibit NK cell activation and hematopoiesis |
| CDw329 | SIGLEC9 | Neutrophils, monocytes | Sialic-acid dependent adhesion molecule |
| CD331 | FGFR1 | Fibroblasts and epithelia | Binds FGF, high-affinity receptor for fibroblast growth factor |
| CD332 | FGFR2 | Fibroblasts and epithelia | Binds FGF, high-affinity receptor for fibroblast growth factor |
| CD333 | FGFR3 | Fibroblasts and epithelia | Binds FGF, high-affinity receptor for fibroblast growth factor |
| CD334 | FGFR4 | Fibroblasts and epithelia | Binds FGF, high-affinity receptor for fibroblast growth factor |
| CD335 | NKp46 | NK cells | Activates NK cells on non-MHC ligand binding |
| CD336 | NKp44 | NK cells | Activates NK cells on non-MHC ligand binding |
| CD337 | NKp30 | NK cells | Activates NK cells on non-MHC ligand binding |
| CDw338 | ABCG2 | Stem cell subset | Multi-drug resistance transporter |
| CD339 | Jagged-1 | Stromal cells, epithelia | Associates with Notch, regulation in hematopoiesis |
| CD340 | HER2/neu | Epidermal growth factor receptor | Associates with over-expression in breast cancer |
| CD344 | FZD4 (frizzled-4) | Receptor for Wnt-2 | Angiogenic molecule |
| CD349 | FZD9 (frizzled-9) | Receptor for Wnt proteins | ? |
| CD350 | FZD10 (frizzled-10) | Receptor for Wnt proteins | ? |

*w (for workshop) designation is used to indicate recently submitted antibodies whose reactivity is incompletely described.

**Mouse only

# INDEX

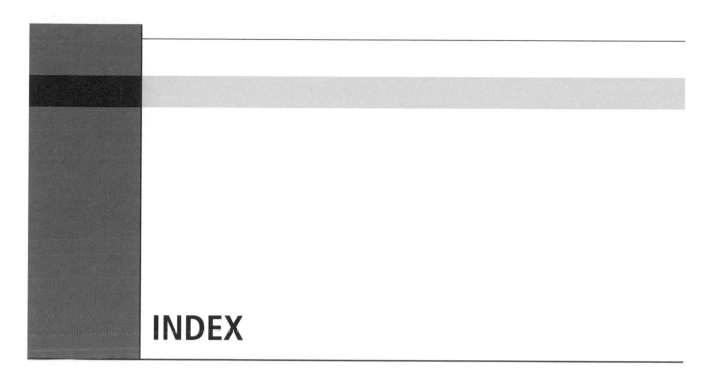